369 0085473

KU-407-174

FETAL AND NEONATAL BRAIN INJURY

Now in its third edition, this is a comprehensive survey of fetal and neonatal brain injury arising from hypoxia, ischemia, or other causes. The publication spans a broad range of areas from epidemiology and pathogenesis, through to clinical manifestations and obstetric care, and then on to diagnosis, long-term outcomes, and medicolegal aspects. An important theme running throughout is to highlight scientific and clinical advances that have a role to play in minimizing risk, improving clinical care and outcomes. The text describes how placental abnormalities, imaging studies, and laboratory measurements can identify the timing and severity of the injury event. Despite these advances, fetal and neonatal brain injury remains a major concern with devastating consequences. It is hoped that this definitive account will provide the clinician not only with a better understanding of the mechanisms involved but also with the best available knowledge necessary to deal with this intractable problem.

David K. Stevenson is the Harold K. Faber Professor of Pediatrics and Chief of the Division of Neonatal and Developmental Medicine at the Stanford University School of Medicine. He also serves as the Director of the Charles B. and Ann L. Johnson Center for Pregnancy and the Newborn Services at Stanford.

William E. Benitz is Associate Chief of and a Professor in the Division of Neonatal and Developmental Medicine at the Stanford University School of Medicine, and Director of Nurseries at the Lucile Packard Children's Hospital at Stanford.

Philip Sunshine is Professor of Pediatrics (Emeritus) in the Division of Neonatal and Developmental Medicine and Department of Pediatrics at the Stanford University School of Medicine.

FETAL AND NEONATAL BRAIN INJURY

Mechanisms, Management, and the Risks of Practice

THIRD EDITION

Edited by

David K. Stevenson, William E. Benitz, and Philip Sunshine

Stanford University Medical Center, Palo Alto, CA, USA

Foreword by Avroy A. Fanaroff

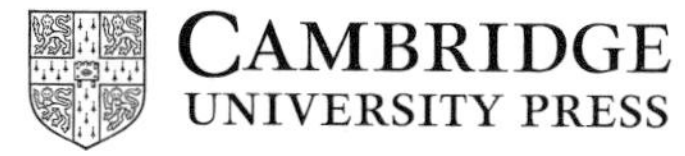

PUBLISHED BY THE PRESS SYNDICATE OF THE UNIVERSITY OF CAMBRIDGE
The Pitt Building, Trumpington Street, Cambridge, United Kingdom

CAMBRIDGE UNIVERSITY PRESS
The Edinburgh Building, Cambridge CB2 2RU, UK
40 West 20th Street, New York, NY 10011–4211, USA
477 Williamstown Road, Port Melbourne, VIC 3207, Australia
Ruiz de Alarcón 13, 28014 Madrid, Spain
Dock House, The Waterfront, Cape Town 8001, South Africa

http://www.cambridge.org

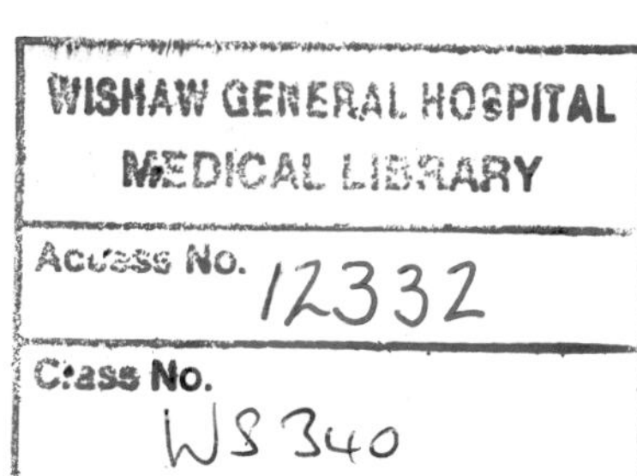

First edition published 1989 by Oxford University Press
Second edition published 1997 by Oxford University Press
Third edition published 2003

Printed in Italy by G. Canale & C. S.p.A

Typeface Minion 8.5/12 pt *System* QuarkXPress™ [SE]

A catalogue record for this book is available from the British Library

Library of Congress Cataloguing in Publication data

Fetal and neonatal brain injury : mechanisms, management, and the risks of practice /
[edited by] David K. Stevenson, Philip Sunshine, William E. Benitz. – 3rd ed.
p. ; cm.
Includes bibliographical references and index.
ISBN 0 521 80691 7 (hardback)
1. Brain – Diseases. 2. Brain-damaged children. 3. Brain – Wounds and injuries. 4. Fetus – Diseases.
5. Fetal brain – Growth. 6. Infants (Newborn) – Diseases. 7. Infants (Newborn) – Wounds and injuries.
I. Stevenson, David K. (David Kendal), 1949– II. Sunshine, Philip, 1930– III. Benitz, William E.
[DNLM: 1. Brain Injuries – Infant, Newborn. 2. Brain Diseases – Infant, Newborn. 3. Fetal Diseases.
4. Infant, Newborn, Diseases. 5. Pregnancy Complications. WS 340 F419 2002]
RG629.B73 F456 2002
618.92′8–dc21 2002073485

ISBN 0 521 80691 7 hardback

Every effort has been made in preparing this book to provide accurate and up-to-date information which is in accord with accepted standards and practice at the time of publication. Nevertheless, the authors, editors and publisher can make no warranties that the information contained herein is totally free from error, not least because clinical standards are constantly changing through research and regulation. The authors, editors and publisher therefore disclaim all liability for direct or consequential damages resulting from the use of material contained in this book. Readers are strongly advised to pay careful attention to information provided by the manufacturer of any drugs or equipment that they plan to use.

Contents

Part II Pregnancy, Labor, and Delivery Complications Causing Brain Injury

Part III Diagnosis of the Infant with Asphyxia

Part IV Specific Conditions Associated with Fetal and Neonatal Brain Injury

Contributors

Reinaldo Acosta
Fetal Maternal Medicine
Department of Gynecology and Obstetrics
Stanford Medical Center
Stanford, CA 94305
reinaldo.acosta@stanford.edu

Geoffrey Altshuler
University of Oklahoma Health Services Center and Children's Hospital of Oklahoma
940 NE 13th St, Room 3, B400
Oklahoma City, OK 73104
galtshuler@home.com

Patrick D. Barnes
Department of Radiology
Lucile Packard Children's Hospital
725 Welch Rd
Palo Alto, CA 94304
pbarnes@stanford.edu

Laura Bennet
Research Center for Developmental Medicine and Biology, Faculty of Medicine and Health Services
University of Auckland
Private Bdg 92019
Auckland
New Zealand
l.bennet@auckland.ac.nz

William E. Benitz
Division of Neonatal and Developmental Medicine
Stanford University Medical Center
750 Welch Rd #315
Palo Alto, CA 94304
benitzwe@stanford.edu

Michael D. Black
CVRB, MC 5407
Stanford, CA 94305
michael.black@stanford.edu

Francis G. Blankenberg
Department of Pediatrics
Lucile Packard Children's Hospital
725 Welch Rd
Palo Alto, CA 94304
blankenb@stanford.edu

David P. Carlton
Division of Neonatology
Department of Pediatrics
University of Wisconsin and Meriter Hospital
202 South Park St
Madison, WI 53715
dpcarlton@facstaff.wisc.edu

Christopher H. Contag
Stanford University Medical Center
Stanford, CA 94305
ccontag@cmgm.stanford.edu

Marvin Cornblath
Johns Hopkins University School of Medicine and University of Maryland School of Medicine
802 The Colonnade
3801 Canterbury Rd
Baltimore, MD 21218-2377
mcornblath@erols.com

Phyllis A. Dennery
Division of Neonatal and Developmental Medicine
Stanford University Medical Center
750 Welch Rd #315
Palo Alto, CA 94304
Dennery@stanford.edu

Maurice L. Druzin
Stanford University Medical Center
300 Pasteur Drive
Stanford, CA 94305
druzin@stanford.edu

Yasser Y. El-Sayed
Stanford University Medical Center
300 Pasteur Drive
Stanford, CA 94305
yasser.elsayed@stanford.edu

Gregory M. Enns
Department of Pediatrics
Stanford Medical Center
300 Pasteur Drive
Stanford, CA 94305
greg.enns@stanford.edu

Andrea M. Enright
Pediatric Infectious Diseases
Department of Pediatrics
Stanford University Medical Center
300 Pasteur Drive
Stanford, CA 94305
hovezoe2@yahoo.com

Hayley A. Gans
Division of Infectious Diseases
Department of Pediatrics
Stanford University Medical Center
300 Pasteur Drive
Stanford, CA 94305
hagans@stanford.edu

Peter D. Gluckman
Research Centre for Developmental Medicine and Biology
Faculty of Medicine and Health Services
University of Auckland
Private Bag 92019
Auckland
New Zealand
pdgluckman@auckland.ac.nz

Jian Guan
Research Centre for Developmental Medicine and Biology
University of Auckland
Private Bag 92019
Auckland
New Zealand
j.guan@auckland.ac.nz

Alistair J. Gunn
Research Centre for Developmental Medicine and Biology
Faculty of Medicine and Health Service
University of Auckland
Private Bag 92019
Auckland
New Zealand
aj.gunn@auckland.ac.nz

Jin S. Hahn
Department of Neurology
Stanford University Medical Center
300 Pasteur Drive
Stanford, CA 94305
jhahn@stanford.edu

Louis P. Halamek
Division of Neonatal and Developmental Medicine
Department of Pediatrics
Stanford University Medical Center
750 Welch Rd #315
Palo Alto, CA 94304
halamek@stanford.edu

Susan R. Hintz
Division of Neonatal and Developmental Medicine
Stanford University Medical Center
750 Welch Rd #315
Palo Alto, CA 94304
srhintz@stanford.edu

Satish Kalhan
c/o Rainbow Babies and Children Hospital
11100 Euclid Ave.
Cleveland, OH 44109-1998
sck@po.cwrv.edu

John A. Kerner, Jr
Division of Gastroenterology and Nutrition
Stanford University Medical Center
750 Welch Rd #315
Palo Alto, CA 94304
md.kenjo@stanford.edu

Tekoa King
Department of Obstetrics and Gynecology
University of California Health Services Center
505 Parnassus Ave.
San Francisco, CA 94143
tking@midwives.org

Anneliese F. Korner
2299 Tasso St
Palo Alto, CA 94301

Ronald J. Lemire
University of Washington School of Medicine
Box 359300
Seattle, WA 98195
rlemir@chmc.org

Deirdre J. Lyell
Department of Gynecology and Obstetrics
Stanford University Medical Center
300 Pasteur Drive
Stanford, CA 94305
dlyell@stanford.edu

Yvonne A. Maldonado
Division of Infectious Diseases
Department of Pediatrics
Stanford University Medical Center
300 Pasteur Drive
Stanford, CA 94305
bonniem@stanford.edu

Lee J. Martin
Johns Hopkins University School of Medicine
Neuropathology Laboratory
720 Rutland Avenue
558 Ross Research Bldg
Baltimore, MD 21205
lmartin@jhmi.edu

William Oh
Department of Pediatrics
Brown University
593 Eddy Street
Providence, RI 02903
william oh@brown.edu

Donald M. Olson
Department of Neurology
Stanford University Medical Center
300 Pasteur Drive
Stanford, CA 94305
donald.olson@stanford.edu

Charles Palmer
Milton S. Hershey Medical Center
PO Box 850
Hershey, PA 17033-0850
cxps@isu.edu

Julian T. Parer
University of California Health Sciences Center
505 Parnassus Ave.
San Francisco, CA 94143
bill-parer@quickmail.ucsr.edu

Alistair G.S. Philip
Division of Neonatal and Developmental Medicine
Stanford University Medical Center
750 Welch Rd #315
Palo Alto, CA 94304

Charles G. Prober
Division of Infectious Diseases
Stanford University Medical Center
300 Pasteur Drive
Stanford, CA 94305
cprober@stanford.edu

William D. Rhine
Division of Neonatal and Developmental Medicine
Stanford University Medical Center
750 Welch Rd #315
Palo Alto, CA 94304
wrhine@stanford.edu

Charlene M.T. Robertson
University of Alberta
Glenrose Rehabilitation Hospital
10230-111 Ave.
Edmonton, Alberta
Canada T5G 0B7
croberts@cha.ab.ca

Ted S. Rosenkrantz
Chief, Division of Neonatology
University of Connecticut Health Center
M/C 2203
Farmington, CT 06030-2203
tedrl@aol.com

Mark S. Scher
Rainbow Babies and Children's Hospital
Case Western Reserve University
11100 Euclid Ave., M/C 6090
Cleveland, OH 44106
mss20@po.cwru.edu

Robert Schwartz
Division of Pediatric Endocrinology and Metabolism
Rhode Island Hospital
593 Eddy Street
Providence, RI 02903
dberger@lifespan.org

Daniel S. Seidman
Department of Obstetrics and Gynecology
Sheba Medical Center, Tel-Hashomer and Sadder Faculty of Medicine
Tel-Aviv University
Israel Chaim Sheba Medical Center
5261 Tel-Hashomer
Israel
dseidman@post.tau.ac.il

Seetha Shankaran
Wayne State University School of Medicine
Children's Hospital of Michigan
3901 Beaubien Blvd
Detroit, MI 48201-2119
sshankaran@wayne.edu

David Sheuerman
Sheuerman, Martini & Tabari Attorneys at Law
111 North Market Street
Suite 700
San Jose, CA 95113
dsheurerman@smtlaw.com

Kimberlee A. Sorem
c/o California Pacific Medical Center
3700 California Street
San Francisco, CA 94118
soremk@sutterhealth.org

David K. Stevenson
Department of Pediatrics
Stanford University Medical Center
750 Welch Rd #315
Palo Alto, CA 94304
dstevenson@stanford.edu

Philip Sunshine
Division of Neonatal and Developmental Medicine
Department of Pediatrics
Stanford University Medical Center
750 Welch Rd #315
Palo Alto, CA 94304
psunshine@stanford.edu

Krisa P. Van Meurs
Division of Neonatal and Developmental Medicine
Department of Pediatrics
Stanford University Medical Center
750 Welch Rd #315
Palo Alto, CA 94304
vanmeurs@stanford.edu

Robert C. Vannucci
Department of Pediatrics
PO Box 850
Milton S. Hersey Medical Center
Hershey, PA 17033-0850

Boaz Weisz
Department of Obstetrics and Gynecology
Chaim Sheba Medical Center
52621 Tel-Hashomer
Israel
boazmd@zahav.net.il

Jenny A. Westgate
Research Center for Developmental Medicine and Biology
University of Auckland
Delivery Suite
North Shore Hospital
Private Bag 93-503
Takapuma
Auckland
New Zealand
ja.westgate@auckland.ac.nz

Thomas E. Wiswell
Division of Neonatology
SUNY Stony Brook
Pediatrics HSC-11-060
Stony Brook, NY 11794-8111
twiswell@notes.cc.sunnysb.edu

Ernlé W.D. Young
Stanford University
701 Welch Rd #1105
Palo Alto, CA 94304
eyoung@stanford.edu

Foreword

Great strides have been taken in the relatively new specialty of neonatal–perinatal Medicine. The evidence upon which neonatal–perinatal medicine is practiced has expanded considerably and the rationale for many interventions is now supported by scientific data. Application of the biochemical and technologic advances to obstetrics and neonatology has improved the immediate and long-term outlook for the majority of neonates. Inspection of the major causes of neonatal mortality reveals that birth defects now head the list and there has been a sharp decline in death from respiratory disorders and immaturity. However, injury to the central nervous system continues to be a major concern. After an apparently normal pregnancy only a brief period of oxygen deprivation or exposure to other noxious stimuli may cause devastating and permanent injury to the central nervous system. Haldane is attributed to have said that "Hypoxia not only stops the motor, but also destroys the machinery." Hypoxia can definitely destroy the developing brain. This edition of *Fetal and Neonatal Brain Injury* is very timely and not only provides comprehensive coverage of the emerging issues and clinical trials in progress but also provides state-of-the-art deliberations on neuroimaging in addition to the infectious and metabolic encephalopathies.

Stevenson, Benitz, and Sunshine have assembled an outstanding group of contributors to tackle comprehensively the accumulating evidence on fetal and neonatal brain injury. No topic worthy of discussion on the developing brain has been omitted and the expert contributors have uniformly excelled in their assigned tasks, providing indepth commentaries and facts in an easy-to-read manner. This book is truly at the cutting edge and the hot topics have been appropriately highlighted, the established information well packaged, and a heroic effort made to cross-link the basic science with the bedside needs. Often neglected topics such as ethics and medicolegal issues are well represented side by side with sophisticated imaging, pathophysiology, and molecular biology.

There is a great deal of anticipation about the use of hypothermia for the treatment of hypoxic–ischemic encephalopathy. This therapy is being carefully evaluated. Regrettably, there is no way to shorten the interval between the intervention and primary outcome, which is long-term neurodevelopmental status. Furthermore these cases occur sporadically so that, despite the fact that there are multicenter – even multinational – trials, recruitment is proceeding slowly and we must patiently await the outcomes. Hopefully the trials have been sufficiently powered so that the results will be definitive.

Modern perinatal care, including fetal surveillance, antenatal administration of glucocorticoids, surfactant administration, and ventilatory assistance, has improved survival rates for very-low-birth-weight infants. There has however been no improvement in the neurodevelopmental outcomes of such infants and handicapping conditions are documented in 20–40%. Unraveling the relationship between chorioamnionitis, cytokines, and periventricular leukomalacia may shed light on this complex problem and provide some clues on when and how to intervene and prevent permanent injury. Perhaps further refinements in imaging and spectroscopy will clarify the sequencing and timing of insults to the brain. There is still much to be learned about the developing brain but the foundations have been expanded and the exponential rate of data acquisition is cause for optimism that solutions to preventing or correcting injuries to the brain will be on the radar screen within a reasonable time period.

Avroy A. Fanaroff
Eliza Henry Barnes Professor of Neonatology
Rainbow Babies and Children's Hospital
Case Western Reserve University
Cleveland, Ohio

Preface

Injury to the fetal and neonatal brain continues to be a major risk in an era when perinatal care has improved significantly and neonatal survival rates have improved steadily. A great deal of emphasis has been placed on the understanding of the pathophysiological and biochemical alterations that occur during the asphyxial episode or episodes, and which continue through the resuscitative and reparative periods. Newer technologies and approaches to therapy have also been developed to maximize the chances of an optimal outcome for the affected patient. There has been a great deal of effort by the American Academy of Pediatrics and the American Heart Association to educate caretakers in order to improve the immediate and follow-up care of the neurologically depressed newborn who is in need of resuscitative management.

In this, the third edition of our text, we have incorporated many of the newer approaches to the understanding of the cellular and molecular bases of hypoxic–ischemic encephalopathy (HIE), as well as the newer approaches to the immediate and continuing care of these infants. We have added new chapters on obstetrical conditions that may be associated with brain injury of the fetus, including chorioamnionitis, various maternal diseases, and obstetrical catastrophes. Metabolic disorders that may have clinical manifestations that mimic HIE have been emphasized as well. The chapters on infectious diseases that can result in brain injury have been enhanced, with particular reference to viral and group B streptococcal infections. The long-term follow-up of the affected infants as well as the ethical considerations involved in the approach to care have also been updated.

We have added a third editor, Dr William E. Benitz, in order to strengthen the recruitment of contributors and to "fine-tune" many of the presentations.

As noted in our previous editions, with any text that has multiple contributors there is a certain amount of overlap and repetition among the various presentations. Rather than editing these chapters to avoid such overlap entirely, we have elected to respect the authors' unique presentations and styles, as different perspectives also reflect the richness of their clinical experiences. We also believe that this allows the contributors to express their opinions more freely, and the variation of opinion on similar topics can thus be appreciated.

We would like to take this opportunity to thank our collaborators, especially those who met their editorial deadlines and the members of Cambridge University Press for their support and expertise in preparing the text. Secretarial help from Jenni Edgar, Christy Stoffel, and Lani Lucente, who spent many hours in preparation of the manuscript, as well as Tonya Gonzales-Clenny, who edited many of the papers to fit the format of the text, is deeply appreciated.

We also wish to thank our respective wives, Joan Stevenson, Andrea Benitz, and Sara Sunshine for their support, encouragement, and patience.

David K. Stevenson
William E. Benitz
Philip Sunshine

PART I

Epidemiology, Pathophysiology, and Pathogenesis of Fetal and Neonatal Brain Injury

1

Perinatal asphyxia: an overview

Philip Sunshine

Department of Pediatrics, Stanford University Medical Center, Palo Alto, CA, USA

Although there has been a marked reduction in perinatal morbidity and mortality rates over the past four decades, asphyxia in the perinatal period, leading to major motor and cognitive disabilities, continues to be a significant health problem worldwide. With a great deal of emphasis being placed on fetal monitoring, the rapid institution of appropriate resuscitative measures in depressed infants, as well as having more precision in the diagnosis and documentation of asphyxia, the mortality rate due to intrauterine hypoxia and birth asphyxia (ICD-9 code 768) has decreased by over 70% since 1979 in the USA.[1] This trend has been noticed in Sweden[2] and in the UK[3] as well.

Despite these advances, a large number of infants with neurological abnormalities manifested by cerebral palsy, hearing or visual impairment, and mental retardation are born each year, many due to problems encountered during the birthing process. For many years, since W. J. Little's initial report linking neurological and mental handicaps in infants and children to abnormalities of labor and delivery, premature birth and asphyxia neonatorum,[4] physicians in general and the lay public in particular have considered that birth trauma and "perinatal asphyxia" were the primary causes of handicaps in children. They also felt that had appropriate obstetrical and neonatal care been provided, the majority of such handicaps could have been prevented. However, over the past 13–15 years, many epidemiological and clinical studies have demonstrated that most cases of cerebral palsy are not related to intrapartum asphyxia, and that if one eliminated infants born prematurely, as few as 7% to as many as 23% of infants born at term who developed cerebral palsy did so because of injuries sustained during this interval.[5–20] Most authorities in the field judge that the incidence is about 10% in developed countries and somewhat higher in developing countries. Nevertheless, it is the single most common cause of neurological/intellectual handicaps in children.

Major difficulties have been encountered in the inability to identify the timing, the type, the duration, and the severity of the insult that are associated with the neurological deficits. Also, the terminology used to describe the depressed or affected infant is often nonspecific and vague. Perinatal asphyxia, intrapartum asphyxia, hypoxemic–ischemic encephalopathy, neonatal neurologic dysfunctional syndrome, and fetal–neonatal acidemia have been used interchangeably to identify the affected newborn.

Several recent and excellent reviews of these problems have been published and have advanced our understanding of the incidence, the clinical manifestations, the laboratory correlates, the electroencephalographic abnormalities, and the imaging findings in infants with neonatal neurological abnormalities.[16–27] These studies have also evaluated infants who have few, if any, neonatal abnormalities but who were later found to be handicapped. While our understanding in these spheres has improved remarkably, we often lack sufficient data to understand thoroughly the mechanism or mechanisms involved in any particular affected newborn. Unfortunately, a thorough investigation attempting to identify the cause or causes of neonatal neurological depression is often not attempted or is incomplete, and the diagnosis of perinatal asphyxia is made by default.[28] The long-term evaluation of the depressed infant is often lacking, and except for a few studies, little is known of the subsequent development of these patients.[3,20,29–32] Although severely affected infants are most likely to be enrolled in interventional and follow-up programs, those who have mild-to-moderate depression usually do not participate in long-term evaluations. Lastly, an infant or child may be identified as having neurologic or intellectual impairment, and then a retrospective analysis is instituted to identify the etiology of the abnormality. In many instances a definitive causative factor is not found, but there are suggestions that some "irregularities" of practice occurred during the perinatal period. Such suggestions sometimes provide the *only* bases for the assumptions that "perinatal asphyxia" was responsible for the child's impairment, and that if alternative approaches had been undertaken in the intrapartum period, little if any damage would have resulted. Unfortunately such reasoning has prevailed over the years despite the lack of substantive supporting data, and numerous litigations have been instituted in the belief that retrospective associations represent cause-and-effect relationships.

We readily recognize those infants who have been subjected to severe intrauterine stress, who are depressed at birth, and who remain obtunded during the neonatal period. These infants often have seizures with aberrant electroencephalographic patterns, have multiorgan abnormalities, and have a high incidence of neonatal death or subsequent neurological handicaps. These infants fit the classic clinical scenario of the neonate with hypoxemic–ischemic encephalopathy. In a number of these infants, this type of encephalopathy may not be due to intrapartum or neonatal difficulties, but may be due to other factors such as sepsis, congenital malformations, chorioamnionitis, congenital metabolic abnormalities, and various types of myotonic conditions.[11]

But what about the neonate who is depressed at birth, but who responds readily to resuscitation and has an uneventful neonatal course? If such an infant is later found to have neurological disabilities, can one implicate abnormalities in the perinatal period as being the "proximate cause" of the sequelae? The currently available data suggest that episodes of mild neonatal depression are not associated with subsequent handicaps, and that even following moderate or severe depressions, most infants, if they survive, develop normally.[29,33]

It is critical that we have a better understanding of those factors that contribute to the development of the "brain-damaged child" and that we not be unduly influenced by circumstantial evidence. It is also critical to recognize that many of the events leading to difficulties in the infant occur long before the mother has the onset of labor. With the improvement of ultrasonographic, computed tomography (CT), and magnetic resonance imaging (MRI) expertise, more and more infants are being recognized with intrauterine abnormalities that have already caused significant damage.[34–50] Careful examination of the placenta can also identify lesions that are associated with infection or anomalies that have been present for a period of time[51–53] (see Chapter 24). We recognize that these infants are often unable to tolerate the stress of labor well, may have fetal heart rate abnormalities either prior to delivery or during the early stages of labor, or have abnormal contraction stress tests or nonstress testing.[34,50] These infants are often difficult to resuscitate and show neurological features that seem excessive considering the problems that occurred during labor or the birthing process. In addition, some infants may have suffered a significant intrauterine catastrophe, recover, and may even be able to tolerate labor well enough not to have abnormalities noted on their fetal heart rate tracings.[54]

We also recognize that events leading to difficulties in the prematurely born infant may be different from those in infants born near or at term. Similarly, the preterm infant may have many more and vastly different difficulties in the postpartum rather than the intrapartum period, and will have different clinical features from those seen in the full-term infant. In attempts to evaluate etiology, pathogenesis, intervention, and management one must be aware that similar events may have different consequences depending upon the patient's capacity to respond to various insults, and some of these are determined by gestational age. In addition, infants with intrauterine growth restriction make up a disproportionate share of infants with neonatal brain injury, suggesting that the underlying cause or causes of the growth restriction may have started in utero and continued through the intrapartum and postpartum periods.

Asphyxia

Asphyxia is defined as progressive hypoxemia and hypercapnea accompanied by the progressive development of metabolic acidosis. The definition has both clinical and biochemical components, and indicates that, unless the process is reversed, it will lead to cellular damage and ultimately death of the patient.[23] As stated by Stanley et al., "Birth asphyxia is a theoretical concept, and its existence in a patient is not easy to recognize accurately by clinical observation."[20] We currently do not have the sophisticated technology of routinely measuring fetal cerebral activity or the response to unfavorable conditions such as hypoxia, ischemia, or acidosis, the compensatory mechanisms that protect the brain cells, or, when such mechanisms are inadequate, the documentation of cell injury and cellular death.

In lieu of direct measurements, we have utilized indirect indicators that have been based on studies carried out in laboratory animals and extrapolated to be used in the human fetus. In a few instances, direct measurements have been possible, but have not been linked well to outcome. Indirect assessments include the biophysical profile, fetal heart rate measurements, evidence of severe metabolic acidosis, depressed Apgar scores, abnormal newborn neurological function, and development of seizures. As mentioned, the timing of the events is often unknown and difficult to ascertain as far as onset, duration, and severity are concerned.

Based on studies in monkeys by Dawes[55] and Brann and Myers,[56,57] and also substantiated to a great extent in fetal lambs by the group in Auckland,[58–62] two major types of intrauterine asphyxial conditions have been recognized. The causes of the acute total asphyxial events are listed in Table 1.1, and have been referred to as "sentinel events" by MacLennan and the International Cerebral Palsy Task Force.[24] In the acute type of asphyxia, there is a catastrophic event, the fetus is suddenly and rapidly deprived of his or her lifeline, and usually does not have the opportunity to protect the brain by "invoking the diving reflex." The conditions most commonly encountered include prolapse of the cord,[63–65] placental abruption, and fetal hemorrhage. With the increasing use of vaginal births after cesarean sections, we are also encountering more and more neonates being born following uterine rupture.[66]

These infants have damage to the deep gray matter of the brain involving the thalamus, basal ganglia, and the brainstem, often with sparing of the cerebral cortex.[67–70] These infants, if successfully resuscitated, often do not have evidence of multisystem or multiorgan dysfunction. Laboratory animals, who were quite healthy prior to the onset of the acute asphyxial event, develop evidence of neurological damage as early as 8 min after the event.[55] Major irreversible lesions were found after 10–11 min,[56,57] and the animals usually succumbed if not resuscitated within 18 min. After 20 min of asphyxia, some animals could be resuscitated, but usually died of cardiogenic shock within 24–48 h even with intensive care.

Table 1.1. Acute causes of fetal brain injury (sentinel events)

Prolapsed umbilical cord
Uterine rupture
Abruptio placentae
Amniotic fluid embolism
Acute neonatal hemorrhage
Vasa previa
Acute blood loss from cord
Acute maternal hemorrhage
Any condition causing an abrupt decrease in maternal cardiac output and/or blood flow to the fetus

Although data in humans are lacking, studies of infants following prolapsed cords suggest similar time frames,[63–65] and those infants who have occult prolapse[65] often have a better outcome than those with overt prolapse. The study from Los Angeles County University of Southern California (LAC/USC) Medical Center noted that if it required greater than 18 min to deliver the fetus after spontaneous rupture of the uterus, neurological sequelae would ensue.[66] Unfortunately, the long-term follow-up of the surviving infants in this study is not available. Thus the 30-min timing of "decision to incision," as recommended by the American College of Obstetricians and Gynecologists (ACOG), is not valid in these situations.

The infants who have suffered this type of acute event will have varying degrees of neurological injury, often manifesting extrapyramidal types of cerebral palsy and with varying degrees of mental impairment depending upon the severity and extent of the injury.[67–70]

Those infants subjected to prolonged partial asphyxial episodes and who have neurological involvement most often have lesions in the cerebral cortex in a watershed type of distribution.[27,71] They often have multiorgan involvement and have pyramidal signs of cerebral palsy.[27] The incidence and severity of cognitive impairment also depend upon the extent and severity of the lesion.

An acute event may also occur in a fetus who has already been subjected to a partial prolonged asphyxial condition or a preexisting neurological insult. That fetus may demonstrate complications of both processes and have both pyramidal and extrapyramidal neurological findings associated with varying degrees of auditory, visual, and/or cognitive abnormalities.

Incidence of asphyxia and correlation with outcome

Most authorities suggest that "perinatal asphyxia" occurs in 3–5 infants per 1000 live births, and that the incidence of encephalopathy occurs in 0.5–1 per 1000 live births.[2,20,27] Various techniques have been used to identify the asphyxiated infant including the time required to initiate spontaneous ventilation, the time that positive-pressure ventilation was required to sustain the infant before spontaneous respirations ensued, and the use of the neonatal scoring system developed by Virginia Apgar.[72–74]

The newborn scoring system which was developed by Apgar has been used in almost every delivery room to identify those infants who are depressed and who require resuscitation efforts. In addition, the use of the scoring system required an "advocate" for the neonate because someone had to evaluate the infant in the immediate neonatal period and provide a numerical score of the baby's condition. Dr Apgar did not design the scoring system to be used to evaluate neurological outcome and to identify infants early on who would subsequently develop neurological handicaps. Unfortunately, the Apgar score has been utilized in many situations for that very purpose.

It was so utilized in the National Collaborative Perinatal Project (NCPP) of the National Institutes for Neurological Disease and Stroke.[75] Unfortunately, there are many factors that can influence the Apgar score, including immaturity, maternal anesthesia and analgesia, fetal or neonatal sepsis, or neuromuscular abnormalities.[75–77] Despite these caveats, the Apgar scoring system remains the standard by which neonates are evaluated immediately after birth as well as their response to appropriate resuscitative techniques.

The long-term neurological outcome, especially in term infants, has not correlated well with low scores at 1 and 5 min, but begins to have better correlation for those infants who have scores of 0–3 for 10, 15, and 20 min after birth.[78]

If one uses an Apgar score of 6 or less at 5 min of age to indicate asphyxia, the incidence of asphyxia in the NCPP study was almost 5% (Table 1.2). Interestingly, Levene and coworkers evaluated two methods of predicting outcome in asphyxiated infants using several different Apgar ratings.[79] They found that a 10-min Apgar score of 5 or less had a sensitivity of 43% and a specificity of 95% in predicting adverse outcomes. This was in a group of infants that had postasphyxial encephalopathy.

Table 1.2. Incidence of perinatal asphyxia, mortality, and handicaps in survivors

						Outcome in survivors (%)		
Authors	Years of study	Definition of asphyxia	Number of patients	Incidence of asphyxia	Deaths (%)	Normal	Mild-to-moderate damage	Severe damage
Neligan et al. 1974:[84] community study	1960–1962	Delay greater than 5 min to establish respiration	13203	27/1000 (includes prematures)	21	95.4	0.05	4
Steiner and Neligan 1975:[87] hospital study	1961–1970	Cardiac arrest or delay greater than 20 min to establish respiration	20793	1.8/1000	52	77		23
Scott 1976[86]	1966–1971	Apparent stillborn or delay greater than 20 min to establish respiration	12389	3.8/1000	52	74		26
Nelson and Ellenberg 1981[78]	1959–1966	Apgar scores 6 or less at 5 min (all weights)	49498	47/1000	24	96.4		3.6
		Apgar scores 0–3 at 5 min (all weights)	49498	15.7/1000	42	94.7		5.3
		Apgar score 0–3 at 10 min (all weights)	49498	7.2/1000	76	76	10	14
Peters et al. 1984[82,83]	4/4–4/11/70	More than 3 min to establish respiration (all weights)	16333	45/1000	6.0	86		14
MacDonald et al.[80] and Mulligan et al 1980[81]	1970–1975	More than 1 min positive-pressure ventilation	38405	11.6/1000	46.1[a]	81.5		18.5
MacDonald et al. 1985[144]	1981–1983	Neonatal seizures	13084	3/1000	23	80		20
Jain et al. 1991[85]	1982–1986	Apparent stillborn (Apgar 0 at 1 min) all weights	81242	7.5/1000	64	61	13	26
Thornberg et al. 1995[2]	1985–1991	Apgar <7 at 5 min	42203	6.9/1000	5.7	93	1.4	5.6
Yeo and Trudehope 1994[89]	1981–1991	Apgar 0 at 1 min	64064	8.4/1000	92	63	12	25
Casalaz et al. 1998[88]	1986–1994	Apgar 0 at 1 min	94511	0.5/1000 (62% term)	7 immediate 42 total	64	16	23

Notes:
[a] 89% <30 weeks, 18% >36 weeks.
Source: Modified from Dennis.[9]

In 1980 MacDonald and coworkers evaluated 38405 consecutive deliveries and defined neonatal asphyxia in infants who required more than 1 min of positive pressure ventilation before sustained respiration occurred.[80,81] They found 447 infants with asphyxia – an overall incidence of 1.15%. The more immature the infant, the greater the incidence, severity, and mortality associated with asphyxial episodes (Table 1.2).

Peters and coworkers evaluated 17196 infants born during the week of 5 April 1970 through 11 April 1970 in the UK. These investigators used the time required for the onset of regular respirations to define asphyxia. The times were less than 1 min, 1–3 min (mild-to-moderate asphyxia), and more than 3 min (severe asphyxia).[82,83] The mortality rates were very low in infants who required either less than 1 min or 1–3 min to breathe; however, there was an increase in mortality in infants who required more than 3 min to institute normal respiration. The incidence of mild-to-moderate asphyxia was 18% and that of severe asphyxia was 4%. The overall mortality was most pronounced in very-low-birth-weight infants. The subsequent follow-up demonstrated an increased incidence of cerebral palsy not only in infants of low birth weight but also in larger infants, especially in those requiring more than 3 min to institute spontaneous respiration (Table 1.2).

Neligan and coworkers, using the criterion of a 5-min delay in establishing respirations, found an incidence of asphyxia of 27/1000 births, including preterm infants.[84] They also noted a mortality rate of 21%, but 95.4% of the surviving infants were normal at follow-up examination.

Jain and coworkers evaluated the outcome of infants who were apparently stillborn (Apgar scores 0 at 1 min).[85] Data from a total of 81242 mother–infant pairs were analyzed and 613 infants were identified. Of these, 520 were classified as fetal deaths and were not resuscitated. Of the remaining 93 infants, 31 did not respond to resuscitative efforts, but 62 patients did. Twenty-six died in the neonatal period, three died after discharge, and 10 infants were lost to follow-up. Of the remainder, 61% were felt to be normal infants, 26% were abnormal, and 13% were suspected of having some neurological damage. None of the infants weighing less than 750 g at birth survived. The survival rate of the infants was 16% if the Apgar score remained 0 at 5 min and only 1.7% if it remained 0 at 10 min. Also, infants who were resuscitated at level II centers had a 50% delivery room mortality rate as compared with 26% cared for in level III centers.

Scott, defining severe asphyxia in infants who were apparently stillborn or who required more than 20 min to establish spontaneous respirations, included both preterm and term infants in the evaluation.[86] Scott also noted that, although half of the infants died, three-quarters of the survivors were apparently normal – a surprising finding considering the dire condition of the infants at birth (Table 1.2).

Steiner and Neligan, evaluating the neonates with cardiac arrest or a delay greater than 20 min for them to establish respiration, noted an incidence of 1.8/1000 births for this type of severe asphyxia. The mortality rate for these infants was 52%, but 77% of the survivors were normal at follow-up examinations.[87]

Casalaz and coworkers described 45 infants who were 24 weeks' gestation or greater who were classified as an unsuspected apparent stillborn – an incidence of 0.5/1000 live births.[88] Of these, 42 were successfully resuscitated, 52% either died or survived severely disabled, but 36% survived apparently intact. In this study, indicators of poor outcome included 5- and 10-minute Apgar scores of 3 or less, an arterial pH within the first 2 hours of life of less than 7.0, and an absent heart beat at 5 min of age.

Yeo and Tudehope described 539 infants with Apgar scores of 0 at 1 min – an incidence of 8.4/1000 births, of whom only 8.3% were successfully resuscitated.[89] Of the survivors who left the hospital, 64% had a normal outcome.

There are a few published reports that have evaluated the outcome of severely depressed infants who have required 30 min or more of assisted ventilation before they were able to initiate spontaneous respiration. Steiner and Neligan reported that all of the four patients they cared for died or had severe handicaps.[87] Scott reported 11 such infants, four of whom were normal or had mild handicaps.[86] Koppe and Kleiverda reported that all 13 of such patients either died or had severe handicaps.[90] De Souza and Richards, on the other hand, had seven infants who required greater than 30 min to establish spontaneous respirations, and all seven survived, and were normal or had minimal disabilities.[91] Amazing.

Correlative signs of asphyxia

Several signs or findings have been correlative to some extent with the severity of asphyxia in the intrapartum period. These have included the presence of meconium in the amniotic fluid, evidence of metabolic acidosis measured either from cord blood or in the immediate neonatal period, the presence and severity of the neonatal neurological assessment, the onset of seizures within the first 3 days of life, supporting laboratory data, findings on electroencephalography, corroborative findings on imaging studies, and evidence of multiorgan dysfunction.

Meconium

The presence of meconium in the amniotic fluid has long been thought to indicate fetal stress (see Chapters 24 and 31). Meconium is found in 8–20% of all deliveries, being uncommonly encountered in preterm gestations and more frequently encountered in the postterm baby. If meconium is recognized in amniotic fluids of infants at 34 weeks' gestation or younger, significant intrauterine stress or intrauterine infection must be suspected. In term and postterm infants, meconium staining is usually light and the fetus and newborn are essentially symptom-free. However, heavy, thick meconium passed early in labor tends to have a more ominous significance than when passed more proximate to delivery.[92] But even this finding has not been substantiated in other studies.[93]

The presence of meconium *per se* in term infants is not predictive of neurological sequelae; in fact, Nelson and Ellenberg noted that fewer than 0.5% of the infants weighing more than 2500 g with meconium staining had neurological sequelae.[94] In studies in the Netherlands, the presence of meconium-stained amniotic fluid had no predictive value in regard to outcome, the development of neurologic symptoms in the newborn period, or acidosis measured by the pH of cord blood.[95–97] Even when the presence of meconium was ascertained and used in conjunction with either Apgar scores or cord pH values or both, the finding did not alter the incidence of subsequent neurological abnormalities. In Chapter 24, Dr Altshuler discusses the factors in meconium that affect the placenta and fetal circulation, and in Chapter 31, Dr Wiswell addresses the significance of meconium in amniotic fluid and its relationship to neonatal problems.

Fetal and neonatal blood gas levels

Steward Clifford was one of the first clinicians to suggest that neurologic abnormalities in the neonate are not necessarily due to birth trauma but rather to the accumulation of lactic and carbonic acids secondary to the hypoxic–anoxic episode.[98] He also noted that, in addition to damage occurring in the central nervous system, every organ and tissue in the body could be affected to some degree. Since his observations, which subsequently have been supported by studies in laboratory animals, it has been postulated that the accumulation of lactic acid is correlated with the abnormalities seen in hypoxic–ischemic encephalopathy.

Since 1967, obstetricians have utilized fetal acid–base measurements as adjuncts to fetal heart rate monitoring to evaluate the well-being of the fetus, and to identify those fetuses who were at risk for intrapartum difficulties.[99,100] However, there is a great deal of debate as to whether or not these techniques are truly helpful in the management of labor.[101,102]

Subsequently, investigators attempted to correlate the fetal acid–base status with subsequent neurological outcome. Initially it was stated that the normal umbilical arterial pH was 7.25–7.35 and defined a pH below 7.20 as acidosis. Then lower levels of pH such as 7.15 or even 7.10 were noted to be indicative of acidosis.

In the study by Sykes and coworkers only 20% of the neonates with Apgar scores of 6 or less had cord pH values of 7.10 or less.[103] Of infants whose cord pH value was 7.10 or less, 22% had Apgar scores of 6 or less. Similar results were obtained by Silverman and coworkers, who noted that the metabolic state of the fetus as measured by the umbilical artery pH level was not closely related to the Apgar score unless a severe degree of biochemical abnormality was encountered, i.e., a pH value less than 7.05.[104] Dijxhoorn and coworkers found similar results in appropriately grown neonates.[95–97] They found that measurements of the arterial or venous pH or the maternal-fetal difference in pH alone could not be used as predictors of neonatal neurological depression. However, in infants who were small-for-gestational-age, the incidence of fetal acidosis was greater than in appropriate-for-gestational-age infants, but was not necessarily correlative with severe neonatal depression.[97]

Correlative data appear when the cord arterial pH is 7.00 or less and when there is evidence of neurological abnormalities in the neonatal period as well. Also, the finding of a low pH in itself is of less prognostic significance if it is due primarily to respiratory acidosis rather than metabolic or even mixed acidosis.[105–113] Low and coworkers, who have written extensively on this subject, noted that "the threshold for significant metabolic acidosis is a base deficit between 12 and 16 mmol/liter."[23,114,115] They have found a base deficit of 12 mmol/l in 2% of all births and a base deficit of 16 mmol/l in 0.5% of the population studied. An increased number of neurological abnormalities were encountered in infants as the degree of acidosis worsened. Also, the longer the acidosis was present, the greater was the correlation with neurological deficits;[23,115–120] and a period of 1 h or greater was a critical time for the metabolic acidosis to have been present.[120]

These studies have more clinical significance and have better correlation with subsequent outcome if the acidosis is associated with abnormal neurological findings in the infant at the time of birth. Interestingly, a group of infants with metabolic acidosis (umbilical arterial base deficit of greater than 12 mmol/l) but who had either none or mild neurological complications were followed for 8 years and were found to have no greater incidence of neurological or cognitive handicaps than a control group of patients.[33]

Table 1.3. Severity of fetal acidosis and hypoxic–ischemic encephalopathy and other organ dysfunction

pH	% with encephalopathy	% with other organ damage
6.61–6.70	80	80
6.71–6.79	60	60
6.80–6.89	33	52
6.90–6.99	12	25

Source: Data from Goodwin et al.[108]

Goodwin and coworkers from LAC-USC Medical Center identified 126 term live-born singleton infants who had no major anomalies over a 4½ year period (total deliveries were 76 548).[108] Of these, 109 infants were evaluated if the blood gas was documented to be arterial. The vast majority of the infants had either mixed or metabolic acidemia and the lower the pH, the greater was the risk of hypoxemic–ischemic encephalopathy (Table 1.3).

In evaluating the outcome in the 126 infants, five died (4%), 8% had major neurological deficits, 4% were suspected of having neurological problems, 6% were lost to follow-up, and 78% were normal.

In a follow-up study, these investigators noted that in the patients with an umbilical arterial pH of 7.00 or less, there was a greater incidence of seizures, hypoxic–ischemic encephalopathy, cardiac, pulmonary, and renal dysfunction and abnormal development at follow-up if the arteriovenous difference in $P\text{CO}_2$ was greater than 25 mmHg. The sensitivities of these clinical findings ranged from 84 to 95% and the specificities ranged from 54 to 60%. The arteriovenous difference in $P\text{O}_2$ correlated to a much lesser extent.[111]

Van den Berg and coworkers found an increased number of neonatal complications in newborns with an umbilical arterial pH below 7.00.[112]

Obtaining routine umbilical arterial and venous cord samples in 14 025 infants over an 8-year period, they found that 1.3% of infants who had reliable cord samples had an arterial cord pH less than 7.00. Only two of these infants died, but 32% had to be admitted to an intensive care nursery and 23% had neurological abnormalities. If the base deficit was 15 mmol/l or greater, 93% had neurological abnormalities. Interestingly, 27% of these infants had no neonatal problems. Unfortunately, the long-term evaluation of these infants is lacking.

Andres et al. found similar data in 93 infants with umbilical arterial pH of less than 7.00.[113] Nine percent of the infants died, 40% required intubation, 5% had seizures and 2% had hypoxic–ischemic encephalopathy. These authors also found a higher base deficit (>19 mmol/l) in the seriously affected infants. This was a retrospective evaluation and long-term outcome is lacking.

In an interesting study, Kruger and coworkers found a better correlation using fetal scalp lactate measurements than scalp pH in predicting low Apgar scores and moderate-to-severe hypoxic–ischemic encephalopathy. Further evaluation of this technique using microquantities of blood is warranted.[121]

Using data from numerous studies, the International Cerebral Palsy Task Force has recommended that in order to determine that an intrapartum hypoxic event has taken place, one of the three major criteria listed is a pH of less than 7.00 and a base deficit of greater than 12 mmol/l.[24]

Laboratory correlates

Various metabolic parameters have been used to identify or verify the severity of the asphyxial insult in addition to the severity of the metabolic acidosis mentioned above (Table 1.4). Goldberg and coworkers described severe hyperammonemia, usually accompanied by elevated activities of aspartate amino transferase and alanine aminotransferase, as a consequence of severe asphyxia.[122] As the condition of the infant improved, the levels of ammonia decreased as well. Table 1.4 lists the various parameters that have been measured in various body fluids. Until recently, most of these products were significantly elevated in patients who had severe and prolonged asphyxia.[123,124] Studies of creatinine kinase brain isoenzyme and neuron-specific enolase[125] in the cerebrospinal fluid (CSF) have a more correlative effect with the severity of the asphyxiated period. Even the elevation of aspartate and glutamate, the neuroexcitatory amino acids, was only increased in the severely asphyxiated infants.[126,127] Similarly, elevations of glial fibrillary acidic protein in the CSF were found in severely asphyxiated infants.[128] Hypoxanthine elevations in plasma and urine have had variable correlative effects with the degree of asphyxia.[129]

Table 1.4. Laboratory studies used to support the diagnosis and severity of perinatal asphyxia

Study	Body fluid
Ammonia	Blood
Lactate	Serum, CSF
Hypoxanthine	Serum, urine
Erythropoietin	Serum, CSF
Creatine kinase brain isoenzyme (CK-BB)	Serum, CSF
Myelin basic protein	CSF
Neuron-specific enolase	CSF
Aspartate	CSF
Glutamate	CSF
Glial fibrillary acidic protein	CSF
Lactate: creatinine ratio	Urine
Carbon monoxide	Plasma
Nitric oxide	Plasma

Notes:
CSF, cerebrospinal fluid.
Source: Modified from Volpe (27)

Similar to the findings of an elevated scalp lactate level as an adjunct to evaluating the severity of intrapartum difficulties, da Silva et al. measured lactic acid levels and base deficit at 30 min of age in 115 term infants who were suspected of having intrapartum asphyxia.[130] They found excellent correlation between the base deficit and plasma lactate levels, and when the lactate level was less than 5 mmol/l and/or the base deficit lower than 10 mmol/l, the infants did not have moderate or severe hypoxic–ischemic encephalopathy. If the plasma lactate level was greater than 14 mmol/l and/or the base deficit greater than 20 mmol/l, severe neonatal encephalopathy was found in 80% and 100% of the infants.

Huang et al. recently reported on the base of the measurement of urinary lactate to creatinine ratio for early detection of infants at risk of developing hypoxic–ischemic encephalopathy, especially if this ratio was measured on urine collected within 6 h of birth.[131] They were able to correlate levels with degrees of hypoxic–ischemic encephalopathy as well as neurological outcome at 1 year of age, with only one infant who had an adverse outcome demonstrating a normal ratio. Although the authors noted that the first urine sample was obtained at a mean of 4 ± 1 h in all groups, many of us who care for such severely depressed infants note no urine output for a much longer period of time in severely depressed neonates.

Juul and colleagues from Florida evaluated erythropoietin levels in the spinal fluid of infants with asphyxia and found it to be elevated in those infants as well.[132] The levels in plasma as well as in the CSF were markedly elevated even in comparison to infants with intraventricular hemorrhage or meningitis and were similar to the findings originally reported by Ruth et al. in plasma.[133]

Lastly, a study evaluating the concentration of nitric oxide and carbon monoxide in plasma has been useful in delineating those infants without hypoxic–ischemic encephalopathy or stage 1 hypoxic–ischemic encephalopathy from those with stage 2 and stage 3 hypoxic–ischemic encephalopathy. These are preliminary data and long-term follow-up is clearly indicated.[134]

(For a more complete listing of laboratory correlates, see Volpe,[27] p. 336.)

Seizures

The onset of seizures within the first 2–3 days of life has been thought to indicate the quality of perinatal care[135,136] (see Chapter 21). More likely, however, seizures have more correlation with long-term neurological handicaps, since these infants are 15–17 times more likely to have neurological sequelae than newborns without seizures.[137] The incidence of neonatal seizures has been reported to vary between 1.3 per 1000 and 14 per 1000 live births, but more recent data suggest that the incidence does not exceed 9 per 1000.[138] Over 60% of neonatal seizures occur within the first 48 h of life, if they are due to intrapartum asphyxia. Except for those seizures occurring secondary to bacterial meningitis, early-onset seizures secondary to asphyxia, have a more ominous outcome, in terms of mortality and neurological sequelae, than those occurring later in the neonatal period.[139,140] The overall mortality rate varies from 9 to 35% (Table 1.5).

The etiology of neonatal seizures varies as well. Even though many investigators suggest that the early onset of seizures is due primarily to intrapartum events, other etiologic factors have been incriminated as well. In a study in Leicester, UK, Levene and Trounce found that, although intrapartum and postnatal asphyxia accounted for 53% of their patients, hemorrhage (15%), infection (8%), metabolic aberrations (5%), hypoglycemia (3%), and stroke (5%) also contribute to the problem.[141] Only 8% of these patients had seizures of unexplained origin, a finding at variance with the incidences reported in Stockholm (29%)[142] and Australia (64%).[138] Typically, infants who suffer from severe hypoxemic–ischemic encephalopathy have seizures beginning in the first 48 h after birth. These seizures are often recurrent and extremely difficult to control. Those that occur within the first 12 h after the insult or those that are difficult to control are more likely to result in significant neurological sequelae.[27] Conversely, patients who have a single seizure of a fleeting nature should have an excellent outcome, especially if the seizures do not recur.

As noted by Niswander and coworkers,[143] even when mothers were managed appropriately during the intrapartum period, early-onset seizures occurred in their offspring. In the Dublin randomized study described by MacDonald et al., the incidence of early-onset seizures was twice as great in

Table 1.5. Incidence and outcome of infants with neonatal seizures

Author	Incidence	Mortality	Incidence of handicaps: survivors
Eriksson and Zetterstrom 1979[142]	1.5/1000 full-term deliveries all infants <4 weeks of age	14%	41%
Finer et al. 1981[148]	3.22/1000 of inborn; total of 6.5 infants inborn and outborn 37 weeks	8%	50% (14% mild, 17% moderate, 19% severe)
Holden et al. 1982 (NCPP data)[137]	5/1000	34.8%; two-thirds died in neonatal period	13% cerebral palsy; 19% mental retardation; 33% epilepsy; 13% mental retardation, cerebral palsy, or epilepsy
Goldberg 1983[138]		33.5%	
1971–1974	2/1000	17.5%	
1975–1977	6/1000	18.5% mortality due to cerebral hypoxia: overall 50%	
1978–1980	8.6/1000		
Derham et al. 1985[136]	1.6/1000 infants >37 weeks; seizures within 48h after birth	35%	36%
Minchom et al. 1987[139]	1.3/1000 live births >37 weeks; seizures within 48h after birth	9.2%	22.4% (4% mild, 8% moderate, 10% severe)
Grant et al. 1989[145]	Electronically monitored, 1.8/1000	25%	25%
MacDonald et al. 1985[144]	Auscultation, 4.1/1000	22	25%
Curtis et al. 1988[146] (101 829 term infants)	0.87/1000	18%	25%
Halligan et al. 1992[151] (total 28 655 infants)			
High-risk group (6251)	0.16/1000	0	28% hypertonic
Low-risk group (22 404)	1.43/1000	28%	6% moderately handicapped, 19% severe

Notes:
NCPP, National Collaborative Perinatal Project

the intermittently monitored population as in those in whom electronic fetal heart rate monitoring was employed.[144,145] However, the mortality and incidence of severe disability in the survivors of neonatal seizures at 1 year of age were identical in the two groups studied.[145]

Curtis and coworkers evaluated seizures in over 100 000 term infants and found the incidence to be 0.87/1000 live births. The infants had a mortality rate of 18%, and 26% of the survivors were handicapped.[146]

Keegan and coworkers identified 66 patients with neonatal seizures, 34 of whom were term births, and retrospectively evaluated the perinatal events that occurred in the infants.[147] The affected infants had lower 1- and 5-min Apgar scores than control infants and had increased incidence of placenta previa, abruptio placentae, and postdatism. Abnormal fetal heart rate patterns were noted in 85% of these patients, with an absence of variability in 59% or an abnormal pattern with absence of variability in 53%. In the patients with aberrant fetal heart rate patterns, there was appropriate intervention in over 80% of cases. Despite intervention, all infants had seizures and almost half (42%) of the survivors had significant neurologic handicaps. Even more disconcerting was the number of infants with seizures who did not demonstrate fetal heart rate patterns suggestive of fetal distress and thus no intervention was indicated. These observations suggest that either the event leading to the seizures occurred prior to the onset of labor or the event (or events) occurred in infants with lesser degrees of fetal heart rate abnormalities than are currently being recognized.

Finer and coworkers reported an incidence of seizures in 3.22/1000 live births with an 8% mortality and a 50% incidence of handicap, of which 19% had severe handicaps.[148]

Neonatal neurologic syndrome

If significant intrapartum asphyxia has occurred, the infant should demonstrate neurologic abnormalities in the neonatal period. It is often difficult to appreciate such abnormalities in preterm infants, especially those who have cardiopulmonary abnormalities and who are being treated with assisted ventilation. Often these infants cannot be distinguished from other prematurely born infants with similar cardiopulmonary abnormalities. However, in the term or near-term infant, signs of encephalopathy are readily discernible. Sarnat and Sarnat developed an infant scoring system that categorizes the patients into three stages of "postasphyxial encephalopathy," identifying mild, moderate, and severe.[149] Although they correlated many of the findings with electroencephalographic changes, one can use their classification even if the electroencephalograms are not evaluated.

Patients with mild encephalopathy often are hyperirritable and have hyperactive reflexes, tachycardia, and poor sucking, but no evidence of seizures. Patients with severe encephalopathy are stuporous, flaccid, and hypotonic; there are no Moro, oculovestibular, or tonic neck reflexes. The infants do not suck and often show decerebrate posturing. These patients are often in need of assisted ventilation and cardiotonic support and remain in this state for days to weeks. The electroencephalographic pattern usually demonstrates burst suppression or is isopotential. Patients with moderate encephalopathy tend to be in the middle of these two extremes, have mild hypotonia and weak or incomplete reflexes, and often have focal or multifocal seizures.

The neurologic outcome in these infants is related to the severity of the neonatal symptoms. Robertson and Finer reported that infants with mild symptoms had no handicaps at follow-up; 76% of those with moderate encephalopathy were without handicap; those with severe encephalopathy either died or had moderate-to-severe neurologic sequelae.[29]

Levene and coworkers, using slightly different criteria to grade severity, also defined three separate classes of postasphyxial encephalopathy.[30] They noted that the overall incidence of postasphyxial encephalopathy was 6 per 1000 live births. Severe encephalopathy was found in 2.1 births per 1000, but only two of the 11 babies who died in this study were in the severe postasphyxial encephalopathy group. In this study, 23% of the infants with postasphyxial encephalopathy had "unremarkable" Apgar scores at 1 and 5 min. In Levene's study, 25% of the patients had evidence of intrauterine growth restriction, whereas 29% of Robertson and Finer's patients were similarly growth-restricted.

Levene and coworkers also commented upon the fact that using the severity of the postasphyxial encephalopathic score was much better than utilizing the Apgar scores of 5 or less at 10 min in predicting aberrant neurological outcome.[79] Table 1.6 lists the major studies evaluating the use of the postasphyxial encephalopathy scoring system in predicting long-term neurological handicaps and death. While Robertson and Finer[29] found an incidence of 3.3 infants/1000 births, Levene et al.[30] and Brown et al.[150] found the incidence of postasphyxial encephalopathy to be approximately 6/1000 live births, the difference being primarily in the number of infants in the mildly affected group of infants found by Robertson and Finer.

Table 1.6. Hypoxemic–ischemic encephalopathy in term or near-term infants (postasphyxia encephalopathy)

		Incidence/1000 live births			Outcome of survivors (%)		
Author	No. of births	Grade I	Grade II	Grade III	Grade II		Grade III
Brown et al.[150]	14020	5.9/1000		(not graded)		Deaths	22
						Handicapped	42
						Normal	36
Robertson and Finer[29]	20155	1.15	1.65	0.5	3	Deaths	50
					21	Handicapped	50
					76	Normal	0
Levene et al.[30,79]	20975	3.9	1.1	1.0	4	Deaths	62
					21	Handicapped	14
					75	Normal	24
Hull and Dodd 1976–1980[3]	24824	5.1	1.6	1.0	6	Deaths	0
					13	Handicapped	100
					77	Normal	0
Hull and Dodd 1984–1988[3]	24265	2.8	1.2	0.6	0	Deaths	80
					17	Handicapped	7
					83	Normal	13
Thornberg et al. 1985–1991[2]	42203	0.85	0.4	0.3	6	Deaths	92
					47	Handicapped	8
					47	Normal	0

Hull and Dodd noted a decrease in the incidence of postasphyxial encephalopathy in their studies from Derby, UK, over two 5-year periods.[3] Similarly, Halligan and coworkers from the Rotunda Hospital in Dublin, using the criterion of seizures in the newborn within the first 48 h of life as a sign of hypoxic–ischemic encephalopathy, noted a decrease in severe encephalopathy or death if the mother was cared for in the fetal assessment unit which was developed for the care of the high-risk maternal–fetal pair[151] (Table 1.6).

As noted by Volpe, "the occurrence of a recognizable neonatal neurological syndrome is the single most useful indicator that a significant hypoxemic–ischemic insult to the brain has occurred . . . In nearly 30 years of study of newborns and children with neurological disorders, I have not encountered a child with documented perinatal asphyxia but no neonatal neurological syndrome and the subsequent development of major neurological abnormalities."[27]

Thus, if a neonate shows evidence of asphyxia as demonstrated by abnormal fetal heart rate patterns, low Apgar scores, or delayed onset of respirations, but has little, if any, evidence of neurologic depression or abnormalities in the immediate neonatal period, it is highly unlikely that the patient will demonstrate significant neurological sequelae. Analyzing the data from the NCPP study, Nelson and Ellenberg substantiated previous observations and stated that infants who are depressed at birth, but who do not demonstrate evidence of neonatal encephalopathy, do not have an increased risk of cerebral palsy as they develop.[152]

When attempting to identify those factors that would predict newborn encephalopathy in term infants, the group from Western Australia evaluated 164 term infants over a 2⅓-year period and reported an incidence of 3.8/1000 live births.[16,18] The mortality rate was 9.1%, and they noted that maternal pyrexia, persistent occipital posterior position, and an acute intrapartum event were all risk factors for the encephalopathy. These authors noted that 69% of the infants had only antepartum risk factors identified, 24% had antepartum and intrapartum risk factors, and 5% had only intrapartum risk factors. Two percent had no factors recognized. These authors question the premise that the risk factors for newborn encephalopathy are found in the intrapartum period alone.

Multiple organ dysfunction in asphyxiated infants

(See Chapters 4 and 20)

In understanding the pathophysiology of intrapartum asphyxia and the fetal response to this problem, the perfusion of the heart, brain, and adrenal glands tends to be preserved at the expense of the other organs of the body.[153] In acute asphyxial events such as a prolapsed cord, this autoregulation may not be in evidence; however, in the usual state of decreased perfusion, the fetus can adapt to preserve cardiac and brain function. Thus, if the newborn has significant neurological obtundation yet there is little, if any, evidence of other organ system involvement, intrapartum asphyxia is unlikely to be the cause of the patient's obtundation. If an acute asphyxial event occurred, such as listed in Table 1.1, then there may be little, if any, evidence of multiorgan abnormalities.

Most often, the renal system will be involved and is the easiest to evaluate.[153–155] Findings may range from mild oligouria (less than 1 ml/kg per h), proteinuria, and hematuria to renal tubular necrosis and acute renal failure. Perlman and coworkers also demonstrated that these affected infants often had elevated urinary secretion of β_2-microglobulin concentrations.[154] Unfortunately, most laboratories do not routinely measure this protein in urine.

Cardiac manifestations of asphyxia vary from minor arrhythmias, ST segment changes on the electrocardiogram, and tricuspid insufficiency to papillary muscle necrosis, poor ventricular contractions, and cardiogenic shock. Patients with moderately severe-to-severe asphyxia may have a fixed, nonvariable rapid heart rate of 140–160 beats/min which may be a prelude to impending failure and cardiogenic shock.

Pulmonary manifestations of asphyxia include increased pulmonary vascular resistance that responds readily to correction of acidosis and hypoxia, to persistent pulmonary hypertension of the newborn, severe pulmonary insufficiency, or pulmonary hemorrhage, that are difficult to manage.

Other organs that are involved and the manifestations of their involvement are listed in Table 1.7. One area often overlooked in the patient with severe asphyxia is damage to the spinal column. Clancy and coworkers described 18 severely asphyxiated newborns, 12 of whom expired.[156] On autopsy, five of the 12 demonstrated severe ischemic necrosis in the spinal cord gray matter. Electromyographic studies in the six survivors were abnormal and consistent with recent injury to the lower motor neurons above the level of the dorsal root ganglion. It is often difficult to distinguish clinically between damage to the cortical motor area and the spinal cord.

Perlman and coworkers reported an acute systemic organ injury in 35 term infants after asphyxia.[154] Twelve of the infants had no evidence of organ involvement, eight infants had an abnormality confined to one organ, 12 had two-organ involvement and three infants had three-organ involvement. Interestingly, of the eight infants with only one-organ involvement, three infants had central nervous system involvement only, but the authors did not describe the specific findings in these three infants as compared with the central nervous system findings in the other affected infants. If an infant with intrapartum asphyxia demonstrates only central nervous system involvement without other organ abnormalities, it may be that there was an acute hypoxic event, that the central nervous system damage did not occur in the intrapartum period, or that it was due to a cerebrovascular event that did not cause profound hypoxia or hypotension to affect other organs.

Table 1.7. Effect of asphyxia on various organs in the newborn

Central nervous system injury
Hypoxic–ischemic encephalopathy
Cerebral necrosis
Cerebral edema
Seizures
Hemorrhage
Spinal cord injury
Renal injury
Oliguria
Hematuria
Proteinuria
Acute renal failure
Pulmonary injury
Respiratory failure
Pulmonary hemorrhage
Persistent pulmonary hypertension of the newborn
Pulmonary edema
Meconium aspiration syndrome
Cardiovascular injury
Decreased ventricular function
Abnormalities of rate and rhythm
Tricuspid regurgitation
Papillary muscle necrosis
Hypotension
Cardiovascular shock
Gastrointestinal injury
Gastrointestinal hemorrhage
Sloughing of mucosa
Necrotizing enterocolitis
Hepatic injury
Hyperammonemia
Elevated liver enzymes
Coagulopathies
Hematological abnormalities
Elevated nucleated red cell count
Neutropenia or neutrophilia
Thrombocytopenia
Coagulopathy
Metabolic abnormalities
Hypoglycemia
Hypocalcemia
Sodium and potassium abnormalities
Hypo- or hypermagnesemia

Source: Modified from Carter et al.[155]

Likewise, Phelan and others reported similar findings in a group of patients with fetal asphyxial brain injury without multiorgan system dysfunction.[157] They described 57 infants with hypoxic–ischemic encephalopathy, of whom 14 had no evidence of multisystem problems. Six infants were delivered following uterine rupture, one had fetal exsanguination, one had a cord proplapse, and one was delivered following maternal cardiopulmonary arrest. Five fetuses had sudden and prolonged fetal heart rate decelerations which persisted until delivery. All of these infants would be classified as having an acute asphyxia or sentinel episode and would not have had the opportunity to develop the "diving reflex" necessary to protect the brain and heart at the expense of other organs.

Electroencephalographic findings in asphyxia

(See Chapter 20)

Neuroimaging findings in asphyxia

(See Chapters 22 and 23)

Use of fetal heart rate monitoring in assessing intrauterine asphyxia

(See Chapters 4 and 11)

Focal brain infarcts (stroke) in neonates

Focal infarcts in the neonatal period are rarely encountered, but with the increasing use of imaging techniques, more of these lesions are being identified.[30] These lesions can occur spontaneously, may be associated with maternal drug abuse (primarily cocaine), antenatal and intrapartum asphyxia, septicemia with or without meningitis, maternal diabetes, and polycythemia.[158–164] These infants usually present with seizures, and next to "perinatal asphyxia," may be the most common cause of neonatal seizures. The middle cerebral artery is most commonly affected and the left side is affected twice as frequently as the right. The overall incidence ranges from 1.5 to 35 per 100 000 live births.

Hypercoagulable status secondary to genetic prothrombotic risk factors has been recognized with increasing frequency and may be associated with these infarcts. Increased levels of lipoprotein a, factor V Leiden mutation, the presence of cardiolipin antibodies, as well as protein C, protein S, and antithrombin III deficiencies, have been linked to cerebral vascular thromboses and infarcts. Often multiple placental thrombi on the fetal side may be present as well.[159,163] It would seem feasible to evaluate an infant for these genetic risk factors if either of placental thrombi and/or neonatal stroke is encountered. The outlook for these infants is usually good unless the infarct is extensive or if it was associated with asphyxia and severe neonatal neurological abnormalities.

Conditions causing neonatal depression and/or neonatal encephalopathy that mimic perinatal asphyxia (Table 1.8)

Nelson and Leviton were among the first to question whether all infants with neonatal encephalopathy had these insults secondary to birth asphyxia.[11] One of the more common problems that can present in this fashion is the infant with neonatal sepsis. Currently, group B streptococcal sepsis is the most common organism involved.[76,165] In many instances, the mother had been pretreated, and an organism was not able to be cultured from the newborn's blood or spinal fluid. Indirect evidence of the disease is encountered, including an abnormally low or elevated white blood cell count, an elevated C-reactive protein, and/or evidence of severe chorioamniotis, if the placenta is examined (see Chapter 24). The infants have severe lactic acidosis, may have pulmonary hypertension or hemorrhage, and are very difficult to manage in the neonatal period. Even with the use of nitric oxide, high-frequency ventilation, and extracorporeal membrane oxygenation (ECMO), the mortality and morbidity rates are great.

Similarly, the infant born of a mother with chorioamnionitis can also behave like the infant with birth asphyxia.[166–170] Placental perfusion has been shown to be decreased in such pregnancies, further subjecting the fetus to increased risk of damage.[166,171–173]

Table 1.8. Conditions causing neonatal depression and/or neonatal encephalopathy that mimic "perinatal asphyxia"

Neonatal sepsis
Chorioamnionitis without documented neonatal sepsis (see Chapter 14)
Congenital infections
Viral
Toxoplasmosis
Neuronal migration disorders
Congenital myotonic disorders, including congenital and transient myesthenia gravis
Metabolic conditions causing lactic acidosis (see Chapter 19)
Genetic disorders associated with thrombotic or thrombolytic abnormalities, including:
Protein C and protein S deficiencies
Factor V Leiden deficiency
Anticardiolipin antibodies, etc. (see Chapter 9)

Although most infants with congenital infection such as cytomegalovirus or toxoplasmosis are asymptomatic at birth and later develop clinical manifestations of their disease, a few will be symptomatic in the neonatal period and behave as if they have suffered from birth asphyxia (see Chapter 17). Infants with congenital parvoviral infection may be born with hydrops and appear to have suffered from intrauterine asphyxia. Newborns with neuronal migration disorders and these with early-onset myotonic disorders have also been mislabeled as infants suffering from intrauterine asphyxia. As mentioned in the previous section on neonatal stroke, genetic prothrombotic factors predispose infants to intrauterine stress not only because of central nervous system thrombi, but because of placental thrombi and poor perfusion as well.

Table 1.8 lists some of these conditions, and the clinician should be aware that not all patients with neonatal depression have had their insult because of asphyxia *per se*.

Cerebral palsy

The relationship between birth asphyxia and cerebral palsy with or without cognitive impairment continues to be elusive and difficult to ascertain. An excellent review of the causes of cerebral palsy has recently been published by Stanley et al.[20] These authors have presented this perplexing problem in an elegant review, based not only on their own experience, but on the data compiled in the literature as well.

The incidence of cerebral palsy varies, and is dependent on the severity of the disorders and the manner by which it is described. In most developed countries, the incidence is remarkably similar and varies between 1.5 and 2.5/1000 live births. In the NCPP study, the incidence of moderate-to-severe cerebral palsy in infants who survived the neonatal period was 3.2/1000 live births.[7,174] The incidence in Liverpool reported by Pharoah et al. varied between 1.18 and 1.97/1000 live births.[175,176] These authors have demonstrated that, in their population, the prevalence of cerebral palsy among infants weighing greater than 2500 g was 1.0–1.4/1000 survivors. In the group weighing between 1500–2499 g, the incidence varied from 4/1000 in the late 1960s to 12/1000 in the late 1970s. The infants weighing less than 1500 g had an incidence of almost 90/1000.

In Sweden, Hagberg et al. have monitored the incidence of cerebral palsy since 1971,[177–180] and noted that it fell from 1.9 to 1.4/1000, but then increased to 2.49/1000 live births. In the last period reported, 1987–1990, the incidence fell slightly to 2.36/1000 live births, with an incidence of 0.98 for preterm births and 1.38 for term infants. The gestational age-specific prevalence was 80.3/1000 for gestational age less than 28 weeks, 53.5/1000 for gestational age 28–31 weeks, 7.8/1000 for gestational age 32–36 weeks and 1.35/1000 live births for gestational age greater than 36 weeks. This is a slight reduction from their previous report in 1993.[179] As in other studies, the risk of cerebral palsy increases with decreasing gestational age and birth weight.

Data from Western Australia are similar to those reported from Sweden, Ireland, and the UK.[20,181,182] In a study from northern California evaluating over 155000 infants born over a 3-year period, the incidence was 1.23 per 1000 infants surviving to the age of 3 years.[183] The incidence again varied from a high of 44.2/1000 of gestational age less than 27 weeks to a low of 0.63/1000 born at 40–42 weeks.

Table 1.9. Correlation of Apgar scores of 0–3 and the risk of death and cerebral palsy in survivors among infants weighing more than 2501 g at birth (National Collaborative Perinatal Project data)

Times for which Apgar scores of 0–3 recorded (min)	Live-born infants	Death (%)	Known to 7 years	% Cerebral palsy
1	1729	3.1	1330	0.7
5	286	7.7	217	0.9
10	66	18.2	43	4.7
15	23	47.8	11	9.1
20	39	59.0	14	57.1

Source: Modified from Nelson and Ellenberg.[78]

In attempting to correlate the development of cerebral palsy with Apgar scores in term infants, Nelson and Ellenberg demonstrated that the incidence increased significantly when the low Apgar scores persisted for more than 10 min[78] (Table 1.9). If the scores were 0–3 at 5 min but increased to 4 or more by 10 min, the incidence of cerebral palsy was less than 1% in the survivors. Only when the score remained low for 15 min or more did the incidence of cerebral palsy increase significantly. Conversely, 55% of the patients who developed cerebral palsy had 1-min Apgar scores of 7–10; 73% of the patients had Apgar scores of 7–10 at 5 min.

In an attempt to identify risk factors that would predict cerebral palsy, Nelson and Ellenberg reviewed the NCPP data and found that 5% of the population at greatest risk contributed 37% of the patients with cerebral palsy.[7] Over two-thirds of the patients with cerebral palsy did not emanate from this group. Even more significant was the fact that over 97% of the patients identified in the high-risk population group did not have cerebral palsy.[7]

These investigators, in focusing on this high-risk cohort, could predict 13% of the patients with cerebral palsy on the basis of prepregnancy factors and 34% on the basis of both prepregnancy and pregnancy factors. The additional information derived from data regarding labor, delivery, and the neonatal period increased this predictability to 37% – a negligible increase.

In the large Dublin randomized trial of electronic versus intermittent auscultation, six infants who had seizures in the neonatal period were found to have cerebral palsy at 4 years of age. Three were from each group of monitored patients. Interestingly, 15 additional patients with cerebral palsy who were diagnosed at 4 years of age did not have neonatal seizures and were not in the high-risk group. Thus, of the total number of patients with cerebral palsy at 4 years of age, 29% had intrapartum difficulties.[145]

If most of the patients with cerebral palsy do not have significant intrapartum or neonatal events that predispose them to brain injury, what were the etiological factors involved in cerebral palsy? Holm was one of the first to point out that more than 50% of her patients with cerebral palsy had prenatal abnormalities, 10% had postnatal problems, and about one-third had perinatal problems.[184]

Using clinical criteria to identify the specific types of cerebral palsy and timing of etiology, Holm suggested that in about 50% of those with spastic diplegia, 37% of those with spastic quadriplegia, 50% of those with athetosis, and 50% of those with mixed findings, the origin was "prenatal complications." In almost all of the patients with ataxia and hypotonia, the problems were the results of prenatal factors. Perinatal problems tended to manifest primarily as spastic diplegia (prematurely born) and quadriplegia in term infants.

Nelson, in a systematic review of the NCPP data, found that the incidence of cerebral palsy associated with intrapartum asphyxia was in the range of 3–15% and that, if all factors were taken into consideration, it would not exceed 20%.[5] Volpe noted that, if preterm births were excluded, 12–23% of children who were born at term had their cerebral palsy related to intrapartum events.[27] Truwit and coworkers, using MRI findings, found that seven of 29 term infants had sufficient findings to conclude that intrapartum events led to the infant's difficulties, although one of these infants also had evidence of prenatal problems.[48]

In 1988, Blair and Stanley stated that in their population of patients with cerebral palsy, only 8% were caused by intrapartum events.[8] Their more recent data[20] support their findings, as do the studies by Yudkin and coworkers.[32] This latter study estimated that the frequency of cerebral palsy associated with birth asphyxia was one in 3700 full-term live births, while their total incidence of cerebral palsy was 2.6 per 1000 live births.

As Stanley and Blair[12,14] have noted, improvements in obstetrical care and appropriate neonatal resuscitation have not had a profound effect in decreasing the overall incidence of cerebral palsy. Nelson and Ellenberg also noted that patients who had significant late pregnancy or birth complications, but who were asymptomatic or had transient symptoms in the neonatal period, did not have an increased incidence of cerebral palsy compared with patients without any risk factors (2.4 per 1000 vs 2.3 per 1000).[152]

Torfs and coworkers followed 19 044 children born of monitored pregnancies for at least 5 years.[185] Significant predictors of cerebral palsy included another major birth defect, low birth weight, small placenta, abnormal fetal position, and premature separation of the placenta. Seventy-eight percent of the children with cerebral palsy had no evidence of birth asphyxia; 22% did, but they had other prenatal factors that could have complicated their courses.

Studying another aspect, Manning et al. evaluated the incidence of cerebral palsy in infants of women with high-risk pregnancies who received antenatal testing to evaluate the fetal biophysical profile.[186] They also evaluated the incidence of cerebral palsy in infants of mothers with no or low-risk pregnancies and who did not have antenatal testing. Although this was a retrospective study, the incidence of cerebral palsy in the tested group was

1.33/1000 live births, and 4.74/1000 in the untested group. These data suggest that, by altering the management of the women based on their test scores, one could recognize potential fetal jeopardy and respond earlier to avoid any further potential damage. As the authors note, "the relationship between the incidence of cerebral palsy and the last test fetal biophysical profile score was inverse, exponential and highly significant."

Whether a prospective randomized study could ever be carried out to document these observations is speculative. Several questions remain unresolved as to whether there was a difference in the number of growth-restricted infants in the two groups, and whether there are increased rates of cesarean sections performed to decrease the number of infants who may have developed birth asphyxia.

A question that still remains unanswered is whether an infant delivered by repeat cesarean section who has no antenatal risk factors would have a decreased incidence of cerebral palsy. Scheller and Nelson suggest not,[187] and studies from the Oxford regional health authority suggest that, although elective repeat cesarean section did not do away with cerebral palsy, none of the infants in their series who were delivered via elective cesarean section had neonatal encephalopathy.[15]

Epidemiology of mental retardation

Using IQ measurements alone, epidemiologists have defined severe mental retardation as an IQ score below 50 and mild mental retardation as a score between 50 and 69. As proposed by Paneth and Stark,[188] the prevalence of severe mental retardation is remarkably consistent and varies between three and four per 1000 school-age children. This type of retardation is often associated with motor handicaps, abnormal features or appearance, and seizures. These patients are generally found with equal frequency in all socioeconomic classes and most commonly are retarded as a result of "biologic insult to the brain."

Patients with mild mental retardation most commonly come from the most disadvantaged socioeconomic classes, have learning problems, and often require special classes or schooling in order to reach their ultimate levels of achievement. Associated neurologic handicaps may be found in as many as 30% of these patients, epilepsy being the most common finding.[189]

The incidence of mild mental retardation has been stated to be 23–30 per 1000 in the school-age population and is closely related to socioeconomic class. In Sweden the incidence of this type of mental retardation was only four per 1000.[189] It appears that alterations in the socioeconomic environments may have a significant effect in lowering the incidence of mild mental retardation.

Hagberg and Kyllerman noted that patients with the fetal alcohol syndrome made up almost 10% of those with mild mental retardation and almost 1% of the patients with severe mental retardation.[189] As more of these patients are being recognized in the USA, it is possible that an increased percentage will be found in both the mild mental retardation and severe mental retardation groups. Similarly, if the number of infants delivered of cocaine-abusing mothers increases, it is possible that these patients may also contribute to the number of mentally retarded infants and children encountered.

Both Paneth and Stark[188] and Hagberg and Kyllerman[189] have studied the etiologic factors in mental retardation and noted that perinatal events could account for 10% of the cases of severe and mild mental retardation. Similarly, postnatal difficulties (after the first month of life) could account for at most 10% of patients with both types of retardation. In most of the patients the origin of severe mental retardation lies in prenatal problems, including chromosomal abnormalities (40%), biochemical inborn errors of metabolism (3–5%), and intrauterine infections (5%). In approximately 30% of patients with severe mental retardation, the cause is unknown.[190]

For many years it has been stated that, if an infant or child has severe mental retardation without severe cerebral palsy, the mental retardation is not due to intrauterine asphyxial problems.[191] In Chapter 41, Dr Robertson has challenged this

Table 1.10. Criteria defining an intrauterine asphyxic event

Acute asphyxic event	Prolonged partial asphyxic event
Evidence of a sentinel asphyxic event (see Table 1.1)	Development of a nonreassuring fetal heart rate pattern where an assuring pattern had been present (weak correlation at best)
Severe metabolic acidosis (arterial pH <7.00; base deficit >12 mmol/l)	Severe metabolic acidosis (arterial pH <7.00; base deficit >12 mmol/l)
Early onset of moderate-to-severe neonatal encephalopathy in infants of 34 weeks gestational age or more	Early onset of moderate-to-severe neonatal encephalopathy in infants of 34 weeks gestational age or more
Apgar score of 0–3 for greater than 5 min	Apgar score of 0–3 for greater than 5 min
Imaging studies showing involvement of thalamus, basal ganglia, putamen, brainstem	Imaging studies showing watershed-type lesions in cerebral cortex
Development of extrapyramidal neurological abnormalities	Development of quadriparesis or dykinesia
May or may not have multiorgan dysfunction	Usually has multiorgan dysfunction

Source: Modified from MacLennan et al.[24]

dictum and has identified a group of patients with severe mental retardation, but without severe cerebral palsy. Interestingly, in these patients who had imaging studies, significant abnormalities of the brain have been noted that correspond to those seen in infants with severe cerebral palsy secondary to intrapartum asphyxia.

Conclusion

Although intrapartum asphyxia contributes in some ways to neurologic and intellectual impairment, the degree to which it contributes has been grossly overstated. By current standards it is estimated that intrapartum difficulties contribute to fewer than 20% of patients with cerebral palsy and fewer than 10% of those with severe mental retardation, and that in most situations both abnormalities are present in the same individual.

Even though physicians, attorneys, and the lay public have often blamed inadequate obstetrical and pediatric care as the basis for cerebral palsy and severe mental retardation, current data do not support this belief. Often a diagnosis of cerebral palsy or severe mental retardation is made and a retrospective evaluation of the perinatal period is accomplished. The neonate may be found to be depressed (low Apgar scores), have abnormal fetal heart tracings, and a retrospective evaluation of intrapartum events ensues. Unfortunately, many cases have been brought to litigation on the basis of these findings, and "experts" in both perinatology and neonatal medicine have lent credence to casual interpretations, even when they are not justified by the data.

In order to implicate intrauterine or, more specifically, intrapartum events causing hypoxia, various criteria have been proposed. More recently, the International Cerebral Palsy Task Force has listed criteria defining such an event.[24] I have modified these criteria in Table 1.10 because of some differences noted in infants following an acute or sentinel event where the presentations might be somewhat different (Table 1.10).

In addition, a thorough search should be conducted to insure that other potential or real causative factors were not present, such as sepsis or metabolic derangements. With the case of improved imaging techniques, structural abnormalities, if present, must be explained on the basis of intrapartum asphyxia and not on developmental aberrations.

Lastly, patients who are small-for-gestational-age contribute significantly to the number of patients with neonatal asphyxia, the neonatal neurologic syndrome, cerebral palsy, and neonatal seizures.[192,193] Attempts to improve early recognition and possible intervention in pregnancies complicated by intrauterine growth restriction could potentially enhance the outcome of patients.

REFERENCES

1 Guyer, B., Hoyert, D.L., Martin, J.A. et al. (1999). Annual summary of vital statistics – 1998. *Pediatrics*, **104**, 1229–46.

2 Thornberg, E., Thiringer, K., Odeback, A. et al. (1995). Birth asphyxia: incidence, clinical course and outcome in a Swedish population. *Acta Paediatr.*, **84**, 927–32.

3 Hull, J. and Dodd, K.L. (1992). Falling incidence of hypoxic–ischemic encephalopathy in term infants. *Br. J. Obstet. Gynaecol.*, **99**, 386–91.

4 Little, W.J. (1862). On the incidence of abnormal parturition, difficult labour, premature birth and asphyxia neonatorum on the mental and physical condition of the child, especially in relation to deformities. *Trans. Obstet. Soc. Lond.*, **3**, 293–344.

5 Nelson, K.B. (1986). Cerebral palsy: what is known regarding cause? *Ann. N.Y. Acad. Sci.*, **477**, 22–6.

6 Freeman, J.M. and Nelson, K.B. (1988). Intrapartum asphyxia and cerebral palsy. *Pediatrics*, **82**, 240–50.

7 Nelson, K.B. and Ellenberg, J.H. (1988). Intrapartum events and cerebral palsy. In *Perinatal Events and Brain Damage in Surviving Children*, ed. F. Kubli, N. Patel, W. Schmidt and O. Linderkamp, pp. 139–48. Berlin: Springer-Verlag.

8 Blair, E. and Stanley, F. J. (1988). Intrapartum asphyxia: a rare cause of cerebral palsy. *J. Pediatr.*, **112**, 515–19.

9 Dennis, J. (1985). The long term effects of intrapartum cerebral damage. In *Risks of Labour*, ed. J. W. Crawford, pp. 157–88. London: Wiley.

10 Hill, A. (1991). Current concepts of hypoxic–ischemic cerebral injury in the term newborn. *Pediatr. Neurol.*, **7**, 317–25.

11 Nelson, K.B. and Leviton, A. (1991). How much of neonatal encephalopathy is due to birth asphyxia? *Am. J. Dis. Child.*, **145**, 1325–31.

12 Stanley, F.J. and Blair, E. (1991). Why have we failed to reduce the frequency of cerebral palsy? *Med. J. Aust.*, **154**, 623–6.

13 Nelson, K.B. and Emery, E.S. III (1993). Birth asphyxia and the neonatal brain: what do we know and when do we know it? *Clin. Perinatol.*, **20**, 327–44.

14 Stanley, F.J. (1994). Cerebral palsy trends: implications for perinatal care. *Acta Obstet. Gynaecol. Scand.*, **73**, 5–9.

15 Gaffney, G., Flavell, V., Johnson, A. et al. (1994). Cerebral palsy and neonatal encephalopathy. *Arch. Dis. Child.*, **70**, F195–200.

16 Adamson, S.J., Alessandri, L.M., Badawi, W. et al. (1995). Predictors of neonatal encephalopathy in full term infants. *Br. Med. J.*, **311**, 598–602.

17 Patel, J. and Edwards, A.D. (1997). Prediction of outcome after perinatal asphyxia. *Curr. Opin. Pediatr.*, **9**, 128–32.

18 Badawi, W., Kurinczuk, J.J., Keogh, J.M. et al. (1998). Antepartum risk factor for newborn encephalopathy: the Western Australian case-control study. *Br. Med. J.*, **317**, 1549–53.

19 Badawi, N., Kurinczuk, J.J., Keogh, J.M. et al. (1998). Intrapartum risk factors for newborn encephalopathy: the Western Australian case-control study. *Br. Med. J.*, **317**, 1554–8.

20 Stanley, F., Blair, E. and Alberman, E. (2000). *Clinics in Developmental Medicine no. 151. Cerebral Palsies: Epidemiology and Causal Pathways.* London: Mac Keith Press.

21 Peliowski, A. and Finer, N.W. (1992). Birth asphyxia in the term infant. In *Effective care of the Newborn Infant*, ed. J.C. Sinclair and M.B. Bracken, pp. 249–79. Oxford; Oxford University Press.

22 Longo, L.D. and Packianathan, S. (1997). Hypoxia–ischaemia and the developing brain: hypotheses regarding the pathophysiology of fetal–neonatal brain damage. *Brit. J. Obstet. Gynaecol.*, **104**, 652–62.

23 Low, J.A. (1998). Fetal asphyxia and outcome. In *Asphyxia and Fetal Brain Damage*, ed. D. Maulik, pp. 21–36. New York: Wiley Liss.

24 MacLennan, A. (for the International Cerebral Palsy Task Force) (1999). A template for defining a causal relationship between acute intrapartum events and cerebral palsy: International consensus statement. *Br. Med. J.*, **319**, 1054–62.

25 Nelson, K.B. (1999). The neurologically impaired child and alleged malpractice at birth. *Neurol. Clin.*, **17**, 283–93.

26 Farrell, T., Mires, G.J., Owen, P., et al. (1998). Antecedents of long-term handicap. In *Asphyxia and Fetal Brain Damage*, ed. D. Maulik, pp. 1–19. New York: Wiley-Liss.

27 Volpe, J.J. (2001). Hypoxic–ischemic encephalopathy. In *Neurology of the Newborn*, 4th edn, ed, J.J. Volpe, pp. 217–394. Philadelphia: W.B. Saunders Co.

28 Freeman, J.M. and Freeman, A.D. (1992). Cerebral palsy and the "bad baby" malpractice crisis. *Am. J. Dis. Child.*, **146**, 725–7.

29 Robertson, C. and Finer, N. (1985). Term infants with hypoxic–ischemic encephalopathy: outcome at 3–5 years. *Dev. Med. Child Neurol.*, **27**, 473–84.

30 Levene, M.L., Kornberg, J. and Williams, T.H.C. (1985). The incidence and severity of post-asphyxial encephalopathy in full-term infants. *Early Hum. Dev.*, **11**, 21–6.

31 Yudkin, P.L., Johnson, A., Clover, L.M. et al. (1994). Clustering of perinatal markers of birth asphyxia and outcome at age five years. *Brit. J. Obstet. Gynaecol.*, **101**, 774–81.

32 Yudkin, P.L., Johnson, A., Clover, L.M. et al. (1995). Assessing the contribution of birth asphyxia to cerebral palsy in term singletons. *Paediatr. Perinatal Epidemiol.*, **9**, 156–70.

33 Handley-Derry, M., Lou, J.A., Burke, S.O. et al. (1997). Intrapartum fetal asphyxia and the occurrence of minor deficits in 4- to 8-year-old children. *Dev. Med. Child Neurol.*, **39**, 508–14.

34 Garite, T.J., Linzey, M., Freeman, R.K. et al. (1979). Fetal heart rate patterns and fetal distress in fetuses with congenital abnormalities. *Obstet. Gynecol.*, **53**, 716–20.

35 Jung, J.H., Graham, J.M. Jr, Schultz N. et al. (1984). Congenital hydranencephaly/porencephaly due to vascular disruption in monozygotic twins. *Pediatrics*, **73**, 467–9.

36 McGahan, J.P., Haesslein, H.C., Meyers, M. et al. (1984). Sonographic recognition of in-utero intraventricular hemorrhage. *Am. J. Radiol.*, **142**, 171–3.

37 Sims, M.E., Turkell, S.B., Halterman, G. et al. (1985). Brain injury and intrauterine death. *Am J. Obstet. Gynecol.*, **151**, 721–3.

38 Gunn, T.R., Mok, P.M. and Becroft, D.M.O. (1985). Subdural hemorrhage in utero. *Pediatrics*, **76**, 605–9.

39 Paul, R.H., Yonekusa, L., Cantrell, C.J. et al. (1986). Fetal injury prior to labor: does it happen? *Am. J. Obstet. Gynecol*, **154**, 1187–93.

40 Ellis, W.G., Goetzman, B.W. and Lindenberg, J.A. (1988). Neuropathologic documentation of prenatal brain damage. *Am. J. Dis. Child.*, **142**, 858–66.

41 Low, J.A., Robertson, D.M. and Simpson, L.L. (1989). Temporal relationships of neuropathologic conditions caused by perinatal asphyxia. *Am. J. Obstet. Gynecol.*, **160**, 608–14.

42 Bejar, R., Vigliocco, G., Gramajo, N. et al. (1990). Antenatal origin of neurologic damage in newborn infants. II. Multiple gestations. *Am. J. Obstet. Gynecol.*, **162**, 1230–6.

43 Nelson, K.B. (1991). Prenatal origin of hemiparetic cerebral palsy: how often and why? *Pediatrics*, **88**, 1059–61.

44 Squier, M. and Keeling, J.W. (1991). The incidence of prenatal brain injury. *Neuropathol. Appl. Neurobiol.*, **17**, 29–38.

45 Scher, M.S., Belfar, H., Martin, J. et al. (1991). Destructive brain lesions of presumed fetal onset: antepartum causes of cerebral palsy. *Pediatrics*, **88**, 898–906.

46 Scheller, J.M. and Nelson, K.B. (1992). Twinning and neurologic morbidity. *Am. J. Dis. Child.*, **146**, 1110–13.

47 Roland, E.H. and Hill, A. (1992). MR and CT evaluations of profound neonatal and infantile asphyxia. *Am. J. Neuroradiol.*, **13**, 973–5.

48 Truwit, C.L., Barkovich, A.J., Kock, T.K. et al. (1992). Cerebral palsy: MR findings in 40 patients. *Am. J. Neuroradiol.*, **13**, 67–78.

49 Barabas, R.E., Barmada, M.A. and Scher, M.S. (1993). Timing of brain insults in severe neonatal encephalopathies with isoelectric EEG. *Pediatr. Neurol.*, **9**, 39–44.

50 Phelan, J.P., and Kim, J.O. (2000). Fetal heart rate observations in the brain-damaged infant. *Semin. Perinatol.*, **24**, 221–9.

51 Benirschke, K. (1990). The placenta in the litigation process. *Am. J. Obstet. Gynecol.*, **162**, 1445–50.

52 Altshuler, G. (1993). Some placental considerations in alleged obstetrical and neonatal malpractice. In *Legal Medicine*, ed. C.H. Wecht, pp. 27–47. Salem, NH: Butterworths Legal Medicine.

53 Benirschke, K. (1994). Placenta pathology: questions to the perinatologist. *J. Perinatol.*, **14**, 371–6.

54 Ahn, M.O., Korst, L.M. and Phelan, J.P. (1998). Normal fetal heart rate pattern in the brain-damaged infant: a failure of intrapartum fetal monitoring? *J. Matern. Fetal Invest.*, **8**, 58–60.

55 Dawes, G.S. (1968). *Foetal and Neonatal Physiology.* Chicago: Year Book Medical.

56 Myers, R.E. (1972). Two patterns of perinatal brain damage and their conditions of occurrence. *Am. J. Obstet. Gynecol.*, **112**, 246–76.

57 Brann, A.W. Jr and Myers, R.E. (1975). Central nervous system findings in the newborn monkey following severe in-utero partial asphyxia. *Neurology*, **25**, 327–38.

58 Mallard, G.C., Williams, C.E., Johnston, B.M. et al. (1995). Repeated episodes of umbilical cord occlusion in fetal sheep lead to preferential damage to the striatum and sensitize the heart to further insults. *Pediatr. Res.*, **37**, 707–13.

59 De Haan, H.H., Gunn, A.J., Williams, C.E. et al. (1997). Brief repeated umbilical cord occlusions cause sustained cytotoxic cerebral edema and focal infarcts in near-term fetal lambs. *Pediatr. Res.*, **41**, 96–104.

60 De Haan, H.H., Gunn, A.J. and Gluckman, P.D. (1997). Fetal heart rate changes do not reflect cardiovascular deterioration during brief repeated umbilical cord occlusions in near-term fetal lambs. *Am. J. Obstet. Gynecol.*, **176**, 8–17.

61 Gunn, A.J., De Haan, H. and Gluckman, P.D. (1997). Experimental models of perinatal brain injury. In *Fetal and Neonatal Brain Injury*, ed. D.K. Stevenson and P. Sunshine, 2nd edn, pp. 59–70. Oxford: Oxford University Press.

62 Gunn, A.J., Maxwell, L., De Haan, H.H. et al. (2000). Delayed hypotension and subendocardial injury after repeated umbilical cord occlusion in near-term fetal lambs. *Am. J. Obstet. Gynecol.*, **183**, 1564–72.

63 Critchlow, C.W., Leet, T.L., Benedetti, T.J. et al. (1994). Risk factors and infant outcomes associated with umbilical cord prolapse: a population-based, case-controlled study among births in Washington state. *Am. J. Obstet. Gynecol.*, **170**, 613–18.

64 Murphy, D.J. and MacKenzie, I.Z. (1995). The mortality and morbidity associated with umbilical cord prolapse. *Br. J. Obstet. Gynaecol.*, **102**, 826–30.

65 Prabulos, A.M. and Philipson, E.H. (1998). Umbilical cord prolapse. Is the time from diagnosis to delivery critical? *J. Reprod. Med.*, **43**, 129–32.

66 Leung, H.S., Leung, E.K. and Paul, R.H. (1993). Uterine rupture after precocious cesarian delivery: maternal and fetal consequences. *Am. J. Obstet. Gynecol.*, **169**, 945–50.

67 Barkovich, A.S. (1992). MR and CT evaluation of profound neonatal and infantile asphyxia. *Am. J. Neuroradiol.*, **13**, 959–72.

68 Roland, E.H., Poskitt, K., Rodriguez, E. et al. (1998). Perinatal hypoxic–ischemic thalamic injury: clinical features and neuroimaging. *Ann. Neurol.*, **44**, 161–6.

69 Pasternak, J. F. and Gorey, M.T. (1998). The syndrome of acute near-total intrauterine asphyxia in the term infant. *Pediatr. Neurol.*, **18**, 391–8.

70 Barkovitch, A.J., Hajnal, B.L., Vigneron, D. et al. (1998). Prediction of neuromotor outcome in perinatal asphyxia: evaluation of MR scoring systems. *Am. J. Neuroradiol.*, **19**, 143–9.

71 Barkovitch, A.J. (2000). *Pediatric Neuroimaging*, 3rd edn. Philadelphia: Lippincott Williams and Wilkins.

72 Apgar, V.A. (1953). A proposal for a new method of evaluation of the newborn infant. *Curr. Res. Anesth. Analg.*, **32**, 260–7.

73 Apgar, V. and James, L.S. (1962). Further observations on the newborn scoring system. *Am. J. Dis. Child.*, **104**, 419–28.

74 Apgar, V., Holaday, D.A., James, L.S. et al. (1958). Evaluation of the newborn infant – second report. *J.A.M.A.*, **168**, 1985–8.

75 Niswander, K.R. and Gordon, M. (1972). *Collaborative Perinatal Study of the National Institute for Neurological Disease and Stroke. The Women and their Pregnancies*, Vol. I. Philadelphia: Saunders.

76 Peevy, K.J. and Chalhub, E.G. (1983). Occult group B streptococcal infection: an important cause of intrauterine asphyxia. *Am. J. Obstet. Gynecol.*, **146**, 989–90.

77 Catlin, E.A., Carpenter, M.W., Brann, B.S. IV et al. (1986). The Apgar score revisited: influence of gestational age. *J. Pediatr.*, **109**, 865–8.

78 Nelson, K.B. and Ellenberg, J.H. (1981). Apgar scores as predictors of chronic neurologic disability. *Pediatrics*, **68**, 38–44.

79 Levene, M.I., Grindulis, H., Sands, C. et al. (1986). Comparison of two methods of predicting outcome in perinatal asphyxia. *Lancet*, **i**, 67–9.

80 MacDonald, H.M., Mulligan, J.C., Allen, A.C. et al. (1980). Neonatal asphyxia. I. Relationship of obstetric and neonatal complications to neonatal mortality in 38405 consecutive deliveries. *J. Pediatr.*, **96**, 898–902.

81 Mulligan, J.C., Painter, M.J., O'Donoghue, P.A. et al. (1980). Neonatal asphyxia. II. Neonatal mortality and long-term sequelae. *J. Pediatr.*, **96**, 903–7.

82 Peters, T., Golding, J., Lawrence, C.J. et al. (1984). Factors associated with delayed onset of regular respiration. *Early Hum. Dev.*, **9**, 209–23.

83 Peters, T.J., Golding, J., Lawrence, C.J. et al. (1984). Delayed onset of regular respiration and subsequent development. *Early Hum. Dev.*, **9**, 225–39.

84 Neligan, G., Prudham, D. and Steiner, H. (1974). *The Formative Years: Birth, Family and Development in Newcastle-upon-Tyne.* London: Oxford University Press.

85 Jain, L., Ferre, C., Vidyasaggar, D. et al. (1991). Cardiopulmonary resuscitation of apparently stillborn infants: survival and long-term outcome. *J. Pediatr.*, **118**, 778–82.

86 Scott, H. (1976). Outcome of very severe birth asphyxia. *Arch. Dis. Child.*, **51**, 712–16.

87 Steiner, N. and Neligan, G. (1975). Perinatal cardiac arrest. Quality of the survivors. *Arch. Dis. Child.*, **50**, 696–702.

88 Casalaz, D.M., Marlow, N. and Speidel, B.D. (1998). Outcome of resuscitation following unexpected apparent stillbirth. *Arch. Dis. Child. Fetal Neonatal Ed.*, **78**, F112–15.

89 Yeo, C.L. and Tudehope, D.I. (1994). Outcome of resuscitated apparently stillborn infants: a ten year review. *J. Paediatr. Child Health*, **30**, 129–33.

90 Koppe, J.G. and Kleiverda, G. (1984). Severe asphyxia and outcome of survivors. *Resuscitation*, **12**, 193–206.

91 De Souza, S.W. and Richards, B. (1978). Neurological sequelae in newborn babies after perinatal asphyxia. *Arch. Dis. Child*, **53**, 564–9.

92 Meis, P.J., Hall, M. III, Marshall, J.R. et al. (1978). Meconium passage: a new classification for risk assessment during labor. *Am. J. Obstet. Gynecol.*, **131**, 509–13.

93 Trimmer, K.J. and Gilstrap, L.C. III (1991). "Meconiumcrit" and birth asphyxia. *Am. J. Obstet. Gynecol.*, **165**, 1010–13.

94 Nelson, K.B. and Ellenberg, J.H. (1984). Obstetric complications as risk factors for cerebral palsy or seizure disorders. *J.A.M.A.*, **251**, 1843–8.

95 Dijxhoorn, M.J., Visser, G.H.A., Huisjes, H.J. et al. (1985). The relationship between pH values and neonatal neurological morbidity in full-term appropriate-for-dates infants. *Early Hum. Dev.*, **11**, 33–42.

96 Dijxhoorn, M.J., Visser, G.H.A., Fidler, V.J. et al. (1986). Apgar score, meconium and acidemia at birth in relation to neonatal neurological morbidity in term infants. *Br. J. Obstet. Gynaecol.*, **93**, 212–22.

97 Dijxhoorn, M.J., Visser, G.H.A. and Touwen, B.C.L. (1987). Apgar score, meconium and acidemia at birth in small for gestational age infants born at term, and their relationship to neonatal neurological morbidity. *Br. J. Obstet. Gynaecol.*, **94**, 873–9.

98 Clifford, S.H. (1941). The effects of asphyxia on the newborn infant. *J. Pediatr.*, **18**, 567–78.

99 Boenisch, H. and Saling, E. (1974). A combined clinical–biochemical scoring of all newborns. Results of the past four years. *J. Perinat. Med.*, **2**, 122–9.

100 Van den Berg, P., Schmidt, S., Gesche, J. et al. (1987). Fetal distress and the condition of the newborn using cardiotocography and fetal blood analysis during labour. *Br. J. Obstet. Gynaecol.*, **94**, 72–5.

101 Parer, J.T. (1980). The current role of intrapartum fetal blood sampling. *Clin. Obstet. Gynecol.*, **23**, 565–82.

102 Clark, S.L. and Paul, R.H. (1985). Intrapartum fetal surveillance: the role of fetal scalp blood sampling. *Am. J. Obstet. Gynecol.*, **153**, 717–20.

103 Sykes, G.S., Molloy, P.M., Johnson, P. et al. (1982). Do Apgar scores indicate asphyxia? *Lancet*, **i**, 494–6.

104 Silverman, F., Suidan, J., Wasserman, J. et al. (1985). The Apgar score: is it enough? *Obstet. Gynecol.*, **66**, 331–6.

105 Ruth, V.J. and Raivio, K.O. (1988). Perinatal brain damage: predictive value of metabolic acidosis and the Apgar score. *Br. Med. J.*, **297**, 24–7.

106 Dennis, J., Johnson, A., Mutch, L. et al. (1989). Acid–base status at birth and neurodevelopmental outcome at four and one-half years. *Am. J. Obstet. Gynecol.*, **161**, 213–20.

107 Winkler, C.L., Hauth, J.C., Tucker, J.M. et al. (1991). Neonatal complications at term as related to the degree of umbilical artery acidemia. *Am. J. Obstet. Gynecol.*, **164**, 637–41.

108 Goodwin, T.M., Belai, I., Hernandez, P. et al. (1992). Asphyxial complications in the term newborn with severe umbilical acidemia. *Am. J. Obstet. Gynecol.*, **167**, 1506–12.

109 Goldaber, K.G. and Gilstrap, L.C. III (1993). Correlations between obstetric clinical events and umbilical cord blood acid–base and blood gas values. *Clin. Obstet. Gynecol.*, **36**, 47–59.

110 Perlman, J.M. and Risser, R. (1993). Severe fetal acidemia: neonatal neurologic features and short-term outcome. *Pediatr. Neurol.*, **9**, 277–82.

111 Belai, Y., Goodwin, T.M., Durand, M. et al. (1998). Umbilical arteriovenous Po_2 and Pco_2 differences and neonatal morbidity in term infants with severe acidosis. *Am. J. Obstet. Gynecol*, **178**, 13–19.

112 Van den Berg, P.P., Nelen, W.L.D.M., Jongsma, H.W. et al. (1996). Neonatal complications in newborns with umbilical artery pH <7.00. *Am. J. Obstet.Gynecol.*, **175**, 1152–7.

113 Andres, R.L., Saade, G., Gilstrap, L.C. et al. (1999). Association between umbilical blood gas parameters and neonatal morbidity and death in neonates with pathologic fetal acidemia. *Am. J. Obstet. Gynecol.*, **181**, 867–71.

114 Low, J.A. (1997). Intrapartum fetal asphyxia: definition, diagnosis and classification. *Am. J. Obstet. Gynecol.*, **176**, 957–9.

115 Low, J.A., Lindsay, B.G. and Derrick, E.J. (1997). Threshold of metabolic acidosis associated with newborn complications. *Am. J. Obstet. Gynecol.*, **177**, 1391–4.

116 Low, J.A., Galbraith, R.S., Muir, D.W. et al. (1985). The relationship between perinatal hypoxia and newborn encephalopathy. *Am. J. Obstet. Gynecol.*, **152**, 256–60.

117 Low, J.A. (1993). Relationship of fetal asphyxia to neuropathology and deficits in children. *Clin. Invest. Med.*, **16**, 133–40.

118 Low, J.A. (1993). The relationship of asphyxia in the mature fetus to long-term neurologic function. *Clin. Obstet. Gynecol.*, **36**, 82–90.

119 Low, J.A., Panagiotopoulos, C. and Derrick, E.J. (1994). Newborn complications after intrapartum asphyxia with metabolic acidosis in the term infant. *Am. J. Obstet. Gynecol.*, **170**, 1081–7.

120 Low, J.A., Victory, R. and Derrick, E.J. (1999). Predictive value of electronic fetal monitoring for intrapartum fetal asphyxia with metabolic acidosis. *Obstet. Gynecol.*, **93**, 285–91.

121 Kruger, K., Hallberg, B., Blennow, M. et al. (1999). Predictive value of fetal scalp blood lactate concentration and pH markers of neurologic disability. *Am. J. Obstet. Gynecol.*, **181**, 1072–8.

122 Goldberg, R.N., Cabal, L.A., Sinatra, F.R. et al. (1979). Hyperammonemia associated with perinatal asphyxia. *Pediatrics*, **64**, 336–41.

123 Fernandez, F., Verder, A., Quero, J. et al. (1987). Serum CPK-

BB isoenzyme in the assessment of brain damage in asphyctic term infants. *Acta Paediatr. Scand.*, **76**, 914–18.

124 de Praeter, C., Vanhaesebrouck, P., Govaert, P. et al. (1991). Creatine kinase isoenzyme BB concentrations in the cerebrospinal fluid of newborns: relationship to short-term outcome. *Pediatrics*, **88**, 1204–10.

125 Garcia-Alix, A., Cabanas, F., Pellicer, A. et al. (1994). Neuron-specific enolase and myelin basic protein: relationship of cerebrospinal fluid concentrations to the neurologic condition of asphyxiated full-term infants. *Pediatrics*, **93**, 234–40.

126 Hagberg, H., Thornberg, E., Blennow, M. et al. (1993). Excitatory amino acids in the cerebrospinal fluid of asphyxiated infants: relationship to hypoxic–ischemic encephalopathy. *Acta Paediatr.*, **82**, 925–9.

127 Blennow, M., Hagberg, H., Ingvar, M. et al. (1994). Neurochemical and biophysical assessment of neonatal hypoxic–ischemic encephalopathy. *Semin. Perinatol.*, **18**, 30–5.

128 Blennow, M., Hagberg, H. and Rosengren, L. (1995). Glial fibrillary acidic protein in the cerebrospinal fluid: a possible indicator of prognosis in full-term asphyxiated newborn infants. *Pediatr. Res.*, **37**, 260–4.

129 Saugstad, O.D. (1988). Hypoxanthine as an indicator of hypoxia: its role in health and disease through free radical production. *Pediatr. Res.*, **23**, 143–50.

130 da Silva, S., Hennebert, N., Denis, R. et al. (2000). Clinical value of a single postnatal lactate measurement after intrapartum asphyxia. *Acta Paediatr.*, **89**, 320–3.

131 Huang, C.C., Wang, S.T., Chang, Y.C. et al. (1999). Measurement of the urinary lactate: creatinine ratio for the early detection of newborn infants at risk for hypoxemic–ischemic encephalopathy. *N. Engl. J. Med.*, **341**, 328–35.

132 Juul, S.E., Stallings, S.A. and Christensen, R.D. (1999). Erythropoietin in the cerebrospinal fluid of neonates who sustained CNS injury. *Pediatr. Res.*, **46**, 543–7.

133 Ruth, V., Widness, J.A., Clemons, G. et al. (1990). Postnatal changes in serum immunoreactive erthropoietin in relation to hypoxia before and after birth. *J. Pediatr.*, **116**, 950–4.

134 Ski, Y., Pan, F., Li, H. et al. (2000). Role of carbon monoxide and nitric oxide in newborn infants with postasphyxial hypoxic–ischemic encephalopathy. *Pediatrics*, **106**, 1447–51.

135 Dennis, J. and Chalmers, I. (1982). Very early neonatal seizure rate: a possible epidemiological indicator of the quality of perinatal care. *Br. J. Obstet. Gynaecol.*, **89**, 418–26.

136 Derham, R.J., Matthews, T.G. and Clarke, T.A. (1985). Early seizures indicate quality of perinatal care. *Arch. Dis. Child.*, **60**, 809–13.

137 Holden, K.R., Mellits, E.D. and Freeman, J.M. (1982). Neonatal seizures. I. Correlation of prenatal and perinatal events with outcome. *Pediatrics*, **70**, 165–76.

138 Goldberg, H.J. (1983). Neonatal convulsions – a 10 year review. *Arch. Dis. Child.*, **58**, 976–8.

139 Minchom, P., Niswander, K., Chalmers, I. et al. (1987). Antecedents and outcome of very early neonatal seizures in infants born at or after term. *Br. J. Obstet. Gynaecol.*, **94**, 431–9.

140 Grant, A. (1988). The relationship between obstetrically preventable intrapartum asphyxia, abnormal neonatal neurological signs and subsequent motor impairment in babies born at or after term. In *Perinatal Events and Birth Damage in Surviving Children*, ed. F. Kubli, N. Patel, W. Schmidt and D. Lindercamp, pp. 149–159. Berlin: Springer-Verlag.

141 Levene, M.I. and Trounce, J.Q. (1986). Cause of neonatal convulsions. Towards a more precise diagnosis. *Arch. Dis. Child.*, **61**, 78–9.

142 Eriksson, M. and Zetterstrom, R. (1979). Neonatal convulsions. Incidence and causes in the Stockholm area. *Acta Paediatr. Scand.*, **68**, 807–11.

143 Niswander, K., Henson, G., Elbourne, D. et al. (1984). Adverse outcome of pregnancy and the quality of obstetric care. *Lancet*, **ii**, 827–31.

144 MacDonald, D., Grant, A., Sheridan-Pereira, M. et al. (1985). Dublin randomized controlled trial of intrapartum fetal heart rate monitoring. *Am. J. Obstet. Gynecol.*, **152**, 524–39.

145 Grant, A., O'Brien, W., Joy, M.T. et al. (1989). Cerebral palsy among children born during the Dublin randomized trial of intrapartum monitoring. *Lancet*, **ii**, 1233–6.

146 Curtis, P.D., Matthews, T.G., Clarke, T.A. et al. (1988). Neonatal seizures: the Dublin collaborative study. *Arch. Dis. Child.*, **63**, 1065–8.

147 Keegan, K.A. Jr, Waffarn, F. and Quilligan, E.J. (1985). Obstetric characteristics and fetal heart rate patterns of infants who convulse during the newborn period. *Am. J. Obstet. Gynecol.*, **153**, 732–7.

148 Finer, N.W., Robertson, C.M., Richards, R.T. et al. (1981). Hypoxic–ischemic encephalopathy in term neonates: perinatal factors and outcome. *J. Pediatr.*, **98**, 112–17.

149 Sarnat, H.B. and Sarnat, M.S. (1976). Neonatal encephalopathy following fetal distress. A clinical and electroencephalographic study. *Arch. Neurol.*, **33**, 696–705.

150 Brown, J.K., Purvis, R.J., Forfar, J.O. et al. (1974). Neurological aspects of perinatal asphyxia. *Dev. Med. Child Neurol.*, **16**, 567–80.

151 Halligan, A., Connolly, M., Clarke, T. et al. (1992). Intrapartum asphyxia in term and post-term infants. *Irish Med. J.*, **85**, 97–100.

152 Nelson, K.B. and Ellenberg, J.H. (1987). The asymptomatic newborn and risk of cerebral palsy. *Am. J. Dis. Child.*, **141**, 1333–5.

153 Iwamoto, H.S., Teitel, D. and Rudolph, A.M. (1987). Effects of birth-related events on blood flow distribution. *Pediatr. Res.*, **22**, 634–40.

154 Perlman, J.M., Tack, E.D., Martin, T. et al. (1989). Acute systemic organ injury in term infants after asphyxia. *Am. J. Dis. Child.*, **143**, 617–20.

155 Carter, B.S., Haverkamp, A.D. and Merenstein, G.B. (1993). The definition of acute perinatal asphyxia. *Clin. Perinatol.*, **20**, 287–304.

156 Clancy, R.R., Sladky, J.T. and Rorke, L.B. (1989). Hypoxic–ischemic spinal cord injury following perinatal asphyxia. *Ann. Neurol.*, **25**, 185–9.

157 Phelan, J.P., Ahn, M.O., Korst, L. et al. (1998). Intrapartum fetal asphyxial brain injury with absent multiorgan system dysfunction. *J. Matern. Fetal Med.*, **7**, 19–22.

158 Allan, W.C. and Riviello, J.J. (1992). Perinatal cerebrovascular disease in the neonate: parenchymal ischemic lesions in term and preterm infants. *Pediatr. Clin. North Am.*, **39**, 621–50.

159 Thorarensen, O., Ryan, S., Hunter, J. et al. (1997). Factor V Leiden mutation: an unrecognized cause of hemiplegic cerebral palsy, neonatal stroke and placental thrombosis. *Ann. Neurol.*, **42**, 372–5.

160 Estan, J. and Hope, P. (1997). Unilateral neonatal cerebral infarction in full term infants. *Arch. Dis. Child*, **76**, F88–93.

161 Kraus, F.T. (1997). Cerebral palsy and thrombi in placental vessels of the fetus: insights from litigation. *Hum. Pathol.*, **28**, 246–8.

162 Jan, M.M.S. and Camfield, P.R. (1998). Outcome of neonatal stroke in full-term infants without significant birth asphyxia. *Eur. J. Pediatr.*, **157**, 846–8.

163 Gunther, G., Junker, R., Strater, R. et al. (2000). Symptomatic ischemic stroke in full-term infants. Role of acquired and genetic prothrombotic risk factors. *Stroke*, **31**, 2437–41.

164 Govaert, P., Matthys, E., Zecic, A. et al. (2000). Perinatal critical infarction within middle cerebral artery trunks. *Arch. Dis. Child Fetal Neonatal Ed.*, **82**, F59–63.

165 Keogh, J.M., Paed, D., Badawi, W. et al. (1999). Group B streptococcus infection, not birth asphyxia. *Aust. N.Z. Obstet. Gynaecol.*, **39**, 108–10.

166 Flagen, N.B., Elias, E.G., Liang, K.C. et al. (1990). Perinatal and neonatal significance of bacteria-related placental villous edema. *Acta. Obstet. Gynecol. Scand.*, **69**, 287–90.

167 Gilstrap, L.C. III and Ramin, S.M. (2000). Infection and cerebral palsy. *Semin. Perinatol.*, **24**, 200–3.

168 Nelson, K.B., Dambrosia, J.M., Grether, J.K. et al. (1998). Neonatal cytokines and coagulation factors in children with cerebral palsy. *Ann. Neurol.*, **44**, 665–75.

169 Perlman, J.M. (1999). Maternal fever and neonatal depression: preliminary observations. *Clin. Pediatr.*, **38**, 287–91.

170 Nelson, K.B. and Willoughby, R.E. (2000). Infection, inflammation and the risk of cerebral palsy. *Curr. Opin. Neurol.*, **13**, 133–9.

171 Safalia, C.M., Weigl, C. and Silberman, L. (1989). The prevalence and distribution of acute placental inflammation in uncomplicated term pregnancies. *Obstet. Gynecol.*, **73**, 383–9.

172 Salafia, C.M., Mangam, H.E., Weigl, C.A. et al. (1989). Abnormal fetal heart rate patterns and placental inflammation. *Am. J. Obstet. Gynecol.*, **160**, 140–7.

173 Salafia, C.M., Ghidini, A., Sherer, D.M. et al. (1998). Abnormalities of the fetal heart rate in preterm deliveries are associated with acute intra-amniotic infection. *J. Soc. Gynecol. Invest.*, **5**, 188–91.

174 Nelson, K.B. and Ellenberg, J.H. (1986). Antecedents of cerebral palsy. Multivariant analysis of risk. *N. Engl. J. Med.*, **315**, 81–6.

175 Pharoah, P.O.D., Cooke, T., Rosenbloom, I. et al. (1987). Trends in birth prevalence of cerebral palsy. *Arch. Dis. Child.*, **62**, 379–84.

176 Pharoah, P.O.D., Platt, M.J. and Cooke, T. (1996). The changing epidemiology of cerebral palsy. *Arch. Dis. Child.*, **75**, F169–73.

177 Hagberg, B., Hagberg, G. and Olow, I. (1984). The changing panorama of cerebral palsy in Sweden. IV. Epidemiological trends 1959–1978. *Acta Paediatr. Scand.*, **73**, 433–40.

178 Hagberg, B., Hagberg, G., Olow, I. et al. (1989). The changing panorama of cerebral palsy in Sweden. V. The birth period 1979–1982. *Acta. Paediatr. Scand.*, **78**, 283–90.

179 Hagberg, B., Hagberg, G., and Olow, I. (1993). The changing panorama of cerebral palsy in Sweden. VI. Prevalence and origin during the birth period 1983–1986. *Acta Paediatr.*, **82**, 387–93.

180 Hagberg, B., Hagberg, G., Olow, I. et al. (1996). The changing panorama of cerebral palsy in Sweden. VII. Prevalence and origin in the birth year period 1987–1990. *Acta Paediatr.*, **85**, 954–60.

181 Stanley, F.J. and Watson, L.D. (1988). Cerebral palsy in Western Australia: trends 1968–1981. *Am. J. Obstet. Gynecol.*, **158**, 89–92.

182 Stanley, F.J. and Watson, L. (1992). Trends in perinatal mortality and cerebral palsy in Western Australia 1967 to 1985. *Br. Med. J.*, **304**, 1658–63.

183 Cummins, S.K., Nelson, K.B., Grether, J.K. et al. (1993). Cerebral palsy in four Northern California countries, births 1983 through 1985. *J. Pediatr.*, **123**, 230–7.

184 Holm, V.A. (1982). The causes of cerebral palsy. A contemporary perspective. *J.A.M.A.*, **247**, 1473–7.

185 Torfs, C.P., van den Berg, B.J., Oechsli, F.W. et al. (1990). Prenatal and perinatal factors in the etiology of cerebral palsy. *J. Pediatr.*, **116**, 615–19.

186 Manning, F.A., Bondaji, W., Harman, C.R. et al. (1998). Fetal assessment based on fetal biophysical profile scoring. VIII The incidence of cerebral palsy in tested and untested perinates. *Am. J. Obstet. Gynecol.*, **178**, 696–706.

187 Scheller, J.M. and Nelson, K.B. (1994). Does cesarian delivery prevent cerebral palsy or other neurologic problems of childhood? *Obstet. Gynecol*, **83**, 624–30.

188 Paneth, W. and Stark, R.I. (1983). Cerebral palsy and mental retardation in relation to indicators of perinatal asphyxia. *Am. J. Obstet. Gynecol.*, **147**, 960–6.

189 Hagberg, B. and Kyllerman, M. (1983). Epidemiology of mental retardation – a Swedish survey. *Brain Dev.*, **5**, 441–9.

190 Crocker, A.C. (1989). The causes of mental retardation. *Pediatr. Ann.*, **18**, 623–36.

191 Low, J.A., Galbraith, R.S., Muir, D.W. et al. (1984). Factors associated with motor and cognitive deficits in children after intrapartum fetal hypoxia. *Am. J. Obstet. Gynecol.*, **148**, 533–9.

192 Soothill, P.W., Nicolaides, K.H. and Campbell, S. (1987). Prenatal asphyxia, hyperlactic acidemia, hypoglycaemia and erythroblastosis in growth retarded fetuses. *Br. Med. J.*, **294**, 1051–3.

193 Uverbeant, P. and Hagberg, G. (1992). Intrauterine growth in children with cerebral palsy. *Acta Paediat.*, **81**, 407–12.

2

Mechanisms of brain damage in animal models of hypoxia–ischemia in newborns

Lee J. Martin

Departments of Pathology, Division of Neuropathology, and Neuroscience, Johns Hopkins University School of Medicine, Baltimore, Maryland, USA

Perinatal hypoxia–ischemia (HI) in newborns is a major cause of pediatric mortality and morbidity and causes brain damage resulting in lifelong neurobehavioral handicaps. Systemic asphyxia resulting from a disruption in placental gas exchange occurs perinatally in 2–4 per 1000 full-term infants.[1] Approximately 15–20% of infants who develop brain damage subsequently die during the newborn period, and up to 25% of survivors exhibit permanent neurological disabilities.[2] Neurologic abnormalities, such as movement disorders (e.g., ataxia, choreoathetosis, diplegia, or dystonia), epilepsy, and developmental delay, are possible lifelong consequences that occur following perinatal HI.[3] Preterm or term HI infants have damage in the forebrain and brain stem,[4–6] with basal ganglia and somatosensory systems showing selective vulnerability.[3,7,8] The mechanisms for this brain damage and the resulting neurologic disorders in newborns are still not understood. Unfortunately, no treatments for the prevention or amelioration of this neurologic injury are available for infants and children who have suffered HI.

Animal models are essential for understanding the mechanisms of hypoxic-ischemic encephalopathy (HIE). These models are important because it is very difficult to study directly the process of nerve cell death by analyzing individuals with HIE. The advanced brain-imaging technologies have insufficient resolution to study directly dying neurons at cellular and molecular levels in living patients. When patients with HIE die and when postmortem brain samples become available for experimentation, neurological and neuropathological associations can be gleaned, but cause-and-effect relationships are difficult to identify. Therefore animal models must be used to provide an in vivo system to delineate the biochemical, molecular, and structural evolution of brain damage and nerve cell degeneration in paradigms that mirror certain neuropathological and possibly clinical features of HIE in humans. Furthermore, experimental manipulations, including surgical and pharmacological, can be performed in animal models in sufficient numbers to draw conclusions on the mechanisms of brain damage and the possible benefits of experimental treatments.

Few models have been developed in newborn animals that mimic neuropathological and clinical outcomes observed in asphyxic near-term humans. Exciting early advances were made using monkeys,[9] but nonhuman primates are not used currently in models of HIE. The commonly used postnatal rat model of HIE has prominent forebrain damage,[10–12] but neuronal vulnerability is not particularly selective and the injury resembles that found with focal ischemia with the formation of cavitary lesions rarely seen in human newborns. Recently, we have developed a very successful animal model of brain injury after HI in newborns.[13–16]

Piglet model of HIE

Our piglet model of HIE causes damage very similar to the pattern of brain injury found in human newborns that have experienced HI.[13–15,17] It is a recovery-survival cardiopulmonary resuscitation (CPR) model (Figure 2.1). One-week-old piglets (~3 kg) are anesthetized with intraperitoneal sodium pentobarbital (65 mg/kg), intubated, ventilated mechanically with a fractional inspired oxygen (Fio_2) of 0.30 in humidified air, and instrumented with femoral artery and vein catheters. Oxygenation, ventilation, and acid–balance are all maintained at normal values. Ventilation is set to maintain end-tidal and $Paco_2$ at 35–40 mmHg. Tympanic membrane temperature is maintained at 38.5–39.5 °C. Piglets receive a maintenance infusion of intravenous lactated Ringer's solution (10 mg/kg per h), with additional analgesia and neuromuscular blockade provided by intravenous fentanyl (10 μg/kg) and pancuronium (0.3 mg/kg), respectively. Baseline arterial blood gases, pH, hemoglobin, glucose, lactate, heart rate, and blood pressure are measured.

The insult is made after a postsurgical stabilization period of 120 min. Piglets are exposed to 30 min of hypoxia by decreasing Fio_2 to 0.1 (saturated oxygen Sao_2 ~30%), followed by 5 min of ventilation with room air to permit partial reoxygenation (Sao_2 ~60%) necessary for later myocardial resuscitation, and then 7 min of airway occlusion (Sao_2 ~5%), resulting in asphyxic cardiac arrest (Figure 2.1). For the first minute of asphyxia, progressive tachycardia and hypertension occur, followed by an abrupt drop in heart rate to about 50% of normal (i.e., normal is ~170 beats/min) during the second minute. Mean arterial blood pressure (MABP) declines progressively until circulation virtually ceases (MABP <25 mmHg) at 5–6 min of asphyxia. Total downtime is 1–2 min. CPR is initiated by unclamping the endotracheal tube, reinstating ventilation with 100% O_2, manual chest compressions (100/min, 50% duty cycle), intravenous epinephrine (10 μg/kg bolus), and intravenous sodium bicarbonate until return of spontaneous circulation, usually within 2–3 min.

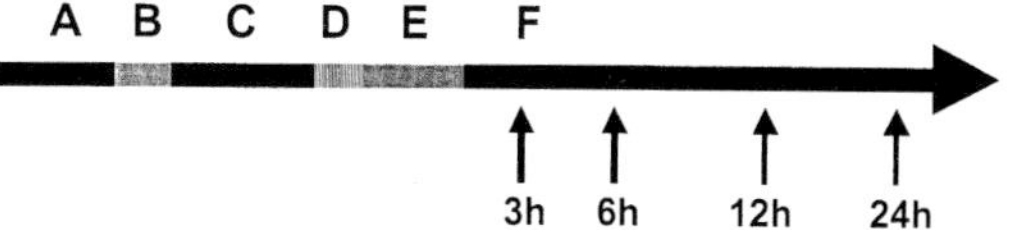

Figure 2.1 Basic design of the piglet model of hypoxia–ischemia. Model of hypoxic–ischemic cardiac arrest in 1-week-old piglets. A, anesthesia induction; B, stabilization; C, hypoxia: 30 min in Fio_2 0.11 l/min; D, room air: 5 min Fio_2 0.21 l/min; E, asphyxia: 7 min; F, cardiopulmonary resuscitation & recovery.

CPR is continued until spontaneous circulation is restored with MABP above 60 mmHg. Approximately 90% of piglets are successfully resuscitated. Piglets are allowed to awaken and are extubated when able to maintain spontaneous oxygenation and ventilation, usually at 6 h. By 12 h after asphyxia piglets are generally able to sit up and drink water. Piglets perambulate and drink formula milk, usually by 24 h recovery. Animals are allowed to survive for designated times dictated by the experimental design (Figure 2.1).

Our piglet model was adopted because of its relevance to HIE in human newborns and children.[17] HI in 1-week-old piglets preferentially damages primary sensory and forebrain motor systems (Figure 2.2). This neuropathology is progressive and is not static. The cerebral cortex and basal ganglia are highly vulnerable (Figure 2.2). The neocortical area that is most vulnerable to HI corresponds to primary somatosensory cortex based on electrophysiological mapping of somatosensory-evoked potentials in newborn pigs.[18,19] The most vulnerable region of piglet striatum (i.e., central putamen) appears to be the sensorimotor-recipient region (Figure 2.2), based on known corticostriatal connectivity in other mammals[20] and our tract-tracing studies in piglets (Figure 2.3). In diencephalon, thalamic relay nuclei for somatosensory (ventral posterior nucleus, Figures 2.2 and 2.3), visual (lateral geniculate nucleus), auditory (medial geniculate nucleus), and motor (ventral anterior/lateral) systems are consistently damaged. In brainstem, visual (superior colliculus) and auditory (inferior colliculus) relay nuclei are predisposed to injury.

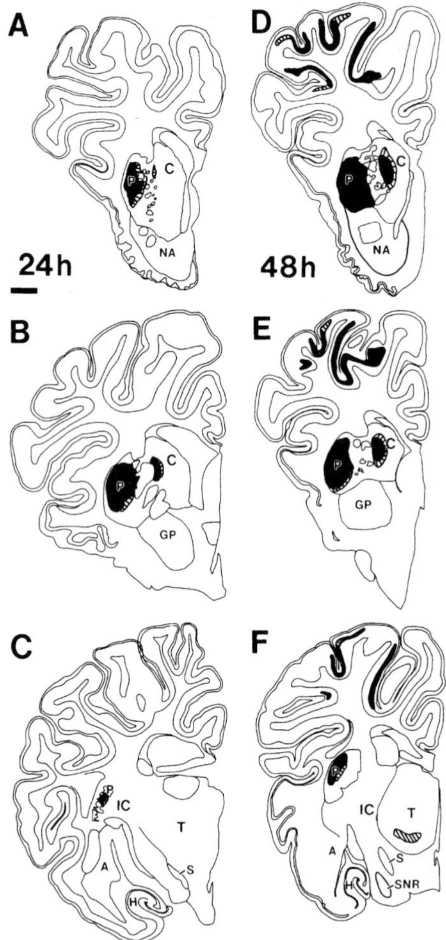

Figure 2.2 Topographic distribution of brain damage in piglets at 24 and 48 h after hypoxia–ischemia (HI). A–C and D–F are representative coronal sections from the forebrain (A and D are most anterior) through rostral midbrain (C and F are most posterior). The midline is to the right. Note the neuroanatomical similarity to the human brain. Solid black denotes areas of necrosis and hatching denotes areas of prenecrosis (i.e., the presence of ischemic neurons and inflammatory changes, but not elimination of neurons as in necrosis). At 24 h after HI, damage is found primarily in the putamen. At 48 h, laminar necrosis and prenecrosis are found in parietal cortex (somatosensory neocortex). Thalamic damage is emerging at 48 h. A, amygdala; C, caudate nucleus; GP, globus pallidus; H, hippocampus; IC, internal capsule; NA, nucleus accumbens; P, putamen; S, subthalamic nucleus; SNR, substantia nigra reticulata; T, thalamus. Scale bar (in A) = 2 mm.

This regional distribution of neocortical and subcortical injury is important conceptually because it indicates that the formation of HIE in newborns is not a random and static process but, rather, is highly organized and topographic, targeting preferentially regions that function in sensorimotor integration and control of movement. This distribution of neonatal brain damage is possibly dictated by regional connectivity (Figures 2.2 and 2.3), function, and mitochondrial activity. This theory has been designated as the connectivity-metabolism hypothesis for brain damage in newborns.[13,14] The pattern of brain damage in HI piglets bears a close resemblance to that found in perinatal asphyxia in humans[4–6] and nonhuman primates.[9]

Neuronal signal transduction mechanisms important for brain damage in HI

Glutamate receptor-mediated excitotoxicity may be responsible for the brain damage in newborns after HI.[21] Glutamate is a primary excitatory neurotransmitter in the central nervous system. Glutamate is released from nerve terminals into the synaptic cleft (Figure 2.4A) by regulated exocytosis of synaptic vesicles. Concentrations of glutamate at the synaptic cleft are estimated to be ~1 mmol/l, whereas the concentration of interstitial glutamate is ~1 μmol/l. Glutamate can bind and activate several types of glutamate receptors (GluRs) on neurons (Figure 2.4A; Table 2.1). These GluRs are classified broadly as either ion channel or metabotropic G protein-coupled receptors. These classes of GluRs have distinct molecular compositions and distinct signal transduction mechanisms.[22]

The ion channel GluRs are the *N*-methyl-D-aspartate (NMDA) receptors and the non-NMDA receptors. The non-NMDA GluRs are further divided into the α-amino-3-hydroxy-5-methyl-4-isoxazole propionate (AMPA) and kainate (KA) receptors (Table 2.1). The ion channel GluRs all form monovalent cation (Na^+, K^+)-conducting channels, but they have differences in their permeabilities to divalent cations (Ca^{2+}). The activation of ion channel GluRs directly changes conductance of specific ions

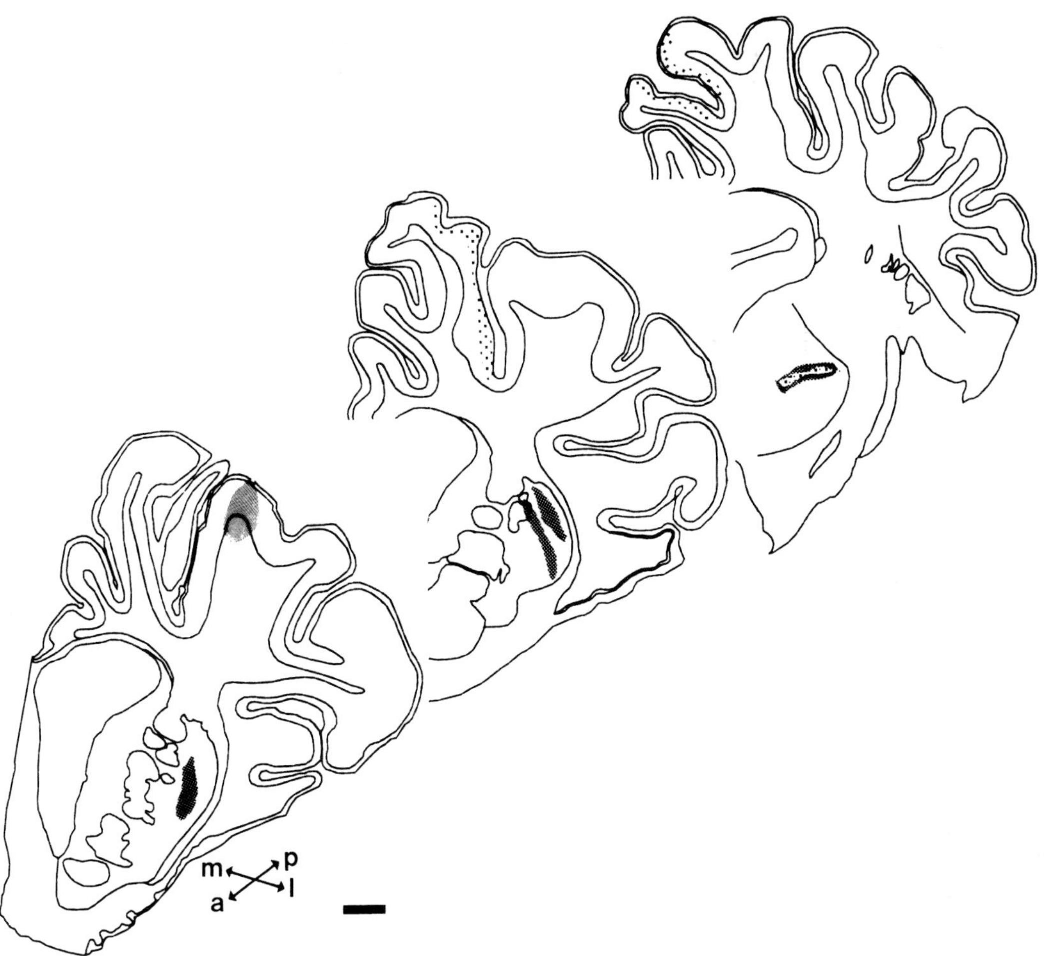

Figure 2.3 Tract-tracing studies in piglet brain show that the region of striatum that is highly vulnerable to hypoxic–ischemia (HI) is innervated by primary somatosensory cortex. Wheatgerm agglutinin-horseradish peroxidase was injected into primary somatosensory cortex (stippling). The central and dorsolateral putamen, the regions of striatum that are damaged by HI, are extensively innervated by the primary somatosensory cortex (identified by the anterograde labeling, hatching in putamen but not in the caudate nucleus). In addition, corticostriatal terminal fields in putamen are organized into diagonal bands. Injection of the primary somatosensory cortex was verified by the retrograde labeling of neuronal cell bodies (dots) and terminals (hatching) in the ventral posterior lateral thalamic nucleus and by the retrograde labeling of neuronal cell bodies (dots) in cortical areas 3a and 3b of more posterior levels. Orientation arrows: a, anterior; p, posterior; m, medial; l, lateral. Scale bar = 5 mm.

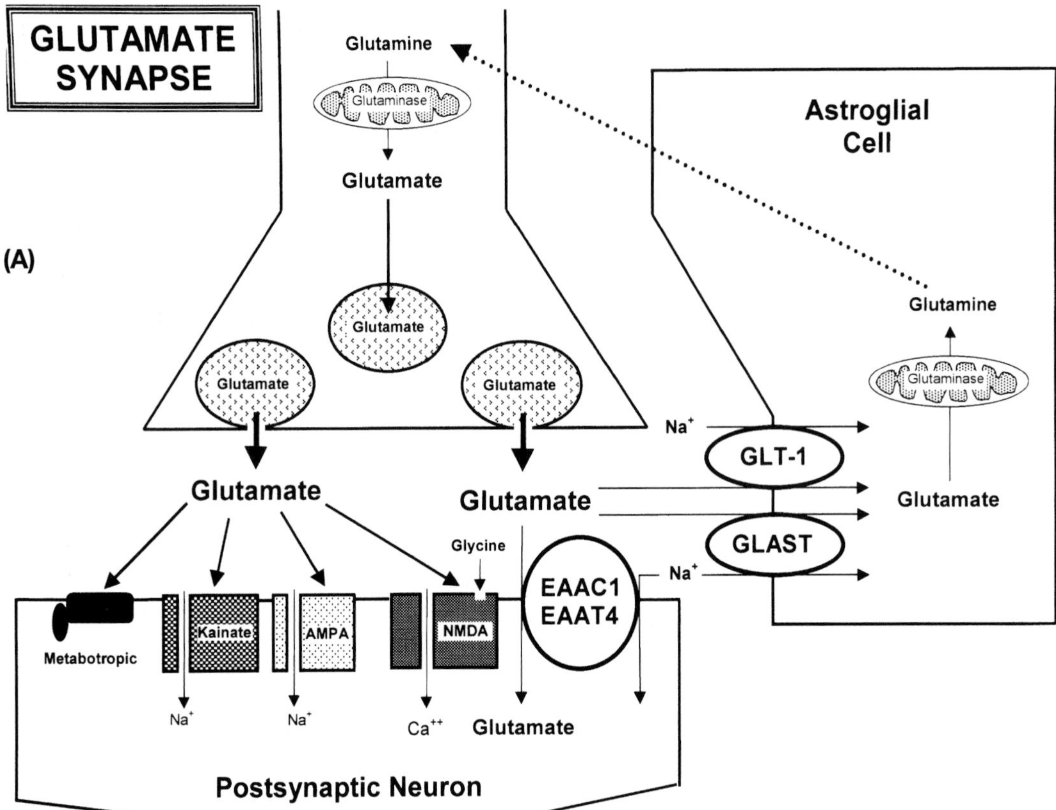

Figure 2.4 Molecular anatomy of a glutamate synapse and excitotoxic activation of a striatal neuron synapse. (A) The synthesis of glutamate (the major excitatory neurotransmitter within the central nervous system) involves glutamine metabolism. Glutamate is packaged within neurotransmitter vesicles and is released from the presynaptic axon terminal in response to axon depolarization. Glutamate can bind and activate ion channel glutamate receptors, including the *N*-methyl-D-aspartate (NMDA) receptors and the non-NMDA receptors which are the α-amino-3-hydroxy-5-methyl-4-isoxazole propionate (AMPA) and kainate (KA) receptors. Removal of glutamate from the synapse occurs either by passive diffusion or by transport involving a family of neuronal and glial glutamate transporter proteins, including GLAST (EAAT1), GLT1 (EAAT2), EAAC1 (EAAT3), EAAT4, and EAAT5. (B) Diagram of signal transduction mechanisms related to excitotoxic and hypoxic–ischemic (HI) neuronal death. The diagram shows a dendritic spine of a striatal neuron and a glutamatergic presynaptic terminal. The prominent postsynaptic intracellular pathways are shown that lead to neuronal injury and death resulting from excitotoxic activation of glutamate receptor. Abbreviations: AMPA/KA-R, α-amino-3-hydroxy-5-methyl-4-isoxazole propionate and kainate receptors; DAG, diacylglycerol; IP_3, inositol trisphosphate; mGluR, metabotropic glutamate receptor; NMDA-R, *N*-methyl-D-aspartate receptor; NO, nitric oxide; NOS, NO synthase; PKC, protein kinase C; PLA_2, phospholipase A_2; V-gated Ca^{2+} Ch, voltage-gated Ca^{2+} channel.

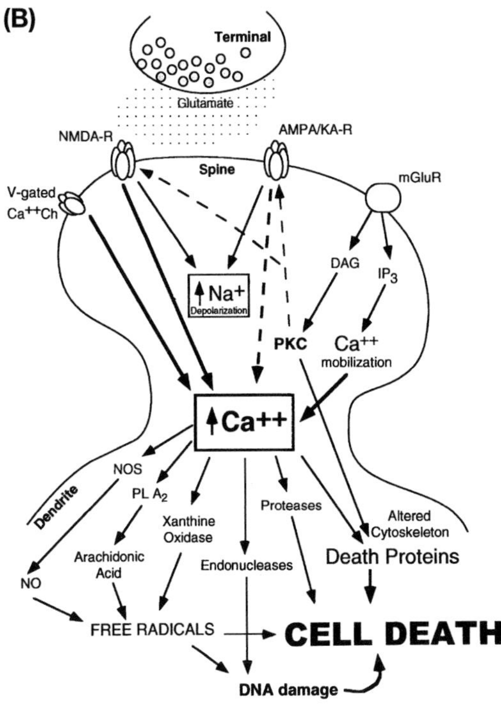

Figure 2.4 (*cont.*)

through the receptor–ion channel complex, thereby inducing membrane depolarization. Fast, short-lived (1–10 ms) excitatory postsynaptic currents in most neurons in the central nervous system are mediated by these receptors. These receptors are oligomers, most likely pentameric heterooligomers, of homologous subunits encoded by distinct genes. The NMDA receptor subunits are NR1, NR2A-NR2D, and NR3; the AMPA receptor subunits are GluR1–GluR4 (or GluRA–GluRD); and the kainate receptor subunits are GluR5–GluR7 and KA1–2 (Table 2.1).

The metabotropic GluRs (mGluRs) are G protein-coupled receptors that are single proteins encoded by single genes. The mGluRs do not form ion channels but are instead linked to signal transduction molecules within the plasma membrane. mGluRs have slower electrophysiological characteristics (latencies >100 ms) than ion channel GluRs. Group I mGluRs (mGluR1 and mGluR5) operate through activation of phospholipase C (PLC) by G_q proteins, phosphoinositide hydrolysis and generation of inositol-1,4,5 triphosphate and diacylglycerol, and subsequent mobilization of Ca^{2+} from nonmitochondrial intracellular stores. Group II mGluRs (mGluR 2 and 3) and group III mGluRs (mGluR 4

Table 2.1. Molecular classification of glutamate receptors

Ion channel (ionotropic) receptors			G Protein-coupled (metabotropic) receptors		
NMDA	Non-NMDA		Group I	Group II	Group III
	AMPA	Kainate	mGluR1	mGluR2	mGluR4
Receptor subunits			mGluR5	mGluR3	mGluR6
					mGluR7
					mGluR8
NR1	GluR1	GluR5			
NR2A	GluR2	GluR6			
NR2B	GluR3	GluR7			
NR2C	GluR4	KA1			
NR2D		KA2			
NR3					

Notes:

NMDA, *N*-methyl-D-aspartate; GluR, glutamate receptor; KA, kainate.

Table 2.2. Molecular classification of glutamate transporters

Transporter subtype	Primary cellular localization	Change within 24 h after HI in newborn brain
GLAST/EAAT1	Astroglia	Unchanged
GLT1/EAAT2	Astroglia; subsets of neurons in developing central nervous system	Unchanged or increased
EAAC1/EAAT3/N1	Neurons	Decreased
EAAT4	Purkinje cells	Unchanged
EAAT5	Retinal cells	?

Notes:
HI, hypoxic ischemia.

and 6–8) function by G_I or G_0 protein-mediated inhibition of adenylyl cyclase and modulation of ion channel activity.

Normal excitatory synaptic neurotransmission mediated by glutamate relies upon active transport of glutamate into cells (Figure 2.4A), thereby preventing extracellular glutamate from reaching neurotoxic concentrations (Figure 2.4B). Accumulation of excitatory amino acids can occur by either increased vesicular or nonvesicular release or impaired removal of glutamate from the synapse, either by passive diffusion or by transport involving a family of neuronal and glial glutamate transporter proteins.[23] To date, five distinct high-affinity, sodium-dependent glutamate transporters have been cloned from animal and human tissue: GLAST (EAAT1), GLT1 (EAAT2), EAAC1 (EAAT3), EAAT4, and EAAT5 (Table 2.2). These proteins differ in structure, pharmacologic properties, and tissue distribution.[23–25] Immunocytochemical studies have shown (Table 2.2) in normal, uninjured brain that GLAST is present in astroglia and in some neurons,[26] but GLT1 is expressed primarily by astrocytes.[26,27] EAAC1 is present widely in neurons but not astroglia.[26] EAAT4 is expressed mainly by cerebellar Purkinje cells,[28] and EAAT5 is found primarily in retina.[25] GLAST, GLT1, and EAAC1 are thus the major glutamate transporter subtypes in forebrain.

Role of excitotoxic mechanisms in HI brain damage in newborns

Although glutamate and GluR activation are critical for normal nervous system function, glutamate is toxic to neurons at abnormally high concentrations, if GluRs on neurons are excessively activated.[21,29] This process is called excitotoxicity (Figure 2.4B). The excessive stimulation of GluRs by presynaptic glutamate or chemical analogs of glutamate can activate voltage-dependent Ca^{2+} channels and produce numerous abnormalities (Figure 2.4B). These cellular alterations include: abnormal intracellular ion (e.g., Na^+ and Ca^{2+}) concentrations and pH; dysregulated protein phosphorylation via kinase activation and phosphatase inactivation; energetic defects from adenosine triphosphate (ATP) depletion and mitochondrial failure; and generation of reactive oxygen species via mitochondrial perturbations, nitric oxide synthase and xanthine oxidase activation, and prostaglandin synthesis. These events can cause perturbations in cell volume control, protein stability, and DNA integrity that can lead to cell death (Figure 2.4B). Acute excitotoxicity causes degeneration in neuronal cultures of animal brain and spinal cord and after intracerebral delivery of GluR activators into the central nervous system of experimental animals. In addition, excitotoxicity participates in the mechanisms of neuronal degeneration in animal models of cerebral ischemia as well as brain and spinal cord trauma.

The contributions of GluR-mediated excitotoxicity to neurodegeneration after cerebral ischemia in adults and newborns continue to be scrutinized for new therapies, while the potential role of glutamate transporter dysfunction in clinically relevant, pediatric animal models of HI are only recently being explored. In newborn piglets, neuronal cell death in striatum after HI closely resembles excitotoxic injury induced by NMDA receptor activation,[30,31] and in newborn rats the NMDA receptor antagonist MK-801 ameliorates brain damage following HI.[32,33] In piglets, however, some antagonists to the NMDA receptor[34] or the AMPA receptor[14,16,35] are not neuroprotective after HI. Extracellular glutamate concentrations in striatum rise acutely during HI in fetal lamb.[36] From the standpoint of glutamate transporters an increase in extracellular glutamate during HI may occur through defective glutamate uptake[37] or from reversed glutamate transport.[38] Glutamate transporter function and expression are altered after cerebral ischemia. In 7-day-old rat pups, high-affinity glutamate transport in striatum falls transiently during HI and through 1 h of recovery.[37] After forebrain ischemia in adult rats, D-[^{3}H]aspartate binding sites in hippocampus increase within 5 min,[39] although hippocampal GLT1 mRNA and protein levels decrease within 3–6 h.[40] Impaired glutamate transport can cause neurodegeneration. In rats, the glutamate transport inhibitor DL-threo-3-hydroxyaspartate (DL-THA) causes neuronal degeneration in striatum after intracerebral injection.[41] In mice, some animals deficient in GLT1 exhibit lethal spontaneous seizures and increased susceptibility to acute cortical injury,[42] and GLAST gene ablation exacerbates ischemic retinal damage.[43] The precise role for GluR excitotoxicity and possible glutamate transporter defects in the pathophysiological mechanisms of neuronal degeneration after HI, therefore, still remain poorly understood. We have examined whether early and sustained abnormalities in glutamate transport occur during the first 24 h after HI and whether any changes coincide with the evolution of striatal neurodegeneration in newborn piglets.

Striatal neuron death after HI in newborns is rapid and progressive over 24 h

Striatal neurons are highly vulnerable to HI in newborns. Profound degeneration of neurons in HI piglet striatum occurs during 3–24 h recovery (Figures 2.5 and 2.6). Neuronal injury is progressive, with percentage neuronal damage increasing with time after HI (Figure 2.5A). At 24 h after HI, neuronal density is decreased significantly (Fig. 2.5B), and ~80% of remaining principal neurons within the putamen are degenerating (Figures 2.5A and 2.6A). The progression of striatal neuron injury revealed by hematoxylin & eosin (H&E) staining (Figure 2.6A,B) is paralleled by loss of cytoskeletal protein (Figure 2.7) and the occurrence of DNA fragmentation (Figures 2.5C and 2.6C). Immunostaining shows that the putamen is profoundly depleted of microtubule-associated protein-2 (MAP2) but the caudate is much less affected (Figure 2.7). In situ end labeling of DNA fragments with TUNEL (Figure 2.6C) shows that nuclear DNA fragmentation in striatal neurons is progressive over 3–24 h after HI (Figure 2.5C). In contrast, during early recovery, astroglia appear to be uninjured based on the levels of the astroglial cytoskeletal protein glial fibrillary acidic protein (Figure 2.5D).

The structural progression of principal striatal neuron death in 1-week-old HI piglets was determined by electron microscopy (EM). The degeneration of these neurons is not apoptosis or a hybrid form of apoptosis and necrosis (see below), based on previously established criteria for neuronal death.[44] Striatal neuron degeneration in newborn piglet brain during the first 24 h after HI is classical necrosis (Figure 2.8).

Glutamate transporter defects do not occur early during the emergence of striatal neurodegeneration after HI

Glutamate transport activity in newborn piglet striatum is decreased after HI,[45] but not until neuronal degeneration is well underway.[31] High-affinity sodium-dependent glutamate uptake into striatal

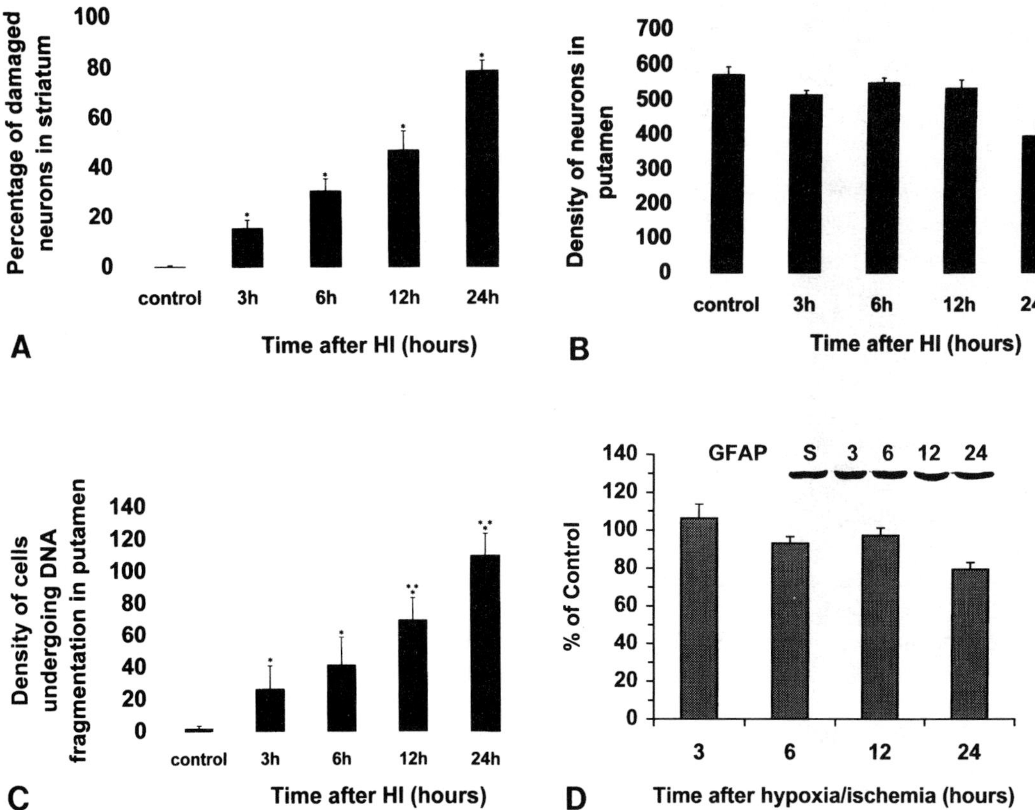

Figure 2.5 Striatal neuropathology after hypoxia–ischemia (HI) in newborns is rapid and progressive over 24 h. (A) The number of degenerating neurons in putamen increases progressively during the first 24 h after HI. Values (% of neurons damaged) are mean ±SEM. Percentage neuronal damage was estimated by identifying the fraction of neurons with ischemic cytopathology relative to the total number of neurons in microscopic fields of the striatum. Single asterisk, significantly different ($P < 0.05$) from control and from preceding recovery time. (B) Neuronal density in the putamen of control and ischemic piglets at 3, 6, 12, and 24 h after HI. Values are mean ±SEM. Asterisk, significantly different ($P < 0.05$) from control. (C) Striatal neuron death (in putamen) in control piglets (C) and piglets at 3, 6, 12, and 24 h after HI. Terminal deoxynucleotidyl transferase-mediated biotin-deoxyuridine triphosphate nick end-labeling (TUNEL)-positive cell densities (cells/mm^2) are mean ±SEM. Asterisk indicates significant difference ($P < 0.05$) from control. Double asterisk indicates significant difference ($P < 0.05$) from control, 3 h and 6 h after HI. (D) Glial fibrillary acidic protein (GFAP) protein levels in newborn piglet striatum are stable after HI. Representative GFAP immunoblot for membrane-enriched (P2) fractions of striatum from control piglets (S) and from piglets recovered for 3, 6, 12, or 24 h after HI. Blots consistently revealed a single prominent band at ~45 kDa. GFAP immunodensity (2–3 piglets per group) was corrected for synaptophysin immunodensity in the same sample, then expressed as percent control. GFAP immunodensity was not significantly different from control at any time point ($P > 0.05$, Wilcoxon signed-ranks test). Values represent mean ±1 SEM.

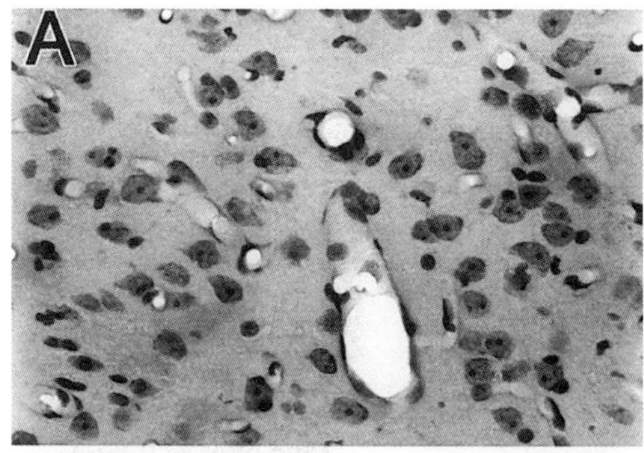

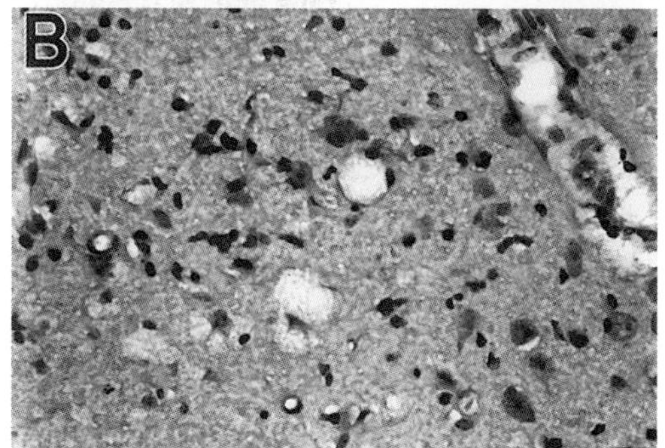

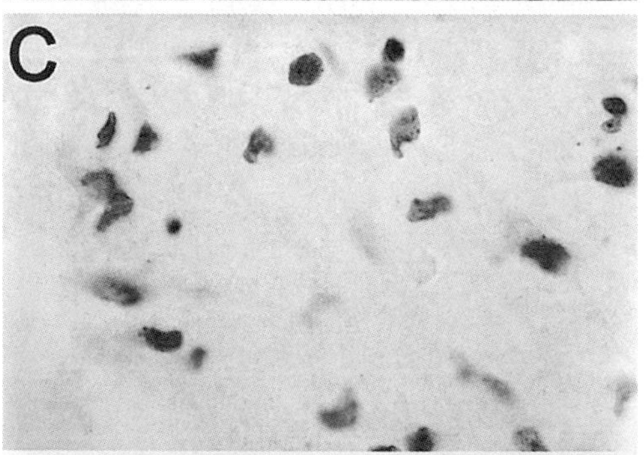

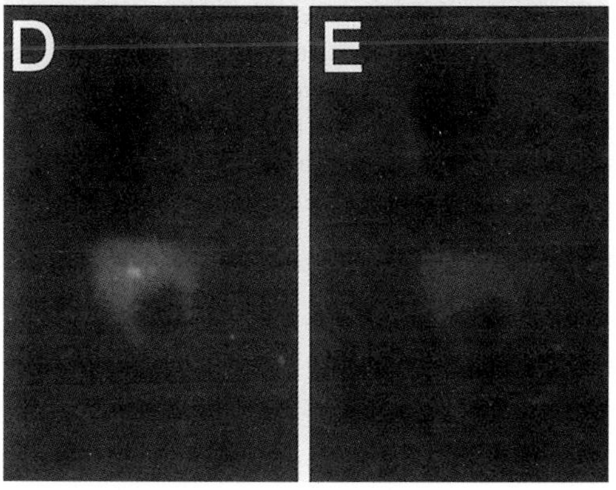

Figure 2.6 Striatal neuron degeneration in piglets after hypoxia–ischemia (HI). (A) In hematoxylin & eosin (H&E) sections of controls, numerous round, medium-sized (10–20 μm) neurons are present. (B) At 24 h after HI, there is severe loss of neurons in putamen, and many remaining principal neurons show ischemic cell injury, as evidenced by the eosinophilic cytoplasm, nuclear pyknosis, and shrinkage of the cell body in H&E sections. Astrocytes are swollen, causing vacuolation of the neuropil and formation of perineuronal spaces. (C) After 24 h after HI, in situ DNA fragmentation assay (terminal deoxynucleotidyl transferase-mediated biotin-deoxyuridine triphosphate nick end-labeling (TUNEL), counterstained with cresyl violet) shows that many principal putaminal neurons are positive (brown nuclear staining). Nearby cells (with only purple nuclear staining) are not TUNEL-positive. (D) and (E) Immunofluorescence for nitrotyrosine (D, green fluorescein isothiocyanate labeling) and Golgi 58K protein (E, red Texas-red labeling) and confocal microscopy demonstrates that nitrotyrosine immunoreactivity (D) occurs at fragments of the Golgi apparatus (E) in striatal neurons at 6 h after HI.

synaptosomes is 100%, 64%, and 52% of control at 3, 6–12, and 24 h after HI (Figure 2.9A), paralleling the progression of striatal neuron degeneration (Figure 2.5). Analysis of transport kinetics by Eadie–Hofstee plots shows that, despite the decrease in overall transport velocity, neither the calculated affinity constant (K_m) nor the number of binding sites (V_{max}) is significantly different from control at any time point during the first 24 hours after HI (Figure 2.10; Table 2.3).

Alterations in glutamate transporter expression can account for decreased glutamate uptake. We measured glutamate transporter proteins in piglet striatum at 3, 6, 12, and 24 h after HI by immunoblotting. Glutamate transporter antibodies detect distinct proteins with molecular weights of 65–73 kDa in piglet striatum. Apparent homomultimers of GLAST and GLT1 are observed. These results are consistent with the demonstration that glutamate transporters can form homomultimers.[46] During the first 24 h after HI, GLT1 and GLAST (primary astroglial transporters) levels do not change significantly (Figure 2.9C,D). However, striatal EAAC1 (neuronal

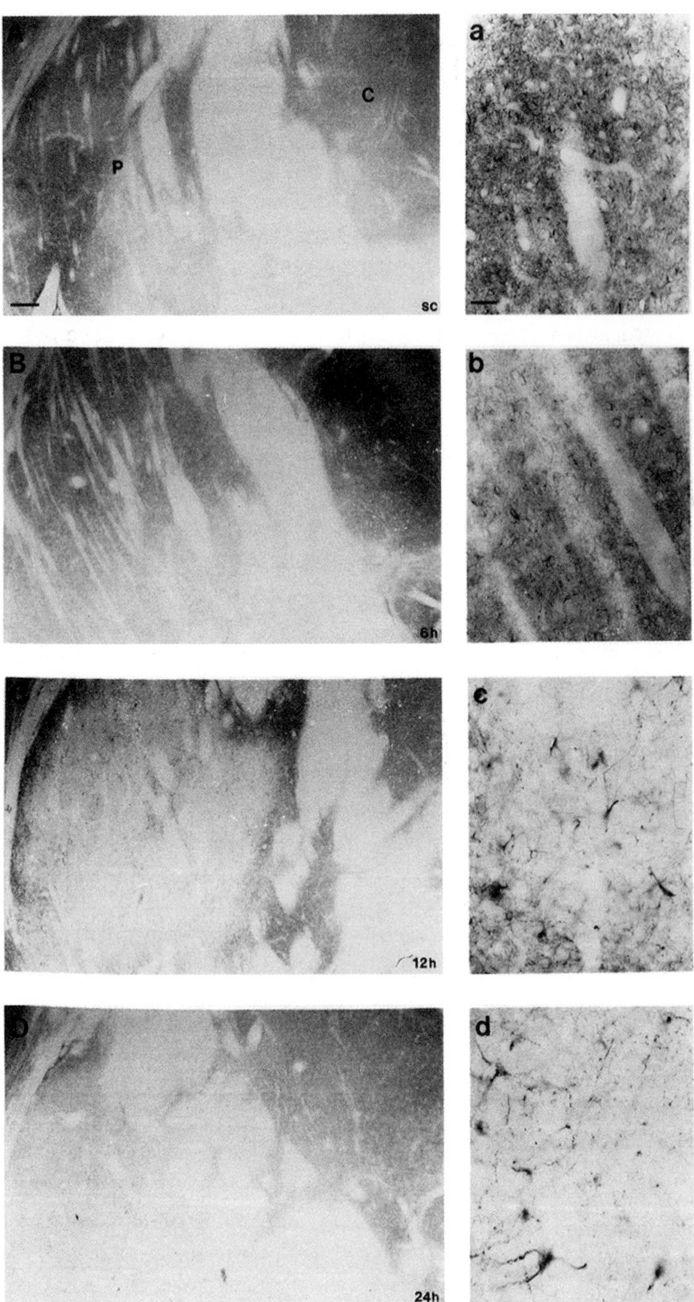

Figure 2.7 Immunolocalization of microtubule-associated protein-2 (MAP-2) in the striatum of sham control (sc) piglets and piglets at 6, 12, and 24 h after hypoxia–ischemia (HI). Low-magnification photographs (A, B, C, D) show the caudate nucleus (C) and the putamen (P) and higher-magnification photographs (a, b, c, d) show the putamen. The high vulnerability of the putamen is illustrated. Immunoreactivity (dark staining) is lost progressively in the putamen. Scale bars = 1000 μm (A); 40 μm (a).

transporter) levels are significantly lower than control at 12 and 24 h after HI (Figure 2.9B).

Our experiments show that glutamate transporter defects do not occur early during the emergence of striatal neurodegeneration after HI. Glutamate transporter defects are detected after the neurodegeneration has already begun. GLAST and GLT1 protein levels in newborn piglet striatum do not change during the first 24 h after HI; however, neuronal glutamate transporter is decreased at 12 and 24 h after HI. We conclude that loss of synaptic glutamate uptake after HI is primarily a consequence of reduced EAAC1 levels secondary to progressive neuronal degeneration. Thus, failure of glutamate transport does not appear to be an early primary mechanism for striatal neurodegeneration after HI in newborns.

Glutamate transporter defects do not occur prior to cortical neurodegeneration after HI

Previous studies from our laboratory have shown that the piglet somatosensory cortex is damaged after HI, with progression to either selective laminar injury or panlaminar degeneration by 96 h.[13,14] Neurons in layers II/III and layers IV/V of somatosensory cortex are vulnerable. Other regions such as the frontal cortex and occipital cortex are relatively spared from neurodegeneration after HI.[13,14] Because of the regional vulnerability of our model of perinatal HI and the potential contribution of glutamate transporters in delayed cortical neurodegeneration, we performed several additional experiments. We determined if defects in glutamate transporter function precede neurodegeneration in the vulnerable somatosensory cortex after HI in newborns, and whether changes in the levels of specific molecular subtypes of glutamate transporter proteins correlate with changes in glutamate transporter function. We found that glutamate transporter activity is increased (rather than decreased) in vulnerable cortex following HI at the onset of neurodegeneration and is coincident with increased levels of GLT1 (Figure 2.11). Specifically, we found that glutamate uptake in controls is greater in occipital cortex (less vulnerable cortex) compared to parietal cortex (highly vulnerable cortex). After HI, glutamate uptake is increased in parietal cortex, with both K_m and V_{max} elevated, but uptake is unchanged in occipital cortex (Figure 2.11B). By immunoblotting, the levels of GLT1, GLAST, EAAC1, and EAAT4 are not changed significantly in homogenates of total somatosensory cortex or occipital cortex (Figure 2.11B), but localization experiments with immunocytochemistry show a cortical layer-selective increase in GLT1 in vulnerable layers of neocortex. Thus, failure of glutamate transport does not precede or coincide with the onset of cortical neurodegeneration in newborn HI.

NMDA receptor phosphorylation is elevated in piglet striatum after HI

We have hypothesized that the mechanisms for the profound degeneration of striatal neurons after HI involve NMDA receptor-mediated excitotoxicity.[30,31] Protein phosphorylation is a major mechanism for regulation of receptor function and plays a role in NMDA receptor modulation and activation.[47–50] We have examined in our newborn piglet model of cardiac arrest the protein levels and phosphorylation status of NMDA receptors after HI.[51]

The levels of NMDA receptor subunit proteins change differentially in the striatum of HI piglets. Western blots of piglet synaptic membrane fractions of total striatum reveal that NMDA receptor subunit 1 (NR1) levels do not change significantly at 3–24 h recovery after HI compared to controls. However, when NR1 levels are related to the evolving neuronal cell injury in the putamen, we discovered an interesting association. NR1 levels are lower than baseline when few neurons are damaged, but levels increase as the number of damaged neurons increases. The highest levels of NR1 protein correlate with the highest number of neurons showing injury.

Because of this apparent relationship between NR1 levels and accumulating neuronal injury, the levels of a phosphorylated form of NR1 were measured to analyze indirectly NR1 activation after HI. Piglet synaptic membrane fractions of total striatum were probed with antibody recognizing phospho-Ser897 NR1. Incremental increases in the number of

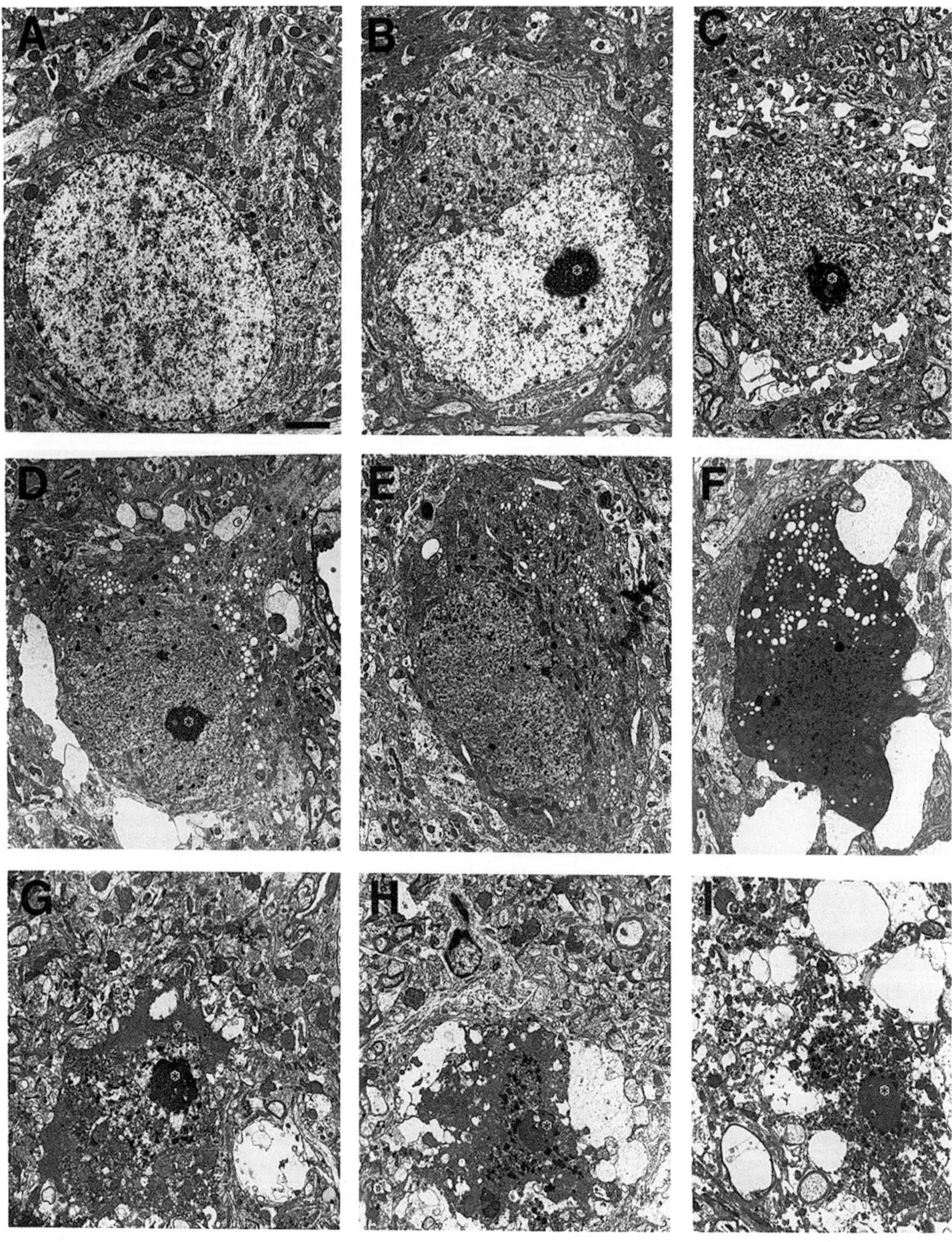
A
B
C
D
E
F
G
H
I

Figure 2.8 (*Left*) Electron microscopic analysis of striatal neuron degeneration in hypoxia–ischemia (HI) piglets. A normal principal striatal neuron from control piglet (A) is shown for comparison with neurons from piglets at 3, 6, 12, and 24 h after HI (B–I) arranged in a temporal sequence to show the predominant ultrastructural evolution of ischemic neuron necrosis. This neuronal death is not completely synchronized, because dying neurons can be found at different stages of degeneration at most times after HI; however, the neuronal profiles shown for each time represent the predominant stage of degeneration. Asterisks identify the nucleolus (when present in the plane of section). By 3 h after HI (B), the neuronal cell body swells and numerous, clear vacuoles are formed within the cytoplasm, increasing progressively over 9–12 h (C–E). At 6 h after HI (C), the arrays of rough endoplasmic reticulum are severely dilated (D, E) and then become fragmented, and the mitochondria become dark and condensed, as the cytoplasmic matrix becomes progressively dark and homogeneously granular. The overall contour of the cell changes from a round shape (A–C) to a fusiform or angular shape (D–E), as the neurons become shrunken 6–12 h after HI (F). Concurrently, during the first 12 h after HI, the nucleus shrinks and the nuclear matrix progressively becomes uniformly dark (C–E) as numerous small, irregular clumps of chromatin are formed throughout the condensing nucleus (F). The nucleolus (asterisks) still remains prominent throughout this process (B–D), even until ultimate neuronal disintegration (G–I). Between 12 and 24 h, injured cells disintegrate as the dark, severely vacuolated cytoplasm, containing few discernible but very swollen mitochondria, undergoes dissolution, while the nucleus progressively forms more chromatin clumps and undergoes karyolysis (G–I). The cytoplasmic and nuclear debris is liberated into the surrounding neuropil (I). This neurodegeneration is structurally necrotic. Scale bar (A) = 1.3 μm (same for B–I). Reproduced from Martin et al.[31] with permission.

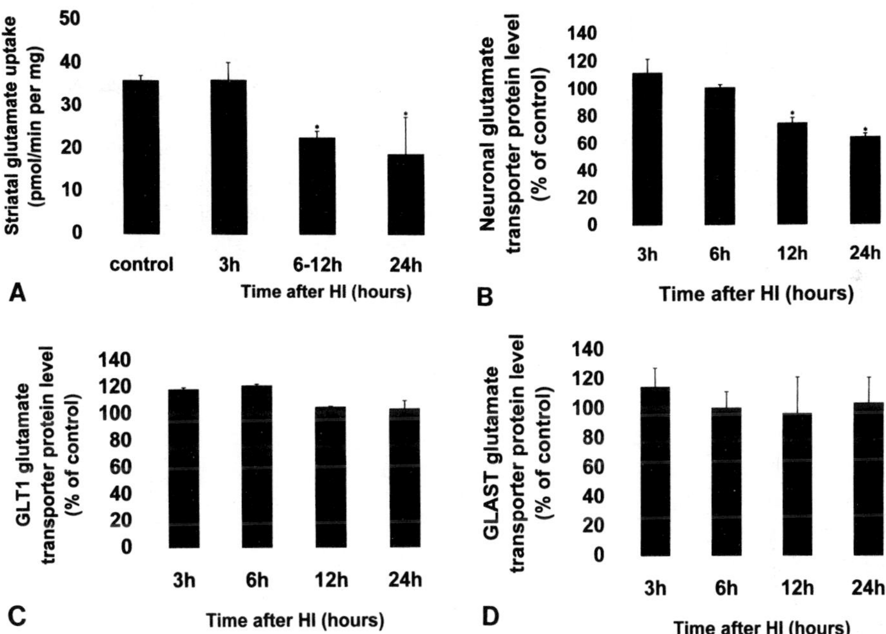

Figure 2.9 (*Above*) Glutamate transporter defects do not occur early during the emergence of striatal neurodegeneration after hypoxia–ischemia (HI). (A) High-affinity glutamate uptake in newborn piglet striatum is decreased after HI. High-affinity Na^+-dependent glutamate uptake into striatal synaptosomes from control piglets, and from piglets recovered for 3, 6, 12, or 24 h after HI. Results from 6 and 12 h were combined. There is no change in high-affinity glutamate transport at 3 h, but at 6–12 h high-affinity glutamate transport is reduced significantly to 64% of control, and at 24 h to 52% of control (Wilcoxon signed-ranks test, $P <$ 0.05 was considered significant). Values represent mean ±1 SEM. (B–D) Immunoblot analyses of the levels of individual glutamate transporter subtypes in the piglet striatum at 3, 6, 12, or 24 h after HI, represented as % of control (values are mean ±SEM). Neuronal glutamate transporter (EAAC1, B) is decreased significantly (asterisk, $P < 0.05$) at 12 and 24 h after HI, coinciding with neurodegeneration (Figure 2.5), but the levels of astroglial glutamate transporters (GLT1 (C) and GLAST (D)) remain normal.

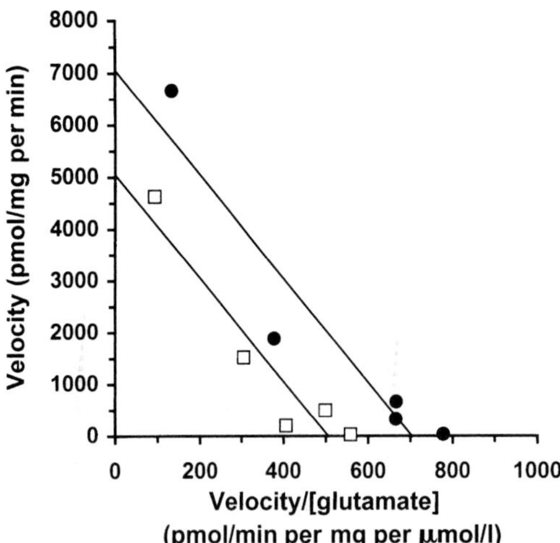

Figure 2.10 Kinetic values of high-affinity glutamate uptake are not changed in newborn piglet striatum after hypoxia–ischemia (HI). Eadie–Hofstee plots of high-affinity Na^+-dependent glutamate uptake into striatal synaptosomes from control piglets (closed circles), and from piglets recovered for 24 h after HI (open squares). Neither the calculated affinity constants ($K_m = -$slope, in μmol/l), nor the number of binding sites ($V_{max} = y$-intercept, in pmol/mg per min) after HI are significantly different after HI compared to control ($P > 0.05$, Wilcoxon signed-ranks test).

Table 2.3. Kinetic analysis of high-affinity glutamate transport in newborn piglet striatum after hypoxia–ischemia (HI)

Group	Affinity (K_m) (μmol/l^{-1})	Number of binding sites ($V_{max} \times 10^{-3}$: pmol/mg per min)
Control	10.9 ± 1.6	7.4 ± 0.4
3 h	9.3 ± 1.3	6.4 ± 0.2
6/12 h	13.6 ± 4.0	6.7 ± 3.3
24 h	11.8 ± 1.5	5.3 ± 2.3

Notes:
Kinetics of high-affinity sodium-dependent glutamate uptake into striatal synaptosomes from control piglets and from HI piglets recovered for 3, 6, 12, or 24 h were analyzed with standard Eadie–Hofstee plots using linear regression analysis. Values are expressed as mean ±1 SEM. Neither the calculated affinity constant ($K_m = -$slope, in μmol/l) nor the number of binding sites ($V_{max} = y$-intercept, in pmol/mg per min) was significantly different from control at any time point after HI ($P > 0.05$, Wilcoxon signed-ranks test).

injured neurons in the putamen correlate with an increase in phosphoNR1 levels, further suggesting an association between evolving neuronal damage and NR1 activation. The increased phosphoNR1 is not clearly associated with the amount of elapsed time after HI but rather with the specific amount of neuronal damage in the putamen. To identify whether changes in NMDA receptors are subunit-specific, selected NR2 subunits were measured. NR2B levels do not change significantly at 3, 6, and 12 h recovery after HI compared to controls but, at 24 h after HI, NR2B levels are elevated significantly above control at 24 h after HI. The levels of NR2B do not relate to the number of damaged putaminal neurons, but the increase is associated with augmented astroglial expression evolving in parallel with the neuronal damage. NR2A levels in striatum of HI piglets are not different from control during the 3–24-h evaluation period. We conclude that NMDA receptor subunits are changed differentially in the striatum after neonatal HI and that abnormal NMDA receptor potentiation through increased NR1 phosphorylation participates in the mechanisms of striatal neuron degeneration after HI.

NMDA receptors function in activity-dependent synaptic plasticity during development[52] and play a central role in synaptic mechanisms of learning and memory, such as long-term potentiation (LTP).[53] NMDA receptors are particularly interesting because of their physiological and pathophysiological duality. They gate Ca^{2+} ions and link Ca^{2+}-dependent intracellular signaling mechanisms for LTP and excitotoxicity (Figure 2.4). The principal striatal neurons (i.e., medium-sized spiny neurons) receive massive glutamatergic corticostriatal inputs[54,55] and express high levels of NMDA receptors that are enriched at dendritic spines.[56] However, under physiological conditions activation of corticostriatal inputs leads to long-term depression (LTD) of synaptic transmission in striatum rather than LTP; but,

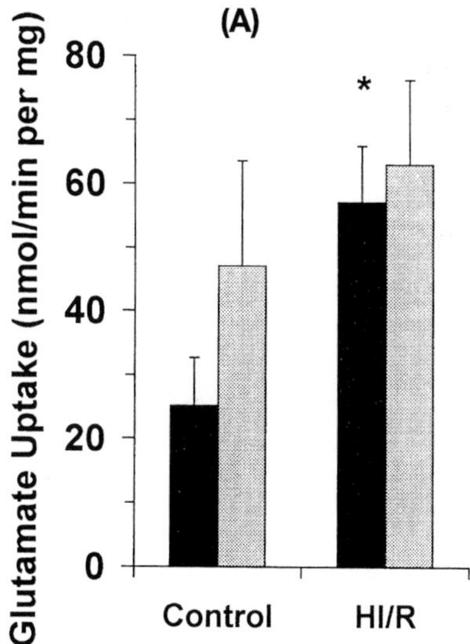

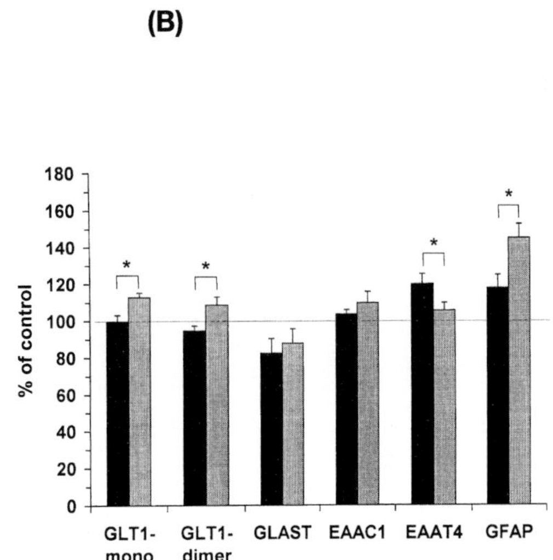

Figure 2.11 Glutamate transporter defects do not occur prior to cortical neurodegeneration after hypoxia–ischemia reperfusion (HI/R). (A) Synaptosomal high-affinity glutamate transport in piglet neocortical regions that are relatively vulnerable (parietal cortex) or insensitive (occipital cortex) to HI. High-affinity Na^{+}-dependent glutamate transport from control ($n=4$) and HI ($n=7$) piglets was assessed in the vulnerable parietal cortex (black columns) and in the spared occipital cortex (gray columns). In control neocortex, baseline glutamate uptake tends to be higher in occipital cortex compared to parietal cortex. After HI, glutamate uptake is increased significantly in parietal cortex compared to control parietal cortex. HI did not elevate glutamate uptake above control levels in occipital cortex. Bars represent 1 SEM. Asterisk indicates $P<0.05$. (B) Glutamate transporter protein levels in occipital cortex and parietal cortex are stable after HI in newborn piglets. Neocortical glial fibrillary acidic protein (GFAP) expression is elevated after HI. Densitometric analysis of glutamate transporter and GFAP protein levels in parietal (black columns, $n=7$) and occipital cortex (gray columns, $n=7$) of newborn piglet striatum after HI. Values are expressed as a percentage of control. In HI piglets, GLT1 (monomer and dimer) and GFAP protein levels increase significantly more in occipital cortex compared to parietal cortex, while EAAT4 expression is increased significantly more in parietal cortex compared to occipital cortex ($P<0.05$). Bars represent 1 SEM.

after removal of the voltage-dependent Mg^{2+} block of NMDA receptors, LTP is induced rather than LTD.[57] Mechanisms that relieve the voltage-dependent Mg^{2+} block are thus relevant to the activation of NMDA receptors. Alterations in resting membrane potential can cause partial depolarization and activation of NMDA receptors. With regard to striatal neurodegeneration after HI in newborns it is interesting that, in addition to increased phosphorylation of NR1, suggesting potentiated or sensitized function, we have found evidence for impaired function of striatal Na,K-ATPase early after HI.[58] In light of these data, it seems that the same properties of NMDA receptors that make them so suitable for LTP, notably the voltage-dependent Mg^{2+} block of the channel and the Ca^{2+} gating, also render striatal neurons in newborns so vulnerable to HI. Thus, it is possible that striatal neuron death after HI in newborn is initiated by aberrant (unmasked) or dysregulated LTP mediated by NMDA receptors.

Na, K-ATPase is defective early after HI in newborn piglets

We have found that regions that are vulnerable to HI in the newborn brain exhibit higher basal levels of oxidative metabolism (identified by high concentrations of cytochrome oxidase and Na, K-ATPase) and

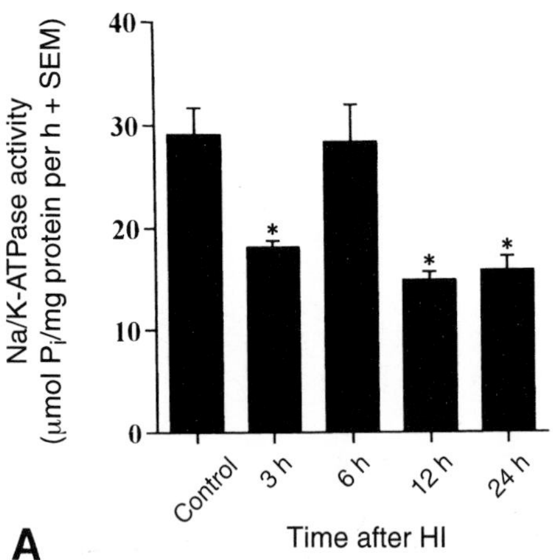

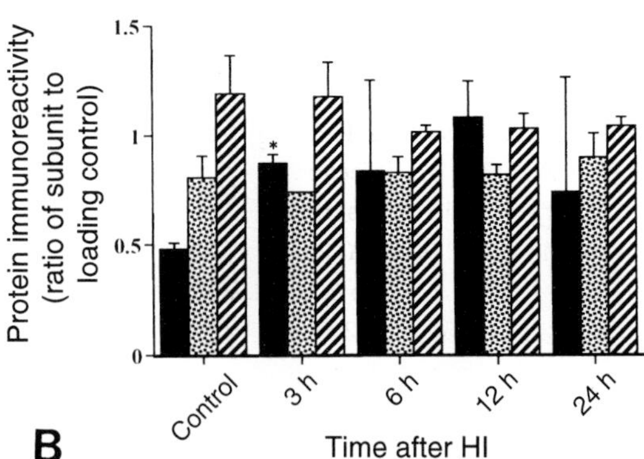

Figure 2.12 Na, K-ATPase activity is impaired early after hypoxia–ischemia (HI) in 1-week-old piglets. (A) Na, K-ATPase activity in striatal membrane fractions of piglets exposed to HI. Each bar represents mean adenosine triphosphatase (ATPase) activity (plus standard error of the mean) as measured by net inorganic phosphate (P_i) production, excluding effects of Mg^{2+}-ATPase and spontaneous adenosine triphosphate (ATP) hydrolysis. Controls are piglets not exposed to HI. An asterisk (*) signifies a statistically significant ($P \leq 0.05$) difference between enzyme activity of animals recovered up to the specific time point and the activity of control animals not exposed to HI. Na, K-ATPase undergoes early inactivation, a short period of recovery, and then sustained dysfunction after HI. (B) Na, K-ATPase subunit immunoreactivity in 20-μg aliquots of striatal membrane fractions from 1-week-old piglets exposed to HI. HI and control samples were subjected to Western blot analysis. Protein levels of the α_3 (dotted bars), β_1 (cross-hatched bars) and α_1 isoforms (solid bars) are represented as the ratio of the mean optical density of the subunit to control (plus standard error of the mean). For each subunit, 3–5 blots were used to measure immunoreactivity. An asterisk (*) represents a statistically significant ($P \leq 0.05$) increase in isoform expression in the HI animals relative to control. Minimal changes in α_3 and β_1 immunoreactivity occur during recovery from HI, while α_1 immunoreactivity in HI animals shows a moderate increase relative to control, which achieves statistical significance at 3 h into recovery.

have particular connections with other brain regions (Figure 2.3).[13,14] These findings suggest that intrinsic metabolic status and connectivity contribute to brain regional vulnerability after HI in newborns. Na, K-ATPase is a ubiquitous cell membrane enzyme that is necessary for cell function because it establishes ion gradients essential for maintenance of the resting membrane potential of neurons.[59] The enzyme contains two major subunits: a larger α protein responsible for the majority of the catalytic activity, and a smaller, glycosylated β protein required for maturation of the enzyme and transport to the cell surface.[60] Multiple α and β isoforms have been identified in mammalian brain,[61,62] likely reflecting cell type-specific expression heterogeneity and diversity in enzyme expression based on tissue-specific requirements.[60] It has been shown that Na, K-ATPase activity is diminished in cortical synaptosomes isolated from animals exposed acutely to hypoxia in a non-survival model.[63] At present, however, it is still uncertain whether Na, K-ATPase is a major molecular target in the mechanisms of selective neuronal death after HI in newborns. We examined whether abnormalities in Na, K-ATPase activity and protein subunit isoform levels occur in newborn piglet striatum during the first 24 h after HI.

We found that Na, K-ATPase function is inactivated in the striatum early after HI (Figure 2.12). This inactivation is selective for the putamen which sustains preferential damage.[58] Na, K-ATPase activity (percent of control) was 60%, 98%, 51%, and 54% at 3, 6, 12, and 24 h after HI, respectively (Figure 2.12A). Intrastriatal differences in enzyme activity occur, as the putamen shows greater loss of Na, K-ATPase activity than caudate after 12 h recovery. We have identified a loss of Na, K-ATPase activity in striatum at 3 h after HI. This defect coincides with the onset of cellular edema in striatal neurons seen by EM (Figure 2.8). The early loss of ATPase activity at this time of recovery occurs prior to appreciable ischemic neurodegeneration (Figure 2.5); thus, we interpret this abnormality as a mechanism, rather than a consequence, of neuronal death. The near complete recovery of activity at 6 h (Figure 2.12A) suggests that a reversible modification of the enzyme (e.g., perhaps phosphorylation or nitration) is at least partially responsible for the early loss of function seen at 3 h. At 12 and 24 h, striatal Na, K-ATPase activity is again decreased, coinciding with the destruction of striatal neurons (Figure 2.5). This alteration in enzyme function appears to be mediated by factors other than reduced levels of its composite subunits, as measured by immunoblotting (Figure 2.12B). Further investigations are necessary to determine the molecular modifications occurring in the specific α and β isoforms and the relationships between different α/β heterodimers and total Na, K-ATPase activity.

Excitotoxic excitatory amino acids (i.e., glutamate) have been implicated as a major contributor to the pathogenesis of HIE.[21,29] Reactive oxygen species (ROS) are generated during excitotoxicity[29] (Figure 2.4) as shown in cultured neurons after activation of the NMDA receptor. One particular signal transduction pathway activated by NMDA receptors is nitric oxide (NO) generation.[29] Na, K-ATPase activity can be inhibited by NO-producing compounds.[64] We hypothesize that Na, K-ATPase is modified at tyrosine residues by mechanisms involving the formation of peroxynitrite ($ONOO^-$) through the combination of superoxide and NO.[65] The possible links between NMDA receptor activation and the generation of NO, superoxide, and $ONOO^-$ need to be explored in greater detail in this clinically relevant animal model of newborn HIE.

Previous experiments from our laboratory using this piglet model have revealed depletion of glutathione stores at 3 h recovery after HI and $ONOO^-$-mediated oxidative damage to intracellular proteins, including β-tubulin and Golgi apparatus-associated protein (Figures 2.6D,C, and 2.13).[31] Given this evidence for oxidative stress, it is plausible that HI-induced ROS modify mature, membrane-associated Na, K-ATPase or nascent enzyme heterodimers during processing through the Golgi apparatus. Transport of mature enzyme from the endoplasmic reticulum to the plasma membrane requires at least 40–60 min,[66] coinciding with the onset of decreased Na, K-ATPase activity seen in striatum at 3 h after HI. Recovery of enzyme function at 6 h may be related to reversal of protein modification, recovery of mitochondrial function (decreasing the ROS production), or rapid turnover of the defective membrane Na, K-ATPase. As cleavage of genomic DNA (Figure 2.5C), loss of cytoskeletal structure (Figure 2.7), and organelle damage progresses between 6 and 24 h,[31] production of cellular enzymes ceases, resulting in the sustained decrease in Na, K-ATPase function seen over the remainder of the time course.

Striatal neurons in HI newborn piglets sustain profound ONOO—mediated damage (Figure 2.13).[31] Several domains in the α and β subunits of Na, K-ATPase may be targets of $ONOO^-$ modification. In rat brain, three additional tyrosine residues occur in the $\alpha 3$ subunit compared to the $\alpha 1$ subunit.[67] The β subunit, known more for its role in Na, K-ATPase trafficking to the cell membrane, facilitates cation occlusion through a specific interaction with a region of the carboxy terminus of the α subunit.[66] The interactive region of the rat β subunit contains tyrosine residues; thus, $ONOO^-$ attack on this region would result in failed heterodimer interaction and enzyme inactivation. Lipid peroxidation in conjunction with loss of Na, K-ATPase activity after HI also has been described;[63,68] thus, damage to membrane phospholipids may potentiate defects in subunit interactions and failure of enzyme function. There is an urgent need to reduce the incidence of HIE and its long-term sequelae. Our work on Na, K-ATPase, NMDA receptors, and oxidative stress may prove

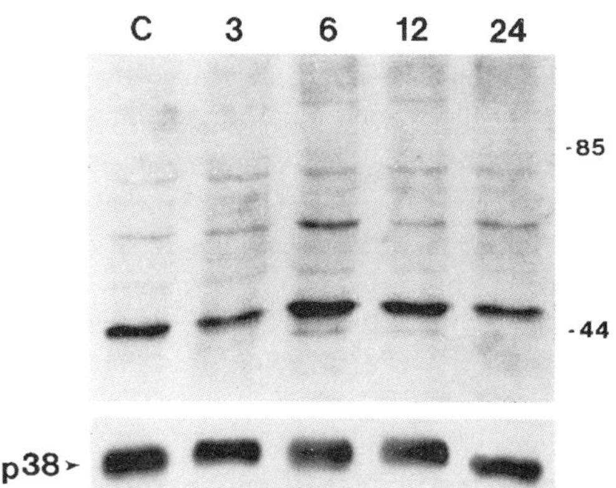

Figure 2.13 Peroxynitrite-mediated oxidative damage to proteins occurs early after hypoxia–ischemia (HI). Immunoblot of nitrotyrosine-modified membrane proteins in striatum from control (C) and HI piglets at 3, 6, 12, and 24 h recovery. Molecular mass markers (in kDa) are indicated at right. Lanes with proteins from HI piglets are darker than the control lane, particularly at 6 h. Blot was reprobed with antibody to synaptophysin (p38) to show approximately equal protein loading in each lane.

valuable in designing therapies to target brain regions vulnerable to neonatal HI.

Neuronal cell death in newborn animal models of HI

Neurons degenerate after HI. It is critical to understand how these neurons die for therapeutic direction. Neurons can die in different ways. The death of cells has been classified generally as two distinct types, called apoptosis and necrosis. These two forms of cellular degeneration are classified differently because they are believed to differ structurally and biochemically.

Apoptosis is an organized programmed cell death (PCD) that is mediated by active, intrinsic mechanisms involving specific molecular pathways. Apoptosis is generally regarded as physiological cell death in developing brain. Several families of genes regulate apoptosis in mammals (Table 2.4): the Bcl-2 family; the caspase family of cysteine-containing, aspartate-specific proteases; the inhibitor of apoptosis protein (IAP) family; the tumor necrosis factor (TNF) receptor family, and the p53 gene family.[44] The *bcl-2* protooncogene family is a group of apoptosis regulatory genes that encode for proteins that function by interactions. These interactions among members of the Bcl-2 family influence cellular survival and death. Caspases (cysteinyl aspartate-specific proteinases) are cysteine proteases that exist as constitutively expressed proenzymes that are activated by regulated proteolysis. Numerous target proteins are cleaved by active caspases, including nuclear proteins, cytoskeletal proteins, and cytosolic proteins. To prevent unwanted apoptosis in normal cells, the activities of proapoptotic proteins are neutralized by IAPs. Cell death by apoptosis can also be initiated at the cell membrane by surface receptors that function as death receptors. The TNF receptor family functions as death receptors. Fas (CD95/Apo-1) and p75 (low-affinity nerve growth factor (NGF) receptor) are family members. With this mechanism, apoptosis is initiated at the cell surface by aggregation (trimerization) of Fas. The activation of Fas is induced by the binding of the multivalent Fas ligand (FasL), a member of the TNF-cytokine family. The oncosuppressor protein p53 and its two homologues, p63 and p73, also induce apoptosis.

In contrast, necrosis is cell death resulting from failure to sustain homeostasis due to extrinsic insults to the cell (e.g., osmotic, thermal, toxic, or traumatic). The process of cellular necrosis involves damage to the structural and functional integrity of the cell plasma membrane, rapid influx of ions and H_2O, and subsequently, dissolution of the cell. Thus, cellular necrosis is induced not by an intrinsic program within the cell *per se* (as in PCD) but by abrupt or slow homeostatic perturbations and departures from physiological conditions. It has been identified recently that an abnormal activation of PCD in nervous system neurons has a role in human neurodegenerative disorders; therefore, deciphering the contributions of the different types of cell death after HI in human newborns and in animal models could help to develop treatments for HIE. These treatments could possibly be drugs that

Table 2.4. Molecular regulation of apoptosis

Bcl-2 family				
Antiapoptotic proteins	Proapoptotic proteins	Caspase family	IAP family	Tumor suppressor family
Bcl-2	Bax	Apoptosis "initiators": caspase-2, -8, -9, -10	NAIP SMN	p53 p63 p73
Bcl-x_L	Bak	Apoptosis "executioners": caspase-3, -6, -7	IAP1	
Boo	Bcl-x_S Bad	Cytokine processors: caspase-1, -4, -5, -11, 12, -14	IAP2	
	Bid		XIAP	
	Bik			

Notes:
IAP, inhibitor of apoptosis protein.

inhibit the actions of key enzymes, ion channels in cell membranes (e.g., NMDA receptors and Ca^{2+} channels), or numerous other proteins, as well as drugs (e.g., antioxidants) that block or inactivate the production of toxic chemicals (e.g., free oxygen radicals) that are generated during the process of neuronal injury.

Neurodegeneration in the immature brain is phenotypically heterogeneous and regionally specific. We have found that the neurodegeneration in specific regions is model- or species-related. For example, compared to HI in piglet which results in prominent neuronal necrosis in striatum,[15,31,58] we have found that neuronal apoptosis is much more prominent in newborn rat after HI.[11,12,69] The notion that selectively vulnerable neurons undergo apoptosis after HI in adults is still very controversial[30,70–72] and, in newborn brain, this idea should be examined more critically because much is at stake. The accurate identification of the contributions of apoptosis and necrosis to neuronal death after HI has critical therapeutic relevance and needs to be clarified soon in animal models, because antiapoptotic therapies have been suggested, possibly prematurely, for human clinical trials for the treatment of brain ischemia in adults.[73]

We have demonstrated that the death of striatal neurons after HI in piglets (10-day-old) is categorically necrosis (Figures 2.6 and 2.8).[30,31,58] This neuronal death evolves over 24 h. It has a specific temporal pattern of subcellular organelle damage and biochemical defects. Damage to the Golgi apparatus and rough endoplasmic reticulum occurs at 3–12 h, while most mitochondria appear intact until 12 h. Mitochondria undergo an early suppression of activity, then a transient burst of activity at 6 h after the insult, followed by mitochondrial failure. Cytochrome c is depleted at 6 h after HI and thereafter. Damage to lysosomes occurs within 3–6 h. Inactivation of Na, K-ATPase is observed at 3 h. By 3 h recovery, glutathione levels are reduced, and $ONOO^-$-mediated oxidative damage to membrane proteins occurs at 3–12 h. The Golgi apparatus and cytoskeleton are early targets for extensive tyrosine nitration. Striatal neurons also sustained hydroxyl radical damage to DNA and RNA within 6 h of HI. Our work demonstrates that neuronal necrosis in the striatum evolves rapidly and is possibly driven by early oxidative stress and inactivation of Na, K-ATPase, NMDA receptor activation, and oxidative damage to protein, DNA, and RNA.

Our experiments demonstrate in piglets that

neuronal apoptosis does not have a major contribution to this degeneration during the first 24 h after HI. Apoptosis of neurons and neuroglia may, however, have a more prominent contribution to the neuropathology after HI in newborns as a form of delayed or secondary cell death that is related to target deprivation of interconnected brain regions.[13,14,30,70]

We have studied neuronal cell death in the neonatal rat (7-day-old) model of HI.[11,12,69] In this model, neurodegeneration occurs as necrosis and apoptosis. We have also discovered a new form of cell death in this model. This novel form of neuronal cell death has mixed characteristics of apoptosis and necrosis. From structural and biochemical evaluations of the injured cerebral hemisphere, neuronal necrosis predominates in cerebral cortex, classical apoptosis is prominent in thalamus and brainstem, and the mixed cell death form occurs in hippocampus and striatum.

The thalamic neuron apoptosis in the neonatal rat brain after HI is structurally identical to the apoptosis of thalamic neurons after cortical injury.[11,69] HI in the neonatal rat causes severe infarction of cerebral cortex,[11] and we speculate that this thalamic neuron apoptosis is caused by neurotrophin withdrawal resulting from target deprivation, similar to the remote neurodegeneration that occurs after injury to the cerebral cortex. Damage to the cerebral cortex causes neuropathology in brain regions distant from the primary cortical lesion. The thalamus is a major site of remote neurodegeneration after cortical damage in humans and experimental animals. For example, severe loss of thalamic neurons occurs in humans after surgical hemidecortication and after head trauma and stroke.[74,75] Ablation of the visual cortex in a variety of adult mammals induces retrograde neuronal degeneration in the lateral geniculate nucleus of thalamus.[76–81] The geniculocortical projection neurons die apoptotically.[79–83] This apoptosis is preceded by the accumulation of mitochondria within the neuron and oxidative damage to nuclear DNA of geniculocortical projection neurons.[80] This neuronal death requires the presence of the *Bax* gene and is modified by the functional *p53* gene, thus it appears to be a form of PCD.[81]

Our laboratory has found that apoptosis in thalamic neurons after HI in neonatal rat is associated with a rapid increase in the levels of the Fas death receptor and caspase-8 cleavage.[69] Concurrently, the levels of Bax in mitochondrial-enriched cell fractions increase and cytochrome c accumulates in the soluble protein compartment. Increased levels of Fas death receptor and Bax, cytochrome c accumulation, and caspase-8 cleavage in the thalamus are upstream to marked cleavage of caspase-3 and the occurrence of neuronal apoptosis.

Discrepancies on the location and occurrence of neuronal apoptosis after HI in newborn animals have been noted by us when comparing our data to other results. This variation in reports is partly due to differences in the criteria for apoptosis, differences in the comprehensiveness of the EM analysis, and to differences in the animal species used for the experimental injury. It was reported that the ultrastructure of neuronal degeneration in hippocampus is apoptosis after HI in 1-week-old rat.[82] However, the EM data shown would be interpreted as necrosis by us and others.[30,70,83] The nuclear pyknosis with condensation of chromatin into many small, irregularly shaped clumps in ischemic neurons contrasts with the formation of few, uniformly dense and regularly shaped chromatin aggregates which occurs in neuronal apoptosis.[30,70,79,83–86] Alternatively, the data from neonatal rats may support our emerging concept of an apoptosis–necrosis continuum for neuronal death[30,44,84,85] in that this neuronal degeneration may be a hybrid of necrosis and apoptosis (see below). DNA fragmentation analyses[82,87,88] would support this interpretation, in view of a structure indicative of necrosis in the presence of internucleosomal laddering. Internucleosomal fragmentation of DNA is not found in HI piglet striatum.[31] Digestion of DNA in an internucleosomal pattern may not be specific for apoptosis, because it occurs in NMDA receptor-mediated excitotoxic neuronal necrosis in adult brain[85] and in neuronal culture,[89] and in cells undergoing necrosis induced by calcium ionophores and heat shock.[90] Moreover, in situ end labeling methods for DNA fail to discriminate among apoptotic and necrotic cell deaths[30,31,85,91] and can also detect DNA fragments during DNA synthesis.[92] Observations demonstrating that a pan-caspase inhibitor is neuroprotective in neonatal rats after HI suggests a possible contribution of neuronal apoptosis[82] to this neuropathology; however, many caspase family members function in the proteolytic processing of proinflammatory cytokines (Table 2.3), thus neuroprotective effects of pharmacological inhibition of all caspases may be mediated by mechanisms other than blocking apoptosis (e.g., antiinflammation and hypothermia).

The rat pup and piglet models of newborn HI are different physiologically and neuropathologically. Rat pups and piglets near the day of birth are at very different stages of maturation with respect to glutamate receptors and glutamate transporters.[15,26–28] The peak of the brain growth spurt occurs near term in pig and human, whereas this peak occurs at about 7 days postnatally in rat.[93] Moreover, the percentage of adult brain weight at birth in pig is much closer to human compared to that of rat.[93] These fundamental neurobiological differences are very important when considering the relevance of experimental animals as models for brain injury in human newborns.

The apoptosis–necrosis cell death continuum

Wyllie proposed that apoptosis could be induced by injurious stimuli of lesser amplitude than insults causing necrosis.[94] Toxicological studies in cultured nonneuronal cells have verified that stimulus intensity influences the mode of cell death,[95,96] although the modes of cell death are still viewed as mechanistically distinct.

We have proposed that neuronal cell death is a continuum of apoptosis and necrosis.[30,44,84–85] In this continuum, cell death occurs as hybrids ranging from apoptosis to necrosis (Figure 2.14). We found that the death of neurons is not always strictly apoptosis or necrosis, according to a traditional binary classification of cell death. Neuronal death also occurs as intermediate or hybrid forms of cell death with coexisting characteristics (Figure 2.14) that lie along a structural continuum with apoptosis and necrosis at the extremes.[30,44,84–85] We have embraced fuzzy logic[97] to develop the concept of the apoptosis–necrosis cell death continuum.

So far we have identified that the maturity of the brain and the subtype of GluR that is activated influence cell death along this continuum. Hence, neuronal death induced by excitotoxicity and HI is not the same in mature and immature brain and may not be identical in every neuron. Different survival and death-signaling mechanisms (Figure 2.14) may modulate neuronal death pathways depending on neuronal maturity[98] and the severity and types of DNA damage.[99,100] In addition, variations in neuronal death may arise from the high diversity in the expression, localization, and function of GluR subtypes (Table 2.1), glutamate transporters (Table 2.2), second messenger systems, and cell death proteins (Table 2.4) in the developing and mature central nervous system.

The structure of the typical apoptosis–necrosis hybrid form of cell death has been revealed in different models of neurodegeneration. Excitotoxic brain injury is one model that reveals the death hybrid (Figure 2.14). They are best seen with non-NMDA GluR receptor excitotoxicity (Figure 2.14) in immature and mature rat brain[30,84,85] and with HI in neonatal rat.[11,12] Hybrid cells undergo progressive compaction of chromatin into few, discrete, large, irregularly shaped clumps (Figure 2.14). This morphology contrasts with the formation of few, uniformly shaped, dense, round masses in classic apoptosis and the formation of numerous, smaller, irregularly shaped chromatin clumps in classic necrosis. The cytoplasmic changes in hybrid cells generally appear more similar to necrosis than apoptosis, but differ in severity. Some of the neurodegeneration after HI might be better classified according to the concept of the apoptosis–necrosis continuum. We have found that the cell death continuum is revealed fully in a neonatal rat (7-day-old)

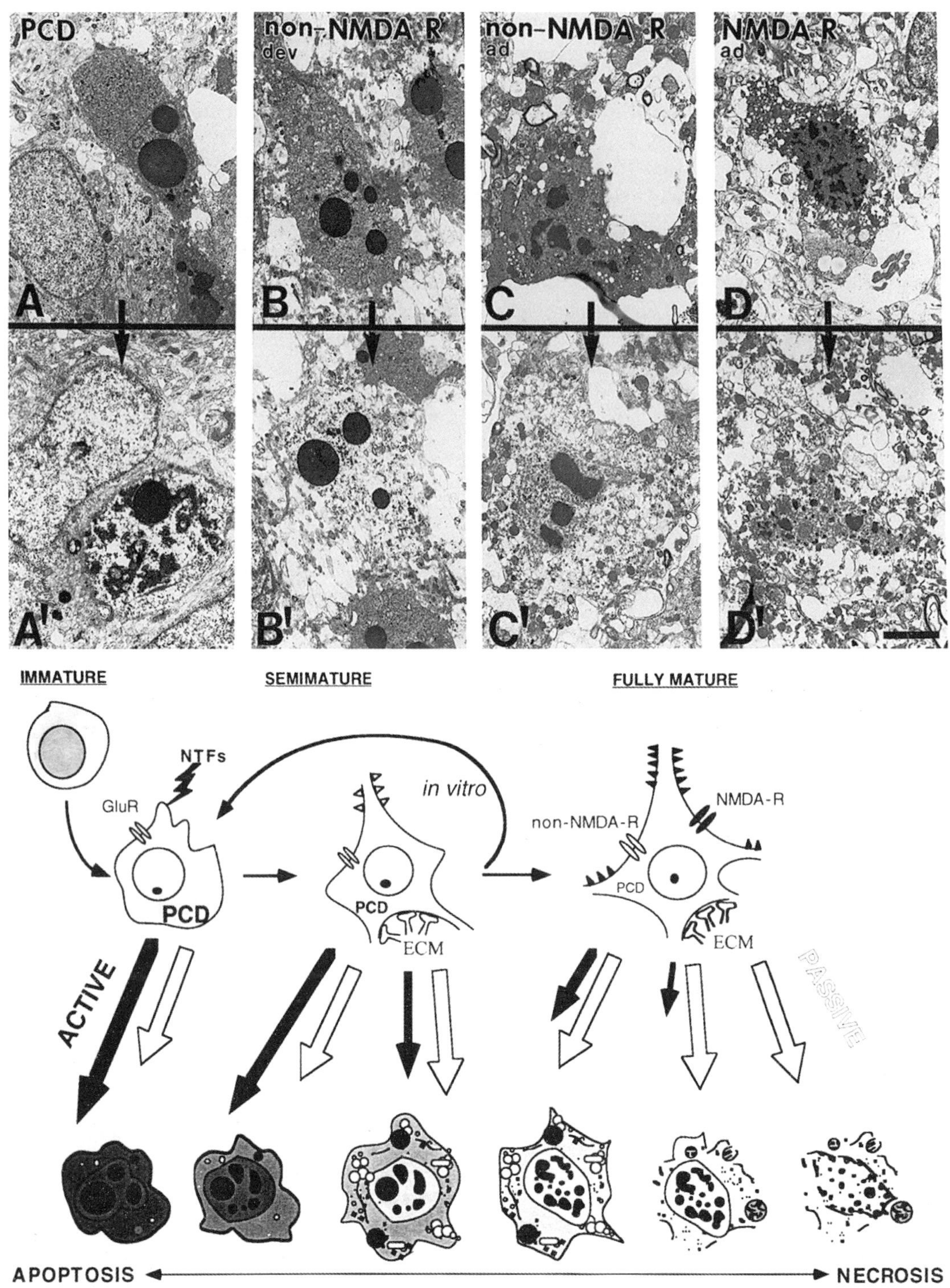
PCD
non-NMDA R
dev
non-NMDA R
ad
NMDA R
ad
A
B
C
D
A'
B'
C'
D'
IMMATURE
SEMIMATURE
FULLY MATURE
NTFs
GluR
in vitro
NMDA-R
non-NMDA-R
PCD
PCD
PCD
ECM
ECM
ACTIVE
PASSIVE
APOPTOSIS
NECROSIS

model of HI. In this model, neuronal cell death occurs as several forms, including necrosis, apoptosis, and hybrids of necrosis and apoptosis.[11,12]

This new concept could be important for understanding neuronal degeneration in human neurological disorders and cell death in general, and thus may be important for the prevention of neuronal loss in neurological disorders in infants, children, and adults. We need to identify better the relationships between mechanisms of neuronal death and the structure of dying neurons in human neuropathology in the developing and adult central nervous system as well as in animal and cell culture models of neurotoxicity in immature and mature neurons. We have found already that apoptosis mechanisms are different in immature neurons compared to mature neurons.[98] These studies are important particularly for addressing hypotheses as to whether PCD and apoptosis are equivalent, whether apoptosis and necrosis are mutually exclusive forms of cell death, and whether neuronal cell death in young and old neurons is the same. If brain maturity dictates how neurons die, as we suspect, then, in humans, neuronal degeneration in adults may be fundamentally different from neuronal degeneration in infants and children.

Acknowledgments

I am eternally grateful for the birth of my beautiful and healthy twin daughters, Gabrielle Ann and Isabella Cecelia (born 24 July 2000). Dr. Martin's research is supported by grants from the US Public Health Service, National Institutes of Health, National Institute of Neurological Disorders and Stroke (NS 34100 and NS 20020) and National Institute on Aging (AG16282) and the US Army Medical Research and Material Command (DAMD17–99–1–9553). I am thankful for the expert assistance of Ann Price, Frank Barksdale, Debora Flock, and Adeel Kaiser and the experimental contributions to my laboratory of Drs Carlos Portera-Cailliau, Nael Al-Abdulla, Frances Northington, JoAnne Natale, Dawn Agnew, Rebecca Ichord, Stephan Hayes, Chris Golden, Anne-Marie Guerguerian, and Ansgar Brambrink.

REFERENCES

1 Vannucci RC and Perlman JM (1997). Interventions for perinatal hypoxic–ischemic encephalopathy. *Pediatrics*, 100:1004–14.

Figure 2.14 (*Left*) The apoptosis–necrosis cell death continuum. Neuronal cell death occurs as an apoptosis–necrosis continuum. (Top) Electron micrographs of striatal neurons at relatively "middle" (A, B, C, D) and "late" (A′, B′, C′, D′) stages of degeneration. Developmental programmed cell death (PCD) of neurons in postnatal day 8 striatum is a "gold standard" for neuronal apoptosis (A, A′). Non-*N*-methyl-D-aspartate (non-NMDA) glutamate receptor (GluR) excitotoxicity induces apoptosis in developing (dev) rat striatum (B, B′). Non-NMDA GluR excitotoxicity induces apoptosis–necrosis hybrids in adult (ad) rat striatum (C, C′). NMDA receptor excitotoxicity induces necrosis in adult (ad) rat striatum (D, D′). A continuous spectrum of cell death morphologies can be identified ranging from classical apoptosis (A) to classical necrosis (D). Scale bar = 3 μm. (Bottom) Diagram showing the potential relationships among naturally occurring PCD and induced neuronal cell death, as mediated by differential contributions of active mechanisms (black arrows) and passive mechanisms (open arrows) along the apoptosis–necrosis continuum. This cell death continuum for neuronal degeneration is influenced by the degree of neuronal maturity and the subtype of GluR that is activated, as well as possibly other factors, including cell type and the composition of the cytoskeleton and extracellular matrix (ECM). The sizes of the arrows vary according to the relative contributions of the different mechanisms. Neurons in the developing central nervous system (CNS) at immature and semimature states undergo PCD in response to neurotrophin (NTF) deprivation, target deprivation, and GluR activation. Semimature neurons that are removed from the developing brain are prone to undergo apoptosis when used for in vitro manipulations. Excitotoxic neuronal death induced by NMDA receptor (NMDA-R) and non-NMDA GluR (non-NMDA-R) in the developing brain can resemble classic apoptosis, classic necrosis, and hybrid forms of cell death. However, in the fully mature adult CNS, excitotoxic cell death can resemble classic necrosis (NMDA receptor toxicity) or a hybrid of apoptosis–necrosis (non-NMDA receptor toxicity), with primarily passive mechanisms operating in the former and a combination of passive and active mechanisms operating in the latter. Depending on the neuronal groups, axotomy and target deprivation in the adult CNS can cause neuronal injury (atrophy but not death) with necrotic-like features or neuronal death that resembles apoptosis.

2 Vannucci RC (1997). Hypoxia–ischemia: clinical effects. In *Neonatal–Perinatal Medicine: Diseases of the Fetus and Infant*, ed. AA Fanaroff and RJ Martin, pp. 877–91. St Louis: Mosby-Year Book.

3 Volpe JJ (1995). *Neurology of the Newborn*. Philadelphia: Saunders.

4 Schneider HL, Ballowitz H, Schachinger F et al. (1975). Anoxic encephalopathy with predominant involvement of basal ganglia, brain stem, and spinal cord in the perinatal period. Report on seven newborns. *Acta Neuropathol.*, 32:287–98.

5 Low JA, Robertson DM and Simpson LL (1989). Temporal relationships of neuropathologic conditions caused by perinatal asphyxia. *Am. J. Obstet. Gynecol.*, 160:608–14.

6 Rorke LB (1992). Perinatal brain damage. In *Greenfield's Neuropathology*, ed. JH Adams and LW Duchen, pp. 639–708. New York: Oxford University Press.

7 Roland EH, Poskitt K, Rodriguez E et al. (1998). Perinatal hypoxic–ischemic thalamic injury: clinical features and neuroimaging. *Ann. Neurol.*, 44:161–6.

8 Maller AI, Hankins LL, Yeakley JW and Butler IJ (1998). Rolandic type cerebral palsy in children as a pattern of hypoxic–ischemic injury in the full-term neonate. *J. Child Neurol.*, 13:313–21.

9 Myers RE (1977). Experimental models of perinatal brain damage: relevance to human pathology. In *Intrauterine Asphyxia and the Developing Fetal Brain*, ed. L Gluck, pp. 37–97. Chicago: Year Book Medical Publishers.

10 Towfighi J, Tager JY, Housman C and Vannucci RC (1991). Neuropathology of remote hypoxic–ischemic damage in the immature rat. *Acta Neuropathol.*, 81:578–87.

11 Northington FJ, Ferriero DM, Graham EM et al. (2001). Early neurodegeneration after hypoxia–ischemia in neonatal rat is necrosis while delayed neuronal death is apoptosis. *Neurobiol. Dis.*, 8:207–19.

12 Nakajima W, Ishida A, Lange MS et al. (2000). Apoptosis has a prolonged role in the neurodegeneration after hypoxic ischemia in the newborn rat. *J. Neurosci.*, 20:7994–8004.

13 Martin LJ, Brambrink A, Koehler RC and Traystman RJ (1997). Primary sensory and forebrain motor systems in the newborn brain are preferentially damaged by hypoxia–ischemia. *J. Comp. Neurol.*, 377:262–85.

14 Martin LJ, Brambrink A, Koehler RC and Traystman RJ (1997). Neonatal asphyxic brain injury is neural system preferential and targets sensory-motor networks. In *Fetal and Neonatal Brain Injury: Mechanisms, Management, and the Risks of Practice*, ed. DK Stevenson and P Sunshine, pp. 374–99. New York: Oxford University Press.

15 Martin LJ, Brambrink AM, Lehmann C et al. (1997). Hypoxia–ischemia causes abnormalities in glutamate transporters and death of astroglia and neurons in newborn striatum. *Ann. Neurol.*, 42:335–48.

16 Brambrink AM, Martin LJ, Hanley DF et al. (1999). Effects of the AMPA receptor antagonist NBQX on the outcome of newborn pigs after asphyxic cardiac arrest. *J. Cereb. Blood Flow Metab.*, 19:927–38.

17 Johnston MV (1998). Selective vulnerability in the neonatal brain. *Ann. Neurol.*, 44:155–6.

18 Woolsey CN and Fairman D (1946). Contralateral, ipsilateral, and bilateral representation of cutaneous receptors in somatic areas I and II of the cerebral cortex of pig, sheep, and other mammals. *Surgery*, 19:684–702.

19 Craner SL and Ray RH (1991). Somatosensory cortex of the neonatal pig: I. Topographic organization of the primary somatosensory cortex (SI). *J. Comp. Neurol.*, 306:24–38.

20 Jones EG, Coulter JD, Burton H and Porter R (1977). Cells of origin and terminal distribution of corticostriatal fibers arising in the sensory-motor cortex of monkeys. *J. Comp. Neurol.*, 173:53–80.

21 Olney JW (1994). Excitatory transmitter neurotoxicity. *Neurobiol. Aging*, 15:259–60.

22 Nakanishi S (1992). Molecular diversity of glutamate receptors and implications for brain function. *Science*, 258:597–603.

23 Danbolt NC (1994). The high affinity uptake system for excitatory amino acids in the brain. *Prog. Neurobiol.*, 44:377–96.

24 Gegelashvili G and Schousboe A (1998). Cellular distribution and kinetic properties of high-affinity glutamate transporters. *Brain Res. Bull.*, 45:233–8.

25 Kanai Y, Smith CP and Hediger MA (1993). The elusive transporters with a high affinity for glutamate. *Trends Neurosci.*, 16:365–70.

26 Furuta A, Rothstein JD and Martin LJ (1997). Glutamate transporter protein subtypes are expressed differentially during rat CNS development. *J. Neurosci.*, 17:8363–75.

27 Furuta A and Martin LJ (1999). Laminar segregation of the cortical plate during corticogenesis is accompanied by changes in glutamate receptor expression. *J. Neurobiol.*, 39:67–80.

28 Furuta A, Martin LJ, Lin C-L G et al. (1997). Cellular and synaptic localization of the neuronal glutamate transporters, excitatory amino acid transporters 3 and 4. *Neuroscience*, 81:1031–42.

29 Choi DW (1992). Excitotoxic cell death. *J. Neurobiol.*, 23:1261–76.

30 Martin LJ, Al-Abdulla NA, Brambrink AM et al. (1998). Neurodegeneration in excitotoxicity, global cerebral ische-

mia, and target deprivation: a perspective on the contributions of apoptosis and necrosis. *Brain Res. Bull.*, 46:281–309.

31 Martin LJ, Brambrink AM, Price AC et al. (2000). Neuronal death in newborn striatum after hypoxia–ischemia is necrosis and evolves with oxidative stress. *Neurobiol. Dis.*, 7:169–91.

32 McDonald JW, Silverstein FS and Johnston MV (1987). MK-801 protects the neonatal brain from hypoxic–ischemic damage. *Eur. J. Pharmacol.*, 140:359–61.

33 Ford LM, Sanberg PR, Norman AB and Fogelson MH (1989). MK-801 prevents hippocampal neurodegeneration in neonatal hypoxic–ischemic rats. *Arch. Neurol.*, 46:1090–6.

34 LeBlanc MH, Vig V, Smith B et al. (1991). MK-801 does not protect against hypoxic–ischemic brain injury in piglets. *Stroke*, 22:1270–5.

35 LeBlanc MH, Li XQ, Huang M et al. (1995). AMPA antagonist LY293558 does not affect the severity of hypoxic–ischemic injury in newborn pigs. *Stroke*, 26:1908–15.

36 Hagberg H, Andersson P, Kjellmer I et al. (1987). Extracellular overflow of glutamate, aspartate, GABA and taurine in the cortex and basal ganglia of fetal lambs during hypoxia–ischemia. *Neurosci. Lett.*, 78:311–17.

37 Silverstein FS, Buchanan K and Johnston MV (1986). Perinatal hypoxia–ischemia disrupts striatal high-affinity [^{3}H]glutamate uptake into synaptosomes. *J. Neurochem.*, 47:1614–19.

38 Szatkowski M and Attwell D (1994). Triggering and execution of neuronal death in brain ischaemia: two phases of glutamate release by different mechanisms. *Trends Neurosci.*, 17:359–65.

39 Anderson KJ, Nellgård B and Wieloch T (1993). Ischemia-induced upregulation of excitatory amino acid transport sites. *Brain Res.*, 662:93–8.

40 Torp R, Lekieffre D, Levy LM et al. (1995). Reduced postischemic expression of a glial glutamate transporter, GLT1, in the rat hippocampus. *Exp. Brain Res.*, 103:51–8.

41 McBean GJ and Roberts PJ (1985). Neurotoxicity of L-glutamate and DL-threo-3-hydroxyaspartate in the rat striatum. *J. Neurochem.*, 44:247–54.

42 Tanaka K, Watase K, Manabe T et al. (1997). Epilepsy and exacerbation of brain injury in mice lacking the glutamate transporter GLT-1. *Science*, 276:1699–702.

43 Harada T, Harada C, Watanabe M et al. (1998). Functions of the two glutamate transporters GLAST and GLT-1 in the retina. *Proc. Natl Acad. Sci. USA*, 95:4663–6.

44 Martin LJ (2001). Neuronal cell death in nervous system development, disease, and injury. *Int. J. Mol. Med.*, 7:455–78.

45 Natale JE, Brambrink AM, Traytsman RJ and Martin LJ (1999). Hypoxia–ischemia in newborn piglets produces early defects in striatal high-affinity glutamate uptake. *Pediatr. Res.*, 45:345A.

46 Haugeto Ø, Ullensvang K, Levy LM et al. (1996). Brain glutamate transporter proteins form homomultimers. *J. Biol. Chem.*, 271:27715–22.

47 Tingley WG, Roche KW, Thompson AK and Huganir RL (1993). Regulation of NMDA receptor phosphorylation by alternative splicing of the C-terminal domain. *Nature*, 364:70–3.

48 Tingley WG, Ehlers MD, Kameyama K et al. (1997). Characterization of protein kinase A and protein kinase C phosphorylation of the *N*-methyl-D-aspartate receptor NR1 subunit using phosphorylation site-specific antibodies. *J. Biol. Chem.*, 272:5157–66.

49 Hisatsune C, Umemori H, Inoue T et al. (1997). Phosphorylation-dependent regulation of the *N*-methyl-D-aspartate receptors by calmodulin. *J. Biol. Chem.*, 272:20805–10.

50 Pisani A, Calabresi P, Centonze D and Bernardi G (1997). Enhancement of NMDA responses by group I metabotropic glutamate receptor activation in striatal neurones. *Br. J. Pharmacol.*, 120:1007–14.

51 Guerguerian AM, Brambrink A, Martin LA, Traystman RJ and Martin LJ (2000). Expression and phosphorylation of NMDA receptors are altered in striatum early after hypoxia–ischemia in piglets. *Soc. Neurosci. Abstr.*, 26:760.

52 Ramoa AS and McCormick DA (1994). Enhanced activation of NMDA receptor responses at the immature retinogeniculate synapse. *J. Neurosci.*, 14:2098–105.

53 Nicoll RA, Kauer JA and Malenka RC (1988). The current excitement in long-term potentiation. *Neuron*, 1:97–103.

54 Somogyi P, Bolam JP and Smith AD (1981). Monosynaptic cortical input and local axon collaterals of identified striatonigral neurons. A light and electron microscopic study using the Golgi-peroxidase transport-degeneration procedure. *J. Comp. Neurol.*, 195:567–84.

55 Kocsis JD, Sugimori M and Kitai ST (1977). Convergence of excitatory synaptic inputs on caudate spiny neurons. *Brain Res.*, 124:403–13.

56 Petralia RS, Wang YX and Wenthold RJ (1994). The NMDA receptor subunits NR2A and NR2B show histological and ultrastructural localization patterns similar to those of NR1. *J. Neurosci.*, 14:6102–20.

57 Calabresi P, Pisani A, Mercuri NB and Bernardi G (1992). Long-term potentiation in the striatum is unmasked by

removing the voltage-dependent magnesium block of NMDA receptor channels. *Eur. J. Neurosci.*, 4:929–35.

58 Golden WC, Brambrink AM, Traystman RJ and Martin LJ (2001). Failure to sustain recovery of Na,K ATPase function is a possible mechanism for striatal neurodegeneration in hypoxic–ischemic newborn piglets. *Mol. Brain Res.*, 88:94–102.

59 Sweadner KJ (1991). Subunit diversity in the Na,K-ATPase. In *The Sodium Pump: Structure, Mechanism, and Regulation*, ed. JH Kaplan and P de Weer, vol. 46, pp. 63–76. New York: Rockefeller University Press.

60 Lingrel JB (1992). Na, K-ATPase: isoform structure, function, and expression. *J. Bioenerg. Biomembr.*, 24:263–70.

61 McGrail KM, Phillips JM and Sweadner KJ (1991). Immunofluorescent localization of three Na, K-ATPase isoenzymes in the rat central nervous system: both neurons and glia can express more than one Na, K-ATPase. *J. Neurosci.*, 11:381–91.

62 Peng L, Martin-Vasallo P and Sweadner KJ (1997). Isoforms of Na, K ATPase α and β subunits in the rat cerebellum and in granule cell cultures. *J. Neurosci.*, 17:3488–502.

63 Razdan B, Marro PJ, Tammela O et al. (1993). Selective sensitivity of synaptosomal membrane function to cerebral cortical hypoxia in newborn piglets. *Brain Res.*, 600:308–14.

64 Sato T, Kamata Y, Irifune M and Nishikawa T (1997). Inhibitory effect of several nitric oxide-generating compounds on purified Na^+, K^+-ATPase activity from porcine cerebral cortex. *J. Neurochem.*, 68:1312–18.

65 Beckman JS, Chen J, Ischiropoulos H and Conger KA (1992). Inhibition of nitric oxide synthesis and cerebral neuroprotection. In *Pharmacology of Cerebral Ischemia*, ed. J Krieglstein and H Oberpichler-Schwen, pp. 383–94. Stuttgart: Wissenschaftliche Verlagsgesellschaft.

66 Chow DC and Forte JG (1995). Functional significance of the β-subunit for heterodimeric P-type ATPases. *J. Exp. Biol.*, 198:1–17

67 Shull GE, Greeb J and Lingrel JB (1986). Molecular cloning of three distinct forms of the Na^+, K^+-ATPase α-subunit from rat brain. *Biochemistry*, 25:8125–32.

68 Jamme I, Barbery O, Trouve' P et al. (1999). Focal cerebral ischemia induces a decrease in activity and a shift in ouabain affinity of Na^+, K^+ ATPase isoforms without modifications in mRNA and protein expression. *Brain Res.*, 819:132–42.

69 Northington FJ, Ferriero DM, Flock DL and Martin LJ (2001). Delayed neurodegeneration in neonatal rat thalamus after hypoxia–ischemia is apoptosis. *J. Neurosci.*, 21:1931–8.

70 Martin LJ, Sieber FE and Traystman RJ (2000). Apoptosis and necrosis occur in separate neuronal populations in hippocampus and cerebellum after ischemia and are associated with alterations in metabotropic glutamate receptor signaling pathways. *J. Cereb. Blood Flow Metab.*, 20:153–67.

71 Colbourne F, Sutherland GR and Auer RN (1999). Electron microscopic evidence against apoptosis as the mechanism of neuronal death in global ischemia. *J. Neurosci.*, 19:4200–10.

72 Yamashima T (2000). Implications of cysteine proteases calpain, cathepsin and caspase in ischemia neuronal death of primates. *Prog. Neurobiol.*, 62:273–95.

73 Schulz JB, Weller M and Moskowitz MA (1999). Caspases as treatment targets in stroke and neurodegenerative diseases. *Ann. Neurol.*, 45:421–9.

74 Powell TPS (1952). Residual neurons in the human thalamus following hemidecortication. *Brain*, 75:571–84.

75 Adams JH, Graham DI and Jennett B (2000). The neuropathology of the vegetative state after an acute brain insult. *Brain*, 123:1327–38.

76 Lashley KS (1941). Thalamo-cortical connections of the rat's brain. *J. Comp. Neurol.*, 75:67–121.

77 Barron KD, Doolin PF and Oldershaw JB (1967). Ultrastructural observations on retrograde atrophy of lateral geniculate body. 1. Neuronal alterations. *J. Neuropathol. Exp. Neurol.*, 26:300–26.

78 Agarwala S and Kalil RE (1998). Axotomy-induced neuronal death and reactive astrogliosis in the lateral geniculate nucleus following a lesion of the visual cortex in the rat. *J. Comp. Neurol.*, 392:252–63.

79 Al-Abdulla NA, Portera-Cailliau C and Martin LJ (1998). Occipital cortex ablation in adult rat causes retrograde neuronal death in the lateral geniculate nucleus that resembles apoptosis. *Neuroscience*, 86:191–209.

80 Al-Abdulla NA and Martin LJ (1998). Apoptosis of retrogradely degenerating neurons occurs in association with the accumulation of perikaryal mitochondria and oxidative damage to the nucleus. *Am. J. Pathol.*, 153:447–56.

81 Martin LJ, Kaiser A, Yu JW et al. (2001). Injury-induced apoptosis of neurons in adult brain is mediated by p53-dependent and p53-independent pathways and requires *Bax. J. Comp. Neurol.*, 433:299–311.

82 Cheng Y, Deshmukh M, D-Costa A et al. (1998). Caspase inhibitor affords neuroprotection with delayed administration in a rat model of neonatal hypoxic–ischemic brain injury. *J. Clin. Invest.*, 101:1992–9.

83 Ishimaru MJ, Ikonomidou C, Tenkova TI et al. (1999). Distinguishing excitotoxic from apoptotic neurodegeneration in the developing rat brain. *J. Comp. Neurol.*, 408:461–76.

84 Portera-Cailliau C, Price DL and Martin LJ (1997). Excitotoxic neuronal death in the immature brain is an apoptosis–necrosis morphological continuum. *J. Comp. Neurol.*, 378:70–87.

85 Portera-Cailliau C, Price DL and Martin LJ (1997). Non-NMDA and NMDA receptor-mediated excitotoxic neuronal deaths in adult brain are morphologically distinct: further evidence for an apoptosis–necrosis continuum. *J. Comp. Neurol.*, 378:88–104.

86 Martin LJ, Kaiser A and Price AC (1999). Motor neuron degeneration after sciatic nerve avulsion in adult rat evolves with oxidative stress and is apoptosis. *J. Neurobiol.*, 40:185–201.

87 Hill IE, MacManus JP, Rasquinha I and Tuor UI (1995). DNA fragmentation indicative of apoptosis following unilateral cerebral hypoxia–ischemia in the neonatal rat. *Brain Res.*, 676: 398–403.

88 Beilharz EJ, Williams CE, Dragunow M et al. (1995). Mechanisms of delayed cell death following hypoxic–ischemic injury in the immature rat: evidence for apoptosis during selective neuronal loss. *Mol. Brain Res.*, 29:1–14.

89 Gwag BJ, Koh JY, DeMaro JA et al. (1997). Slowly triggered excitotoxicity occurs by necrosis in cortical cultures. *Neuroscience*, 77:393–401.

90 Collins RJ, Harmon BV, Gobé VC and Kerr JFR (1992). Internucleosomal DNA cleavage should not be the sole criterion for identifying apoptosis. *Int. J. Radiat. Biol.*, 61:451–3.

91 Grasl-Kraupp B, Ruttkay-Nedecky B, Koudelka H et al. (1995). In situ detection of fragmented DNA (TUNEL assay) fails to discriminate among apoptosis, necrosis, and autolytic cell death: a cautionary note. *FASEB J.*, 21:1465–8.

92 Lockshin RA and Zakeri A (1994). Programmed cell death: early changes in metamorphosing cells. *Biochem. Cell Biol.*, 72:589–96.

93 Dobbing J and Sands J (1979). Comparative aspects of the brain growth spurt. *Early Hum. Devel.*, 3:79–83.

94 Wyllie AH (1987). Apoptosis: cell death under homeostatic control. *Arch. Toxicol.*, 11(suppl.):3–10.

95 Lennon SV, Martin SJ and Cotter TG (1991). Dose-dependent induction of apoptosis in human tumour cell lines by widely diverging stimuli. *Cell Prolif.*, 24:203–14.

96 Fernandes RS and Cotter TG (1994). Apoptosis or necrosis: intracellular levels of glutathione influence mode of cell death. *Biochem. Pharmacol.*, 48:675–81.

97 Kosko B (1994). *Fuzzy Thinking.* London: HarperCollins.

98 Lesuisse C and Martin LJ (2001). Apoptosis is mediated differentially by MAP kinase and caspase pathways during development of mouse cortical neurons in culture. *Soc. Neurosci. Abstr.*, 27:126.

99 Liu Z and Martin LJ (2001). Motor neurons rapidly accumulate DNA single strand breaks after in vitro exposure to nitric oxide and peroxynitrite and in vivo axotomy. *J. Comp. Neurol.*, 432:35–60.

100 Liu Z and Martin LJ (2001). Isolation of mature spinal motor neurons and single cell analysis using the comet assay of early low-level DNA damage induced in vitro and in vivo. *J. Histochem. Cytochem.*, 49:957–72.

3

Cellular and molecular biology of perinatal hypoxic–ischemic brain damage

Charles Palmer and Robert C. Vannucci

Pennsylvania State University College of Medicine, Hershey, PA, USA

Perinatal cerebral hypoxia–ischemia (asphyxia) typically is initiated by compromised placental or pulmonary gas exchange, leading to systemic hypoxia/anoxia with or without concurrent acidosis (asphyxia).[1] Hypoxia/hypercapnic acidosis increases cerebral blood flow (CBF) to an extent which is adequate to maintain cerebral oxidative metabolism stable until cerebral ischemia supervenes owing to cardiac depression with secondary bradycardia and systemic hypotension. With the cerebral oxygen and substrate (glucose) debt arising from ischemia, oxidative metabolism shifts to anaerobic glycolysis with its inefficient generation of high-energy phosphate reserves necessary to maintain cellular ionic gradients and other metabolic processes. Ultimately, cellular energy failure occurs, which, in association with other processes, ultimately results in death of the tissue.

Over the past several years, a wealth of basic and clinical research has expanded our knowledge of those critical cellular and molecular events which eventually lead to brain damage arising from hypoxia–ischemia. Investigations have shown that hypoxia–ischemia sets in motion a cascade of biochemical alterations that are initiated during the course of the insult and proceed well into the recovery period after resuscitation (reperfusion injury). This chapter will highlight those cellular and molecular processes involved in this metabolic cascade and how they evolve into perinatal hypoxic–ischemic brain damage.

Cellular energy transformations

Adenosine triphosphate (ATP) is the primary energy modulator of essentially all cells within the body, including neurons and glia.[2,3] Its two ~P exists at an energy level capable of providing the necessary driving force for innumerable biochemical reactions and physiologic processes. Accordingly, ATP not only promotes energy-consuming reactions but also drives critical physiologic processes, especially ion pumping, by acid hydrolysis. As such, the compound provides the cellular chemical energy necessary to maintain neuronal viability with its specialized function.

Under physiologic conditions, cellular ATP is maintained remarkably stable, as the rate of energy consumption by endergonic reactions is exactly balanced by the rate of ATP production. The cell's ability to maintain ATP constant, even under situations of increased energy expenditure, is dependent upon those biochemical processes that generate ATP. The first and most important biochemical process is the oxidative phosphorylation of nicotinamide adenine dinucleotide – reduced (NADH) and flavine adenine dinucleotide – reduced (FADH), and this process takes place within mitochondria. Mitochondrial oxidation is a highly efficient process which couples molecular oxygen to the hydrogen ion of NADH and FADH to form water coincident with the phosphorylation of adenosine diphosphate (ADP) to form ATP. A small amount of ATP is also produced by substrate phosphorylation, which occurs within mitochondria as well as the cytosol.[2,4]

In addition to substrate and oxidative phosphorylation, which are net energy-producing processes, two other mechanisms exist to maintain cellular ATP constant.[2,3] These include the creatine phosphokinase (CPK) and adenylate kinase (AK) equilibria, biochemical reactions that simply transfer energy (~P) from one compound to another. CPK catalyzes a reversible transfer of ~P between phosphocreatine (PCr) and ATP, while the AK reaction catalyzes the conversion of two molecules of ADP to one molecule each of ATP and adenosine monophosphate (AMP). Owing to their equilibrium constants, both reactions serve to maintain an optimal intracellular concentration of ATP even under situations of reduced ATP synthesis by oxidative phosphorylation or of increased ATP expenditure exceeding the capacity of oxidative phosphorylation to generate adequate ATP.

Tissue hypoxia denotes a cellular oxygen debt, owing typically to inadequate oxygen delivery (CBF × saturated oxygen or Sao_2) via nutrient arteries. When the mitochondrial partial pressure of oxygen falls below a critical value (<0.1 mmHg), the cytochrome system becomes unsaturated, and the reducing equivalents (NADH and FADH) begin to accumulate.[5,6] ATP production by oxidative phosphorylation is curtailed, with concurrent increases in cellular ADP and AMP as cytosolic ATP hydrolysis continues to drive endergonic reactions. The elevations in ADP and AMP stimulate glycolysis, through activation of its key regulatory enzyme, phosphofructokinase (PFK). Unlike oxidative phosphorylation, which produces 36 mol of ATP for every mole of glucose consumed, anaerobic glycolysis generates only 2 mol of ATP per mol of glucose consumed by substrate phosphorylation – an obviously inefficient method to generate ATP. Indeed, to produce the amount of ATP equivalent to that of oxidative phosphorylation, glycolysis would need to increase to a rate 18 times its basal flux. In reality, glycolysis, even when maximally stimulated by total cerebral ischemia, is capable of increasing only four- to fivefold, owing in part to the concurrent accumulation of H^+ ions derived from the accumulated NADH, which serves to inhibit PFK activity.[7,8] Thus, anaerobic glycolysis can never completely substitute for mitochondrial oxidation, although its stimulation can supplement oxidative phosphorylation under conditions of partial oxygen debt.

Cerebral hypoxia–ischemia severe enough to produce irreversible tissue injury is always associated with major perturbations in the energy status of the brain.[2,9,10] Alterations occur not only in the adenine nucleotides but also in PCr, and these changes actually precede those of ATP, ADP, and AMP. During cerebral hypoxia–ischemia in perinatal animals, changes in the tissue concentrations of the high-energy phosphate reserves occur early during the course of the metabolic insult, with lingering alterations proceeding well into the recovery period[11–13] (Figure 3.1). As anticipated, greater depletions in PCr occur relative to ATP as the cell attempts to maintain optimal levels of ATP through the CPK equilibrium reaction, driven also by the accumulation of ADP and H^+ ions. With the eventual decline in tissue ATP, ADP and AMP accumulate in proportion to the loss of ATP. Ultimately, the total adenine nucleotide pool (ATP + ADP + AMP) also decreases, as AMP is catabolized slowly to adenosine and other breakdown products (see below).

Of necessity, the loss of cellular ATP during hypoxia–ischemia severely compromises those metabolic processes that require energy for their completion. Thus, ATP-dependent Na^+ extrusion through the plasma membrane in exchange for K^+ is curtailed with the resultant intracellular accumulation of Na^+ and Cl^+ as well as water (cytotoxic edema). Equally vital to cellular function is the prompt restoration of the high-energy phosphate reserves during and after resuscitation. Without regeneration of ATP, endergonic reactions cannot resume, especially those involving ion pumping at cellular and intracellular membranes. Intracellular Na^+ and Cl^+ ions and water will continue to accumulate, and electrochemical gradients cannot be reestablished. Just how long the cell can survive under this situation is not entirely known, but other factors are called into play which adversely influence ultimate cellular integrity.

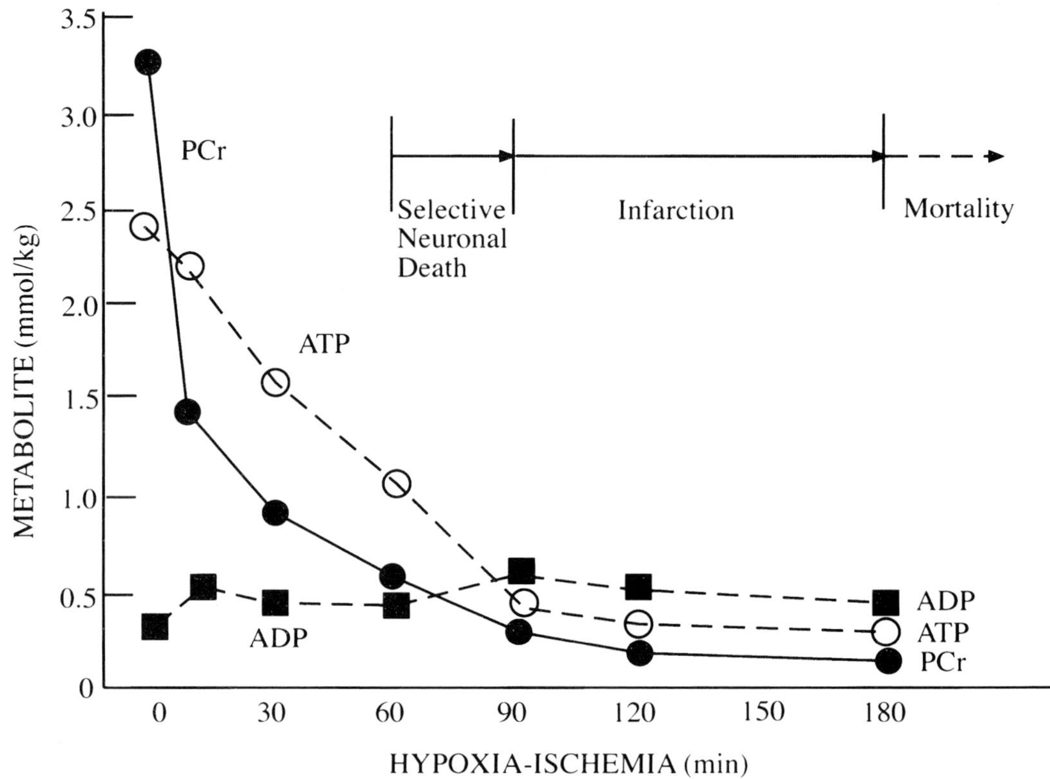

Figure 3.1 The alterations which occur in high-energy phosphate reserves during cerebral hypoxia–ischemia in the immature rat. Seven-day postnatal rats were subjected to unilateral common carotid artery ligation followed thereafter by exposure to hypoxia with 8% oxygen at 37 °C. Symbols represent means for phosphocreatine (PCr), adenosine triphosphate (ATP), and adenosine diphosphate (ADP). Note the immediate decrease in PCr, followed thereafter by a decrease in ATP. ADP accumulates slightly. Histologic brain damage commences after 60 min of hypoxia–ischemia, with increasing severity thereafter. Derived from data of Welsh et al.[11]

Originally it was thought that when hypoxia–ischemia is severe enough to produce brain damage, the depletion of high-energy phosphate reserves which occur during the course of the insult persist throughout the recovery interval.[11] Indeed, there is a close correlation between the level of ATP and the severity of brain edema at 4 h of recovery from hypoxia–ischemia; the edema reflects the ultimate tissue injury.[13] However, more recently, it has been proposed that the high-energy phosphate reserves are at least partially restored during the early phase of recovery from hypoxia–ischemia and that a delayed or secondary energy failure occurs later on, which causes or accentuates the ultimate brain damage. Hope and his research colleagues[14,15] have championed the proposal of a delayed energy failure, initially based on research in human newborn infants. In this regard, ^{31}P-magnetic resonance (MR) spectroscopy measurements of newborn human brain have shown an early restitution of the phosphorus spectra (PCr, ATP) upon resuscitation from asphyxia followed thereafter by a secondary decline in energy status. More recently, the same research group has demonstrated a similar delayed cerebral energy failure following hypoxia–ischemia in the newborn piglet, again using MR spectroscopy.[16,17] In these animal experiments, the investigators showed that PCr/inorganic phosphate ratios initially are depressed by hypoxia–ischemia, only to normalize in the early recovery interval. Thereafter, a secondary decrease in the ratio occurs at 24 and 48 h of recovery. From these human and animal studies, these investigators have concluded that the secondary failure in cerebral energy status following hypoxia–ischemia is a significant contributor to the ultimate brain damage and neurologic compromise. The phenomenon of a secondary depletion of high-energy phosphate reserves has also been observed in adult experimental animals subjected to hypoxia–ischemia and heralds the onset of delayed neuronal death.[18–20]

Secondary depletions in both PCr and ATP at 24 h of recovery from hypoxia–ischemia have also been observed in the fetal and early postnatal rat.[12,13,21] Based on sequential neuropathologic analyses of immature rats during the early recovery interval following hypoxia–ischemia,[22] it is likely that the secondary depletion in high-energy reserves follows rather than precedes brain tissue injury, at least in the rat. Furthermore, the secondary decreases in both PCr and ATP do not denote a delayed energy failure of the brain but rather reflect a loss of total creatine and adenine nucleotides from the tissue and their conversion to creatinine and adenosine and other metabolites, respectively (Figures 3.2 and 3.3). The reduction in PCr appears to occur as a mass action effect of the CPK equilibrium reaction, while the reduction in ATP appears to occur as a mass action effect of the AK equilibrium reaction. It has been speculated that the loss of creatine from the brain or its conversion to creatinine, which also would be lost, should result in detectable or increased concentrations of one or both metabolites in cerebrospinal fluid (CSF). Possibly, the presence of these compounds in CSF would serve as a biochemical marker for prior cerebral hypoxia–ischemia, in a manner similar to and perhaps more sensitive than the adenine nucleotide derivatives, xanthine and hypoxanthine.[23] Clearly, more experiments are required, especially in experimental perinatal animals, to resolve the issue of the contribution of the observed secondary energy failure following hypoxia–ischemia to the ultimate brain damage.

The mechanism(s) by which ATP disruption persists into the recovery period, whether or not a temporary restitution occurs, presumably relates to a lingering alteration in the function of mitochondria. In this regard, the classic pathologic studies of Brown and Brierley[24,25] indicate that the earliest morphologic alteration of the neuron arising from hypoxia–ischemia is a dilation of mitochondria with an accompanying separation of their cristae (see below). Biochemical studies support the morphologic alterations to the extent that following hypoxia–ischemia in vitro analysis of mitochondria reveals a disturbance in substrate oxidation, suggesting an "uncoupling of oxidative phosphorylation."[26–28] It is assumed that reducing equivalents (NADH, FADH) are oxidized in the presence of oxygen but ATP is not formed from the energy generated; such energy is consumed internally (not transferred to the cytosol) or is lost as heat. That oxidative phosphorylation is compromised after hypoxia–ischemia is also confirmed by studies that show that the brain can be well oxygenated concurrent with a persisting depletion in ATP.[11,29–31] Studies in the immature rat also suggest that an uncoupling of oxidative phosphorylation occurs following cerebral hypoxia–ischemia.[32] The issue remains as to what factors perpetuate the condition of uncoupled oxidative phosphorylation (see below).

Excitatory neurotransmitter neurotoxicity

To establish neuronal development and function requires a delicate balance between excitatory and inhibitory neurotransmitter activity. Well-established excitatory neurotransmitters include acetylcholine and the monoamines dopamine, norephinephrine and serotonin, whereas transmitters known to inhibit neuronal activity include (γ-aminobutyric acid and glycine. There is evidence that the amino acid glutamate also functions as an endogenous excitatory

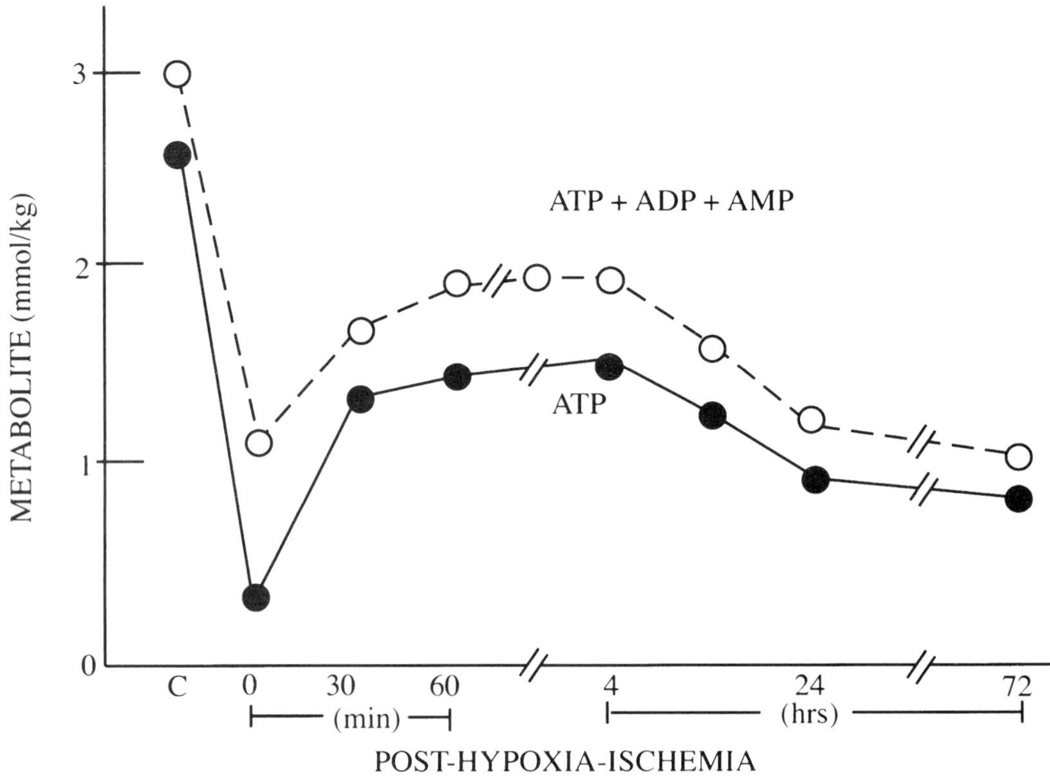

Figure 3.2 The alterations in adenine nucleotides which occur during recovery from cerebral hypoxia–ischemia in the immature rat. Shown are the changes in adenosine triphosphate (ATP) and total adenine nucleotides (ATP + adenosine diphosphate (ADP) + adenosine monophosphate (AMP)) which occur in the first 72 h of recovery from hypoxia–ischemia. Note the partial restoration of ATP and total adenine nucleotides for up to 12 h of recovery with secondary depletions at 24 and 72 h. Derived from data of Palmer et al.[12] and Yager et al.[13]

neurotransmitter and is especially important during development of the brain.[33–35]

The manner in which glutamate exerts its action on neurons has been elucidated. The presence of specialized receptors responsive to glutamate has been identified in specific regions of immature and adult brain, including the middle layers of cerebral cortex, the striatum, and the CA1 sector of the hippocampus.[36,37] Investigations have shown that at least three membrane receptors can be activated by glutamate. They are named after derivatives that individually excite them: kainic acid (KA), quisqualic acid (QA), and *N*-methyl-D-aspartate (NMDA) (Figure 3.4). A more recently discovered receptor site, which is either identical to or a subtype of the QA receptor, is the (α-amino-3-hydroxy-5-methyl-4-isoxazole proprionate (AMPA-QA) receptor site.[35,38] These receptors and their subunits subserve agonist-operated channels through which ions can pass either dependent upon or independent of the electrochemical (voltage) gradient across the cellular membrane (ionotropic receptors).[34,39] The AMPA-QA receptor also contains a subtype that stimulates cellular membrane phosphoinositide hydrolysis and the production of intracellular secondary messengers (metabotropic receptors).[35,38]

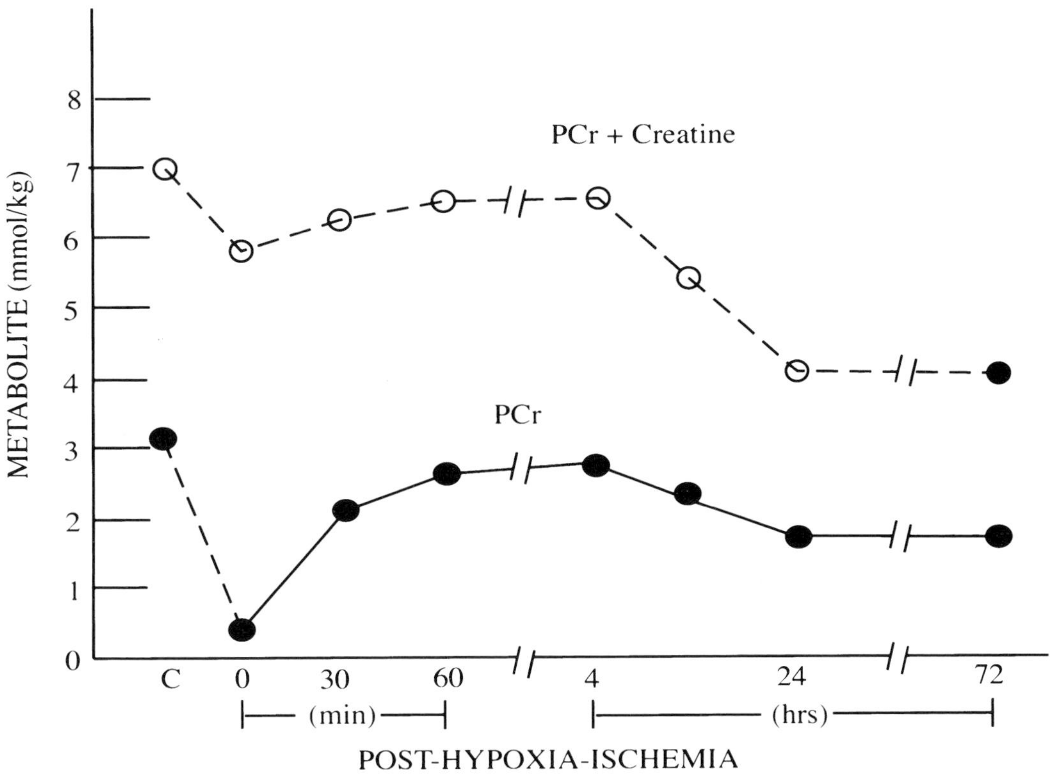

Figure 3.3 The alterations which occur in phosphocreatine (PCr) and PCr + creatine during recovery from hypoxia–ischemia in the immature rat. Note the early restitution in PCr and PCr + creatine for up to 12 h of recovery, followed thereafter by secondary depletions at 24 and 72 h. Derived from data of Palmer et al.[12] and Yager et al.[13]

Many years ago it was proposed that glutamate is toxic to neurons when present in high concentrations. Olney[40] championed the "excitotoxic" nature of glutamate and its analogs. In vitro and in vivo studies have confirmed early experiments, with glutamate toxicity as a major factor in the production of hypoxic–ischemic injury of selectively vulnerable neurons, i.e., those nerve cells predominantly innervated by glutaminergic neurons. First, glutamate is directly toxic to mature neurons in culture.[34] Second, neurons in culture and hippocampal slices die upon exposure to anoxia, but death can be prevented or attenuated by the presence of Mg^{2+}, which blocks a specific site on the glutamate receptor, or by glutamate antagonists.[41–45] Third, direct injection of glutamate or glutamate agonists into specific regions of the brain produce neuronal injury identical to that seen after hypoxia–ischemia,[46–48] to which the immature brain appears especially vulnerable.[38,49,50] Fourth, deafferentation of the glutaminergic excitatory input into the hippocampus causes damage produced by hypoxia–ischemia.[44,51] Fifth, the topography of hypoxic–ischemic brain damage in the immature animal roughly corresponds to the distribution of excitatory amino receptors in the brain, although the correspondence is not precise, especially in the hippocampus.[35] Finally, specific glutamate antagonists ameliorate hypoxic–ischemic brain damage.[52]

The role of glutamate in the susceptibility of the

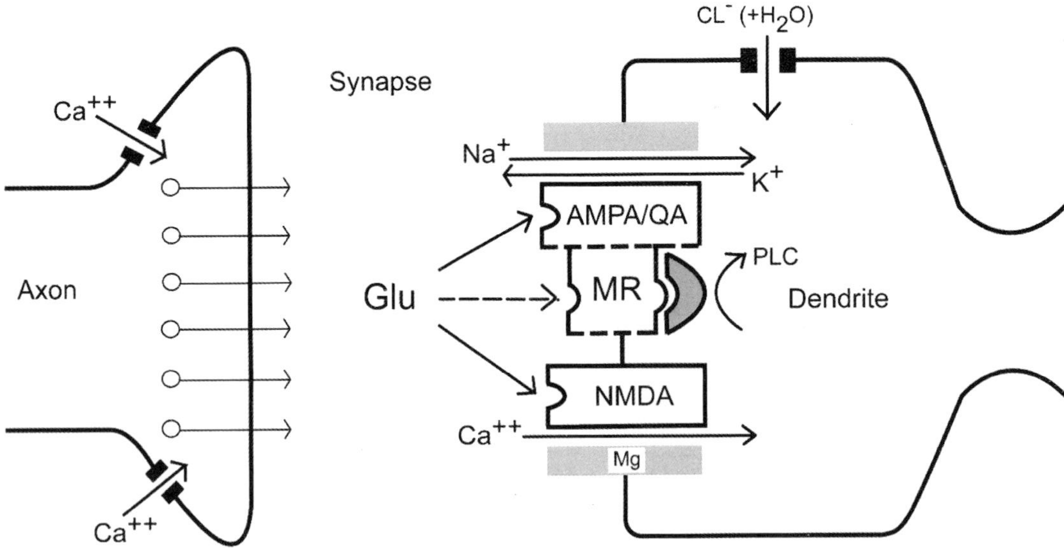

Figure 3.4 Schematic representation of the cell surface glutamate (Glu) receptor. Two distinct channels have been proposed to be gated by the subtypes of the glutamate receptors: one for monovalent ions (Na^+ in K^+ out) gated by the α-amino-3-hydroxy-5-methyl-4-isoxazole propionic acid/quisqualic acid (AMPA/QA) receptor, and one which allows predominantly Ca^{2+} entry into cells, gated by the *N*-methyl-D-aspartate (NMDA) receptor. Despite the fact that the Ca^{2+} channel is agonist-operated, it can be blocked by Mg^{2+} in a voltage-dependent manner. Depolarization reverses the block, whereupon glutamate activation of the receptor leads to Ca^{2+} influx. Glycine potentiates the action of glutamate at the NMDA receptor. Closely linked to the AMPA/QA receptor is a metabotrophic receptor, and this stimulation leads to secondary intracellular activation of phospholipase C (PLC).

immature brain to hypoxic–ischemic damage has undergone extensive investigation. Researchers have shown that glutamate receptor agonists exhibit preferential toxic effects on specific regions of the brain (see above) that is dependent on the age of the animal. In the immature rat, the hierarchy of neurotoxicity is NMDA>AMPA-QA>KA, while that of the adult rat is KA>NMDA>AMPA-QA.[38,49,50] Furthermore, intracerebral injections of NMDA produce far greater damage in immature rat brain than equivalent or larger doses of the analog in adult rat brain.[50] These age-specific differences in the sensitivity of the brain to excitatory neurotransmitter toxicity presumably relates to developmental alterations in the density and distribution of glutamate receptor subtypes, in glutamate binding to its receptors, or in transmembrane biochemical events (cation fluxes or signal transduction initiated by receptor activation).[36,37]

The mechanism by which glutamate exerts its toxic effect relates primarily to altered ion fluxes across the neuronal cellular membrane.[39,53] Based on their investigations in neuronal cell cultures, Rothman and Olney [34] have proposed two mechanisms of ion-mediated neuronal injury. The first or early toxicity relates to glutamate-induced Na^+ influx into neurons during depolarization, the Na^+ influx occurring probably through the AMPA-QA receptor.[38] Depolarization, which occurs during hypoxia–ischemia, disrupts the intracellular–extracellular balance of Cl^-, and the anion flows down its electrochemical gradient into the neuron. The entry of Na^+ and Cl^- increases cell osmolality, necessitating the influx of water. Subcellular edema ensues, which, if severe enough, leads to lysis of the neuron. A delayed neurotoxicity also occurs, as has been observed in vivo in selected neurons of the hippocampus in both adult and immature animals.[54–56] This delayed neuronal death presumably relates to excessive Ca^{2+} entry into the cell via NMDA receptor-mediated channels which, in turn, sets in motion a cascade of biochemical events that culminate in the death of the neuron (see below).

In an immature rat model of hypoxic–ischemic brain damage, alterations in glutamate homeostasis occur during the course of and following the insult. Silverstein and her research colleagues[57,58] employed microdialysis to measure extracellular glutamate concentrations in striatum and hippocampus during the course of hypoxia–ischemia. Significant increases in glutamate were first noted at 90 min of hypoxia–ischemia, an interval that corresponds temporally to the onset of tissue infarction in this model.[22,59] Infarction denotes destruction of all cellular elements, including neurons, glia, and blood vessels. Using our immature rat model, we measured glutamate concentrations in CSF as a reflection of the concentration in extracellular fluid.[60] During the course of hypoxia–ischemia, CSF glutamate did not increase above control values until 105 min, at which time the concentration was 240% of control. By 120 min, CSF glutamate had increased over twofold above the control value (Figure 3.5).[60] Based on the previously published microdialysis and our CSF experiments, we concluded that an elevation in extracellular glutamate is a late event during hypoxia–ischemia in the immature rat, which corresponds better temporally to cerebral infarction than to selective neuronal death. A secondary elevation in CSF glutamate, observed at 6 h of recovery from 2 h of hypoxia–ischemia, occurs coincident with the onset of tissue necrosis.

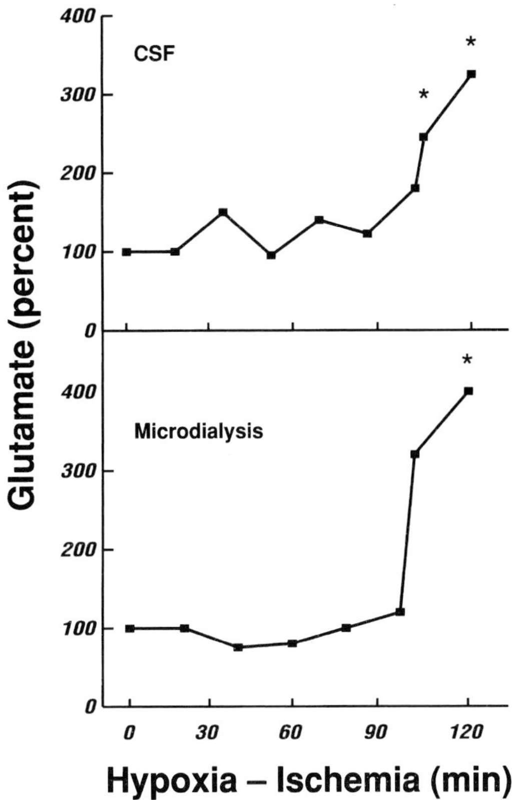

Figure 3.5 Cerebrospinal fluid (CSF) and extracellular glutamate during cerebral hypoxia–ischemia in the immature rat. Samples of CSF were obtained from the cisterna magna at specific intervals during hypoxia–ischemia and in control animals (0 time point). Extracellular fluid glutamate was obtained via microdialysis. Note the close temporal correspondence between the increases in CSF glutamate and extracellular glutamate, obtained via microdialysis, beginning after 90 min of hypoxia–ischemia.CSF data derived from Vannucci et al.;[60] microdialysis data derived from Gordon et al.[57]and Silverstein et al.[58]

Intracellular calcium overload

Owing to its ubiquitous functions, calcium (Ca^{2+}) is considered an intracellular second messenger. The divalent cation is intimately involved as a cofactor in numerous cellular reactions. Therefore, it is not surprising that a disruption of intracellular Ca^{2+} homeostasis has wide-ranging effects on neuronal metabolism and function.

Given the cation's strategic role in metabolic regulation, it is important that concentrations of Ca^{2+} are tightly regulated within the cell (Figure 3.6). Nearly 100% of intracellular Ca^{2+} is tightly bound within subcellular organelles, and the free Ca^{2+} normally exists in very low concentrations ($<10^{-7}$ mol/l). Given the physiologic extracellular

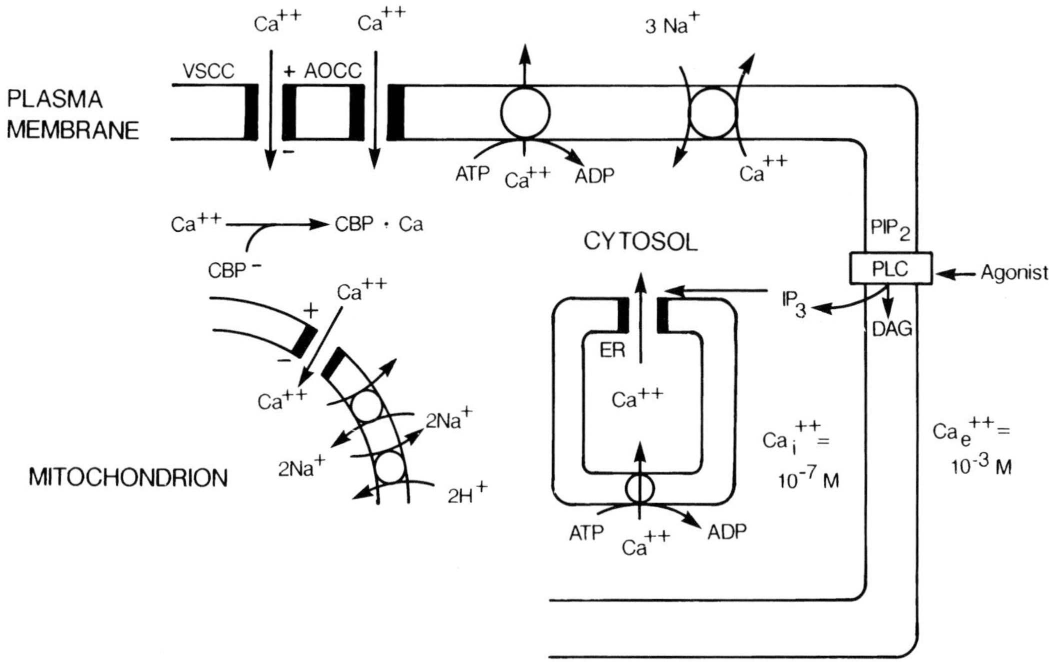

Figure 3.6 Transcellular and intracellular calcium fluxes. Ca^{2+} influx from the extracellular space into the cytosol occurs via both voltage-sensitive Ca^{2+} channels (VSCC) and agonist-operated Ca^{2+} channels (AOCC). Ca^{2+} efflux from the cytosol into extracellular space occurs via an energy-dependent uniport system and an antiport system involving Na^+. Intracellular Ca^{2+} sequestration occurs primarily within mitochondria and the endoplasmic reticulum (ER). Ca^{2+} is also bound via specific calcium-binding proteins (CBP^-). Ca^{2+} release from the ER occurs upon stimulation by inducible NOSitol-1,4,5–trisphosphate (IP_3), an intracellular second messenger. Ca^{2+} release from mitochondria involves an antiport system with Na^+, influenced by H^+. ATP, adenosine triphosphate; ADP, adenosine diphosphate; PIP_2, phosphatidylinositol-4,5-bisphosphate; PLC, phospholipase C; DAG, diacylglycerol. From Vannucci[64] with permission.

concentration of Ca^{2+} (10^{-3} mol/l), there is an enormous gradient for free Ca^{2+} across the cellular membrane that tends to drive the ion into cells. The sites of intracellular Ca^{2+} binding include primarily mitochondria and the endoplasmic reticulum, and to a lesser extent the nucleus and cellular membrane of the neuron. Binding occurs by both energy-dependent (ATP) and independent processes, which are also influenced by the intracellular pH. Specific Ca^{2+}-binding proteins, dispersed within the cytosol, also serve to maintain free Ca^{2+} concentrations low.[39,61–63] In addition to Ca^{2+} sequestration into subcellular organelles, the free cytosolic concentration of the cation is closely regulated by fluxes across the cellular membrane (Figure 3.6). Specific ion channels exist for Ca^{2+} exist in all cells, which are either voltage-sensitive Ca^{2+} channels or agonist-operated Ca^{2+} channels at membrane receptors predominantly of the NMDA (glutamate) type. These channels allow for Ca^{2+} flux into the cell under conditions of membrane depolarization or receptor activation. A network of ion channels also exists for the extrusion of intracellular Ca^{2+}; these channels operate via either Ca^{2+}-ATPase or a NA^+/Ca^{2+} exchange (antiport) system with energy derived from the transmembrane Na^+ gradient.[64] Accordingly, free intracellular Ca^{2+} concentrations can be maintained extremely low under physiologic

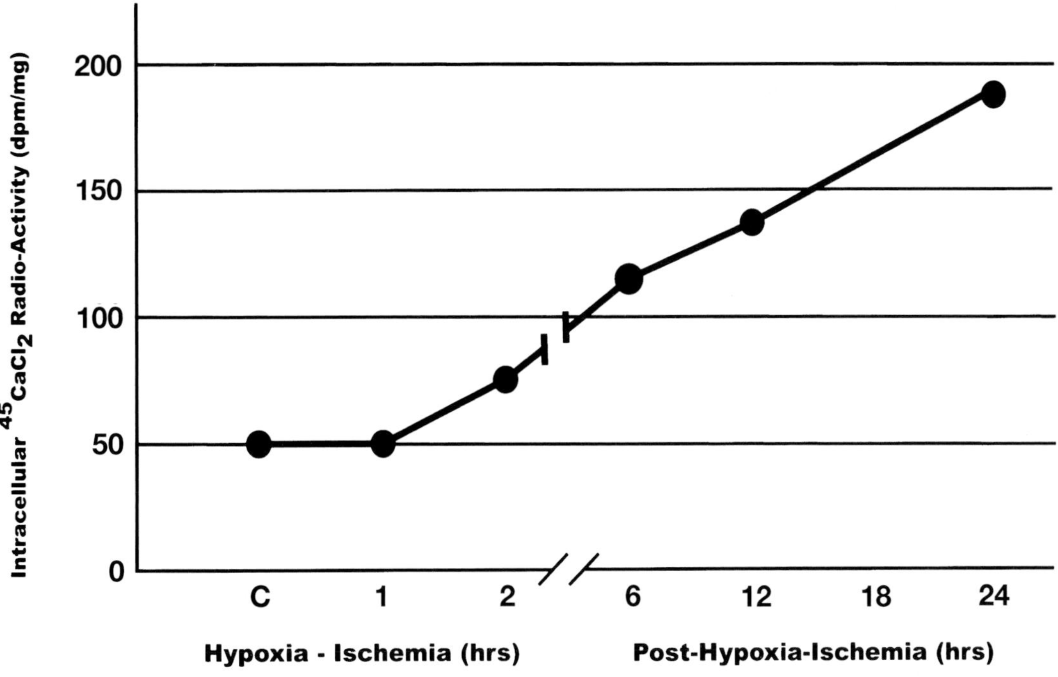

Figure 3.7 Brain intracellular $^{45}CaCl_2$ radioactivity during and following hypoxia–ischemia in the immature rat. Brain $^{45}CaCl_2$ radioactivity, as a reflection of Ca^{2+} tissue accumulation, was unchanged from control (C) during the first hour of hypoxia–ischemia, with a slight but significant increase at 2 h. During recovery, Ca^{2+} progressively accumulates for up to 24 h. Derived from data of Vannucci et al.[69]

conditions, owing to the ion's sequestration into subcellular organelles or to extrusion from the cell through ion channels.

Hypoxia–ischemia increases the free cytosolic concentration of Ca^{2+}.[65–67] It is presumed that the elevation arises from two sources, specifically, release of intracellular stores and increased influx (or decreased efflux) across the cellular membrane. The release of intracellular bound Ca^{2+} into the cytosol occurs predominantly from mitochondria and the endoplasmic reticulum, and is favored by the development of metabolic acidosis which occurs during hypoxia–ischemia. Increased Ca^{2+} influx across the cellular membrane occurs in response to depolarization, opening voltage-sensitive Ca^{2+} channels, as well as by a stimulation of the NMDA receptor-operated Ca^{2+} channels by glutamate. Finally, Ca^{2+} efflux through the cellular membrane is disrupted by the energy failure which accompanies hypoxia–ischemia, upon which Ca^{2+}-ATPase is dependent and by a curtailment or even reversal of the Na^+/Ca^{2+} antiport system. These events, occurring in concert, serve to increase free cytosolic Ca^{2+} to a potentially toxic level.

Relevant to the immature brain, we have conducted experiments to ascertain the presence and extent of altered Ca^{2+} homeostasis in an experimental model of perinatal cerebral hypoxia–ischemia.[68,69] Using the radioactive tracer, $^{45}CaCl_2$, we have shown that, during hypoxia–ischemia, calcium flux into brain occurs predominantly in cerebral cortex, hippocampus, striatum, and thalamus. Like glutamate (see above), calcium flux is most prominent during the latter phase of hypoxia–ischemia, especially after 90 min, when infarction is eminent (Figure 3.7). During the recovery phase, Ca^{2+} radioactivity in all brain regions increases progressively over 24 h. From the experiments, we have concluded that hypoxia–ischemia is associated with enhanced but late calcium uptake into the immature brain, which temporarily dissipates but then progressively accumulates during the recovery interval. The findings implicate a disruption of intracellular Ca^{2+} homeostasis as a major factor in the evolution of perinatal hypoxic–ischemic brain damage.

The mechanisms by which altered Ca^{2+} balance threatens the cell is undoubtedly related to disturbances in those biochemical reactions subserved by the cation. As mentioned previously, Ca^{2+} activates numerous intracellular reactions, the continued stimulation of which severely compromises the viability of the neuron.[64] These reactions include the activation of several lipases, proteases, and endonucleases, all of which attack the structural integrity of the cell. Also important is the continued activation of phospholipase C, which promotes a progressive breakdown in the phospholipid components of the cellular (and possibly subcellular) membrane. Ca^{2+} also contributes to the formation of reactive oxygen species via the formation of xanthine and prostaglandins. Such radicals peroxidize the free fatty acid moiety of membranes. Finally, high concentrations of intracellular free Ca^{2+} lead to an uncoupling of oxidative phosphorylation within mitochondria, since the energy formed during recovery from hypoxia–ischemia is immediately consumed in an attempt to reverse and then maintain the electrochemical (ion) gradient across the mitochondrial membrane. This "futile" cycling of ions restricts the production and transfer of ATP into the cytosol to be used for structural repair and the reestablishment of ion gradients across the cellular membrane. Taken together, the toxic effects of excessive intracellular Ca^{2+} accumulation are adequate to cause membrane disintegration and death of the neuron. Thus, altered Ca^{2+} homeostasis might represent a "final common pathway" not only for hypoxia–ischemia, but for other forms of acute brain damage as well.[62]

Reactive oxygen species, iron, and nitric oxide

A free radical is a chemical species with one or more unpaired electrons in its outer orbital. This makes the species unstable, as most biologic species have their electrons arranged in pairs. Free radicals donate (reducing radical) or take (oxidizing radical) electrons from other biomolecules in an attempt to pair their electron and generate a more stable species. In this way, radicals generate new radicals and destroy the chemical structure of their target molecules, which include DNA, protein, and most common membrane lipids. The brain, being particularly rich in polyunsaturated phospholipids, is susceptible to free radical attack. Free iron and nitric oxide are important collaborators in oxidative injury as they transform mildly reactive oxygen species to more damaging free radicals.[70–75]

Free radicals and reactive oxygen species (superoxide and hydrogen peroxide) are formed during normal metabolism and only cause injury when they exceed the brain's antioxidant defenses. The recent availability of transgenic and mutant mice with an excess or deficiency in antioxidant enzymes has confirmed the role they play in neuroprotection.[76] Oxygen is paradoxically the basis of most free radical species generated during reperfusion. Following cerebral hypoxia–ischemia excessive free radicals are formed and antioxidant defenses are diminished.[77] The human newborn, especially the preterm newborn infant, may be particularly susceptible to free radical injury because of deficiencies in brain superoxide dismutase,[78] glutathione peroxidase,[79] plasma glutathione,[80] and the ability to sequester iron.[81] Some newborn infants have detectable free iron in cord blood.[79,82]

During cerebral reperfusion, potentially damaging amounts of superoxide, hydrogen peroxide, and the hydroxyl radical can be produced by free fatty acid and prostaglandin metabolism.[83–85] Other sources included dysfunctional mitochondria, the respiratory burst of activated neutrophils, macrophages[86] and endothelial cell xanthine oxidase.[87] During cerebral hypoxia–ischemia mitochondrial oxidative phosphorylation is impaired, causing ATP degradation and accumulation of hypoxanthine.[88] During reperfusion,hypoxanthine is metabolized by xanthine oxidase to xanthine and uric acid in reactions that produce superoxide and hydrogen peroxide. Xanthine oxidase is concentrated within the endothelial cell lining of the cerebral microvasculature,[89] thus targeting the blood–brain barrier for oxidative attack. An additional source of xanthine oxidase can be found circulating in the blood derived originally from liver and intestine after systemic hypotension or ischemia.[90,91] Consequently, circulating xanthine oxidase may generate free radicals at sites distal to its release into the circulation.

The contribution of reactive oxygen species to cell death in cerebral ischemia has been demonstrated by the protection that can be achieved by the administration of antioxidant molecules or enzymes, even during reperfusion. Allopurinol, and its active metabolite, oxypurinol, are inhibitors of the enzyme xanthine oxidase. When used in adult animal models of ischemic brain injury they are neuroprotective.[51,92–97] In the immature rat, we found that hypoxic–ischemic brain injury could be prevented with allopurinol pretreatment (135 mg/kg s.c.).[98] In a separate study we showed that allopurinol pretreatment (200 mg/kg s.c.) preserved cerebral energy metabolism of the 7-day postnatal rat during hypoxia–ischemia.[99]

While the neuroprotective mechanism of allopurinol has usually been attributed to its ability to inhibit xanthine oxidase, studies have shown that doses in excess of that required to inhibit xanthine oxidase are needed to produce neuroprotection.[92,95] We have found in our immature rat model that pretreatment with allopurinol was more effective at doses above 100 mg/kg, with no protection seen at 50 mg/kg.[100] In addition, we found that allopurinol can reduce brain damage even when it is administered 15 min after the hypoxic–ischemic insult, as a "rescue therapy."[101] We have since determined that allopurinol is protective even if given 4 h after recovery but not at 24 h after recovery.[102]

There are several lines of evidence that support a role for oxygen radicals in vascular injury after cerebral ischemia. Asphyxia and cerebral ischemia in the piglet[103] and the cat[104] result in the generation of superoxide anion during early reperfusion.[85] Cytochemical studies show that superoxide formation is located primarily in the extracellular space associated with blood vessels and occasionally in endothelial cells.[105] Phillis and Sen[106] used electron spin resonance spectroscopy to study the temporal profile of hydroxyl radicals formed on the pial surface in adult rats subjected to 30 min transient cerebral ischemia. These measurements revealed that, while some hydroxyl radicals were generated during ischemia, production peaked after 10 min of reperfusion and declined to nondetectable levels over the subsequent 90 min of reperfusion.

Oxygen-derived radicals cause increased blood–brain barrier permeability,[107–109] abnormal arteriolar reactivity,[110] and altered transport activity.[111,112] Reactive oxygen species also enhance neutrophil[113] and platelet adhesion to endothelium, promote phospholipase A_2 activation, platelet-activating factor (PAF) production, and postischemic hypoperfusion.[114,115] Yet free radical injury is not confined to the perivascular region. Microdialysis probes placed into the cerebral hemispheres have recorded evidence of hydroxyl radical production for hours following recovery from cerebral ischemia, especially in the periinfarct region.[116,117]

Although reactive oxygen species can injure cells or macromolecules directly, new evidence implicates free radicals in the promotion of proapoptotic genes and stimulation of damaging signal transduction pathways.The build-up of superoxide in mitochondria is thought to stimulate release of cytochrome c which initiates a cascade of intracellular events that includes activation of caspase 3, committing the cell to apoptosis. Apoptosis is also promoted because of the inhibitory effect of free radicals on DNA repair enzymes. Reactive oxygen species activate many transcription factors, including NFκB, which in turn stimulates a number of target genes that contribute to inflammation and brain injury following reperfusion. These genes include cyclooxygenase 2, inducible nitric oxide synthase, adhesion molecules and inflammatory cytokines.[76]

Iron

The toxicity of iron is attributed to its ability to transfer electrons and catalyze formation of more reactive species, specifically hydroxyl radicals and other iron–oxygen compounds like the ferryl and perferryl ions. Iron-dependent stimulation of lipid peroxidation can occur independently of hydroxyl radicals. Iron can initiate peroxidation by subtracting a hydrogen atom from fatty acids to form alkoxy and peroxy radicals. Propagation of this process follows as these radicals remove hydrogen atoms from adjacent fatty acids.[71,118] When exogenous iron is injected into the brain in the form of hemoglobin, heme, or ferric chloride, it causes lipid peroxidation with inhibition of the membrane-bound enzyme Na^+/K^+-ATPase.[119–123] These deleterious effects are blocked by the iron chelator desferroxamine.[123]

Brain regions with high iron contents are more susceptible to peroxidative brain injury.[124,125] We have discovered that blood vessels of the 3–7-day-old rat stain strongly positive for iron and stain progressively less as the rat ages.[126] This may make the blood vessels of the immature rats particularly susceptible to iron-mediated oxidant injury. As a consequence of hypoxia–ischemia, there is an increase in those agents that can reduce iron to the ferrous state and free it from carrier proteins. These include xanthine oxidase,[127] superoxide, nitric oxide,[128] and metabolic acidosis.[129] In the immature rat pup model of cerebral hypoxia–ischemia we showed that there is a rapid (within 2–4 h) increase in histochemically detectable iron in brain regions that undergo injury.[130] In a preliminary report van Bel et al. reported measuring free iron and increased products of lipid peroxidation in the plasma of severely asphyxiated newborns.[131] Elimination of transition metals like free iron is fundamental for the development of an effective antioxidant strategy. It can be achieved with chelators like deferoxamine or by preventing the delocalization of iron from carrier proteins.[71,132] We found that hypoxic–ischemic brain damage in immature rats could be markedly reduced by deferoxamine, even when we administered deferoxamine (100 mg/kg s.c.) 5 min after the insult.[133] For a review of the role of iron in cerebral ischemia, see Palmer.[134]

Nitric oxide

Nitric oxide (NO), also known as endothelial-derived relaxation factor, is a free radical gas that is produced by NO synthase (NOS) from L-arginine and oxygen. It is produced in fetal rabbit brain during sustained hypoxia–ischemia and is associated with the production of reactive nitrogen species and lipid peroxidation.[135] Its production is enhanced during reperfusion when replenishment of its key substrates occurs. NO binds irreversibly to hemoglobin so it is removed by neighboring blood flow. However, during hypoperfusion states, its removal may be impaired.

NO is produced in cerebral endothelial cells, astrocytes, and neurons constitutively in response to an increase in intracellular calcium. Another isoform of NOS is also present in macrophages and astrocytes. It is calcium-independent, inducible by cytokines, and is capable of producing large amounts of NO for days.[136] It is likely that neuronal NOS can also be upregulated in injured neurons. In rat brain only a few select cells and neurons have NOS activity; the distribution of the NOS isoenzymes changes with maturation.[137,138]

In the setting of cerebral ischemia, NO has both protective and cytotoxic effects.[139,140,141] Beneficial effects of endothelial-derived NO include vasodilation, inhibition of neutrophil and platelet aggregation, and the scavenging of superoxide.[136,142] Inhibition of endothelial NO production initiates superoxide-mediated leukocyte adhesion to postcapillary venules and increased extravasation. Clearly, inhibition of these mechanisms is undesirable during reperfusion. How then do NO inhibitors reduce ischemic brain injury?

The pathophysiological role of NO has been reviewed recently.[143–145] The neuronal and inducible forms of NO secreted by activated macrophages or produced in large quantities by stimulated neurons, endothelial cells, and astrocytes can be cytotoxic. NO impairs energy metabolism in cells by causing iron loss from enzymes essential for mitochondrial respiration.[146] NO causes DNA damage, which stimulates the enzyme poly-ADP-ribose polymerase, promoting DNA repair but also depletion of nicotinamide adenine dinucleotide and ATP.[147] Toxic mechanisms include mono ADP-ribosylation and *S*-nitrosylation of glyceraldehyde-3-phosphate dehydrogenase.[148] These cytotoxic effects cause depletion of energy metabolites secondary to alteration of glycolytic enzymes and depletion of energy substrates after stimulation of ADP-ribosylation.[149] Inhibitors of poly-ADP ribosylation protect neurons in culture from NO-mediated injury.[150] Hence it is possible that NO could contribute to delayed energy failure following cerebral ischemia.

In cocultures of immunostimulated microglia and cerebellar granule neurons, neuronal cell death is mediated via reactive nitrogen oxides produced by the microglia.[151] Oligodendrocytes are also susceptible to being killed via microglial-produced NO.[152,153] Palmer et a.l[154] have shown that NO synthesized by inducible NOS in endothelium reduces the viability of endothelial cells. Thus, while large amounts of cytotoxic inducible NOS can be stimulated by cytokines, in vivo this mechanism does not occur for hours. In the 7-day-old rat model of cerebral hypoxia–ischemia inducible NOS mRNA appeared from 6 to 24 h after hypoxia–ischemia. The inducible NOS protein and its activity increased significantly from 12 h and reached a maximum level at 48 h after the insult.[155] Specific inhibitors of the neuronal (7-nitroindazole)[139] (or ARL17477),[156] and the inducible (aminoguanidine)[157] isoforms of NOS provide selective protection against NO-mediated brain injury.

NO may be produced in the vicinity of superoxide during reperfusion, especially in microvessels. This is important because NO reacts so rapidly with superoxide that it even outcompetes superoxide dismutase for superoxide.[144] Beckman et al.[75] have shown that the reaction product of superoxide and NO is peroxynitrite, which decomposes when protonated to form potent oxidants with reactivity similar to the hydroxyl radical and nitrogen dioxide.[75,144,158,159] Peroxynitrite can nitrate or hydroxylate protein tyrosine residues. Possible cytotoxic mechanisms of peroxynitrite involve DNA damage and activation of poly ADP-ribose synthase, with subsequent depletion of NAD and ATP,[148] or mitochondrial damage.[160]

A useful footprint of peroxynitrite toxicity is the identification of nitrated proteins, especially nitrotyrosine. Coeroli et al.[161] induced transient cerebral ischemia in 7-day-old rat pups by bilateral carotid artery occlusion and used an antibody to nitrotyrosine to identify tyrosine nitration in blood vessels close to the infarct at 48–72 h of recovery. Other investigators have used a high-performance liquid chromatography (HPLC) method to measure nitrotyrosine in the periinfarct region of rats following brain ischemia.[162] Similar findings were shown by Ikeno et al.[155] who demonstrated that inducible NOS enzymatic activity peaked at 48 h of recovery following cerebral ischemia in 7-day-old rats: this was coincident with the peak of 3-nitrotyrosine formation. When the investigators inhibited inducible NOS with a specific inhibitor administered starting before reperfusion, brain injury was reduced from 31.9% to 10.6%.[155] This indicates that inducible NOS is significantly damaging. What makes it even more interesting from the therapeutic standpoint is the fact that it takes around 12 h before the enzyme activity is enhanced.[133] Preliminary studies in my laboratory indicate that NOS inhibition, started many hours after recovery from cerebral hypoxia–ischemia in 7-day-old rats, is a rewarding therapeutic strategy. We administered L-nitroargininemethylester (L-NAME), a nonselective NOS inhibitor, 15 h after the hypoxic–ischemic insult to 7-day-old rats and significantly reduced cerebral atrophy.[163]

Thus NO, like free iron, may substantially increase the toxicity of superoxide. Excess NO and superoxide can be generated in concert from the injured brain parenchyma and microvessels during ischemia/reperfusion. Accordingly, strategies for limiting NO- and peroxynitrite-mediated injury to both compartments are necessary. There are dangers however in depleting vascular NO because it protects against vascular injury. As discussed above, attempts to prevent neuronal toxicity should ideally

Table 3.1. Functional distinctions between necrosis and apoptosis

Necrosis	Apoptosis
Cellular homeostasis lost	Cellular homeostasis intact
Increased membrane ion fluxes (Na^+, Ca^{2+})	Membrane ion fluxes maintained
Swelling of organelles	Cytosol condensation
Energy depletion	Energy reserves maintained
Decreased macromolecular synthesis	Macromolecular synthesis activation
Loose aggregation of chromatin	Condensed aggregation of chromatin
Passive atrophy	**Active degeneration**

Source: Modified from Sastry and Rao.[169]

not inhibit the important vasodilatory and antiadhesive properties of endothelial NO.

Another approach to investigating the significance of the different NOS isoforms is to use animals in which one of the isoenzymes has been genetically removed. When mutant mice deficient in neuronal NOS were subjected to middle cerebral artery occlusion, the infarct volumes and neurological deficits were significantly less.[164] However, the infarct size in the mutant increased after endothelial NOS was inhibited with nitro-L-arginine. Ferriero et al.[165] showed that prior destruction of NOS neurons with quisqualate protected the 7-day-old rat from hypoxic–ischemic injury. These studies emphasize the importance of developing selective strategies to conserve the constitutive endothelial isoforms of NOS and inhibit the neuronal and inducible isoforms. The correct timing of specific NOS inhibition is important, as endothelial NOS and even neuronal NOS help to maintain cerebral blood flow. Inhibition of NOS activity in the microvasculature during the early hours of reperfusion may be harmful. In reflecting on the place for NO-based strategies for neuroprotection, Iadecola[141] suggested that NO *donors* may be indicated for patients within the first few hours of the onset of ischemia; *inhibitors* of neuronal NOS may be also indicated early (once reperfusion of the previously ischemic brain is established). At later times of reperfusion (>12 h) then inducible NOS *inhibitors* would be indicated. Clearly these strategies place the emphasis on the clinician in recognizing the stage of recovery in order to select the appropriate therapy.

Necrosis vs apoptosis

Tissue injury arising from hypoxia–ischemia in the immature and adult brain takes the form of either selective neuronal death or infarction. Infarction implies destruction of all cellular elements, including neurons, glia, and blood vessels. It is now known that selective neuronal death takes two forms: specifically, necrosis and apoptosis. It is generally believed that neuronal necrosis is a relatively rapid process, occurring over minutes to hours, while apoptosis requires hours to days to develop. Both forms of selective neuronal death have been observed in the perinatal brain suffering hypoxia–ischemia, having been best characterized in the immature rat.[166–168]

Notable functional and anatomic distinctions exist between neuronal necrosis and apoptosis (Table 3.1). As previously discussed, the metabolic alterations which occur during a hypoxic–ischemic insult severe enough to produce tissue injury involve numerous biochemical alterations (Figure 3.8). These biochemical events commence with a shift from oxidative to anaerobic metabolism, which leads to an accumulation of NADH, FADH, and lactic acid plus H^+ ions. Anaerobic glycolysis cannot keep pace with cellular energy demands, resulting in a depletion of high-energy phosphate reserves,

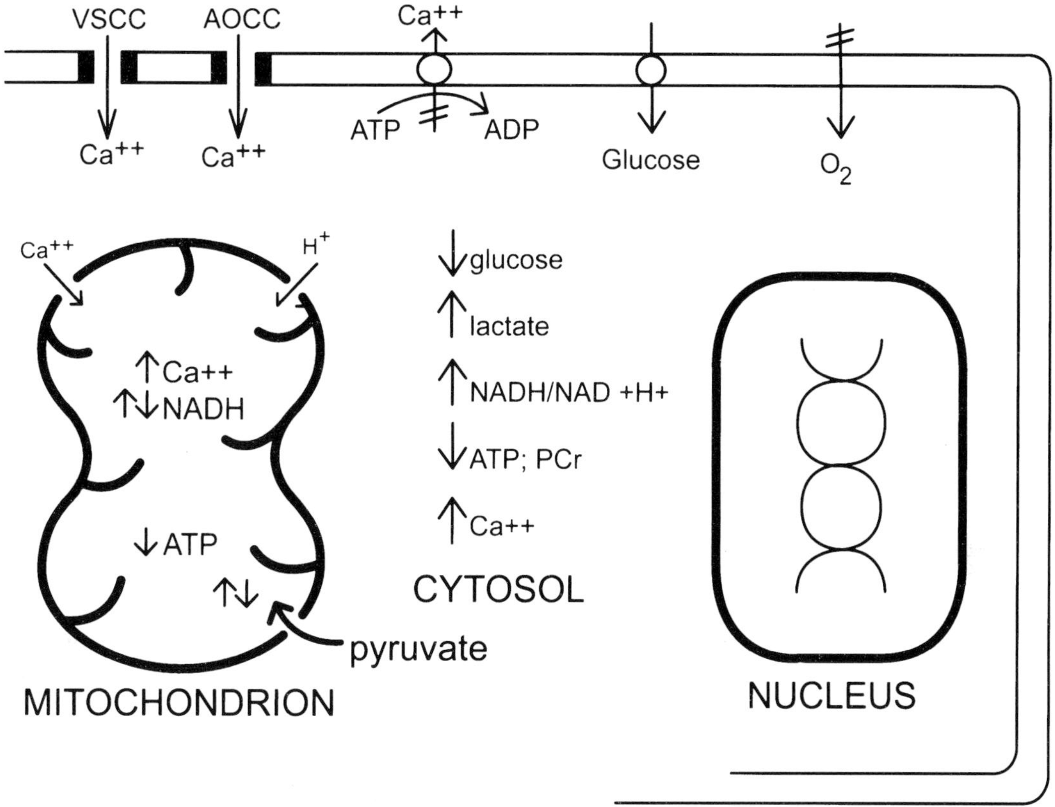

Figure 3.8 Schematic representation of those metabolic alterations which occur during the course of perinatal hypoxia–ischemia. Hypoxia–ischemia sets in motion a cascade of metabolic events which occur during the course of the insult. Such alterations include an increase in anaerobic glycolysis with a secondary depletion in intracellular glucose stores. Anaerobic glycolysis leads to an increase in lactic acid formation with associated H^+ accumulation. Reducing equivalents (nicotinamide adenine dinucleotide – reduced (NADH); flavine adenine dinucleotide – reduced (FADH)) accumulate in the cytosol and at least initially in mitochondria. Ca^{2+} influx is accentuated with a curtailment of Ca^{2+} efflux. Accordingly, Ca^{2+} accumulates within mitochondria and the cytosol. High-energy phosphate reserves are depleted. VSCC, voltage-sensitive Ca^{2+} channels; AOCC, agonist-operated Ca^{2+} channels; ATP, adenosine triphosphate; ADP, adenosine diphosphate; PCr, phosphocreatine.

including ATP and PCr. Transcellular ion pumping fails, leading to an accumulation of intracellular Na^+, Cl^-, and water (cytotoxic edema). Hypoxia–ischemia also stimulates the release of excitatory amino acids (glutamate) from axon terminals. The glutamate release into the synaptic cleft, in turn, activates AMPA-QA and NMDA cell surface receptors on dendrites, resulting in an influx of Na^+ and Ca^{2+} ions. Ca^{2+} ions accumulate within the cytosol as a consequence of increased cellular membrane influx and decreased efflux, combined with release from mitochondria and the endoplasmic reticulum. The combined effects of cellular energy failure, acidosis, and Ca^{2+} accumulation set in

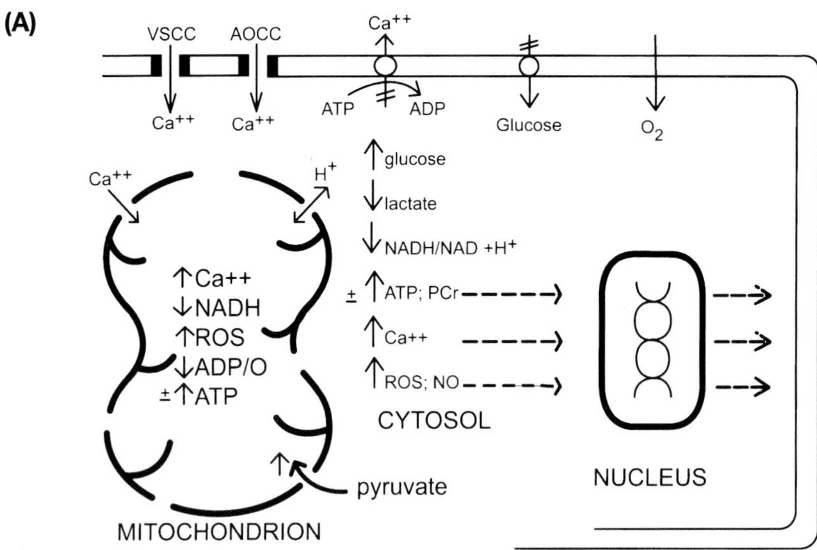

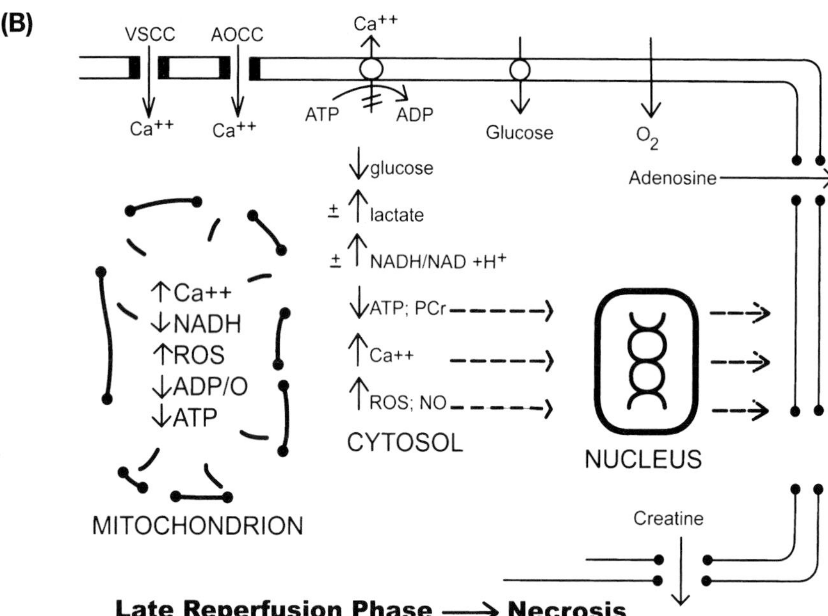

Figure 3.9 The metabolic alterations which occur during the reperfusion phase of cerebral hypoxia–ischemia leading ultimately to necrosis. Shown are the metabolic alterations which occur during (A) the early and (B) late phases of reperfusion following hypoxia–ischemia. The sequence of the metabolic events is described in detail in the text, as also are the abbreviations. Depicted morphologically is swelling and ultimate lysis of the mitochondrion as well as lysis of the cellular membrane. Also depicted is ultimate shrinkage (pyknosis) of the nucleus.

motion a cascade of additional biochemical events during the reperfusion phase which, if severe enough, leads to death of the neuron.

Distinctive differences in the functional and anatomic integrity of the neuron exist during the reperfusion phase in those neurons undergoing either necrosis or apoptosis. When a neuron is destined to undergo necrosis, lingering metabolic disturbances include a reversal of at least some biochemical processes, owing to the now ready availability of oxygen and substrate (glucose) to the cell (Figure 3.9). Glycolysis is inhibited by the initial cellular acidosis, and lactate becomes the preferred fuel for oxidative metabolism. As a consequence, glucose consumption is curtailed, leading to increased intracellular glucose concentrations. Once oxidative metabolism is reestablished, NADH and FADH are consumed within mitochondria, and both mitochondria and the cytosol become oxidized. However, there is a continued intracellular accumulation of Ca^{2+} ions, owing possibly to continued activation of voltage-sensitive and agonist-operated Ca^{2+} channels by glutamate; the Ca^{2+} continues to accumulate in mitochondria and the cytosol. With reoxygenation, free radicals are formed through a variety of metabolic processes, including the production of NO (see above). The mitochondrial Ca^{2+} and free radical accumulation lead to an uncoupling of oxidative phosphorylation, which, in turn, causes a persisting or secondary energy failure. At the morphologic level, cellular and subcellular membranes begin to disintegrate with resultant swelling of organelles, especially mitochondria. The nucleus undergoes aggregation of its chromatin, which microscopically appears as pyknosis. Ultimately the neuron undergoes total lysis and death.

The functional and anatomic alterations which characterize apoptosis differ in many ways from that of necrosis (Figure 3.10). The most prominent disturbances occur within mitochondria, with secondary effects on the nucleus.[169–173] During the early reperfusion phase of a neuron destined to undergo apoptosis, oxidative metabolism is reestablished with consequent increases in intracellular glucose and decreases in intracellular lactate and mitochondrial NADH. Ca^{2+} influx into the neuron is curtailed, while Ca^{2+} efflux is stimulated. Within mitochondria, oxidative phosphorylation is reestablished with replenishment of high-energy phosphate reserves. However, in at least some mitochondria, an uncoupling of oxidative phosphorylation occurs, owing presumably to a continued mitochondrial Ca^{2+} overload combined with the production of reactive oxygen species. In addition, the conversion of NADH to NAD^+ leads to a further decrease in mitochondrial pH which adversely influences the mitochondrial membrane potential. Ultimately, permeability transition pores (PTP) form within the mitochondrial membrane, which allow for the release of cytochrome c into the cytosol. It has been found that cytochrome c is equivalent to apoptotic protease-activating factor 2 (Apaf-2). Apaf-2 then binds to Apaf-1, which in the presence of Apaf-3 (caspase-9) activates caspase-3 in the presence of deoxyATP. Caspases are a family of cystein proteases involved in the apoptotic cascade. Finally, within the cytosol, a DNA fragmentation factor is cleaved by caspase-3, which initiates DNA degradation within intact nuclei. Intranuclear DNA fragmentation is also attributed to the activation of endonucleases, which leads to DNA cleavage at internucleosomal linker areas, resulting in a ladder formation of DNA noted on agarose gel electrophoresis. At the morphologic level, apoptosis is characterized predominantly by nuclear DNA alterations, which histologically is identified by specific staining techniques (terminal deoxynucleotidyl transferase-mediated biotin-deoxyuridine triphosphate nick end-labeling or TUNEL). Consequently, cell shrinkage, membrane blebbing, and chromatin condensation occur with death of the neuron.

It should be mentioned that apoptosis also occurs physiologically in all developing nervous systems. When neurons commit suicide as part of a physiologic process, the cells are undergoing "programmed cell death." The process occurs in all developing nervous systems as a method of pruning unneeded neurons, which typically proliferate in excessive numbers. This pruning process allows for the ultimate normal constituent number of neurons to be present in the adult brain.

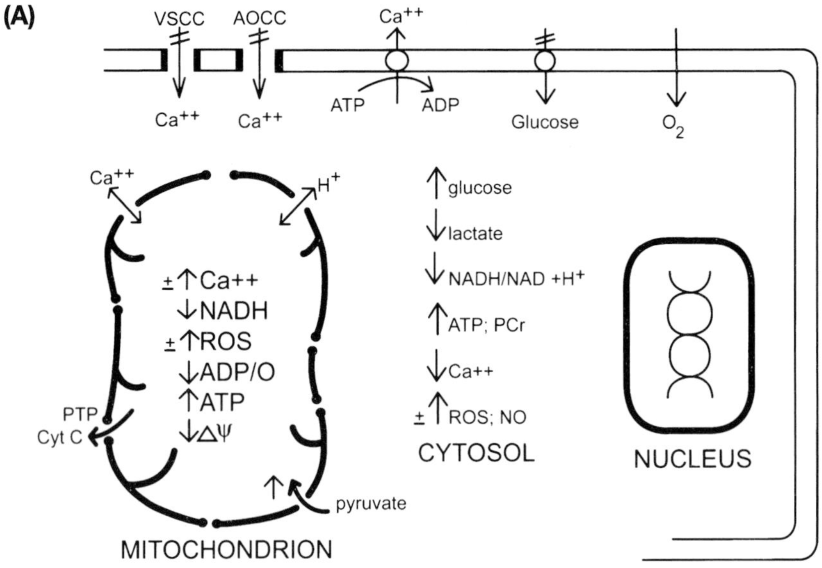

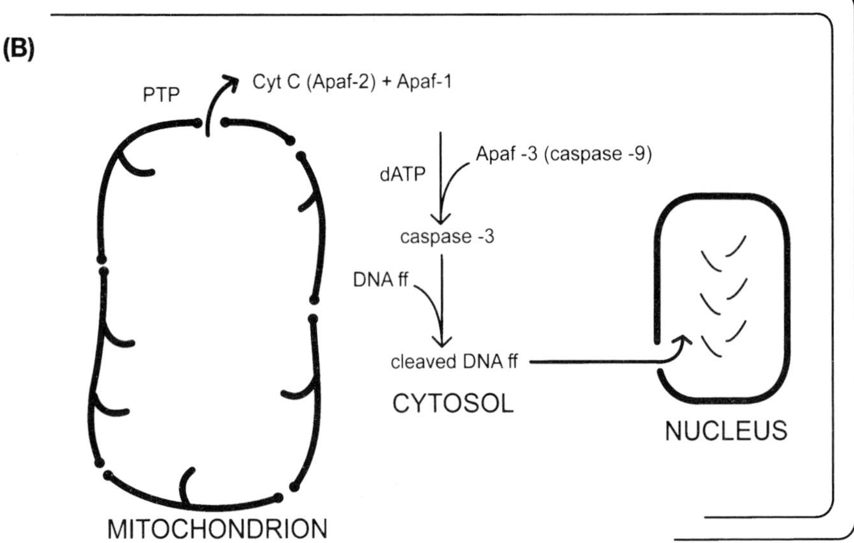

Figure 3.10 The metabolic alterations which occur during the reperfusion phase of cerebral hypoxia–ischemia leading ultimately to apoptosis. Shown are the metabolic alterations which occur during (A) the early and (B) late phases of reperfusion following hypoxia–ischemia. The sequence of the metabolic events is described in detail in the text, as are the abbreviations. Depicted morphologically is the development of permeability transition pores (PTP) of the mitochondrial membrane as well as intranuclear DNA fragmentation.

Acknowledgment

Drs Palmer and Vannucci's research currently is supported by the National Institute of Child Health and Human Development grant P01 HD30704.

REFERENCES

1 Vannucci, R. C. & Palmer, C. (1997). See 125 In *Neonatal–Perinatal Medicine*, ed. A. A. Fanaroff & R. J. Martin, pp. 856–77. Philadelphia: Mosby-Yearbook.

2 Siesjo, B. (1978). *Brain Energy Metabolism*. Chichester: Wiley.

3 Erecinska, M. & Silver, I. (1989). ATP and brain function. *J. Cereb. Blood Flow & Metab.*, 9, 2–19.

4 Hawkins, R. (1985). Cerebral energy metabolism. In *Cerebral Energy Metabolism and Metabolic Encephalopathy*, ed. D. McCandless, pp. 3–23. New York: Plenum Press.

5 Sugano, T., Oshino, N. & Chance, B. (1974). Mitochondrial functions under hypoxic conditions. The steady states of cytochrome c reduction and of energy metabolism. *Biochim. Biophys. Acta*, 347, 340–58.

6 LaManna, J., Light, A., Peretsman, S. et al. (1984). Oxygen insufficiency during hypoxic hypoxia in rat brain cortex. *Brain Res.*, 293, 313–18.

7 Lowry, O., Passonneau, J., Hasselberger, F. et al. (1964). Effect of ischemia on known substrates and cofactors of the glycolytic pathway in brain. *J. Biol. Chem.*, 239, 18–30.

8 Duffy, T. E., Kohle, S. J. & Vannucci, R. C. (1975). Carbohydrate and energy metabolism in perinatal rat brain: relation to survival in anoxia. *J. Neurochem.*, 24, 271–6.

9 Hossmann, K. (1982). Treatment of experimental cerebral ischemia. *J. Cereb. Blood Flow Metab.*, 2, 275–97.

10 Raichle, M. E. (1983). The pathophysiology of brain ischemia. *Ann. Neurol.*, 13, 2–10.

11 Welsh, F. A., Vannucci, R. C. & Brierley, J. B. (1982). Columnar alterations of NADH fluorescence during hypoxia–ischemia in immature rat brain. *J. Cereb. Blood Flow Metab.*, 2, 221–8.

12 Palmer, C., Brucklacher, R. M., Christensen, M. A. et al. (1990). Carbohydrate and energy metabolism during the evolution of hypoxic–ischemic brain damage in the immature rat. *J. Cereb. Blood Flow Metab.*, 10, 227–35.

13 Yager, J. Y., Brucklacher, R. M. & Vannucci, R. C. (1992). Cerebral energy metabolism during hypoxia–ischemia and early recovery in immature rats. *Am. J. Physiol.*, 262, H672–7.

14 Hope, P. L., Cady, E. B., Tofts, P. S. et al. (1984). Cerebral energy metabolism studied with phosphorus NMR spectroscopy in normal and birth-asphyxiated infants. *Lancet*, 2, 366–70.

15 Azzopardi, D., Wyatt, J. S., Cady, E. B. et al. (1989). Prognosis of newborn infants with hypoxic–ischemic brain injury assessed by phosphorus magnetic resonance spectroscopy. *Pediatr. Res.*, 25, 445–51.

16 Lorek, A., Takei, Y., Cady, E. B. et al. (1994). Delayed ("secondary") cerebral energy failure after acute hypoxia–ischemia in the newborn piglet: continuous 48-hour studies by phosphorous magnetic resonance spectroscopy. *Pediatr. Res.*, 36, 699–706.

17 Penrice, J., Lorek, A., Cady, E. et al. (1997). Proton magnetic resonance spectroscopy of the brain during acute hypoxia–ischemia and delayed cerebral energy failure in the newborn piglet. *Pediatr. Res.*, 41, 795–802.

18 Munekata, K. & Hossmann, K. (1987). Effect of 5-minute ischemia on regional pH and energy state of the gerbil brain: relation to selective vulnerability of the hippocampus. *Stroke*, 18, 412–17.

19 Pettigrew, L., Grotta, J., Rhoades, H. et al. (1988). Regional depletion of adenosine triphosphate, phosphocreatine, and glucose in ischemic hippocampus. *Metab. Brain Dis.*, 3, 185–99.

20 Selman, W., Ricci, A., Crumrine, R. et al. (1990). The evolution of focal ischemic damage: a metabolic analysis. *Metab. Brain Dis.*, 5, 33–44.

21 Nakai, A., Asakura, H., Taniuchi, Y. et al. (2000). Effect of alpha-phenyl-*N*-tert-butyl nitrone (PBN) on fetal cerebral energy metabolism during intrauterine ischemia and reperfusion in rats. *Pediatr. Res.*, 47, 456.

22 Towfighi, J., Zec, N., Yager, J. et al. (1995). Temporal evolution of neuropathologic changes in an immature rat model of cerebral hypoxia: a light microscopic study. *Acta Neuropathol. (Berl.)*, 90, 375–86.

23 Saugstad, O. D. (1996). Role of xanthine oxidase and its inhibitor in hypoxia: reoxygenation injury. *Pediatrics*, 98, 103–7.

24 Brown, A. W. & Brierley, J. B. (1973). The earliest alterations in rat neurones and astrocytes after anoxia–ischaemia. *Acta Neuropathol.*, 23, 9–22.

25 Brown, A. W. (1977). Structural abnormalities in neurones. *J. Clin. Pathol.*, 11, 155–69.

26 Rehncrona, S., Mela, L. & Siesjo, B. K. (1979). Recovery of brain mitochondrial function in the rat after complete and incomplete cerebral ischemia. *Stroke*, 10, 437–46.

27 Linn, F., Paschen, W., Ophoff, B. G. et al. (1987). Mitochondrial respiration during recirculation after prolonged ischemia in cat brain. *Exp. Neurol.*, 96, 321–33.

28 Sims, N. R. & Pulsinelli, W. A. (1987). Altered mitochondrial respiration in selectively vulnerable brain subregions following transient forebrain ischemia in the rat. *J. Neurochem.*, 49, 1367–74.

29 Kogure, K., Busto, R., Schwartzman, R. et al. (1980). The dissociation of cerebral blood flow, metabolism, and function in the early stages of developing cerebral infarction. *Ann. Neurol.*, 8, 278–90.

30 Dora, E., Tanaka, K., Greenberg, J. et al. (1986). Kinetics of microcirculatory, NAD/NADH, and electrocorticographic changes in cat brain cortex during ischemia and recirculation. *Ann. Neurol.*, 19, 536–44.

31 Yager, J. Y., Brucklacher, R. M. & Vannucci, R. C. (1991). Cerebral oxidative metabolism and redox state during hypoxia–ischemia and early recovery in immature rats. *Am. J. Physiol.*, 261, H1102–8.

32 Vannucci, R. C., Yager, J. Y. & Vannucci, S. J. (1994). Cerebral glucose and energy utilization during the evolution of hypoxic–ischemic brain damage in the immature rat. *J. Cereb. Blood Flow Metab.*, 14, 279–88.

33 Fonnum, F. (1984). Glutamate: a neurotransmitter in mammalian brain. *J. Neurochem.*, 42, 1–11.

34 Rothman, S. M. & Olney, J. W. (1986). Glutamate and the pathophysiology of hypoxic–ischemic brain damage. *Ann. Neurol.*, 19, 105–11.

35 McDonald, J. & Johnston, M. (1990). Physiological and pathophysiological roles of excitatory amino acids during central nervous system development. *Brain Res. Rev.*, 15, 41–70.

36 Greenamyre, J., Olson, J. & Penney, J. (1985). Autoradiographic characterization of *N*-methyl-D-aspartate-, quiaqualate- and kainate-sensitive glutamate binding sites. *J. Pharmacol. Exp. Ther.*, 233, 254–63.

37 Greenamyre, J., Penney, J. & Young, A. (1987). Evidence for transient perinatal glutamatergic innervation of globus pallidus. *J. Neurosci.*, 7, 1022–30.

38 McDonald, J., Trescher, W. & Johnston, M. (1992). Susceptibility of brain to AMPA induced excitotoxicity transiently peaks during early postnatal development. *Brain Res.*, 583, 54–70.

39 Siesjo, B. & Bengtsson, F. (1989). Calcium fluxes, calcium antagonists, and calcium-related pathology in brain ischemia, hypoglycemia, and spreading depression: a unifying hypothesis. *J. Cereb. Blood Flow Metab.*, 9, 127–40.

40 Olney, J. (1969). Brain lesions, obesity, and other disturbances in mice treated with monosodium glutamate. *Science*, 164, 719–21.

41 Kass, I. & Lipton, P. (1982). Mechanisms involved in irreversible anoxic damage to the in vitro rat hippocampal slice. *J. Physiol.*, 332, 459–72.

42 Rothman, S. M. (1983). Synaptic activity mediates death of hypoxic neurons. *Science*, 220, 536–7.

43 Rothman, S. (1984). Synaptic release of excitatory amino acid neurotransmitter mediates anoxic neuronal death. *J. Neurosci.*, 4, 1884–91.

44 Clark, G., Samaie, M. & Rothman, S. (1985). Blockade of synaptic transmission protects rat hippocampal slices from hypoxia. *Ann. Neurol.*, 18, 385–6.

45 Novelli, A., Reilly, J. & Lysko, P. (1988). Glutamate becomes neurotoxic via the *N*-methyl-D-aspartate receptor when intracellular energy levels are reduced. *Brain Res.*, 451, 205–12.

46 Coyle, J., Bird, S. & Evans, R. (1981). Excitatory amino acid neurotoxins: selectivity, specificity and mechanism of action. *Neurosci. Res. Progr. Bull.*, 19, 329–427.

47 McBean, G. & Roberts, P. (1984). Chronic infusion of L-glutamate causes neurotoxicity in rat striatum. *Brain Res.*, 290, 372–5.

48 Steiner, H., McBean, G. & Kohler, C. (1984). Ibotenate-induced neuronal degeneration in immature rat brain. *Brain Res.*, 307, 117–24.

49 Silverstein, F., Chen, R. & Johnston, M. (1986). The glutamate analogue quisqualic acid is neurotoxic in striatum and hippocampus of immature rat brain. *Neurosci. Lett.*, 71, 13–18.

50 McDonald, J., Silverstein, F. & Johnston, M. (1988). Neurotoxicity of *N*-methyl-D-aspartate is markedly enhanced in developing rat central nervous system. *Brain Res.*, 459, 200–3.

51 Pulsinelli, W. A. (1985). De-afferentation of the hippocampus protects CA1 pyramidal neurons against ischemic injury. *Stroke*, 16, 144.

52 Vannucci, R. C. & Perlman, J. M. (1997). Interventions for perinatal hypoxic-ischemic encephalopathy. *Pediatrics*, 100, 1004–14.

53 Meldrum, B. (1985). Excitatory amino acids and anoxic–ischemic brain damage. *Trends Neurosci.*, 8, 47–8.

54 Kirino, T. (1982). Delayed neuronal death in the gerbil hippocampus following ischemia. *Brain Res.*, 239, 57–69.

55 Pulsinelli, W. A., Brierley, J. B. & Plum, F. (1982). Temporal profile of neuronal damage in a model of transient forebrain ischemia. *Ann. Neurol.*, 11, 491–8.

56 Hattori, H., Morin, A. M., Schwartz, P. H. et al. (1989). Post-hypoxic treatment with MK-801 reduces hypoxic–ischemic damage in the neonatal rat. *Neurology*, 39, 713–18.

57 Gordon, K. E., Simpson, J., Statman, D. et al. (1991). Effects of perinatal stroke on striatal amino acid efflux in rats studied with in vivo microdialysis. *Stroke*, 22, 928–32.

58 Silverstein, F., Naik, B. & Simpson, J. (1991). Hypoxia–ische-

mia stimulates hippocampal glutamate efflux in perinatal rat brain: an in vivo microdialysis study. *Pediatr. Res.*, 30, 587–90.

59 Vannucci, R., Rossini, A., Towfighi, J. et al. (1997). Measuring the accentuation of the brain damage that arises from perinatal cerebral hypoxia–ischemia. *Biol. Neonate*, 72, 187–91.

60 Vannucci, R., Brucklacher, R. & Vannucci, S. (1999). CSF glutamate during hypoxia–ischemia in the immature rat. *Dev. Brain Res.*, 118, 147–51.

61 Alberts, B., Bray, D., Lewis, J. et al. (1983). Chemical signalling between cells. In *Molecular Biology of the Cell*, eds B. Alberts, D. Bray, J. Lewis et al., pp. 743–4. New York: Garland Publishing.

62 Siesjo, B. K. (1981). Cell damage in the brain: a speculative synthesis. *J. Cereb. Blood Flow Metab.*, 1, 155–85.

63 Greenberg, D. A. (1987). Calcium channels and calcium channel antagonists. *Ann. Neurol.*, 21, 317–30.

64 Vannucci, R. C. (1990). Experimental biology of cerebral hypoxia–ischemia: relation to perinatal brain damage. *Pediatr. Res.*, 27, 317–26.

65 Simon, R., Griffiths, T. & Evans, M. (1984). Calcium overload in selectively vulnerable neurons of the hippocampus during and after ischemia: an electron microscopy study in the rat. *J. Cereb. Blood Flow Metab.*, 4, 350–61.

66 Chen, S. T., Hsu, C. Y., Hogan, E. L. et al. (1987). Brain calcium content in ischemic infarction. *Neurology*, 37, 1227–9.

67 Deshpande, J., Siesjo, B. & Wieloch, T. (1987). Calcium accumulation and neuronal damage in the rat hippocampus following cerebral ischemia. *J. Cereb. Blood Flow Metab.*, 7, 89–95.

68 Stein, D. T. & Vannucci, R. C. (1988). Calcium accumulation during the evolution of hypoxic–ischemic brain damage in the immature rat. *J. Cereb. Blood Flow Metab.*, 8, 834–42.

69 Vannucci, R. C., Brucklacher, R. M. & Vannucci, S. J. (2001). Intracellular calcium accumulation during the evolution of hypoxic–ischemic brain damage in the immature rat. *Dev. Brain Res.*, 126, 117–20.

70 Aruoma, O. I. & Halliwell, B. (1987). Superoxide-dependent and ascorbate-dependent formation of hydroxyl radicals from hydrogen peroxide in the presence of iron. *Biochem. J.*, 241, 273–8.

71 Halliwell, B. (1991). Reactive oxygen species in living systems: source, biochemistry and role in human disease. *Am. J. Med.*, 91, 14S–22S.

72 Nowicki, J. P., Duval, D., Poignet, H. et al. (1991). Nitric oxide mediates neuronal death after focal cerebral ischemia in the mouse. *Eur. J. Pharmacol.*, 204, 339–40.

73 Reilly, P. M., Schiller, H. J. & Bulkley, G. B. (1991). Pharmacologic approach to tissue injury mediated by free radicals and other reactive oxygen metabolites. *Am. J. Surg.*, 161, 488–503.

74 Traystman, R. J., Kirsch, J. R. & Koehler, R. C. (1991). Oxygen radical mechanisms of brain injury following ischemia and reperfusion. *J. Appl. Physiol.*, 71, 1185–95.

75 Beckman, J. S., Beckman, T. W., Chen, J. et al. (1990). Apparent hydroxyl radical production by peroxynitrite: implications for endothelial injury from nitric oxide and superoxide. *Proc. Natl Acad. Sci. USA*, 87, 1620–4.

76 Chan, P. H. (2001). Reactive oxygen radicals in signaling and damage in the ischemic brain. *J. Cereb. Blood Flow Metab.*, 21, 2–14.

77 Liu, X. H., Kato, H., Araki, T. et al. (1994). An immunohistochemical study of copper/zinc superoxide dismutase and manganese superoxide dismutase following focal cerebral ischemia in the rat. *Brain Res.*, 644, 257–66.

78 Takashima, S., Kuruta, H., Mito, T. et al. (1990). Immunohistochemistry of superoxide dismutase-1 in developing human brain. *Brain Dev.*, 12, 211–13.

79 Inder, T. E., Graham, P., Sanderson, K. et al. (1994). Lipid peroxidation as a measure of oxygen free radical damage in the very low birthweight infant. *Arch. Dis. Child. Fetal Neonatal*, 70, F107–11.

80 Smith, C. V., Hansen, T. N., Martin, N. E. et al. (1993). Oxidant stress responses in premature infants during exposure to hyperoxia. *Pediatr. Res.*, 34, 360–5.

81 Sullivan, J. L. (1992). *Iron Metabolism and Oxygen Radical Injury in Premature Infants.* Boca Raton: CRC Press.

82 Evans, P. J., Evans, R., Kovar, I. Z. et al. (1992). Bleomycin-detectable iron in the plasma of premature and full-term neonates. *FEBS*, 303, 210–12.

83 Chan, P. H. & Fishman, R. A. (1980). Transient formation of superoxide radicals in polyunsaturated fatty acid-induced brain swelling. *J. Neurochem.*, 35, 1004–7.

84 Kukreja, R. C., Kontos, H. A., Hess, M. L. et al. (1986). PGH synthase and lipoxygenase generate superoxide in the presence of NADH or NADPH. *Circ. Res.*, 59, 612–19.

85 Pourcyrous, M., Leffler, C. W., Bada, H. S. et al. (1993). Brain superoxide anion generation in asphyxiated piglets and the effect of indomethacin at therapeutic dose. *Pediatr. Res.*, 34, 366–9.

86 Babior, B. M. (1978). Oxygen-dependent microbial killing by phagocytes. *N. Engl. J. Med.*, 298, 659–68.

87 McCord, J. M. (1885). Oxygen-derived free radicals in post-ischemic tissue injury. *N. Engl. J. Med.*, 312, 159–63.

88 Hagberg, H., Andersson, P., Lacarewicz, J. et al. (1987). Extracellular adenosine, inosine, hypoxanthine, and xan-

thine in relation to tissue nucleotides and purines in rat striatum during transient ischemia. *J. Neurochem.*, 49, 227–31.

89 Betz, A. L. (1985). Identification of hypoxanthine transport and xanthine oxidase activity in brain capillaries. *J. Neurochem.*, 44, 574–9.

90 Tan, S., Yokoyama, Y., Dickens, E. et al. (1993). Xanthine oxidase activity in the circulation of rats following hemorrhagic shock. *Free Radic. Biol. Med.*, 15, 407–14.

91 Tan, S., Gelman, S., Wheat, J. K. et al. (1995). Circulating xanthine oxidase in human ischemia reperfusion. *South Med. J.*, 88, 479–82.

92 Betz, A. L., Randall, J. & Martz, D. (1991). Xanthine oxidase is not a major source of free radicals in focal cerebral ischemia. *Am. J. Physiol.*, 260, H563–8.

93 Itoh, T., Kawakami, M., Yamauchi, Y. et al. (1986). Effect of allopurinol on ischemia and reperfusion-induced cerebral injury in spontaneously hypertensive rats. *Stroke*, 17, 1284–7.

94 Lin, Y. & Phillis, J. W. (1991). Oxypurinol reduces focal ischemic brain injury in the rat. *Neurosci. Lett.*, 126, 187–90.

95 Lindsay, S., Liu, T. H., Xu, J. et al. (1991). Role of xanthine dehydrogenase and oxidase in focal cerebral ischemic injury to rat. *Am. J. Physiol.*, 261, H2051–7.

96 Martz, D., Rayos, G., Schielke, G. P. et al. (1989). Allopurinol and dimethylthiourea reduce brain infarction following middle cerebral artery occlusion in rats. *Stroke*, 20, 488–94.

97 Mink, R. B., Dutka, A. J. & Hallenbeck, J. M. (1991). Allopurinol pretreatment improves evoked response recovery following global cerebral ischemia in dogs. *Stroke*, 22, 660–5.

98 Palmer, C., Vannucci, R. C. & Towfighi, J. (1990). Reduction of perinatal hypoxic–ischemic brain damage with allopurinol. *Pediatr. Res.*, 27, 332–6.

99 Williams, G. D., Palmer, C., Heitjan, D. F. et al. (1992). Allopurinol preserves cerebral energy metabolism during perinatal hypoxia–ischemia: a ^{31}P NMR study in unanesthetized immature rats. *Neurosci. Lett.*, 144, 103–6.

100 Palmer, C., Smith, M. B., Williams, G. D. et al. (1991). Allopurinol preserves cerebral energy metabolism during perinatal hypoxic–ischemic injury and reduces brain damage in a dose dependent manner. *J. Cereb. Blood Flow Metab.*, 11, S144.

101 Palmer, C., Towfighi, J., Roberts, R. L. et al. (1993). Allopurinol administered after inducing hypoxia–ischemia reduces brain injury in 7-day-old rats. *Pediatr. Res.*, 33, 405–11.

102 Palmer, C. & Roberts, R. L. (1997). Delayed administration of allopurinol after cerebral hypoxia–ischemia reduces brain injury in neonatal rats. *Pediatr. Res.*, 41, 294A.

103 Armstead, W. M., Mirro, R., Busija, D. W. et al. (1988). Postischemic generation of superoxide anion by newborn pig brain. *Am. J. Physiol.*, 255, H401–3.

104 Nelson, C. W., Wei, E. P., Povlishock, J. T. et al. (1992). Oxygen radicals in cerebral ischemia. *Am. J. Physiol. Heart Circ. Physiol.*, 263, H1356–62.

105 Kontos, C. D., Wei, E. P., Williams, J. I. et al. (1992). Cytochemical detection of superoxide in cerebral inflammation and ischemia in vivo. *Am. J. Physiol. Heart Circ. Physiol.*, 263, H1234–42.

106 Phillis, J. W. & Sen, S. (1993). Oxypurinol attenuates hydroxyl radical production during ischemia/reperfusion injury of the rat cerebral cortex: an ESR study. *Brain Res.*, 628, 309–12.

107 Chan, P. H., Schmidley, J. W., Fishman, R. A. et al. (1984). Brain injury, edema and vascular permeability changes induced by oxygen-derived free radicals. *Neurology*, 34, 315–20.

108 Schleien, C. L., Koehler, R. C., Shaffner, D. H. et al. (1990). Blood–brain barrier integrity during cardiopulmonary resuscitation in dogs. *Stroke*, 21, 1185–91.

109 Wei, E. P., Ellison, M. D., Kontos, H. A. et al. (1986). O_2 radicals in arachidonate-induced increased blood–brain barrier permeability to proteins. *Am. J. Physiol.*, 251, H693–9.

110 Leffler, C. W., Busijia, D. W., Armstead, W. M. et al. (1990). Activated oxygen and arachidonate effects on newborn cerebral arterioles. *Am. J. Physiol.*, 259, H1230–8.

111 Elliot, S. J. & Schilling, W. P. (1992). Oxidant stress alters Na^+ pump and Na^+-K^+-Cl^- cotransporter activities in vascular endothelial cells. *Am. J. Physiol.*, 263, H96–102.

112 Lo, W. D. & Betz, A. L. (1986). Oxygen free-radical reduction of brain capillary rubidium uptake. *J. Neurochem.*, 46, 394–8.

113 Gasic, A. C., McGuire, G., Drater, S. et al. (1991). Hydrogen peroxide pretreatment of perfused canine vessels induces ICAM-1 and CD18-dependent neutrophil adherence. *Circulation*, 84, 2154–66.

114 Rosenberg, A. A., Murdaugh, E. & White, C. W. (1989). The role of oxygen free radicals in postasphyxia cerebral hypoperfusion in newborn lambs. *Pediatr. Res.*, 26, 215–19.

115 Thiringer, K., Hrbek, A., Karlsson, K. et al. (1987). Postasphyxial cerebral survival in newborn sheep after treatment with oxygen free radical scavengers and a calcium antagonist. *Pediatr. Res.*, 22, 62–6.

116 Ste-Marie, L., Vachon, P., Vachon, L. et al. (2000). Hydroxyl radical production in the cortex and striatum in a rat model of focal cerebral ischemia. *Can. J. Neurol. Sci.*, 27, 152–9.

117 Solenski, N. J., Kwan, A. L., Yanamoto, H. et al. (1997).

Differential hydroxylation of salicylate in core and penumbra regions during focal reversible cerebral ischemia. *Stroke*, 28, 2545–51.

118 Halliwell, B. (1992). Iron and damage to biomolecules. In *Iron and Human Disease*, ed. R. B. Lauffer, pp. 210–30. Boca Raton, FL: CRC Press.

119 Ciuffi, M., Gentilini, G., Franchi-Micheli, S. et al. (1991). Lipid peroxidation induced "in vivo" by iron–carbohydrate complex in the rat brain cortex. *Neurochem. Res.*, 16, 43–9.

120 Sadrzadeh, S. M. H., Anderson, D. K., Panter, S. S. et al. (1987). Hemoglobin potentiates central nervous system damage. *J. Clin. Invest.*, 79, 662–4.

121 Sadrzadeh, S. M. H. & Eaton, J. W. (1992). Hemoglobin-induced oxidant damage to the central nervous system. In *Free Radical Mechanisms of Tissue Injury*, ed. M. T. Moslen & C. V. Smith, pp. 23–32. Boca Raton, FL: CRC Press.

122 Sadrzadeh, S. M. H. & Eaton, J. W. (1988). Hemoglobin-mediated oxidant damage to the central nervous system requires endogenous ascorbate. *J. Clin. Invest.*, 82, 1510–15.

123 Sadrzadeh, S. M. H., Graf, E., Panter, S. S. et al. (1984). Hemoglobin: a biological Fenton reagent. *J. Biol. Chem.*, 259, 14354.

124 Subbarao, K. V. & Richardson, J. S. (1990). Iron-dependent peroxidation of rat brain: a regional study. *J. Neurosci. Res.*, 26, 224–32.

125 Zaleska, M. M. & Floyd, R. A. (1985). Regional lipid peroxidation in rat brain in vitro: possible role of endogenous iron. *Neurochem. Res.*, 10, 397–410.

126 Connor, J. R., Pavlick, G., Karli, D. et al. (1995). A histochemical study of iron-positive cells in the developing rat brain. *J. Comp. Neurol.*, 355, 111–23.

127 Bolann, B. J. & Ulvik, R. J. (1987). Release of iron from ferritin by xanthine oxidase. *Biochem. J.*, 243, 55–9.

128 Reif, D. W. & Simmons, R. D. (1990). Nitric oxide mediates iron release from ferritin. *Arch. Biochem. Biophys.*, 283, 537–41.

129 Bralet, J., Schreiber, L. & Bouvier, C. (1992). Effect of acidosis and anoxia on iron delocalization from brain homogenates. *Biochem. Pharmacol.*, 43, 979–84.

130 Palmer, C., Menzies, S. L., Roberts, R. L. et al. (1999). Changes in iron histochemistry after hypoxic–ischemic brain injury in the neonatal rat. (Erratum appears in *J. Neurosci. Res.*, 1999; 58, 349–55). *J. Neurosci. Res.*, 56, 60–71.

131 van Bel, F., Dorrepaal, C. A., Benders, M. J. N. L. et al. (1994). Neurologic abnormalities in the first 24h following birth asphyxia are associated with increasing plasma levels of free iron and TBA-reactive species. *Pediatr. Res.*, 35, 388A.

132 Hedlund, B. E. & Hallaway, P. E. (1993). High-dose systemic iron chelation attenuates reperfusion injury. *Biochem. Soc. Trans.*, 21, 340–3.

133 Palmer, C., Roberts, R. L. & Bero, C. (1994). Deferoxamine posttreatment reduces ischemic brain injury in neonatal rats. *Stroke*, 25, 1039–45.

134 Palmer, C. (1997). Iron and oxidative stress in neonatal hypoxic–ischemic brain injury. In *Metals and Oxidative Damage in Neurological Disorders*, ed. J. R. Connor, pp. 205–236. New York: Plenum Press.

135 Tan, S., Zhou, F., Nielsen, V. G. et al. (1998). Sustained hypoxia–ischemia results in reactive nitrogen and oxygen species production and injury in the premature fetal rabbit brain. *J. Neuropathol. Exp. Neurol.*, 57, 544–53.

136 Nathan, C. (1992). Nitric oxide as a secretory product of mammalian cells. *FASEB J*, 6, 3051–64.

137 Tomic, D., Zobundzija, M. & Meáugorac, M. (1994). Postnatal development of nicotinamide adenine dinucleotide phosphate diaphorase (NADPH-d) positive neurons in rat prefrontal cortex. *Neurosci. Lett.*, 170, 217–20.

138 Bertini, G., Savio, T., Zaccheo, D. et al. (1996). NADPH-diaphorase activity in brain macrophages during postnatal development in the rat. *Neuroscience*, 70, 287–93.

139 Dalkara, T., Yoshida, T., Irikura, K. et al. (1994). Dual role of nitric oxide in focal cerebral ischemia. *Neuropharmacology*, 33, 1447–52.

140 Dalkara, T. & Moskowitz, M. A. (1994). The complex role of nitric oxide in the pathophysiology of focal cerebral ischemia. *Brain Pathol.*, 4, 49–57.

141 Iadecola, C. (1997). Bright and dark sides of nitric oxide in ischemic brain injury. *Trends Neurosci.*, 20, 132–9.

142 Davenpeck, K. L., Gauthier, T. W. & Lefer, A. M. (1994). Inhibition of endothelial-derived nitric oxide promotes P-selectin expression and actions in the rat microcirculation. *Gastroenterology*, 107, 1050–8.

143 Dalkara, T. & Moskowitz, M. A. (1998). Nitric oxide vascular and parenchymal roles. In *Cerebrovascular Disease: Pathology, Diagnosis and Management*, ed. M. D. Ginsberg & J. Bogousslavsky, pp. 471–480. Malden: Blackwell Science.

144 Beckman, J. S. (1998). Interactions of oxidants, nitric oxide, and antioxidant defenses in cerebral ischemia and injury. In *Cerebrovascular Disease: Pathophysiology, Diagnosis, and Management*, ed. M. D. Ginsberg & J. Bogousslavsky, pp. 455–470. Malden: Blackwell Science.

145 Gross, S. S. & Wolin, M. S. (1995). Nitric oxide: pathophysiological mechanisms. *Annu. Rev. Physiol.*, 57, 737–69.

146 Drapier, J. C. & Hibbs, J. (1988). Differentiation of murine macrophages to express nonspecific cytotoxicity for tumor cells results in L-arginine-dependent inhibition of mito-

chondrial iron-sulfur enzymes in the macrophage effector cells. *J. Immunol.*, 140, 2829–38.

147 Schraufstatter, I. U., Hyslop, P. A., Hinshaw, D. B. et al. (1986). Hydrogen peroxide-induced injury of cells and its prevention by inhibitors of poly(ADP-ribose) polymerase. *Proc. Natl Acad. Sci. USA*, 83, 4908–12.

148 Zhang, J., Dawson, V. L., Dawson, T. M. et al. (1994). Nitric oxide activation of poly(ADP-ribose) synthetase in neurotoxicity. *Science*, 263, 687–9.

149 Brüne, B., Dimmeler, S., Molina y Vedia, L. et al. (1994). Nitric oxide: a signal for ADP-ribosylation of proteins. *Life Sci.*, 54, 61–70.

150 Wallis, R. A., Panizzon, K. L., Henry, D. et al. (1993). Neuroprotection against nitric oxide injury with inhibitors of ADP-ribosylation. *Neuroreport*, 5, 245–8.

151 Boje, K. M. & Arora, P. K. (1992). Microglial-produced nitric oxide and reactive nitrogen oxides mediate neuronal cell death. *Brain Res.*, 587, 250–6.

152 Merrill, J. E. & Zimmerman, R. P. (1991). Natural and induced cytotoxicity of oligodendrocytes by microglia is inhibitable by TGF beta. *Glia*, 4, 327–31.

153 Merrill, J. E., Ignarro, L. J., Sherman, M. P. et al. (1993). Microglial cell cytotoxicity of oligodendrocytes is mediated through nitric oxide. *J. Immunol.*, 151, 2132–41.

154 Palmer, R. M. J., Foxwell, N. A. & Moncada, S. (1992). The role of nitric oxide in endothelial cell damage and its inhibition by glucocorticoids. *Br. J. Pharmacol.*, 105, 11–12.

155 Ikeno, S., Nagata, N., Yoshida, S. et al. (2000). Immature brain injury via peroxynitrite production induced by inducible nitric oxide synthase after hypoxia–ischemia in rats. *J. Obstet. Gynaecol. Res.*, 26, 227–34.

156 Zhang, Z. G., Reif, D., MacDonald, J. et al. (1996). ARL 17477, a potent and selective neuronal NOS inhibitor decreases infarct volume after transient middle cerebral artery occlusion in rats. *J. Cereb. Blood Flow Metab.*, 16, 599–604.

157 Cross, A. H., Misko, T. P., Lin, R. F. et al. (1994). Aminoguanidine, an inhibitor of inducible nitric oxide synthase, ameliorates experimental autoimmune encephalomyelitis in SJL mice. *J. Clin. Invest.*, 93, 2684–90.

158 Beckman, J. S., Ischiropoulos, H., Chen, J. et al. (1991). Nitric oxide as a mediator of superoxide-dependent injury. In *Oxidative Damage and Repair. Chemical, Biological and Medical Aspects*, ed. K. Davies, pp. 251–5. Oxford: Pergamon Press.

159 Radi, R., Beckman, J. S., Bush, K. M. et al. (1991). Peroxynitrite-induced membrane lipid peroxidation: the cytotoxic potential of superoxide and nitric oxide. *Arch. Biochem. Biophys.*, 288, 481–7.

160 Dalkara, T., Endres, M. & Moskowitz, M. A. (1998). Mechanisms of NO neurotoxicity. *Prog. Brain Res.*, 118, 231–9.

161 Coeroli, L., Renolleau, S., Arnaud, S. et al. (1998). Nitric oxide production and perivascular tyrosine nitration following focal ischemia in neonatal rat. *J. Neurochem.*, 70, 2516–25.

162 Fukuyama, N., Takizawa, S., Ishida, H. et al. (1998). Peroxynitrite formation in focal cerebral ischemia–reperfusion in rats occurs predominantly in the peri-infarct region. *J. Cereb. Blood Flow Metab.*, 18, 123–9.

163 Palmer, C. & Roberts, R. L. (1997). Delayed inhibition of nitric oxide production reduces post hypoxic–ischemic brain injury in neonatal rats. *Pediatr. Res.*, 41, 294A.

164 Huang, Z., Huang, P. L., Panahian, N. et al. (1994). Effects of cerebral ischemia in mice deficient in neuronal nitric oxide synthase. *Science*, 265, 1883–5.

165 Ferriero, D. M., Sheldon, R. A., Black, S. M. et al. (1995). Selective destruction of nitric oxide synthase neurons with quisqualate reduces damage after hypoxia–ischemia in the neonatal rat. *Pediatr. Res.*, 38, 912–18.

166 Hill, I. E., MacManus, J. P., Rasquinha, I. et al. (1995). DNA fragmentation indicative of apoptosis following unilateral cerebral hypoxia–ischemia in the neonatal rat. *Brain Res.*, 676, 398–403.

167 Dell'Anna, E., Chen, Y., Engidawork, E. et al. (1997). Delayed neuronal death following perinatal asphyxia in rat. *Exp. Brain Res.*, 115, 105–15.

168 Renolleau, S., Aggoun-Zouaoui, D., Ben-Ari, Y. et al. (1998). A model of transient unilateral focal ischemia with reperfusion in the P7 neonatal rat: morphological changes indicative of apoptosis. *Stroke*, 29, 1454–61.

169 Sastry, P. & Rao, K. (2000). Apoptosis and the nervous system. *J. Neurochem.*, 74, 1–20.

170 Fiskum, G., Murphy, A. N. & Beal, M. F. (1999). Mitochondria in neurodegeneration: acute ischemia and chronic neurodegenerative diseases. *J. Cereb. Blood Flow Metab.*, 19, 351–69.

171 Murphy, A., Fiskum, G. & Beal, M. (1999). Mitochondria in neurodegeneration: bioenergetic function in cell life and death. *J. Cereb. Blood Flow Metab.*, 19, 231–45.

172 Nicotera, P. & Lipton, S. (1999). Excitotoxins in neuronal apoptosis and necrosis. *J. Cereb. Blood Flow Metab.*, 19, 583–91.

173 Siesjo, B., Hu, B. & Kristian, T. (1999). Is the cell death pathway triggered by the mitochondrion or the endoplasmic reticulum? *J. Cereb. Blood Flow Metab.*, 19, 19–26.

4

Fetal responses to asphyxia

Laura Bennet, Jenny A. Westgate, Peter D. Gluckman, and Alistair J. Gunn

The Departments of Paediatrics, Obstetrics and Gynaecology and the Liggins Institute, Faculty of Medical and Health Sciences, University of Auckland, New Zealand

For most of the twentieth century the concept of perinatal brain damage centered around cerebral palsy and intrapartum asphyxia. It is only in the last 20 years that this view has been seriously challenged by clinical and epidemiological studies which have demonstrated that approximately 70–90% or more of cerebral palsy is unrelated to intrapartum events.[1] Many term infants who subsequently develop cerebral palsy are believed to have sustained asphyxial events in midgestation. In some cases, prenatal injury may lead to chronically abnormal heart rate tracings, and impaired ability to adapt to labor which may be confounded with an acute event.[2,3]

Furthermore, it has become clear that the various abnormal fetal heart rate patterns that have been proposed to be markers for potentially injurious asphyxia are consistently only very weakly predictive for cerebral palsy.[4] Although metabolic acidosis is more strongly associated with outcome, more than half of babies born with severe acidosis (base deficit (BD) >16 mmol/l and pH <7.0) do not develop even mild encephalopathy, while conversely encephalopathy can still occur, although at low frequency, in association with relatively modest acidosis (BD 12–16 mmol/l).[5] These data contrast with the presence of very abnormal fetal heart rate tracings and severe metabolic acidosis in those infants who *do* develop neonatal encephalopathy.[6]

The key factor underlying all of these observations is the effectiveness of fetal adaptation to asphyxia. The fetus is, in fact, spectacularly good at defending itself against such insults, and injury occurs only in a very narrow window between intact survival and death. These adaptations work sufficiently well in the majority of cases that even the concept of "birth asphyxia" itself has been controversial. However, recent studies where cerebral function has been monitored from birth in infants with clinical evidence of compromise during labor have shown that many such children did have a precipitating episode in the immediate peripartum period, with evidence of acute evolving cerebral injury,[6–8] and long-term cognitive or functional sequelae.[7] In those infants with evidence for acute, perinatal asphyxial event(s), the link between asphyxia and long-term problems is the severity of early-onset encephalopathy. Newborns with mild encephalopathy are completely normal during follow-up, while all of those with severe (stage III) encephalopathy die or have severe handicap. In contrast, only half of those with moderate (stage II) hypoxic–ischemic encephalopathy develop handicap; however even those who do not develop neurological impairment are at risk of future academic failure.[9]

Causes of pathological asphyxia

A number of events, some peculiar to labor, may result in asphyxia, and fetal compromise both antenatally, and during labor. Broadly these may be grouped as chronic, acute catastrophic, and repeated hypoxia.[6] Chronic hypoxia may be caused by decreased fetal hemoglobin (e.g., fetomaternal or fetofetal hemorrhage), infection and maternal causes such as systemic hypoxia and reduced uteroplacental blood flow due to hypotension.

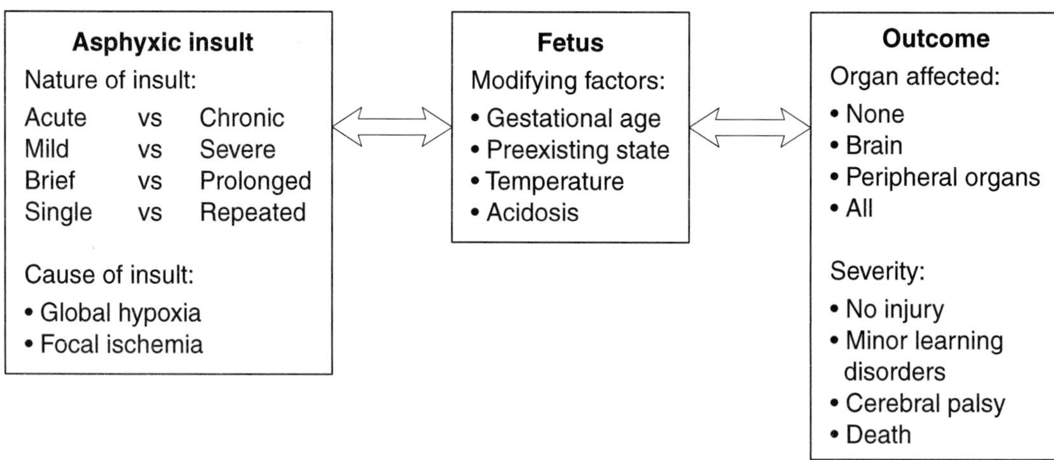

Figure 4.1 Schema of the factors influencing the development of cerebral injury after perinatal asphyxia.

Immediate catastrophic events include cord prolapse and to some extent cord entanglements and true knots in the cord, vasa previa, placental abruption, uterine rupture and finally entrapment, such as shoulder dystocia. The impact of asphyxia during placental abruption may be potentiated by fetal blood loss with fetal volume contraction. Finally, in labor, the fetus may be exposed to shorter but frequent episodes during labor which may lead to a progressive decompensation over time.[6]

Characteristics of perinatal asphyxial encephalopathy

The fetal response to asphyxia is not stereotypical. Both the fetal responses and the ability of the fetus to avoid injury depend upon both the type of the insult, as above, the precise environmental conditions, and the condition of the fetus (Figure 4.1). This review focuses on recent developments in our understanding of the factors that determine whether the brain is damaged after an asphyxial insult. We will briefly review the fundamental cellular mechanisms of cerebral damage and discuss in detail the systemic adaptations of the fetus to asphyxia in relation to the factors which can modulate the evolution of cerebral injury.

The pathogenesis of cell death

What initiates neuronal injury?

At the most fundamental level, injury requires a period of insufficient delivery of oxygen and substrates such as glucose (and other substances such as lactate in the fetus) such that neurons (and glia) cannot maintain homeostasis. Once the neuron's supply of high-energy metabolites such as adenosine triphosphate (ATP) can no longer be maintained during hypoxia–ischemia, there is failure of the energy-dependent mechanisms of intracellular homeostasis such as the Na^+/K^+-ATP-dependent pump. Neuronal depolarization occurs, leading to sodium and calcium entry into cells. This creates an osmotic and electrochemical gradient that in turn favors further cation and water entry, leading to cell swelling (cytotoxic edema). If sufficiently severe, this may lead to immediate lysis.[10] The swollen neurons may still recover, at least temporarily, if the hypoxic insult is reversed or the osmotic environment is manipulated. Evidence suggests that several additional factors act to increase cell injury during and following depolarization. These include the extracellular accumulation of excitatory amino acid neurotransmitters due to impairment of energy dependent reuptake, which promote further receptor-mediated cell swelling and intracellular calcium entry,[11] and the generation of oxygen free radicals.[12,13] Nevertheless, these factors appear to be injurious mainly in the presence of hypoxic cell depolarization.

If oxygen is reduced, but substrate delivery is effectively maintained (i.e., pure or nearly pure hypoxia), the cells will adapt in two ways to avoid or delay depolarization. First, they can use anaerobic metabolism to support their production of high-energy metabolites for a time. The use of anaerobic metabolism is of course very inefficient since anaerobic glycolysis produces lactate and only two ATP, whereas aerobic glycolysis produces 38 ATP. Thus glucose reserves are rapidly consumed, and a metabolic acidosis develops, which, as discussed further below, may have local and systemic consequences. In some circumstances, the fetus may be able to benefit from increased circulating lactate. Because many fetal tissues such as the heart get a high proportion of their substrate from sources other than glucose, particularly lactate, if hypoxia is intermittent the circulating lactate may help support systemic metabolism during normoxic intervals.[14,15]

Second, the brain can to some extent reduce non-obligatory energy consumption. This is clearly seen in neurons, where moderate hypoxia typically induces a switch to a high-voltage low-frequency electroencephalographic (EEG) state requiring less oxygen consumption.[16,17] As an insult becomes more severe, neuronal activity ceases completely at a threshold above that which causes actual neuronal depolarization.[18] It is the total duration of neuronal depolarization, rather than the duration of suppression of the EEG *per se*, which ultimately determines the severity of injury.[19] Thus the brain remains protected as long as depolarization is avoided.

In contrast, under conditions where levels of both oxygen and substrate are reduced, the options for the neuron are much more limited, since not only is there less oxygen, but there is also much less glucose available to support anaerobic metabolism. This may occur during either pure ischemia (reduced tissue blood flow), but even more critically during conditions of hypoxia–ischemia, i.e., the combination of reduced oxygen content with reduced tissue blood flow. In the fetus hypoxia–ischemia commonly occurs due to hypoxic cardiac compromise. Under these conditions depletion of cerebral high-energy metabolites will occur much more rapidly and profoundly, while at the same time, there may actually be *less* acidosis, both because there is much less glucose available to be metabolized to lactate, and because the insult is evolving more quickly.

These concepts help to explain the consistent observation, discussed later in this chapter, that most cerebral injury after acute insults occurs in association with hypotension and consequent tissue hypoperfusion or ischemia. In contrast, although asphyxial brain injury by definition requires exposure to an anaerobic environment, there is only a very weak correlation between the severity of systemic acidosis and the severity of injury in any paradigm, at any age. Asphyxia is defined as the combination of impaired respiratory gas exchange (i.e., hypoxia and hypercapnia) accompanied by the development of metabolic acidosis. When we think about the impact on the brain of clinical asphyxia it will be critical to keep in mind that this definition tells us much about things that are relatively easily measured (fetal blood gases and systemic acidosis) and essentially nothing about the fetal blood pressure and perfusion of the brain, the key factors which contribute directly to the pathogenesis of brain injury.

Systemic and cardiovascular adaptation to asphyxia

The systemic adaptations of the fetus to whole-body asphyxia are critical to outcome. Although the focus of most of the classic studies in this area was to delineate the cardiovascular and cerebrovascular responses, more recently the relationship between particular patterns of asphyxia and neural outcome has been examined. The great majority of studies of the pathophysiology of asphyxia have been performed in the chronically instrumented fetal sheep, studied in utero.

Fetal adaptations and defense mechanisms

The fetus is highly adapted to intrauterine conditions, which include low partial pressures of oxygen and relatively limited supply of substrates compared with postnatal life. Although tissue myoglobin could in theory act as an oxygen store, in practice the fetus does not have appreciable tissue myoglobin levels except in the heart.[20] Myocardial myoglobin concentrations do increase in hypoxic fetuses, consistent with previous observations in postnatal animals. This appears to represent an intracellular compensatory mechanism for sustaining short-term mitochondrial oxygen delivery in a critical organ with a high rate of oxygen consumption.[21] Thus the fetus is almost entirely dependent on a steady supply of oxygen.

For the fetus, hypoxia is perhaps the greatest challenge to its well-being in utero and consequently it has many adaptive features, some unique to the fetus, which help it to maximize oxygen availability to its tissues. Thanks to these adaptations, it normally exists with a surplus of available oxygen relative to its metabolic needs. This surplus provides a significant margin of safety when oxygen delivery is impaired. These adaptive features include: higher basal blood flow to organs, left shift of the oxygen dissociation curve which increases the capacity of blood to carry oxygen and the amount of oxygen that can be extracted at typical fetal oxygen tensions, the capacity to reduce significantly energy-consuming processes, greater anaerobic capacity in many tissues, and the capacity to redistribute blood flow towards essential organs away from the periphery.

Additional structural features of the fetal circulation also augment these adaptive features including the systems of "shunts," such as the ductus arteriosus, and preferential blood flow streaming in the inferior vena cava to avoid intermixing of oxygenated blood from the placenta and deoxygenated blood in the fetal venous system. These features insure maximal oxygen delivery to essential organs such as the brain and heart. The preferential streaming patterns may be augmented during hypoxia to help maintain oxygen delivery to these organs. Thus, during hypoxia the fetus can maintain normal oxygen consumption down to the equivalent of approximately 50% of uterine artery blood flow. Under these conditions, it is able to maintain the removal of waste products of metabolism, mainly carbon dioxide and water, and thus avoids any oxygen debt and does not become acidotic.

Fetal responses to hypoxia

The response of the fetal sheep to moderate, stable hypoxia has been extensively evaluated and reviewed.[22–25] Fetal isocapnic hypoxia is typically induced by reduction of maternal inspired oxygen fraction to 10–12%. This model permits the fetal responses to changes in oxygenation to be studied separately from the effects of hypercapnia and acidosis. In the late-gestation fetus the response to this degree of hypoxia is characterized by an initial transient, moderate bradycardia followed by tachycardia and an increase in blood pressure. There is a rapid redistribution of combined ventricular output (CVO), the sum of right and left ventricular outputs, in favor of the cerebral, myocardial and adrenal vascular beds (central or vital organs) at the expense of the gastrointestinal tract, renal, pulmonary, cutaneous and skeletal beds (i.e., the periphery; Figure 4.2).[22,24] The magnitude of the hemodynamic changes largely depends upon the extent to which the arterial pH and blood gases change.[26]

The relationship between uteroplacental oxygen delivery and fetal oxygen consumption is well described, with overall fetal oxygen consumption only falling when uteroplacental blood flow falls below 50%.[27] Cerebral oxygen consumption is even more protected, and is little changed, even if arterial oxygen content falls as low as 1.5 mmol/l (compared with about 4 mmol/l in the normal fetus), thanks to the compensating increases in both cerebral blood flow (CBF) and oxygen extraction.[28] Within the brain there is a greater increase in blood flow to the brainstem compared with the cerebrum, such that oxygen delivery is fully maintained to the brainstem, but not

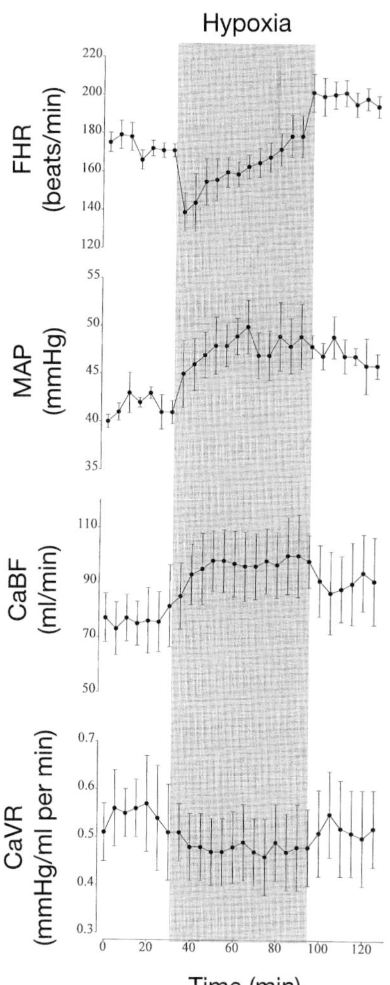

Figure 4.2 The responses in the near-term fetal sheep to moderate isocapnic hypoxia for 60 min induced by altering the maternal inspired gas mixture, showing changes in fetal heart rate (FHR), mean arterial blood pressure (MAP), carotid blood flow (CaBF), and carotid vascular resistance (CaVR). Moderate hypoxia is associated with a sustained redistribution of blood flow away from peripheral organs to essential organs such as the brain. Data derived from Bennet et al.[61]

to the cerebrum.[29] Nitric oxide (NO) has been shown to play a role in mediating the local increase in CBF.[30]

The fetal cardiovascular response to hypoxia is initially mediated via reflex responses, which are rapid in onset, and via endocrine responses, which augment these reflexes but which take much longer to become fully active. The afferent component of the reflex arc causing the initial bradycardia and increase in peripheral vasoconstriction during hypoxia is mediated by carotid chemoreceptors (chemoreflex). Hypoxia stimulates the carotid chemoreceptors, which are known to be functional in utero.[31–35] The aortic chemoreceptors do not appear to play a role in these responses, during hypoxia at least.[36] The efferent limb of the fall in fetal heart rate is mediated by muscarinic (parasympathetic) pathways as demonstrated by vagotomy[37] and blockade (atropine) studies.[38] The fall in fetal heart rate is then followed by a progressively developing tachycardia which is mediated by the increase in circulating catecholamines.[24,25]

The reflex vasoconstriction is mediated in part by α-adrenergic efferent mechanisms, since it is depressed by sympathectomy[39] and α-adrenergic blockade.[40–43] The significant increase in peripheral vasoconstriction in turn mediates the rise in blood pressure observed during hypoxia and this is augmented by circulating catecholamines released from the adrenal medulla. The rise in blood pressure during hypoxia is also at least partly mediated by increased release of other vasopressors such as arginine vasopressin[44] and angiotensin II.[45] There is also a large adrenocorticotropic and cortisol response to hypoxia.[46,47] Their role in the cardiovascular response to hypoxia is unclear, but cortisol has been shown to modulate the actions of other vasopressors.[48]

In addition to the cardiovascular responses, the fetus can also make changes to its behavior to help conserve energy. The fetus expends considerable energy making fetal breathing movements (FBMs), particularly in late gestation. In contrast to the neonate and adult, where hypoxia stimulates breathing, in the fetus hypoxia abolishes FBMs.[49]

This inhibition is mediated through activation of neural networks which either arise from, or pass through the upper pons,[50,51] and thalamus.[52] The fetus also preferentially switches to a high-voltage low-frequency electrocortical state (nonrapid eye movement sleep (NREM)) in which cerebral oxygen consumption is lower compared to the low-voltage high-frequency state or rapid eye movement (REM) sleep.[53] Similarly, the fetus suspends other energy-consuming activities such as body and limb movements.

Prolonged hypoxia

The effect of prolonged hypoxemia on cerebral metabolism in near-term fetal sheep has been studied during stepwise reductions of the maternal inspired oxygen concentration from 18% to 10–12% over four successive days.[54] Until the fetal arterial oxygen saturation was reduced to less than 30% of baseline, cerebral oxidative metabolism remained stable. At the lowest inspired oxygen concentration (with 3% CO_2) a progressive metabolic acidemia was induced. Initially, CBF increased, thus maintaining cerebral oxygen delivery as seen in acute hypoxia studies. Eventually, when the pH fell below 7.00, cerebral oxygen consumption fell to less than 50% of control values.

If mild-to-moderate hypoxia is continued, the fetus may be able to adapt fully, as measured by normalization of fetal heart rate and blood pressure and there is a return to making FBMs and body movements, but redistribution of blood flow is maintained.[54] This is consistent with the clinical situation of "brain sparing" in growth retardation. These fetuses can improve tissue oxygen delivery to near baseline levels by increasing hemoglobin synthesis, mediated by greater erythropoietin release.[55]

Maturational changes in response to hypoxia

The cardiovascular response to fetal hypoxia appears to be age-related. In the premature fetal sheep before 100 days (0.7) gestation, isocapnic hypoxia and hemorrhagic hypotension were not associated with hypertension, bradycardia, or peripheral vasoconstriction.[56,57] Thus it has been suggested that peripheral vasomotor control starts to develop at 0.7 of gestation, coincident with maturation of neurohormonal regulators and chemoreceptor function.[24,29] However, when interpreting these results it is also important to consider the degree of hypoxia in relation to the much greater anerobic capacity of the premature fetus. This is discussed below in the section on premature brain injury. It is likely that the degree of hypoxia attained in these studies did not reduce tissue oxygen availability below the critical threshold for this developmental stage.

Fetal responses to asphyxia

Studies of asphyxia by definition involve both hypoxia and hypercapnia with metabolic acidosis. It is important to appreciate that these studies of asphyxia also involve a greater depth of hypoxia than is possible using maternal inhalational hypoxia. Further, asphyxia can be induced relatively abruptly, limiting the time available for adaptation. Brief, total clamping of the uterine artery or umbilical cord leads to a rapid reduction of fetal oxygenation within a few minutes, with massive hemodynamic changes and rapid metabolic deterioration.[25,58] In contrast, gradual partial occlusion induces a slow fetal metabolic deterioration without the initial fetal cardiovascular responses of bradycardia and hypertension; this is a function of the relative hypoxia attained.[59]

The responses to moderate asphyxia are similar to those described above for hypoxia, with redistribution of blood flow to essential organs.[25] During profound asphyxia, corresponding with a severe reduction of uterine blood flow to 25% or less and a fetal arterial oxygen content of less than 1 mmol/l, the cardiovascular responses of the normal fetus are substantially different. Bradycardia is sustained and there is a generalized vasoconstriction involving essentially all organs.[25] CBF does not increase or

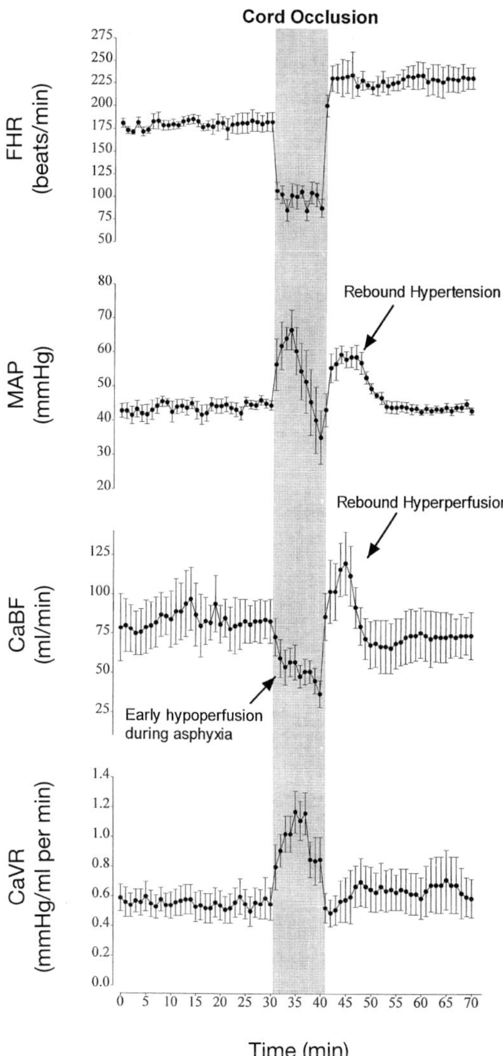

Figure 4.3 The responses in the near-term fetal sheep to complete umbilical cord occlusion for 10 min. In contrast to the response to moderate hypoxia, the profound fall in fetal heart rate (FHR) is maintained throughout the occlusion. Fetal mean arterial blood pressure (MAP) was initially elevated but then fell to below normal just prior to release. Carotid blood flow (CaBF) did not increase, and this was associated with a large increase in carotid vascular resistance (CaVR). Hypotension and hypoperfusion develop in the second half of the occlusion. Data derived from Bennet et al.[61]

may even fall despite a marked initial increase in fetal blood pressure and this is due to significantly increased cerebral vasoconstriction. Partial cord compression for 90 min, titrated to induce severe asphyxia in near-term fetal sheep, had effects similar to those following a correspondingly severe reduction of uterine perfusion.[25,60] Both methods produced similar levels of asphyxia and cerebral injury.[60] In the near-term sheep, within the brain blood flow is preferentially redirected during asphyxia to protect structures important for survival, such as the brainstem. Speculatively, this redirection may maintain autonomic function at the expense of the cerebrum.[29] Furthermore, the reduced oxygen content limits oxygen extraction from the blood. The combination of these two factors, restricted CBF and reduced oxygen extraction, profoundly restricts cerebral oxygen consumption.[25]

Figure 4.3 shows the cardiovascular and cerebrovascular responses of a near-term fetus to severe asphyxia of rapid onset. This figure demonstrates the failure of carotid blood flow (CaBF, used as an index of CBF) to increase during asphyxia in contrast to the rise seen during moderate isocapnic hypoxia (Figure 4.2). CaBF is instead briefly maintained around control values before falling. The failure of CBF to increase is not due to hypotension but rather is a function of a significant rise in cerebral vascular resistance, as demonstrated by the increase in carotid vascular resistance (Figure 4.3).[25,61] During asphyxia blood pressure initially increases markedly but as asphyxia proceeds the fetus becomes hypotensive (Figure 4.3).

The initial bradycardia and increased peripheral resistance in the late-gestation fetus during asphyxia are mediated via afferent input from the carotid chemoreceptors, leading to activation of the efferent sympathetic and parasympathetic systems respectively. Selective chemodenervation attenuates the initial rate of fall in heart rate during asphyxia, but does not abolish the bradycardia and has little effect on blood pressure,[62] providing further evidence for the operation of the vagal

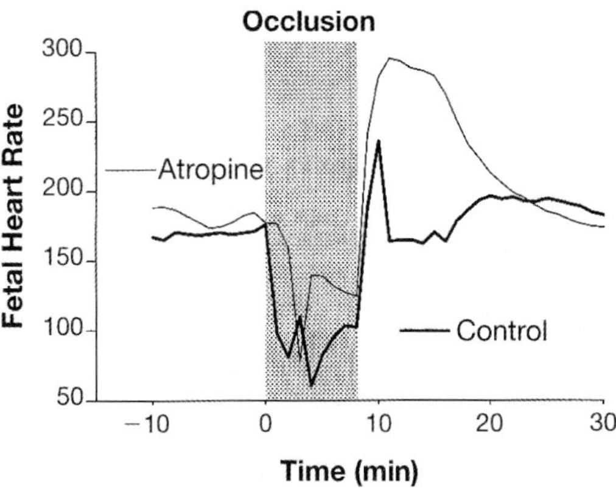

Figure 4.4 An example showing the contribution of the parasympathetic system to bradycardia during 8 min of severe asphyxia in near-term sheep fetuses. Pretreatment with atropine delayed the fall in heart rate until the third minute after the start of umbilical occlusion, in contrast with the immediate bradycardia seen in the control fetus. This abrupt, delayed fall in fetal heart rate in the atropine-treated fetus was due to transient atrioventricular blockade. This was followed by partial recovery due to resolution of the atrioventricular block, but a progressive fall from the fourth minute onward. Similar results are seen with vagotomy. Thus, the typical variable deceleration which lasts for approximately 1 min is entirely chemoreflexly mediated, whereas prolonged decelerations involve an increasing proportion of true hypoxic myocardial depression.

chemoreflexes during oxygen deprivation, but demonstrating that they are less important during profound asphyxia than moderate hypoxemia. Nevertheless, complete vagal blockade significantly delays the onset of bradycardia during umbilical cord occlusion, as shown in Figure 4.4. These data suggest that there are substantial additional afferent inputs which are not well understood at present, for example, from more significant recruitment of aortic chemoreceptors during severe hypoxia. Ultimately, with sustained severe hypoxia, fetal bradycardia does develop, despite full parasympathetic blockade or vagotomy;[24] this is consistent with clinical observations made by Caldeyro-Barcia and colleagues that late decelerations during labor are not abolished by atropine, indicating that these must be related to severe myocardial hypoxia with depletion of myocardial anaerobic stores such as glycogen.[38] Unlike moderate hypoxia where there is a progressive later rise in fetal heart rate during the insult, bradycardia is maintained. This occurs despite the logarithmic rise in circulating catecholamines and reflects both the preferential recruitment of parasympathetic input and the degree of myocardial hypoxia. Although it does not significantly alter heart rate during severe asphyxia, the sympathetic neural activation initiates the intense peripheral vasoconstriction during asphyxia and is further augmented by the subsequent rise in circulating catecholamine levels.[24]

These data indicate that the chemoreflexes which mediate the early fetal heart rate deceleration are highly sensitive indicators of hypoxemia. However, except in the case of very prolonged periods of bradycardia, they are poor indicators of fetal well-being or tolerance to hypoxia. Decelerations due to true myocardial hypoxia do not occur unless hypoxia is continued for a pathologically long time or, we may speculate, unless the fetus is chronically hypoxic with low reserves of myocardial glycogen. The depth to which fetal heart rate falls is broadly related to the severity of the hypoxia.[63] Shallow decelerations indicate a modest reduction in uteroplacental flow, while a deep deceleration indicates near total or total abolition of uteroplacental flow.[63] Unfortunately, once deep decelerations are established, there is relatively little further change in the shape of the deceleration despite repeated decelerations and the consequent development of hypotension.[64] Thus all we can say from inspecting the typical variable deceleration is that the fetus has been exposed to a brief period of deeper hypoxia.

Hypotension during profound asphyxia may occur partly as a function of loss of peripheral vasoconstriction during profound hypoxia or asphyxia (see discussion below), but is primarily related to asphyxial impairment of myocardial contractility. This is due to a direct inhibitory effect of profound acidosis and depletion of myocardial glycogen stores.[65] Once glycogen is depleted, there is rapid loss of high-energy metabolites such as ATP in mitochondria.[66] During a shorter episode, e.g., 5 min, of asphyxia, the fetus may not become hypotensive. If the insult is repeated before myocardial glycogen can be replenished, successive periods of asphyxia will be associated with increasing duration of hypotension.[67]

Another possible factor leading to impaired contractility during asphyxia is myocardial injury, which has been found after severe birth asphyxia and with congenital heart disease in limited case series.[68] Studies in adult animals have shown that there may be a significant delay in recovery of cardiac contractility after reperfusion from brief ischemia in the absence of necrosis. This delayed recovery has been termed "myocardial stunning."[69] There is some evidence that this contributes to the progressive myocardial dysfunction and to delayed recovery of heart rate after exposure to a series of repeated umbilical cord occlusions in the fetal lamb.[70]

Progressive asphyxia

During gradually induced asphyxia, even to arterial oxygen contents of less than 1 mmol/l, fetal adaptation may be closer to that seen with hypoxia. Progressive reduction of uterine perfusion over a 3–4-h period in near-term fetal sheep led to a mean pH <7.00, and serum lactate levels >14 mmol/l, with a fetal mortality of 53%. Surviving animals remained normotensive and normoglycemic, and CBF was more than doubled. Interestingly, in surviving fetuses neuronal damage was limited to selective loss of the very large, metabolically active cerebellar Purkinje cells.[59]

Uterine contractions and brief repeated asphyxia

Although the fetus can be exposed to a wide range of insults during labor, the key distinctive characteristic of labor is the development of brief intermittent, repetitive episodes of asphyxia, which is almost entirely related in some way to uterine contractions. In turn, the effects of repeated hypoxia may be amplified by fetal vulnerability, for example, due to intrauterine growth retardation and/or chronic hypoxia or by greater severity of contractions, as discussed next. Even a normal fetus, with normal placental function, may not be able to adapt fully to hyperstimulation causing brief but severe asphyxia repeated at an excessive frequency.

Uterine contractions have such a significant impact on fetal gas exchange during labor that it is worth examining their effect in detail. Contraction patterns preceding and during labor have been well described.[71] Prelabor contractions occur infrequently and reach pressures of 20–30 mmHg. Contraction frequency and intensity increase progressively during labor until contractions of up to 60 mmHg can occur every 2.5–3 min in the normal second stage. During labor maternal blood supply to the placenta has been shown to be normally reduced by uterine contractions[72] so that oxygen levels in fetal blood fall during contractions and recover once placental flow resumes.[73] Human Doppler studies have shown an almost linear relationship between the fall in uterine artery flow and a rise in intrauterine pressure from 0 to 60 mmHg. Median flow was reduced by 60% (range 48–73%) when intrauterine pressure increased by 60 mmHg.[74] The direct effect of increased pressure may be augmented by compression of the umbilical cord. Normally the cord is cushioned by amniotic fluid; however, during oligohydramnios or after rupture of the membranes the cord may be compressed between the fetus and the abdominal wall.[75,76]

Although contraction strength is important, once labor is established contraction frequency and duration are the key factors which determine the rate at which fetal asphyxia develops during labor. The proportion of time the uterus spends at resting tone compared with contracting tone will determine the extent to which fetal gas exchange can be restored between contractions.[77] Studies using near-infrared spectroscopy showed a progressive fall in cerebral oxygen saturation when contractions occurred more frequently than every 2.3 min.[78] Any intervention which increases the frequency and/or duration of uterine contractions clearly places the fetus at increased risk of asphyxia. The impact of uterine hyperstimulation or prolonged tonic contractions with oxytocin infusion used for induction or augmentation is well established.[72] Similarly, the use of prostaglandin preparations to induce labor also carries a risk of excessive uterine activity.[79,80]

During even normal labor the intermittent impairment of placental gas exchange results in a fall in pH and oxygen tension, and a rise in carbon dioxide and base deficit.[77,81] Typically, the second stage of normal labor will be the time of greatest asphyxic stress for the fetus and is accompanied by a more rapid decline in pH[81–83] and transcutaneous oxygen tension[77,83] and a rise in transcutaneous carbon dioxide tension.[83]

Thus, technically, during labor essentially all fetuses may be said to be exposed to "asphyxia." Fortunately it is usually mild and well tolerated by the fetus. Unfortunately, both the lay public and many clinicians associate the term "asphyxia" with the development of severe metabolic acidosis, post-asphyxial encephalopathy, and other end-organ damage or death. In our haste to avoid using the term, the normal nature of labor and its effects on the fetus are often not fully appreciated.

Experimental studies of brief repeated asphyxia

Brief repeated asphyxia has been produced in the fetal sheep by repeated occlusions of the umbilical cord at frequencies chosen to represent different stages of labor. For example, recent studies compared the effect of 1 min of umbilical cord occlusion repeated every 5 min (1:5 group, consistent with early labor) and 1-min occlusions repeated every 2.5 min (1:2.5 group, consistent with late first-stage and second-stage labor). Occlusions were continued for 4 h or until fetal hypotension (<20 mmHg) occurred.[64,84–88] The fetal heart rate and blood pressure changes for these two occlusion groups are shown in Figure 4.5.

1:5 occlusions series (Figure 4.5)

The onset of each occlusion was accompanied by a variable fetal heart rate deceleration and a return to baseline levels between occlusions.[88] Fetal mean arterial blood pressure (MAP) rose at the onset of each occlusion and never fell below baseline levels during the occlusions. There was a sustained elevation in baseline MAP between occlusions. A small fall in pH and rise in BD and lactate occurred in the first 30 min of occlusions (pH 7.34 ± 0.07, BD 1.3 ± 3.9 mmol/l, and lactate 4.5 ± 1.3 mmol/l), but no subsequent change occurred despite a further 3.5 h of occlusions. This experiment demonstrated the capacity of the healthy fetus to adapt fully to repeated episodes of asphyxia.

1:2.5 occlusion series (Figure 4.5)

Although this again produced a series of variable decelerations, the outcome in this group was substantially different.[64,88] The rapid occlusion frequency provided only a brief period of recovery between occlusions, which was inadequate to allow fetal reoxygenation and replenishment of glycogen stores.[66] Three phases in fetal response to occlusions were seen, as follows.

1 Initial adjustment phase, first 30 min: a progressive tachycardia developed in the interval between occlusions. During the first three occlusions, there was a sustained rise in MAP during occlusions, followed by recovery to baseline once the occlusion ended. After the third occlusion, all fetuses developed a biphasic blood pressure response to successive occlusions, with initial hypertension followed by a fall in MAP reaching a nadir a few seconds after release of the occluder. However, minimum MAP did not fall below baseline values. Over this initial 30 min pH fell from 7.40 ± 0.01 to 7.25 ± 0.02, BD rose from -2.6 ± 0.6 to 3.3 ± 1.1 mmol/l and lactate rose from 0.9 ± 0.1 to 3.9 ± 0.6 mmol/l.
2 Stable compensatory phase, mid 30 min: minimum fetal heart rate during occlusions fell ($P < 0.001$ compared to first 30 min) and interocclusion baseline rose ($P < 0.01$ compared to first 30 min). Although minimum MAP did fall at the end

of each occlusion, it never fell below baseline levels. Despite a stable blood pressure response, without hypotension, the metabolic acidosis slowly worsened: pH fell from 7.14±0.03 to 7.09±0.03, BD rose from 11.8±1.1 to 13.6±1.2 mmol/l and lactate rose from 8.2±0.8 to 9.9±0.7 mmol/l.

3 Decompensation, last 30 min: minimum fetal heart rate during decelerations continued to fall ($P<0.001$ compared to mid 30 min) but there was no further rise in interocclusion baseline fetal heart rate. Minimum MAP fell below baseline levels and the degree of hypotension became greater with successive occlusions. During the last 30 min all animals developed a severe metabolic acidosis, with pH 6.92±0.03, BD 19.2±1.46 mmol/l and lactate 14.6±0.8 mmol/l, by the end of occlusions. The studies were stopped after a mean of 183±43 min (range 140–235 min).

The key difference in outcome between the two groups was that the 1 in 2.5 group developed focal neuronal damage in the parasagittal cortex, the thalamus, and the cerebellum,[84] whereas no damage was seen in the 1 in 5 group.

Maturational changes in fetal responses to asphyxia

The fetal lambs at 90 days' gestation, prior to the onset of cortical myelination, can tolerate extended periods of up to 20 min of umbilical cord occlusion without neuronal loss.[89] The very prolonged cardiac survival (up to 30 min; Figure 4.6[90]) corresponds with the maximal levels of cardiac glycogen which are seen near midgestation in the sheep and other species, including humans.[66] Interestingly, while the premature fetal response to hypoxia appears to be different to that seen at term, the overall cardiovascular and cerebrovascular response during asphyxia was similar to that seen in more mature fetuses, with sustained bradycardia, accompanied by circulatory centralization, initial hypertension, then a progressive fall in pressure.[61,90] As also reported in the term fetus, there was no increase in blood flow to the brain during this initial phase, and again this was due to a significant increase in vascular resistance rather than to hypotension.[90] The mechanism mediating this remains speculative. As shown in Figures 4.3 and 4.6, once blood pressure begins to fall, CaBF falls in parallel. The fall in pressure is partly a function of the loss of redistribution of blood flow, as seen in Figure 4.6 with a rise in femoral blood flow (FBF). The mechanisms mediating this loss of redistribution are unknown, but are likely to relate to profound local peripheral acidosis. A similar phenomenon is also seen at term near the end of occlusion.[91]

In the latter half of a maximal interval of asphyxia in the preterm fetus, there is progressive failure of CVO, with a fall in both central and peripheral perfusion. This phase is much less likely to be seen for any significant duration in the term fetus as glycogen stores in the term fetus are depleted more quickly.[66] The term fetus is unable to survive such prolonged periods of sustained hypotension, and typically will recover from a maximum of 10–12 min of cord occlusion[61] compared with up to 30 min at 0.6 gestation.[90] As a consequence of this extended survival the premature fetus is exposed to profound and prolonged hypotension and hypoperfusion. It may be speculated that during this final phase of asphyxia in the premature fetus there is a catastrophic failure of redistribution of blood flow within the fetal brain which places previously protected areas of the brain such as the brainstem at risk of injury,[92] consistent with clinical reports.[93] Postasphyxia, a brief period of arterial hypertension and hyperperfusion is followed by a prolonged period of hypoperfusion, despite normalization of blood pressure, with a reduction in cerebral oxygenation as measured by near-infrared spectroscopy (Figure 4.7).[90] This postasphyxial hypoperfusion and reduced cerebral oxygenation may contribute to further cerebral injury.

Acute-on-chronic asphyxia

In addition to its potential impact on neurodevelopment (as outlined below), chronic asphyxia may also adversely affect the ability of the fetus to adapt to acute insults.[94] Chronic placental insufficiency leads

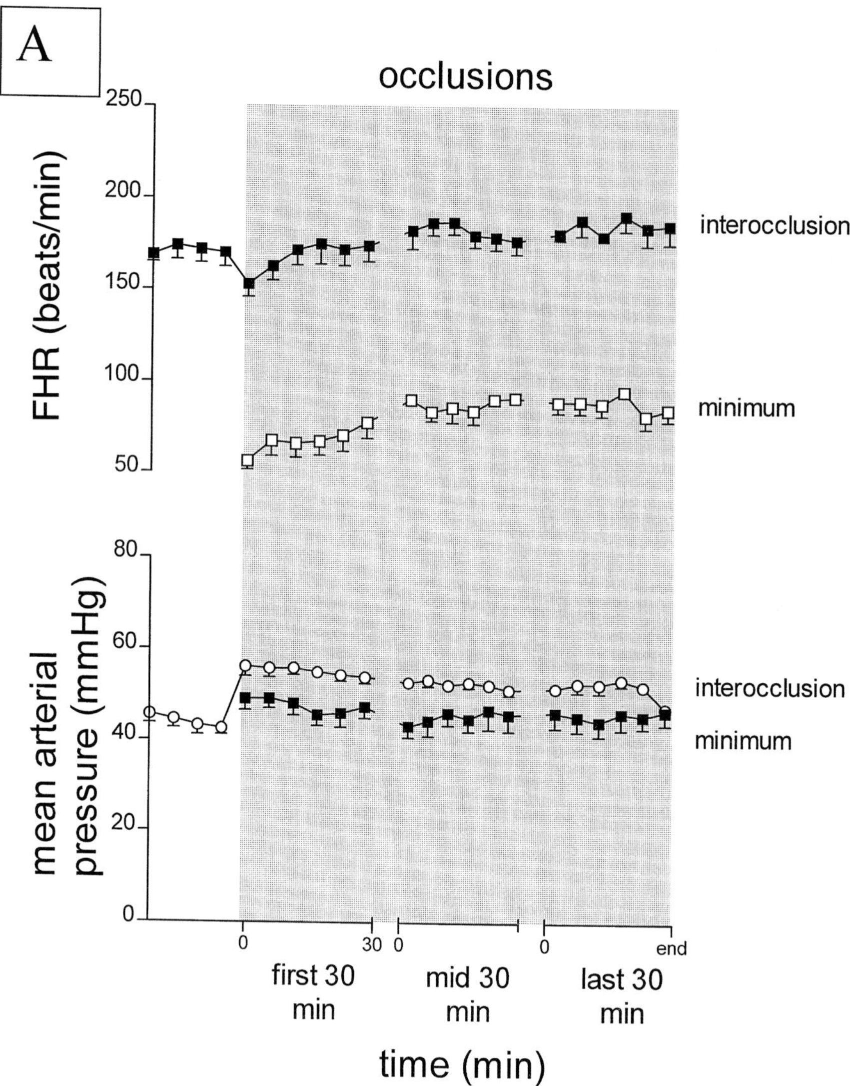

Figure 4.5 Fetal heart rate (FHR) and mean arterial pressure (MAP) changes occurring in near-term fetal sheep exposed to (A) 1 min umbilical cord occlusion repeated every 5 min for 4 h (1:5 group) and (B) 1 min occlusions repeated every 2.5 min (1:2.5 group) until fetal MAP fell <20 mmHg. The minimum FHR and MAP during each occlusion and the interocclusion FHR and MAP are shown. As the individual experiments in the 1 in 2.5 group were of unequal duration, the data in both groups are presented for three time intervals: the first 30 min, the middle 30 min (defined as the median ±15 min), and the final 30 min of occlusions.

In the 1:5 group there was no significant change in interocclusion baseline FHR, and minimum MAP during occlusions never fell below preocclusion levels. A small fall in pH and rise in base deficit (BD) and lactate occurred in the first 30 min of occlusions (pH 7.34 ± 0.07, BD 1.3 ± 3.9 mmol/l and lactate 4.5 ± 1.3 mmol/l), but no subsequent change occurred despite a further 3.5 h of occlusions. In the 1:2.5 group interocclusion FHR rose in the first and mid 30 min. Minimum MAP fell steadily in the first 30 min, stabilized in the mid 30 min, and fell progressively in the last 30 min. All animals developed a severe metabolic acidosis, with pH 6.92 ± 0.03, BD 19.2 ± 1.46 mmol/l, and lactate 14.6 ± 0.8 mmol/l by the end of occlusions. Data derived from Westgate et al.[86–88]

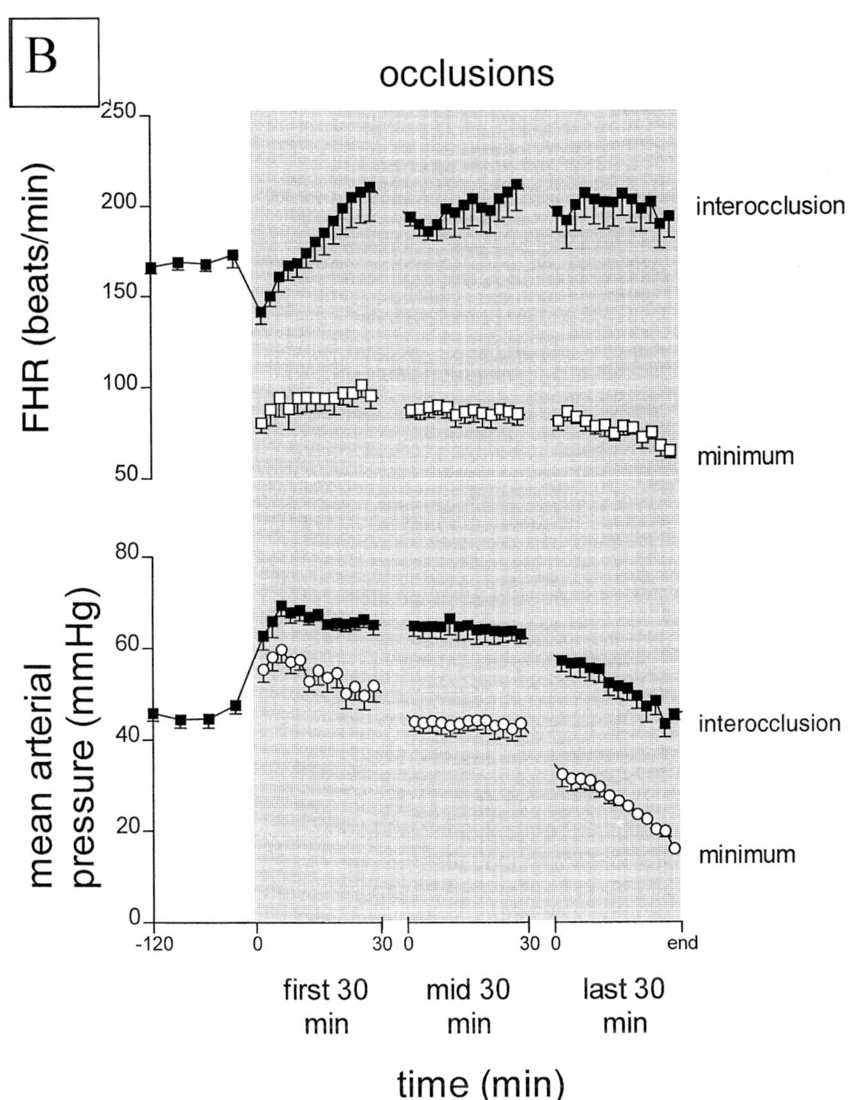
B
occlusions
FHR (beats/min)
250
200
150
100
50
interocclusion
minimum
mean arterial pressure (mmHg)
80
60
40
20
0
interocclusion
minimum
-120
0
30
0
30
0
end
first 30 min
mid 30 min
last 30 min
time (min)

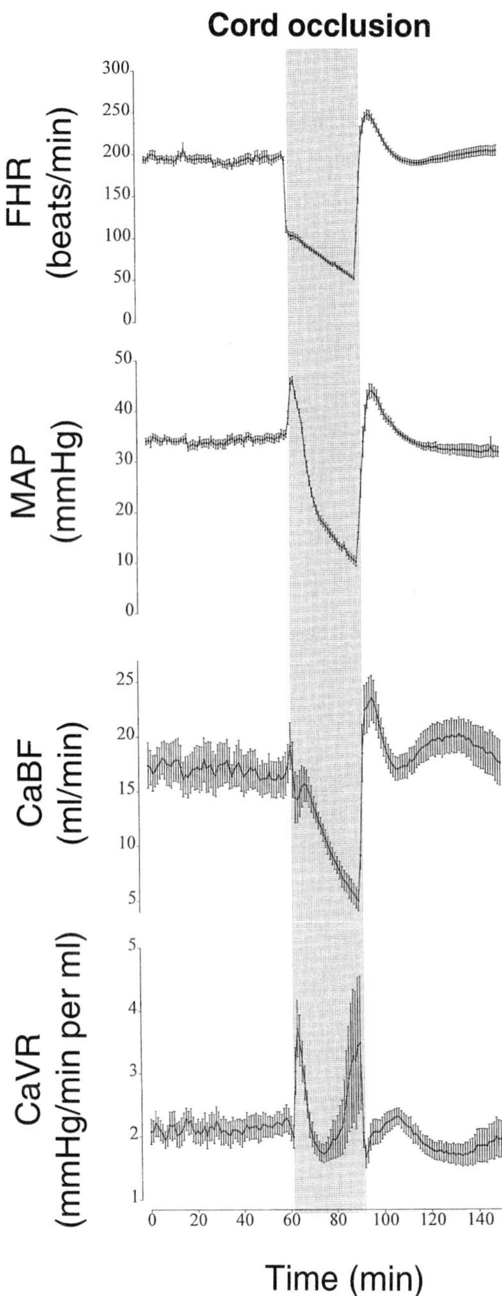

Figure 4.6 The responses of the midgestation (0.6 gestation) fetal sheep to complete umbilical cord occlusion for 30 min, showing fetal heart rate (FHR), mean arterial blood pressure (MAP), carotid blood flow (CaBF), and carotid vascular resistance (CaVR). Contrary to early reports, the overall response of the premature fetus was similar to that of the near-term fetus, with sustained bradycardia and redistribution of blood flow away from the periphery to essential organs, with initial hypertension. With continued asphyxia there was failure of adaptation with profound hypotension and hypoperfusion. The major difference with the near-term fetus (Figure 4.3) was that the premature fetus was able to survive such a prolonged period of cord occlusion. Data derived from Bennet et al.[90]

to fetal arterial hypertension and myocardial hypertrophy with increased umbilical artery resistance. Experimentally growth-retarded fetuses exhibit sustained elevation of plasma catecholamines, cortisol and prostaglandin E_2, with a significant fall in corticotropin, and when challenged with hypoxia have a blunted rise in plasma catecholamines, and cardiovascular responses in general.[94] In contrast, despite exposure to chronic hypoxia, the llama fetus does not show blunted chemoreflex responses; additional mechanisms such as increased vasopressin act to produce an intense vasoconstrictor response.[31] There are surprisingly few systematic data on the effect of chronic hypoxia on the response to labor-like insults. However, we can reasonably predict that such fetuses will have limited oxygen-carrying capacity and reduced glycogen levels, and thus will decompensate more quickly during repeated hypoxia.

Acidosis: friend or foe?

The systemic acidosis caused by asphyxia is both associated with and can exacerbate systemic fetal compromise, primarily by impairing cardiac contractility.[95] The contribution of the local tissue acidosis to neural injury however remains unclear. In vitro, acidosis limits both hypoxic and excitotoxic neuronal injury in hippocampal neurons.[96,97] It is a striking observation that in experimental studies in the fetal sheep the dorsal horn of the hippocampus

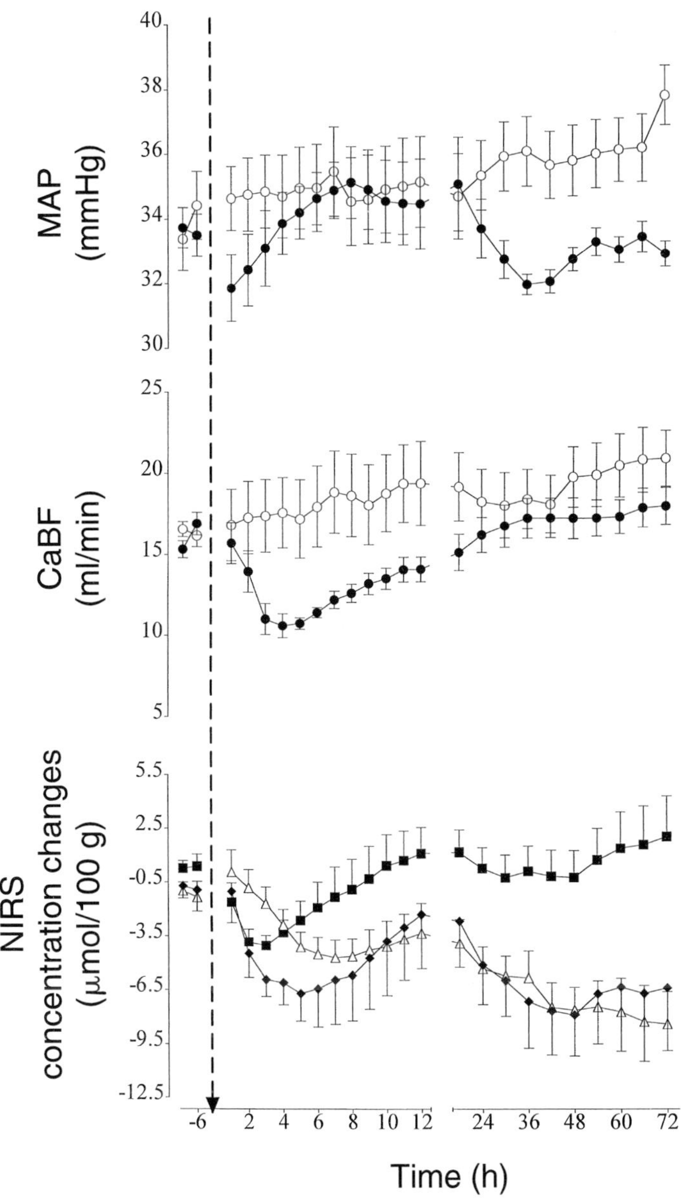

Figure 4.7 The recovery of the near-midgestation (0.6 gestation) fetal sheep following 30 min of complete umbilical cord occlusion (denoted by the heavy dashed line; for occlusion data, see Figure 4.6). In the top and middle panels, open symbols are control fetuses and closed symbols are asphyxiated fetuses. Postasphyxia carotid blood flow (CaBF) showed a secondary fall, with a nadir after 4–6 h. This secondary change was not due to a fall in mean arterial blood pressure (MAP). The near-infrared spectroscopy (NIRS) data (bottom panel) include only the asphyxia group. A similar secondary fall was seen in total cerebral hemoglobin (diamonds), which is the combination of oxyhemoglobin (squares) and deoxyhemoglobin (triangles), and provides an index of total cerebral blood volume. Significantly, this fall was mainly due to a significant reduction in cerebral oxyhemoglobin around 2–4 hours postasphyxia, suggesting a true impairment of cerebral perfusion. This may have contributed to the final injury. Data derived from Bennet et al.[90]

is very vulnerable to short periods of dense ischemia or asphyxia which cause only modest acidosis, but has been reported to be spared after both brief repeated asphyxia and prolonged partial asphyxia which are associated with profound acidosis.[84] Consistent with the hypothesis that local acidosis may protect this region, there was only a mild metabolic acidosis after 10 min of umbilical cord occlusion with severe selective loss in the cornu ammonis fields of the hippocampus (5 min after reperfusion the mean pH was >7.10),[58] whereas a very profound acidosis developed during brief repeated cord occlusions (pH 6.83 ± 0.03) but little or no hippocampal injury.[84] Further studies are clearly required to clarify the impact of acidosis on hypoxic–ischemic encephalopathy.

Pathophysiological determinants of asphyxial injury

Recent studies using well-defined experimental paradigms of asphyxia in the near-term fetal sheep have explored the relationship between the distribution of neuronal damage and the type of insult. These studies suggest that, while local cerebral hypoperfusion due to hypotension is required to cause injury, a number of factors, including the pattern of repetition of insults as well as fetal factors such as maturity, preexisting metabolic state, and cerebral temperature (Figure 4.1) markedly alter the impact of the insult on the brain.

Hypotension and the "watershed" distribution of neuronal loss

The development of hypotension appears to be the critical factor precipitating neural injury during acute asphyxia. This is readily understood, since reduced perfusion will reduce supply of glucose for anerobic metabolism, compounding the reduction in oxygen delivery and concentration. The real-life importance of hypotension is supported by both the correlation of injury with arterial blood pressure across multiple paradigms, and by the common patterns of neural damage.

The close relationship between changes in CaBF and blood pressure during asphyxia is shown in Figures 4.3, 4.6 and 4.8. In these fetuses, MAP initially rose with intense peripheral vasoconstriction. At this time CaBF was maintained. As cord occlusion was continued, MAP eventually fell, probably as a function of impaired cardiac contractility and failure of peripheral redistribution. When MAP fell below baseline, carotid blood flow fell in parallel. It appeared that there was a small window during which flow was maintained as pressure was falling (Figure 4.8), suggesting that autoregulation was intact. This is consistent with the known relatively narrow low range of fetal cerebrovasculature autoregulation.[25]

In the term fetus, neural injury has been commonly reported in areas such as the parasagittal cortex, the dorsal horn of the hippocampus, and the cerebellar neocortex after a range of insults, including pure ischemia, prolonged single complete umbilical cord occlusion, and prolonged partial asphyxia and repeated brief cord occlusion (e.g., as illustrated in the left panel of Figure 4.9).[58,59,84,98,99] These areas are "watershed" zones within the borders between major cerebral arteries, where perfusion pressure is least, and clinically lesions in these areas in adults and children are typically seen after systemic hypotension.[100]

There are some data suggesting that limited or localized white- or gray-matter injury may occur even when significant hypotension is not seen,[59,60] particularly when hypoxia is very prolonged.[101] Clearly there may have been some relative hypoperfusion in these studies. Nevertheless, there is a strong correlation between either the depth or duration of hypotension and the amount of neuronal loss within individual studies of acute asphyxia.[60,67,84,99] This is also seen between similar asphyxial paradigms causing severe fetal acidosis which have been manipulated either to cause fetal hypotension[60,99] or not.[59] In fetal lambs exposed to prolonged severe partial asphyxia, as judged by the degree of metabolic compromise, neuronal loss occurred only in those in whom one or more episodes of acute hypotension occurred.[99] In contrast,

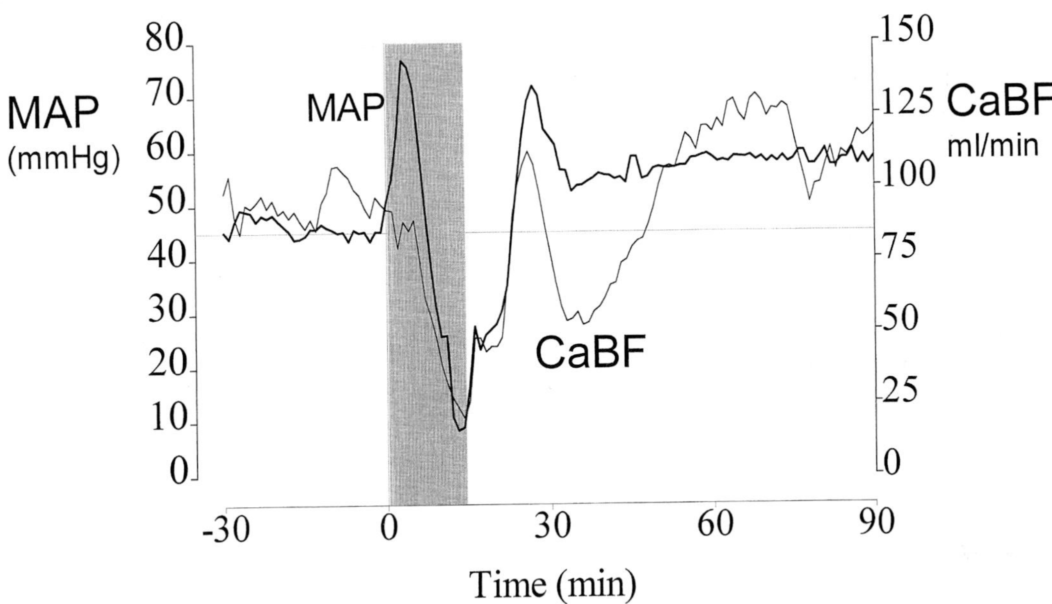

Figure 4.8 An example of the close relationship between the development of hypotension during complete umbilical cord occlusion and carotid blood flow (CaBF) during cord occlusion in a near-term fetal sheep. The period of occlusion starts at time zero, and is shown by the shaded area. Note that CaBF began to fall only when mean arterial blood pressure (MAP) was below baseline levels (shown by the dotted horizontal line), and thereafter paralleled the changes in MAP very closely.

in a similar study where an equally severe insult was induced gradually and titrated to maintain normal or elevated blood pressure throughout the insult, no neuronal loss was seen except in the cerebellum.[59]

The pattern of injury: repeated insults

The one apparent exception to a general tendency to a "watershed" distribution after global asphyxial insults in the near-term fetus is the selective neuronal loss in striatal nuclei (putamen and caudate nucleus, Figure 4.9, right panel) which develops when relatively prolonged periods of asphyxia or ischemia are repeated.[67,102] Whereas 30 min of continuous cerebral ischemia leads to predominantly parasagittal cortical neuronal loss, with only moderate striatal injury, when the insult was divided into three episodes of ischemia, a greater proportion of striatal injury was seen relative to cortical neuronal loss (Figure 4.10).[102] Intriguingly, significant striatal involvement was also seen after prolonged partial asphyxia in which distinct episodes of bradycardia and hypotension occurred.[99]

The striatum is not in a watershed zone but rather within the territory of the middle cerebral artery. It is thus likely that the pathogenesis of striatal involvement in the near-term fetus is related to the precise timing of the relatively prolonged episodes of asphyxia and not to more severe local hypoperfusion. The vulnerability of the medium-sized neurons of the striatum to this type of insult may be related to a greater release of glutamate into the striatal extracellular space after repeated insults compared with a single insult of the same cumulative duration. Consistent with this, immunohistochemical techniques have shown that inhibitory striatal neurons were primarily affected.[103]

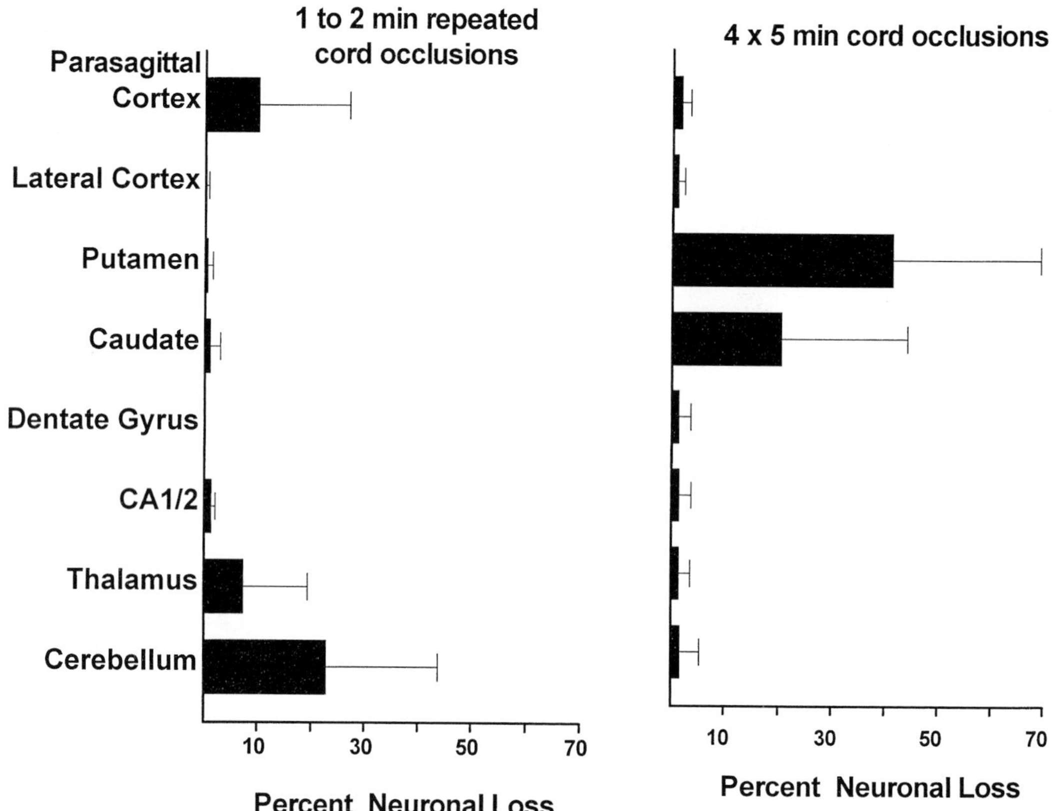

Figure 4.9 The distribution of neuronal loss assessed after 3 days' recovery from two different patterns of prenatal asphyxia in near-term fetal sheep. The left panel shows the effects of brief (1 or 2 min) cord occlusions repeated at frequencies consistent with established labor. Occlusions were terminated after a variable time, when the fetal blood pressure fell below 20 mmHg for two successive occlusions. This insult led to damage in the watershed regions of the parasagittal cortex and cerebellum.[84] The right-hand panel shows the effect of 5-min episodes of cord occlusion, repeated four times, at intervals of 30 min. This paradigm is associated with selective neuronal loss in the putamen and caudate nucleus, which are nuclei of the striatum.[67] CA1/2 and the dentate gyrus are regions of the hippocampus. Mean ± SD.

Premature brain injury: the effect of maturation

Surprisingly little work has been done to resolve the effect of maturation on sensitivity to injury. This is of critical importance, for two reasons. First, in recent years improvements in obstetric and pediatric management have resulted in significantly increased survival of preterm infants from 24 weeks of gestation, with an associated increase in later handicap.[104] Second, many infants may sustain neural injuries well before birth, including a significant number of infants with cerebral palsy.[105] The characteristic patterns of cerebral injury in the preterm fetus differ from those seen at term or after birth. Key features include preferential injury of subcortical structures and white matter.

Cortical vs subcortical grey matter

Clinical imaging data suggest that profound asphyxia before 32 weeks' gestation is associated

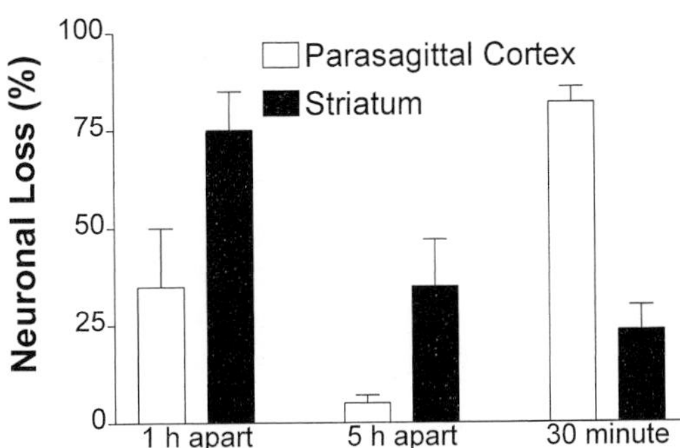

Figure 4.10 The effects of different intervals between insults on the distribution of cerebral damage after ischemia in the near-term fetal sheep. Cerebral ischemia was induced by carotid occlusion for 10 min repeated three times, at intervals of either 1 h or 5 h, compared with a single continuous episode of 30 min occlusion. The divided insults were associated with a preponderance of striatal injury, whereas a single episode of 30 min of carotid occlusion was associated with severe cortical neuronal loss. Increasing the interval to 5 h nearly completely abolished cortical injury, but was still associated with significant neuronal loss in the striatum. Data derived from Mallard et al.[102]

with injury to subcortical structures, particularly the diencephalon (including the thalamus), basal ganglia, and brainstem.[93] This is consistent with the patterns observed in infants with cerebral palsy of prenatal origin who show predominantly diencephalic lesions, variably associated with periventricular white matter damage or leukomalacia (PVL), cortical or subcortical lesions and ventricular dilatation.[106] Similarly, in fetal sheep at 0.65–0.7 gestation (96–102 days), a maturation comparable to the 28-week gestation human fetus, 30 min of cerebral ischemia induced by reversible carotid occlusion led to the development of subcortical infarction involving the deeper layers (V and VI) of the cortex, and underlying white-matter tracts.[107] In contrast, the same insult in the near-term fetal sheep leads to neuronal loss which is greatest in the superficial layers (II, II, and IV) of the cortex.

This difference is consistent with the stages of anatomical maturation. As neurons migrate into the cortex during development, the deeper layers are populated first and thus mature first, while the superficial layers include immature, migrating neurons which are less metabolically active and are still using primarily anaerobic pathways.[108] Another factor may be progressive maturation of the neuronal glutamate receptors during and after migration.[109] This is an area requiring considerably greater attention.

White-matter injury

In the very-low-birth-weight infant the distinctive white-matter lesion PVL is the major pathological associate of later developmental handicap. Key factors that have been identified include vascular development, the intrinsic vulnerability of the oligodendrocyte to neurotoxic factors, and exposure to maternal/chorionic membrane infection. PVL classically occurs in areas that represent arterial end zones or border zones.[110] Prolonged hypoperfusion due to hypotension or associated with hypocapnia may expose these areas to overt ischemia, as discussed above.

The immaturity of oligodendrocyte precursors is clearly critical, since the period of greatest risk for PVL is before myelination has begun, at a time when oligodendrocyte precursors are actively proliferating and differentiating. Such actively differentiating cells have an increased metabolic demand and are sensitive to substrate limitation. It has been suggested that developing oligodendroglia are very sensitive to the excitatory neurotransmitter glutamate and to free radical toxicity because of a developmental lack of antioxidant enzymes to mediate oxidative stress.[111]

Finally, compelling evidence has recently linked prenatal inflammation or infection to later cerebral palsy.[112] Exposure to maternal or placental infection is associated both with increased risk of preterm birth and also with brain lesions predictive of cerebral palsy.[113] It is proposed that the effect of infection is mediated by systemic inflammation since fetal plasma interleukin levels, including interleukins-1, -8, -9, tumor necrosis factor-α, and the interferons, are strongly and independently associated with PVL.[112,113]

Intraventricular hemorrhage

Intraventricular hemorrhage (IVH) with extension into the periventricular regions is also associated with adverse outcome. The white-matter injury appears to be a venous infarction with hemorrhage occurring as a secondary phenomenon. Further, there is evidence of prolonged loss of cerebrovascular autoregulation postasphyxia, which may leave the fetal brain vulnerable to factors causing fluctuations in blood pressure and thus CBF; this is proposed to be a key mechanism in the pathogenesis of IVH. Other factors that may contribute to IVH include the fragility of immature germinal matrix capillaries, deficient vascular support, and a limited vasodilatory capacity impairing perfusion during asphyxia. In this regard, the antenatal administration of glucocorticoids has been associated with a significant reduction in the sonographic incidence of severe IVH and the associated white-matter involvement. Postnatal administration of indometacin to high-risk infants has promise for reducing IVH, apparently by increasing cerebrovascular resistance.[110]

Preexisting metabolic status, and chronic hypoxia

While the original studies of factors influencing the degree and distribution of brain injury, primarily by Myers,[92] focused on metabolic status, the issue remains controversial. It has been suggested, for example, that hyperglycemia is protective against hypoxia–ischemia in the infant rat,[114] but not in the piglet.[115] The extreme differences between these neonatal species in the degree of neural maturation and activity of cerebral glucose transporters may underlie the different outcomes.[114] The most common metabolic disturbance to the fetus is intrauterine growth retardation (IUGR) associated with placental dysfunction. Although there is reasonable clinical information that IUGR is usually associated with a greater risk of brain injury, recent studies have suggested a greatly reduced rate of encephalopathy in this group over time.[6] This would suggest that the apparently increased sensitivity to injury is mostly due to reduced aerobic reserves, leading to early onset of systemic compromise during labor.

Neural maturation is markedly altered in IUGR with some aspects delayed and others advanced.[116,117] This is likely to influence the response to asphyxia but also to introduce a confounding independent effect on neural development. Severe growth retardation has been associated with altered neurotransmitter expression, reduced cerebral myelination, altered synaptogenesis, and smaller brain size.[118] The effect of the timing and severity of placental restriction has been examined in a range of studies in fetal sheep.[101] Chronic mild growth retardation due to periconceptual placental restriction was associated with delayed formation of neuronal connections in the hippocampus, cerebellum, and visual cortex, but did not alter neuronal migration or numbers. In contrast, in studies in the near-midgestation fetus, hypoxia induced by a variety of methods was associated with a reduction in numbers of Purkinje cells in the cerebellum and delayed development of neural processes. With more severe hypoxia the cortex and hippocampus were also affected and there was reduced subcortical myelination. The cerebellum develops later in gestation than the hippocampus, and thus appears to be more susceptible to the effects of hypoxia at this stage of development.[101]

Temperature and hypoxia–ischemia

Hypothermia during experimental cerebral ischemia is consistently associated with potent, dose-related,[119] long-lasting neuroprotection.[120–122] Conversely, hyperthermia of even 1–2 °C extends and markedly worsens damage,[119,123–129] and promotes pan-necrosis.[119,124] Although the majority of studies of hyperthermia have involved ischemia in adult rodents, similar results have been reported from studies of ischemia or hypoxia–ischemia in the newborn piglet and 7-day-old rat respectively.[130,131]

The impact of cerebral cooling or warming the brain by only a few degrees is disproportionate to the known changes in brain metabolism (approximately a 5% change in oxidative metabolism per °C[132]), suggesting that changes in temperature modulate the secondary factors that mediate or increase ischemic injury.[119,133] Mechanisms that are likely to be involved in the worsening of ischemic injury by hyperthermia include greater release of oxygen free radicals and excitatory neurotransmitters such as glutamate, enhanced toxicity of glutamate on neurons,[134] increased dysfunction of the blood–brain barrier,[135] and accelerated cytoskeletal proteolysis.[136]

Pyrexia in labor: chorioamnionitis and hyperthermia

These data logically lead to the concept that, although mild pyrexia during labor might not necessarily be harmful in most cases, in those fetuses also exposed to an acute hypoxic–ischemic event it would be expected to accelerate and worsen the development of encephalopathy. Case-control and case series studies strongly suggest that maternal pyrexia is indeed associated with an approximately fourfold increase in risk for unexplained cerebral palsy,[137] or newborn encephalopathy.[138–140] Similar associations are reported in premature infants.[141–143]

Clearly, this association could potentially be mediated by maternal infection or by the fetal inflammatory reaction. However, maternal pyrexia was a major component of the operational definition of chorioamnionitis in all of these studies, and in several studies pyrexia was either considered sufficient for diagnosis even in isolation, or was the only criterion used.[137–139] The most common cause of pyrexia in low-risk patients is epidural analgesia.[144] Consistent with this hypothesis, in a case-control study of 38 term infants with early-onset neonatal seizures, in whom sepsis or meningitis was excluded, and 152 controls, intrapartum fever was associated with a comparable 3.4-fold increase in the risk of unexplained neonatal seizures in a multifactorial analysis.[145]

Finally, it is very interesting to note that, although exposure to lipopolysaccharide at the time of hypoxia–ischemia in adult rats worsened injury, this effect was not seen when the lipopolysaccharide-induced hyperthermia was prevented.[129] Thus it is highly likely that at least part of the adverse effects of chorioamnionitis are simply mediated by hyperthermia.

Concluding thoughts

One of the most important issues in perinatology is to identify the fetus at risk of decompensation at an early enough stage that we may intervene and prevent actual injury or death. The ability to measure fetal pH or oxygenation at any single point in time generally provides little information about how well maintained fetal heart or brain function is at that point. Impaired gas exchange and mild asphyxia are a normal part of labor and the normal fetus has an enormous ability to respond to the consequent intervals of hypoxia/asphyxia while maintaining the function of essential organs such as the brain and the heart.

What sort of fetal problem are we trying to detect? If the fetus is being monitored in any way, there is no difficulty in detecting the prolonged bradycardia that accompanies an acute, catastrophic event of whatever cause, such as abruption or prolapse of the umbilical cord. Such events account for approximately 25% of cases of moderate-to-severe post-asphyxial encephalopathy and are seldom predictable or even potentially preventable.[6]

The major clinical problem is to identify the fetuses whose adaptation to repeated asphyxia is beginning to fail. Conceptually, the fetus can be thought of as being on a "slippery slope," as illustrated in Figure 4.11. The fetal condition or reserve determines the fetus's position on the slope, while the effectiveness of the primary defenses and the severity of the insults determine how quickly the fetus moves down the slope (decompensation). Healthy fetuses are at the very top of the slope, with considerable reserves for initial adaptation before significant hypoperfusion develops, while others start further down, closer to the final catastrophic failure of adaptation that leads to death or injury. When compensation begins to fail the pattern of the insult, modified by fetal maturity, aerobic reserve, and environmental temperature interact to determine both how serious the decompensation is, and

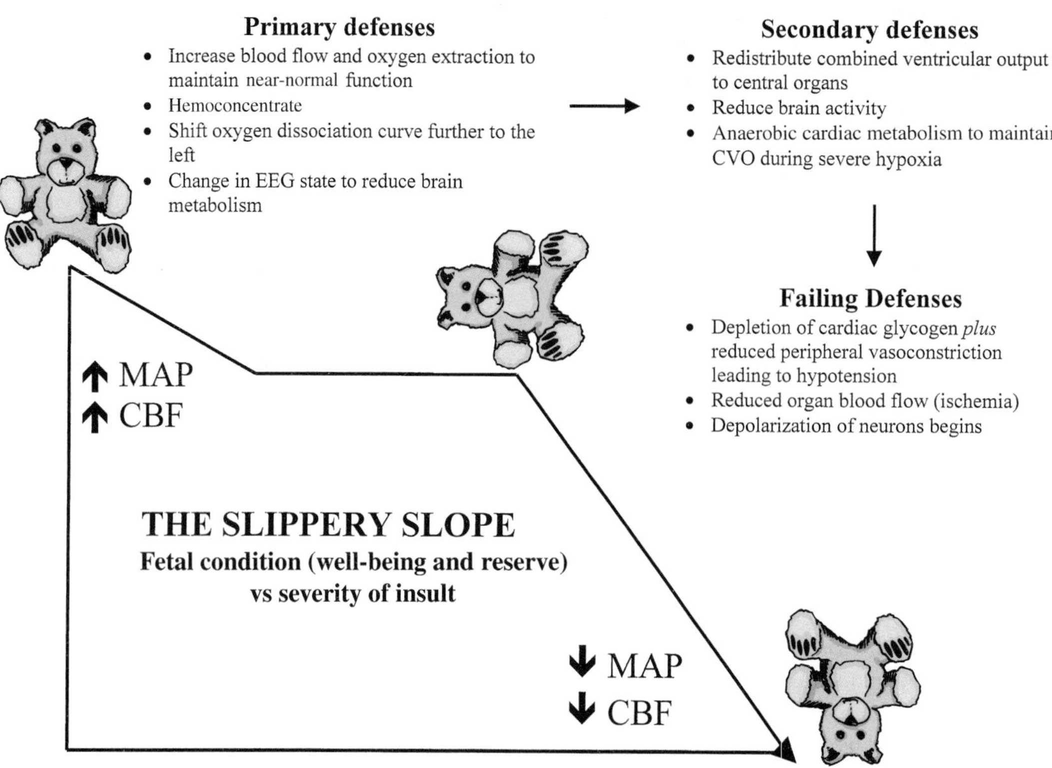

Figure 4.11 The slippery slope. A conceptual outline of fetal adaptations to episodes of asphyxia. The impact of asphyxia on the fetus depends greatly on the quality of fetal adaptation, which certainly depends partly on the severity of the insult, and how long it has continued for, but also where the fetus starts on the slope, i.e., its preexisting reserves. With a sufficiently severe insult, e.g., very frequent, more prolonged contractions, even a very healthy fetus will ultimately become profoundly acidotic and develop intermittent hypotension, but only after a prolonged period where cerebral and cardiac perfusion are maintained. In contrast, a chronically hypoxic fetus, or one that has recent exposure to hypoxia that has depleted its cardiac glycogen, may develop hypotension from very shortly after the start of the insult. EEG, electroencephalogram; CVO, combined ventricular output; MAP, mean arterial blood pressure; CBF, cerebral blood flow.

to localize any injury. With sufficient spacing between short (1-minute) periods of profound asphyxia, a healthy fetus may be able to defend its central organs almost indefinitely. In contrast, and not surprisingly, a growth-retarded or previously hypoxic fetus may have almost no reserve and begin to decompensate very early on, and yet show a similar pattern of variable decelerations to the healthy fetus.

How can we identify the fetus whose adaptations are failing? The options are limited because access to the fetus is limited. Traditionally, we try to assess fetal condition by assessing changes in fetal heart rate and occasionally fetal scalp pH measurements. Although fetal heart rate changes have an excellent negative predictive value, the positive predictive value of heart rate changes in isolation is very low. As we discuss above, the development of severe variable decelerations simply indicates transient exposure to hypoxia, regardless of whether the fetus is still in the initial stage of adaptation, or is beginning to decompensate. Delayed recovery from the decelerations with continued occlusions occurs only in a minority of fetuses, at a time that is very close to terminal hypoxic cardiac arrest.[64] Other features of decelerations may have utility. For example, overshoot of the fetal heart rate after a variable deceleration occurs invariably after longer periods of occlusion: however with more typical decelerations (up to 1 min), overshoot did not occur until fetal hypotension and acidosis had begun to develop.[85]

Similarly, both the experimental studies reviewed above and clinical experience[5] show there is, and can be, no close, intrinsic pathophysiological relationship between the severity of metabolic acidosis, and fetal compromise. Peripheral acidosis is primarily a consequence of peripheral vasoconstriction, and reflects peripheral oxygen debt which occurs during redistribution of combined ventricular output. Thus severe acidosis may accompany both successful protection of the brain and catastrophic failure.[84] Indeed, brief intense insults such as complete cord occlusion may cause brain injury with a comparatively modest acidosis.[58]

In contrast, there are very strong relationships both within and between paradigms between the development and severity of fetal blood pressure and impairment of cerebral perfusion, and the development of subsequent cerebral injury. The impact of hypotension is directly related to both its depth and cumulative duration in relationship to the brain's metabolic requirements given its developmental stage. Thus, ideally we would like to measure fetal blood pressure, but this is not feasible at present. Newer methods for fetal surveillance include fetal pulse oximetry,[146] NIRS,[61,78] more detailed analysis of the fetal electrocardiogram[86,88] and assessment of Doppler velocity waveforms.[147] Systolic time intervals, as measured by ultrasonography, are good indicators of myocardial contractility, and preliminary studies have suggested that these correlate with fetal acid–base status.[148,149] However, at present these techniques still provide only indirect measurements of the key variables, fetal blood pressure and perfusion, and require considerable further validation. As the critical events which lead to clinically significant perinatal hypoxic–ischemic encephalopathy are clarified by innovative experimental approaches, our ability to recognize significant prenatal events and to intervene appropriately will also improve.

Acknowledgments

The authors' work reported in this review has been supported by National Institutes of Health grant RO-1 HD32752, and by grants from the Health Research Council of New Zealand, Lottery Health Board of New Zealand, and the Auckland Medical Research Foundation.

REFERENCES

1 MacLennan, A. (1999). A template for defining a causal relation between acute intrapartum events and cerebral palsy: international consensus statement. *Br Med J* **319**: 1054–1059.

2 Shields, J.R. and Schifrin, B.S. (1988). Perinatal antecedents of cerebral palsy. *Obstet Gynecol* **71**: 899–905.

3 Phelan, J.P. and Kim, J.O. (2000). Fetal heart rate observations in the brain-damaged infant. *Semin Perinatol* **24**: 221–229.

4 Nelson, K.B., Dambrosia, J.M., Ting, T.Y. et al. (1996). Uncertain value of electronic fetal monitoring in predicting cerebral palsy. *N Engl J Med* **334**: 613–618.

5 Low, J.A. (1997). Intrapartum fetal asphyxia: definition, diagnosis, and classification. *Am J Obstet Gynecol* **176**: 957–959.

6 Westgate, J.A., Gunn, A.J. and Gunn, T.R. (1999). Antecedents of neonatal encephalopathy with fetal acidaemia at term. *Br J Obstet Gynaecol* **106**: 774–782.

7 Roth, S.C., Baudin, J., Cady, E. et al. (1997). Relation of deranged neonatal cerebral oxidative metabolism with neurodevelopmental outcome and head circumference at 4 years. *Dev Med Child Neurol* **39**: 718–725.

8 Hellstrom Westas, L., Rosen, I. and Svenningsen, N.W. (1995). Predictive value of early continuous amplitude integrated EEG recordings on outcome after severe birth asphyxia in full term infants. *Arch Dis Child Fetal Neonat Ed* **72**: F34–F38.

9 Robertson, C.M. and Finer, N.N. (1993). Long-term follow-up of term neonates with perinatal asphyxia. *Clin Perinatol* **20**: 483–500.

10 Rothman, S.M. and Olney, J.W. (1995). Excitotoxicity and the NMDA receptor – still lethal after eight years. *Trends Neurosci* **18**: 57–58.

11 Choi, D.W. (1995). Calcium: still center-stage in hypoxic–ischemic neuronal death. *Trends Neurosci* **18**: 58–60.

12 Bagenholm, R., Nilsson, U.A. and Kjellmer, I. (1997). Formation of free radicals in hypoxic–ischemic brain damage in the neonatal rat, assessed by an endogenous spin trap and lipid peroxidation. *Brain Res* **773**: 132–138.

13 Kuroda, S. and Siesjo, B.K. (1997). Reperfusion damage following focal ischemia: pathophysiology and therapeutic windows. *Clin Neurosci* **4**: 199–212.

14 Fowden, A.L., Forhead, A.J., Silver, M. et al. (1997). Glucose, lactate and oxygen metabolism in the fetal pig during late gestation. *Exp Physiol* **82**: 171–182.

15 Fisher, D.J., Heymann, M.A. and Rudolph, A.M. (1980). Myocardial oxygen and carbohydrate consumption in fetal lambs in utero and in adult sheep. *Am J Physiol* **238**: H399–H405.

16 Harding, R., Rawson, J.A., Griffiths, P.A. et al. (1984). The influence of acute hypoxia and sleep states on the electrical activity of the cerebellum in the sheep fetus. *Electroencephalogr Clin Neurophysiol* **57**: 166–173.

17 Koos, B.J., Sameshima, H. and Power, G.G. (1987). Fetal breathing, sleep state, and cardiovascular responses to graded hypoxia in sheep. *J Appl Physiol* **62**: 1033–1039.

18 Astrup, J., Symon, L., Branston, N.M. et al. (1977). Cortical evoked potential and extracellular K^+ and H^+ at critical levels of brain ischemia. *Stroke* **8**: 51–57.

19 Li, J., Takeda, Y. and Hirakawa, M. (2000). Threshold of ischemic depolarization for neuronal injury following four-vessel occlusion in the rat cortex. *J Neurosurg Anesthesiol* **12**: 247–254.

20 Longo, L.D., Koos, B.J. and Power, G.G. (1973). Fetal myoglobin: quantitative determination and importance for oxygenation. *Am J Physiol* **224**: 1032–1036.

21 Guiang, S.F.3, Widness, J.A., Flanagan, K.B. et al. (1993). The relationship between fetal arterial oxygen saturation and heart and skeletal muscle myoglobin concentrations in the ovine fetus. *J Dev Physiol* **19**: 99–104.

22 Giussani, D.A., Spencer, J.A.D. and Hanson, M.A. (1994). Fetal cardiovascular reflex responses to hypoxaemia. *Fetal Maternal Med Rev* **6**: 17–37.

23 Jensen, A., Garnier, Y. and Berger, R. (1999). Dynamics of fetal circulatory responses to hypoxia and asphyxia. *Eur J Obstet Gynecol Reprod Biol* **84**: 155–172.

24 Hanson, M.A. (1997). Do we now understand the control of the fetal circulation? *Eur J Obstet Gynecol Reprod Biol* **75**: 55–61.

25 Parer, J.T. (1998). Effects of fetal asphyxia on brain cell structure and function: limits of tolerance. *Comp Biochem Physiol A Mol Integr Physiol* **119**: 711–716.

26 Cohn, H.E., Sacks, E.J., Heymann, M.A. et al. (1974). Cardiovascular responses to hypoxemia and acidemia in fetal lambs. *Am J Obstet Gynecol* **15**: 817–824.

27 Wilkening, R.B. and Meschia, G. (1983). Fetal oxygen uptake, oxygenation, and acid–base balance as a function of uterine blood flow. *Am J Physiol* **244**: H749–H755.

28 Peeters, L.L., Sheldon, R.E., Jones, M.D.J. et al. (1979). Blood flow to fetal organs as a function of arterial oxygen content. *Am J Obstet Gynecol* **135**: 637–646.

29 Jensen, A. (1996). The brain of the asphyxiated fetus – basic research. *Eur J Obset Gynecol Reprod Biol* **65**: 19–24.

30 Green, L.R., Bennet, L. and Hanson, M.A. (1996). The role of nitric oxide synthesis in cardiovascular responses to acute hypoxia in the late gestation sheep fetus. *J Physiol (Lond)* **497**: 271–277.

31 Giussani, D.A., Riquelme, R.A., Moraga, F.A. et al. (1996). Chemoreflex and endocrine components of cardiovascular responses to acute hypoxemia in the llama fetus. *Am J Physiol* **271**: R73–R83.

32 Blanco, C.E., Dawes, G.S., Hanson, M.A. et al. (1984). The response to hypoxia of arterial chemoreceptors in fetal sheep and new-born lambs. *J Physiol (Lond)* **351**: 25–37.

33 Siassi, B., Wu, P.Y., Blanco, C. et al. (1979). Baroreceptor and chemoreceptor responses to umbilical cord occlusion in fetal lambs. *Biol Neonate* **35**: 66–73.

34 Itskovitz, J. and Rudolph, A.M. (1982). Denervation of arterial chemoreceptors and baroreceptors in fetal lambs in utero. *Am J Physiol* **242**: H916–H920.

35 Boekkooi, P.F., Baan, J.J., Teitel, D. et al. (1992). Chemoreceptor responsiveness in fetal sheep. *Am J Physiol* **263**: H162–H167.

36 Bartelds, B., van Bel, F., Teitel, D.F. et al. (1993). Carotid, not aortic, chemoreceptors mediate the fetal cardiovascular response to acute hypoxemia in lambs. *Pediatr Res* **34**: 51–55.

37 Barcroft, J. (1947). *Researches on Prenatal Life*, pp. 260–272. Oxford: Blackwell Scientific Publications.

38 Caldeyro-Barcia, R., Medez-Bauer, C., Poseiro, J. et al. (1966). Control of the human fetal heart rate during labour. In *The Heart and Circulation in the Newborn and Infant*, ed. D. Cassels, pp. 7–36. New York: Grune & Stratton.

39 Iwamoto, H.S., Rudolph, A.M., Mirkin, B.L. et al. (1983). Circulatory and humoral responses of sympathectomized fetal sheep to hypoxemia. *Am J Physiol* **245**: H767–H772.

40 Giussani, D.A., Spencer, J.A., Moore, P.J. et al. (1993). Afferent and efferent components of the cardiovascular reflex responses to acute hypoxia in term fetal sheep. *J Physiol (Lond)* **461**: 431–449.

41 Paulick, R.P., Meyers, R.L., Rudolph, C.D. et al. (1991).

Hemodynamic responses to alpha-adrenergic blockade during hypoxemia in the fetal lamb. *J Dev Physiol* **16**: 63–69.

42 Lewis, A.B., Donovan, M. and Platzker, A.C. (1980). Cardiovascular responses to autonomic blockade in hypoxemic fetal lambs. *Biol Neonate* **37**: 233–242.

43 Reuss, M.L., Parer, J.T., Harris, J.L. et al. (1982). Hemodynamic effects of alpha-adrenergic blockade during hypoxia in fetal sheep. *Am J Obstet Gynecol* **142**: 410–415.

44 Giussani, D.A., Riquelme, R.A., Sanhueza, E.M. et al. (1999). Adrenergic and vasopressinergic contributions to the cardiovascular response to acute hypoxaemia in the llama fetus. *J Physiol (Lond)* **515**: 233–241.

45 Green, L.R., McGarrigle, H.H., Bennet, L. et al. (1998). Angiotensin II and cardiovascular chemoreflex responses to acute hypoxia in late gestation fetal sheep. *J Physiol (Lond)* **507**: 857–867.

46 Green, J.L., Figueroa, J.P., Massman, G.A. et al. (2000). Corticotropin-releasing hormone type I receptor messenger ribonucleic acid and protein levels in the ovine fetal pituitary: ontogeny and effect of chronic cortisol administration. *Endocrinology* **141**: 2870–2876.

47 Fraser, M., Braems, G.A. and Challis, J.R. (2001). Developmental regulation of corticotrophin receptor gene expression in the adrenal gland of the ovine fetus and newborn lamb: effects of hypoxia during late pregnancy. *J Endocrinol* **169**: 1–10.

48 Tangalakis, K., Lumbers, E.R., Moritz, K.M. et al. (1992). Effect of cortisol on blood pressure and vascular reactivity in the ovine fetus. *Exp Physiol* **77**: 709–717.

49 Dawes, G.S. (1984). The central control of fetal breathing and skeletal muscle movements. *J Physiol (Lond)* **346**: 1–18.

50 Gluckman, P.D. and Johnston, B.M. (1987). Lesions in the upper lateral pons abolish the hypoxic depression of breathing in unanaesthetized fetal lambs in utero. *J Physiol (Lond)* **382**: 373–383.

51 Dawes, G.S., Gardner, W.N., Johnston, B.M. et al. (1983). Breathing in fetal lambs: the effect of brain stem section. *J Physiol (Lond)* **335**: 535–553.

52 Koos, B.J., Chau, A., Matsuura, M. et al. (1998). Thalamic locus mediates hypoxic inhibition of breathing in fetal sheep. *J Neurophysiol* **79**: 2383–2393.

53 Richardson, B.S. (1992). The effect of behavioral state on fetal metabolism and blood flow circulation. *Semin Perinatol* **16**: 227–233.

54 Richardson, B.S. and Bocking, A.D. (1998). Metabolic and circulatory adaptations to chronic hypoxia in the fetus. *Comp Biochem Physiol A Mol Integr Physiol* **119**: 717–723.

55 Kitanaka, T., Alonso, J.G., Gilbert, R.D. et al. (1989). Fetal responses to long-term hypoxemia in sheep. *Am J Physiol* **256**: R1348–R1354.

56 Iwamoto, H.S., Kaufman, T., Keil, L.C. et al. (1989). Responses to acute hypoxemia in fetal sheep at 0.6–0.7 gestation. *Am J Physiol* **256**: H613–H620.

57 Szymonowicz, W., Walker, A.M., Yu, V.Y. et al. (1990). Regional cerebral blood flow after hemorrhagic hypotension in the preterm, near-term, and newborn lamb. *Pediatr Res* **28**: 361–366.

58 Mallard, E.C., Gunn, A.J., Williams, C.E. et al. (1992). Transient umbilical cord occlusion causes hippocampal damage in the fetal sheep. *Am J Obstet Gynecol* **167**: 1423–1430.

59 de Haan, H.H., Van Reempts, J.L., Vles, J.S. et al. (1993). Effects of asphyxia on the fetal lamb brain. *Am J Obstet Gynecol* **169**: 1493–1501.

60 Ikeda, T., Murata, Y., Quilligan, E.J. et al. (1998). Physiologic and histologic changes in near-term fetal lambs exposed to asphyxia by partial umbilical cord occlusion. *Am J Obstet Gynecol* **178**: 24–32.

61 Bennet, L., Peebles, D.M., Edwards, A.D. et al. (1998). The cerebral hemodynamic response to asphyxia and hypoxia in the near- term fetal sheep as measured by near infrared spectroscopy. *Pediatr Res* **44**: 951–957.

62 Jensen, A. and Hanson, M.A. (1995). Circulatory responses to acute asphyxia in intact and chemodenervated fetal sheep near term. *Reprod Fertil Dev* **7**: 1351–1359.

63 Itskovitz, J., LaGamma, E.F. and Rudolph, A.M. (1983). Heart rate and blood pressure responses to umbilical cord compression in fetal lambs with special reference to the mechanism of variable deceleration. *Am J Obstet Gynecol* **147**: 451–457.

64 de Haan, H.H., Gunn, A.J. and Gluckman, P.D. (1997). Fetal heart rate changes do not reflect cardiovascular deterioration during brief repeated umbilical cord occlusions in near-term fetal lambs. *Am J Obstet Gynecol* **176**: 8–17.

65 Rosen, K.G., Hrbek, A., Karlsson, K. et al. (1986). Fetal cerebral, cardiovascular and metabolic reactions to intermittent occlusion of ovine maternal placental blood flow. *Acta Physiol Scand* **126**: 209–216.

66 Shelley, H.J. (1961). Glycogen reserves and their changes at birth and in anoxia. *Br Med Bull* **17**: 137–143.

67 de Haan, H.H., Gunn, A.J., Williams, C.E. et al. (1997). Magnesium sulfate therapy during asphyxia in near-term fetal lambs does not compromise the fetus but does not reduce cerebral injury. *Am J Obstet Gynecol* **176**: 18–27.

68 Donnelly, W.H. (1987). Ischemic myocardial necrosis and papillary muscle dysfunction in infants and children. *Am J Cardiovasc Pathol* **1**: 173–188.

69 Ferrari, R. (1995). Metabolic disturbances during myocardial ischemia and reperfusion. *Am J Cardiol* **76**: 17B–24B.
70 Gunn, A.J., Maxwell, L., de Haan, H.H. et al. (2000). Delayed hypotension and subendocardial injury after repeated umbilical cord occlusion in near-term fetal lambs. *Am J Obstet Gynecol* **183**: 1564–1572.
71 Caldeyro-Barcia, R., Medez-Bauer, C., Poseiro, J. et al. (1966). Control of the human fetal heart rate during labour. In *The Heart and Circulation in the Newborn and Infant*, ed. D. Cassels, pp. 7–36. New York: Grune & Stratton.
72 Brotanek, V., Hendricks, C.H. and Yoshida, T. (1969). Changes in uterine blood flow during uterine contractions. *Am J Obstet Gynecol* **103**: 1108–1116.
73 Jansen, C.A., Krane, E.J., Thomas, A.L. et al. (1979). Continuous variability of fetal Po_2 in the chronically catheterized fetal sheep. *Am J Obstet Gynecol* **134**: 776–783.
74 Janbu, T. and Nesheim, B.I. (1987). Uterine artery blood velocities during contractions in pregnancy and labour related to intrauterine pressure. *Br J Obstet Gynaecol* **94**: 1150–1155.
75 Grubb, D.K. and Paul, R.H. (1992). Amniotic fluid index and prolonged antepartum fetal heart rate decelerations. *Obstet Gynecol* **79**: 558–560.
76 Shields, L.E. and Brace, R.A. (1994). Fetal vascular pressure responses to nonlabor uterine contractions: dependence on amniotic fluid volume in the ovine fetus. *Am J Obstet Gynecol* **171**: 84–89.
77 Huch, A., Huch, R., Schneider, H. et al. (1977). Continuous transcutaneous monitoring of fetal oxygen tension during labour. *Br J Obstet Gynaecol* **84**: 1–39.
78 Peebles, D.M., Spencer, J.A., Edwards, A.D. et al. (1994). Relation between frequency of uterine contractions and human fetal cerebral oxygen saturation studied during labour by near infrared spectroscopy. *Br J Obstet Gynaecol* **101**: 44–48.
79 Gunn, T.R. and Wright, I.M. (1996). The use of black and blue cohosh in labour. *N Z Med J* **109**: 410–411.
80 Winkler, M. and Rath, W. (1999). A risk–benefit assessment of oxytocics in obstetric practice. *Drug Safety* **20**: 323–345.
81 Modanlou, H., Yeh, S.Y. and Hon, E.H. (1974). Fetal and neonatal acid–base balance in normal and high-risk pregnancies: during labor and the first hour of life. *Obstet Gynecol* **43**: 347–353.
82 Weber, T. and Hahn-Pedersen, S. (1979). Normal values for fetal scalp tissue pH during labour. *Br J Obstet Gynaecol* **86**: 728–731.
83 Katz, M., Lunenfeld, E., Meizner, I. et al. (1987). The effect of the duration of the second stage of labour on the acid–base state of the fetus. *Br J Obstet Gynaecol* **94**: 425–430.
84 de Haan, H.H., Gunn, A.J., Williams, C.E. et al. (1997). Brief repeated umbilical cord occlusions cause sustained cytotoxic cerebral edema and focal infarcts in near-term fetal lambs. *Pediatr Res* **41**: 96–104.
85 Westgate, J.A., Bennet, L., de Haan, H.H. et al. (2001). Fetal heart rate overshoot during repeated umbilical cord occlusion in sheep. *Obstet Gynecol* **97**: 454–459.
86 Westgate, J.A., Bennet, L., Brabyn, C. et al. (2001). ST waveform changes during repeated umbilical cord occlusions in near-term fetal sheep. *Am J Obstet Gynecol* **184**: 743–751.
87 Westgate, J.A., Bennet, L. and Gunn, A.J. (1999). Fetal heart rate variability changes during brief repeated umbilical cord occlusion in near term fetal sheep. *Br J Obstet Gynaecol* **106**: 664–671.
88 Westgate, J.A., Gunn, A.J., Bennet, L. et al. (1998). Do fetal electrocardiogram PR-RR changes reflect progressive asphyxia after repeated umbilical cord occlusion in fetal sheep? *Pediatr Res* **44**: 297–303.
89 Keunen, H., Blanco, C.E., Van Reempts, J.L. et al. (1997). Absence of neuronal damage after umbilical cord occlusion of 10, 15, and 20 minutes in midgestation fetal sheep. *Am J Obstet Gynecol* **176**: 515–520.
90 Bennet, L., Rossenrode, S., Gunning, M.I. et al. (1999). The cardiovascular and cerebrovascular responses of the immature fetal sheep to acute umbilical cord occlusion. *J Physiol (Lond)* **517**: 247–257.
91 Jensen, A., Hohmann, M. and Kunzel, W. (1987). Dynamic changes in organ blood flow and oxygen consumption during acute asphyxia in fetal sheep. *J Dev Physiol* **9**: 543–559.
92 Myers, R.E. (1977). Experimental models of perinatal brain damage: relevance to human pathology. In *Intrauterine Asphyxia and the Developing Fetal Brain*, ed. L. Gluck, pp. 37–97. Chicago: Year Book Medical.
93 Barkovich, A.J. and Sargent, S.K. (1995). Profound asphyxia in the premature infant: imaging findings. *Am J Neuroradiol* **16**: 1837–1846.
94 Hanson, M.A. (1998). Role of chemoreceptors in effects of chronic hypoxia. *Comp Biochem Physiol A Mol Integr Physiol* **119**: 695–703.
95 Fisher, D.J. (1986). Acidemia reduces cardiac output and left ventricular contractility in conscious lambs. *J Dev Physiol* **8**: 23–31.
96 Tombaugh, G.C. (1994). Mild acidosis delays hypoxic spreading depression and improves neuronal recovery in hippocampal slices. *J Neurosci* **14**: 5635–5643.
97 Giffard, R.G., Monyer, H., Christine, C.W. et al. (1990). Acidosis reduces NMDA receptor activation, glutamate neurotoxicity, and oxygen-glucose deprivation neuronal injury in cortical cultures. *Brain Res* **506**: 339–342.

98 Gunn, A.J., Gunn, T.R., de Haan, H.H. et al. (1997). Dramatic neuronal rescue with prolonged selective head cooling after ischemia in fetal lambs. *J Clin Invest* **99**: 248–256.

99 Gunn, A.J., Parer, J.T., Mallard, E.C. et al. (1992). Cerebral histological and electrophysiological changes after asphyxia in fetal sheep. *Pediatr Res* **31**: 486–491.

100 Torvik, A. (1984). The pathogenesis of watershed infarcts in the brain. *Stroke* **15** : 221–223.

101 Rees, S., Mallard, C., Breen, S. et al. (1998). Fetal brain injury following prolonged hypoxemia and placental insufficiency: a review. *Comp Biochem Physiol* **119**: 653–660.

102 Mallard, E.C., Williams, C.E., Gunn, A.J. et al. (1993). Frequent episodes of brief ischemia sensitize the fetal sheep brain to neuronal loss and induce striatal injury. *Pediatr Res* **33**: 61–65.

103 Mallard, E.C., Waldvogel, H.J., Williams, C.E. et al. (1995). Repeated asphyxia causes loss of striatal projection neurons in the fetal sheep brain. *Neuroscience* **65**: 827–836.

104 Kiely, J.L. and Susser, M. (1992). Preterm birth, intrauterine growth retardation and perinatal mortality. *Am J Public Health* **82**: 343–344.

105 Stanley, F.J. (1992). Survival and cerebral palsy in low birthweight infants: implications for perinatal care. *Paediatr Perinatal Epidemiol* **6**: 298–310.

106 Volpe, J.J. (1995). Hypoxic–ischemic encephalopathy: neuropathology and pathogenesis. In *Neurology of the Newborn*, ed. J.J. Volpe, pp. 279–313. Philadelphia: W.B. Saunders Company.

107 Reddy, K., Mallard, C., Guan, J. et al. (1998). Maturational change in the cortical response to hypoperfusion injury in the fetal sheep. *Pediatr Res* **43**: 674–682.

108 Hansen, A. (1977). Extracellular potassium concentration in juvenile and adult rat brain cortex during anoxia. *Acta Physiol. Scand.* **99**: 412–420.

109 Gressens, P., Marret, S. and Evrard, P. (1996). Developmental spectrum of the excitotoxic cascade induced by ibotenate: a model of hypoxic insults in fetuses and neonates. *Neuropathol Appl Neurobiol* **22**: 498–502.

110 Perlman, J.M. (1998). White matter injury in the preterm infant: an important determination of abnormal neurodevelopment outcome. *Early Hum Dev* **53**: 99–120.

111 Rivkin, M.J., Flax, J., Mozell, R. et al. (1995). Oligodendroglial development in human fetal cerebrum. *Ann Neurol* **38**: 92–101.

112 Nelson, K.B., Dambrosia, J.M., Grether, J.K. et al. (1998). Neonatal cytokines and coagulation factors in children with cerebral palsy. *Ann Neurol* **44**: 665–675.

113 Dammann, O. and Leviton, A. (1997). Maternal intrauterine infection, cytokines, and brain damage in the preterm newborn. *Pediatr Res* **42**: 1–8.

114 Vannucci, S.J., Maher, F. and Simpson, I.A. (1997). Glucose transporter proteins in brain: delivery of glucose to neurons and glia. *Glia* **21**: 2–21.

115 LeBlanc, M.H., Huang, M., Vig, V. et al. (1993). Glucose affects the severity of hypoxic–ischemic brain injury in newborn pigs. *Stroke* **24**: 1055–1062.

116 Cook, C.J., Gluckman, P.D., Williams, C.E. et al. (1988). Precocial neural function in the growth retarded fetal lamb. *Pediatr Res* **24**: 600–604.

117 Stanley, O., Fleming, P. and Morgan, M. (1989). Abnormal development of visual function following intrauterine growth retardation. *Early Hum Dev* **19**: 87–101.

118 Kramer, M.S., Olivier, M., McLean, F.H. et al. (1990). Impact of intrauterine growth retardation and body proportionality on fetal and neonatal outcome. *Pediatrics* **86**: 707–713.

119 Busto, R., Dietrich, W.D., Globus, M.Y. et al. (1987). Small differences in intraischemic brain temperature critically determine the extent of ischemic neuronal injury. *J Cereb Blood Flow Metab* **7**: 729–738.

120 Green, E.J., Dietrich, W.D., Van Dijk, F. et al. (1992). Protective effects of brain hypothermia on behavior and histopathology following global cerebral ischemia in rats. *Brain Res* **580**: 197–204.

121 Nurse, S. and Corbett, D. (1994). Direct measurement of brain temperature during and after intraischemic hypothermia: correlation with behavioral, physiological, and histological endpoints. *J Neurosci* **14**: 7726–7734.

122 Dietrich, W.D., Busto, R., Alonso, O. et al. (1993). Intraischemic but not postischemic brain hypothermia protects chronically following global forebrain ischemia in rats. *J Cereb Blood Flow Metab* **13**: 541–549.

123 Dietrich, W.D., Busto, R., Valdes, I. et al. (1990). Effects of normothermic versus mild hyperthermic forebrain ischemia in rats. *Stroke* **21**: 1318–1325.

124 Minamisawa, H., Smith, M.L. and Siesjo, B.K. (1990). The effect of mild hyperthermia and hypothermia on brain damage following 5, 10, and 15 minutes of forebrain ischemia. *Ann Neurol* **28**: 26–33.

125 Chen, H., Chopp, M. and Welch, K.M. (1991). Effect of mild hyperthermia on the ischemic infarct volume after middle cerebral artery occlusion in the rat. *Neurology* **41**: 1133–1135.

126 Chen, Q., Chopp, M., Bodzin, G. et al. (1993). Temperature modulation of cerebral depolarization during focal cerebral ischemia in rats: correlation with ischemic injury. *J Cereb Blood Flow Metab* **13**: 389–394.

127 Haraldseth, O., Gronas, T., Southon, T. et al. (1992). The effects of brain temperature on temporary global

ischaemia in rat brain. A 31-phosphorous NMR spectroscopy study. *Acta Anaesthesiol Scand* **36**: 393–399.

128 Wass, C.T., Lanier, W.L., Hofer, R.E. et al. (1995). Temperature changes of > or = 1 degree C alter functional neurologic outcome and histopathology in a canine model of complete cerebral ischemia. *Anesthesiology* **83**: 325–335.

129 Thornhill, J. and Asselin, J. (1998). Increased neural damage to global hemispheric hypoxic ischemia (GHHI) in febrile but not nonfebrile lipopolysaccharide *Escherichia coli* injected rats. *Can J Physiol Pharmacol* **76**: 1008–1016.

130 Laptook, A.R., Corbett, R.J., Sterett, R. et al. (1994). Modest hypothermia provides partial neuroprotection for ischemic neonatal brain. *Pediatr Res* **35**: 436–442.

131 Yager, J., Towfighi, J. and Vannucci, R.C. (1993). Influence of mild hypothermia on hypoxic-ischemic brain damage in the immature rat. *Pediatr Res* **34**: 525–529.

132 Laptook, A.R., Corbett, R.J.T., Sterett, R. et al. (1995). Quantitative relationship between brain temperature and energy utilization rate measured in vivo using ^{31}P and ^{1}H magnetic resonance spectroscopy. *Pediatr Res* **38**: 919–925.

133 Towfighi, J., Housman, C., Heitjan, D.F. et al. (1994). The effect of focal cerebral cooling on perinatal hypoxic–ischemic brain damage. *Acta Neuropathol Berl* **87**: 598–604.

134 Suehiro, E., Fujisawa, H., Ito, H. et al. (1999). Brain temperature modifies glutamate neurotoxicity in vivo. *J Neurotrauma* **16**: 285–297.

135 Dietrich, W.D., Busto, R., Halley, M. et al. (1990). The importance of brain temperature in alterations of the blood–brain barrier following cerebral ischemia. *J Neuropathol Exp Neurol* **49**: 486–497.

136 Ginsberg, M.D. and Busto, R. (1998). Combating hyperthermia in acute stroke: a significant clinical concern. *Stroke* **29**: 529–534.

137 Grether, J.K. and Nelson, K.B. (1997). Maternal infection and cerebral palsy in infants of normal birth weight. *JAMA* **278**: 207–211.

138 Adamson, S.J., Alessandri, L.M., Badawi, N. et al. (1995). Predictors of neonatal encephalopathy in full-term infants. *Br Med J* **311**: 598–602.

139 Badawi, N., Kurinczuk, J.J., Keogh, J.M. et al. (1998). Intrapartum risk factors for newborn encephalopathy: the Western Australian case-control study. *Br Med J* **317**: 1554–1558.

140 Lieberman, E., Lang, J., Richardson, D.K. et al. (2000). Intrapartum maternal fever and neonatal outcome. *Pediatrics* **105**: 8–13.

141 Alexander, J.M., Gilstrap, L.C., Cox, S.M. et al. (1998). Clinical chorioamnionitis and the prognosis for very low birth weight infants. *Obstet Gynecol* **91**: 725–729.

142 O'Shea, T.M., Klinepeter, K.L., Meis, P.J. et al. (1998). Intrauterine infection and the risk of cerebral palsy in very low-birthweight infants. *Paediatr Perinat Epidemiol* **12**: 72–83.

143 Grether, J.K., Nelson, K.B., Emery, E.S.3 et al. (1996). Prenatal and perinatal factors and cerebral palsy in very low birth weight infants. *J Pediatr* **128**: 407–414.

144 Lieberman, E., Lang, J.M., Frigoletto, F.J. et al. (1997). Epidural analgesia, intrapartum fever, and neonatal sepsis evaluation. *Pediatrics* **99**: 415–419.

145 Lieberman, E., Eichenwald, E., Mathur, G. et al. (2000). Intrapartum fever and unexplained seizures in term infants. *Pediatrics* **106**: 983–988.

146 Luttkus, A.K. and Dudenhausen, J.W. (1996). Fetal pulse oximetry. *Baillieres Clin Obstet Gynaecol* **10**: 295–306.

147 Damron, D.P., Chaffin, D.G., Anderson, C.F. et al. (1994). Changes in umbilical arterial and venous blood flow velocity waveforms during late decelerations of the fetal heart rate. *Obstet Gynecol* **84**: 1038–1040.

148 Lewinsky, R.M. (1994). Cardiac systolic time intervals and other parameters of myocardial contractility as indices of fetal acid–base status. *Baillieres Clinical Obstet Gynaecol* **8**: 663–681.

149 Koga, T., Athayde, N. and Trudinger, B. (2001). The fetal cardiac isovolumetric contraction time in normal pregnancy and in pregnancy with placental vascular disease: the first clinical report using a new ultrasound technique. *Br J Obstet Gynaecol* **108**: 179–185.

5

Congenital malformations of the brain

Ronald J. Lemire

University of Washington School of Medicine, Seattle, WA, USA

Embryonic stages and brain malformations

The central nervous system (CNS) is one of the earliest to begin development in the human embryo and does not complete maturation until several years after birth when myelination is complete. The embryonic period encompasses 23 stages that are completed approximately 2 months following fertilization. These developmental stages, frequently referred to as the Carnegie stages, provide a precise morphological framework for following development and are helpful in determining the timing of many abnormalities of the brain and spinal cord in humans. The definitive account of embryonic development was published by O'Rahilly and Müller[1] who refined and updated previous work on the Carnegie embryo collection. Additional clarification of staging and prenatal ages has also been provided.[2] They have recently added a detailed account of the development of the human brain during the embryonic period[3] and this reference, along with the older work of Lemire et al.,[4] provides specific information about the development of the human CNS. Table 5.1 outlines a general framework of features related to the embryonic stages and Table 5.2 provides selected information on brain development.

A useful concept in assessing the timing of human malformations is that of a "termination period,"[5] a point in time beyond which a specific malformation cannot occur. For example, in humans the rostral neuropore closes in embryonic stage 11. Anencephaly is felt to arise in most cases when the neuropore fails to close. The termination period for anencephaly is therefore stage 11 (24 days after fertilization) and as such suspected teratogenic agents acting at a later time (e.g., radiation at 35 days) should be held responsible for the defect. When possible it is helpful to relate such concerns to the stage of development to eliminate them as causation.

Closure of the neural tube

The manner in which the neural tube closes in the human embryo has been of interest to clinicians and scientists. It was always thought that there was one site of initial closure over the hindbrain and that the closure then proceeded rostrally and caudally. In 1993 Van Allen et al.[6] raised the question of multisite closure based on clinical observations. The importance of resolving this issue is directed toward being able to determine the timing of onset of neural tube defects. O'Rahilly and Müller recently stated that "there is at present no embryological evidence in the human that a specific pattern of multiple sites of closure exists, such as has been described in the mouse."[7] This has been largely supported by a recent review of the Japanese human embryo collection by Nakatsu and Shiota,[8] although they did propose a variation of initial fusion sites.

Anencephaly and neural tube defects

Anencephaly encompasses the spectrum of the most severe malformations of the brain.[9] There are many different forms of anencephaly phenotypically but all stem from problems arising before or

Table 5.1. Stages of human embryonic development

Stage	Size (mm)	Age (days)	Representative features
1		1	Fertilization
2		2–3	Two- to 16-cell stage
3		4	Blastocyst
4		5–6	Blastocyst attaching to uterine wall
5	0.1–0.2	7–12	Implantation
6	0.2	13	Primitive streak
7	0.4	16	Notochordal process
8	1.0–1.5	18	Neural plate, neurenteric canal
9	1.5–2.5	20	One to 3 somites, neural folds
10	2–3.5	22	Four to 12 somites, first fusion of neural folds
11	2.5–4.5	24	13–20 somites, rostral neuropore closes
12	3–5	26	21–29 somites, caudal neuropore closes
13	4–6	28	Arm and leg limb buds
14	5–7	32	Optic cup, lens invagination
15	7–9	33	Cerebral vesicles, hand developing
16	8–11	37	Retinal pigment, foot developing
17	11–14	41	Finger rays
18	13–17	44	Toe rays, nipples appear
19	16–18	48	Trunk straightening, limbs extend straight
20	18–22	50	Elbows bent
21	22–24	52	Vascular plexus on head one-half distance
22	23–28	54	Hand overlap
23	27–31	56	Hand erect, scalp plexus near vertex

Table 5.2. Selected features in the development of the human embryonic brain

Stage	Brain
7–8	Neural plate/groove
9	Neural folds, three rhombomeres
10	Optic primordium; fusion of rhombencephalic folds; cranial flexture
11	Rostral neuropore closes; acousticofacial complex; optic vesicle; primordium of corpus striatum
12	Hindbrain roof thins; cerebellar plate
13	Three divisions of trigeminal nerve; pontine flexture; olfactory placode
14	Oculomotor nerve; hypothalamic sulcus; roots of CN5–10 formed
15	Cerebral vesicles appear; striatal ridge; CN-4 decussate
16	Infundibulum; subthalamic nucleus
17	Frontal and parietal lobe areas; choroid fissure closes; posterior commissure
18	Choroid plexus in fourth ventricle; superior and inferior colliculi; caudate nucleus
19	Choroid plexus in lateral ventricle; putamen; occipital pole area present; first fibers in internal capsule
20	Tentorium begins laterally; nerve fiber layer in retina
21	Choroid plexus in third ventricle
22	Anlage of denate nucleus; superior colliculus
23	Temporal pole area present

during human embryonic stage 11. To understand its importance, anencephaly must be viewed within the spectrum of neural tube defects (NTDs) which have been the subject of intensive epidemiologic investigations for many years.

There are three general types of NTDs that arise during primary neurulation in the human embryo (Table 5.3).[10] In the event that there is failure of the initial fusion of the neural folds during embryonic stage 10, the result is termed craniorachischisis. If the neural tissue of both the brain and spinal cord are completely exposed there is usually early fetal demise. However some cases of craniorachischisis are born and then undergo postnatal death, usually within hours. Because of the appearance of the face and brain they are usually diagnosed as anencephaly and from the taxonomic standpoint are indeed considered within this spectrum. The second primary neurulation defect is anencephaly where the cranium is open but not the spine. Anencephaly is subdivided into meroacrania where only the cranial vault is open and holoacrania in which the defect extends through the foramen magnum. This distinction is of questionable importance. The final

Table 5.3. Primary neurulation neural tube defects (NTDs) in humans

Stage(s)	Normal event	Mechanism	Resulting NTD
8	Neural plate	Nonfolding	Craniorachischisis
9	Neural folds	Nonfolding	Craniorachischisis
10	First fusion of neural folds	Nonfusion	Craniorachischisis
11	Closure of rostral neuropore	Failure of closure	Anencephaly
12	Closure of caudal neuropore	Failure of closure	Meningomyelocele

NTD that arises during primary neurulation is the myelocele (meningomyelocele) which arises if the caudal neural folds or neuropore fail to close before or during stage 12.

Some infants with anencephaly are born alive and live for days, occasionally even weeks. This usually presents a problem for parents, nursery personnel, and neonatologists because the outcome is hopeless. Some of these infants have purposeful movements, regular respiratory and cardiovascular patterns, crying sounds, and the ability to swallow. In some instances these infants' organs have been used for transplantation. However, a significant proportion of these organs are malformed or hypoplastic.[11,12]

The neuropathology of anencephaly is variable depending on gestational age and extent of the lesion. The cerebral hemispheres may be absent or rudimentary and tissue is softened with blood infiltration. Islands of choroid plexus and neuroglial cells can be present. The brainstem has variable preservations of nuclei; the pyramidal tracts are absent or markedly reduced. While the eyes may have a normal appearance, externally they frequently lack a central connection.

Until recently the prevalence of NTDs has averaged about 1/1000 deliveries but geographically wide variations exist.[13] The highest rates were found in Ireland (4.6–6.7/1000), South Wales (3.55), Liverpool (3.15), Scotland (2.59), Egypt (3.75), and Lebanon (3.05). Low prevalence rates occurred in Colombia (0.1), Norway (0.2), France (0.5), and Japan (0.6). There has been an ongoing search for the factors responsible for anencephaly. Penrose[14] described eight different genetic mechanisms that might be considered. Most studies show a predominance of females. Infectious agents have been suspected based on an increase in NTDs associated with influenza epidemics but in most such epidemics no increase occurred. Blighted potatoes, religion, hardness of water, migration–ethnic factors, and intergenerational influences have all been investigated. Seasonal and secular trends have provided no important answers. There seems to be an association of NTDs in people of lower socioeconomic status within a given population. Of clinical importance is the association of the anticonvulsant valproic acid with spina bifida but not anencephaly. Maternal hyperthermia has been suspected as being associated with some cases.[15,16]

Although the prevalence of anencephaly is approximately 1/2000 live births, there is as much as a 100-fold increase in risk among mothers who have had a previous child with this condition. Early prenatal screening programs were initially directed toward this latter group. Mothers who had a previous child with an NTD received an amniocentesis during the 14th–16th week of pregnancy for amniotic fluid α-fetoprotein determination. This glycoprotein is produced by the fetal liver, is in high concentration during that period of gestation, and gains access to the amniotic fluid by vessels in the exposed neural tissue. Now the more widespread use of ultrasound and maternal serum α-fetoprotein determinations have extended the prenatal NTD diagnostic capabilities to a larger population. In recent years there has been a successful effort to eradicate NTDs with periconceptional dietary supplementation of folic acid. The Medical Research Council Vitamin Study Research Group in the UK showed that there was a 72% protective effect if folic acid supplementation was started before pregnancy[17] and presently there is a recommendation that all women who are planning to get pregnant supplement their diet with 0.4 mg of folic acid daily.[18,19] A recent study reviewed regulations in 12 countries and found the recommended daily consumption of folates to be between 0.4 and 1.0 mg when planning a pregnancy.[20] Efforts to identify genes that predispose to NTDs have been made through linkage analysis and candidate gene analysis of families with increased risk for NTDs. Early studies have not been successful but this approach is regarded as promising.[21,22]

Encephalocele

Cephalocele, cranium bifidum, and cranial meningoceles have all been used to describe what is more commonly referred to as encephalocele. In the usual case there is herniation of intracranial structures through a defect in the skull to form a sac covered by intact skin. When the prolapse involves meninges only the term cranial meningocele is used whereas when cerebral or cerebellar tissue is present, it is called encephalocele. Other terms are found in the literature but are variations on this theme. These include meningoencephalocele, encephalocystocele, ventriculocele, hydranencephalocele, and encephalocystomeningocele.

The classification of encephaloceles undergoes further division based on location such as occipital, parietal, or anterior. Anterior encephaloceles are classified as sincipital (if they are visible) or basal (if prolapse is through the base of the skull and cannot be seen). Division of encephaloceles is important because of the varying etiologies, prevalence, prognosis, and associated malformations.[23]

Unfortunately many epidemiological studies have included encephalocele within the classification of NTD that are associated with anencephaly and meningomyelocele. As previously mentioned, the latter two arise during primary neurulation whereas encephaloceles occur later. This has clouded some of the data relative to prevalence but it is probable that they occur in 1/2000 to 1/5000 live births. They are more common in oriental and African countries.[24] Topographical distributions are observed, with the ratio of frontal to occipital being about 1:6 in the USA but 1:1 in Africa. In spontaneous abortions the prevalence of encephalocele was 1/154 fetuses (17 in 2620 cases) but there were probably some artifacts.[25] Nevertheless, it is reasoned that a large number of cases with encephalocele undergo fetal demise. There appears to be a female predominance in occipital encephalocele.

Occipital encephalocele

There is still a question as to the pathogenesis of encephalocele. An experimental study in stage 26 chick embryos made a strong argument that decompression of the ventricle in a postneurulation period of rapid brain growth did not allow mesodermal repair and was associated with a high prevalence of encephalocele.[26] Regarding occipital encephalocele, Emery and Kalhan[27] proposed that a focal blowout of cerebral tissue occurs following development of mesoderm tissue overlying a closed neural tube. Based on pathological observations a small amount of cerebral tissue is initially prolapsed with a larger herniation occurring later in gestation. In an experimental study where encephalocele was induced in hamster embryos, Marin-Padilla[28] found fenestrations of the neuroectoderm associated with cranial changes and proposed that a primary mesodermal deficiency is the fundamental defect – that this arises because of an insufficient amount of supporting mesodermal tissue.

Occipital encephalocele has varying clinical presentations from a very small aperture in the skull to one that is extremely large encompassing the foramen magnum and the posterior arch of the atlas. There may be enough cerebral contents prolapsed into the sac that the head is microcephalic with the size of the encephalocele exceeding that of the skull. Cortical tissue within the sac may show hemorrhagic infarction and portions of lateral ventricles may be prolapsed. The cerebellum may be partly within the sac or even absent.[29] Some cases of iniencephaly apertus are associated with occipital encephalocele. This fatal condition has enlargement of the foramen magnum, retroflexion of the head on the spine and spina bifida of numerous vertebrae. These infants are either stillborn or die early in the neonatal period.

Symptoms are variable depending on the size and nature of the defect. Occipital encephalocele may be asymptomatic but if the ventricular system is involved, hydrocephalus can occur. Seizures, blindness, ocular palsies, laryngeal stridor, and weakness are common.

A well-known condition with occipital encephalocele is Meckel syndrome (Meckel–Gruber syndrome). Associated malformations include polydactyly, polycystic kidneys, congenital heart defects, eye defects, cleft palate, and ambiguous genitalia. The pituitary gland may be absent and adrenal hypoplasia is common. Additional features include microcephaly, absence of the corpus callosum and septum pellucidum, and craniosynostosis. This monogenic condition can be differentiated from trisomy 13 (which it can resemble) by normal karyotype. Eye abnormalities include microphthalmos, cryptophthalmos, microcornea, partial aniridia, and cataract.[30] Frequently patients with Meckel syndrome die shortly after birth.

Other conditions associated with occipital encephalocele include dyssegmental dysplasia, Knobloch syndrome, pseudo-Meckel syndrome, warfarin embryopathy, and associations with clefting, ectrodoctyly, hemifacial microsomia, holoprosencephaly, and meningomyelocele.[31]

The mortality rates vary according to the size of the lesion and contents of the sacs. If no hydrocephalus is present and the sacs only have a small amount of glial tissue there is 2% mortality, but with hydrocephalus it is 29%.[32] Nearly all patients who have a massive encephalocele and microcephaly die. The presence of brain tissue within the sac and hydrocephalus are also adverse factors in those patients that live. Mental retardation, seizures, blindness, deafness, and spasticity are all more common in this group than those with minor lesions.

Aside from a careful neurological examination, the diagnosis of these lesions can be enhanced by the use of computed tomography (CT) and magnetic resonance imaging (MRI) studies. Consideration of the condition of the infant and the results of the imaging studies permits an approach to therapy to be formulated. In the case of a massive encephalocele with a large amount of cerebral tissue and associated hydrocephalus there may be no attempt to resect the lesion, especially if the infant is experiencing neonatal distress. In contrast there is no urgency to resect small encephaloceles unless there is hydrocephalus, and ventriculoperitoneal shunting is needed. Careful neurological follow-up and developmental assessment are needed in all cases.

Anterior encephalocele

As previously mentioned anterior, encephaloceles are referred to as sincipital if visible, and basal if they cannot be seen. Sincipital encephaloceles are of three types:

1 frontoethmoidal, which can be in the midline at the root of the nose (nasofrontal), on one or both sides of the nose (nasoethmoidal), or at the superior medial angle of the orbital cavity displacing the eye laterally (nasoorbital)
2 interfrontal (between the frontal bones) or
3 appearing as a craniofacial cleft

There are five types of basal encephalocele:

1 sphenoorbital, which enters the orbit causing exophthalmous
2 sphenomaxillary, which presents in the pterygopalatine fossa
3 transethmoidal, presenting in the anterior nasal fossae
4 sphenoethmoidal, presenting in the posterior nasal fossae and
5 sphenopharyngeal, in the rhinopharynx and sphenoid sinus[24]

Sincipital encephalocele is common in Burma, India, and Thailand with a prevalence of about 1/3500 to 1/6000 live births. The frequency in the USA is much less but has not been accurately determined presumably because occipital encephalocele is more common. In addition the pathogenesis of these lesions is poorly understood but they probably arise because of insufficient mesodermal tissue in the areas of prolapse. Unusual associations are found, such as with a large lipoma overlying the corpus callosum.[33] Basal encephalocele is even less well understood as many can remain undetected for long periods after birth. One such case of a 29-year-old was recently reported with associated moyamoya disease.[34] A prevalence of 1/35 000 live births has been given[35] and there are varying theories of pathogenesis depending on the location.[36] A frequent clinical presentation is a small swelling at the base of the nose which may progress in size and can be cystic or solid. Ocular hypertelorism is sometimes present and problems with breathing or vision may be accompanying symptoms. Swelling of the eyelids can occur as well as sixth-nerve palsies. Clinically an enlarged metopic fontanel can be confused with encephalocele, as can congenital subgaleal cysts over the anterior fontanel. Diagnosis can be clarified by CT scan or MRI.

Holoprosencephaly

Holoprosencephaly encompasses a spectrum of CNS anomalies that result from impaired midline cleavage of the embryonic forebrain.[37] The prosencephalon fails to cleave into cerebral hemispheres (sagittally), into telencephalon and diencephalon (transversely), and into olfactory and optic bulbs (horizontally). Depending upon the severity, most holoprosencephaly cases are classified into alobar, semilobar, or lobar. Clinicians dealing with newborns over the past 30 years have been quicker to recognize the significance of certain facies and the correlation with holoprosencephaly because of the classic publication of DeMyer et al.[38] These facies are currently classified as cyclopia, ethmocephaly, cebocephaly, median cleft facies, and less severe facial dysmorphism.

The prevalence of holoprosencephaly is about 0.6/10000 live births[39,40] and among induced abortions is about 40/10000.[41] However, the live birth data are open to questions as the study by Roach et al.[42] concerns only nonchromosomal holoprosencephaly and therefore is probably an underestimate.[37] Interestingly, the sex ratio for alobar holoprosencephaly is a 3:1 female predilection but for lobar holoprosencephaly it is 1:1. Holoprosencephaly is associated with trisomy 13 syndrome, deletion 13q and deletion 18p syndromes, as well as autosomal recessive and autosomal dominant inheritance. Although several teratogens have been suggested to be associated with holoprosencephaly none have been widely accepted. Infants of diabetic mothers seem to be at a greater risk.[43] A curious association exists between the facies of holoprosencephaly and anencephaly.[44,45]

The neurological examination of infants with holoprosencephaly has wide variations. Muscle tone may be normal, decreased, or increased: spasticity and opisthotonus can be present. Deep tendon reflexes may be normal, absent, or increased; the Moro reflex has similar variability. Sensation is usually normal. Except for a weak suck in some patients, most cranial nerves can be normal. The exception is the eyes, which can have nystagmus, variable pupillary response, and dysconjugate movements. Patients on the more severe end of the spectrum of holoprosencephaly tend to have more abnormalities.

Examinations (physical and roentgenological) of the child may show many malformations, especially when associated with trisomies. Umbilical hernia, omphalocele, polydactyly, abnormal dermatoglyphics, abnormal lobation of lungs, numerous anomalies of the cardiovascular system (especially ventricular and atrial septal defects), malrotation of the intestine, and renal malformations are all found. The pituitary gland may be absent or hypoplastic and hypoplasia of the thyroid and adrenal glands is common.

Atelencephaly and aprosencephaly

Atelencephaly is a rare condition in which derivatives of the telencephalon are absent or dysplastic. When a more extensive form occurs involving the diencephalon, the term aprosencephaly is applied. The latter can be associated with holoprosencephalic facies and when it occurs in a syndromic form it is termed XK-aprosencephaly.[46–48] Atelencephaly was extensively studied in a 21-week human fetus.[49,50] This condition is usually fatal and can be diagnosed prenatally by ultrasound.

Microcephaly

Microcephaly is a term that is applied to heads whose circumference is smaller than three standard deviations (SD) below the mean for age and sex,[24] although some studies have used 2 SD.[51,52] Corrections must also take intrauterine growth retardation[53] and low birth weight into account.[54] Plotting the head circumference can be misleading if it is not corrected for body length. The reason for concern about microcephaly is that there can be a correlation with future intelligence. Classifications of microcephaly have been made, but for the purposes of clinical medicine there only needs to be a distinction between primary (microcephalia vera) and secondary (microcephalia spuria). In the former the brain is damaged during prenatal life whereas the secondary microcephalies reflect an unfound event during the neonatal period or infancy.

Over the past 60 years it has been accepted that genetic and environmental factors can cause microcephaly (small skull) and micrencephaly (small brain). Chromosomal and gene aberrations are both associated with small brains. Nearly every chromosome has been identified with deletions or trisomies that are associated with microcephaly.[24,55] Down syndrome is a well-known part of this grouping.

Historically the true microcephalies were attributed to autosomal recessive inheritance. In these cases the brain and skull are abnormally small but the remainder of the body and organ systems are normal. Parental consanguinity has been a conspicuous part of this literature.

Environmental factors associated with microcephaly include prenatal radiation, maternal rubella, cytomegalic inclusion disease, toxoplasmosis, herpes simplex virus (type 2), fetal alcohol syndrome, and fetal hydantoin syndrome. Microcephaly is also found associated with many syndromes; most are genetic as previously noted, but also in others such as deLange syndrome. It is the conspicuous finding in atelencephalic microcephaly where the frontal lobes are absent in an intact calvarium.[49,50]

Hydrocephalus

Hydrocephalus has been defined in many ways and clinicians are familiar with the terms "communicating versus noncommunicating" (depending on whether the cerebrospinal fluid (CSF) flow passes out of the ventricular system or not) or "obstructive" (when CSF resorption is impaired by hemorrhage of infection). Other designations include "internal hydrocephalus" (CSF is within the ventricular space) or "external" (when the abnormal fluid is within the subdural space around the brain). When there has been cerebral hypoplasia or atrophy the phrase "hydrocephaly ex vacuo" is frequently used.

The prevalence of neonatal hydrocephalus around the world varies from 1/256 to 1/9000 live births. Stevenson et al.[56] made a study of 24 centers for the World Health Organization and provided an overall estimate of 1/1150 live births. These data are old, and with diagnosis now being made with prenatal ultrasound, and elective termination of pregnancy, new prevalence figures are needed. Many cases of hydrocephalus are associated with myelomeningocele. With prenatal ultrasound, α-fetoprotein (amniotic fluid and maternal serum) determinations, and periconceptional folic acid supplementation there appears to be a reduced prevalence in cases of myelomeningocele. Two more recent studies have cited a prevalence of hydrocephalus of 0.81/1000 live births[57] and 0.70/1000,[58] which are close to Stevenson's numbers.

When the intrauterine diagnosis of hydrocephalus is made it requires careful coordination between the obstetrician and the postnatal care providers. In earlier times sacrificing the fetus to save the mother was occasionally practiced, although there were strong ethical objections. Today many couples choose to have the child delivered by cesarean section (if the head is too large to deliver vaginally).

Hydrocephalus can be hereditary and the X-linked recessive form with aqueductal stenosis is perhaps the best known, although it accounts for a very small percentage of cases. There have been cases where dominant inheritance is suspected and hydrocephalus is also associated with some known autosomal dominant conditions (e.g., achondroplasia, tuberous sclerosis). There have been many reports of families in which hydrocephalus is present but no clear pattern of inheritance was determined.[24] Concordance of hydrocephalus has been reported in both monozygotic and dizygotic twins. Among the environmental factors responsible for hydrocephalus are toxoplasmosis and cytomegalic inclusive disease, both of which can also cause microcephaly.

Chiari II malformation

There is nearly a constant association of hydrocephalus in patients with meningomyelocele and Chiari II malformations. Many hypotheses have been set forth to explain the link between the intracranial abnormalities and the spinal lesion but none has been universally accepted. Hydrocephalus is but one part of a complicated malformation complex that involves forebrain, midbrain, and hindbrain. The underlying abnormality in Chiari II malformation is caudal displacement of the posterior lobe of the vermis of the cerebellum into the foramen magnum and upper cervical spinal canal. Forebrain abnormalities consist of abnormal cortex with polymicrogyria, thinning of white matter, anomalous septum pellucidum, and an enlarged massa intermedia. Midbrain anomalies include beaked tectum fusion of the colliculi and stenosis or atresia of the cerebral aqueduct. The hindbrain anomalies include kinking of the medulla and with the caudal displacement there is upward angulation of cranial and upper cervical nerves. Cysts and nodules in the roof of the fourth ventricle have recently been reported.[59] The fourth ventricle is slit-like and there are no lateral recesses. Syringobulbia, hydromyelia, syringomyelia, and disordered myelination patterns are frequently present. The cranium usually has a small posterior fossa with loss of the inner table and craniolacunae. There is vernicomyelia in the leptomeninges and heterotopias. The dural reflections have hypoplasia of the tentorium and falx cerebri. This is in addition to the spinal lesion, which includes the meningomyelocele, hemivertebrae, and diastematomyelia.[60–65] Hydrocephalus is a major part of the Chiari II malformation and postnatally about 80% of these infants require a ventriculoperitoneal shunt to decrease the intracranial pressure and provide a route for the flow of CSF that cannot be adequately drained from the ventricular system. Some patients required surgical bony decompression of the hindbrain because of apnea, cranial nerve palsies, and dysphagia.[66]

Meningomyelocele occurs at embryonic stage 12 and there is no real definition of hindbrain and cerebellum at that stage. It is therefore difficult to explain the strong association with Chiari II malformation.[67] Several hypotheses have been postulated regarding the pathogenesis of this malformation. A "traction theory" proposed that there is tethering of the dysplastic spinal cord to the vertebrae and as the fetus develops the hindbrain structures are caudally displaced through the foramen magnum. Observations of the angulations of cervical and thoracic nerves in fetuses with Chiari II malformation have shown that, if traction does occur, it is dissipated within a few segments.[68] An experimental study testing this hypothesis also failed to produce this malformation.[69]

Another popular hypothesis is that hydrocephalus causes pressure from above and pushes the cerebellum through the foramen magnum. Some patients with Chiari II do not develop significant hydrocephalus and also the presence of squamous cells and lanugo hair in the central canal and subarachnoid spaces in cases with meningomyelocele and Chiari II malformations – implying an upward flow of CSF – would be against the above idea.[70] Leakage from the meningomyelocele has also been proposed as the pathogenetic factor[58] and, with the cervical medullary kinking, this provides another possibility.[63] Daniel and Strich[61] felt that the primary problem might be a failure of the pontine flexure to form, and Peach[64] expanded this hypothesis to include a developmental arrest prior to the formation of the pontine flexure. Barry et al.[68] postulated that overgrowth of the cerebellum and medulla in a small posterior fossa caused their protrusion through the foramen magnum, whereas Padget[71] believed the Chiari II to arise from a premature approximation of the primordia of the cerebellum in a small posterior fossa. A new hypothesis was proposed by Jennings et al.[72] who felt the initial event was caudal displacement of the initial site of fusion of the neural folds such that the brain cord transition zone would be displaced caudally. None of these hypotheses explains all of the findings in Chiari II and the pathogenesis remains unknown. As previously mentioned, the strange dissociation in the timing of onset of meningomyelocele and Chiari II and their nearly constant associations in the newborn is of extreme interest to those who have attempted to solve this problem.

Dandy–Walker malformations

Some newborns with Dandy–Walker malformation present with hydrocephalus and an increased head circumference while others may appear externally normal. Other cystic lesions of the posterior fossa can be confused with Dandy–Walker malformation. These include cerebellar hypoplasia, agenesis of the cerebellar vermis, and retrocerebellar arachnoid cyst.[73]

Dandy–Walker malformation is a cystic dilation of the fourth ventricle associated with hypoplasia and lateral displacement of the cerebellar hemispheres. It may or may not be associated with atresia of the foramina of Luschka or Magendie. Clinical presentation depends on the severity of the associated hydrocephalus and among the more severe cases there can be associated malformations in over 50%.[74] These include microcephaly, encephalocele, syringomyelia, gyral malformations, agenesis of the corpus callosum, and a variety of anomalies besides the nervous system. It is found in association with Aase–Smith, Coffin–Siris, cryptophthalmos, Ehlers–Danlos, Jones, Joubert and Walker-Warburg syndromes.[75]

Other associations

Many other conditions are associated with neonatal hydrocephalus but will not be discussed. These include tumors such as retinoblastoma and cystic teratoma,[76] teratomas, astrocytomas, medulloblastomas, and choroid plexus papillomas,[77] and craniopharyngioma.[78] Vascular malformations such as aneurysms of the vein of Galen compressing the cerebral aqueduct can cause hydrocephalus.

Megalencephaly

An infant's head can be enlarged because the brain is too big and this can cause a problem during delivery. In some cases such as Sotos syndrome (cerebral gigantism) the large head is associated with a large body.[79] The terms megalencephaly and macrencephaly are synonymous and can be applied to large brains, as contrasted with macrocephaly, which denotes a large head from whatever cause (such as in hydrocephalus). Dekaban and Sakuragawa[80] reviewed previous classifications and then divided megalencephaly into three main categories and various subgroups:

I Primary megalencephaly
- (i) with normal body build and no systemic disease
- (ii) associated with specific endocrine disorders
- (iii) associated with achondroplasia
- (iv) familial

II Secondary megalencephaly, associated with
- (i) specific storage disease or disturbance of metabolism
- (ii) degenerative CNS disease
- (iii) intoxications (lead)
- (iv) neurocutaneous disorders

III Unilateral megalencephaly, either with or without body asymmetry

Megalencephaly is therefore a heterogeneous condition associated with many syndromes or metabolic problems. To standardize the definition the head circumference must be over 2.5 SD above the mean corrected for age and sex. Some have included achondroplasia among their classifications while others have not.[80] Because of the numerous other conditions that can cause the brain to be of abnormal size (e.g., storage diseases) there is a high incidence of mental retardation associated with a large head in addition to spasticity, seizures, and failure to thrive. Familial megalencephaly has an excellent prognosis in most cases.

There are a number of syndromes with megalencephaly. Riley and Smith[81] described a family in which the mother and two children had macrocephaly, pseudopapilledema, and multiple hemangiomas; two others had the macrocephaly and pseudopapilledema only. Bannayan[82] described a similar syndrome with megalencephaly, angiomatosis, and lipomatosis. It differs from the previous syndrome by the presence of lipomatosis and absence of pseudopapilledema. Other syndromes have been recorded by Salmon and Flanigan[83] and DeMyer.[84] There was an association of a case of megalencephaly with 47XYY karyotype.[85] While not present at birth, megalencephaly is also present in Tay–Sachs disease, Canavan disease, Alexander disease and Shilder disease. A large number of cases of unilateral megalencephaly have been reported and a case was diagnosed in a fetus of 20 weeks' gestation.[86] It has also been found associated with linear sebaceous nevus syndrome.[87] Powell et al.[88] reported 27 children with a dominant inheritance of megalencephaly which was associated with a carnitine-deficient myopathy.

Hydranencephaly

Hydranencephaly is a severe brain malformation in which the cerebral hemispheres are absent but the meninges are intact and the skull appears normal. CSF fills the void left by the absent cerebrum. Hydranencephaly arises from destruction of brain that is formed and the skull is intact. This frequently happens late in fetal life and the infant can appear completely normal at birth. Other newborns with hydranencephaly will have severe neurological devastation characterized by seizures, decerebrate rigidity, and respiratory failure.[89]

Vascular lesions have been suspected of being a causative factor in hydranencephaly, although they could merely be the result of the destruction. This hypothesis is based on the findings of small but patent anterior and middle cerebral arteries. There is also experimental evidence to suggest this mechanism.[24] Infectious causes such as toxoplasmosis,[90,91] syphilis, mucormycosis,[92] cytomegalic inclusion disease,[93,94] and Herpes simplex[95] have been found in some cases. Attempted abortions and maternal trauma have also been reported to be associated with hydranencephaly.

Newborns with hydranencephaly do poorly and frequently die during the first 2 years. Others live for years with no hope for improvement in neurological status.

Porencephaly

Porencephaly is a term used for cavities within the cerebral hemispheres that communicate with the subarachnoid space (external porencephaly), the ventricles (internal porencephaly), neither (central porencephaly), or both. There is an overlap between porencephaly and hydranencephaly and another defect called schizencephaly, which arises as a result of an arrest in development of the wall of the cerebral hemisphere. Destruction of cerebral tissue can arise from prenatal, perinatal, or postnatal events and is termed encephaloclastic porencephaly – as opposed to schizencephaly, which is always prenatal.[24,96]

Vascular malformations

Vascular anomalies within the cranium are uncommon in the newborn period. When they occur and are symptomatic they can cause a difficult management problem depending on their location. Elaborate classifications have been proposed and were reviewed by Warkany et al.[24] A simple way to categorize vascular malformations is the following: (1) arteriovenous malformations; (2) malformations of the vein of Galen; (3) hemangioblastoma of the cerebellum; (4) congenital aneurysms of the circle of

Willis; and (5) anomalies of the carotid artery system. In many cases of intracranial hemorrhage in the term newborn consideration is given to whether or not a vascular malformation may be the underlying cause. Usually this is not the case. The manner in which vascular anomalies arise is uncertain in most cases because of lack of an adequate experimental model.[97]

Arteriovenous malformations

In arteriovenous malformations (AVMs) the arteries and veins are abnormal and have no capillaries between them. Most are located in the cerebral hemispheres but some are found in the deep midline structures. There is a hereditary component that is not well defined and a male sex preponderance exists.[98]

The pathogenesis of AVMs is poorly understood because of their many variations. It is suspected that they arise early in embryonic development because of the fact that there are arterial and venous contributions, which are readily found at this time when there is continuous development and regression of primitive vessels. The fact that arteries and veins frequently cross each other at right angles probably prevents more AVMs from occurring. Padget[99] felt that AVMs probably occur before 40-mm length, which is prior to thickening of arterial walls. At 20-mm length, sinusoidal channels connect some large veins and arteries. Abnormal arterial influx may cause permanent fistulae, secondary dilations, and spread to adjacent vessels. Pathologic features of AVM have been described by Anonson,[100] Lagos,[101] and McCormick.[102] Twisted, dilated veins and arteries exist with multiple communications such that arterial blood is shunted through venous channels. Hemorrhage can occur because the vessels are thin-walled and may contain calcifications. Depending on the location and compression by vessels, brain tissue adjacent to the AVM may have necrosis, atrophy, and gliosis.

While AVMs may be present at birth they are usually asymptomatic until a later time, most commonly the third decade. Size in some way predicts symptoms, with large AVMs being associated with seizures and smaller lesions with bleeding (headache, loss of consciousness). Heart failure can also be the presenting problem but rarely occurs after 5 months of age.[103] The diagnosis is confirmed in a variety of ways, including standard radiograph of the skull (which may reveal streak calcifications), CT, and MRI. The first clue is sometimes red blood cells in the CSF if bleeding has occurred. An intracranial bruit is frequently present.

Surgical intervention can provide excellent results in selected patients. More recently the gamma knife and arterial endovascular embolization techniques have been used successfully in the treatment of AVMs that have been inaccessible to surgery and are small (up to 3 cm).

Vein of Galen malformation

The varying clinical presentations of malformation of the vein of Galen were first published by Gold et al.[104] In the neonatal period infants with cyanosis and respiratory distress who are in congestive failure can have blood abnormally shunted to the venous system by this malformation. Intracranial bruits, seizures, and intracranial hemorrhage may also be present. In contrast, those cases presenting during infancy usually have progressive hydrocephalus, although intracranial bruits and seizures can occur. Paralysis of upward gaze is frequent and proptosis can be found. Subarachnoid hemorrhage occurs in one-third of cases. The third phase of onset of symptoms is during late childhood or adulthood. Headache is the main symptom and occurs with or without subarachnoid hemorrhage. Vertigo, fatigue, epistaxis, and distended head veins are common but usually no bruit is present.

Usually the vein of Galen is dilated and branches of the posterior cerebral, superior cerebellar, and middle cerebral arteries communicate with it. When the vein of Galen enlarges it can compress the quadrigeminal plate and aqueduct, causing hydrocephalus. Because blood can be shunted to the vein, bypassing the capillary network, ischemic damage can be caused to cerebral tissue.

Over 400 cases had been reported by 1993.[105,106] Onset of symptoms can occur from the neonatal period to 55 years of age.[107] Vein of Galen malformation is usually sporadic and a male predominance exists. In recent years it has been possible to make the diagnosis prenatally with combinations of real-time ultrasound, pulsed Doppler, electrocardiogram-phonocardiogram, and MRI.[108–110] In spite of these advances and prenatal diagnosis, fetal demise has occurred[111] and in other cases prenatal cerebral atrophy of a severe nature was present at birth.[112]

There has been a grave prognosis in cases of neonatal onset with congestive heart failure and intracranial hemorrhage, whereas those who developed symptoms during teenage or adult years did better. In the past the only approach to therapy was surgical, consisting of extracranial carotid ligations, clipping of feeder vessels, or total excision. Those patients that had these approaches had variable results, with up to 50% mortality and about 25% of the patients who lived were normal. In recent years there has been success in using transcatheter embolization techniques, with Friedman et al.[113] reporting no mortality in 11 patients, and none in 12 patients by Rodesch et al.[114] Embolization was undertaken in a 16-day-old with hydrocephalus and severe congestive heart failure and the child developed normally and had no neurological problems at 5 years of age.[115] Careful case selection is necessary.[116]

Hemangioblastoma

Hemangioblastoma of the cerebellum has a distinct cellular pattern that distinguishes it from other vascular malformations. It can be associated with angiomas of the spinal cord and retina, and is referred to as Lindau (von Hippel–Lindau) syndrome if there are multiple cysts of the kidney and pancreas. The prevalence of this malformation is not known but it accounts for about 7% of posterior fossa tumors.[117] There is a small male predominance and they are present from early childhood to over 70 years of age, most commonly presenting in the third and fifth decades.[118–120]

The etiology and pathogenesis of this malformation are unknown, but when associated with Lindau syndrome it is autosomal dominant. The lesion may be solid or cystic, single or multiple, and located in the cerebellar hemispheres or vermis. There is also an occasional association with both pheochromocytoma and syringomyelia and a constant association with polycythemia. Renal cell carcinoma has occurred in a few patients.

Congenital aneurysms

In the term newborn with intracranial hemorrhage the question of whether it is a ruptured congenital aneurysm sometimes arises. Many previously doubted the existence of these lesions but many cases in infants have now been reported.[121,122] There is still a question as to whether or not those adults with symptoms have a pre-existing lesion from fetal development. Familial cases have been reported as well as concordance in identical twins.[123,124] Most aneurysms are symptomatic until they rupture and no characteristic neurological picture has been found. An arteriogram done on a 9-month-old child who had ophthalmoplegia and quadriparesis since age 2 weeks revealed an aneurysm.[125]

It is of interest that there are a variety of associations with congenital aneurysms. These include other intracranial vascular anomalies, coarctation of the aorta, polycystic kidneys, and agenesis of the corpus callosum. They have also been present in patients with Marfan, Ehlers–Danlos, and pseudoxanthoma elasticum syndromes.[24]

Carotid artery malformations

Anomalies of the carotid artery system have been discussed in a monograph by Lie.[126] The most important problems arise in anomalies of the internal carotid, as those involving the external and common carotid arteries usually cause no trouble.

Famial hypoplasia of both internal carotids has been seen.[127] Complete absence of the artery is probably a primary malformation when associated with absence of the foramen. If collateral circulation is not adequate in either case there can be adverse neurological sequelae. Other malformations that occur are carotid–basilar artery anastomoses, in which case there is a persistence of one of six primitive vessels that connect the dorsal and ventral circulation in the embryo, although these may not cause problems.

Diagnostic approach to newborn malformations of the brain

This chapter has discussed selected malformations of the brain. The clinician faced with an infant with visible malformations has a different problem from that of seeing a normal-appearing infant who has an underlying brain malformation of significance (e.g., hydranencephaly). Fortunately, with the availability of CT scanners and MRI, answers are provided sooner than they have been in the past. It is of considerable comfort to parents if physicians have a reasoned approach to these patients because of the intense emotion arising from the birth of a malformed infant.

Perhaps the most difficult situation is that of a newborn who is requiring assisted ventilation and has a dysmorphic condition which includes a severe brain malformation. Frequently, the management decisions will be made (at least in part) on the basis of whether or not the infant has a "lethal" syndrome or whether the brain malformation precludes any chance of a meaningful existence. In most tertiary-care neonatal intensive care units these decisions are shared between the health-care providers, consultants, and parents, but in some cases these decisions are extended to others such as ethics committees and sometimes the courts. With maximum supportive care even the most severely malformed infants can be kept alive indefinitely. There is no simple way to approach these situations except that as soon as possible, the attending physician should initiate appropriate consultation and imaging studies to acquire rapidly accurate information. With the birth of such infants in more rural areas it may be necessary to transport the patient to the nearest referral center which has the experience to make such decisions.

With regard to specific brain malformations discussed in this chapter, some comments will be presented that may be helpful diagnostically and prognostically. The infant with a mild form of anencephaly (meroacrania) can appear like one with aprosencephaly, severe microcephaly, or microcephaly with an attenuated encephalocele. These can be differentiated by whether or not the lesion is skin-covered. If there is no skin covering it is anencephaly, no matter how small the aperture, and this lesion arises in embryonic stage 11. The typical case of anencephaly can be easily diagnosed by anyone in newborn nurseries. No imaging studies are necessary and no immediate prognosis should be rendered. Such infants may live for days or weeks with gavage feedings and usually die of no apparent cause. Most infants with anencephaly are stillborn. Supportive care and counseling for the parents should be undertaken. Many parents choose to take the infant home.

The newborn with an encephalocele presents a different type of problem. When the lesion is small and the sac not under pressure the resection can be delayed to allow neonatal adaptation. Two things should be initiated: address the question as to whether or not a syndrome exists and obtain a CT scan to see whether or not there are associated malformations of the brain. Parents frequently want to know whether or not their child will be handicapped and/or have mental retardation. Obviously this cannot be answered in a completely "normal" newborn so it shouldn't be answered about the infant with minor malformations of the brain. Parents are not likely to forget the careless clinician's comment that their child will be retarded. In contrast, the newborn with microcephaly and a large encephalocele containing cerebral cortex, ventricles, and cerebellum presents a difficult management decision. Immediate determinations of syndromic status and neuroimaging are necessary to make decisions prior to the necessity to provide assisted ventilation. Sometimes these lesions are unresectable or at best carry an unacceptable operative risk.

Finally, the infants with abnormal head size need

an approach to diagnosis and management. These patients should all have some type of imaging, whether that is ultrasound, CT scans, or MRI. When a newborn is born with a large head it is important to determine whether this is secondary to hydrocephalus or just a large brain. The presence of distended veins, "setting sun" eyes, and bulging fontanels is indicative of increased intracranial pressure but it is still necessary to determine the ratio of ventricular distension to cortex. Neurosurgical intervention with ventriculoperitoneal shunting of CSF is usually indicated within the first week after birth. In contrast, the infant with a large brain requires no surgery and efforts can be directed toward finding out whether a syndrome exists.

Infants with severe microcephaly present a different problem in that there is usually not any hopeful therapy that can be offered. A diagnostic approach to syndrome identification and other causation is necessary before formulating a plan with the family.

Clearly malformations of the brain represent one of the most challenging problems to deal with in the newborn. While respiratory and feeding issues may be the most critical elements of management during early weeks, the brain problems are present for the lifetime of the individual. An early and reasoned approach to diagnosis and counseling can set the stage for a smooth transition to optimal growth and development.

REFERENCES

1 O'Rahilly R and Müller F. (1987). *Developmental Stages in Human Embryos.* Baltimore, MD: Carnegie Institutions of Washington.

2 O'Rahilly R and Müller F. (2000). Mini-review: Prenatal ages and stages – measures and errors. *Teratology,* **61**, 382–384.

3 O'Rahilly R and Müller F. (1999). *The Embryonic Human Brain. An Atlas of Developmental Stages,* 2nd edn. New York: Wiley-Liss.

4 Lemire RJ, Loeser JD, Leech RW, et al. (1975). *Normal and Abnormal Development of the Human Nervous System.* Hagerstown: Harper and Row.

5 Warkany J. (1971). *Congenital Malformations: Notes and Comments.* Chicago: Yearbook.

6 Van Allen MI, Kalousek DK, Chernoff GF, et al. (1993). Evidence for multi-site closure of the neural tube in humans. *Am J Med Genet,* **47**, 723–743.

7 O'Rahilly R and Müller F. (1999). Mini-review: Summary of the initial development of the human nervous system. *Teratology,* **60**, 39–41.

8 Nakatsu T and Shiota K. (2000). Neurulation in the human embryo revisited. *Congen Anom,* **40**, 93–96.

9 Lemire RJ, Beckwith JB and Warkany J. (1978). *Anencephaly.* New York: Raven.

10 Lemire RJ. (1988). Neural tube defects. *JAMA,* **259**, 558–562.

11 Lemire RJ and Siebert JR. (1990). Anencephaly: its spectrum and relationship to neural tube defects. *J Craniofac Gen,* **10**, 163–174.

12 Melnick M and Myrianthopoulos NC. (1987). Studies in neural tube defects II. Pathological findings in a prospectively collected series of anencephalics. *Am J Med Genet,* **26**, 797–810.

13 Elwood JM, Little J and Elwood JH. (1992). *Epidemiology and Control of Neural Tube Defects.* Oxford: Oxford University Press.

14 Penrose LS. (1957). Genetics of anencephaly. *J Mental Defic Res,* **1**, 4–15.

15 Chambers CD, Johnson KA, Dick LM, et al. (1998). Maternal fever and birth outcome: a prospective study. *Teratology,* **58**, 251–257.

16 Shaw GM, Todoroff K, Velie EM, et al. (1998). Maternal illness, including fever, and medication use as risk factors for neural tube defects. *Teratology,* **57**, 1–7.

17 Wald N. (1991). Prevention of neural tube defects: results of the Medical Research Council vitamin study. *Lancet,* **ii**, 131–137.

18 Centers for Disease Control. (1992). *MMWR.* **41**, 1–7. Available online at http://www.cdc.gov/mmwr.

19 Wald NJ and Bower C. (1994). Folic acid, pernicious anaemia, and prevention of neural tube defects. *Lancet,* **343**, 307.

20 Cornel MC and Erickson JD. (1997). Comparison of national policies on periconceptional use of folic acid to prevent spina bifida and anencephaly (SBA). *Teratology,* **55**, 134–137.

21 Melvin EC, George TM, Worley G, et al. (2000). Genetic studies in neural tube defects. *Pediatr Neurosurg,* **32**, 1–9.

22 Trembath D, Sherbondy AL, VanDyke DC, et al. (1999). Analysis of select folate pathway genes, PAX 3, and human T in a midwestern neural tube defect population. *Teratology,* **59**, 331–341.

23 Cohen MM Jr and Lemire RJ. (1982). Syndromes with cephaloceles. *Teratology,* **25**, 161–172.

24 Warkany J, Lemire RJ and Cohen MM Jr. (1981). *Mental Retardation and Congenital Malformations of the Central Nervous System.* Chicago: YearBook.

25 Creasy MR and Alberman ED. (1976). Congenital malformations of the central nervous system in spontaneous abortions. *J Med Genet,* **13**, 9–16.

26 Gluckman TJ, George TM and McLone DG. (1996). Postneurulation rapid brain growth represents a critical time for encephalocele formation: a chick model. *Pediatr Neurosurg,* **25**, 130–136.

27 Emery JL and Kalhan SC. (1970). The pathology of exencephalus. *Dev Med Child Neurol,* **12**, 51–64.

28 Marin-Padilla M. (1980). Morphogenesis of experimental encephalocele (cranioschisis occulta). *J Neurol Sci,* **24**, 83–99.

29 Karch SB and Urich H. (1972). Occipital encephalocele: a morphological study. *J Neurol Sci,* **15**, 89–112.

30 MacRae DW, Howard RO, Albert DM, et al. (1972). Ocular manifestations of the Meckel syndrome. *Arch Ophthalmol,* **88**, 106–113.

31 Gorlin RJ, Cohen MM Jr and Levin LS. (1990). *Syndromes of the Head and Neck,* 3rd edn. New York: Oxford University Press.

32 Guthkelch AN. (1970). Occipital cranium bifidum. *Arch Dis Child,* **45**, 104–109.

33 Warkany J, Lemire RJ and Cohen MM Jr. (1981). *Mental Retardation and Congenital Malformations of the Central Nervous System.* Chicago: YearBook.

34 Komiyama M, Yasui T, Sakamoto H, et al. (2000). Basal meningoencephalocele, anomaly of optic disc and panhypopituitarism in association with Moya Moya disease. *Pediatr Neurosurg,* **33**, 100–104.

35 Van Nouhuys JM and Bruyn GW. (1964). Nasopharyngeal transsphenoidal encephalocele, crater-like hole in the optic disc and agenesis of the corpus callosum; pneumoencephalographic visualization in a case. *Psychiatry Neurol Neurochirurg,* **67**, 243–258.

36 Pollack JA, Newton TH and Hoyt WF. (1968). Transsphenoidal and transethmoidal encephaloceles. *Radiology,* **90**, 442–453.

37 Siebert JR, Cohen MM Jr, Sulik KK, et al. (1990). *Holoprosencenphaly: An Overview and Atlas of Cases.* New York: Wiley-Liss.

38 DeMyer WE, Zeman W and Palmer CG. (1964). The face predicts the brain: diagnostic significance of median facial anomalies for holoprosencephaly (arhinencephaly). *Pediatrics,* **34**, 256–263.

39 Roach E, DeMyer W, Palmer K, et al. (1975). Holoprosencephaly: birth data, genetic and demographic analysis of 30 families. *Birth Defects,* **XI**, 294–313.

40 Urioste M, Valcarcel E, Gomez MA, et al. (1988). Holoprosencephaly and trisomy 21 in a child born to a non-diabetic mother. *Am J Med Genet,* **30**, 925–928.

41 Matsunaga E and Shiota K. (1977). Holoprosencephaly in human embryos: epidemiologic studies of 150 cases. *Teratology,* **16**, 261–272.

42 Roach E, DeMyer W, Palmer C, et al. (1975). Holoprosencephaly: birth data, genetic and demographic analysis of 30 families. *Birth Defects,* **XI**, 294–313.

43 Barr M, Hansen JW, Currey K, et al. (1983). Holoprosencephaly in infants of diabetic mothers. *J Pediatr,* **102**, 565–568.

44 Lemire RJ, Cohen Jr MM, Beckwith JB, et al. (1981). The facial features of holoprosencephaly in anencephalic human specimens. I. Historical review and associated malformations. *Teratology,* **23**, 297–303.

45 Siebert JR, Kokich VG, Beckwith JB, et al. (1981). The facial features of holoprosencephaly in anencephalic human specimens. II. Craniofacial anatomy. *Teratology,* **23**, 305–315.

46 Kim TS, Cho S and Dickson DW. (1990). Aprosencephaly: review of the literature and report of a case with cerebellar hypoplasia, segmented epithelial cyst and Rathke's cleft cyst. *Acta Neuropathol,* **79**, 424–431.

47 Blackburn BL and Fineman RM. (1994). Epidemiology of congenital hydrocephalus in Utah, 1940–1979: report of an iatrogenically related 'epidemic'. *Am J Med Genet,* **52**, 123–129.

48 Lurie IW, Nedzved MK, Lazjuk GI, et al. (1979). Brief clinical reports: aprosencephaly-atelencephaly and the aprosencephaly (XK) syndrome. *Am J Med Genet,* **3**, 303–309.

49 Siebert JR, Kokich VG, Warkany J, et al. (1987). Atelencephalic microcephaly: craniofacial anatomy and morphologic comparisons with holoprosencephaly and anencephaly. *Teratology,* **36**, 279–285.

50 Siebert JR, Warkany J and Lemire RJ. (1986). Atelencephalic microcephaly in a 21-week human fetus. *Teratology,* **34**, 9–19.

51 Avery GB, Meneses L and Lodge A. (1972). The clinical significance of "measurement microcephaly." *Am J Dis Child,* **119**, 128–131.

52 Martin HP. (1970). Microcephaly and mental retardation. *Am J Dis Child,* **119**, 128–131.

53 Davies PA and Davis JP. (1970). Very low birth weight and subsequent head growth. *Lancet,* **ii**, 1216–1219.

54 Illingworth RS and Eid EE. (1971). The head circumference in infants and other measurements to which it may be related. *Acta Paediatr Scand,* **60**, 333–337.

55 Jones KL. (1997). *Smith's Recognizable Patterns of Human Malformation,* 5th edn. Philadelphia: Saunders.

56 Stevenson AC, Johnston HA, Stewart ML, et al. (1966). Congenital malformations. A report of a study of series of consecutive births in 24 centers. *Bull World Health Org,* **34** (suppl.), 9–127.

57 Stoll C, Alembik Y, Dott B, et al. (1992). An epidemiologic study of environmental and genetic factors in congenital hydrocephalus. *Eur J Epidemiol,* **8**, 797–803.

58 Cameron AH. (1957). The Arnold–Chiari and other neuroanatomical malformations associated with spina bifida. *J Pathol Bacteriol,* **73**, 195–211.

59 Piatt JH Jr and D'Agostino A. (1999). The Chiari II malformation: lesions discovered within the fourth ventricle. *Pediatr Neurosurg,* **30**, 79–85.

60 Cameron AH. (1957). The Arnold–Chiari and other neuroanatomical malformations associated with spina bifida. *J Pathol Bacteriol,* **73**, 195–211.

61 Daniel PM and Strich SJ. (1958). Some observations in the congenital deformity of the central nervous system known as the Arnold–Chiari malformation. *J Neuropathol Exp Neurol,* **17**, 255–266.

62 Emery JL and Gadson DR. (1975). A quantitative study of the cell population of the cerebellum in children with myelomeningocele. *Dev Med Child Neurol,* **17**, 20–25.

63 Emery JL and MacKenzie N. (1973). Medullo-cervical dislocation deformity (Chiari II deformity) related to neurospinal dysraphism (meningomyelocele). *Brain,* **96**, 155–162.

64 Peach B. (1965). The Arnold–Chiari malformation. Morphogenesis. *Arch Neurol,* **12**, 527–535.

65 Variend S and Emery JL. (1974). The pathology of the central lobes of the cerebellum in children with myelomeningocele. *Dev Med Child Neurol,* **16**, 99–106.

66 Teo C, Parker EC, Aureli S, et al. (1997). The Chiari malformation: a surgical series. *Pediatr Neurosurg,* **27**, 223–229.

67 Lemire RJ, Shepard TH and Alvord EC Jr. (1965). Caudal myeloschisis (lumbo-sacral spina bifida cystica) in a five millimeter (Horizon XIV) human embryo. *Anat Rec,* **152**, 9–16.

68 Barry A, Patten BM and Stewart BR. (1957). Possible factors in the development of the Arnold–Chiari malformation. *J Neurosurg,* **14**, 285–301.

69 Goldstein F and Kepes JJ. (1966). The role of traction in the development of the Arnold–Chiari malformation. An experimental study. *J Neuropathol Exp Neurol,* **25**, 654–666.

70 Jacobs EB, Landing BH and Thomas W Jr. (1961). Vernicomyelia: its bearing on theories of genesis of the Arnold–Chiari complex. *Am J Pathol,* **39**, 345–353.

71 Padget DH. (1972). Development of so-called dysraphism: with embryologic evidence of clinical Arnold–Chiari and Dandy–Walker malformations. *Johns Hopkins Med,* **130**, 127–165.

72 Jennings MT, Clarren SK, Kokich VG, et al. (1982). Neuroanatomic examination of spina bifida aperta and the Arnold–Chiari malformation in a 130-day human fetus. *J Neurol Sci,* **54**, 325–338.

73 Gilles FH and Rockett FX. (1971). Infantile hydrocephalus: retrocerebellar 'arachnoidal' cyst. *J Pediatr,* **79**, 436–443.

74 Hart MN, Malamud N and Ellis WG. (1972). The Dandy–Walker malformation syndrome. *Neurology,* **22**, 771–780.

75 Gorlin RJ, Cohen MM Jr and Levin LS. (1990). *Syndromes of the Head and Neck,* 3rd edn. New York: Oxford University Press.

76 Larson SL and Banner EA. (1966). Hydrocephalus: a 30-year survey. *Obstet Gynecol,* **28**, 571–577.

77 Solitare GB and Krigman MR. (1964). Congenital intracranial neoplasm. A case report and review of the literature. *J Neuropathol Exp Neurol,* **23**, 280–292.

78 Milhorat TH. (1972). *Hydrocephalus and the Cerebrospinal Fluid.* Baltimore: Williams and Wilkins.

79 Jones KL. (1997). *Smith's Recognizable Patterns of Human Malformation,* 5th edn. Philadelphia: Saunders.

80 Dekaban AS and Sakuragawa N. (1977). Megalencephaly. In *Handbook of Clinical Neurology,* vol. 30, ed. Vinken PJ and Bruyn GW, pp. 647–660. North Holland, Amsterdam.

81 Riley HD and Smith WR. (1960). Macrocephaly, pseudopapilledema and multiple hemangromata. A previously undescribed heredofamilial syndrome. *Pediatrics,* **26**, 293–300.

82 Bannayan GA. (1971). Lipomatosis, angiomatosis and macrocephalia. A previously undescribed congenital syndrome. *Arch Pathol,* **92**, 1–5.

83 Salmon JH and Flanigan S. (1964). Megalencephaly. A clinical study with chromosomal analysis. *J Neurosurg,* **21**, 409–412.

84 DeMyer W. (1972). Megalencephaly in children. Clinical syndromes, genetic patterns, and differential diagnosis from other causes of megalocephaly. *Neurology,* **22**, 634–643.

85 Brun A and Gustavson KH. (1972). Cerebral malformations in the XYY syndrome. *Acta Pathol Microbiol Scand,* **80**, 627–633.

86 Ramirez M, Wilkins I, Kramer L, et al. (1994). Prenatal diagnosis of unilateral megalencephaly by real-time ultrasonography. *Am J Obstet Gynecol,* **170**, 1384–1385.

87 Cavenagh EC, Hart BL and Rose D. (1993). Association of linear sebaceous nevus syndrome and unilateral megalencephaly. *Am J Neuroradiol,* **14**, 405–408.

88 Powell BR, Budden SS and Buist NR. (1993). Dominantly inherited megalencephaly, muscle weakness, and myoliposis: a carnitine-deficient myopathy within the spectrum of the Ruvalcaba–Myhre–Smith syndrome. *J Pediatr*, **123**, 70–75.

89 Halsey JH Jr. (1987). Hydranencephaly. In *Handbook of Clinical Neurology*, vol. 50: *Malformations*, ed. PJ Vinken, GW Bruyn and JL Klawans, pp. 337–353. Amsterdam: Elsevier.

90 Altshuler G. (1973). Toxoplasmosis as a cause of hydroanencephaly. *Am J Dis Child*, **125**, 251–252.

91 Dambska M, Krasnicka Z and Michalowicz R. (1966). Hydroanencephalia in the course of congenital toxoplasmosis. *Pol Med J*, **5**, 432–446.

92 Liss L, Knoblich RR and Wolter JR. (1967). Cerebral mucornycosis with hydrencephaly and primary optic atrophy: in a 4-month-old child. *J Pediatr Ophthalmol*, **4**, 36.

93 Arey JB and Baird HW III. (1954). Hydranencephaly. *Am J Pathol*, **30**, 645.

94 McElfresh AE and Arey JB. (1957). Generalized cytomegalic inclusion disease. *J Pediatr*, **51**, 146–156.

95 Herzen JL and Benirschke K. (1977). Unexpected disseminated herpes simplex infection in a newborn. *Obstet Gynecol*, **50**, 728.

96 Gross H and Grisold W. (1987). Porencephaly. In *Handbook of Clinical Neurology*, vol. 50: *Malformations*, ed. PJ Vinken, GW Bruyn and HL Klawans, pp. 355–363. Amsterdam: Elsevier.

97 Warkany J and Lemire RJ. (1984). Arteriovenous malformations of the brain: a teratologic challenge. *Teratology*, **29**, 333–353.

98 Amin-Hanjani S, Robertson R, Arginteanu MS, et al. (1998). Familial intracranial arteriovenous malformations. Case report and review of the literature. *Pediatr Neurosurg*, **29**, 208–213.

99 Padget DH. (1956). The cranial venous system in man in reference to development, adult configuration and relation to the arteries. *Am J Anat*, **98**, 307–355.

100 Anonson SM. (1971). Vascular malformation. In *Pathology of the Nervous System*, vol. 2, ed. J. Mincker, pp. 1884–1897. New York: McGraw Hill.

101 Lagos JC. (1977). Congenital aneurysms and arteriovenous malformations. Congenital malformations of the brain and skull (pt 2). In *Handbook of Clinical Neurology*, vol. 31, ed. PJ Vinken and GW Bruyn, pp. 137–209. Amsterdam: North Holland.

102 McCormick WF. (1966). The pathology of vascular ('arteriovenous') malformations. *J Neurosurg*, **28**, 807–816.

103 Lagos JC. (1977). Congenital aneurysms and arteriovenous malformations. Congenital malformations of the brain and skull (pt 2). In *Handbook of Clinical Neurology*, vol. 31, ed. PJ Vinken and GW Bruyn, pp. 137–209. Amsterdam: North Holland.

104 Gold A, Ramsohoff J and Carter S. (1964). Vein of Galen malformation. *Acta Neurol Scand*, **40**, 3–31.

105 Lylyk P, Vinuela F, Dion JE, et al. (1993). Therapeutic alternatives for vein of Galen vascular malformation. *J Neurosurg*, **78**, 438–445.

106 Zerah M, Garcia-Monaco R, Rodesch G, et al. (1992). Hydrodynamics in vein of Galen malformations. *Childs Nerv Syst*, **8**, 111–117.

107 Mylonas C and Booth AE. (1992). Vein of Galen aneurysm presenting in middle age. *Br J Neurosurg*, **6**, 491–494.

108 Strauss S, Weintraub Z and Goldberg M. (1991). Prenatal diagnosis of vein of Galen arteriovenous malformation by duplex sonography. *J Perinat Med*, **19**, 227–230.

109 Yamaguchi M, Kaneko M, Miyakawa I, et al. (1991). Prenatal diagnosis of the aneurysm of the vein of Galen by pulsed Doppler unit. *Am J Perinatol*, **8**, 244–246.

110 Yamashita Y, Abe T, Ohara N, et al. (1992). Successful treatment of neonatal aneurysmal dilatation of the vein of Galen: the role of prenatal diagnosis and transarterial embolization. *Neuroradiology*, **34**, 457–459.

111 Ballester MJ, Raga F, Serra-Serra V, et al. (1994). Early prenatal diagnosis of an ominous aneurysm of the vein of Galen by color Doppler ultrasound. *Acta Obstet Gynecol Scand*, **73**, 592–595.

112 Baenziger O, Martin E, Willi U, et al. (1993). Prenatal brain atrophy due to a giant vein of Galen malformation. *Neuroradiology*, **35**, 105–106.

113 Friedman DM, Verma R, Madrid M, et al. (1993). Recent improvement in outcome using transcatheter embolization techniques for neonatal aneurysmal malformations of the vein of Galen. *Pediatrics*, **91**, 583–586.

114 Rodesch G, Hui F, Alvarez H, et al. (1994). Prognosis of antenatally diagnosed vein of Galen aneurysmal malformations. *Childs Nerv Syst*, **10**, 79–83.

115 Hamasaki T, Kai Y, Hamada J, et al. (2000). Successful treatment of a neonate with vein of Galen aneurysmal malformation. *Pediatr Neurosurg*, **32**, 200–204.

116 Swanstrom S, Flodmark O and Lasjaunias P. (1994). Conditions for treatment of cerebral arteriovenous malformation associated with ectasia of the vein of Galen in the newborn. *Acta Paediatr*, **83**, 255–257.

117 Rubenstein LJ. (1972). *Tumors of the Central Nervous System*, pp. 235–256. Bethesda: Armed Forces Institute of Pathology.

118 Mondkar VP, McKissock W and Russell RW. (1967). Cerebellar hemangioblastomas. *Br J Surg*, **54**, 45–49.

119 Palmer JJ. (1972). Hemangioblastomas. A review of 81 cases. *Acta Neurochirurg*, **27**, 125–148.
120 Silver ML and Hennigar GR. (1952). Cerebellar hemangioma (hemangioblastoma). A clinicopathological review of 40 cases. *J Neurosurg*, **9**, 484–494.
121 Lagos JC. (1977). Congenital aneurysms and arteriovenous malformations. Congenital malformations of the brain and skull (pt 2). In *Handbook of Clinical Neurology*, vol. 31, ed. PJ Vinken and GW Bruyn, pp. 137–209. Amsterdam: North Holland.
122 Lipper S, Morgan D, Krigman MR, et al. (1978). Congenital saccular aneurysm in a 19-day-old neonate. Case report and review of the literature. *Surg Neurol*, **10**, 161–165.
123 Bannerman RM, Ingall GB and Graf CJ. (1970). The familial occurrence of intracranial aneurysms. *Neurology*, **20**, 283–292.
124 Fairburn B. (1973). 'Twin' intracranial aneurysms causing subarachnoid haemorrhage in identical twins. *Br J Med*, **1**, 210–211.
125 Thompson RA and Pribram HFW. (1969). Infantile cerebral aneurysms associated with ophthalmoplegia and quadriparesis. *Neurology*, **19**, 785–789.
126 Lie TA. (1968). *Congenital Anomalies of the Carotid Arteries*, pp. 1–143. New York: Excerpta Medica.
127 Austin JH and Stears JC. (1971). Familial hypoplasia of both internal carotid arteries. *Arch Neurol*, **24**, 1–10.

6

Prematurity and complications of labor and delivery

Yasser Y. El-Sayed and Maurice L. Druzin

Stanford University Medical Center, Stanford, CA, USA

Introduction

Prematurity is a major contributor to perinatal morbidity and mortality in the USA and around the world. Preterm birth is officially defined as delivery occurring prior to 37 completed weeks from the first day of the last menstrual period.[1] The term "low-birth-weight" is used to describe infants weighing less than 2500 g at birth. This includes neonates who are born after 37 weeks' gestational age, of which approximately one-third are in the category of "growth restriction." This group of neonates is distinct from the group of premature infants and is the subject of another chapter (see Chapter 7). This discussion will be confined to the preterm fetus, that which is delivered between 20 and 37 completed weeks of gestation (140–259 days gestation).

Complications of labor and delivery in both preterm and term gestations have been implicated in adverse neonatal outcomes. Traditionally, cerebral palsy and "brain damage" have been linked to intrapartum events that resulted in "birth asphyxia" and subsequent neurologic damage. This association has continued to be proposed in spite of the fact that current evidence suggests that only about 10% of patients with cerebral palsy, about 1–2 per 10 000 births, experience serious birth asphyxia.[2] Most studies in this field refer to the term fetus. The preterm neonate has its own unique complications resulting from being born prematurely and the resultant sequelae.

The incidence of preterm birth is approximately 10% in the USA.[3] There are significant ethnic differences and differences between socioeconomic groups. Blacks have twice the incidence of preterm birth of whites. Preterm births account for the majority of perinatal deaths around the world.[4] Birth weight is the best predictor of survival after 30 weeks' gestation while gestational age predicts survival prior to 30 weeks. The lower limits of viability are changing and recent studies have demonstrated survival and improved short-term outcome at gestational ages of 24 weeks.[5] However, delivery prior to 27 weeks has a high incidence of serious long-term impairment.[6] Major improvements in survival occur with each completed week of gestation from 24 weeks to 33 weeks' gestation, after which time minimal increases in survival occur, although morbidity may be decreased. Neonatal morbidity in terms of respiratory distress syndrome, necrotizing enterocolitis, sepsis, intraventricular hemorrhage, hyperbilirubinemia, and hypoglycemia are also inversely related to gestational age, i.e., the lower the gestational age the higher the incidence of complications.[7]

Factors associated with prematurity

A history of preterm birth is associated with a 20–40% recurrence risk.[8] Preterm delivery is a result of either preterm labor, preterm premature rupture of membranes (PROM), and labor or maternal or fetal conditions requiring intervention for maternal or fetal reasons. The majority of preterm births result from preterm labor and PROM with approximately 20% resulting from maternal/fetal indications for delivery. The cause of premature birth may vary according to socioeconomic status, with PROM being higher in the lower socioeconomic group.[9]

Demographic factors

Lower socioeconomic status,[10] ethnicity, and maternal age all have been associated with increased incidence of preterm birth. Black women have an incidence of preterm birth that is about double that of Caucasian women. Even if socioeconomic status is accounted for, this disparity remains apparent.[11] The incidence of preterm birth is higher in women under the age of 20 years irrespective of whether they have their first or subsequent pregnancies before age 20 years. First pregnancies after age 35 years are also at increased risk for preterm birth.[12] Poor nutritional status and inadequate weight gain during pregnancy are associated with an increased incidence of preterm birth.[13]

Substance abuse

Cocaine abuse,[14] alcohol use, and cigarette smoking[15] have all been associated with increased rates of preterm birth. The confounding variables of poor nutrition, inadequate weight gain, and associated medical problems seen commonly in patients suffering substance abuse makes it difficult to pinpoint the exact etiology of preterm delivery.

Obstetrical factors

A history of preterm birth is one of the most important risk factors for subsequent preterm delivery. The risk increases with the number of preterm births and decreases with the number of term deliveries.[16] There is some debate over whether legal abortions in the first trimester increase the rate of preterm delivery.[17,18] There seems to be an increased incidence in women who have had second-trimester terminations.[12]

Multiple gestation is associated with an increased incidence of preterm birth. Between 30 and 50% of multiple gestations deliver prior to 37 weeks with the higher order of multiple gestation delivering the earliest.[19,20] Multiple gestations account for about 10% of all preterm births in the USA. Assisted reproductive technologies (ART) lead to multiple gestation in about 20% of cases but the incidence of preterm delivery in singleton pregnancies resulting from ART is also higher – about 15%. The overall incidence of preterm delivery from ART is approximately 27%.[21]

Fetal anomalies such as renal agenesis,[22] anencephaly,[23] multiple congenital anomalies, anomalies leading to polyhydramnios, oligohydramnios, or fetal hydrops will also precipitate preterm labor. First-trimester bleeding[24] and third-trimester bleeding from placental abnormalities also increase the risk of preterm delivery, either by precipitating preterm labor or because of maternal/fetal compromise.[12,25]

Uterine abnormalities lead to an increased risk of preterm delivery. These abnormalities are often congenital or may be related to in utero exposure to diethylstilbestrol (DES). Preterm birth rates of 15–30% have been reported in these cases. The greatest incidence is noted in patients with demonstrable abnormalities of the genital tract, such as T-shaped uterus or cervical abnormalities.[26,27]

Cervical incompetence is often associated with DES exposure but is sometimes iatrogenic, secondary to trauma, and is also seen with no known predisposing factors. The diagnosis is difficult to ascertain and is most often made following a history of rapid painless cervical dilatation in the second or early third trimester or repetitive premature deliveries with minimal uterine activity. The gold standard is the documentation of cervical effacement, shortening, or dilatation in the absence of obvious premature contractions.[28] Ultrasonographic evaluation of the length of the cervix has been proposed as a method of diagnosing cervical incompetence and/or risk of preterm labor.[29] Treatment with cervical cerclage has reported success rates of 75–90% but most studies are retrospective[16,30] and only a few prospective studies are available.[31–33] The rate of preterm birth following cerclage is still as high as 30%.[34,30]

Medical and surgical complications of pregnancy lead to iatrogenic preterm delivery in up to 20% of cases of preterm labor. These include conditions such as hypertensive disorders of pregnancy, renal disease, systemic lupus erythematosus, cardiac disease, acute infections, acute appendicitis, and other surgical and medical conditions.

Preterm labor with intact membranes may often be a result of intraamniotic infection which is unrecognized.[35,36] These patients often do not have overt evidence of chorioamnionitis but the preterm labor is often refractory to tocolysis.[37–40] The possible mechanism of infection causing preterm labor has been elaborated by Romero and others.[41–43]

Preterm premature rupture of the amniotic membranes (PPROM) is defined as rupture of the amniotic membranes prior to term (less than 37 weeks' gestation). The interval between PROM and onset of labor is the latency period and is inversely related to gestational age. Pediatricians are concerned about the latency period in term gestations and often refer to "prolonged" rupture of membranes when the latency period exceeds 18–24 h. PROM accounts for up to 30% of all preterm deliveries and thus is a major concern in perinatal medicine.[44] The causes of PROM are not clearly understood but weakening of the chorioamniotic membrane has been demonstrated as the pregnancy progresses.[45,46] Local infection from vaginal flora ascending through the cervix has been implicated as the etiology in a substantial number of cases.[47] Carriers of certain sexually transmitted organisms such as group B beta-hemolytic streptococcus (GBS), *Chlamydia*, *Trichomonas*, *Gonococcus*, and bacterial vaginosis, have a higher incidence of PROM than those who are not carriers.[48]

Some bacteria release proteases which cause membrane weakening and probably early rupture.[49] There are host factors and immune activation mechanisms that probably account for the great variation in incidence of PROM between populations. Polyhydramnios, cervical cerclage procedures, amniocentesis, smoking and multiple gestation have all been implicated as etiological factors in PROM.[50] However, in the majority of cases the etiology is unknown. The major complications of PROM are premature labor and preterm delivery. The latency period is inversely related to gestational age with 50% of patients with PROM prior to 26 weeks being in labor within 1 week.[51] When PROM occurs between 28 and 34 weeks, 50% are in labor within 24 h and 80–90% within 1 week.[52,53] The other significant risk of PROM is maternal/fetal/neonatal sepsis.

Chorioamnionitis occurs in 15–25% of PROM cases.[54] Incidence of neonatal sepsis at term is in the range of 1 in 500 deliveries. This incidence increases dramatically with PPROM and even more significantly in the presence of chorioamnionitis.[55–57] Umbilical cord compression and prolapse occur more often in cases of PROM with the associated complications of hypoxia and even asphyxia leading to fetal death or neonatal compromise.[58–61] Fetal deformation syndrome from PROM prior to 26 weeks is seen in approximately 3–4% of cases. This syndrome includes compression malformations and lethal pulmonary hypoplasia.[62,63]

Management of preterm labor

The diagnosis of preterm labor is important in order to initiate appropriate tocolytic therapy to prolong gestation and thus decrease the incidence of neonatal complications. The criteria for the diagnosis of preterm labor seem deceptively simple, i.e., gestational age of 20–37 weeks and documented uterine contractions of four in 20 min or eight in 60 min. In addition, there should be ruptured membranes, or intact membranes and documented cervical change in either dilatation or effacement. Cervical effacement of 80% or dilation of 2 cm or greater with contractions are additional criteria.[64] The major problem with the diagnosis is interobserver variability in documentation of cervical change, dilatation, and effacement. This is often subjective and may lead to a false diagnosis of preterm labor. Strict adherence to criteria for the diagnosis of preterm labor will allow meaningful comparison of studies in the management of this condition. Awaiting cervical change in order to diagnose preterm labor accurately does not compromise the efficacy of tocolysis.[65]

Initial assessments of the patient in suspected preterm labor include confirming the diagnosis and careful fetal evaluation by both sonography and continuous electronic fetal monitoring (EFM). Fetal anomalies must be ruled out and evidence of fetal compromise such as intrauterine growth restriction (IUGR) detected prior to consideration of tocolytic therapy. Maternal condition should be evaluated to detect any medical or surgical problems that may contraindicate tocolysis or in fact require preterm delivery. Urinary tract infection should be ruled out and cervical–vaginal cultures taken. GBS prophylaxis should be administered. Fetal fibronectin may help rule out preterm labor by virtue of its high negative predictive value.[66] The patient is placed at bedrest with a left lateral tilt and cervical evaluation performed (with intact membranes). If signs and symptoms of chorioamnionitis are present, tocolysis is contraindicated. With PPROM in the absence of clinical chorioamnionitis, antibiotic prophylaxis helps prolong latency, and should be administered for a period of 7–10 days.[67,68] Other absolute contraindications to the use of tocolytic therapy include severe pregnancy-induced hypertension, severe bleeding from abruptio placentae or placenta previa, and fetal conditions such as fetal death, growth restriction, or anomalies incompatible with life. Relative contraindications include maternal hypertensive disorders, cardiac disease, and diabetes as well as mild abruptio placentae, stable placenta previa, and mild fetal growth restriction. If cervical change is noted and there are no contraindications to tocolytic therapy, a decision must be made concerning the use of tocolytic medication. There is still debate about whether any tocolytic agent is justified because only about 20% of cases of preterm labor are truly idiopathic. In the majority of cases, an identifiable cause of preterm labor or a maternal/fetal condition precludes the use of tocolytic therapy. Reports of excellent neonatal outcome in preterm labor without the use of tocolytic agents[69] are contrasted with reports of the cost-effectiveness of the use of β-adrenergic agents.[70] A more recent study [71] demonstrated the efficacy of β-agonist tocolysis for at least 48 h. This allowed the administration of antenatal steroids, although the overall perinatal outcome was not significantly improved.

Bedrest, hydration, and often sedation may lead to a decrease in uterine activity.[72,73] Hydration should not be rigorous as fluid balance is important if tocolytic therapy is subsequently used.

Management of delivery of the preterm fetus

Initial approach

The most important factors to consider in cases in which preterm delivery will occur is availability of resources to deliver optimal care to both the neonate and the mother. Preterm neonates delivered in a perinatal center specializing in providing care for these patients have a much improved prognosis compared to neonates who are transported after birth.[74–76] Prior to arranging for maternal transport the gestational age and birth weight need to be determined. The use of real-time sonography will reliably estimate fetal weight and gestational age with a small margin of error in the preterm fetus.[77,78] The clinical estimation of gestational age and birth weight is subject to many errors, including inaccurate menstrual history, oligo- or polyhydramnios, fetal presentation, maternal body habitus, and other pathology such as myomata uteri. The tendency is often to underestimate fetal weight.[79] The gestational ages at which maternal transfer would not be indicated will vary according to the level of neonatal care available in most circumstances. At gestational ages of 36 weeks or greater, and birth weights of ≥2500 g, most obstetrical/pediatric facilities would have the resources to care for these neonates. If the gestation is previable, then transport may not confer an advantage in terms of neonatal survival. In practical terms, many community hospitals are uncomfortable with the possibility that a supposedly previable gestation may turn out to be larger than anticipated and delivery will have occurred without adequate facilities. The philosophy of "When in doubt, ship them out" is often the most prudent approach. Most maternal transports will be made for gestational ages of 24–36 weeks. However, diagnosis of fetal anomalies or serious maternal illness may require transfer at any gestational age.

Close communication between referring physicians, accepting maternal–fetal physicians, neonatologists, and other appropriate pediatric staff is essential. The patient and her family need to be given a realistic and consistent evaluation of the situation, including risks, benefits, alternatives, and ultimately, prognosis. Survival rates and follow-up data need to be known for the institution and counseling should be initiated by both obstetrics and neonatology staff as soon as is feasible. The type of transportation used will be quite region-specific but, as a general rule, transports from less than 100 miles (160 km) can be accomplished by ground ambulance while air transport is often used for greater distances. Mountains, road conditions, and weather will all influence the choice of method of transport. Once the decision to transport is made it is advantageous to have a transport team available. At many institutions, physicians and nurse teams are specially trained to transport either the pregnant mother or the neonate. These are two distinctly different types of health professionals and maternal–fetal transport is done by personnel trained in obstetrics while neonatal transports are done by persons trained in care of the sick neonate.

Communication is vital between all the parties involved in caring for maternal–fetal and neonatal transports. There must be an efficient mechanism of initiating a request for transport. One phone call to the referring center or regional dispatch center should set in motion a chain of events leading to appropriate transportation. Medical staff at the referring hospital will need to contact the accepting institution's staff without difficulty in order to provide appropriate information concerning the patient. The obstetricians accepting a maternal–fetal transport will need to contact their neonatology group to inform them of the impending transport and confirm availability of a neonatal bed. If there is a problem with this, alternative strategies need to be devised.

The referring institution needs to provide as much information as possible so that adequate resources can be mobilized to deal with specific problems. Examples would be availability of pediatric surgical specialties or availability of blood for transfusion. There are cases in which a maternal–fetal transport team may arrive after an unexpected delivery or find that transport would be inadvisable and delivery preparations undertaken. In this type of situation, close communication between the maternal–fetal and neonatal teams is vital.

Discussion needs to be instituted concerning the use of medications or other interventions prior to initiation of transport. When there is a maternal–fetal transport, discussion usually centers around the use of tocolytic agents, antihypertensive and antiseizure medications in cases of hypertensive disorders of pregnancy, and sometimes the use of antibiotics in cases of preterm labor and/or PPROM. The use of pharmacologic agents given to the pregnant patient in order to improve neonatal outcome is an extremely important consideration. The most effective and well-studied therapy is the use of antenatal corticosteroid administration. The most commonly used regimens are either dexamethasone 5 mg i.m. every 12 h for four doses or betamethasone 12 mg intramuscularly and repeated in 24 h.

Currently, the consensus conference of the National Institute of Health[80] recommends that all women between 24 and 34 weeks of pregnancy at risk for preterm delivery be considered candidates for antenatal corticosteroid therapy. Optimal therapeutic benefits begin 24 h after initiation of therapy and last 7 days. Because there is evidence suggesting that mortality, respiratory distress syndrome, and intraventricular hemorrhage are reduced even when treatment lasts for less than 24 h, steroids should be given unless delivery is imminent.

Management of labor and delivery in the preterm gestation

Once delivery is imminent, optimal management of the delivery process is important. Pain relief is an essential element in the management of patients in preterm labor. It should be accepted that all analgesic medications commonly used in obstetrics cross the placenta. The long-held misconception about neonatal depression secondary to analgesic medication continues to prevent physicians from administering adequate pain relief in labor. Some medications may indeed lead to temporary respiratory depression of the neonate but other causes for the problem must be sought. There is evidence that central nervous system depressants may in fact protect the central nervous system of the fetus from the effects of hypoxia.[81]

Continuous epidural anesthesia is a safe and effective method of pain relief in preterm labor. Avoidance of maternal hypotension is important to prevent in utero placental insufficiency. General anesthesia for emergency operative delivery poses no threat to the fetus provided maternal oxygenation is maintained and hypotension avoided.

Fetal monitoring

Intrapartum hypoxia and acidosis in the preterm fetus may be a significant factor in subsequent complication of prematurity.[82] Possible mechanisms include the absence of autoregulation of cerebral blood flow, which makes the preterm fetus more vulnerable to the consequences of rapid redistribution of blood flow in response to hypoxia. Continuous EFM appears to predict fetal hypoxia in the preterm fetus with some degree of accuracy.[83,84]

Skilled auscultation may also be used.[85] However, this is often not practical because of the more labor-intensive nature of surveillance by auscultation. Amnioinfusion has been demonstrated to reduce the incidence of cord compression and cesarean delivery in patients with PROM.[86]

Route of delivery

Vertex presentation

There has been some controversy over the method of delivery of the premature fetus. Enthusiasm for liberal use of cesarean delivery has been tempered by the findings of several retrospective studies showing no difference in mortality between cesarean and vaginal delivery.[87–89] The current accepted approach is to allow labor with intensive fetal monitoring. Indication for cesarean section is very similar to that of the term fetus. The difference is that the preterm fetus probably tolerates hypoxia less effectively than at term and prompt atraumatic delivery should be considered early in the process. Delivery "in caul" (membranes intact) has been advocated to decrease risk of trauma and fluctuations of cerebral blood flow in response to cord compression.[90] The use of "prophylactic forceps" for preterm delivery has been proven to be potentially hazardous.[91,92] Use of episiotomy should be evaluated on an individual basis. Umbilical cord blood gases, particularly arterial, are more accurate in assessing fetal condition in the preterm neonate than are Apgar scores, which are quite unreliable at early gestational ages.[93]

Malpresentation, multiple gestations

Malpresentations are common in the preterm fetus. The incidence of breech presentation at 28 weeks' gestation approaches 25%. The incidence of fetal abnormalities is increased with breech presentation, including neuromuscular deficits. The risk of the lower extremities, abdomen, and thorax delivering through an incompletely dilated cervix, leaving the relatively larger fetal head trapped behind the cervix prior to 32 weeks has led to a liberal policy of cesarean delivery for the premature fetus. The increased risk of cord prolapse also supports this approach. There have been conflicting reports in the literature regarding cesarean section for breech.[94–96] The very-low-birth-weight fetus (less than 1500 g) is at greatest risk for head entrapment, and thus may benefit most from a cesarean section. However, even with term breech, a study did show greater morbidity with the vaginal approach.[94]

Atraumatic cesarean delivery must be accomplished and this will often require a vertical uterine incision in a poorly developed lower uterine segment. A wide transverse incision is preferable but an adequate incision must be employed. The splint technique[97] is often helpful in assisting with atraumatic delivery of a malpresentation.

Multiple gestations of a higher order (greater than two) are generally delivered by cesarean section. In twin gestations, with the leading twin presenting as a breech, cesarean delivery is indicated. If the lead twin is vertex and twin B is either concordant or smaller than twin A, vaginal delivery of twin A and either external version or breech delivery of twin B may be undertaken. Clinical judgment is important and there should be no hesitation in abandoning difficult vaginal delivery and performing cesarean section if indicated. Real-time sonography should be used to help determine the position and route of delivery. Availability of both obstetric and neonatal expertise is important in decisions on the location of delivery. Obstetrical management is often not a problem but expertise in resuscitation and stabilization of the preterm fetus is crucial in optimizing subsequent outcome.[98,99] This will often require maternal–fetal transportation.

Labor and delivery

The influence of events of labor and delivery on perinatal "brain damage" has been the focus of both obstetricians and pediatricians since the early nineteenth century. Little[100] and Freud[101] stated that the major cause of cerebral palsy (CP) and mental retardation (MR) was intrapartum "brain damage." Prolonged labors and traumatic deliveries supported this impression and it is has only recently been proved that only about 10% of cases of CP and MR can be attributed to events of labor and delivery.[102–104] However, this group of patients is one in which some type of intervention may have a meaningful impact on perinatal outcome. Fetal heart rate (FHR) patterns, determined by continuous EFM, may be of value in predicting hypoxemia and acidosis during labor, thus allowing potentially beneficial therapy. FHR patterns may be obtained through EFM or by auscultation. Continuous EFM may be a less labor-intensive and more practical method of monitoring compared to auscultation, which is more labor-intensive. FHR monitoring is only one parameter of fetal condition and must be evaluated along with the total clinical picture. Transient and repetitive episodes of fetal hypoxemia are extremely common during normal labor. These episodes are usually well tolerated by the fetus. Only when hypoxia and resultant metabolic acidemia reach extreme levels is the fetus at risk for long-term neurologic damage.[105] Terminology must be appropriately used and the following definitions reflect current thinking:[106]

Hypoxemia	Decreased oxygen content in blood
Hypoxia	Decreased level of oxygen in tissue
Acidemia	Increased concentration of hydrogen ions in the blood
Acidosis	Increased concentration of hydrogen ions in tissue
Asphyxia	Hypoxia with metabolic acidosis

The fetus is well adapted to tolerating intermittent episodes of decreased oxygen delivery in labor that occur with contractions. However, numerous factors can lead to significant hypoxemia and eventually to metabolic acidemia. Decreased uterine blood flow will influence the level of fetal oxygenation. Contractions, maternal position, and blood pressure will all have an effect on uterine blood flow. The umbilical cord is also vulnerable during labor. Intermittent cord compression is common and normally well tolerated by the fetus but prolonged compression may lead to hypoxemia, acidosis, and asphyxia. The premature fetus and those with growth disorders are more susceptible to effects of hypoxemia in the intrapartum period and the onset of metabolic acidosis may occur more rapidly. This may lead to fetal or neonatal death or poor long-term outcome.[107,108] Alterations in the FHR are under central nervous system control and may be sensitive indicators of fetal hypoxia.[109,110] A normal FHR is reassuring and is almost always associated with a healthy newborn. The term "reassuring" thus implies normal oxygenation and acid–base status. On the other hand nonreassuring patterns have a wider range of predictability. In many cases nonreassuring patterns are a result of early gestational age, fetal rest cycles, and medications. These patterns may be difficult to distinguish from patterns resulting from hypoxia and early acidosis. The term "fetal distress" should be abandoned and the type of heart-rate pattern should be described.

The FHR should be evaluated systematically, a mechanism for changes in FHR proposed, and the clinical situation assessed. Judgment concerning further management of labor should be made with all relevant information.

FHR is evaluated in the following sequence:

1 Initial assessment of uterine activity. Hyperstimulation can be spontaneous, as a result of abruptio placentae or secondary to labor-inducing medication. FHR abnormalities as a result of hyperstimulation may simply be managed by reducing excessive uterine activity. An example would be decreasing or discontinuing oxytocin stimulation.

2 Evaluation of baseline FHR (rate between contractions). The FHR at term ranges from 110 to 160 beats/min. Greater than 160 beats/min is called tachycardia and less than 110 beats/min is bradycardia (baseline). Causes of tachycardia include maternal fever, intraamniotic infection, and congenital heart disease. Hypoxia that is either chronic or prolonged and severe may also lead to fetal tachycardia. Fetal tachyarrhythmias may also present as tachycardia.

   The initial response of the FHR to hypoxia is deceleration. Change of the baseline to bradycardiac ranges must be carefully evaluated to detect hypoxia.

3 Variability. FHR variability is one of the most reliable indicators of fetal well-being. This can only be detected by continuous electronic FHR monitoring. Short-term variability (STV) is the beat-to-beat variation of every R-R interval of the fetal electrocardiogram. Normal variability is greater than 6 beats/min. Long-term variability (LTV) has a cyclicity of 3–5 cycles per minute. Normal FHR variability represents one of the best indicators of intact integration between the fetal central nervous systems and the cardiovascular system. Loss of variability may suggest fetal hypoxia and acidosis. Medications, fetal sleep cycles, and congenital anomalies also decrease variability. The presence or absence of variability (both STV and LTV) is often subjective, which may lead to differences of opinion concerning the optimal management in a particular clinical situation.

4 Periodic changes. Periodic changes of the FHR are those associated with either uterine activity or fetal movement and will indicate the mechanism of FHR changes.

   (a) Accelerations. These are periodic accelerations above the baseline. They are usually defined as 15 beats/min above the baseline for 10–15 s. These are an indicator of fetal health and nonacidosis.[111]

   (b) Early decelerations. These are decelerations that are U-shaped and coincident with contractions (mirror image). They represent head compression and reflect altered cerebral blood flow and are not indicative of acidosis.

   (c) Variable decelerations. These may begin before, at the onset of, or following the onset of a uterine contraction. The onset is abrupt with a sharp downward limb, plateau, and sharp recovery limb (inverted square). This pattern represents differential cord compression and variable decelerations are classified as mild if less than 30 s duration, moderate if 30–60 s and severe if lasting greater than 60 s and below 70 beats/min.[112] These correlate with acid–base status.

   (d) Late decelerations. These are transient slowing of the FHR that occur after the onset of the contraction or late in the contraction phase of uterine activity. Repetitive late decelerations (following more than three successive contractions) are required for there to be clinical significance. Late decelerations may indicate uteroplacental insufficiency with subsequent hypoxia. There are two types of late decelerations:

      (i) Reflex late decelerations. These are seen

when a sudden acute insult (hypoxia) is superimposed on a previously normally oxygenated fetus. There is normal variability and thus normal central nervous system control.[113] There is no significant acidosis with this pattern.

(ii) Nonreflex late decelerations. There is again an acute insult but there is some preexisting myocardial hypoxic depression. There is decreased variability and this indicates inadequate fetal cerebral and myocardial oxygenation. It is seen more commonly in states of decreased placental reserve, such as IUGR or following prolonged asphyxial stresses, such as a long period of severe reflex late decelerations. There is often significant acidosis associated with this pattern. Late decelerations are classified as mild at ≤15 beats/min, moderate at 15–45 beats/min, or severe at <45 beats/min. Correlation of FHR patterns with fetal acid–base status has been well characterized in numerous studies.[112,114] In summary, a normal FHR baseline with accelerations, early decelerations, mild and moderate variable decelerations, reflex late decelerations, and normal variability will indicate an intact fetal central nervous system. This will be demonstrated by normal neural control of FHR and is correlated with normal fetal acid–base status. Severe variable decelerations, nonreflex late decelerations, and/or loss of variability may indicate fetal acidosis. A sinusoidal heart rate (sine-wave FHR) is often associated with fetal anemia, which may or may not lead to acidemia. The fetus with unexplained loss of variability with no periodic changes may have extremely severe asphyxia with inability of the heart to demonstrate periodic changes. This may also indicate some type of congenital anomaly.[115]

Management of FHR patterns

After evaluation of the FHR in labor by using the sequential approach previously outlined, a preliminary impression of fetal health is obtained. The first question to be answered is whether the fetus has a normal FHR. This will be accurate in predicting a normal outcome in the vast majority of cases. If the sequential approach is strongly suggestive of fetal acidosis, further fetal evaluation and assessment of the clinical situation are necessary. If there is an impression of significant acidosis, delivery by the most expedient method may be indicated. If there are conflicting data and evidence of acidosis is not overwhelming, further evaluation of the fetus and strategies to improve uterine blood flow, fetal oxygenation, and acid–base status must be undertaken.

Standard measures to improve fetal status include maintenance of normal maternal cardiac output, maximizing maternal and fetal oxygenation, and control of uterine activity. Fluid administration and occasionally medication may be required to correct maternal hypotension. Avoidance of the supine position will prevent aortocaval compression. Maternal position change may alleviate cord compression. Discontinuation of oxytocin administration will treat uterine hyperstimulation. Amnioinfusion may ameliorate cord compression in states of oligohydramnios and may improve the outcome of labor complicated by meconium passage.

Evaluation and management of nonreassuring FHR patterns have been outlined in the American College of Obstetricians and Gynecologists technical bulletin, number 207 of July 1995 and can be summarized as follows:

1 Determine the etiology of the pattern.
2 Attempt correction of the pattern by correcting the primary problem or by instituting general measures aimed at improving fetal oxygenation and placental perfusion.
3 If attempts to correct the patterns are not successful, further evaluation of fetal acid–base status is required. Fetal scalp capillary blood sampling will enable direct measurement of acid–base status.

This is invasive and somewhat cumbersome. Fetal scalp stimulation[116] or vibroacoustic stimulation[117] have been shown to be reliable in determining normal fetal acid–base status noninvasively if accelerations of the FHR occur. However, if accelerations do not occur, up to 60% of fetuses are nonacidotic.

4 Determine whether operative intervention is warranted, and if so, how urgently.

Other specific measures to attempt to improve fetal condition include amnioinfusion to decrease the frequency and severity of variable decelerations.[118,119] There may be an advantage to using amnioinfusion in cases of meconium passage to dilute the meconium and possibly prevent fetal gasping.[120–122] However, reports of amniotic fluid embolism in such cases should lead to caution about infusing fluid under pressure.[123]

Another potentially valuable tool in the management of intrapartum events is the use of tocolytic agents to decrease uterine activity. Terbutaline,[124] magnesium sulfate,[125] and nitroglycerin[126] have all been used. Use of these agents is usually temporary while preparing for expeditious delivery.

It should be emphasized that individual circumstances in each case must be considered. Decisions on whether to continue labor or expedite delivery will be dictated by the complete clinical picture and not isolated pieces of information. The overriding principle must be optimal outcome for both the mother and the fetus. Giving the fetus the benefit of the doubt in confusing situations is often the most prudent approach.

Operative vaginal delivery

Normal spontaneous vaginal delivery is considered a physiological process and complications with spontaneous delivery are relatively uncommon. Acute events in the late second stage of labor, prior to anticipated delivery, may cause fetal and neonatal complications. These include abruptio placentae, umbilical cord prolapse, ruptured uterus, ruptured vasa previa, and shoulder dystocia. Diagnosis of these complications may lead to operative vaginal delivery. Instruments for operative vaginal delivery include forceps and vacuum extraction. Cesarean section is classified as operative abdominal delivery.

Shoulder dystocia

Shoulder dystocia is a relatively uncommon complication but is one of the most serious acute obstetrical events facing the obstetrician. The diagnosis is made following vaginal delivery of the head, with immediate retraction of the head against the perineal body. The supposed mechanism is impingement of the anterior shoulder against the symphysis pubis. There is a correlation between birth weight and an increased incidence of shoulder dystocia, but methods of estimating fetal weight have not been reliable in predicting shoulder dystocia. Similarly, maternal obesity, postdates pregnancy, gestational diabetes,[127] prolonged second stage of labor, and midpelvic delivery[128] have all been associated with an increased risk of shoulder dystocia. Neonatal complications of shoulder dystocia include brachial plexus injuries, fractured humerus, fractured clavicle, and fetal hypoxia and acidosis. Once the diagnosis is made a well-rehearsed sequence of actions such as the following needs to be implemented.[129]

1 Call for additional help and obstetric anesthesia.
2 The initial attempt at traction should coincide with McRoberts maneuvers, flexion of the maternal thighs towards the abdomen, and suprapubic pressure in an oblique plane to attempt to disimpact the anterior shoulder. Fundal pressure should not be used.
3 A generous episiotomy may help to increase space for manipulation.
4 The initial attempt at traction with maternal expulsive efforts and the above procedures should be abandoned if this does not effect delivery.
5 Perform a Woods screw maneuver, where the anterior shoulder is converted to the posterior shoulder through 180°.
6 Alternatively, delivery of the posterior arm can be attempted by placing a hand posterolaterally in

the vagina, splinting the humerus and delivering the arm. This can lead to fracture of the humerus. Deliberate fracture of the clavicle can be attempted but is often difficult.

7 Cephalic replacement (Zavanelli maneuver) with subsequent cesarean section is an option when all other methods have failed.[130]

Instrumental deliveries

The role of midforceps operations in causing increased perinatal morbidity has been controversial, with older literature painting a more ominous picture[131,132] than more recent literature.[133,134] There was a correlation noted between a second stage of labor exceeding 2 h and fetal morbidity and mortality prior to the 1970s. Currently, the length of the second stage, provided that intrapartum fetal monitoring demonstrates fetal tolerance of labor, does not correlate with increased neonatal morbidity. However, a prolonged second stage of (1) more than 2 h in a nulliparous patient without regional anesthesia; (2) 3 h with regional anesthesia; (3) more than 2 h in a parous patient with regional anesthesia; or (4) 1 h without anesthesia should prompt reassessment of the clinical situation. Length of the second stage alone should not be used as an indication for operative delivery provided fetal well-being is assured and other indications for delivery are not present. Instrumental delivery, like any other medical procedure, is appropriately used after evaluation of the indications for, risk of, and alternatives to the procedure.

Indications for operative vaginal delivery

Maternal

There are certain medical conditions in which the mother needs to avoid or cannot perform voluntary expulsive efforts such as certain cardiovascular, cerebral, gastrointestinal, or neuromuscular diseases. Maternal exhaustion, lack of cooperation, and excessive analgesia may affect the patient's ability to assist adequately in the expulsion of the fetus.

Fetal

Nonreassuring FHR pattern is a major indication for operative delivery. Second-stage FHR monitoring patterns are frequently misinterpreted as nonreassuring with subsequent intervention. These patterns are often confusing and need to be evaluated carefully to determine whether there is fetal intolerance of labor.[111] Failure of spontaneous vaginal delivery following an appropriately managed second stage is another major indication for operative vaginal delivery. The use of "prophylactic" forceps for the delivery of a preterm fetus is generally discouraged and standard obstetrical indications should be used in making decisions on whether forceps should be used in these circumstances.

Selective shortening of the second stage of labor with outlet forceps is considered appropriate when the fetal head is on the perineum and rotation does not exceed 45°. There is no difference in perinatal outcome compared to spontaneous deliveries.[132,135]

After determination of the indications for instrumental delivery, appropriate anesthesia and patient positioning are required. The most important factors to consider are pelvic adequacy, fetal station, and fetal rotation. Criteria of forceps deliveries are outlined in Table 6.1.

The choice of instrument is influenced by the training of the operator and the clinical situation. For example, Elliot forceps are used for the unmolded head while Simpsons forceps are used for the molded head. Specialized forceps include rotational forceps such as Kielland, Barton, and Piper forceps (for the after-coming head of a breech). The vacuum extractor is an alternative to forceps and the same sound judgment needs to be exercised when using this instrument. The ease of application of a vacuum cup sometimes leads to inappropriate use. If the clinical situation is such that a forceps instrument would be contraindicated, then a vacuum extractor should not be used. An advantage of a vacuum over forceps is the potential avoidance of maternal soft-tissue trauma, but both maternal and fetal complications have been reported.[129]

Careful documentation in the medical record of

Table 6.1. Criteria of forceps deliveries according to station and rotation

Type of procedure	Criteria
Outlet forceps	1. Scalp is visible at the introitus without separating labia 2. Fetal skull has reached pelvic floor 3. Sagittal suture is in anteroposterior diameter or right left occiput anterior or posterior position 4. Fetal head is at or on perineum 5. Rotation does not exceed 45°
Low forceps	Leading point of fetal skull is at station ⩾+2 cm and not on the pelvic floor: 1. Rotation ⩽45° (left or right occiput anterior to occiput anterior, or left or right occiput posterior to occiput posterior) 2. Rotation >45°
Mid forceps	Station above +2 cm but head engaged
High forceps	Not included in classification[129]

the indication for the procedure, the position and station of the vertex, the degree of difficulty of the procedure, and any maternal and neonatal complications is essential. There should be no hesitation in abandoning attempts at operative vaginal delivery and resorting to abdominal delivery if satisfactory progress is not made. Knowledge of physiology and pathophysiology, intelligent application of technology, and sound clinical judgment will all help to optimize perinatal outcome

REFERENCES

1 World Health Organization. (1969). *Prevention of Perinatal Morbidity.* Public health papers, 42. Geneva: WHO.

2 Nelson KB and Ellenberg JH. (1986). Antecedents of cerebral palsy: multivariate analysis of risk. *N Engl J Med,* **315**, 81–86.

3 Monthly Vital Statistics Report. (1991). *Advance Report on Fetal Natality Studies,* **40** (suppl), 8.

4 Cooper RK, Goldenberg RL, Creasy RK, et al. (1993). A multicenter study of preterm birth weight and gestational age specific mortality. *Am J Obstet Gynecol,* **168**, 78–84.

5 Ferrara TB, Hoekstra RE, Couser RS, et al. (1994). Survival and follow-up of infants born at 23–26 weeks gestational age: effects of surfactant therapy. *J Pediatr,* **124**, 119–124.

6 Nwasi CG, Young DC, Byrne JM, et al. (1987). Preterm birth at 23 to 26 weeks gestation: is active management justified? *Am J Obstet Gynecol,* **157**, 890–897.

7 Robertson PA, Sniderman SH, Laros RK Jr, et al. (1992). Neonatal morbidity according to gestational age and birth weight from five tertiary centers in the United States, 1983 through 1986. *Am J Obstet Gynecol,* **166**, 1629–1645.

8 Papiernik E and Kaminski M. (1974). Multifactional study of the risk of prematurity at 32 weeks of gestation. *J Perinat Med,* **2**, 30–36.

9 Meis PJ, MacErnest J and Moore ML. (1987). Causes of low birth weight births in public and private patients. *Am J Obstet Gynecol,* **156**, 1165–1168.

10 Fedrick J and Anderson ABM. (1976). Factors associated with spontaneous preterm birth. *Br J Obstet Gynaecol,* **83**, 342–350.

11 US Department of Health and Human Services. (1985). *Report of the Secretary's Task Force on Black and Minority Health,* publication 0-487-637 (QL3), vol. 6. *Infant mortality and low birth weight.* Hyattsville, Maryland: National Center for Health Statistics.

12 Bakketeig LS and Hoffman HJ. (1981). Epidemiology of preterm birth: results from longitudinal study of births in Norway. In *Preterm Labour,* ed. MG Elder and CH Dendricks, pp. 17–46. London: Butterworths.

13 Abrams B, Newman V, Key T, et al. (1989). Maternal weight gain and preterm delivery. *Obstet Gynecol,* **74**, 577–583.

14 MacGregor SW, Keith LG, Chasnoff IJ, et al. (1987). Cocaine use during pregnancy: adverse perinatal outcome. *Am J Obstet Gynecol,* **57**, 686–690.

15 Shiono PH, Klebanoff MA and Rhoads GG (1986). Smoking and drinking during pregnancy. *JAMA,* **255**, 82–84.

16 Keirse M, Rush R, Anderson A, et al.(1978). Risk of preterm delivery in patients with previous preterm delivery and/or abortion. *Br J Obstet Gynaecol,* **85**, 81–85.

17 Linn S, Schoenbaum S, Monson R, et al. (1983). The relationship between induced abortion and outcome of subsequent pregnancies. *Am J Obstet Gynecol,* **146**, 136–140.

18 Chung C, Smith R, Steinhoff P, et al. (1982). Induced abortion and spontaneous fetal loss in subsequent pregnancies. *Am J Public Health,* **72**, 548–554.

19 US Department of Health and Human Services, Public Health Service (1986). *Vital Statistics of the United States, 1982,* vol. I. *Natality.* Hyattsville, Maryland: US Department of Health.

20 Neilson JP, Verkuyl DAA, Crowther CA, et al. (1988). Preterm labor in twin pregnancies: prediction by cervical assessment. *Obstet Gynecol*, **72**, 719–723.

21 Australian Institute of Health and Welfare National Perinatal Statistics Unit. (1992). *Assisted Conception in Australia and New Zealand.* Sydney: AIHW.

22 Ratten GJ, Beischer NA and Fortune DIO. (1973). Obstetric complications when the fetus has Potter's syndrome. *Am J Obstet Gynecol*, **115**, 890–896.

23 Honnebier WJ and Swaab DF. (1973). The influence of anencephaly upon intrauterine growth of fetus and placenta and upon gestational length. *J Obstet Gynaecol, Br Commonwlth*, **80**, 577–588.

24 Williams MA, Millendorf R, Liererman E, et al. (1991). Adverse infant outcomes associated with first trimester vaginal bleeding. *Obstet Gynecol*, **78**, 14–18.

25 Roberts, G. (1970). Unclassified antepartum haemorrhage incidence and perinatal mortality in a community. *J Obstet Gynaecol, Br Commonwlth*, **77**, 492–495.

26 Herbst AL, Hubby MM, Blough RR, et al. (1980). A comparison of pregnancy experiment in DES exposed and DES-unexposed daughters. *J Reprod Med*, **24**, 62–69.

27 Kaufman RH, Noller K, Adam E, et al. (1985). Upper genital tract abnormalities and pregnancy outcome in diethylstilbestrol-exposed progeny. *Am J Obstet Gynecol*, **148**, 973–984.

28 Harger JH. (1983). Cervical cerclage: patient selection, morbidity and success rates. *Clin Perinatol*, **10**, 321–341.

29 Zemlyn S. (1981). The length of the uterine cervix and its significance. *J Clin Ultrasound*, **9**, 267–269.

30 Rush RLO. (1979). Incidence of preterm delivery in patients with previous preterm delivery and/or abortion. *S Afr Med J*, **56**, 1085–1087.

31 Rush RW, Issacs S, McPherson K, et al. (1984). A randomized controlled trial of cervical cerclage in women at moderate risk of preterm delivery. *Br J Obstet Gynaecol*, **91**, 724–730.

32 Lazar P, Gueguen S, Dreyfuss J, et al. (1984). Multicentre controlled trial of cervical cerclage in women at moderate risk of preterm delivery. *Br J Obstet Gynaecol*, **91**, 731–735.

33 Grant A. (1986). *Cervical Cerclage: Evaluation Studies. Proceedings of a Workshop on Prevention of Preterm Birth.* Paris: INSERM.

34 Medical Research Council and Royal College of Obstetricians and Gynaecologists Working Party on Cervical Cerclage. (1988). Interim report of the Medical Research Council and Royal College of Obstetricians and Gynaecologists multicentre randomized trial on cervical cerclage. *Br J Obstet Gynaecol*, **95**, 437–445.

35 Bobbitt JR and Ledger WJ. (1977). Unrecognized amnionitis and prematurity: a preliminary report. *J Reprod Med*, **19**, 8–12.

36 Bobbitt JR and Ledger WJ. (1978) Amniotic fluid analysis: its role in maternal and neonatal infection. *Obstet Gynecol*, **51**, 56–62.

37 Leigh J and Garite TJM. (1986). Amnionitis and the management of premature labor. *Obstet Gynecol*, **67**, 500–506.

38 Gravett MG, Hummel D, Eschenbach DA, et al. (1986). Preterm labor associated with subclinical amniotic infection and with bacterial vaginosis. *Obstet Gynecol*, **67**, 229–237.

39 Hameed C, Teiane N, Verma UL, et al. (1984). Silent chorioamnionitis as a cause of preterm labor refractory to tocolytic therapy. *Am J Obstet Gynecol*, **149**, 726–730.

40 Duff P and Kopelman JN. (1987). Subclinical intraamniotic infection in asymptomatic patients with refractory preterm labor. *Obstet Gynecol*, **69**, 756–769.

41 Romero R and Mazor M. (1988). Infection and preterm labor. *Clin Obstet Gynecol*, **31**, 553–584.

42 Gibbs RS, Romero R, Hillier SL, et al. (1992). A review of premature birth and subclinical infection. *Am J Obstet Gynecol*, **166**, 1515–1528.

43 Gomez R, Romero R, Ghezzi F, et al. (1998). The fetal inflammatory response syndrome. *Am J Obstet Gynecol*, **179**, 194–202.

44 Kaltreider DF and Kohl S. (1980). Epidemiology of preterm delivery. *Clin Obstet Gynecol*, **23**, 17–31.

45 Artal JP, Sokol RJ, Newman M, et al. (1976). The mechanical properties of prematurely and non-prematurely ruptured membranes. *Am J Obstet Gynecol*, **125**, 655–659.

46 Lavery JP, Miller CE and Knight RD. (1982). The effect of labor on the rheologic response of chorioamniotic membranes. *Obstet Gynecol*, **60**, 87–91.

47 Lonky NN and Hayashi RH. (1988). A proposed mechanism for premature rupture of membranes. *Obstet Gynecol Surv*, **43**, 22–28.

48 Minkoff H, Grunebaum AN, Schwarz RH, et al. (1984). Risk factors for prematurity and premature rupture of membranes; a prospective study of vaginal flora in pregnancy. *Am J Obstet Gynecol*, **150**, 965–972.

49 Iams JD and McGregor JA. (1990). Cervicovaginal microflora and pregnancy outcome: results of a double blind, placebo-controlled trial of erythromycin treatment. *Am J Obstet Gynecol*, **163**, 1580–1591.

50 Naeye RL. (1982). Factors that predispose to premature rupture of the fetal membranes. *Obstet Gynecol*, **60**, 93–98.

51 Taylor J and Garite TJ (1984). Premature rupture of membranes before fetal viability. *Obstet Gynecol*, **64**, 615–620.

52 Mead, P.B. (1980). Management of the patient with premature rupture of the membranes. *Clin Perinatol*, **7**, 243–255.
53 Kennedy KA and Clark SL. (1992). Premature rupture of infant morbidity after preterm premature rupture of the membranes: management controversies. *Clin Perinatol*, **19**, 385–397.
54 Garite TJ, Freeman RK, Linzy EM, et al. (1981). Prospective randomized study of corticosteroids in the management of premature rupture of membranes and the premature gestation. *Am J Obstet Gynecol*, **141**, 508–515.
55 Gibbs RS, Blanco JD, St Clair PJ, et al. (1982). Quantitative bacteriology of amniotic fluid from patients with clinical intra-amniotic infection at term. *J Infect Dis*, **145**, 1–8.
56 Yoder PR, Gibbs RS, Blanco JD, et al. (1983). A prospective controlled study of maternal and perinatal outcome after intra-amniotic infection at term. *Am J Obstet Gynecol*, **145**, 695–701.
57 Garite TJ. (1994). Premature rupture of the membranes. In *Maternal–Fetal Medicine: Principles and Practices*, ed. RK Creasy and R Resnick, pp. 625–638. Philadelphia: Saunders.
58 Garite TJ and Freeman RK. (1982). Chorioamnionitisin the preterm gestation. *Obstet Gyneco*l, **54**, 539–545.
59 Gabbe SG, Ettinger BB, Freeman RK, et al. (1976). Umbilical cord compression associated with amniotomy: laboratory observations. *Am J Obstet Gynecol*, **126**, 353–356.
60 Wilson JC, Levy DC and Wilds PL. (1982). Premature rupture of membranes prior to term. Consquences of non-intervention. *Obstet Gynecol*, **60**, 601–606.
61 Moberg LJ and Garite TJ. (1987). Antepartum fetal heart rate testing in PROM. *Seventh Annual Meeting of the Society of Perinatal Obstetricians*.
62 Morretti M and Sibai BM. (1988). Maternal and perinatal outcome of expectant management of premature rupture of membranes in the mid-trimester. *Am J Obstet Gynecol*, **159**, 390–396.
63 Major CA and Kitzmiller JL. (1990). Perinatal survival with expectant management of mid-trimester rupture of membranes. *Am J Obstet Gynecol*, **163**, 838–844.
64 Creasy RK. (1985). Preterm labor and delivery. In *Disorders of Parturition*, Part III, ed. LJ Moberg and TJ Garite, pp. 494–520.
65 Utter GO, Dooley SL, Tamura RK, et al. (1990). Awaiting cervical change for the diagnosis of preterm labor does not compromise the efficacy of ritodrine tocolysis. *Am J Obstet Gynecol*, **163**, 882–886.
66 Peaceman AM, Andrews WW, Thorp JM, et al. (1997). Fetal fibronectin as a predictor of preterm birth in patients with symptoms: a multicenter trial. *Am J Obstet Gynecol*, **177**, 13–18.
67 Mercer BM and Arheart KL. (1995) Antimicrobial therapy in expectant management of preterm premature rupture of the membranes. *Lancet*, **346**, 1271–1279.
68 Mercer BM, Miodovnik M, Thurnau GR, et al. (1997). Antibiotic therapy for reduction of infant morbidity after preterm premature rupture of the membranes: a randomized controlled trial. *JAMA*, **278**, 989–995.
69 Boylan T and O'Driscoll K. (1983). Improvement in perinatal mortality rate attributed to spontaneous pre term labor without use of tocolytic agents. *Am J Obstet Gynecol*, **145**, 781–783.
70 Korenbroit CC, Aalto LH and Laros J. (1984). The cost effectiveness of stopping preterm labor with beta adrenergic treatment. *N Engl J Med*, **310**, 691–696.
71 Canadian Preterm Labor Investigators Group. (1992). The treatment of preterm labor with the beta-adrenergic agonist ritodrine. *N Engl J Med*, **327**, 308–312.
72 Valenzuela C, Kline S and Hayashi RH. (1983) Follow up of hydration and sedation in the pre-therapy of premature labor. *Am J Obstet Gynecol*, **147**, 396–398.
73 Sica-Blanco Y, Rozada H and Remedio MR. (1967). Effects of meperidine on uterine contractability of pregnancy and prelabor. *Am J Obstet Gynecol*, **97**, 1096–1100.
74 Usher R. (1977). Changing mortality rates with perinatal intensive care and regionalization. *Semin Perinatol*, **1**, 309–319.
75 Gortmaker S, Sobol A, Clark C, et al. (1985). The survival of very low-birth weight infants by level of hospital of birth. A population study of perinatal systems in four states. *Am J Obstet Gynecol*, **152**, 517–524.
76 Kitchen W, Ford G, Orgill A, et al. (1984). Outcome in infants with birth weight 500–999 grams. A regional study of 1979 and 1980 births. *J Pediatr*, **104**, 921–927.
77 Hadlock FP, Harrist RB, Carpenter RJ, et al. (1984). Sonographic estimation of fetal weight. The value of fetal length in addition to head and abdominal measurements. *Radiology*, **152**, 497–501.
78 Seeds JW, Cefalo RL and Bowes WA. (1984). Femur lengths in the estimation of fetal weight less than 1500 grams. *Am J Obstet Gynecol*, **149**, 233–235.
79 Paul RH and Hon EH. (1974). Clinical fetal monitoring. V. Effect on perinatal outcome. *Am J Obstet Gynecol*, **118**, 529–533.
80 National Institute of Health Consensus Statement. (1994). Effect of antenatal steroids for fetal maturation on perinatal outcomes. *NIH Consensus Statement*, **12**, 1–24.
81 Myers RE and Myers SE. (1979). Use of sedative, analgesic and anesthetic drugs during labor and delivery: bane or boon. *Am J Obstet Gynecol*, **133**, 83–108.

82 Low JA, Gallbraith RS, Muir DW, et al. (1984). Factors associated with motor and cognitive deficits in children after intrapartum fetal hypoxia. *Am J Obstet Gynecol*, **148**, 533–539.

83 Bowes WA Jr, Gabbe S and Bowes C. (1980). Fetal heart rate monitoring in premature infants weighing 1500 grams or less. *Am J Obstet Gynecol*, **137**, 791–796.

84 Westgren LMR, Malcus P and Sveningsen NW. (1986). Intrauterine asphyxia and longterm outcome in preterm fetuses. *Obstet Gynecol*, **67**, 512–516.

85 Luthy DA, Kirkwood KS, van Belle G, et al. (1987). A randomized trial of electronic fetal monitoring in preterm labor. *Obstet Gynecol*, **69**, 637–695.

86 Nageotte MP, Freeman RK, Garite TJ, et al. (1985). Prophylactic intrapartum amnioinfusion in patients with preterm premature rupture of membranes. *Am J Obstet Gynecol*, **153**, 557–562.

87 Olshan AF, Shy KK and Luthy DA. (1984). Cesarean birth and neonatal mortality in very low birth weight infants. *Obstet Gynecol*, **64**, 267–270.

88 Yu VYH, Bajak B, Cutting D, et al. (1984). Effect of mode of delivery on outcome of very low birthweight infants. *Br J Obstet Gynaecol*, **91**, 633–639.

89 Kithen W, Ford GW, Doyle LW, et al. (1985). Cesarean section or vaginal delivery at 24 to 28 weeks' gestation: comparison of survival and neonatal and two year morbidity. *Obstet Gynecol*, **66**, 149–157.

90 Goldenberg RL and Davis RO. (1983). In caul delivery of the very premature infant. *Am J Obstet Gynecol*, **145**, 645–646.

91 Schwarz DB, Miodovnik MK and Lavin JP Jr. (1983). Neonatal outcome among low birth weight infants delivered spontaneously or by low forceps. *Obstet Gynecol*, **62**, 283–286.

92 Kriewall TJ. (1982). Structural, mechanical, and material properties of fetal cranial bone. *Am J Obstet Gynecol*, **143**, 707–714.

93 Goldenberg RL, Huddlestone JF and Nelson KG. (1984). Apgar scores and umbilical arterial pH in preterm newborn infants. *Am J Obstet Gynecol*, **149**, 651–654.

94 Bowes WA Jr, Taylor ES, O'Brien M, et al. (1979). Breech delivery: evaluation of the method of delivery on perinatal results and maternal morbidity. *Am J Obstet Gynecol*, **135**, 965–973.

95 Bodmer B, Benjamin A, McLean FH, et al. (1986). Has use of cesarean section reduced the risk of delivery in the preterm breech presentation? *Am J Obstet Gynecol*, **154**, 244–250.

96 Rosen G and Chick L. (1984). The effect of delivery route on outcome in breech presentation. *Am J Obstet Gynecol*, **148**, 909–914.

97 Druzin ML. (1986). Atraumatic delivery in cases of malpresentation of the very low birth weight fetus at cesarean section: the splint technique. *Am J Obstet Gynecol*, **154**, 941–942.

98 Harris TR, Isman J and Giles HR. (1978). Improved neonatal survival through maternal transport. *Obstet Gynecol*, **52**, 294–300.

99 Paneth N, Kiely JL, Wallenstein S, et al. (1987). The choice of place of delivery: effect of hospital level on mortality in all singleton births in New York City. *Am J Dis Child*, **141**, 60–64.

100 Little WJ. (1862). On the influence of abnormal parturition, difficult labors, premature birth, and asphyxia neonatorum on the mental and physical condition of the child, especially in relation to deformities. *Trans Obstet Soc Lond*, **2**, 293–344.

101 Freud S. (1897). Infantile cerebrallhhmung. *Notbnagel's Specielle Pathologic and Tberapie*, vol. 12. Vienna: Holder.

102 Blair E and Stanley FJ. (1988). Intrapartum asphyxia: a rare cause of cerebral palsy. *J Pediatr*, **112**, 515–519.

103 Committee on Obstetrics, Maternal and Fetal Medicine. (1992). *Fetal and Neonatal Neurologic Injury*. ACOG Technical Bulletin 163. Washington, DC: ACOG.

104 Naeye RL, Peters EC, Bartholomew M and Landis JR. (1989). Origins of cerebral palsy. *Am J Dis Child*, **143**, 1154–1156.

105 Stanley FJ and Blair E. (1991). Why have we failed to reduce the frequency of cerebral palsy? *Med J Aust*, **154**, 623–626.

106 American College of Obstetricians and Gynecologists. (1995). *Fetal Heart Rate Patterns: Monitoring, Interpretation, and Management*. ACOG Technical Bulletin 207. Washington, DC: ACOG.

107 Low JA, Boston RW and Pancham FR. (1972). Fetal asphyxia during the intrapartum period in intrauterine growth retarded infants. *Am J Obstet Gynecol*, **113**, 351–357.

108 Westgran LMR, Malcus P and Svenningsen NW. (1986). Intrauterine asphyxia and longterm outcome in preterm fetuses. *Obstet Gynecol*, **67**, 512–516.

109 Myers RE, Mueller-Huebach E and Adamson K. (1992). Predictability of the state of fetal oxygenation from quantitative analysis of the components of late decelerations. *Am J Obstet Gynecol*, **115**, 1083–1094.

110 Watasuki A, Murata Y, Ninomiya Y, et al. (1992). Autonomic nervous system regulation of baseline heart rate in the fetal lamb. *Am J Obstet Gynecol*, **167**, 519–523.

111 Clark SL, Gimovsky ML and Miller FC. (1982). Fetal heart rate response to scalp blood sampling. *Am J Obstet Gynecol*, **44**, 706–708.

112 Kubli FW, Hon EH, Khazin AF, et al. (1969). Observations on heart rate and pH in the human fetus during labor. *Am J Obstet Gynecol*, **104**, 1190–1206.

113 Parer JT. (1983). *Handbook of Fetal Heart Rate Monitoring.* Philadelphia: Saunders.

114 Low JA, Cox MJ, Karchmar EJ, et al. (1981). The prediction of intrapartum fetal metabolic acidosis by fetal heart rate monitoring. *Am J Obstet Gynecol,* **139**, 299–305.

115 Kero P, Antila K, Ylitalo V, et al. (1978). Decreased heart rate variation in deceleration syndrome: quantitative clinical criterion of brain death? *Pediatrics,* **62**, 307–311.

116 Clark SL, Gimovsky ML and Miller FC. (1984). The scalp stimulation test: a clinical alternative to fetal scalp blood sampling. *Am J Obstet Gynecol,* **148**, 274–277.

117 Edersheimm TG, Hutson JM, Druzin ML, et al. (1987). Fetal heart rate response to vibroacoustic stimulation predicts fetal pH in labor. *Am J Obstet Gynecol,* **157**, 1557–1560.

118 Strong TH Jr. (1992). Amnioinfusion with preterm, premature rupture of membranes. *Clin Perinatol,* **19**, 399–409.

119 Strong TH Jr, Hetzler G, Sarno AP, et al. (1990). Prophylactic intrapartum amnioinfusion: a randomized clinical trial. *Am J Obstet Gynecol,* **162**, 1370–1375.

120 Sadovsky Y, Amon E, Bade ME, et al. (1989). Prophylactic amnioinfusion during labor complicated by meconium: a preliminary report. *Am J Obstet Gynecol,* **141**, 613–617.

121 Wenstrom KD and Parsons MT. (1989). The prevention of meconium aspiration in labor using amnioinfusion. *Obstet Gynecol,* **73**, 47–51.

122 Marci CJ, Schrimmer DB, Leung A, et al. (1992). Prophylactic amnioinfusion improves outcome of pregnancy complicated by thick meconium and oligohydramnios. *Am J Obstet Gynecol,* **167**, 117–121.

123 Maher E, Wenstrom K, Hauth J, et al. (1994). Amniotic fluid embolism after saline amnioinfusion: two cases and review of the literature. *Obstet Gynecol,* **83**, 851–854.

124 Arias F. (1978). Intrauterine resuscitation with terbutaline: a method for the management of acute intrapartum fetal distress. *Am J Obstet Gynecol,* **131**, 139–143.

125 Reece EA, Chervenak FA, Romero R, et al. (1984). Magnesium sulfate in the management of acute intrapartum fetal distress. *Am J Obstet Gynecol,* **148**, 104–107.

126 Riley ET, Flanagan B, Cohen SE, et al. (1996). Intravenous nitroglycerin: a potent uterine relaxant for emergency obstetric procedures. Review of the literature and report of three cases. *Int J Obstet Anesth,* **5**, 264–268.

127 Spellacy WN, Miller MS, Winegar A, et al. (1985). Macrosomia, maternal characteristics and infant complications. *Obstet Gynecol,* **66**, 158–161.

128 Benedetti TJ and Gabbe SG. (1978). Shoulder dystocia: a complication of fetal macrosomia and prolonged second stage of labor with mid-pelvic delivery. *Obstet Gynecol,* **52**, 526–529.

129 American College of Obstetricians and Gynecologists. (1994). *Operative Vaginal Delivery.* Technical Bulletin 196. Washington: ACOG.

130 Sandberg EC. (1985). Zavanelli maneuver: a potentially revolutionary method for the resolution of shoulder dystocia. *Am J Obstet Gynecol,* **152**, 479–484.

131 Taylor ES. (1953). Can mid-forceps operations be eliminated? *Obstet Gynecol,* **2**, 302–307.

132 Friedman EA, Sachtleben-Murray MR, Dahrouge D, et al. (1984). Long-term effects of labor and delivery on offspring: a matched pair analysis. *Am J Obstet Gynecol,* **150**, 941–945.

133 Gilstrap LC III, Hauth JC, Schiano S, et al. (1984). Neonatal acidosis and method of delivery. *Obstet Gynecol,* **63**, 681–685.

134 Dierker LJ Jr, Rosen MG, Thompson K, et al. (1986). Midforceps deliveries: long-term outcome of infants. *Am J Obstet Gynecol,* **151**, 54–58.

135 Nyiriesy I and Pierce WE. (1964). Perinatal mortality and maternal morbidity in spontaneous and forceps vaginal deliveries. *Am J Obstet Gynecol,* **89**, 568–578.

7

Intrauterine growth retardation (restriction)

Alistair G. S. Philip

Division of Neonatal and Developmental Medicine, Stanford University Medical Center, Palo Alto, CA, USA

Introduction

There are several terms that are frequently used interchangeably for intrauterine growth retardation (IUGR). These include fetal growth retardation, fetal mal- or undernutrition, small-for-gestational-age (SGA), small- or light-for-dates, dysmature, placental insufficiency syndrome, "runting" syndrome and hypotrophy. More recently, there has been a move towards using "restriction" instead of "retardation," because parents tend to link "retardation" with mental retardation.[1,2] Unfortunately, these terms do not all mean the same thing,[3] which has led to some confusion, both with regard to etiologic classification and also with regard to follow-up and outcome. In interpreting studies dealing with IUGR, it is important to know how the term has been defined for the particular study.

Even for studies dealing with infants who are called SGA, it is important to know the normative data used for comparison. For many years, the growth curves developed in Denver, Colorado,[4] were used as the basis for comparison by many authors. It should be appreciated that these data were gathered from infants born at an altitude of 5000 ft (1525 m) and altitude may have an effect upon birth weight for gestational age.[5,6] Thus, infants classified as below the 10th percentile by birth weight for gestational age in Colorado probably represent infants below the third percentile at sea level, for example using Montreal curves.[7] More recent data from Sweden, also at sea level, indicate that birth weights in recent years may be even higher than noted in an earlier era.[8] This may be partially related to the extreme limitation on weight gain during pregnancy that was imposed by most obstetricians in North America during the 1950s and 1960s, when these data were being gathered.

The use of the term intrauterine growth retardation (or restriction) implies that the infant (fetus) has failed to achieve his or her full growth potential. While it is true that the majority of SGA infants will have some degree of IUGR, some SGA infants were predestined to fall below the 10th percentile on a genetic or racial basis. On the other hand, some infants who have a birth weight which is appropriate-for-gestational-age (AGA: between the 10th and 90th percentiles) may be suffering from the effects of IUGR. These infants will usually display some evidence of wasting or appear scrawny.

Although the concept has been around for many years, the use of ponderal index or weight–length ratio seems to be gaining favor in helping to describe the wasted appearance that some of these babies have. The ponderal index was described by Röhrer[9] and attracted the attention of Lubchenco and her colleagues[4] as well as Miller and Hassanein.[10] This was derived by taking the weight (in grams) and multiplying by 100 and dividing by the length (in centimeters) cubed. Although the Colorado curves were widely distributed and used to plot weight, length, and head circumference, few bothered to plot the ponderal index, at least in the 1970s. Different authors used the ponderal index to classify infants, mostly for research purposes.[10–13] Unfortunately, this may lead to multiple subgroups within the total population of IUGR infants.[14] While this may reflect the great heterogeneity of this group of infants, it can also lead to confusion.

The simplest classification is to consider infants with IUGR as either proportionally (symmetrically) or disproportionally (asymmetrically) grown. Most proportionally grown infants will have a normal ponderal index, whereas the disproportionally grown will have a decreased ponderal index. However, such clearcut distinctions are not always possible.[14,15] Proportionally grown infants are likely to have had a chronic insult (e.g., a chromosomal problem such as trisomy 18), whereas the disproportionally grown infants are likely to have suffered a subacute or acute insult (e.g., decreased uteroplacental blood flow with maternal toxemia). For many years it was believed that a chronic insult resulted in a decrease in cell number, but a subacute or acute insult produced a decrease in cell size.[16] Work by Sands et al.[7] indicated that cell size increased much earlier than originally believed and that cell multiplication continues unabated throughout tissue growth. They stated: "The hypothesized early circumscribed phase of cell division, which is said to be particularly vulnerable to permanent stunting, does not appear to exist."[17] This helps to explain the difficulty in predicting subsequent growth based on birth weight.[18]

Further support for an earlier onset of growth restriction, even in asymmetric IUGR, comes from a prospective study using prenatal ultrasound at 17, 25, 33, and 37 weeks' gestation.[19] The investigators evaluated the hypothesis that symmetrical IUGR would start in the first trimester and asymmetrical IUGR would start in the third trimester. The hypothesis was disproved, with both groups starting in the second trimester.[19] Furthermore, the authors were unable to distinguish different patterns of growth.

With asymmetrical growth retardation, the concept of "brain sparing" has been proposed, but this may be misleading, because, although the head circumference may appear to be relatively large, it is frequently below the 10th percentile for gestational age,[20,21] and a study could not support evidence of "brain sparing" when asymmetric SGA were compared to symmetric SGA.[19] Thus, although redistribution of blood flow may favor brain growth, this "adaptation" may be incomplete and result in deficient growth of the brain. Supporting evidence comes from studies using magnetic resonance imaging, which showed decreases in brain volume, although this was less affected than body weight.[22] It has been noted that in many instances of IUGR, decrease in size may represent an appropriate adaptive response to the availability of nutrients, but extreme IUGR may represent pathology.[23] Indeed, this adaptation to adverse nutrient transfer may also result in long-term sequelae (see later).[24] Mild IUGR may allow for "catch-up growth," whereas severe IUGR is more likely to result in permanent growth restriction. One intriguing aspect is that, although the overall growth of the brain may be deficient, there may be acceleration of brain maturation, with neurobehavioral development at birth.[25] However, this may not result in long-term benefit (see later).

Factors affecting fetal growth

While there is a substantial amount of information regarding the regulation of growth in the postnatal period, there is limited knowledge of factors that affect fetal growth. The maternal phenotype probably exerts the greatest influence on fetal size at birth.[26] This was clearly demonstrated in the classic studies of Walton and Hammond in 1938 when they bred the Shetland pony with the Shire horse.[27] If the mother was the pony, the offspring was smaller by far than if the mother was the Shire. This discrepancy in size persisted for at least the first 3 years and probably throughout the lives of the animals.

The nutritional state of the mother, both in the pre- and intragestational periods, the intrauterine capacity, the function of the uteroplacental unit, and various growth factors also affect the rate of fetal growth and development. As noted by Gluckman and Harding,[26] there are numerous and active interactions between maternal factors, placental factors, and the growth-promoting factors elaborated by the fetus.

Fetal growth factors

The major growth factor elaborated by the fetus is insulin. Overproduction of insulin leads to macrosomia,[28] while underproduction, as found in congenital agenesis of the pancreas,[29,30] or in transient or persistent neonatal diabetes mellitus, is associated with growth restriction.[31]

Insulin-like growth factors IGF-1 and IGF-2, especially IGF-1, are also important growth factors in the fetus, and circulating levels of IGF-1 in fetal and cord blood correlate well with fetal size.[32] The mechanisms involved are beginning to be better understood[33] and there is evidence for genetic control, which may go awry.[34] Additionally, IGF-1 seems to play an important role in brain development.[33,34]

Maternal IGF-1 and IGF-2 and insulin do not cross the placenta and have little direct effect on the fetus. They interact with the placenta and are instrumental in maintaining an intact fetoplacental unit. Similarly, the IGF-binding proteins and proteases that affect the binding proteins function to modulate the delivery of IGF to the placenta.

For many years it was thought that fetal growth hormone (GH) had little effect on the intrauterine growth of the fetus, but more recent data demonstrate that fetuses with GH deficiency tend to be short at birth.[35] Some infants with IUGR have hypersecretion of GH, but there may be a reduction or delayed development of receptor sites for GH or in the amount of GH-binding protein.[36] Certainly, most infants with IUGR will not respond to GH soon after birth,[37] although some children demonstrate linear growth in response to GH at a later age.[38,39] Thyroid hormones have little effect on fetal growth, and the absence or abundance of the various sex hormones also does not affect fetal growth. However, the male fetus is usually 100–150 g heavier than the female.

In recent years there has been considerable interest in the hormone leptin, which has been linked to fetal growth. Although early results were somewhat confusing, it appears that leptin concentrations are significantly lower in IUGR than in AGA fetuses after 34 weeks' gestation.[40] However, significantly higher levels of leptin per kilogram fetal weight were found in IUGR fetuses with more severe signs of fetal distress.[40]

Placental growth factors

The placenta elaborates various hormones that maintain the fetoplacental unit, including chorionic gonadotropins, placental growth hormone, and placental somatropins. Placental growth hormone and placental lactogen are important in maintaining increased concentrations of glucose and amino acids in the mother, which are then available for transplacental passage to the fetus.[41]

In addition, the placenta also seems to be capable of producing leptin, although the contributions of the fetus and placenta have not yet been clearly delineated. It is believed that leptin may also be linked to the transfer of glucose and amino acids.[40]

Incidence of IUGR

The true incidence of IUGR on a worldwide basis is difficult to ascertain. While a close approximation can be made in developed countries, it is not known in many developing nations because many women in these countries give birth at home and often the weight, gestational age, and follow-up evaluations of the infants are not known. Using the World Health Organization classification of low birth weight as newborns weighing less than 2500 g, 16% of the infants born worldwide in 1982 were of low birth weight.[42] Many of these infants were most likely growth-retarded. These data were similar to those reported by Villar and Belizan for 1979.[43]

Chiswick noted that up to 10% of all live-born infants and at least 30% of low-birth-weight infants suffered from IUGR.[44] He also noted that the perinatal mortality rate in these infants was 4–10 times that of appropriately grown infants.

Villar and Belizan noted that 90% of low-birth-weight infants were born in developing countries, where the incidence of low-birth-weight infants could be as great as 45%. They also stated that when the incidence of low birth weight exceeds 10%, it is almost always due to the increase in the number of infants with IUGR, since the rate of preterm births tends to remain between 5 and 7%.[43] It has been proposed that chest circumference could be used as a proxy for birth weight in developing countries. At term gestation, a chest circumference of equal to or less than 29 cm indicates IUGR.[45]

Etiology of IUGR

Gluckman and Harding stated that IUGR is a result of one of three general mechanisms:[26] (1) chromosomal/genetic abnormalities; (2) fetal infection/toxicity; or (3) compromised substrate delivery to the fetus. The last group accounts for the majority of infants with IUGR. However, the etiology is clearly multifactorial[15,46] and in this section, factors are classified as fetal, maternal, placental, and environmental causes.

Fetal factors

These include genetic factors leading to low birth weight, chromosomal abnormalities, nonchromosomal syndromes, congenital malformations, and intrauterine infections.

Infectious agents causing or associated with IUGR are listed in Table 7.1. Klein and Remington state that there is evidence to establish a causal relationship for IUGR for only rubella, cytomegaloviral infection, and toxoplasmosis.[47] These agents directly inhibit cell division which may lead to cellular death and a decreased number of fetal cells. However, intrauterine infections with other organisms, including syphilis, varicella-zoster, human immunodeficiency virus (HIV), *Trypanosoma*, and malaria have also been associated with IUGR. Placental infection without affecting the neonate directly has been demonstrated in tuberculosis, syphilis, malaria, and coccidiomycosis. Congenital infection is implicated in less than 10% of patients with IUGR and the incidence may be as low as 3%.

Chromosomal abnormalities include infants with trisomy 21, 13, and 18. In addition, infants with triploidy, various deletion syndromes and those with super X syndromes (XXY, XXXY, XXXX) tend to be of

Table 7.1. Infectious agents causing or associated with intrauterine growth retardation

Viral	Cytomegalovirus
	Rubella
	Varicella-zoster
	Human immunodeficiency virus
Bacterial	Syphilis
Protozoal	*Toxoplasma gondii*
	Plasmodium malariae
	Trypanosoma cruzi

low birth weight.[48] Another recent association with IUGR is maternal uniparental disomy 7 (where both chromosomes come from the same parent – in this case, the mother).[49] Only 2–5% of infants with IUGR have chromosomal abnormalities, but the incidence may be much greater if both IUGR and mental retardation are present.[50]

As many as 5–15% of fetuses with growth retardation have congenital malformation and/or dysmorphic syndromes such as thanatophoric dwarfing, leprechaunism, or Potter's, Cornelia de Lange, Smith–Lemli–Opitz, Seckel, Silver, or Williams syndromes, and VATER or VACTERL (vertebral, anal, cardiovascular, tracheoesophageal, renal, radial, and limb) associations.[51]

Infants with varying types of congenital heart disease, those with single umbilical arteries, and monozygotic twins also frequently suffer from IUGR. Donors of twin-to-twin transfusions tend to be growth-retarded, while the recipient twin is often normally grown. These factors account for less than 2% of infants with IUGR.[44]

Certain metabolic and endocrine disorders are associated with low birth weight and growth retardation. These include infants with transient neonatal diabetes mellitus, neonatal thyrotoxicosis, Menkes syndrome, hypophosphatasia, and I-cell disease.[51] Recently, a form of iron-overload disease has been associated with fetal growth retardation, in a report from Finland.[52]

The role of race also cannot be ignored, with consistent increases in the number of low-birth-weight infants born to black women in the USA, which is not all explained by increased rates of preterm delivery.[53,54] However, environmental factors (see later) may be more important than genetic factors in this regard.[53,54] "Race very often serves as a proxy for poverty"[54] so that undernutrition, malnutrition, poor prenatal care, and other factors may be important etiologic considerations.

Placental factors

Abnormalities of placental function leading to IUGR are listed in Table 7.2.[55] The placenta has a great reserve capacity and may lose up to 30% of its function without affecting fetal growth.[44] Placental abnormalities such as hemangiomata, circumvallate placentas, or infarctions account for less than 1% of infants with IUGR.[44] It has also been stated that no single lesion of the placenta accounts for IUGR, but rather that it is an accumulation (or total burden) of placental injury that produces growth restriction.[55]

When multiple gestation is present, there is an increased incidence of IUGR, and it is most likely due to the inability of the placentas to meet the growth needs of the fetuses. As many as 15–25% of twins suffer from IUGR, and the incidence increases with triplets and quadruplets. Monochorionic twinning contributes disproportionately to intrauterine growth restriction.[57] Increasing discordance in size also contributes to an increase in preterm delivery before 32 weeks' gestation, with the discordance attributable to fetal growth restriction (most often in the second-born twin).[58]

Table 7.2. Placental factors associated with intrauterine growth retardation

Decreased placental mass
Absorption
Infarction
Partial separation
Multiple gestation
Intrinsic placental disorders
Poor implantation
Placental malformation
Vascular disease
Villitis
Decreased placental blood flow
Maternal vascular disease
Hypertension
Hyperviscosity

Source: Modified from Gabbe.[54]

Table 7.3. Maternal factors associated with intrauterine growth retardation (IUGR)

Maternal malnutrition
Disordered eating prior to pregnancy
Decreased maternal prepregnancy weight and height
Decreased weight gain during pregnancy
Labor-intensive occupation
Decreased plasma volume
Prior poor obstetrical history
Previous stillborn
Previous infant with IUGR
Low socioeconomic status
Maternal illness
Maternal drug use and abuse

Maternal factors

Maternal factors are the most common causes of IUGR, and many of them are listed in Table 7.3. The state of maternal nutrition is a major factor in determining fetal growth and size at birth. Significant maternal malnutrition will mitigate conception, as demonstrated in the seige of Leningrad during World War II.[59] If the malnourished woman does conceive, the adequacy of maternal nutrition tends to affect the fetus primarily during the last trimester of pregnancy. This was clearly delineated in the studies of women during the Dutch famine in 1944–45 when food intake was severely curtailed. This reduction resulted in a 10% decrease in birth weights of their infants and a 15% reduction in the weights of the placentas.[60,61] Interestingly, data from the Netherlands also demonstrate that female fetuses exposed to starvation in the first trimester of pregnancy subsequently gave birth to growth-retarded infants themselves.[62]

Similarly, dietary supplementation of malnourished pregnant women, especially if the supplementation is provided for greater than 13 weeks during gestation, increased the birth weight of the infants significantly.[63] Prentice and coworkers working with Gambian women reported that when women were in negative energy balance and had a high energy workload, dietary supplementation reduced the incidence of low-birth-weight infants from 28.2% to 4.7%.[64] However, when the women were in positive energy balance, dietary supplementation had little effect on birth weight. There are conflicting data regarding the effect of supplemental nutrition in various populations, and not all have shown beneficial effects.[63,65]

Specific deficiencies of micronutrients may also contribute to reduced fetal growth even if the mother's diet appears to be adequate as far as caloric and protein intake is concerned. Deficiency of zinc in pregnant women has been associated with increased rates of prematurity, perinatal death, and growth retardation of the fetus.[66] Zinc supplementation in such women has improved perinatal outcome. Thiamine deficiency in pregnancy has also been associated with the growth-retarded newborn, and has been found in mothers with inadequate nutritional intake, hyperemesis, alcohol abuse, and various infections, including HIV.[67]

Although severe maternal malnutrition is uncommon in developed countries, it can still exist in population areas where appropriate nutrition, nutritional supplementation, or nutritional consultation is lacking. It can also be seen in pregnant women with severe gastrointestinal disease, such as Crohn's disease or ulcerative colitis, women with hyperemesis, or in women who utilize excessive energy in labor-intensive occupations. Recently, it has been documented that among women delivering SGA infants at term, there was a much higher incidence (32%) of disordered eating in the 3 months prior to pregnancy, compared to controls (5%) or those delivering prematurely (9%).[68]

Maternal illness, especially toxemia of pregnancy, not only has an adverse effect on the growth of the fetus, but it may also predispose the infant to premature birth, especially if the mother's or infant's condition necessitates early delivery. The presence of IUGR adversely affects survival in these preterm infants.[69] It is of interest to note that multiparous women with preeclampsia have a greater risk of having an infant with IUGR than does a nulliparous mother.[70] During gestation, the mother's plasma volume and cardiac output increase primarily because of increased uterine blood flow. Studies by Rosso and coworkers showed that women who had infants with fetal growth retardation had much lower plasma volumes and decreased cardiac outputs as compared to women who had normally grown fetuses.[71] It has also been demonstrated that hypertensive women with growth-retarded fetuses have decreased plasma volumes as compared to hypertensive women whose fetuses were normally grown.[72]

Chronic illnesses in the mother including those listed in Table 7.4 are associated with the birth of growth-retarded infants. The more common of these are women with chronic hypertension and chronic anemias, such as sickle-cell disease, sickle-C disease, and thalassemia. Women who have antiphospholipid antibodies, even if they are not diagnosed as having systemic lupus erythematosus, have an increased risk of giving birth to infants with IUGR.[50] When studying subgroups, it is important to evaluate carefully the total population, because some controls will have high rates of SGA infants. A recent study documented that 21% of infants born to mothers with antiphospholipid antibodies were SGA, but control mothers had an incidence of 13% SGA infants.[73]

Wolfe and coworkers have reported that women with a history of poor outcome in pregnancy have an increased risk of having a subsequent birth of a growth-retarded infant. A woman who had a growth-retarded infant doubled her risk of having a second infant with IUGR. After two such outcomes, the risk

Table 7.4. Maternal illness associated with intrauterine growth retardation

Acute illness
Preeclampsia
Eclampsia
HELLP syndrome
Chronic illness
Chronic hypertension
Chronic renal disease
Collagen vascular disease
Cyanotic heart disease
Chronic pulmonary disease
Diabetes mellitus (classes B–F)
Thyrotoxicosis
Chronic anemia
Maternal phenylketonuria

Notes:
HELLP, hemolysis, elevated liver enzymes, and low platelet count.

of having a fetus with IUGR is quadrupled.[74] These authors urge that women who have growth-retarded infants should have a thorough search for an underlying maternal disorder if the reason for the IUGR is otherwise not apparent. Ounsted and Ounsted also noted that mothers of infants with IUGR were often growth-retarded at birth themselves.[75]

Environmental factors

It is difficult to separate maternal factors from some factors that might be considered to be environmental factors such as tobacco usage. Therefore, these are discussed together in the ensuing section.

Medications and drugs taken by mothers can not only lead to various congenital malformations, but can also be associated with the birth of growth-retarded newborns.[76,77] Maternal smoking is one of the most prevalent causes of IUGR in their offspring. Birth weight may be reduced by a significant amount as compared to infants of nonsmoking mothers.[78] Haddow and coworkers assayed serum cotinine, the major metabolite of nicotine, in smoking and non-smoking women, and correlated the concentration of the metabolite with the birth weight of their offspring.[79] The infants of women with the highest concentrations of serum cotinine were over 440 g lighter at birth as compared to the infants of women who did not smoke. The mechanism by which smoking affects the fetus is not completely understood, but factors such as decreased maternal nutrition, decreased uterine blood flow, increased production of carbon monoxide, and impaired fetal oxygenation have all been implicated in the overall equation. If the mother stops smoking before she enters the second trimester of pregnancy, her fetus tends to have normal intrauterine growth.[78] Of particular concern is a recent report from Sweden which showed a highly significant association between smoking and a small head circumference for gestational age,[80] since decreased head circumference has been associated with neurodevelopmental deficits (see later).

Table 7.5. Drugs taken by mothers that are associated with intrauterine growth retardation

Tobacco	Cocaine
Alcohol	LSD
Marijuana	Coumadin
Heroin	Hydantoin
Methadone	Trimethadione

Other drugs taken by the mother which have been implicated in causing growth retardation are shown in Table 7.5. Alcohol not only causes fetal growth impairment, but may lead to permanent damage to the fetus and newborn. The quantity of alcohol ingested, maternal size, and the ability of the mother to metabolize alcohol all determine how much alcohol is transported to the fetus.[81] Although the incidence of fetal alcohol effects is not known in the USA, the incidence in Sweden is 1 in 300 births, and 1 in 600 have recognizable features of the fetal alcohol syndrome.[82]

The incidence of illicit drug use by pregnant women in the USA can only be surmised, and accurate follow-up data are not available for the infants delivered from such women.[83] The consensus is that 15–40% of infants of drug-abusing mothers are growth-retarded,[83] and in some infants of cocaine-abusing mothers, the decrease in head circumference is more pronounced than is the decrease in length and weight.[84] Similar data regarding the use of marijuana in pregnant women have also been described.[85,86]

Caffeine, especially if taken in quantities of greater than 300 mg/day, has been associated with decreased fetal growth.[87,88] Lesser intakes of caffeine do not seem to have an adverse effect on fetal growth, but high caffeine intake may be related to smoking[89] and this has not always been considered. Specific syndromes such as fetal hydantoin, fetal warfarin, and fetal trimethadione syndromes are associated with an increased incidence of growth retardation.[77]

It has long been stated that infants born to mothers who live at 10000 ft (3000 m) or greater above sea level weigh approximately 250 g less at birth than do infants born to mothers who live at sea level.[5,6] Kruger and Arias-Stella reported that women who live in the Peruvian Andes at levels of over 15000 ft (4500 m) had infants whose birth weights were 15% less than those who live in Lima, Peru (elevation 500 ft or 150 m), but the placentas of these infants weighed 15% more than those near sea level.[90] This would suggest that the placentas were working at greater energy expenditure to provide adequate nutrients and oxygen to the fetus at the high altitudes.

In evaluating data obtained from deliveries in Leadville, Colorado, a community located about 10000 ft (3000 m) above sea level, Cotton and coworkers classified infants carefully by gestational age, and found no infants who were undergrown or suffering from IUGR. In fact, the average birth weight was almost identical to those infants born in Denver, Colorado, whose elevation was 5280 ft (1600 m).[91] These data are at variance with those of Yip[5] and Unger and coworkers[6] who documented decreased birth weights of infants born at higher altitudes.

Along somewhat similar environmental lines, the workplace may prove detrimental under certain circumstances. In a study from Thailand, it was shown recently that the risk of delivering an SGA infant was increased for women working more than 50 hours per week, for those whose work involved protracted squatting, and for those having high psychological job demands.[92] In Australia, both unemployment and depressive or stress symptomatology were associated with infants being SGA.[15]

Mercury toxicity in pregnant women and their fetuses was highlighted during the 1950s to the 1970s when three separate epidemics of mercury poisoning occurred in Minamoto, Japan, Niigata, Japan, and in Iraq. Koos and Longo reviewed the problem in depth and noted that, while all mercury compounds can cause harm to the fetus, methyl mercury has the greatest toxicity.[93] These compounds cross the placenta readily and have teratogenic and adverse growth effects in the fetus.

Mothers exposed to radiation, other pollutants, and contaminated food or water over a period of time appear to be at risk for delivery of infants with IUGR. The incidence and severity of these factors are not known at present.

Other associations with IUGR

Despite the numerous recognizable factors that cause or are associated with the births of infants with IUGR, up to 30% of these infants have no discernible cause for their growth retardation. Nieto and coworkers analyzed numerous determinants of fetal growth retardation in the central area of Spain.[94] The most important factors that were encountered were maternal smoking, low prepregnancy weight, and low socioeconomic status. Two other important factors were decreased weight gain during pregnancy and maternal urinary tract infections.

Kramer, performing a metaanalysis of almost 900 publications, found that in developed countries by far the most important factor associated with IUGR was maternal cigarette smoking.[42] This was followed by poor gestational nutrition, low prepregnancy weight, primiparity, female sex of the infant, and maternal short stature. In developing countries, the most important factors were nonwhite race, poor gestational nutrition, low prepregnancy weight, short maternal stature, and infection with malaria.[42]

Detection of the fetus with IUGR

Increased awareness of the risk factors in the pregnant patient will alert the clinician to the possibility of her fetus being growth-retarded.[95,96] Several authors have stated that with this increased awareness of risks and accurate measurement of the symphysis–fundus height (SFH) one can detect up to 85% of infants who are at risk of having IUGR.[97,98] This measurement is noninvasive, inexpensive, simple, rapid, and requires little training to be utilized. Many other investigators have noted that the SFH measurement is of limited value as a screening method to detect abnormal size at birth.[99,100] Not only are growth-retarded fetuses not identified, but there is an increased incidence of false positives, with up to 18% of infants identified incorrectly as having IUGR. Pearce and Campbell noted that decreased SFH measurements can identify the 28% of the population that has 75% of the infants with IUGR.[101]

Currently, ultrasound is the preferred method of evaluating fetal growth and, in many instances, fetal well-being as well. Ultrasound in obstetrics has been used extensively, and several excellent reviews have been published evaluating its use in identifying the undergrown fetus.[102–106] In populations where routine ultrasound is not available, careful review of risk factors, physical examination, and measurements of SFH must be used to screen for IUGR. In populations where ultrasound is readily available, initial studies are often performed at 8–10 weeks' gestation. This examination documents fetal viability, the presence of multiple gestation, and gross fetal malformation, and can confirm the gestational age of the fetus. This early examination is not used to determine abnormalities of intrauterine growth.[106] The biparietal diameter (BPD), the abdominal circumference (AC), and the femur length (FL) are the usual biometric measurements taken during the ultrasonographic examination.[104] Measurements of the BPD between 12 and 18 weeks' gestation are accurate in detecting gestational age within 5–6 days. However, measurements of individual parameters are not very good predictors of IUGR. To predict appropriateness of intrauterine growth more accurately, the ultrasound examination should be performed in the third trimester. The estimated fetal weight (EFW) at that time relies on multiple measurements, including the abdominal circumference and ratios of head circumference (HC)/AC or FL/AC. The optimal time to perform the examination is not clear, but it is estimated that over 50% of infants with IUGR will be detected at or about 32 weeks' gestation. Thus, several ultrasounds may have to be performed in order to monitor the growth of the fetus and to determine the optimal time of delivery of these infants. In pregnancies with multiple gestations, more frequent serial ultrasonographic examinations should be carried out during the last trimester.

Other studies to evaluate fetal well-being, especially in the growth-retarded infants, are shown in Table 7.6. Few, if any, centers are currently using endocrine measurements of estrogens, pregnanediol, or placental lactogen in maternal serum or urine. Decreased amounts of amniotic fluid were found to correlate well with IUGR, but subsequent studies have not confirmed this observation.[104]

Assessment of fetal well-being with the biophysical profile (BPP), while not used to detect IUGR, has been found to be more useful in predicting an abnormal fetal outcome than either the contraction stress test (CST) or the nonstress test (NST) alone.[96,104,107,108] Vibroacoustic stimulation may also help in evaluation.[107]

Doppler flow velocity waveforms of the fetal circulation have also been used as adjuncts in evaluating fetal well-being and appropriate growth. The fetal umbilical artery, aorta, and cerebral arteries have been studied and varying indices have been evaluated, including the resistance index (RI), the pulsatility index (PI), and the systolic-to-diastolic ratio (S/D) of these vessels.[105] Abnormalities of these indices have been evaluated as to their capabilities in detecting the

Table 7.6. Techniques to evaluate fetal growth and well-being

Measurements of symphysis-to-fundus height
Ultrasound examination
Endocrine measurements of maternal serum or urine
Estriol
Placental lactogen
Pregnanediol
Biophysical profile (including measurement of amniotic fluid index)
Contraction and noncontraction stress tests
Vibroacoustic stimulation
Doppler flow velocity waveforms
Cordocentesis

growth-retarded fetus and in evaluating the state of well-being of the fetus. The most accurate predictor of poor neonatal outcome was shown to be umbilical cord Doppler waveform abnormalities,[109] which have been associated with abnormal blood flow in the fetal middle cerebral artery in IUGR.[110] However, Doppler assessment of the middle cerebral artery may reveal blood flow redistribution even when umbilical artery Doppler is normal, especially when the HC/AC ratio is elevated.[111] Lastly, cordocentesis, which has an increased risk-to-benefit ratio, can be utilized to document hypoxemia, lactic acidemia, and increased numbers of nucleated red cells in the fetal circulation and to identify those infants who are in need of immediate delivery.[112–115]

These improved techniques of diagnosing and evaluating the status of the infant with IUGR have also resulted in improved management of the fetus and newborn.[116] Specific interventions, such as maternal hyperoxygenation,[117] have been undertaken on a more rational basis, and decisions about delivery are based on what is optimal for the fetus. At times it is difficult to decide on what the best management may be; in many cases it may be "better out than in" for the fetus.[96] These decisions should involve a combined obstetrical–pediatric approach.

Table 7.7. Clinical problems commonly encountered with intrauterine growth retardation

Fetal and neonatal asphyxia
Fetal heart rate abnormalities
Require resuscitation in delivery room
Persistent pulmonary hypertension
Glucose disorders
Hypoglycemia
Hyperglycemia
Hypocalcemia
Hypothermia
Hematologic problems
Neutropenia
Thrombocytopenia
Increased nucleated red blood cells
High hematocrit/hyperviscosity
Susceptibility to infection
Necrotizing enterocolitis
Pulmonary hemorrhage
Large anterior fontanel

Associated problems and complications (Table 7.7)

Fetal and neonatal asphyxia

The infant with IUGR is much more likely to experience difficulties during labor and delivery, although this is primarily related to the etiology of IUGR. Since many cases result from uteroplacental insufficiency, it is hardly surprising that a partially compromised fetus becomes a severely compromised fetus during labor. Particularly as labor progresses, the frequency and strength of contractions increase, minimizing blood flow to the fetus, and this does not allow the fetus to recover between contractions. Lack of blood flow leads to decreased oxygen delivery and development of metabolic acidosis. The ability to remove carbon dioxide may also be compromised and the combination results in fetal asphyxia, frequently manifest by late decelerations on fetal heart rate monitoring. In addition, there may be variable decelerations (or cord-compression patterns) because decreased blood flow to the fetus may have produced a decrease in the quantity of amniotic fluid surrounding the fetus. This increases the probability that uterine contractions will be transmitted to the umbilical cord (especially the umbilical vein), further compromising blood flow to the fetus. An additional factor that may contribute to compromise is that, in fetuses with IUGR, the umbilical cord is frequently very thin, so that the umbilical vessels lack the protection of Wharton's jelly.

At the time of delivery, the asphyxiated, acidotic fetus becomes an asphyxiated, acidotic neonate and prompt attention is required in the delivery room and early neonatal period to prevent further compromise. Those infants with a low ponderal index are more likely to have problems, including asphyxia.[118] If the fetus has been subjected to a chronic intrauterine insult there is the potential for structural change in the pulmonary vasculature, with muscularization of the walls of arterioles and capillaries.[119] Particularly when combined with neonatal asphyxia, the potential for developing persistent pulmonary hypertension is great.

Hypoglycemia (see Chapter 26)

The majority of infants who are born with IUGR demonstrate a lack of subcutaneous fat and those with asymmetrical IUGR usually have a decreased abdominal circumference documented before and after delivery.[120] This suggests that the liver size is diminished and that glycogen stores may be depleted. For many years it has been recognized that preterm infants and SGA infants are prone to develop hypoglycemia, with the highest risk occurring in those infants born preterm and SGA.[121–123] It is generally believed that the predisposition to develop hypoglycemia results from depletion of the glycogen stores; however, infants with IUGR and hypoglycemia are able to respond to the administration of glucagon and increase their concentrations of glucose in serum.[124] It is also known that infants with IUGR have limited capabilities to utilize 3-carbon precursors to make glucose via the gluconeogenic pathways.[122] Additionally, hyperinsulinemia has been documented in some infants with IUGR, with hypoglycemia developing after 48 h or so.[125,126] An association of hypoglycemia with Rubinstein–Taybi syndrome (including IUGR) has also been reported.[127]

It is certainly true that the supply of nutrients to IUGR infants has been less than optimal prior to delivery, so that glucose levels at delivery are comparatively low[128] and may not be maintained because of altered homeostatic mechanisms, including inability to mobilize fat and glycogen stores, since both may be depleted. The brain is relatively large in many infants with IUGR (especially when it is asymmetrical) and since the brain relies heavily on glucose metabolism, it may be necessary to calculate glucose requirements (oral or intravenous) based on what the weight *should* have been, rather than the actual weight.

Hyperglycemia

Somewhat paradoxically, treatment of hypoglycemia with "normal" amounts of glucose may lead to hyperglycemia.[129] This may be because the IUGR fetus is exposed to relative hypoglycemia in utero, which suppresses the production of insulin (the major hormone involved in growth) before delivery[130] and cannot be "turned on" after delivery. Further support for this idea comes from the condition of transient diabetes mellitus of the newborn, which seems to be the result of hypoinsulinism, or insulin dependence. Although this is a relatively uncommon condition, neonates with this problem may have hyperglycemia lasting from days to weeks, or even months.[31] Almost always, infants with this condition are born SGA,[31] as they are with congenital agenesis of the pancreas.[29,30] On the other hand, as previously mentioned, some infants with IUGR have been shown to have hyperinsulinism and to develop later-onset (at approximately 48 h) hypoglycemia.[125,126]

Hypocalcemia

Most categories of infant prone to develop hypoglycemia are also prone to develop hypocalcemia. This is certainly true for those infants with IUGR.[131] Hypocalcemia may be due to transient hypoparathyroidism or possibly to an overproduction of calcitonin, which is increased in stressed neonates. With modern-day neonatal intensive care, it would be unusual to encounter the more severe clinical manifestations of hypocalcemia such as seizure activity. The problem is anticipated, looked for, and treated.[132]

Hypothermia

Another problem that used to be encountered with some frequency, but which is now anticipated and usually prevented, is hypothermia. The increased surface-area-to-body-weight ratio of the IUGR infant promotes heat loss more rapidly than in the appropriately grown infant.[133] The ability to produce heat may also be compromised in IUGR infants[133] for three reasons: (1) there is decreased insulation from adipose tissue (white fat); (2) the stores of brown fat, used for nonshivering thermogenesis, are markedly depleted; and (3) the tendency to develop hypoglycemia means that oxidative metabolism of glucose to produce heat is deficient. For all these reasons, it is more likely that IUGR infants will not be able to maintain their body temperature and will develop hypothermia.[134] One study of hypothermic infants (80% of whom were neonates) indicated that all 51 infants had weights less than the 10th percentile for age.[135] In the most extreme cases, when appropriate management is not provided, one may encounter neonatal cold injury syndrome.[136]

The end result of cooling is metabolic acidosis, because peripheral vasoconstriction decreases the delivery of oxygen to the tissues and increases anaerobic metabolism, with the accumulation of lactic acid. In extreme circumstances, the resultant decrease in pH may have wide-reaching effects, including altered metabolism of the brain.

Hematologic problems

There are several problems concerning the hematologic system in IUGR infants. Some of them may be interrelated and seem to be stimulated by chronic hypoxemia. It has been recognized for many years that infants with IUGR are more likely to be born with a high hematocrit. This has been likened to the fetus living at altitude and attempting to increase oxygen-carrying capacity by stimulating erythropoiesis. More recently, particularly in infants born to hypertensive mothers, thrombocytopenia and neutropenia have been observed.[137,138] It is believed that the pluripotent stem cell is stimulated to produce the erythroid series at the expense of neutrophils and platelets.[137] More recently, these same authors have demonstrated that there is an inhibitor of neutrophil production which is elaborated by the placenta and which is present in the infant's serum.[139]

Overproduction of erythropoietin was noted in SGA infants 20 years ago.[140] More recently, there have been studies in the fetus, utilizing cordocentesis, documenting asphyxia and lactic acidemia.[112] It was also noted that the number of erythroblasts (nucleated red blood cells or NRBC) was markedly increased in some of these fetuses.[112] Very similar findings have also been documented immediately after birth in very-low-birth-weight infants who were born SGA.[141] Cordocentesis has also demonstrated that levels of erythropoietin are increased in those IUGR fetuses displaying erythroblastosis,[142] and it may be possible to distinguish IUGR from the small but healthy fetus.[143] Thus, in the neonate with a marked increase in the number of nucleated red blood cells and a normal to high hematocrit, the most likely explanation is chronic intrauterine hypoxemia (although infection may also stimulate NRBC production). It is not clear what the duration of the hypoxemic insult needs to be, to produce a significant elevation of NRBC,[144] although an estimate of the duration of insult can be provided based on numbers of NRBC, which were more elevated with fetal heart rate abnormalities of longer duration.[145]

High hematocrit, especially a venous hematocrit

over 65%, may lead to hyperviscosity syndrome,[146,147] which includes several clinical manifestations involving the central nervous system. The presence of lethargy, jitteriness, or seizures should initiate the consideration of hyperviscosity as a possible explanation. Although it is generally believed that partial exchange transfusion is indicated to treat the hyperviscosity syndrome, it is not clear that this intervention prevents sequelae.[148,149]

At the opposite end of the spectrum, some infants with IUGR are anemic. This occurs in the twin-to-twin transfusion syndrome, where the donor twin is inadequately perfused, and has compromise of intrauterine growth, in association with anemia.[57,150] This too may result in decreased availability of oxygen and damage to the developing brain.[57]

Susceptibility to infection

It was noted earlier that the IUGR fetus and infant are more likely to develop asphyxia, which may predispose to bacterial infection.[151] It is also known that total T cells, helper and inducer T lymphocytes, as well as B cells, are all deficient in number in infants who are SGA.[152,153] Such immunologic handicap seems to predispose to severe infection, including meningitis. Infants with a low ponderal index may have increased susceptibility. In one study,[154] infection was four times more common in IUGR infants with low ponderal index compared to those with appropriate ponderal index. Hypothermia (see earlier) has also been associated with a predisposition to develop bacterial infection.[135] Lastly, since the infants may also be neutropenic, they may not respond to infectious agents as do normally grown infants.[137,139]

Necrotizing enterocolitis

There is continuing debate about the exact etiology of necrotizing enterocolitis, but it has been believed for many years that two important elements in its production are ischemia of the bowel and susceptibility to infection. From the previous paragraphs documenting the increased incidence of asphyxia, acidosis, and hyperviscosity, it is easy to understand why blood flow to the intestine of infants with IUGR might be compromised.[155] The increased susceptibility to infection adds an additional risk. It is therefore not surprising that an increased incidence of necrotizing enterocolitis has been seen in IUGR infants,[156] which may be predictable based on absent end-diastolic frequencies on fetal Doppler studies.[157]

Pulmonary hemorrhage

Another commonly encountered problem of IUGR infants in former years, which seems to be decreasing in frequency, is pulmonary hemorrhage. The pathogenesis is probably related to perinatal asphyxia, with hypothermia (neonatal cold injury) also implicated. As noted earlier, both asphyxia and hypothermia are more common in IUGR infants. In severe IUGR, pulmonary hemorrhage has been reported to produce sudden, unexpected death.[158]

Delayed ossification and large fontanels

For many years it has been known that infants subjected to fetal malnutrition (i.e., IUGR) have delay in the ossification of the epiphyses about the knee.[159] In many cases, term babies were noted to have radiographic absence of ossification of both the distal femoral and proximal tibial epiphyses, despite clinical maturity.[159] Further observations in neonates with IUGR suggested that it is common to observe a large anterior fontanel and that this frequently accompanies markedly reduced epiphyseal ossification.[160,161] This retardation of both enchondral and membranous ossification is quite reminiscent of the findings in congenital hypothyroidism, where large fontanels and decreased bone age are seen.[162] Decreased skeletal maturation seems to be more prominent in those with decreased ponderal indices.[163]

The possibility that thyroid function might be compromised was supported by findings at postmortem study of infants with IUGR (hypotrophy).[164] Their thyroid glands had colloid-filled vesicles, suggesting a failure to release thyroid hormone.[164] This was followed by the finding of significantly lower thyroxine (T_4) levels in SGA infants aged 7–49 days.[165] More recently, SGA fetuses have been evaluated for their thyroid function and found to have significantly lower T_4 and free T_4 levels, as well as significantly higher thyroid-stimulating hormone levels.[166] In addition, the increase in thyroid-stimulating hormone and decrease in free T_4 were associated with the degrees of fetal hypoxemia and acidemia respectively.[166]

Although the data to support the following hypotheses are rather limited, it seems possible first, that those infants with delayed ossification may have a greater potential for catch-up growth[14] and second, that some of the deficits seen in IUGR infants may relate to relative hypothyroidism. As noted earlier, the presence or absence of thyroid function in the fetus had little effect on intrauterine growth, as infants with congenital absence of the thyroid grew normally in utero. The patients reported by Thorpe-Beeston and coworkers[166] document decreased thyroid function in a select group of infants with IUGR. It is possible that these latter infants have decreased thyroid function as a result of them being IUGR rather than causing the IUGR. In the preterm infant, hypothyroxinemia has been documented and there is increasing concern that this should be treated to minimize neurodevelopmental abnormalities.[167]

Ossification may now be assessed with ultrasound, rather than needing radiographs. The lack of ossification has been used to predict IUGR fetuses using ultrasound evaluation. The ossification center of the femur was detectable in 202 of 208 AGA infants, but undetectable in 15 of 18 SGA infants.[168]

Neurobehavioral abnormalities

Accelerated neurological development

It has been stated for some time that preterm infants with IUGR or who are SGA have accelerated lung maturity, and that some of these infants may have accelerated neurological development as well. The link between these developmental changes was first described in 25 infants by Gould et al.[169] However, the concept of accelerated lung maturation has been challenged more recently by Tyson et al.[170] These investigators have carefully compared infants who were SGA and those who were AGA and evaluated the outcome of the infants of similar gestational ages, race, and sex. Their studies documented that the SGA infants actually had increased rates of respiratory distress syndrome, respiratory failure, and death as compared to the infants who were AGA.

Acceleration of neurological maturation was confirmed by Amiel-Tison[171] in other high-risk pregnancies, some of which (but not all) resulted in infants with growth retardation. This acceleration of maturation was at least 4 weeks in 16 infants and may relate to the intensity of placental insufficiency, with the benefits being lost as intensity increases. Maternal hypertension was implicated in approximately half of the cases in the two studies.

Further observations have been made more recently and confirm the acceleration of maturation in stressed pregnancies. Although many of these infants are born SGA, this is not always the case and suggests that the effects on the nervous system may precede the effects on overall growth.[25] The exact mechanism for accelerated maturation remains to be elucidated. Additional support comes from neurophysiological studies, where brainstem auditory evoked responses were more rapid in SGA infants than AGA infants.[172] Further documentation has been provided in growth-retarded fetal lambs.[173] On the other hand, development of visual evoked potentials may be delayed.[174] Whether the accelerated maturational effects are documented when infants are evaluated by methods similar to those used by Tyson et al.[170] remains to be seen.

Furthermore, although accelerated neurological maturation would seem to provide an unanticipated benefit, when infants with IUGR are followed for longer periods of time they do not sustain this advantage. Indeed, by school age, they may be at a disadvantage.[175]

Altered behavior

The preceding section indicates that *some* infants with IUGR have accelerated neurological development, but this is not always the case. With increasing severity of insult, it is likely that the behavior of the baby will be altered. Data from the 1980s indicated that fetal behavioral states may be delayed in IUGR fetuses, with fetal movements being particularly involved,[176–178] but more recently, with increasing experience, the assessment of fetal behavioral organization is not considered to be of great clinical value.[179]

Increasing severity of fetal asphyxia will have a marked effect on the biophysical profile,[107,180] one aspect of which is fetal movement. In uncomplicated IUGR, there is no clear effect on the quality of general movements.[179,181] However, it is commonly observed that infants with IUGR behave differently soon after delivery. In particular, they may feed poorly. Inevitably, this will affect parental perceptions of the baby. Low et al.[134] documented lower activity scores in IUGR infants compared to controls, with a trend to less visual fixation and visual pursuit. Studies using the Brazelton Behavioral Assessment Scale have documented less muscle tone, decreased activity, less responsiveness, but more difficulty in modulating state.[182] A high-pitched cry tends to take longer to be stimulated.[183] Most behavioral studies have been performed in term IUGR infants. Little is known about differences in preterm IUGR infants.

Parental interaction

Many infants with IUGR appear scrawny (especially those with low ponderal index) and are less attractive to parents than the expectation of what their baby "should" look like.[182] In addition, as noted above, the baby's behavior may be distorted and provide less interaction between baby and parents. The cry may be particularly aversive to adults.[184] This lack of "positive reinforcement" was believed to place these infants at particular risk for child abuse or neglect, but more recently this idea seems to have been disproved.[185]

There are quite limited data available about subsequent parent–infant interaction and, although there may be some differences early in the first year,[186] these differences in interaction seem to resolve by 6 months, even though the infants may behave differently.[187]

Outcome

Historical perspective

After the recognition that not all small infants were born preterm, but could be growth-retarded,[188] it was realized that it was important to consider the etiologic heterogeneity of IUGR.[46,189] Not only did infants with chronic intrauterine infection need to be excluded, but it was recognized that those with associated congenital abnormalities probably skewed the follow-up in some early studies,[189] and that in order to discuss outcome appropriately, we need to provide good definitions and standards.[190]

One group of infants that could be evaluated, which even retrospectively could be accurately categorized, was twins with markedly discordant birth weights. These follow-up studies (few in number) were largely performed on preterm twin infants, but continued growth retardation was usually the case in the smaller of discordant twins.[191] This was accompanied by a disadvantage in intellect, persisting into adulthhood.[192] However, it was observed that head circumference was less affected than other measures.[191] Some years later, in a small sample of discordant twins, continued weight deficit in the smaller twin was noted, but without height or IQ deficit at 6 years of age.[193]

The ability to have "catch-up" growth in the smaller twin was also reported.[194,195] Indeed, in a remarkable report, Buckler and Robinson described a female twin pair with marked disparity in birth weights (2.99 vs 1.35 kg), where the smaller had very rapid "catch-up" after birth. By 1 year of age, there was essentially no difference in physical measurements and evaluation at 10 years of age showed no difference in intelligence quotients.[196]

In contrast to the twin studies, most studies of singletons with IUGR involved babies born at term. In singleton IUGR infants, there has been considerable variability in the ability for growth to catch up,[14] leading to the conclusion that appropriate classification at birth is needed, together with categorization by etiology of IUGR. Some of the older studies may have been complicated by problems such as hypoglycemia. Nevertheless, despite the tendency to remain smaller than average in physical dimensions, the intellectual deficits of infants with IUGR described in the 1970s were not always striking and major neurological deficits were considered to be uncommon. For instance, Fitzhardinge and Steven followed 95 full-term SGA infants and noted cerebral palsy in only 1% and seizures in 6%.[197] On the other hand, although the average IQ was normal, a large percentage (50% of boys and 36% of girls) had poor school performance.[197] In other studies, the IQ did not seem to be impaired, although it was somewhat higher in those with normal head circumference, described by Babson and Henderson.[198] They concluded that "severe fetal undergrowth, not complicated by severe asphyxia at birth, or congenital disease, may not severely impair later mental development, even in those whose head size remained at the 3rd percentile."[198]

Although it is now less common to see infants with IUGR born at term, Strauss has recently provided follow-up on two large national cohorts born many years ago.[199,200] The first group were those followed in the US National Collaborative Perinatal Project (1959–76), with a 7-year follow-up. IUGR had little impact on intelligence and motor development, except when associated with large deficits in head circumference at birth.[199] The second group were those enrolled in the 1970 British Birth Cohort Study, where follow-up was available until 1996.[200] Although 93% had been followed at 5 years of age, only 53% were seen at 26 years of age. Among 489 SGA infants (of the original 1064 SGA infants) born at term and assessed as adults, academic achievement and professional attainment were significantly lower than the adults who had normal birth weight (n=6981). However, there appeared to be no long-term social or emotional consequences of being born SGA.[200]

One study of preterm SGA infants indicated that approximately 50% had a developmental handicap, with 20% having major neurologic sequelae.[201] Handicap could not be related to the degree of IUGR or the rate of postnatal head or linear growth. However, it did seem to be related to perinatal asphyxia. These infants were all born in outlying hospitals and referred to a center.[201] When more aggressive obstetrical intervention was undertaken, the outlook seems to have been improved (in a different setting). Cesarean section at 28–33 weeks' gestation for suspected growth retardation and abnormal unstressed cardiotocograms resulted in 17 survivors among 25 infants. Only two survivors were neurologically abnormal.[202]

As obstetrical evaluation and intervention changed, more infants with IUGR were delivered at earlier stages of gestation. The Oxford group demonstrated that attempting to prolong gestation beyond about 36 weeks may not benefit the fetus, but earlier delivery seemed to enhance the chances of compromised fetuses, with IUGR achieving their full developmental potential later.[203] More recently, planned delivery at even earlier gestations has occurred. It seems likely that some of these fetuses would have died in utero, but others might have suffered severe neurological injury. It is therefore important to know about these IUGR fetuses delivered at early gestational ages. A number of studies have been reported in recent years, most of which provide reasonably encouraging data about long-term outcome (see section on follow-up of very-low-birth-weight (VLBW) infants born SGA).

Mortality and morbidity

Short-term outcome involves both mortality and morbidity. The morbidity in these infants has been described in the section on clinical problems. The frequency of problems is in large measure dependent upon the etiology. The same holds true for mortality. It is clear that if there are many infants with chromosomal abnormalities (e.g., trisomy 18) or chronic intrauterine infections (e.g., congenital rubella syndrome) in the population being evaluated, mortality rates are likely to be high. Nevertheless, Lubchenco et al. have shown that the more severe the degree of growth retardation, the higher is the mortality risk.[204] In a separate analysis, morbidity was found to increase progressively as birth weight fell below the 10th percentile at each gestational age.[205]

In contrast, a few years later, it was found that SGA infants had a lower risk for neonatal death than AGA infants, but had a higher risk of problems manifest during the first year.[206] Recent evidence confirms the original findings that both mortality and morbidity are increased in term infants born SGA (<third percentile).[207]

Physical growth

In the last 15–20 years, reports of the subsequent growth of infants with IUGR have included modifiers that might influence the outcome. For instance, disproportionate IUGR (with a low ponderal index) seems to persist as underweight-for-length at 3 years of age, despite catch-up growth in the first 6 months.[208] It was shown earlier that decreased ossification may predispose to catch-up in linear growth.[14] In a different study, term infants with a low ponderal index had larger head circumferences and were taller than those with adequate ponderal index, when evaluated at age 24 months.[209] There appeared to be no effect of the degree of IUGR on later growth in preterm infants.[209]

Catch-up growth in the first 6 months has been noted by others,[210] and adequate ponderal index at birth predicted being smaller at 12 months of age than those with low ponderal index.[211] In a more recent study of long-term follow-up, SGA infants were shorter at age 17 years.[212]

One factor shown to make a large contribution to measurements of SGA infants at follow-up is parental measurements.[213] Although intuitively it makes a lot of sense, most studies do not take this into consideration. These investigators have also shown that SGA babies with high head-to-chest ratios at birth grew faster during the first 6 months, with a sustained effect to 7 years in girls.[214]

One study that may have important implications, but has not been further evaluated, showed variability of response to insulin at 6 months of age.[215] Those SGA infants that had increased incremental linear growth demonstrated insulin release.[215] Given the variability of insulin levels in IUGR infants noted earlier, this is an area that deserves further study. It may also be linked to later evidence of glucose intolerance.[24]

A recent study reported 3-year follow-up of infants with IUGR, the majority of whom were born at term. Although there was considerable catch-up growth in some infants, statistically significant differences in lower weight, height, and head circumference remained at 3 years compared to control infants.[216]

Development and intelligence quotient

While physical growth may have some practical implications, since many parents are concerned about short stature, neurobehavioral and intellectual development are of more concern. These have been examined in a number of studies published in the last 15–20 years. Allen has reviewed data prior to 1984, documenting that most term SGA infants go on to have normal IQs.[76] One study documented that in nonasphyxiated SGA newborns, despite residual physical deficits at age 13–19 years, neurologic and cognitive testing demonstrated scores well within the normal range, although somewhat lower than controls.[217]

In a comparison of SGA infants born to hypertensive mothers with those whose mothers were normotensive, it was found that the former performed better on developmental tests at 4–7 years of age, but had more major neurological problems.[218] In another 7-year follow-up study, neurological problems were detected in 9.5% of growth-retarded infants and in 8.5% of control infants.[219] Others have described surprisingly little difference in developmental status at 4 years of age between small- and average-for-dates infants.[220]

More recent evidence tends to confirm these findings, although lower IQ scores and poorer neurodevelopmental outcome were noted in IUGR infants with neonatal complications.[216] Nevertheless, these neurodevelopmental problems might be characterized as minor, with no cerebral palsy, and no severe hearing or visual impairment.[216]

Using a slightly different approach, when ponderal index at birth was taken into consideration, one study showed that term IUGR infants with adequate ponderal index (symmetric IUGR) had lower developmental scores than those with low ponderal index (asymmetric IUGR), which in turn were lower than those with normal birth weight.[221] Preterm infants with asymmetric or symmetric IUGR have also been compared to AGA infants. In the asymmetric SGA group there were more children with low visuoauditory perception scores and social abilities scores at 18 months than in controls. The symmetric SGA group had deficits in all developmental areas except visuoauditory perception.[222] There were also more neurological abnormalities in both SGA groups.[222]

Follow-up of VLBW infants born SGA

When VLBW (<1500 g) infants born more than 20 years ago were evaluated, SGA infants had significantly lower developmental performance at 9 months through 3 years of age, but differences were not observed at 4 and 5 years.[223] A decade later, results from the same authors were similar with VLBW and SGA infants.[224] At 3 years of age, development of SGA infants was significantly less than that of gestation-matched controls, but did not differ from that of weight-matched controls.[224]

Others have described cohorts born more recently. For instance, Amin et al., reporting from Calgary, Alberta, evaluated 52 IUGR infants (with birth weight <1250 g) at 3 years of age. They were compared with groups of birth weight and gestational age-matched controls and had no significant differences in neurodevelopmental outcome, although all three groups had major disabilities of approximately 15%.[1] Head sparing correlated with a good outcome (35 of 37 were normal).[1]

In a large cohort of even smaller babies, followed for 4–18 years, the majority of SGA babies with birth weight less than 1000 grams had catch-up of head circumference, although this was more likely in the asymmetrical SGA group (85%) than the symmetrical group (73%).[225] Although developmental outcome was not completely addressed in this report, normal head circumference was usually associated with a good outcome, as noted elsewhere.

It should also be remembered that there are difficulties in extrapolating results of follow-up to current VLBW populations, since management of such neonates continues to change (and, we hope, improve). For instance, exogenous surfactant has only been commercially available since 1990 and prenatal use of corticosteroids to accelerate fetal maturity increased considerably after the National Institute of Health consensus conference in 1994. As a result, certain complications of the VLBW infant (e.g., pneumothorax and intraventricular hemorrhage) have decreased, which could influence neurodevelopmental outcome.

Cerebral palsy

Most of the early follow-up studies did not specifically address the issue of cerebral palsy, although a low incidence was mentioned earlier.[197] However, in Sweden, trends in the incidence of cerebral palsy have been followed over several years by Uvebrant and Hagberg. In 1992, it was noted that in 519 children with cerebral palsy born in 1967 to 1982, compared to 445 control children born during the same years, in term and moderately preterm infants the risk of cerebral palsy in SGA infants was significantly increased.[226] Similar data have been reported from Western Australia by Blair and Stanley in growth-retarded infants of 34 weeks' gestation or older.[227]

More recently, in a large cohort of preterm singletons with cerebral palsy born in 1971–82 ($n=191$) in Denmark, the association of SGA with cerebral palsy was observed *only* in preterm infants born at greater than 33 weeks' gestation.[228] The comparison group consisted of all preterm live born singletons born in 1982 ($n=2203$). Cerebral palsy risk was highest at

28–30 weeks gestation, but lower in the SGA group at this gestation.[228]

Learning deficits

It is also the case that most follow-up studies until recently did not extend into the school years, or at least not very far. This began to change in 1984 when a study of term infants with intrauterine malnutrition (not all were SGA) followed from birth to 12–14 years of age was reported.[229] Lower IQ scores were seen in malnourished infants compared to well-nourished infants (104 ± 15 vs 121 ± 13) and more required special education.[229] A study from England looked at boys weighing below the 2nd percentile at birth and controls at age 10–11 years. When two profoundly disabled light-for-dates boys were excluded there were no differences in IQ or school achievement.[230] In another study, from Canada, outcome at 9–11 years of age was measured.[231] A wide range of learning deficits was evaluated in 216 high-risk newborns, 77 of whom had IUGR. Learning deficits were encountered in 35% of the total, but 50% of preterm SGA and 46% of term SGA infants were affected.[231]

A study from England evaluated infants born in 1980–81, with a gestational age of less than 32 weeks or birth weight less than 2 kg, at 8–9 years of age.[232] They concluded that those with fetal growth restriction in the first two trimesters did less well. Both cognitive ability (measured by IQ testing and reading comprehension) and motor ability were negatively associated with the degree of fetal growth restriction.

A study from the Netherlands looked at a 1983 cohort, born with gestational age of less than 32 weeks or birth weight less than 1500 g, at both 5 and 9 years of age.[233] Of an original cohort of 134 SGA infants, 85 were seen at 5 years and 73 at 9 years, compared to 410 AGA infants, of whom 274 and 249 were seen at 5 and 9 years respectively. Cognitive outcome was worse in the SGA group. When neurological disorders were excluded, 16.4% of SGA needed special education at 9 years compared to 11.9% of AGA. When no exclusions were made, only 31.5% of SGA infants were in mainstream education vs 43.2% of AGA.[233]

On a more encouraging note, data from the Jerusalem Perinatal Study showed that long-term follow-up (at age 17) produced minimal differences in IQ tests and no differences in academic achievement, when term SGA and AGA were evaluated.[234]

Some of these recent studies are summarized in Table 7.8.

Effect of fetal malnutrition on disease in adult life

Several studies in the past decade have alluded to the relationship of IUGR with the subsequent increased incidence of cardiovascular disease when these patients reach adult life.[24,235–237] Both hypertension and ischemic heart disease are increased in IUGR infants,[24] and the risk of stroke is also increased.[238] Barker and coworkers[237] suggest that undernutrition during gestation alters the relationships between substrates and hormones, such as between glucose and insulin, and between growth hormone and IGF. Since IGF-1 is decreased in many growth-retarded fetuses and since fetal undernutrition may induce insulin resistance in various tissues and organs, these infants might also become insulin-resistant as adults. Indeed, there is an increased incidence of diabetes mellitus and glucose intolerance.[239,240] While the fetus may adapt to nutritional deprivation in utero, such adaptation may lead to an increased incidence of cardiovascular disease and other problems in adulthood.

Prevention

Although outcome in the nonasphyxiated infant appears to be good, the potential for developing fetal asphyxia in the growth-retarded fetus is high.[112] Indeed, the risk of intrauterine demise drives many obstetrical decisions. For this reason, a number of techniques have been used to improve placental perfusion.

The first of these, which was originally reported from South Africa to produce "superbabies," was intermittent abdominal decompression. The technique was evaluated in a controlled trial reported in 1973.[241] Negative pressure is applied to the abdomen

Table 7.8. Neurodevelopmental and cognitive outcome in infants with intrauterine growth restriction

Authors	Category	Age at evaluation	Method of evaluation	Number evaluated	Outcome		
					Impaired		*Disabled*
Roth et al. 1999[253]	Term infants	1 year	Neurological exam	49 SGA	37%		6%
	Fetal abdominal circumference		Developmental assessment	18 IUGR	33%		6%
					CP		*Major disability*
Amin et al. 1997[1]	Birth weight <1250 g	3 years	Neurodevelopmental assessment	52 IUGR	7.7%		15.4%
				55 BW-matched	9.1%		16.4%
				56 GA-matched	12.5%		16.1%
					Neuro-development	*IQ*	
Fattal-Valevski, et al. 1999[216]	Term/preterm	3 years	Neurodevelopmental assessment and IQ test	85 IUGR	89.0	94.9	
				42 Controls	93.2	94.9	
Scherjon et al. 2000[174]	<34 weeks GA U/C ratio	5 years	IQ test	73 IUGR	Lower IQ with raised U/C ratio (87 vs 96)		
					Special education	*CP*	*Normal development*
Kok et al. 1998[233]	<32 weeks GA and BW <1500 g	9 years	Speech–language development. Need for special education. Neurological exam	73 SGA	16.4%	7%	48%
				149 AGA	11.9%	15%	63%
					Cognitive outcome worse in SGA		
				Males	*IQ*		
Paz et al. 2001[234]	Term	17 years	IQ test, academic achievement	154 severe SGA	100.7		
				431 moderate SGA	102.8		
				5928 AGA	105.1		
				Females			
				86 severe SGA	102.6		
				273 moderate SGA	102.4		
				3664 AGA	103.9		
					No differences in academic achievements		

Notes:
U/C ratio, umbilical artery to middle cerebral artery pulsatility index ratio; GA, gestational age; BW, birth weight; CP, cerebral palsy; SGA, small-for-gestational-age; AGA, appropriate-for-gestational-age; IUGR, intrauterine growth restriction; IQ, intelligence quotient.

to encourage blood flow in the uterus and hence the placenta. In 70 treated vs 70 controls there were some striking differences, with improved growth of fetal biparietal diameter in the treated group and only 26% light-for-dates babies in the treated group compared to 83% in the controls.[241] Fetal distress, low 1-min Apgar scores and perinatal deaths were also lower in the treated group.[241] Further support for the technique was provided in 64 pregnant women with identified placental insufficiency.[242] Abdominal decompression applied over 4 weeks or so improved placental perfusion measurements and serum unconjugated estriol and human placental lactogen levels.[242] To date, this approach has not gained widespread support, although a recent review provided considerable support for this methodology.[243]

As mentioned earlier, another approach to the fetus with IUGR is to evaluate fetal oxygenation using cordocentesis. In situations where fetal hypoxia is documented, the use of maternal oxygen therapy to produce maternal hyperoxygenation may allow fetal oxygenation to be markedly improved.[117,244] However, a recent metaanalysis revealed only two studies using randomized controls, which involved only 62 women and did not provide enough evidence to evaluate adequately the benefits and risks of maternal oxygen therapy.[245]

Another approach that has been tested in a randomized, placebo-controlled, double-blind trial is the use of low-dose aspirin.[246] Women were chosen on the basis of previous fetal growth retardation and/or fetal death or abruptio placentae. The frequency of fetal growth retardation in the placebo group was twice (26% vs 13%) that in the treated group.[246] The benefits of low-dose aspirin were greater in patients with two or more previous poor outcomes. More recent evaluation of low-dose aspirin showed no evidence of improved uteroplacental or fetoplacental hemodynamics,[247] although another study supported the use of a combination of aspirin and glyceryl trinitrate.[248] This too has not been adequately evaluated, to date.

A specific cause of IUGR is severe maternal nutritional deprivation. The role of dietary supplementation and specific deficiencies has been discussed previously.[63–67] It is possible, under certain adverse circumstances, to support adequate fetal growth using total parenteral nutrition.[249] Extending this approach to other situations of less severe nutritional deprivation might allow supplemental parenteral nutrition to prevent fetal growth retardation.[249] However, a recent metaanalysis revealed only three studies, involving 121 women, which did not provide enough evidence to allow an adequate evaluation of nutrient supplementation.[250] Two other analyses from the Cochrane Database also showed insufficient evidence to demonstrate a conclusive effect of either plasma volume expansion[251] or bedrest in hospital on fetal growth.[252]

Prevention remains an area for careful evaluation with randomized trials, and it is hoped that many cases of IUGR will be prevented in the future.[253]

Conclusion

Major advances have been made in our understanding of infants who are growth-retarded in utero. Many of the factors that lead to IUGR have been recognized, and many of the women who are at risk of giving birth to such infants can be identified. In many instances, problems can be avoided by altering the intrauterine environment, by improving maternal nutrition, by improving care of chronic illness in the mother, through immunization programs, and by improved counseling of pregnant women regarding smoking and alcohol and drug abuse.

Infants can also be classified according to the types of growth retardation that are present, and it is recognized that many of these infants do not thrive in a hostile intrauterine environment, do not tolerate the stresses of labor well, and do not have an appropriate transitional period from the fetal to the newborn state.

These infants also have markedly different problems in the neonatal period than do prematurely born infants of the same size or normally grown infants of the same gestational age. Unfortunately, many of these IUGR fetuses are still not being identified early enough to alter these environments, and we are still late in responding to their problems in the neonatal period rather than anticipating and preventing them from developing.

Although significant strides have been made in our understanding of the problems of IUGR infants, we need to focus attention on prevention, early detection, and appropriate management of their problems, in order to produce the best outcome possible.

REFERENCES

1 Amin H, Singhal N and Sauve RS. (1997). Impact of intrauterine growth restriction on neurodevelopmental and growth outcomes in very low birth weight infants. *Acta Paediatr,* **86**, 306–314.

2 Louey S, Cock M, Stevenson KM, et al. (2000). Placental insufficiency and fetal growth restriction lead to postnatal hypotension and altered postnatal growth in sheep. *Pediatr Res,* **48**, 808–814.

3 Metcoff J. (1994). Clinical assessment of nutritional status at birth: fetal malnutrition and SGA are not synonymous. *Pediatr Clin North Am,* **41**, 875–891.

4 Lubchenco LO, Hansman C and Boyd E. (1966). Intrauterine growth in length and head circumference as estimated from live births at gestational ages from 26 to 42 weeks. *Pediatrics,* **37**, 403–408.

5 Yip R. (1987). Altitude and birth weight. *J Pediatr,* **111**, 869–876.

6 Unger C, Weiser JK, McCullough RE, et al. (1988). Altitude, low birth weight, and infant mortality in Colorado. *JAMA,* **259**, 3427–3432.

7 Usher R and McLean F. (1969). Intrauterine growth of live born Caucasian infants at sea level: standards obtained from measurements in 7 dimensions of infants born between 25 and 44 weeks of gestation. *J Pediatr,* **74**, 901–910.

8 Niklasson A, Ericson A, Fryer JG, et al. (1991). An update of the Swedish reference standards for weight, length and head circumference at birth for given gestational age (1977–1981). *Acta Paediatr Scand,* **80**, 756–762.

9 Röhrer R. (1921). Der Index der Körperfülle als Mass des Ernährungszustandes. *Münchener Medizinische Wochenschrift,* **68**, 580–595.

10 Miller HC and Hassanein K. (1971). Diagnosis of impaired fetal growth in newborn infants. *Pediatrics,* **48**, 511–522.

11 Lubchenco LO. (1970). Assessment of gestational age and development at birth. *Pediatr Clin North Am,* **17**, 125–145.

12 Urrusti J, Yoshida P, Velasco L, et al. (1972). Human fetal growth retardation: I. Clinical features of sample with intra-uterine growth retardation. *Pediatrics,* **50**, 547–558.

13 Rosso P and Winick M. (1974). Intrauterine growth retardation: a new systematic approach based on the clinical and biochemical characteristics of this condition. *J Perinat Med,* **2**, 147–160.

14 Philip AGS. (1978). Fetal growth retardation: femurs, fontanels and follow-up. *Pediatrics,* **62**, 446–453.

15 O'Callaghan MJ, Harvey JM, Tudehope DI, et al. (1997). Aetiology and classification of small for gestational age infants. *J Paediatr Child Health,* **33**, 213–218.

16 Winick M. (1970). Cellular growth in intrauterine malnutrition. *Pediatr Clin North Am,* **17**, 69–78.

17 Sands J, Dobbing J and Gratrix CA. (1979). Cell number and cell size: organ growth and development and the control of catch-up growth in rats. *Lancet,* **ii**, 503–505.

18 Ounsted M and Ounsted C. (1973). *On Fetal Growth Rate. Clinical Developmental Medicine,* no. 46. London: Spastics International Publications.

19 Vik T, Vatten L, Jacobsen G, et al. (1997). Prenatal growth in symmetric and asymmetric small-for-gestational age infants. *Early Hum Dev,* **48**, 167–176.

20 Crane JP and Kopta MM. (1980). Comparative newborn anthropometric data in symmetric versus asymmetric intrauterine growth retardation. *Am J Obstet Gynecol,* **138**, 518–522.

21 Kramer MS, McLean FH, Olivier M, et al. (1989). Body proportionality and head and length "sparing" in growth-retarded neonates: a critical reappraisal. *Pediatrics,* **84**, 717–723.

22 Toft PB, Leth H, Ring PB, et al. (1995). Volumetric analysis of the normal infant brain and in intrauterine growth retardation. *Early Hum Dev,* **43**, 15–29.

23 Warshaw JB. (1985). Intra-uterine growth retardation: adaptation or pathology? *Pediatrics,* **76**, 998–999.

24 Barker DJP. (1998). In utero programming of chronic disease. *Clin Sci,* **95**, 115–128.

25 Amiel-Tison C and Pettigrew A. (1991). Adaptive changes in the developing brain during intrauterine stress. *Brain Dev,* **13**, 67–76.

26 Gluckman PD and Harding JE. (1994). Nutritional and hormonal regulation of fetal growth-evolving concepts. *Acta Paediatr Suppl,* **399**, 60–63.

27 Walton A and Hammond J. (1938). The maternal effects on growth and conformation in Shire horse–Shetland pony crosses. *Proc R Soc Lond Biol,* **125**, 311–335.

28 Cornblath M and Schwartz R. (1991). Infant of the diabetic mother. In *Disorders of Carbohydrate, Metabolism in*

Infancy, 3rd edn, ed. M Cornblath and R Schwartz, pp. 125–174. Boston: Blackwell.

29 Lemons JA, Ridenour R and Orsini EN. (1979). Congenital absence of the pancreas and intrauterine growth retardation. *Pediatrics,* **64**, 255–257.

30 Howard CP, Go VLW, Infante AJ, et al.(1980). Long-term survival in a case of functional pancreatic agenesis. *J Pediatr,* **97**, 786–789.

31 Cornblath M and Schwartz R. (1991). Hyperglycemia in the neonate. In *Disorders of Carbohydrate, Metabolism in Infancy,* 3rd edn, ed. M Cornblath and R Schwartz, pp. 225–246. Boston: Blackwell.

32 Evain-Brion D. (1994). Hormonal regulation of fetal growth. *Horm Res,* **42**, 207–214.

33 Guevara-Aguirre J. (1996). Insulin-like growth factor I – an important intrauterine growth factor. *N Engl J Med,* **335**, 1389–1391.

34 Woods KA, Camacho-Hübner C, Savage MO, et al. (1996). Intrauterine growth retardation and postnatal growth failure associated with deletion of the insulin-like growth factor I gene. *N Engl J Med,* **335**, 1363–1367.

35 Gluckman PD, Gunn AJ, Wray A, et al. (1992). Congenital idiopathic growth hormone deficiency associated with prenatal and early postnatal growth failure. *J Pediatr,* **121**, 920–923.

36 Fisher DA. (1984). Intrauterine growth retardation: endocrine and receptor aspects. *Semin Perinatol,* **8**, 37–41.

37 Lafeber HN and Gluckman PD. (1997). Nutritional management and growth hormone treatment of preterm infants born small for gestational age. *Acta Paediatr,* **86**, 202–205.

38 Chernausek SD, Breen TJ and Frank GR. (1996). Linear growth in response to growth hormone treatment in children with short stature associated with intrauterine growth retardation: the National Cooperative Growth Study experience. *J Pediatr,* **128**, 522–527.

39 Fjellestad-Paulsen A, Czernichow P, Brauner R, et al (1998). Three-year data from a comparative study with recombinant human growth hormone in the treatment of short stature in young children with intrauterine growth retardation. *Acta Paediatr,* **87**, 511–517.

40 Cetin I, Morpurgo PS, Radelli T, et al. (2000). Fetal plasma leptin concentrations: relationship with different intrauterine growth patterns from 19 weeks to term. *Pediatr Res,* **48**, 646–651.

41 Stein ZA and Susser M. (1984). Intrauterine growth retardation: epidemiological issues and public health significance. *Semin Perinatol,* **8**, 5–14.

42 Kramer MS. (1987). Determinants of low birth weight: methodological assessment and meta-analysis. *Bull WHO,* **65**, 669–737.

43 Villar J and Belizan JM. (1982). The relative contribution of prematurity and fetal growth retardation to low birth weight in developing and developed societies. *Am J Obstet Gynecol,* **143**, 793–798.

44 Chiswick ML. (1985). Intrauterine growth retardation. *Br Med J,* **291**, 845–848.

45 Rondo PHC and Tomkins AM. (1996). Chest circumference as an indicator of intrauterine growth retardation. *Early Hum Dev,* **44**, 161–167.

46 Bernstein PS and Divron MY. (1997). Etiologies of fetal growth restriction. *Clin Obstet Gynecol,* **40**, 723–729.

47 Klein JO and Remington JS. (2001). Current concepts of infection of the fetus and newborn infants. In *Infectious Diseases of the Fetus and Newborn Infant,* 5th edn, ed. JS Remington and JO Klein, pp. 1–23. Philadelphia: Saunders.

48 Droste S. (1992). Fetal growth in aneuploid conditions. *Clin Obstet Gynecol,* **35**: 119–125.

49 Kalousek DK and Harrison K. (1995). Uniparental disomy and unexplained intrauterine growth retardation. *Contemp Ob/Gyn,* September, pp. 41–52.

50 Creasy RK and Resnick R. (1994). Intrauterine growth restriction. In *Maternal Fetal Medicine,* 3rd edn, ed. RK Creasy and R Resnick, pp. 558–574. Philadelphia: Saunders.

51 Kleigman RM. (1992). Intrauterine growth retardation: determinants of aberrant fetal growth. In *Neonatal-Perinatal Medicine: Diseases of the Fetus and Infant,* 5th edn., ed. AA Fanaroff and RJ Martin, pp. 149–185. St Louis: Mosby.

52 Fellman V, Rapola J, Pihko H, et al. (1998). Iron-overload disease in infants involving fetal growth retardation, lactic acidosis, liver haemosiderosis, and aminoaciduria. *Lancet,* **351**, 490–493.

53 David RJ and Collins JW. (1997). Differing birth weight among infants of U.S.-born blacks, African-born blacks, and U.S.-born whites. *N Engl J Med,* **337**, 1209–1214.

54 Foster HW. (1997). The enigma of low birth weight and race. *N Engl J Med,* **337**: 1232–1233.

55 Gabbe SG. (1991). Intrauterine growth retardation. In *Obstetrics: Normal and Problem Pregnancies,* 2nd edn, ed. SG Gabbe, JR Nieby and JL Simpson, pp. 923–944. New York: Churchill Livingstone.

56 Salafia CM. (1997). Placental pathology of fetal growth restriction. *Clin Obstet Gynecol,* **40**, 740–749.

57 Gaziano EP, De Lia JE and Kuhlman RS. (2000). Diamnionic monochorionic twin gestation: an overview. *J Matern Fetal Med,* **9**, 89–96.

58 Cooperstock MS, Tummaru R, Blackwell J, et al. (2000).

Twin birth weight discordance and risk of preterm birth. *Am J Obstet Gynecol*, **183**, 63–67.

59 Antonov AN. (1947). Children born during the siege of Leningrad in 1942. *J Pediatr*, **30**, 250–259.

60 Stein Z and Susser M. (1975). The Dutch famine, 1944/1945 and the reproduction process. I. Effects in six indices at birth. *Pediatr Res*, **9**, 70–76.

61 Stein Z and Susser M. (1975). The Dutch famine, 1944/1945 and the reproduction process. II. Inter-relations of caloric rations and six indices at birth. *Pediatr Res*, **9**, 76–83.

62 Lumey LH. (1992). Decreased birthweights in infants after maternal in utero exposure to the Dutch famine of 1944–1945. *Pediatr Perinat Epidemiol*, **6**, 240–253.

63 Suescun J and Mora JO. (1989). Food supplements during pregnancy. *Intrauterine Growth Retardation*, In Nestle Nutrition Workshop Series, vol. 18, ed. J Senterre, pp. 223–241. New York: Vevey/Raven.

64 Prentice AM, Whitehead RG, Watkinson M, et al. (1983). Prenatal dietary supplementation of African women and birth weight. *Lancet*, **i**, 489–492.

65 Rush D, Stein Z and Susser M. (1980). A randomized controlled trial of prenatal nutritional supplementation in New York City. *Pediatrics*, **65**, 683–697.

66 Jameson S. (1993). Zinc status in pregnancy: the effect of zinc therapy on perinatal mortality, prematurity and placental ablation. *Ann NY Acad Sci*, **678**, 178–192.

67 Butterworth F. (1993). Maternal thiamin deficiency. A factor in intrauterine growth retardation? *Ann NY Acad Sci*, **678**, 325–329.

68 Conti J, Abraham S and Taylor A. (1998). Eating behavior and pregnancy outcome. *J Psychosom Res*, **44**, 465–477.

69 Witlin AG, Sande GR, Mattar F, et al. (2000). Predictors of neonatal outcome in women with severe preeclampsia or eclampsia between 24 and 33 weeks gestation. *Am J Obstet Gynecol*, **182**, 607–611.

70 Eskenazi B, Fenster L, Sidney S, et al. (1993). Fetal growth retardation in infants of multiparous and nulliparous women with preeclamspia. *Am J Obstet Gynecol*, **169**, 1112–1118.

71 Rosso P, Donoso E, Braun S, et al. (1993). Maternal hemodynamic adjustments in idiopathic fetal growth retardation. *Gynecol Obstet Invest*, **35**, 162–165.

72 Hays PM, Cruikshank DP and Dunn LJ. (1985). Plasma volume determination in normal and preeclamptic pregnancies. *Am J Obstet Gynecol*, **151**, 958–966.

73 Brewster JA, Shaw NJ and Farquharson RG. (1999). Neonatal and pediatric outcome of infants born to mothers with antiphospholipid syndrome. *J Perinat Med*, **27**, 183–187.

74 Wolfe HM, Gross TL and Sokol RS. (1987). Recurrent small for gestational age birth: perinatal risks and outcome. *Am J Obstet Gynecol*, **157**, 288–293.

75 Ounsted M and Ounsted C. (1966). Maternal regulation of intra-uterine growth. *Nature*, **212**, 995–997.

76 Allen MC. (1984). Developmental outcome and follow-up of the small for gestational age infant. *Semin Perinatol*, **8**, 123–156.

77 Crouse DT and Cassady G. (1994). The small for gestational age infant. In *Neonatology: Pathophysiology and Management of the Newborn*, 4th edn, ed. GB Avery, MA Fletcher and MG MacDonald, pp. 369–398. Philadelphia: Lippincott.

78 Butler R, Goldstein H and Ross EM. (1972). Cigarette smoking in pregnancy: its influence on birth weight and perinatal mortality. *Br Med J*, **I**, 127–130.

79 Haddow JE, Knight GJ, Palomaki GE, et al. (1987). Cigarette consumption and serum cotinine in relation to birth weight. *Br J Obstet Gynaecol*, **94**, 678–681.

80 Kallen K. (2000). Maternal smoking during pregnancy and infant head circumference at birth. *Early Hum Dev*, **58**, 197–204.

81 Mills JL, Graubard BI, Harley EE, et al. (1984). Maternal alcohol consumption and birthweight: how much drinking during pregnancy is safe? *JAMA*, **252**, 1875–1879.

82 Olegard R, Sabel K-G, Aronsson M, et al. (1979). Effects on the child of alcohol abuse during pregnancy. Retrospective and prospective studies. *Acta Paediatr Scand Suppl*, **275**, 112–121.

83 Das G. (1994). Cocaine abuse and reproduction. *Int J Clin Pharmacol Ther*, **32**, 7–11.

84 Little BB and Snell LM. (1991). Brain growth among fetuses exposed to cocaine in utero: asymmetric growth retardation. *Obstet Gynecol*, **77**, 361–364.

85 Zuckerman B, Frank DA, Hingson R, et al. (1989). Effects of maternal marijuana and cocaine use on fetal growth. *N Engl J Med*, **320**, 762–765.

86 Frank DA, Bauchner H, Parker S, et al. (1990). Neonatal body proportionality and body composition after in utero exposure to cocaine and marijuana. *J Pediatr*, **117**, 622–626.

87 Fortier I, Marcoux S and Beaulac-Baillargeon L. (1993). Relation of caffeine intake during pregnancy to intrauterine growth retardation and preterm birth. *Am J Epidemiol*, **137**, 931–940.

88 Mills JL, Holmes LB, Aarons JH, et al. (1993). Moderate caffeine use and the risk of spontaneous abortion and intrauterine growth retardation. *JAMA*, **269**, 593–597.

89 Golding J. (1995). Reproduction and caffeine consumption – a literature review. *Early Hum Develop*, **43**, 1–14.

90 Kruger H and Arias-Stella J. (1970). The placenta and the newborn infant at high altitudes. *Am J Obstet Gynecol*, **106**, 586–591.

91 Cotton EK, Hiestand M, Philbin GE, et al. (1980). Re-evaluation of birthweight at high altitudes: study of babies born to mothers living at an altitude of 3100 meters. *Am J Obstet Gynecol*, **138**, 220–222.

92 Tuntiserance P, Geater A, Chongsuvivatwong V, et al. (1998). The effect of heavy maternal workload on fetal growth retardation and preterm delivery. A study among southern Thai women. *J Occup Environ Med*, **40**, 1013–1021.

93 Koos BJ and Longo LD. (1976). Mercury toxicity in the pregnant woman, fetus, and newborn infant. A review. *Am J Obstet Gynecol*, **126**, 390–409.

94 Nieto A, Matorras R, Serra M, et al. (1994). Multivariate analysis of determinants of fetal growth retardation. *Eur J Obstet Gynecol*, **53**, 107–113.

95 Galbraith RS, Karchmar EJ, Piercy WN, et al. (1979). The clinical prediction of intrauterine growth retardation. *Am J Obstet Gynecol*, **133**, 281–286.

96 Peleg D, Kennedy CM and Hunter SK. (1998). Intrauterine growth restriction: identification and management. *Am Fam Physician*, **58**, 453–460, 466–467.

97 Villar J and Belizan JM. (1986). The evaluation of the methods used in the diagnosis of intrauterine growth retardation. *Obstet Gynecol Surv*, **41**, 187–199.

98 Cnattingius S, Axelsson O and Lindmark G. (1984). Symphysis–fundus measurements and intrauterine growth retardation. *Acta Paediatr Scand*, **63**, 335–340.

99 Cronjé HS, Bam RH and Muir A. (1993). Validity of symphysis fundus growth measurements. *Int J Gynecol Obstet*, **43**, 157–161.

100 Persson B, Stangenberg M, Lunell NO, et al. (1986). Prediction of size of infants at birth by measurement of symphysis fundus height. *Br J Obstet Gynaecol*, **93**, 206–211.

101 Pearce JM and Campbell SA. (1987). A comparison of symphysis–fundal height and ultrasound as screening tests for light-for-gestational age infants. *Br J Obstet Gynaecol*, **93**, 206–211.

102 Jacobsen G. (1992). Detection of intrauterine growth retardation. A comparison between symphysis–fundus height and ultrasonic measurements. *Int J Technol Assess Health Care*, **8** (suppl. 1), 170–175.

103 Skupski DW, Cehrvenak FA and McCullough LB. (1994). A routine ultrasound screening for all patients? *Clin Perinatol*, **21**, 707–722.

104 Craigo SD. (1994). The role of ultrasound in the diagnosis and management of intrauterine growth retardation. *Semin Perinatol*, **18**, 292–304.

105 Gaziano EP. (1995). Antenatal ultrasound and fetal Doppler. Diagnosis and outcome in intrauterine growth retardation. *Clin Perinatol*, **22**, 111–140.

106 Kennedy A. (2000). Fetal ultrasound. *Curr Probl Diagn Radiol*, **29**, 109–140.

107 Vintzileos AM, Campbell WA, Ingardia CJ, et al. (1983). The fetal biophysical profile and its predictive value. *Obstet Gynecol*, **62**, 271–278.

108 Weiner Z, Peer E and Zimmerman EZ. (1997). Fetal testing in growth restriction. *Clin Obstet Gynecol*, **40**, 804–813.

109 Dubinsky T, Lau M, Powell F, et al. (1997). Predicting poor neonatal outcome: a comparative study of non-invasive antenatal testing methods. *Am J Roentgenol*, **168**, 827–831.

110 Forouzan I and Tian ZY. (1996). Fetal middle cerebral artery blood flow velocities in pregnancies complicated by intrauterine growth restriction and extreme abnormality in umbilical artery Doppler velocity. *Am J Perinatol*, **13**, 139–142.

111 Harshkovitz R, Kingdom JC, Geary M, et al. (2000). Fetal cerebral blood flow redistribution in late gestation: identification of compromise in small fetuses with normal umbilical artery Doppler. *Ultrasound Obstet Gynecol*, **15**, 209–212.

112 Soothill PW, Nicolaides KH and Campbell S. (1987). Prenatal asphyxia, hyperlacticaemia, hypoglycaemia, and erythroblastosis in growth retarded fetuses. *Br Med J*, **294**, 1051–1053.

113 Nicolaides KH, Economides DL and Soothill PW. (1989). Blood gases, pH and lactate in appropriate- and small-for-gestational-age fetuses. *Am J Obstet Gynecol*, **161**, 996–1001.

114 Weiner CP and Williamson RA. (1989). Evaluation of severe growth retardation in using cordocentesis-hematologic and metabolic alternatives by etiology. *Obstet Gynecol*, **161**, 996–1001.

115 Shalev E, Blondhein O and Peleg D. (1995). Use of cordocentesis in the management of preterm or growth-restricted fetuses with abnormal monitoring. *Obstet Gynecol Surv*, **50**, 839–844.

116 Lin CC and Santolaya-Fargas J. (1999). Current concepts of fetal growth restriction: Part II. Diagnosis and management. *Obstet Gynecol*, **93**, 140–146.

117 Nicolaides KH, Bradley RJ, Soothill PW, et al. (1987). Maternal oxygen therapy for intrauterine growth retardation. *Lancet*, **i**, 942–945.

118 Walther FJ and Ramaekers LHJ. (1982). Neonatal morbidity of SGA infants in relation to their nutritional status at birth. *Acta Paediatr Scand*, **71**, 437–440.

119 Murphy JD, Rabinovitch M, Goldstein JD, et al. (1981). The

structural basis of persistent pulmonary hypertension of the newborn. *J Pediatr*, **98**, 962–967.

120 Warsof SL, Cooper DJ, Little D, et al. (1986). Routine ultrasound screening for antenatal detection of intrauterine growth retardation. *Obstet Gynecol*, **67**, 33–39.

121 Usher RH. (1970). Clinical and therapeutic aspects of fetal malnutrition. *Pediatr Clin North Am*, **17**, 169–183.

122 Cornblath M and Schwartz R. (1991). Hypoglycemia in the neonate. In *Disorders of Carbohydrate Metabolism in Infancy*, 3rd edn, ed. M. Cornblath and R Schwartz, pp. 155–205. Philadelphia: W.B. Saunders.

123 Cornblath M and Ichord R. (2000). Hypoglycemia in the neonate. *Semin Perinatol*, **24**, 136–149.

124 Hawdon JM, Aynsley-Green A and Ward Platt MP. (1993). Neonatal blood glucose concentrations: metabolic effects of intravenous glucagon and intragastric medium chain triglyceride. *Arch Dis Child*, **68**, 255–261.

125 Collins JE and Leonard JV. (1984). Hyperinsulinism in asphyxiated and small-for-dates infants with hypoglycemia. *Lancet*, **ii**, 311–313.

126 Collins JE, Leonard JV, Teale D, et al. (1990). Hyperinsulinaemic hypoglycaemia in small for dates babies. *Arch Dis Child*, **65**, 1118–1120.

127 Wyatt D. (1990). Transient hypoglycemia with hyperinsulinism in a newborn infant with Rubinstein–Taybi syndrome. *Am J Med Genet*, **37**, 103–105.

128 Hawdon JM and Ward Platt MP. (1993). Metabolic adaptation in small for gestational age infants. *Arch Dis Child*, **68**, 262–268.

129 Chance GW and Bower BD. (1966). Hypoglycaemia and temporary hyperglycaemia in infants of low birth weight for maturity. *Arch Dis Child*, **41**, 279–285.

130 Economides DL, Proudler A and Nicolaides KH. (1989). Plasma insulin in appropriate- and small-for-gestational-age fetuses. *Am J Obstet Gynecol*, **160**, 1091–1094.

131 Tsang RC, Gigger M, Oh W, et al. (1975). Studies in calcium metabolism in infants with intrauterine growth retardation. *J Pediatr*, **86**, 936–941.

132 Kramer MS, Olivier M, McLean FH, et al. (1990). Impact of intrauterine growth retardation and body proportionality on fetal and neonatal outcome. *Pediatrics*, **85**, 707–713.

133 Sinclair JC. (1970). Heat production and thermoregulation in the small-for-date infant. *Pediatr Clin North Am*, **17**, 147–158.

134 Low JA, Galbraith RS, Muir D, et al. (1978). Intrauterine growth retardation: a preliminary report of long-term morbidity. *Am J Obstet Gynecol*, **130**, 534–545.

135 Dagan R and Gorodischer R. (1984). Infections in hypothermic infants younger than 3 months old. *Am J Dis Child*, **138**, 483–485.

136 Jackson R and Yu JS. (1973). Cold injury of the newborn in Australia: a study of 31 cases. *Med J Aust*, **2**, 630–633.

137 Koenig JM and Christensen RD. (1989). Incidence, neutrophil kinetics, and natural history of neonatal neutropenia associated with maternal hypertension. *N Engl J Med*, **321**, 557–562.

138 Fraser SH, Tudehope DI. (1996). Neonatal neutropenia and thrombocytopenia following maternal hypertension. *J Pediatr*, **32**, 31–34.

139 Koenig JM and Christensen RD. (1991). The mechanism responsible for diminished neutrophil production in neonates delivered of women with pregnancy induced hypertension. *Am J Obstet Gynecol*, **165**, 467–473.

140 Meberg A, Jakobsen E and Halvorsen KJ. (1982). Humoral regulation of erythropoiesis and thrombopoiesis in appropriate and small for gestational age infants. *Acta Paediatr Scand*, **71**, 769–773.

141 Philip AGS and Tito AM. (1989). Increased nucleated red blood cell counts in small for gestational age infants with very low birth weight. *Am J Dis Child*, **143**, 164–169.

142 Snijders RJM, Abbas A, Melybe O, et al. (1993). Fetal plasma erythropoietin concentration in severe growth retardation. *Am J Obstet Gynecol*, **168**, 615–619.

143 Minior VK, Shatzkin E and Divon MY. (2000). Nucleated red blood cell count in the differentiation of fetuses with pathologic growth restriction from healthy small-for-gestational-age fetuses. *Am J Obstet Gynecol*, **182**, 1107–1109.

144 Benirschke K. (1994). Placenta pathology questions to the perinatologists. *J Perinatol*, **14**, 371–375.

145 Korst LM, Phelan JP, Ahn MO, et al. (1996). Nucleated red blood cells: an update on the marker for fetal asphyxia. *Am J Obstet Gynecol*, **175**, 843–846.

146 Hakanson DO and Oh W. (1980). Hyperviscosity in the small-for-gestational age infant. *Biol Neonate*, **37**, 109–112.

147 Black VD and Lubchenco LO. (1982). Neonatal polycythemia and hyperviscosity. *Pediatr Clin North Am*, **29**, 1137–1148.

148 Oh W. (1986). Neonatal polycythemia and hyperviscosity. *Pediatr Clin North Am*, **33**, 523–532.

149 Black VD. (1987). Neonatal hyperviscosity syndromes. *Curr Probl Pediatr*, **17**, 73–130.

150 Elliott JP, Urig MA and Clewell WH. (1991). Aggressive therapeutic amniocentesis for treatment of twin–twin transfusion syndrome. *Obstet Gynecol*, **77**, 537–540.

151 Töllner U and Pohlandt F. (1976). Septicemia in the newborn due to Gram-negative bacilli: risk factors, clinical symptoms and hematologic changes. *Eur J Pediatr*, **123**, 243–254.

152 Chandra RK. (1981). Serum thymic hormone activity and

cell-mediated immunity in healthy neonates, preterm infants and small-for-gestational age infants. *Pediatrics*, **67**, 407–411.

153 Thomas RM and Linch DC. (1983). Identification of lymphocyte subsets in the newborn using a variety of monoclonal antibodies. *Arch Dis Child*, **58**, 24–38.

154 Villar J, de Onis M, Kestler E, et al. (1990). The differential neonatal morbidity of the intrauterine growth retardation syndrome. *Am J Obstet Gynecol*, **163**, 151–157.

155 Hakanson DO and Oh W. (1977). Necrotizing enterocolitis and hyperviscosity in the newborn infant. *J Pediatr*, **90**, 458–461.

156 Wiswell TE, Robertson CF, Jones TA, et al. (1988). Necrotizing enterocolitis in full-term infants: a case control study. *Am J Dis Child*, **142**, 532–535.

157 Hackett GA, Campbell S, Gamsu H, et al. (1987). Doppler studies in the growth retarded fetus and prediction of neonatal necrotizing enterocolitis, haemorrhage and neonatal morbidity. *Br Med J*, **294**, 13–16.

158 Sly PD and Drew JH. (1981). Massive pulmonary hemorrhage: a cause of sudden unexpected deaths in severely growth retarded infants. *Aust Paediatr J*, **135**, 944–948.

159 Scott KE and Usher R. (1964). Epiphyseal development in fetal malnutrition syndrome. *N Engl J Med*, **270**, 822–824.

160 Philip AGS. (1974). Fontanel size and epiphyseal ossification in neonates with intra-uterine growth retardation: preliminary communication. *J Pediatr*, **84**, 204–207.

161 Philip AGS. (1975). Fontanel size and epiphyseal ossification in neonatal twins discordant by weight. *J Pediatr*, **86**, 417–419.

162 Smith DW and Popich G. (1972). Large fontanels in congenital hypothyroidism: a potential clue toward earlier recognition. *J Pediatr*, **80**, 753–756.

163 Roord JJ, Ramaekers LHJ and van Engelshoven JMA. (1978). Intra-uterine malnutrition and skeletal retardation. *Biol Neonate*, **34**, 167–169.

164 Larroche JC. (1976). Histological structure of the thyroid gland in the newborn: with special reference to hypotrophy, hydrops fetalis and Cesarean section delivery. *Biol Neonate*, **28**, 118–124.

165 Jacobsen BB and Hummer L. (1979). Changes in serum concentrations of thyroid hormones and thyroid hormone-binding proteins during early infancy. Studies in healthy full-term, small-for-gestational age and preterm infants aged 7 to 240 days. *Acta Paediatr Scand*, **68**, 411–418.

166 Thorpe-Beeston JG, Nicolaides KH, Snijders RJM, et al. (1991). Thyroid function in small for gestational age fetuses. *Obst Gynecol*, **77**, 701–706.

167 Vulsma T and Kok JH. (1996). Prematurity-associated neurologic and developmental abnormalities and neonatal thyroid function. *N Engl J Med*, **334**, 857–858.

168 Zilianti M, Fernandez S, Azuaga A, et al. (1987). Ultrasound evaluation of the distal femoral epiphyseal ossification center as a screening test for intrauterine growth retardation. *Obstet Gynecol*, **70**, 361–364.

169 Gould JB, Gluck L and Kulovich MV. (1977). The relationship between accelerated pulmonary maturity and accelerated neurological maturity in certain chronically stressed pregnancies. *Am J Obstet Gynecol*, **127**, 181–186.

170 Tyson JE, Kennedy K, Broyles S, et al. (1995). The small for gestational age infant: accelerated or delayed pulmonary maturation? Increased or decreased survival? *Pediatrics*, **95**, 534–538.

171 Amiel-Tison C. (1980). Possible acceleration of neurological maturation following high-risk pregnancy. *Am J Obstet Gynecol*, **138**, 303–306.

172 Pettigrew AG, Edwards DA and Henderson-Smart DJ. (1985). The influence of intrauterine growth retardation on brainstem development of preterm infants. *Dev Med Child Neurol*, **27**, 467–472.

173 Cook CJ, Gluckman PD, Williams C, et al. (1988). Precocial neural function in the growth-retarded fetal lamb. *Pediatr Res*, **24**, 600–604.

174 Stanley OH, Fleming PJ and Morgan MH. (1991). Development of visual evoked potentials following intrauterine growth retardation. *Early Hum Dev*, **27**, 79–91.

175 Scherjon S, Briet J, Oosting H, et al. (2000). The discrepancy between maturation of visual-evoked potentials and cognitive outcome at five years in very preterm infants with and without hemodynamic signs of fetal brain-sparing. *Pediatrics*, **105**, 385–391.

176 Van Vliet MAT, Martin CB Jr, Nijhuis JC, et al. (1985). Behavioral states in growth-retarded human fetuses. *Early Hum Dev*, **12**, 183–197.

177 Bekedam DJ, Visser GHA, De Vries JJ, et al. (1985). Motor behavior in the growth retarded fetus. *Early Hum Dev*, **12**, 155–165.

178 Bekedam DJ, Visser GHA, Mulder EJH, et al. (1987). Heart rate variation and movement incidence in growth retarded fetuses: the significance of antenatal late heart rate decelerations. *Am J Obstet Gynecol*, **157**, 126–133.

179 Nijhuis IJ, ten Hof J, Nijhuis JG, et al. (1999). Temporal organization of fetal behavior from 24-weeks gestation onwards in normal and complicated pregnancies. *Dev Biol*, **34**, 257–268.

180 Vintzileos AM, Fleming AD, Scorza WE, et al. (1991). Relationship between fetal biophysical activities and

umbilical cord blood gas values. *Am J Obstet Gynecol*, **165**, 707–713.

181 Sival DA, Visser GHA and Prechtl HFR. (1992). The effect of intrauterine growth retardation on the quality of general movements in the human fetus. *Early Hum Dev*, **28**, 119–132.

182 Als H, Tronick E, Adamson L, et al. (1976). The behavior of the full-term but underweight newborn infant. *Dev Med Child Neurol*, **18**, 590–602.

183 Zeskind PS and Lester BM. (1981). Analysis of cry features in newborns with differential fetal growth. *Child Dev*, **52**, 207–212.

184 Lester BM and Zeskind PS. (1978). Brazelton scale and physical size correlates of neonatal cry features. *Infant Behav Dev*, **1**, 393–402.

185 Leventhal JM, Berg A and Egerter SA. (1987). Is intrauterine growth retardation a risk factor for child abuse? *Pediatrics*, **79**, 515–519.

186 Watt J and Strongman KT. (1985). Mother–infant interactions at 2 and 3 months in preterm, small-for-gestational age, and full-term infants; their relationship with cognitive development at 4 months. *Early Hum Dev*, **11**, 231–246.

187 Watt J. (1986). Interaction and development in the first year. II. The effects of intrauterine growth retardation. *Early Hum Dev*, **13**, 211–223.

188 Warkany J, Monroe BB and Sutherland B.S. (1961). Intrauterine growth retardation. *Am J Dis Child*, **102**, 249–279.

189 Drillien CM. (1970): The small-for-date infant: etiology and prognosis. *Pediatr Clin North Am*, **17**, 9–24.

190 Goldenberg RL and Cliver SP. (1997). Small for gestational age and intra-uterine growth restriction: definitions and standards. *Clin Obstet Gynecol*, **40**, 704–714.

191 Babson SG, Kangas J, Young N, et al. (1964). Growth and development of twins of dissimilar size at birth. *Pediatrics*, **33**, 327–333.

192 Babson SG and Phillips DS. (1973). Growth and development of twins dissimilar in size at birth. *N Engl J Med*, **289**, 937–940.

193 Wilson RS. (1979). Twin growth: initial deficit, recovery and trends in concordance from birth to nine years. *Ann Hum Biol*, **6**, 205–220.

194 Falkner F. (1978). Implications for growth in human twins. In *Human Growth*, ed. F Falkner and JM Tanner, pp. 379–413. New York: Plenum Publishing.

195 Philip AGS. (1981). Term twins with discordant birth weights: observations at birth and one year. *Acta Genet Med Gemellol (Roma)*, **30**, 203–212.

196 Buckler JMH and Robinson AH. (1974). Matched development of a pair of monozygous twins of grossly different size at birth. *Arch Dis Child*, **49**, 472–476.

197 Fitzhardinge PM and Steven EM. (1972). The small-for-date infant. II: Neurological and intellectual sequelae. *Pediatrics*, **50**, 50–57.

198 Babson SG and Henderson NB. (1974). Fetal undergrowth: relation of head growth to later intellectual performance. *Pediatrics*, **53**, 890–894.

199 Strauss RS and Dietz WH. (1998). Growth and development of term children born with low birth weight: effects of genetic and environmental factors. *J Pediatr*, **133**, 67–72.

200 Strauss RS. (2000). Adult functional outcome of those born small for gestational age: twenty-six year follow-up of the 1970 British Birth Cohort. *JAMA*, **283**, 625–632.

201 Commey JOO and Fitzhardinge PM. (1979). Handicap in the preterm small-for-gestational age infant. *J Pediatr*, **94**, 779–786.

202 Huisjes HJ, Baarsma R, Hadders-Algra M, et al. (1985). Follow-up of growth-retarded children born by elective Cesarean section before 33 weeks. *Gynecol Obstet Invest*, **19**, 169–173.

203 Ounsted M, Moar VA and Scott A. (1989). Small-for-dates babies, gestational age, and developmental ability at 7 years. *Early Hum Dev*, **19**, 77–86.

204 Lubchenco LO, Searls DT and Brazie JV. (1972). Neonatal mortality rate: relationship to birth weight and gestational age. *J Pediatr*, **81**, 814–822.

205 Lubchenco LO. (1976). Intrauterine growth and neonatal morbidity and mortality. In *The High Risk Infant*, ed. LO Lubchenco, pp. 99–124. Philadelphia: W.B. Saunders.

206 Starfield B, Shapiro S, McCormick M, et al. (1982). Mortality and morbidity in infants with intrauterine growth retardation. *J Pediatr*, **101**, 978–983.

207 McIntire DD, Bloom SL, Casey BM, et al. (1999). Birth weight in relation to morbidity and mortality among newborn infants. *N Engl J Med*, **340**, 1234–1238.

208 Walther FJ and Ramaekers LHJ. (1982). Growth in early childhood of newborns affected by disproportionate intrauterine growth retardation. *Acta Paediatr Scand*, **71**, 651–656.

209 Tenovuo A, Kero P, Piekkala P, et al. (1987). Growth of 519 small for gestational age infants during the first two years of life. *Acta Paediatr Scand*, **76**, 636–646.

210 Fitzhardinge PM and Inwood S. (1989). Long-term growth in small-for-date children. *Acta Paediatr Scand Suppl*, **78/349**, 27–33.

211 Adair LS. (1989). Low birth weight and intrauterine growth retardation in Filipino infants. *Pediatrics*, **84**, 613–622.

212 Paz I, Seidman DS, Danon YL, et al. (1993). Are children born small for gestational age at increased risk for short stature? *Am J Dis Child*, **147**, 337–339.

213 Ounsted M, Moar VA and Scott A. (1985). Children of deviant birth weight: the influence of genetic and other factors on size at seven years. *Acta Paediatr Scand*, **74**, 707–712.

214 Ounsted M, Moar VA and Scott A. (1986). Proportionality of small-for-gestational age babies at birth: perinatal associations and post-natal sequelae. *Early Hum Dev*, **14**, 77–88.

215 Colle E, Schiff D, Andrew G, et al. (1976). Insulin responses during catch-up growth in infants who were small for gestational age. *Pediatrics*, **57**, 363–371.

216 Fattal-Valevski A, Leitner Y, Kutai M, et al. (1999). Neurodevelopmental outcome in children with intrauterine growth retardation: a 3-year follow-up. *J Child Neurol*, **14**, 724–727.

217 Westwood M, Kramer MS, Munz D, et al. (1983). Growth and development of full-term non-asphyxiated small-for-gestational-age newborns: follow-up through adolescence. *Pediatrics*, **71**, 376–382.

218 Winer EK, Tejani NA, Atluru VL, et al. (1982). Four-to-seven-year evaluation in two groups of small-for-gestational age infants. *Am J Obstet Gynecol*, **143**, 425–429.

219 Drew JH, Bayly J and Beischer NA. (1983). Prospective follow-up of growth retarded infants and of those from pregnancies complicated by low oestriol excretion – 7 years. *Aust N Z J Obstet Gynaecol*, **23**, 150–154.

220 Ounsted MK, Moar VA and Scott A. (1983). Small-for-dates babies at the age of four years: health, handicap and developmental status. *Early Hum Dev*, **8**, 243–258.

221 Villar J, Smeriglio V, Martorell R, et al. (1984). Heterogeneous growth and mental development of intrauterine growth-retarded infants during the first 3 years of life. *Pediatrics*, **74**, 783–791.

222 Ameli Martikainen M. (1992). Effects of intrauterine growth retardation and its subtypes on the development of the preterm infant. *Early Hum Dev*, **28**, 7–17.

223 Vohr BR and Oh W. (1983). Growth and development in preterm infants small for gestational age. *J Pediatr*, **103**, 941–945.

224 Sung I-K, Vohr B and Oh W. (1993). Growth and neurodevelopmental outcome of very low birth weight infants with intrauterine growth retardation: comparison with control subjects matched by birth weight and gestational age. *J Pediatr*, **123**, 618–624.

225 Monset-Couchard M and de Beehmann O. (2000). Catch-up growth in 166 small-for-gestational age premature infants weighing less than 1000 g at birth. *Biol Neonate*, **78**, 161–167.

226 Uvebrant P and Hagberg G. (1992). Intrauterine growth in children with cerebral palsy. *Acta Paediatr*, **81**, 407–412.

227 Blair E and Stanley F. (1990). Intrauterine growth and cerebral palsy. I. Association with birthweight for gestational age. *Am J Obstet Gynecol*, **162**, 229–237.

228 Topp M, Langhoff-Roos J, Uldall P, et al. (1996). Intrauterine growth and gestational age in preterm infants with cerebral palsy. *Early Hum Dev*, **44**, 27–36.

229 Hill RM, Verniaud VM, Deter RL, et al. (1984). The effect of intrauterine malnutrition on the term infant: a 14-year progressive study. *Acta Paediatr Scand*, **73**, 482–487.

230 Hawdon JM, Hey E, Kolvin I, et al. (1990). Born too small – is outcome still affected? *Dev Med Child Neurol*, **32**, 943–953.

231 Low JA, Handley-Derry MH, Burke SO, et al. (1992). Association of intra-uterine fetal growth retardation and learning deficits at age 9 to 11 years. *Am J Obstet Gynecol*, **167**, 1499–1505.

232 Hutton JL, Pharoah POD, Cooke RWI, et al. (1997). Differential effects of preterm birth and small (for) gestational age on cognitive and motor development. *Arch Dis Child*, **76**, F75–F81.

233 Kok JH, den-Ouden AL, Verloove-Vanhorick SP, et al. (1998). Outcome of the very preterm small for gestational age infants: the first nine years of life. *Br J Obstet Gynaecol*, **105**, 162–168.

234 Paz I, Laor A, Gale R, et al. (2001). Term infants with fetal growth restriction are not at increased risk for low intelligence scores at age 17 years. *J Pediatr*, **138**, 87–91.

235 Barker DJP, Bull AR, Osmond C, et al. (1990). Fetal and placental size and risk of hypertension in adult life. *Br Med J*, **301**, 259–262.

236 Barker DJP, Hales CN, Fall CHD, et al. (1993). Type 2 (non-insulin-dependent) diabetes mellitus, hypertension and hyperlipidemia (syndrome X): relation to reduced fetal growth. *Diabetologia*, **36**, 62–67.

237 Barker DJP, Gluckman PD, Godfrey KM, et al. (1993). Fetal nutrition and cardiovascular disease in adult life. *Lancet*, **341**, 938–941.

238 Eriksson JG, Forsen T, Tuomilehto J, et al. (2000). Early growth, adult income, and risk of stroke. *Stroke*, **31**, 869–874.

239 Poulsen P, Vaag AA, Kyvik KO, et al. (1997). Low birth weight is associated with NIDDM in discordant monozygotic and dizygotic twin pairs. *Diabetologia*, **40**, 439–446.

240 Forsen T, Eriksson J, Tuomilehto J, et al. (2000). The fetal

and childhood growth of persons who develop type 2 diabetes. *Ann Intern Med*, **133**, 176–182.

241 Varma TR and Curzen P. (1973). The effects of abdominal decompression on pregnancy complicated by the small-for-dates fetus. *J Obstet Gynaecol Br Commonwealth*, **80**, 1086–1094.

242 Pavelka R and Salzer H. (1981). Abdominal decompression: an approach towards treating placental insufficiency. *Gynecol Obstet Invest*, **12**, 317–324.

243 Pollack RN, Yaffe H and Divon MY. (1997). Therapy for intrauterine growth restriction: current options and future directions. *Clin Obstet Gynecol*, **40**, 824–842.

244 Battaglia C, Artini PC, D'Ambrogio G, et al. (1992). Maternal hyperoxygenation in the treatment of intrauterine growth retardation. *Am J Obstet Gynecol*, **167**, 430–435.

245 Gulmezoglu AM and Hofmeyr GJ. (2000). Maternal oxygen administration for suspected impaired fetal growth. *Cochrane Database Syst Rev*, **2**, CD000137.

246 Uzan S, Beaufils M, Breart G, et al. (1991). Prevention of fetal growth retardation with low-dose aspirin: findings of the EPREDA trial. *Lancet*, **337**, 1427–1431.

247 Grab D, Paulus WE, Erdmann M, et al. (2000). Effects of low-dose aspirin on uterine and fetal blood flow during pregnancy: results of a randomized, placebo-controlled, double-blind trial. *Ultrasound Obstet Gynecol*, **15**, 19–27.

248 Oyelese KO, Black RS, Lees CC, et al. (1998). A novel approach to the management of pregnancies complicated by utero-placental insufficiency and previous stillbirth. *Aust N Z J Obstet Gynecol*, **38**, 391–395.

249 Rivera-Alsina ME, Saldaria LR and Stringer CA. (1984). Fetal growth sustained by parenteral nutrition in pregnancy. *Obstet Gynecol*, **64**, 138–141.

250 Gulmezoglu AM and Hofmeyr GJ. (2000). Maternal nutrient supplementation for suspected impaired fetal growth. *Cochrane Database Syst Rev*, **2**, CD000148.

251 Gulmezoglu AM and Hofmeyr GJ. (2000). Plasma volume expansion for suspected impaired fetal growth. *Cochrane Database Syst Rev*, **2**, CD000167.

252 Gulmezoglu AM and Hofmeyr G.J. (2000). Bed rest in hospital for suspected impaired fetal growth. *Cochrane Database Syst Rev*, **2**, CD000034.

253 Roth S, Chang TC, Robson S, et al. (1999). The neurodevelopmental outcome of term infants with different intrauterine growth characteristics. *Early Hum Dev*, **55**, 39–50.

8

Hemorrhagic lesions of the central nervous system

Seetha Shankaran

Wayne State University School of Medicine, Children's Hospital of Michigan, Detroit, MI, USA

Neonatal intracranial hemorrhage in the full-term infant

Intracanial hemorrhage (ICH) in the full-term infant is less common than in the premature infant. The incidence and site of ICH in healthy, term neonates have been reported by sonographic evaluation to be 3.5%, with a subependymal location in 2.0%, choroid plexus locus in 1.1%, and a parenchymal locus in 0.4%. Clinically significant ICH in term infants, although uncommon, occurs in the subdural, intraventricular, and parenchymal areas, or in multiple sites.[1]

Subdural hemorrhage in term infants

Subdural hemorrhage usually occurs secondary to birth trauma. These hemorrhages are relatively uncommon currently because of improvements in obstetric care. The pathogenesis is secondary to mechanical injury to the cranium associated with instrumental delivery with forceps or vacuum extraction of the head, abnormal presentation (face or brow), precipitous delivery, and a large infant resulting in a difficult delivery.[1–3] There are shearing forces on the tentorium and the deep venous system. Tearing of the tentorium occurs, usually at the junction with the falx. Tearing of the falx or the superior cerebral veins occurs with less frequency. Tearing of the tentorium causes rupture of the straight sinus, the vein of Galen, transverse sinus, and infratentorial veins. Tearing of the falx involves the inferior sagittal sinus. Osteodiastasis of the occipital bones can produce tentorial tears and laceration of the inferior surface of the cerebellum.

The clinical presentation of infants is related to the extent of subdural hemorrhage. A massive subdural hemorrhage is associated with symptoms of midbrain compression (stupor, coma) followed by brainstem compression (fixed dilated pupils, bradycardia, and respiratory arrest). Minor subdural hemorrhages may be associated with irritability and seizures. Rarely, subdural hemorrhage presents as prenatal hydrocephalus. Imaging studies should be performed to evaluate extent of involvement. Sonography is not recommend for evaluation of the subdural space: magnetic resonance imaging or computed tomography (CT) scanning is preferable. The prognosis is good for small hemorrhages (in the posterior fossa) with or without surgical intervention while the prognosis for large, rapidly progressive lesions is poor, with a high mortality rate.

Intraventricular hemorrhage in the full-term infant

Intraventricular hemorrhage (IVH) is an uncommon problem in full-term as compared to preterm neonates. Origins of the IVH can be the germinal matrix, choroid plexus, or parenchyma. In term infants only remnants of the germinal matrix remain. The incidence of germinal matrix hemorrhage is therefore low, and infants are often asymptomatic. The mechanism of IVH in term infants has been attributed to trauma at birth (precipitous delivery) or hypoxia; however, no etiology is detected in many cases. Recently, extension of thalamic hemorrhage into the ventricles has been reported as the most common cause of IVH in term infants.[3] The pathogenesis of thalamic hemorrhage is a hemorrhagic infarction of the large venous channels that are in close proximity to the ventricular walls. In the majority of infants none of the previously associated risk factors for thalamic hemorrhage were noted, such as coagulation disorders or hypoxic–ischemic birth injury.

Predisposing factors noted by Roland et al.[3] included sepsis, cyanotic heart disease, and polycythemia. Symptomatology (irritability, seizures, apnea, bulging fontanel) occurred later than that seen in infants with IVH from choroid plexus or germinal matrix hemorrhage.

Management of IVH in term infants is supportive. Prognosis depends on the location and extent of the underlying insult. As a rule, among infants for whom no etiology of the IVH is detected, outcome appears to be good. In infants with IVH secondary to a germinal matrix hemorrhage, prognosis is also good. Neurodevelopmental sequelae are seen in infants with IVH with parenchymal involvement.[4] When bilateral thalamic hemorrhage is associated with birth asphyxia, mortality is high and sequelae in survivors are high. Thalamic hemorrhage with IVH seen in infants with an uneventful birth history is associated with a greater risk for cerebral palsy than IVH from other sites.

ICH in other specific conditions in term infants

Arteriovenous malformations

Arteriovenous malformations occur commonly in the vein of Galen. Other sites include the cerebral hemisphere, third ventricle, choroid plexus, and spinal cord. Vein of Galen arteriovenous malformations usually present with a cranial bruit and congestive cardiac failure while IVH is the presentation with arteriovenous malformations originating from other sites.[1] Diagnosis is by pulsed Doppler sonography, CT, or digital subtraction angiography to define the lesion. Management is based on the size and location of the feeding vessels. Large arteriovenous malformations are associated with a high mortality. Small accessible lesions can be surgically removed. Deeper lesions require pre- and perioperative embolization to occlude the deep feeding vessels, thus reducing dissection of brain tissue during resection of the lesion. Prognosis is poor if there is cerebral tissue damage (seen as calcification or lucencies on diagnostic imaging studies). Minor neuromotor sequelae are reported following surgical resection.[1]

Neonatal alloimmune thrombocytopenia

In neonatal alloimmune thrombocytopenia, fetal and neonatal thrombocytopenia results from the formation of a maternal antiplatelet antibody to a paternally derived platelet antigen, usually platelet surface antigen (PLAI), expressed on the surface of the fetal platelets. Neonatal alloimune thrombocytopenia occurs in 1 in 2000 to 1 in 5000 fetuses and up to 30% of infants with this condition have ICH secondary to thrombocytopenia. With the advent of improving fetal surveillance, as many as 25% of cases of ICH observed among infants with alloimmune thrombocytopenia have occurred antenatally. The platelet count in the cord blood in fetuses with this condition has been reported as low as 20 000.[5] Management in the antenatal period includes administration of intravenous gammaglobulin to the mother with or without corticosteroids prior to delivery. Transfusion of matched compatible platelets to the fetus may safeguard against ICH during the birthing process.[6] Abdominal delivery is suggested if cordocentesis reveals fetal thrombocytopenia. After birth, transfusion with antigen-negative platelets (maternal platelets) is recommended.

Extracorporeal membrane oxygenation (ECMO)

ECMO is the treatment of choice in infants with persistent pulmonary hypertension and cardiorespiratory failure unresponsive to inhaled nitric oxide. In term infants, ICH following ECMO occurs in 13% of infants.[7] The lesions are hemorrhagic with ischemia (60%) or hemorrhage alone (40%). The pathogenesis of ICH following ECMO is multifactorial. The underlying disease process (commonly, severe respiratory failure) contributes to the risk of ICH.[8] Ligation of the jugular vein can lead to increase in central venous pressure. Hemorrhagic infarcts can occur secondary to vessel obstruction from microemboli. Animal studies suggest that venoarterial ECMO (VA ECMO) results in alteration of autoregulation of cerebral blood flow, thus contributing to the risk of ICH.[8] Lastly, heparinization during ECMO is a major risk factor for ICH. These hemorrhagic lesions can be predominantly in one hemisphere[9] or in both cerebral hemispheres.[10]

Sonography is the best imaging technique to evaluate ICH in term infants on ECMO. CT of the head may be performed to evaluate the extent of the lesion after decannulation. Single-photon emission computed tomography is a useful predictor of outcome only when it is normal.[11] It has recently been demonstrated by positron emission tomography that, in infants who have no cerebral injury and have undergone successful ECMO, hemispheric cerebral blood flow is symmetric.[12]

Infants who have undergone ECMO and who have hemorrhagic lesions are at a higher risk for abnormalities of neurodevelopmental outcome than infants who have no ICH.[13,14] Attempts at decreasing risk of ICH with ECMO include venovenous (VV) ECMO where integrity of blood flow to the brain is maintained and cannulation and sacrifice of only the internal jugular vein occur. In VV ECMO, the pulmonary vessels serve as filters for the ECMO circuit. Aminocaproic acid is an antithrombolytic agent administered in infants at risk for bleeding.[15] Lastly, heparin-bonded membranes and tubing that would obviate the need for systemic heparinization are being developed.

Neonatal intracranial hemorrhage in preterm infants

In preterm infants ICH occurs in the subependymal germinal matrix, in the periventricular area, in the choroid plexus, within the ventricular system, in the cerebral parenchyma, and in the cerebellar region. The most common site of ICH is the subependymal germinal matrix region. Cerebellar hemorrhages are relatively uncommon. The emergence of superior imaging techniques may allow for distinction between hemorrhagic and ischemic lesions within the parenchyma, hence the detection of hemorrhagic lesions in preterm infants continues to evolve.

The germinal matrix area is highly vascularized and is described as an "immature vascular rete." It is contiguous with the deep venous system draining blood from the cerebral white matter, choroid plexus, striatum, and the thalamus. It should be noted that the direction of venous drainage changes at the site of the germinal matrix in a peculiar U-turn (contributing to the risk of venous congestion). The integrity of the capillaries in the germinal matrix is tenuous, with lack of supportive tissue. The capillaries are readily injured, leading to rupture when venous congestion occurs. Free oxygen activity may also injure the endothelial cells of the capillaries. The microcirculation of the germinal matrix (not arteries or arterioles) is the site of hemorrhage. The germinal matrix involutes by 34 weeks' gestation. The germinal matrix, therefore, is the most common site of ICH because of these hemodynamic and structural factors.

Germinal matrix hemorrhage (GMH) may be unilateral or bilateral and occurs in isolation in most preterm infants. In some infants GMH may be followed by or occur simultaneously with an IVH. This IVH probably occurs when the vessels in the germinal matrix rupture.

IVH is usually bilateral and the blood is seen throughout the ventricular system, with the ventricles being filled to a varying extent, ranging from minimal blood to a "cast" of the ventricles. Blood clots can be visualized in the ventricular system for as long as 6 weeks following onset of IVH. Fifteen percent (15%) of infants with an IVH have an associated intraparenchymal hemorrhage (IPH). Choroid plexus hemorrhage occurs in infants with GMH and IVH. In older preterm infants, the choroid plexus may be the only site of hemorrhage.

Hemorrhage within the parenchyma (intracerebral hemorrhage) occurs usually with less frequency than GMH alone and occurs usually with GMH and IVH.[16] The frequency of IPH with IVH ranges from 15 to 80% of infants. However, it can occur as an isolated lesion. IPH does not always reflect progression or extension of IVH or GMH. It may reflect venous circulatory abnormalities resulting in hemorrhagic and/or ischemic injury. This lesion is seen as a periventricular or intraparenchymal echodensity on sonography. On microscopic study there is hemorrhagic venous infarction, secondary to obstruction to the medullary veins and the terminal veins by the germinal matrix clot and the IVH. IPH is usually located dorsal and lateral to the external angles of the lateral ventricles. It is usually a unilateral lesion that can be localized or involve the entire periventricular white matter of the parenchyma from the frontal to the parietooccipital regions. If the lesions are bilateral, they are often asymmetric in size. IPH evolves into a cystic lesion following necrosis of affected cerebral tissue, forming a posthemorrhagic or a porencephalic cyst.

Periventricular leukomalacia

Periventricular leukomalcia (PVL) is the most common ischemic injury in the premature infant. The incidence is noted to be high at autopsy. Since most neonatal units perform screening by cranial sonography, PVL among preterms has decreased to 5% (range between National Institute of Child Health and Human Development (NICHD) Network sites, 2–13%).[17] The lesion occurs in areas representing arterial border zones or watershed areas. Based on the development of both the penetrating cerebral and periventricular vasculatures, in the 24–28-week gestation infant the border zones may exist in cerebral white matter relatively distant from the periventricular region. In the older preterm infant, these border zones may exist in both the subcortical and periventricular white matter. The hemodynamic and structural factors that make the preterm infant at risk for ICH also contribute to risk of ischemic injury; hypotension is the greatest underlying risk factor. ICH is observed in 25% of cases of PVL studied on autopsy; hence the two lesions coexist.

PVL can be diffuse or extensive. Tissue necrosis from ischemia leads to cavitation. The two most common sites are at the level of occipital radiation at the trigone of the lateral ventricles and at the level of the cerebral white matter around the foramen of Monro.

Clinical risk factors for PVL include any condition associated with decrease in systemic blood pressure (perinatal asphyxia, respiratory distress syndrome, myocardial failure, sepsis, and apnea). A clear association has been shown between chronic intrauterine hypoxia and damage to cerebral white matter.[18] Chorioamnionitis and fetal inflammation have also been noted to be related to an increased risk for PVL.[19]

Diagnosis of PVL is made by serial sonographic studies. PVL appears initially as an echodense lesion followed by cavitation. In extensive PVL these cavities can coalesce. When ICH occurs with PVL, it is difficult to distinguish this lesion sonographically from intraparenchymal venous infarction.

Pathogenesis of ICH

Alteration in cerebral blood flow in the preterm neonate, further accentuation of impaired autoregulation of cerebral blood flow, increase in central venous pressure, endothelial injury, and reperfusion injury have all been implicated in the pathogenesis of ICH. These hemodynamic characteristics and the presence of a subependymal matrix make the premature infant at risk for ICH. Fluctuations in cerebral blood flow have been documented in infants with respiratory distress syndrome. Infants with an increase in cerebral blood flow are at highest risk for ICH. Hypercarbia, hypoxemia, and acidosis, seen in infants with hyaline membrane disease, increase cerebral blood flow. Rapid volume expansion, pneumothorax, and seizures have been noted to be associated with ICH, probably by increasing cerebral blood flow. A decrease in cerebral blood flow has been documented in infants with systemic hypertension, large patent ductus arteriosus with a ductal "steal" and infants with perinatal asphyxia. ICH occurs in infants with a decrease in cerebral blood flow[20] when reperfusion occurs (usually following aggressive therapy). Fluctuations in systemic blood pressure, observed during clinical care practice, are reflected rapidly in the cerebral circulation because of the pressure-passive state of cerebral blood flow. Elevation of central venous pressure occurs in infants with pneumothorax and birth asphyxia, those infants subjected to labor, and delivery by the vaginal route. Vascular endothelial injury occurs following hypoxic–ischemic events and may be associated with lack of antioxidant activity or release of free oxygen radicals.

Incidence of ICH

The incidence of neonatal ICH has changed over the past decade. Earlier, the incidence was reported to be 40–60%. In a prospective series evaluating ICH from 1987 to 1990–91 in 4795 infants with birth weight <1500 g, infants with no hemorrhage detected by cranial sonography increased from 53% in 1987–88 to 59% in 1991, and infants with grade I hemorrhage remained essentially the same between the two periods (18–19%). The incidence of severe ICH (maximum grade III–IV) decreased significantly over the time period from 19% in 1988 (11% grade III and 8% grade IV) to 15% in 1990 (8% grade III and 7% grade IV).[21] The current incidence of grade III and IV ICH in 4438 neonates 501–1500 g is 6% and 5%, respectively.[17] The majority of hemorrhages are detected within the first week of age. Routine sonography performed after birth has demonstrated ICH within 6 h of age in up to 40% of infants.[22] Few infants have onset of ICH beyond 14 days of age.

Risk and protective factors for ICH

Risk and protective factors associated with ICH can be characterized as prenatal, perinatal, and postnatal factors. Prenatal characteristics associated with a lower risk of ICH in preterm infants include hypertension–preeclampsia in the mother, maternal race, and infant gender.[21] Hypertension–preeclampsia has been found to be protective against all grades of ICH as well as the most severe grades of hemorrhage.[23,24] Infants born to women with hypertension–preeclampsia are often of more advanced gestational age than infants born to women without this diagnosis. Female infants have a lower incidence of ICH as compared to male infants, regardless of race. In a large prospectively collected data registry, the lowest incidence of severe ICH occurred in black female infants.[21]

Prenatal factors associated with ICH include antenatal steroid administration, presentation of fetus, mode of delivery, labor, gestational age, and birth weight.[25,26] Antenatal steroid administration is a therapeutic intervention and the most powerful perinatal factor associated with a decreased risk for ICH.[27] This protective effect of steroids has been demonstrated in observational data, prospective single-center or multicenter trials, and metaanalysis of trials.[21,27–30] The additive effect of antenatal steroid administration and cesarean section delivery in protecting against ICH has been documented.[31] Increasing birth weight and gestational age are associated with a decreasing rate of all grades of ICH as well as severe ICH.[32] Gestational age category (whether an infant was appropriate-for-gestational-age or small-for-gestational-age) influences the risk of grade III–IV ICH. When impact of race on gestational age category was examined, a decrease in grade III–IV ICH was noted in small-for-gestational-age infants, with a greater protective effect in nonblack infants as compared to black infants. The presentation of the fetus (vertex or breech) has been found to be a risk factor for early hemorrhage as well as for all grades of hemorrhage.[33] The role of both labor and mode of delivery as risk factors for ICH have been debated.[23] Although a lack of effect of labor on the incidence of ICH was noted in very-low-birth-weight infants, a lower incidence of overall ICH and grade II–IV ICH was noted in neonates delivered by cesarean section across each 2-year period from 1980 to 1987.[25] In a prospective study evaluating the incidence of ICH with cranial sonograms performed within 2 h of birth, it was noted that the mode of delivery did not influence the incidence of ICH, but vaginal delivery was associated with a high risk for early hemorrhage (<2 h of age), while cesarean delivery was associated with a risk for later hemorrhage.[26] Active-phase labor increased the risk of early ICH, while forceps delivery or abdominal delivery decreased this risk for early ICH.

In a multivariate analysis of prenatal and perinatal factors influencing risk of grade III–IV ICH, presentation of the fetus, labor, and mode of delivery failed to achieve significance in the final model of characteristics affecting risk of grade III–IV ICH.[21] The adjusted odds ratios (OR) of risk for severe ICH corrected for year of birth and prenatal and perinatal characteristics using multivariate logistic regression modeling in this series were as follows: completed course of antenatal steroid therapy, OR=0.44 (95% confidence interval=0.30–0.65); partial course of antenatal steroid therapy, OR=0.74 (0.50–1.99); hypertension–preeclampsia in the absence of antepartum hemorrhage, OR=0.44 (0.33–0.59); black maternal race, OR=0.71(0.60–0.84); female gender of the infant, OR=0.72(0.60–0.85); gestational age per week, OR=0.86 (0.81–0.90), and birth weight per 100g OR=0.86 (0.82–0.90).

Postnatal factors associated with risk of ICH include outborn birth, delivery room resuscitation, low Apgar scores, the presence of respiratory distress syndrome, need for mechanical ventilation, hypercarbia, hypoxemia, acidosis, pneumothorax, and patent ductus arteriosus.[34] Postnatal risk and protective factors should be evaluated with caution, as their temporal relationship to ICH was often not determined in these studies.

It is clinically difficult to distinguish between risk factors for severe IVH and IPH. These lesions often occur together. Ischemic lesions, commonly PVL, may be associated with IVH and IPH. There appear to be clinical associations between intraparenchymal echodensities, probably reflecting hemorrhage, and emergent cesarean section, surfactant therapy, pulmonary hemorrhage, and patent ductus arteriosus.[16]

Diagnosis of ICH

Clinical diagnosis of ICH has become difficult because of aggressive care of high-risk infants. Infants do not present with apnea, shock, or collapse when severe hemorrhage occurs as they are often receiving ventilatory and pressor support. A rapid fall in hematocrit, lack of restoration of the hematocrit after a transfusion, and/or a full fontanel may occasionally be seen following massive ICH. The majority of infants with GMH remain asymptomatic, hence the need for screening by cranial sonography of all infants with a high risk of ICH (infants who are ≤32 weeks). At a minimum, scans should be performed at 5–7 days of age (to detect ICH), and at 2 weeks (to detect onset of ventriculomegaly in the periventricular area or parenchyma and to monitor ventricular size). When ICH is detected, additional sonographic studies should be performed as clinically indicated.

Cranial sonography remains the most useful and cost-effective method of detection of neonatal ICH. GMH can be detected as echodensities in the periventricular area, superior to the caudothalamic groove. There is less concordance between central reading of sonograms and local readers when evaluating these hemorrhages, with a higher incidence reported by local readers. GMH should be diagnosed only when detected in both coronal and sagittal sections of the sonographic studies. IVH should be separated from bleeding into the choroid plexus.

In very preterm infants a diffuse periventricular echodensity or "blush" is seen sonographically, which is often a transient finding. Periventricular echodensities that persist sonographically beyond 2 weeks (and do not become lucent) probably reflect hemorrhagic injury.[35] IPH cannot be distinguished sonographically from a hemorrhagic PVL. It should be noted that IPH is surrounded by a large area of ischemia, as demonstrated by positron emission tomography.

ICH has been classified by investigators using differing systems. The most frequently used is the Papile classification of grade I–IV based on diagnosis by CT at 2 weeks of age.[36] ICH has also been graded as mild, moderate, and severe based on serial sonographic studies.[37] Hemorrhage within the ventricular system has been graded and attempts at assessing ventricular size are now being made.[38]

There is a close relationship between neurologic disability at 2–3 years of age and abnormal cranial sonographic findings in the neonatal period.[39,40] ICH is a dynamic process and echodensities may be transient or persistent. Echodensities may reflect hemorrhage or a hemorrhagic infarction. It is clinically more relevant, therefore, to describe ICH by its location, extent (whether localized or diffuse), and persistence of lesions or complications (persistence of echodensities or ventriculomegaly).

Complications of ICH[41]

The complications of ICH in preterm neonates are related to the location and severity of hemorrhage. Hemorrhage in the subependymal region resolves with no residual effects. The resolution of hemorrhage in the parenchymal region is based on location of the hemorrhage. Over the course of weeks, parenchymal hemorrhage evolves either into posthemorrhagic cysts or porencephalic dilatation of the ventricular system. Among infants with IVH, progressive posthemorrhagic ventricular dilation is the most frequent and serious complication. Ventricular size can increase from blood clots, at the time of the occurrence of the IVH during the first week of life. This acute ventricular distension often subsides; however, in 60–70% of infants with IVH, progressive increase in ventricular size occurs within 2 weeks of the occurrence of IVH due to accumulation of cerebrospinal fluid (CSF). Posthemorrhage ventriculomegaly (PHVM) can progress either slowly or rapidly. In the majority of cases (65%) slowly progressive PHVM is followed by spontaneous arrest. In the remaining 30–35% of infants with PHVM, ventricular size increases rapidly over the course of days to weeks.

Evolution of posthemorrhagic ventriculomegaly

PHVM occurs due to obstruction of the CSF pathway by blood clots, usually at the posterior fossa cisterns and less commonly at the aqueduct of Sylvius or the foramen of Monro. Occlusion to the pathways often results in PHVM that rapidly progresses. Posthemorrhagic inflammatory changes in the arachnid villi may contribute to delayed absorption and, thus, slowly progressive ventriculomegaly. The evolution of PHVM is related to the severity of the ventricular hemorrhage, with larger ventricular hemorrhages associated with greater risk of progressive ventriculomegaly. Brain injury can occur both at the time of IVH as well as during the development of ventricular distension. The injury at the time of IVH is often compounded by the periventricular and parenchymal hemorrhagic injury that may occur concurrently, as well as ischemic white-matter injury that may also be present. The ventricular distension that occurs in neonates with PHVM may increase cerebral vascular resistance, decrease cerebral perfusion, distort developing pathways, and accentuate hypoxic–ischemic injury they had already sustained. Early decompression of enlarged ventricles has demonstrated reversal of these efforts by Doppler sonography while positron emission tomography has shown improvement in cerebral oxygenation after treatment of PHVM. The periventricular white-matter region is especially vulnerable to hypoperfusion. PHVM is not always associated with an increase in intracranial pressure; the ventriculomegaly may result from a passive dilation from atrophy secondary to ischemic or hemorrhagic periventricular brain injury.

Diagnosis of posthemorrhagic ventriculomegaly

The clinical diagnosis of PHVM is challenging since criteria are not specific. An increase in head circumference >2 cm/week, a bulging fontanel, inability to wean from the ventilator, and increase in episodes of apnea and bradycardia are indicative of severe ventriculomegaly and/or increase in intracranial pressure. There is a 2–4-week lag time between increase in ventricular size and a detectable rapid increase in the head circumference since premature neonates have relative excess of water in cerebral white matter, a decrease in myelin, large subarachnoid space, and open sutures.

Cranial sonography is the best bedside diagnostic tool for monitoring ventricular size. Sonograms should be performed every 5–7 days following an IVH. The frequency of studies can be decreased if serial evaluations demonstrate stability of ventricular size. Progressive PHVM is defined as increasing ventricular size on consecutive sonographic scans performed 5–7 days apart. It should be noted that standardized criteria for measurement of ventricular size have not been developed. The posterior horn of the lateral ventricles appears to be disproportionately enlarged in most cases of PHVM with a deleterious effect on the optical pathway. PHVM may coexist with and should be distinguished from PVL. PVL is associated with "blunted" ventricular contours and lucencies in the periventricular regions. Acute PHVM with transependymal CSF accumulation may appear as hyperechoic areas around the distended ventricles. It is essential to perform serial sonographic scans to monitor progression of ventricular and parenchymal hemorrhages, PVL, and ventricular size, since parenchymal and ventricular hemorrhage can occur concurrently.

Diagnostic techniques under investigation to evaluate PHVM not available in a routine clinical setting include Doppler sonography, magnetic resonance imaging and spectroscopy, near-infrared spectroscopy, and positron emission tomography.

Prevention of PHVM

Attempts to prevent PHVM by serial lumbar punctures initiated immediately after IVH has occurred appeared to be encouraging when first reported. The rationale was to remove CSF containing blood and protein so that blocked CSF pathways may be reopened and fibrotic and inflammatory reactions may be reduced. These uncontrolled studies were followed by a randomized controlled trial where serial lumbar punctures were performed in the intervention group within 2 weeks of age and continued for 3 weeks. There was no benefit of serial lumbar punctures in preventing progressive PHVM requiring permanent CSF drainage. Thus, early repeated lumbar punctures cannot be recommended for the prevention of PHVM after neonatal IVH.

Management of PHVM

Since the natural history of ventriculomegaly following neonatal IVH has been described, the management of PHVM depends on the rate of progression of the ventriculomegaly. The definitive intervention for rapidly progressive PHVM is permanent drainage of CSF by ventricular shunt placement. The optimum age for shunt placement is when the preterm neonate is clinically stable, free of respiratory disease and infection, and has gained adequate weight. Interventions that have been used while awaiting clinical stability (or spontaneous arrest of ventriculomegaly) include drugs that decrease CSF production, drugs that increase fibrinolytic activity and clot lysis, and nonpharmacologic therapy such as serial lumbar punctures and ventricular drainage.

Outcome following ICH

Infants with mild grades of hemorrhage (in the germinal matrix or small amount of ventricular blood) perform as well in cognitive and motor developmental outcome as preterm infants with no ICH; however, their global performance may be impaired. Infants with periventricular echodensities persisting beyond 2 weeks have been found to have a cognitive outcome similar to children with normal scans, but with a risk for minor neurologic abnormalities of lower-limb function. Infants with major IVH or IPH have been reported to have 40–60% incidence of neurologic deficits (spastic diplegia, triplegia, hemiplegia). The outcome of infants with IPH varies based on whether the IPH is localized or extensive. Extensive IPH is associated with a higher mortality rate (81% compared to 37%), major motor deficits (100% compared to 80%), and more cognitive delays (86% compared to 53%) than localized IPH.

The neurologic and cognitive outcome following progressive PHVM is discouraging.[41] Only 25% of neonates with PHVM are normal at follow-up; 50–75% of children have moderate-to-severe neuromotor handicap at 5 years of age. The most important determinant of outcome remains the severity of hemorrhage in the neonatal period. Neonates with parenchymal (grade IV) hemorrhage in addition to PHVM have a higher risk for neurodevelopmental deficits. Other prognostic indicators include the concentration of CSF protein at diagnosis of progressive PHVM, the persistence of ventriculomegaly after intervention, the number of shunt revisions, the presence of PVL, seizure disorder, and lower birth weight. Recent studies have demonstrated that deficits in the visual motor and visual spatial areas are pronounced in children with ventriculomegaly following IVH, raising the possibility of ventriculomegaly causing injury to the optic tracts. Neuroimaging with magnetic resonance imaging (at approximately 8.5 years) in children with arrested or shunted hydrocephalus has revealed persistence of enlarged lateral ventricles, enlarged occipital horns, hypoplastic corpus callosum, and atrophy or dysplasia of the cerebral cortex. When preterm infants with no hydrocephalus are compared to those with arrested hydrocephalus, shunted hydrocephalus, and a term comparison group, the children with shunted hydrocephalus have the lowest verbal and perceptual IQ scores. Visual–spatial–motor scores are lower in the shunted compared to the arrested hydrocephalus group, and even lower in the arrested compared to the no hydrocephalus group. Tests of academic skills (arithmetic, science, writing) also demonstrate poorer performance in children with shunted hydrocephalus as compared to those with arrested hydrocephalus.

The presence of severe IVH and the occurrence of progressive PHVM requiring shunting should alert the clinicians to the high risk of subsequent neurodevelopmental morbidity. Since the survival rate of the very-low-birth-weight neonate has increased, the likelihood of neonates surviving with intracranial hemorrhage and complications of ICH increases. The accurate diagnosis and management of neonatal ICH continue to be a challenge to the clinician.

Infants with PVL have neurodevelopmental outcome that varies based on the location of the ischemic injury. In infants with localized PVL in the frontal region, neurodevelopmental outcome is normal. Sequelae occur with frontoparietal and frontoparietooccipital lesions. Parasagittal measurements of the anteroposterior dimension of cystic PVL best predict which infants will have quadriplegia and the more severe cognitive and sensory impairments. In infants with PVL in the occipital area, the incidence of visual disturbances is high.

Prevention of neonatal ICH in the preterm infant

Prevention of ICH should be the focus of management of ICH in preterm infants. The incidence of ICH has decreased over time in most studies evaluating this diagnosis over a period in the same clinical setting. It is difficult to specify the exact causes for this reduction, other than overall improvements in the care of the high-risk mother in preterm labor and the care of the preterm neonate.[42] Prevention of premature birth will prevent ICH, and, currently, tocolytics are used to prevent premature birth. However, they may not delay labor beyond 48 h. Concern has been raised by an increase in ICH incidence noted after indometacin and β-sympathomimetic tocolysis.[43,44]

Pharmacologic prevention of ICH has been the focus of many studies. Initial attempts were aimed at postnatal prevention of ICH. Phenobarbital, tranexamic acid, pancuronium, etamsylate, vitamin E, and indometacin have been the agents utilized postnatally to prevent or decrease the incidence and severity of ICH.

Phenobarbital

The rationale for phenobarbital use was sedation of the preterm infant to prevent the fluctuations of blood pressure that occur with clinical care of high-risk infants. The effects of postnatal phenobarbital therapy in preventing ICH have been reviewed by Whitelaw.[45] Phenobarbital was administered to preterm neonates in a controlled trial shortly after birth and a decrease in the overall incidence as well as severity of ICH was observed in the first report of its use. The dosage used aimed at achieving levels of 20–25 mg/ml. In the seven controlled studies that were subsequently reported, the results were not uniform. One study demonstrated a decrease in severe ICH in infants in the phenobarbital group as compared to the control group, whereas two studies demonstrated an increase in the incidence of ICH in the phenobarbital group. However there were differences in clinical characteristics between the two groups of infants in both studies. Four studies showed no change in the incidence of ICH between the infants in the phenobarbital and the control groups. Hence, current evidence does not warrant the routine use of phenobarbital postnatally in the prevention of ICH.

Tranexamic acid

Tranexamic acid is an inhibitor of plasminogen activators that have fibrinolytic properties.[46] It has been shown to reduce fibrolytic activity of germinal matrix extracts in vitro. In a randomized controlled trial, tranexamic acid failed to prevent neonatal IVH in preterm infants.

Pancuronium

Muscle paralysis using pancuronium bromide to stabilize fluctuating cerebral blood flow patterns in preterm ventilated infants resulted in a decrease in any ICH and severe ICH.[47] These investigators have continued their experience using muscle paralysis in this selected group of infants and found a decrease in both the incidence and severity of ICH. It should be noted that complications of muscle paralysis are edema and electrolyte imbalance.

Etamsylate

The rationale for the use of etamsylate includes its ability to inhibit the production of prostaglandin, a potent cerebral vasodilator. Etamsylate stabilizes capillary membranes and also promotes platelet aggregation and adhesiveness. The initial study utilizing etamsylate demonstrated a decrease in the incidence of ICH in the treated group as compared to the control group.[48] Two subsequent studies, one of which was a large, prospective multicenter randomized controlled trial, demonstrated a reduction in the incidence and severity of ICH.[49,50] Etamsylate is not available for clinical use in the USA.

Indometacin

Indometacin has been used to prevent ICH because of a demonstrated ability to inhibit prostaglandin synthesis and also inhibit free oxygen radical production generated as a byproduct of prostaglandin biosynthesis. Another mechanism may be acceleration of the maturation of the germinal matrix microvasculature. Bada[51] has reviewed the effects of indometacin on ICH. Eight studies have reported on the efficacy of indometacin in reducing the incidence and severity of ICH. Only one of these studies did not demonstrate a reduction of overall ICH or severe ICH. A recent prospective multicenter, randomized controlled trial ($n = 1202$ infants) has conclusively demonstrated that prophylaxis with indometacin did reduce the frequency of patent ductus arteriosus and severe ICH; however there was no improvement in the rate of survival without neurosensory impairment at 18 months of age.[52]

Vitamin E

Vitamin E has been used in an attempt to prevent neonatal ICH because of its ability to scavenge free oxygen radicals that can damage the germinal matrix endothelium. The review by Bada[51] of all four reports of vitamin E use did find a decrease in incidence of ICH and/or severity of ICH. However, in a study evaluating the role of vitamin E in the prevention of retinopathy of prematurity, a high incidence of ICH was noted in a subgroup of infants in the vitamin E-treated group.

Antenatal prevention

The focus of pharmacologic intervention of ICH has moved to the prenatal arena since ICH has pre- and perinatal risks. The pharmacological agents include phenobarbital, vitamin K, and antenatal steroids.

Phenobarbital[53]

The role of antenatal phenobarbital therapy in preventing neonatal ICH has recently been reviewed by Crowther and Henderson-Smart.[53] All five studies demonstrated a decrease in ICH or severe ICH in the phenobarbital-treated group or in subgroups of infants in the phenobarbital group as compared to infants in the control group. The serum levels achieved were lower than those achieved in the studies using phenobarbital postnatally. However, there were differences in clinical characteristics between groups, all infants were not accounted for in the analyses, and products of multiple gestations were included in the analysis in these studies. A large, randomized controlled trial evaluating antenatal phenobarbital and risk of ICH or early death with 610 women participating in the study demonstrated no benefit of antenatal phenobarbital therapy in reducing frequency of neonatal ICH or early death.[54]

Vitamin K

Vitamin K was used antenatally to prevent neonatal ICH, as vitamin K-dependent factors are deficient in preterm infants.[55,56] Although the two studies using vitamin K demonstrated a decrease in incidence of ICH, two subsequent studies did not demonstrate any benefit.[57,58] One of these two studies evaluated combined antenatal use of vitamin K and phenobarbital, and demonstrated no protective effect of these two agents.[58]

Antenatal steroids

In 1990, Crowley et al., while performing a metaanalysis of controlled trials evaluating the effect of corticosteroids before preterm delivery, noted that antenatal corticosteroid administration reduced the risk of neonatal ICH in preterm infants.[27] Secondary analyses of recent trials evaluating the impact of antenatal corticosteroids on neonatal respiratory distress syndrome have also revealed a reduction in incidence of ICH.[28,59] Investigators have noted that a complete course of steroids was protective against early GMH, and a report demonstrates that antenatal steroids and cesarean delivery have independent roles in lowering risk of early-onset IVH.[31] The NICHD Multicenter Neonatal Research Network found that antenatal corticosteroid administration was associated with a reduced incidence of grades III and IV ICH in neonates with a birth weight of 500–1500 g after adjusting for potential prenatal and perinatal characteristics and for date of birth in a prospective registry of 4665 infants.[60]

The precise mechanism of action of antenatal corticosteroids in reducing neonatal ICH is unclear.[61] Because glucocorticoids promote the maturation of all organ systems, stabilization of arterial blood pressure and acceleration of the maturation of neuronal cells and germinal matrix vessels may contribute to their protective effect as well as increased lung maturation and decreased severity of respiratory distress syndrome.

The safety of antenatal corticosteroid use has been well documented in long-term studies.[62,63] Because impairment of neurodevelopmental outcome is associated with severe IVH and IPH, antenatal steroid therapy that is protective against severe ICH should be widely used. A partial course of antenatal steroids has been shown to offer consistent protection against severe ICH,[60] hence, a single course of antenatal steroids should be initiated to all women at 24–34 weeks' gestation, before delivery, even if the duration of treatment is less than 24 h. The safety of repeated courses of antenatal steroids has not been established.

REFERENCES

1 Volpe JJ (ed.). (2001). Intracranial hemorrhage: subdural, primary subarachnoid, intracerebellar, intraventricular (term infant), and miscellaneous. In *Neurology of the Newborn*, ed. JJ Volpe, pp. 397–427. Saunders: Philadelphia.

2 Hanigan WC, Morgan AM, Stahlberg LK et al. (1990). Tentorial hemorrhage associated with vacuum extraction. *Pediatrics*, 85, 534–9.

3 Roland EH, Flodmark O and Hill A. (1990). Thalamic hemorrhagic with intraventricular hemorrhage in the full term newborn. *Pediatrics*, 85, 737–42.
4 Jocelyn LJ and Casiro OG. (1992). Neurodevelopmental outcome of term infants with intraventricular hemorrhage. *Am J Dis Child*, 146, 194–7.
5 Burrows RF and Kelton JG. (1993). Fetal thrombocytopenia and its relation to maternal thrombocytopenia. *N Engl J Med*, 329, 1463–9.
6 Burrows RF and Kelton JG. (1990). Alloimmune neonatal thrombocytopenia associated with incidental maternal thrombocytopenia. *Am J Hematol*, 35, 43–4.
7 Registry of the Extracorporeal Life Support Organization (ELSO). (1996). *Neonatal ECMO Registry*. Ann Arbor, Michigan: ELSO.
8 Short BL, Walker LK, Bender KS et al. (1993). Impairment of cerebral autoregulation during extracorporeal membrane oxygenation in newborn lambs. *Pediatr Res*, 33, 289–94.
9 Campbell LR, Banyapen C, Holmes GL et al. (1998). Right common carotid artery ligation in extracorporeal membrane oxygenation. *J Pediatr*, 113, 110–13.
10 Mendoza JC, Shearer LL and Cook LN. (1991). Lateralization of brain lesions following extracorporeal membrane oxygenation. *Pediatrics*, 88, 1004–9.
11 Kumar P, Bedard MP, Shankaran S et al. (1994). Post extracorporeal membrane oxygenation single photon emission computed tomography (SPECT) as a predictor of neurodevelopmental outcome. *Pediatrics*, 93, 951–5.
12 Perlman JM and Altman DI. (1992). Symmetric cerebral blood flow in newborns who have undergone successful extracorporeal membrane oxygenation. *Pediatrics*, 89, 235–9.
13 Schumacher RE. (1993). Extracorporeal membrane oxygenation. Will this therapy continue to be as efficacious in the future? *Pediatr Clin North Am*, 40, 1005–17.
14 Kanto WP. (1994). A decade of experience with neonatal extracorporeal membrane oxygenation. *J Pediatr*, 124, 335–47.
15 Wilson JM, Bower LK, Fackler JC et al. (1993). Aminocaproic acid decreases the incidence of intracranial hemorrhage and other hemorrhagic complications of ECMO. *J Pediatr Surg*, 28, 536–41.
16 Perlman JM, Rollins N, Burns D et al. (1993). Relationship between periventricular intraparenchymal echodensities and germinal matrix-intraventricular hemorrhage in the very low birth weight neonate. *Pediatrics*, 91, 474–80.
17 Lemons JA, Bauer CR, Oh W et al. (2001). Very-low-birth-weight (VLBW) outcomes of the NICHD Neonatal Research Network, January 1995 through December 1996. *Pediatrics*, 107, e1.
18 Gaffney G, Squier MV, Johnson A et al. (1994). Clinical associations of prenatal ischemic white matter injury. *Arch Dis Child*, 70, F101–6.
19 Gomez R, Romero R, Ghezzi F et al. (1998). The fetal inflammatory response syndrome. *Am J Obstet Gynecol*, 179, 194–202.
20 Bada HS, Korones SB, Perry EH et al. (1990). Mean arterial blood pressure changes in premature infants and those at risk for intraventricular hemorrhage. *J Pediatr*, 117, 607–14.
21 Shankaran S, Bauer C, Bain R et al. (1996). Prenatal and perinatal risk factors for grade III–IV intracranial hemorrhage in singleton 4795 <1500 g infants. *Arch Pediatr Adolesc Med*, 150, 491–7.
22 Paneth N, Pinto-Martin J, Gardiner J et al. (1993). Incidence and timing of germinal matrix/intraventricular hemorrhage in low birth weight infants. *Am J Epidemiol*, 137, 1167–76.
23 Leviton A, Pagano M, Kuban KCK et al. (1991). The epidemiology of germinal matrix hemorrhage during the first half-day of life. *Dev Med Child Neurol*, 33, 138–45.
24 Kuban KCK, Leviton A, Pagano M et al. (1992). Maternal toxemia is associated with reduced incidence of germinal matrix hemorrhage in premature infants. *J Child Neurol*, 7, 70–6.
25 Philip AGS and Allan WC. (1991). Does cesarean section protect against intraventricular hemorrhage in preterm infants? *J Perinatol*, 11, 3–9.
26 Shaver DC, Bada HS, Korones SB et al. (1992). Early and late intraventricular hemorrhage: the role of obstetric factors. *Obstet Gynecol*, 80, 831–7.
27 Crowley P, Chalmers I and Keirse MJNC. (1990). The effects of corticosteroid administration before preterm delivery: an overview of the evidence from controlled trials. *Br J Obstet Gynaecol*, 97, 11–25.
28 Garite TJ, Rumney PJ, Briggs GG et al. (1992). A randomized, placebo-controlled trial of betamethasone for the prevention of respiratory distress syndrome at 24 to 28 weeks' gestation. *Am J Obstet Gynecol*, 166, 646–51.
29 Leviton A, Kuban KC, Pagano M et al. (1993). Antenatal corticosteroids appear to reduce risk of postnatal germinal matrix hemorrhage in intubated low birth weight newborns. *Pediatrics*, 91, 1083–8.
30 Maher JE, Cliver SP, Goldenberg RL et al. (1994). The effects of corticosteroid therapy in the very premature infant. *Am J Obstet Gynecol*, 170, 869–73.
31 Ment LR, Oh W, Ehrenkranz RA et al. (1995). Antenatal steroids, delivery mode, and intraventricular hemorrhage in preterm infants. *Am J Obstet Gynecol*, 172, 795–800.
32 Batton DG, Holtrop P, DeWitte D et al. (1994). Current gesta-

tional age-related incidence of major intraventricular hemorrhage. *J Pediatr*, 125, 623–5.
33 Ment LR, Oh W, Philip AGS et al. (1992). Risk factors for early intraventricular hemorrhage in low birth weight infants. *J Pediatr*, 121, 776–83.
34 Wallin LA, Rosenfeld CR, Laptook AR et al. (1990). Neonatal intracranial hemorrhage: II. Risk factor analysis in an inborn population. *Early Hum Dev*, 23, 129–37.
35 Jongmans M, Henderson S, deVries L et al. (1993). Duration of periventricular densities in preterm infants and neurological outcome at 6 years of age. *Arch Dis Child*, 69, 9–13.
36 Papile L, Burstein J, Berstein R et al. (1978). Incidence and evolution of subependymal and intraventricular hemorrhage: a study of infants with birth weight less than 1500 g. *J Pediatr*, 92, 529–34.
37 Shankaran S, Slovis TL, Bedard MP et al. (1982). Sonographic classification of intracranial hemorrhage: a prognostic indicator of mortality, morbidity and short-term neurologic outcome. *J Pediatr*, 100, 469–75.
38 Brann BS, Qualls C, Wells L et al. (1991). Asymmetric growth of the lateral cerebral ventricle in infants with posthemorrhagic ventricular dilation. *J Pediatr*, 118, 108–12.
39 Aziz K, Vickar DB, Sauve RS et al. (1995). Province-based study of neurologic disability of children weighing 500 through 1249 grams at birth in relation to neonatal cerebral ultrasound findings. *Pediatrics*, 95, 837–44.
40 Pinto-Martin JA, Riolo S, Cnaan A et al. (1995). Cranial ultrasound prediction of disabling and nondisabling cerebral palsy at age two in a low birth weight population. *Pediatrics*, 95, 249–54.
41 Shankaran S. (2000). Complications of neonatal intracranial hemorrhage. *NeoReviews*, 21, e44–7.
42 Strand C, Laptook AR, Dowling S et al. (1990). Neonatal intracranial hemorrhage: I. Changing pattern in inborn low-birth-weight infants. *Early Hum Dev*, 23, 117–28.
43 Groome LJ, Goldenberg RL, Cliver SP et al. (1992). Neonatal periventricular-intraventricular hemorrhage after maternal β-sympathomimetic tocolysis. *Am J Obstet Gynecol*, 167, 873–9.
44 Norton ME, Merrill J, Cooper BAB et al. (1993). Neonatal complications after the administration of indomethacin for preterm labor. *N Engl J Med*, 329, 1602–7.
45 Whitelaw A. (2000). Postnatal phenobarbitone for the prevention of intraventricular hemorrhage in preterm infants. *Cochrane Database Syst Rev*, 2, CDOO1691.
46 Hensy OJ, Morgan MEI and Cooke RWI. (1984). Tranexamic acid in the prevention of periventricular haemorrhage. *Arch Dis Child*, 59, 719–21.
47 Perlman JM, Coodman S, Kreusser KL et al. (1985). Reduction in intraventricular hemorrhage by elimination of fluctuating cerebral blood-flow velocity in preterm infants with respiratory distress syndrome. *N Engl J Med*, 312, 1353–7.
48 Morgan MEI, Benson JWT and Cooke RWI. (1981). Ethamsylate reduces the incidence of periventricular haemorrhage in very low birth-weight babies. *Lancet*, 2, 830–1.
49 Cooke RWI and Morgan MEI. (1984). Prophylactic ethamsylate for periventricular haemorrhage. *Arch Dis Child*, 59, 82–3.
50 Benson JW, Drayton MR, Hayward C et al. (1986). Multicenter trial of ethamsylate for prevention of periventricular haemorrhage in very low birthweight infants. *Lancet*, 2, 1297–300.
51 Bada HS. (2000). Prevention of intracranial hemorrhage. *NeoReviews*, 1, e48–52.
52 Schmidt B, David P, Moddemann D et al. (2001). Long-term effects of indomethacin prophylaxis in extremely-low-birth-weight infants. *N Engl J Med*, 344, 1966–72.
53 Crowther CA and Henderson-Smart DJ. (2001). Phenobarbital prior to preterm birth for preventing neonatal periventricular haemorrhage. *Cochrane Database Syst Rev*, 2, CDOO0164.
54 Shankaran S, Papile L, Wright LL et al. (1997). The effect of antenatal phenobarbital therapy on neonatal intracranial hemorrhage in preterm infants. *N Engl J Med*, 337, 466–71.
55 Morales WJ, Angel JL, O'Brien WF et al. (1988). The use of antenatal vitamin K in the prevention of early neonatal intraventricular hemorrhage. *Am J Obstet Gynecol*, 159, 774–9.
56 Pomerance JJ, Teal JG, Gogolok JF et al. (1987). Maternally administered antenatal vitamin K_1: effect on neonatal prothrombin activity, partial thromboplastic time, and intraventricular hemorrhage. *Obstet Gynecol*, 70, 235–41.
57 Kazzi NJ, Ilagan NB, Liang KC et al. (1989). Maternal administration of vitamin K does not improve the coagulation profile of preterm infants. *Pediatrics*, 84, 1045–50.
58 Thorp JA, Parriott J, Ferrette-Smith D et al. (1994). Antepartum vitamin K and phenobarbital for preventing intraventricular hemorrhage in the premature newborn: a randomized, double-blind, placebo-controlled trial. *Obstet Gynecol*, 83, 70–6.
59 Kari MA, Hallman M, Eronen M et al. (1994). Prenatal dexamethasone treatment in conjunction with rescue therapy of human surfactant: a randomized placebo-controlled multicenter study. *Pediatrics*, 93, 730–6.
60 Shankaran S, Bauer CR, Bain R et al. (1995). The relationship between antenatal steroid administration and grade III–IV intracranial hemorrhage in low birth weight infants. *Am J Obstet Gynecol*, 173, 305–12.

61 Patrias K, Wright LL and Merenstein GB. (1994). Effect of corticosteroids for fetal maturation on perinatal outcomes. In NIH Consensus Statement, pp. 1–24. Bethesda, MD: National Library of Medicine.

62 Schmand B, Neuvel J, Smolder-de Haas H et al. (1990). Psychological development of children who were treated antenatally with corticosteroids to prevent respiratory distress syndrome. *Pediatrics*, 86, 58–64.

63 Smolder-de Haas H, Neuvel J, Schmand B et al. (1990). Physical development and medical history of children who were treated antenatally with corticosteroids to prevent respiratory distress syndrome: a 10-to-12 year follow-up. *Pediatrics*, 86, 65–70.

PART II

Pregnancy, Labor, and Delivery Complications Causing Brain Injury

9

Maternal diseases that affect fetal development

Kimberlee A. Sorem[1] and Maurice L. Druzin[2]

[1] University of California San Francisco, CA, USA
[2] Stanford University Medical Center, Stanford, CA, USA

Introduction

Fetal development is affected by intrinsic (genetic) and environmental (intrauterine) factors. Studies at the molecular level as well as at the epidemiologic level are helpful in determining possible etiologies of diseases that affect not only the developing fetus but also the growing and adult human organism. Complex diseases once thought to be mainly "adult" in onset, such as hypertension and cardiac disease, have recently been linked to low birth weight,[1] suggesting an intriguing "adaptation" of the fetus to a hostile or suboptimal metabolic environment. Genetic diseases, present from conception, may not be apparent at birth, childhood, or even middle age. Although this chapter will focus on specific maternal diseases that are known to affect fetal growth and development, a vast array of genetic programming and metabolic factors are known to influence normal and abnormal fetal development.

Certain maternal systemic diseases affect multiple organ systems in the fetus. The most common endocrine disease in the female reproductive age group is diabetes mellitus: type 1, type 2, and gestational diabetes. From glucose-induced embryo toxicity to cardiac hypertrophy of the newborn, the hyperglycemia (and other metabolic derangements) of uncontrolled diabetes causes wide-ranging birth defects and multiple metabolic abnormalities in the newborn. Likewise, thyroid disease and other maternal endocrine disorders may have an untoward effect on the fetus. Neurological diseases of the mother may have an adverse effect on the development of the fetal nervous system. Not only are genetic influences or genetically determined sensitivities present within the developing cells, but also potential toxicities from psychotropic or antiepileptic drugs may have direct teratogenic effects or even suspected "behavioral" teratogenicity.

An inherited metabolic disorder in the mother, such as phenylketonuria (PKU), can have a profound effect on fetal neurological development, even if the mother's disease was controlled in childhood by appropriate dietary restrictions. Elevated phenylalanine levels in PKU associated with dietary indiscretion during pregnancy can cause permanent developmental delays in the otherwise normal fetus. Other genetic metabolic disorders need to be carefully managed in pregnancy to avoid fetal damage. Some maternal hematologic disorders can affect the fetus either directly or indirectly, as a result of either platelet or red blood cell dysfunction. Finally, genetic diseases either fully or partially expressed by the mother may affect the fetus. This group contains diseases which are autosomal dominant, autosomal recessive, and X-linked. Respiratory, cardiac, and hypertensive disorders as well as hypertension specific to pregnancy (preeclampsia) all affect the fetus by playing a role in uteroplacental perfusion, a topic that will be covered in Chapter 12. Infectious diseases may have differential effects on the mother and fetus, and specific perinatal infections will be highlighted in Chapter 14.

Early malnutrition of the mother may have an effect on the developing fetus, although the confounding variables (poverty, socioeconomic class, drug use, chronic maternal disease, access to prenatal care) are difficult to analyze systematically. One review by Rizzo et al.[2] confirms a general hypothesis that poor maternal nutrition correlates with poorer child performance on standardized tests. Although the most obvious correlations between maternal nutrition and neonatal neurological outcome relate to demonstrable perturbations in the maternal plasma glucose, β-hydroxybutyrate (β-OHB) and free fatty acids (FFA) in maternal diabetes, the potential for other "fuel-mediated teratogenesis" related to other nutritional disorders (e.g., malnutrition) remains unknown.

In one categorization of causes of mental deficiency,[3] category I, which includes approximately 44% of cases, is defined as "prenatal onset of problem in morphogenesis." This group includes single brain defects, as well as multiple inborn brain defects, whether chromosomal, syndromic or unknown. Category II (~3%) includes perinatal insults to the brain, such as infectious, traumatic, hypoxic, or metabolic. Category III (~12%) includes postnatal problems, environmental, and metabolic, whereas a final category (IV) includes those with an unknown time of onset, cases that are perplexing to pediatrician, geneticist, and parents alike. Evaluating a newborn or child for possible causes of neurological defects involves complex methods that are beyond the scope of this chapter.

Maternal endocrine diseases

Diabetes mellitus

The most devastating effect of uncontrolled diabetes and hyperglycemia in the preconception and embryonic period is direct embryo toxicity. Women with type 1 diabetes are at highest risk for this complication, although fetal defects are observed in the more common type of diabetes in reproductive-age women – type 2 diabetes – as well.[4] Gestational diabetes, which has an onset in the third trimester, is not associated with an increase in fetal malformations, unless the mother is an unrecognized type 2 diabetic with poor glucose control prior to conception.

Several studies have documented a two- to sixfold increase in congenital malformations in the infants of insulin-dependent diabetic mothers.[5] The most common birth defects are in the central nervous system (CNS), cardiac, renal, and skeletal systems.[6,7] Diabetic hyperglycemia causes aberrant glucose, amino acid, and fatty acid homeostasis, which leads to "fuel-mediated teratogenesis" in the human as well as in animal models.[8] Although excess glucose is thought to be the primary teratogenic factor, circulating ketones, growth factors, and hypoglycemia have all been suggested.[9] Several proposed pathways for disordered morphogenesis include deficiencies of arachadonic acid,[10,11] altered oxidative metabolism, and excess free oxygen radicals.[12] An increased risk of birth defects is associated with the degree of early-gestation hyperglycemia in both the rat model and in human clinical studies. It appears that fetal anomalies increase with increasing hyperglycemia, and that a glycemic threshold (elevated glycohemoglobin concentration greater than 12%,[13] or a mean daily glucose concentration of 120–130 mmol/dl[14]) correlates with a clinically significant increase in fetal abnormalities. Early embryonic losses (first-trimester miscarriages) are also increased among diabetic women with poor glucose control, presumably due to direct toxicity or lethal malformations.[15]

Beyond the early embryonic period, the developing fetus remains susceptible to adverse effects of hyperglycemia, hypoglycemia, and diabetic ketoacidosis in type 1 diabetics. In diabetic ketoacidosis, hypovolemia and hypotension may result in direct reduction of uteroplacental blood flow, as well as in increased circulating fetal ketones. Although the fetus has a remarkable ability to adapt to changes in the intrauterine metabolic environment, these changes alter the physical and neurodevelopment of the fetus and, if severe, may even result in fetal asphyxia. Chronic and acute hyperglycemia in the fetus lead to hyperinsulinemia, which is linked to fetal hypoxia. Fetal hyperinsulinemia increases the metabolic rate and oxygen demands, which leads to decreased arterial oxygen content and acidemia. Among insulin-dependent diabetics, stillbirths are most common in the last month of pregnancy because of a number of factors. The combination of decreased placental blood flow, acidemia, and hypoxia (along with other potential complications such as polyhydramnios, hydropic swelling of placental villi, and preeclampsia) may lead to intrauterine demise.

Abnormal glucose regulation in pregnancy (hyperglycemia) leading to an increase in fetal birth weight via disturbed metabolic adaptations is known as the Pederson hypothesis.[16] According to Pederson, fetal hyperglycemia stimulates the fetal pancreas to secrete excess insulin, leading to an increase in fetal adipose tissue, as well as fetal organomegaly. Fetal macrosomia, as defined as birth weight greater that 90%, is present in 25–42% of diabetic pregnancies compared with approximately 10% of nondiabetic pregnancies.[17] Macrosomia is associated with an increase in birth trauma and asphyxia in infants of diabetic mothers as well as prolonged labors and increased cesarean section rates. The association of poor maternal glucose control and macrosomia occurs among type 1 and type 2 diabetics, as well as in gestational diabetics. Although the mechanisms of successful adaptation of the fetus to an abnormal metabolic environment are incompletely understood, this "adaptation" poses health risks to the individual during intrauterine development, contributes to intrapartum stress, increases the risks of neonatal metabolic aberrations,[18] and influences lifelong risks for obesity and diabetes.[19]

In addition to macrosomia at birth, neonatal complications in the infant from a mother with diabetes include metabolic derangements, delayed fetal lung maturity, polycythemia, and hypertrophic cardiomyopathy. Immediately after birth, neonatal glucose levels fall, and a level below 35–40 mmol/dl during the first 12 hours of life is considered to be abnormal. The fetal pancreas in the pregnancy with uncontrolled diabetes secretes excessive insulin, leading to an exaggerated glucose response after delivery. Without supplementary glucose, the infant may display abnormal neurological responses, including hypoglycemic seizures. These infants have been found to have elevated umbilical cord C-peptide, high free insulin levels, and an exaggerated pancreatic response to glucose loading.[20] The incidence and severity of neonatal hypoglycemia often correspond with both antepartum and intrapartum maternal glucose levels.

Delayed fetal lung maturity is a complication of the diabetic pregnancy that is poorly understood. Both hyperglycemia and hyperinsulinemia may play a role in pulmonary surfactant secretion,[21] by interfering with either substrate availability or glucocorticoid-induced pulmonary maturation.[22] Current obstetrical management of planned vaginal delivery at term, combined with optimal glycemic control and a fetus that is appropriate for gestational age, minimizes the incidence of this complication. However, an increased incidence of respiratory distress is still observed in fetuses delivered by cesarean section prior to the onset of labor. Other metabolic complications, such as hypocalcemia and hypomagnesemia, occur more frequently in the neonates of diabetic pregnancies. Polycythemia, presumably as a result of intrauterine hypoxia, may be present with or without hyperbilirubinemia, although prematurity and intrapartum factors may modify these risks.

The neurological effects of maternal diabetes on the fetus remain incompletely understood. Although some of the fetal metabolic responses to hyperglycemia are regulated by genetic influences, a prolonged abnormal metabolic environment appears to affect adversely the neurodevelopment of the fetal brain. In 1991, Rizzo et al. reported a correlation between antepartum maternal metabolism and intelligence in the offspring of diabetic mothers.[23] The 223 children of diabetic mothers had Stanford–Binet scores that correlated inversely with maternal β-OHB and free fatty acid levels in the third trimester. Although the mean group IQ differences in children of diabetic mothers compared with non-diabetic mothers was not significantly different, and the association of lower performance scores with increasing maternal ketonemia was relatively small, this report nevertheless emphasizes the potential adverse consequences of maternal diabetes on the developing fetal brain. Further psychomotor studies of the cohort of children at 6, 8, and 9 years of age (using the Bruininks–Oseretsky test) demonstrated a similar inverse correlation to β-OHB levels.[24] It is unknown to what extent the association between maternal ketonemia and the delayed fetal brain development depends on other metabolic, genetic, and hormonal factors. Early teratogenic effects may also influence CNS sensitivities to metabolic derangements or developmental abnormalities in pregnancies with poorly controlled pregestational diabetes.

Significantly more reproductive-age women have type 2 diabetes compared with type 1 diabetes. Several pregnancy issues in women with type 2 diabetes, therefore, deserve specific attention. Because women with type 2 diabetes are not insulin-dependent and not prone to diabetic ketoacidosis, many may be undiagnosed prior to pregnancy, thus increasing the incidence of congenital malformations related to hyperglycemia. Furthermore, those who are taking hypoglycemic agents may have an increase in fetal malformations, not necessarily as a result of direct teratogenicity, but because oral agents often limit the ability of the patient to achieve excellent glycemic control (as measured by mean blood glucose or glycosylated hemoglobin). The incidence of macrosomia and increased cesarean section rate is at least as high as with type 1 diabetes. Finally, as type 2 diabetes increases with increasing maternal age, certain comorbid conditions such as obesity and hypertension contribute to excess fetal risk among these women. The disturbing association of increased incidence of type 2 diabetes and childhood obesity is strongest in the offspring of women who have type 2 diabetes during pregnancy.

Gestational diabetes is defined as glucose intolerance first identified during pregnancy. This definition leaves room for many previously undiagnosed type 2 diabetics, but glucose intolerance that did not exist before the pregnancy and does not exist after the pregnancy is not associated with an increase in congenital malformations. Women with gestational diabetes are likely to have glycosylated hemoglobin in the normal range. Therefore, fetal consequences of gestational diabetes are primarily macrosomia (rates in the same range as type 2 diabetics), birth trauma, and neonatal metabolic complications. Close monitoring of antepartum maternal glucose levels in patients with gestational diabetes as well as pregestational diabetes minimizes the risk of hypoxia and intrauterine fetal demise.

Current obstetrical management of patients with diabetes includes dietary and medical therapy (insulin) as necessary to achieve glucose levels comparable to the nondiabetic gravida. In addition, fetal ultrasound, antepartum testing, intrapartum glucoregulation and appropriate timing and mode of delivery have contributed to perinatal morbidity and mortality rates that approach that of the normal population.

Thyroid disease

Normal function of both the maternal and fetal thyroid glands is critical for normal neurodevelopment of the fetus. Thyroid disease is not uncommon, and both hypothyroidism and hyperthyroidism occur in reproductive-age women. Although severe hypothyroidism may interfere with fertility, mild-to-moderate hypothyroidism may be relatively asymptomatic, yet still require treatment. Among women with untreated hypothyroidism in pregnancy, both the severity and timing of maternal thyroid hormone deficiency influence the degree of impaired neurological function in the newborn. Finally, hypothyroxemia sufficient to affect fetal neural development occurs when low levels of maternal iodine intake induce hypothyroidism and goiter. This condition is rare in the USA and Japan but may be found worldwide where iodine is deficient in the maternal diet. The goiter that results from maternal iodine deficiency is due to glandular hypertrophy in response to increased thyroid-stimulating hormone (TSH) when circulating thyroxine is low.

Most cases of hypothyroidism are autoimmune or idiopathic in origin. The incidence is increased in women with insulin-dependent diabetes and among patients with infertility. It is unclear whether or not the fetus requires (maternal) thyroid hormone in the first trimester, but thyroid deficiency in the second and third trimesters of pregnancy may result in developmental delays and other neurological deficits. Although the fetal thyroid gland is functioning during the mid- and late trimester of pregnancy, the mother largely supplies circulating thyroid hormone in the fetus. This has been shown in cases of congenital neonatal hypothyroidism (cretinism) in which the fetal cord thyroxine levels are up to 50% of normal[25] in the presence of a nonfunctional fetal thyroid gland. If untreated after birth, congenital neonatal hypothyroidism leads to profound and permanent neurological impairment.

Several studies have also shown that isolated maternal hypothyroidism is associated with a milder degree of mental impairment in offspring.[26,27] Haddow et al. reported that a group of children whose mothers had elevated TSH levels during pregnancy had lower performances on the Wechsler Intelligence Scale for children compared with matched controls. Although the average IQ difference was 4% lower overall in the children of hypothyroid mothers, the discrepancy increased to seven points if the mothers received no treatment during pregnancy. Furthermore, 15% overall and 19% in the untreated group had IQ scores less than 85.[28] The pathophysiology of fetal neurologic impairment with maternal hypothyroidism is uncertain, but studies have suggested that placental passage of maternal thyroid hormone may be important in the first trimester of pregnancy,[26] as well as later in fetal life, when neuronal migration and organization associated with complex brain function occur (intelligence, attention, language, and visual motor performance).[29] Regardless of whether or not the maternal thyroid hormone deficiency results from inadequate iodine in the diet or autoimmune hypothyroidism, it appears that treatment (iodine supplementation or thyroid hormone replacement, respectively) will have a significant positive impact on fetal brain development. From a global perspective, iodine supplementation will have the greatest impact; however, the issue of whether all pregnant women should be screened for hypothyroidism remains controversial.

In addition to neonatal and antepartum effects of hypothyroidism, intrapartum events may also be influenced by maternal hypothyroidism. In one case-control study by Badawi et al., maternal hypothyroidism appeared to be a risk factor for newborn encephalopathy. Based on this finding, the authors hypothesize that developmental pathways established during gestation may enhance the sensitivity of the fetal brain to hypoxia.[30]

Unlike hypothyroidism, hyperthyroidism is less likely to be associated with infertility but may also require treatment during pregnancy. Mild maternal hyperthyroidism is generally well tolerated, but severe disease has adverse consequences for both the mother and infant. If untreated prior to pregnancy, hyperthyroidism is associated with an increased incidence of minor congenital anomalies in the neonate.[31]

The most common form of hyperthyroidism is Graves disease, an autoimmune disorder that is mediated by antibodies that bind to the TSH receptor. These antibodies, which are generally stimulating but may also be blocking, cross the placenta and bind to fetal thyroid receptors. The fetal thyroid becomes sensitive to maternal-stimulating antibodies at 20–24 weeks' gestation, and fetal thyrotoxicosis is a rare but serious disorder. Tachycardia and growth restriction in the fetus, as well as advanced bone age and craniosynostosis in the infant, are associated with fetal thyroid response to excessive maternal thyroid-stimulating antibodies. Two cases of fetal death reported by Page et al. described pathologic findings at necropsy, including pulmonary hypertension, organomegaly, generalized adenopathy, and enlarged thyroid.[32] Treatment for maternal hyperthyroidism includes thionamide therapy (propylthiouracil or PTU), which crosses the placenta and enters the fetal circulation, minimizing the fetal thyroid response in some cases.

Neonatal thyrotoxicosis is a relatively rare disease, occurring in approximately 1% of newborns from women with Graves disease or Hashimoto's thyroiditis. Although the level of maternal disease does not correlate well with neonatal thyrotoxicosis, very high levels of maternal TSH (greater than five times normal) are associated with a high-risk newborn. Other newborns at increased risk include those whose mothers have had a thyroidectomy prior to pregnancy and are euthyroid. TSH may be extremely high and cross the placenta without the benefit of PTU for the fetus. Complications of neonatal thyrotoxicosis include poor weight gain, hyperkinesis, ophthalmopathy, cardiac failure, pulmonary and systemic hypertension, and hyperviscosity.

Adrenal disorders

Adrenal disease may coincide with pregnancy and includes Cushing's disease, Addison's disease and congenital adrenal hyperplasia (CAH). Complications associated with Cushing's disease, which is a state of excess cortisol secretion, include increased incidence of fetal loss before 20 weeks, increased prematurity, and increased intrauterine growth restriction. Neonatal adrenal insufficiency has also been reported due to suppression of the fetal hypothalamic–pituitary–adrenal axis. Primary adrenocortical insufficiency (Addison's disease), which may be autoimmune, traumatic, infectious or infiltrative, is a disease that is primarily a risk for the mother. Although maternal adrenal antibodies do cross the placenta, fetal and neonatal adrenal function appear to be minimally affected. Neither Cushing's disease nor Addison's disease is associated with an increase in congenital malformations, and treatment of maternal disease is always indicated.

Congenital adrenal hyperplasia

CAH is caused by an inherited deficiency of one of several enzymes in the steroidogenic pathway. The enzymes involved may include 21-hydroxylase, 11-hydroxylase, and 3-β-hydroxysteroid dehydrogenase, although 95% of cases involve 21-hydroxylase with an incidence of 1/14 000 newborns.[33] In cases of CAH, the fetus receives from each parent one recessive allele, which may be a large gene conversion, large gene deletion, small gene deletions or de novo point mutations. The allelic variability accounts for variability in the severity of the disease,[34] with the most severe forms resulting in salt wasting from significant mineralocorticoid deficits. Lacking sufficient enzymes in the cortisol pathway, the fetus with CAH produces excess C-19 precursors and hypersecretes androgens, including testosterone. The female fetus may be virilized in utero, including persistent urogenital sinus, labial fusion, and clitoromegaly, but the exposed male fetus will be unaffected. Several studies have also examined the effect of excess androgens on brain development and subsequent psychosexual development.[35–37]

Genital ambiguity in the female fetus may be prevented or reduced by maternal treatment with dexamethasone, which crosses the placenta and suppresses androgen production.[38–40] Although it has been recommended that the treatment begin before 7 weeks,[41] in one case report a normal female newborn with classical 21-hydroxylase deficiency was not treated until 16 weeks.[42] Prenatal diagnosis is available for families in which both parents are known carriers, but as is often the case with autosomal recessive disorders, this may occur only after the birth of an affected female infant.

Since effective fetal treatment with dexamethasone for the at-risk pregnancy would have to begin at 6–7 weeks, patients may choose to have a chorionic villus sampling at 11–14 weeks or amniocentesis at 16–20 weeks for DNA analysis on the fetus. Since only one of four pregnancies at risk for this recessive disorder will be affected and only female fetuses will receive potential benefit from dexamethasone, seven out of eight pregnancies would be treated during embryogenesis for at least 5–6 weeks to improve the outcome for one female fetus. In the case of the affected female fetus the treatment would then continue through gestation, whereas in unaffected females and males the treatment would cease. Miller has raised the question of treating the fetus via the mother for a potential benefit with unproven risks.[43] The pharmacology of dexamethasone in the first-trimester fetus and its potential teratogenicity have not been well studied; moreover, the dose that is generally used (20 μg/kg of maternal body weight) is supraphysiological, well above that needed to suppress the adult adrenal gland. Potential maternal complications include hypertension, excessive weight gain, and hyperglycemia.[44] Potential fetal effects of high doses of corticosteriods in utero based on laboratory animals include intrauterine growth restriction, renal and brain abnormalities, sodium retention, and hypertension.[45] In humans, growth restriction, psychomotor delays, and emotional disturbances have been reported, [46] but no major teratogenic malformations have consistently appeared.

Pregnancy in women who are themselves affected with CAH has been reported.[47] Clinically, CAH diagnosed in early infancy is characterized by female pseudohermaphroditism, in addition to salt wasting, dehydration, and electrolyte abnormalities. Measurement of elevated levels of urinary pregnanetriol and 17-keto-steroids in genetic females with genital virilization establishes the diagnosis of CAH. Subsequently, these females require treatment with oral steroids and one or more surgical procedures in order to menstruate and achieve pregnancy. High levels of circulating maternal androgens in women with CAH are potentially teratogenic (i.e., virilizing) to the female fetus. Because placental aromatase effectively converts androgens to estrogens, women with hyperandrogenism not due to a tumor secretion and who are treated in pregnancy are unlikely to deliver virilized females. Nevertheless, serum androgen levels should be monitored throughout pregnancy. In a reported series of four pregnant women with CAH, all of whom had normal female infants, Lo et al. describe guidelines for management of these patients during pregnancy.[47] These guidelines include glucocorticoid therapy, frequent monitoring of circulating androgens (17-hydroxy progesterone, testosterone, and androstenedione), genetic counseling, ultrasound, stress-dose steroids in delivery, and evaluation of the neonate. Furthermore, if genital reconstructive surgery has been extensive, elective cesarean section should be considered.

Neurologic and psychiatric disorders

Women of reproductive age are subject to neurologic and psychiatric disorders and generally need to continue some form of treatment during pregnancy and lactation. Seizure disorders are complex and require continuous treatment with antiepileptic drugs (AED). In addition to the potential teratology of AEDs, genetic influences and other comorbid disorders need to be considered. Migraine headaches are frequent in reproductive-age women, and strategies for pain control during pregnancy may need to be tailored to the hormonal changes during pregnancy and the postpartum period. Psychiatric disorders, including depression, bipolar disease, and schizophrenia, may complicate pregnancy and require comanagement by the patient's psychiatrist and obstetrician, as well as social services involvement. Finally, pregnancy in women with mental retardation or developmental delays, with or without a partner also affected by mental retardation, is not rare. Depending on whether or not other medical conditions exist, a number of specialists, including a neurologist, social worker, genetics specialist, and community/family involvement, may need to work in concert.

Seizure disorder

Approximately 0.5% of pregnant women have a seizure disorder. Although it is difficult to predict the effect of pregnancy on seizure frequency, overall approximately 45% of women with epilepsy experience an increase in seizures. The seizures that occur in pregnancy do not differ clinically from the seizures that the patient experienced before pregnancy, and seizures that appear for the first time during pregnancy tend to be focal. Blood levels of AED tend to fall in pregnancy, and both free and total drug levels need to be monitored in pregnancy to maximize the effect.[48]

Annegers et al. showed that children of epileptic mothers have a higher incidence of seizure disorders than the offspring of epileptic fathers.[49] Patients with a seizure disorder are generally counseled that the incidence of seizure disorder in the infant is approximately 2–3% when the mother is affected. The teratogenic effect of maternal epilepsy is a significant additional concern that has been attributed to AEDs, as well as to the presence of seizures during pregnancy and the multiple factors, including genetic, which caused the mother to have epilepsy in the first place. A number of reports have suggested that AEDs are teratogenic, and none of the drugs currently used to treat seizure disorder is without potential risk.[50]

Dilantin has been associated with fetal hydantoin syndrome in approximately 10% of exposed infants.[51] This disorder consists of fetal growth restriction, microcephaly, dysmorphic facies, and developmental delay. It is difficult to predict which infants will show any of these effects. There have been similar effects noted in infants exposed to carbamazepine, as well as valproate, and the phenotype resembles many features of fetal alcohol syndrome (FAS). In a recent study of congenital malformations and AEDs, most major AEDs were associated with an increase in congenital malformations. Specifically, valproate was associated with CNS malformations and limb deficiencies, in a dose-dependent relationship,[52] carbamazepine monotherapy, benzodiazepines in combination therapy, and caffeine plus phenobarbital all appeared to be associated with increased risks.[53] Dansky et al. reported that low folate blood levels before conception are associated with the occurrence of pregnancy loss and anomalies.[54] Although the US Public Health Service (USPHS) recommends ingestion of folic acid in the preconception period and in early pregnancy for the prevention of neural tube defects, the dose of phenytoin may have to be monitored for a decrease in plasma level with folate treatment. Furthermore, since a case of neural tube defect has been reported in a patient on valproate and folic acid during the preconception period and throughout early pregnancy, folic acid cannot be relied upon to eliminate entirely the risk of CNS defects.[55]

Neonatal coagulopathy may occur in infants of mothers who have been on AEDs. In affected cases, factors II, VII, IX, and X are decreased, whereas factors V and VII as well as fibrinogen are normal. Prevalence rates are 10–30%, and bleeding may even occur in utero.[56] Current recommendations are that the mother receive vitamin K_1 during the last month of pregnancy and that the newborn receive vitamin K as well. Cord blood levels of prothrombin time and partial thromboplastin time should also be measured at the time of delivery, when the mother was receiving treatment with AEDs.

Migraine headache

Among those who suffer with migraine headaches, 80% are women. Although migraine may improve during pregnancy (60–70% improve in the second and third trimesters), some women experience them for the first time during pregnancy. Evaluation of new-onset severe headaches requires a complete neurologic examination, as well as evaluation of teeth, paranasal sinuses, eyes, and urine. If focal signs suggest intracranial disease, imaging such as magnetic resonance imaging (MRI), evaluation by electrocardiogram (EEG), or lumbar puncture may be indicated.

Although migraine headaches that do not improve during pregnancy may require treatment for maternal pain relief, migraine headaches are not associated with adverse perinatal complications. The incidence of preeclampsia, spontaneous pregnancy loss, congenital anomalies, and fetal death are the same as in the general population.[57] Treatment options include acetaminophen and nonsteroidal antiinflammatory agents, as well as chlorpromazine, dimenhydrinate and diphenhydramine. Meperidine and other opioids may be used in severe refractory cases, with concern for neonatal withdrawal if prolonged in the third trimester of pregnancy. Finally, medications such as beta-blockers or tricyclic antidepressants may be safely used for prophylactic therapy in the patient with frequency of migraine greater than three times per week.

Psychiatric disorders in pregnancy

Pregnant women are not protected from major psychiatric disorders, and the treatment of these disorders has consequences for the developing fetus and newborn. Nine percent of pregnant women fulfill the diagnostic criteria for depression, making it the most common major psychiatric disorder.[58] Bipolar disease is less frequent, but may be difficult to control in pregnancy because of limited medication options. Schizophrenia is also difficult to control because of comorbid conditions, a higher percentage of socioeconomic disadvantages, and poor compliance with medications. Other disorders such as anorexia and bulimia may be underrecognized and little studied in pregnancy. Finally, drug abuse, while widespread, is a disorder of long-standing consequences for the mother and offspring and one that requires prolonged and complex treatment. The lack of psychiatric facilities, community resources, and practitioners who treat pregnant women with major psychiatric illness is a significant barrier to adequate control of these diseases.

Effective therapies for depression include psychotherapy, antidepressant medication, and electroconvulsive therapy. Exposure of the fetus to antidepressant medication is a significant concern of the patient and the focus of several review articles. Wisner et al. presented a metaanalysis of the reproductive effects of pharmacologic treatment of depression in women.[59] Reproductive risks examined in this analysis include: (1) fetal deaths; (2) physical malformations; (3) growth impairment; (4) behavioral teratology; and (5) neonatal toxicity. No increase in fetal deaths or major malformations was noted with exposure to tricyclic antidepressant medication or selective serotonin reuptake inhibitors (SSRIs).[59] Using major congenital malformations as an outcome measure, one metaanalysis of 414 infants exposed to tricyclics showed no increase.[60] Several prospective studies of antidepressant exposure including both tricyclics and SSRIs are likewise reassuring;[61,62] however, one report by Chambers et al. showed an increase in minor malformations with fluoxetine. [63] Likewise, most of the studies to date show no increase in intrauterine growth restriction or low birth weight, except the study by Chambers et al., which showed an increased incidence of lower birth weight in association with poor maternal weight gain.[63]

The potential behavioral teratology of many drugs used to treat psychiatric and neurological disorders during pregnancy is an area that is little studied and poorly understood. Examples of behavioral effects include developmental delays, learning disabilities, hyperactivity, and conduct disorders. Studies of behavioral teratology are difficult because of the long time period over which the effects may be seen in human development and because of the variability of genetic, family, and social influences. Nulman et al. found no differences in cognitive function, temperament, and general behavior in children prenatally exposed to tricyclics and SSRIs compared with controls.[64]

Neonatal toxicity of tricyclics and SSRIs has been reported in some, but not all of the above studies. The described neonatal withdrawal syndrome may include irritability, jerky movements, feeding difficulties, profuse sweating, tachycardia, and tachypnea. The relative risk of poor neonatal adaptation reported by Chambers et al. was 8.7 (confidence interval 2.9–26.6).[63] Because of the relatively long half-life of fluoxetine, tapering or stopping this medication near delivery may be considered; however, the risk of profound maternal depression in the postpartum period must be weighed against potential benefit to the newborn.[65]

Treatment of bipolar disease involves mood-stabilizing medications, some of which have fetal and neonatal effects. Carbamazepine and valproic acid, commonly used as AEDs as well as in bipolar disorder, have potential teratogenic effects as listed above. Lithium carbonate has been reported to produce excess cardiac malformations, specifically Ebstein's anomaly; however, the risk to the fetus is likely to be lower than originally reported.[66] Treatment of schizophrenia during pregnancy involves antipsychotic drugs, which are unlikely to cause an increase in fetal malformation rate. Haloperidol, perphenazine, thiothixene, and trifluoperazine do not have known teratogenic effects in animal models or in humans,[67] and studies of these drugs in humans have found no evidence of behavioral teratogenicity, including emotional or cognitive deficits.[68]

Maternal drug and alcohol abuse are common comorbid factors in women with psychiatric disorders or may exist independently as risks to maternal and fetal health. Abel and Sokol reported in 1986 that FAS is the leading (preventable) cause of mental retardation,[69] with an estimated incidence of 1/3000 live births.[70] Maternal alcohol ingestion exposes the fetus to a category X teratogen. According to the US Food and Drug Administration, category X substances are "contraindicated in pregnancy. Studies in animals or humans, or investigational or post-marketing reports have shown that fetal risk clearly outweighs any possible benefit to the patient."[71] Alcohol exposure in humans and in animals during fetal development causes alterations of the CNS. FAS is a constellation of characteristics including prenatal and postnatal growth abnormalities, physical (craniofacial) abnormalities, and CNS abnormalities. These abnormalities include microcephaly, microophthalmia, poorly developed philtrum, mild-to-moderate mental retardation, and hypotonia. Social deficits in children with FAS are more severe than those observed in children with similar cognitive deficits, and social impairment has been noted even among adolescents and adults exposed to alcohol in utero but without the full FAS diagnosis.[72] Lastly, long-term studies of children of alcoholics indicate that these offspring are at increased risk for a variety of behavioral, cognitive, and neuropsychologic deficits, including a possible genetic vulnerability to alcoholism.[73] A more extensive review of substance abuse and pregnancy is beyond the scope of this chapter.

In summary, treatment of psychiatric disorders with medication may involve some increased risks to the fetus, but failing to treat may involve losing control of a difficult mental illness in the pregnant woman. Particularly in the treatment of major depression and schizophrenia, drug options with minimal teratogenicity are available, although long-term outcome data are lacking. In general, using the least toxic agent at the lowest effective dose is recommended, with the option for discontinuing medication during embryogenesis (less than 10 weeks) in some women. However, for women with severe psychiatric disease, changing an effective medical treatment at any time in pregnancy may be ill advised.

Reproductive effects of metabolic disorders

The reproductive effects of maternal metabolic disorders may result in a variety of outcomes. One example of a metabolic disorder causing infertility is galactosemia in association with ovarian failure. A second category of reproductive risks includes maternal metabolic disorders such as ornithine transcarbamylase deficiency, maternal maple syrup urine disease, and maternal homocystinuria, which may either precipitate maternal metabolic crises postpartum or lead to thromboembolic complications. Both methyl malonic aciduria and hyper-homocystinuria may also be associated with an increased risk of neural tube defects in offspring. Finally, parallel to prolonged exposure of other known fetal neurotoxins, elevated maternal levels of phenylalanine in maternal PKU may lead to CNS deficits in the fetus.

An autosomal recessive disorder, PKU is a metabolic disease that in homozygotes causes profound deteriorating cognitive and neurological development after birth if untreated by a diet low in phenylalanine. Newborn screening programs have allowed early identification and treatment of affected individuals with a diet low in phenylalanine, but the length of time that the individual must stay on a severely restrictive diet is unclear. It is now evident, however, that affected homozygous women must obtain good metabolic control prior to pregnancy and throughout gestation in order to minimize the neurologic damage to the fetus.[74] Studies have shown that offspring of untreated maternal PKU have a 92% risk of mental retardation, a 40% risk of low birth weight, and a 12% risk of congenital cardiac disease.[75] The extent of fetal damage correlates with maternal blood levels of phenylalanine, with levels above 10 mg/dl placing the fetus at very high risk of cognitive delay.[76] Mildly affected offspring show delays in language, memory, and quantitative abilities, while behavior and motor skills appear less affected. Interestingly, if infants of maternal PKU are compared with affected homozygote PKU infants, the phenotype is strikingly dissimilar. Affected homozygotes with PKU, who were exposed to a normal intrauterine environment but an abnormal postnatal metabolic milieu, were deficient in visual and motor skills and developed a profound degree of mental retardation in addition to severe autistic behaviors. In contrast, children who were exposed in utero to an abnormal maternal/fetal metabolic environment but normal phenylalanine levels as infants tend to show mild developmental delay, not unlike FAS. Like FAS, a dose-dependent relationship appears to influence the severity of disease in the infant,[77] with long-term follow-up still in process for offspring of mothers with PKU.

The Maternal PKU Collaborative Study (2000)[76] reported on a cohort of 149 women and 253 total offspring using multiple tests of cognitive ability and behavior on the children at 4 years of age. This study, in which data were collected from a total of 78 metabolic clinics in the USA, Canada, and Germany, showed that the cohort of women with PKU experienced considerable difficulty in planning pregnancies, following dietary guidelines, and maintaining metabolic control. The children with the highest scores were those from higher socioeconomic groups whose mothers maintained metabolic control prior to conception. Unfortunately, 47% of children whose mothers did not achieve metabolic control by 20 weeks' gestation had a general cognitive index score 2 standard deviations below the mean for that age. Yet even late treatment (past 20 weeks) improved the cognitive tests compared with reports of untreated pregnancies, in which the percentage of children with mental retardation exceeds 90%.[76] Providing the medical and social resources for reproductive-age women with PKU to plan pregnancies when their metabolic control is excellent will minimize the exposure of fetuses to a known neurotoxin.

Hematologic disease

Some maternal hematologic disorders can affect the fetus as a result or either platelet or red blood cell abnormalities. When a pregnant woman has been sensitized (i.e., produces antibodies) to fetal antigens on the red cell membrane, hemolytic disease of the newborn may result. Erythroblastosis fetalis is most commonly caused by sensitization of the Rh(negative) mother to the D antigen on the fetus, but may also be caused by other more rare antibodies to other red cell antigens such as Kell, Duffy c, and E. If untreated, alloimmunization may cause severe fetal anemia, hydrops, and intrauterine death. In a parallel disorder, maternal platelet alloimmunization to fetal platelet antigens may cause fetal thrombocytopenia and intracranial hemorrhage. As with Rh disease, the first pregnancy is rarely affected, and it is usually a fetal maternal hemorrhage that causes sensitization.

Inherited blood disorder, including sickle-cell disease, thalassemias, and disorders of red cell membranes are usually asymptomatic in the heterozygous maternal carrier. These diseases are primarily a concern when both parents are known carriers, and prenatal diagnosis should be offered early in pregnancy. Occasionally women with sickle-cell disease, sickle-beta thalassemia, or other hemoglobinopathies become pregnant. Their offspring are obligate carriers, but the perinatal issues generally concern maternal health, maintenance of adequate hemoglobin levels, prevention of infectious diseases, and pain control. Fetal growth restriction is increased in fetuses of mothers with sickle-cell disease.

Genetic disorders

Maternal genetic diseases that can affect the development of the fetal or neonatal brain deserve attention because of our increasing ability to provide prenatal diagnosis for couples who are either affected by or carriers of a genetic disease. The list of disorders for which prenatal diagnosis is available by DNA testing is expanding rapidly, and the practical as well as ethical issues surrounding the detection and potential treatment of genetic diseases are complex.

One category of maternal genetic disease that affects the development of offspring is the group of autosomal dominant disorders. This group includes diseases characterized by variable expressivity and penetrance when passed from one generation to the next. Examples in this category include hamartoses such as tuberous sclerosis, neurofibromatosis, and von Hippel–Lindau. These diseases may be mild in the mother, who will pass on the defective gene to 50% of her offspring, but unpredictable in the infant and child. Another autosomal dominant disorder in the mother, Diamond–Blackfan anemia, has been reported to cause congenital anomalies including craniofacial dysmorphism, growth restriction, thumb and neck abnormalities, as well as non-immune hydrops in an affected infant.[78] Other autosomal dominant disorders include diseases such as Huntington's, which may not be identified until well into adulthood in the children of affected mothers.

A second category of diseases includes autosomal recessive disorders with a carrier mother. In the vast majority of autosomal recessive disorders, the carrier mother is not affected, such as in sickle-cell disease or cystic fibrosis, in which both the parents contribute a defective gene to yield an affected child. However, in a few rare autosomal recessive disorders both the carrier and the offspring exhibit disorders. Examples of this are ataxia telangectasia, where the carrier mother experiences increased cancer risks but the affected offspring experience ataxia and degenerative CNS changes and Fanconi's anemia, which may result in microcephaly and mental retardation in the affected offspring. There may be other cases where heterozygosity for well-known autosomal recessive diseases is associated with disorders of "unknown" or "multifactorial" origin.[79] Enhanced identification of carriers for genetic diseases would expand the population that might benefit from prenatal counseling and diagnosis.

Finally, some X-linked disorders exist in mildly affected carrier females who may then pass on the defective X gene to a son who will be severely affected. Fragile X syndrome, the most common form of inherited mental retardation, causes severe mental deficiency in the sons via expansion of a trinucleotide sequence (CGG) inherited from the mother.[80] The dynamics of expansion of the abnormal gene when passed on from mother to son are complex, with maternal premutation size positively correlated with the risk of having a full mutation offspring.[81] The cognitive performance of full mutation mothers is lower than the premutation carrier mothers, but not as severe as the full mutation expression in males. Fragile X syndrome is most accurately described as an X-linked disorder with variable penetrance. Myotonic dystrophy and spinal and bulbar muscular atrophy are other genetic disorders that have been found to result from triplet repeat amplification.

Autoimmune disorders, including systemic lupus erythematosus

Systemic lupus erythematosus (SLE) is the most common autoimmune condition primarily affecting females in their reproductive years. In the past, women with SLE were advised against childbearing. Termination of pregnancy and permanent sterilization were often recommended. Advances in medical management of SLE, improved understanding of pregnancy complications, and advances in neonatal medicine have allowed females with SLE to have successful pregnancies. Complications of SLE and pregnancy are common and careful collaboration between rheumatologists, internists, and obstetricians is essential for optimal outcome.

The following discussion, while specifically addressing problems related to SLE, can be applied to most of the autoimmune disorders such as rheumatoid arthritis (RA), mixed connective tissue diseases (MCTD), undifferentiated connective tissue disease (UCTD), Sjögren's syndrome, juvenile rheumatoid arthritis (JRA), and systemic sclerosis. Rheumatoid arthritis tends to improve during pregnancy with reversion to the prepregnancy state after delivery while the other conditions behave similar to SLE during pregnancy. Approximately one-third of patients will have exacerbations of the disease, one-third will have no change in disease activity, and one-third will improve during the course of pregnancy. These figures are rough estimates and there is some controversy in the literature concerning the effect of pregnancy on the disease.

The effect of pregnancy on the course of SLE

Lupus flares in pregnancy are relatively common but are most often not in critical organ systems and can usually be managed by altering medication.[82] Lupus activity at the time of conception is an important predictor of incidence of flare. If SLE is active at conception, flare is more likely than if the disease is in remission.[83–85] It is essential to continue the appropriate medication to maintain remission. Renal disease in SLE deserves special attention because of the possible effect of pregnancy on renal function. Patients with lupus nephritis that are in remission and stable will do relatively well during pregnancy.[84,86–87] However transient and reversible worsening of renal function will occur in 8–30% of cases and permanent, irreversible renal deterioration may occur in some patients.[86–88] The presence of proteinuria makes the diagnosis of renal lupus flare difficult to distinguish from preeclampsia or pregnancy-induced hypertension. Various clinical characteristics have been reported to be helpful in distinguishing preeclampsia from renal disease.[87,89,90] Quantity of proteinuria, thrombocytopenia, hyperuricemia, and hypertension will not differentiate preeclampsia from renal disease as a result of SLE. However, red blood casts are rare in preeclampsia and onset of proteinuria is usually abrupt, in contrast to the chronic proteinuria in SLE nephritis. In addition, liver functions are rarely abnormal in SLE and are more likely to be so in preeclampsia. These clinical features may aid the clinician establishing the diagnosis in many cases.

Medications during pregnancy

SLE presents with a wide spectrum of disease activity, ranging from minimal symptomatology and serologic abnormalities requiring little or no medication to life-threatening illness requiring large doses of immunosuppressive agents and multiple other medications. Prednisone and azathioprine are considered relatively safe in pregnancy[91,92] although intrauterine growth retardation has been reported.[93,94] However, the use of prednisone in the absence of clear medical indications for its use is discouraged because of the potential for serious maternal complications. There is an increased risk of glucose intolerance, hypertension, coronary artery disease, and osteopenia in patients exposed to high-dose corticosteroids for prolonged periods of time. In addition, there is evidence that corticosteroids may lead to higher rates of fetal loss,[95] and an increased incidence of preterm premature rupture of the membranes.[96] Prednisone should be used when there is a clear medical indication; it should not be used solely for the presence of an antiphospholipid antibody.

Antihypertensive medications, anticoagulants, and low-dose aspirin (LDA) are other medications often used in SLE pregnancy. Antihypertensive agents in chronic hypertension are primarily indicated for maternal health with some suggestion of a decrease in the incidence of superimposed preeclampsia,[97,98] an increase in gestational age and fewer maternal and fetal complications.[99] This is controversial.

Calcium channel blockers have been used as treatment for preterm labor and are considered relatively safe in pregnancy.[100,101] Angiotensin-converting enzyme (ACE) inhibitors are widely used for the management of hypertension and renal disease. Many patients with SLE and renal involvement are using these agents. ACE inhibitors are not teratogenic. Patients who have inadvertently remained on ACE inhibitors during the first trimester of pregnancy should not be counseled about termination. ACE inhibitors are contraindicated in the second and third trimester because of reports of neonatal compromise and renal failure in newborns exposed to these agents.[102]

Anticoagulation is often indicated in pregnancy. Heparin is used in pregnancy to treat thromboembolic disease and the antiphospholipid syndrome, which is often associated with SLE. Coumadin crosses the placenta, affects fetal hemostasis and is not generally used in pregnancy.[103] Low-molecular-weight heparin (LMWH) is safe in pregnancy[104] but the increased cost compared to standard heparin may limit its use. LMWH may have a lower incidence of excessive bleeding and heparin-induced thrombocytopenia (HIT).

LDA, 150 mg/day or less, has been extensively used in pregnancy. Aspirin dosages of greater than 150 mg/day have been reported to cross the placenta and be associated with fetal malformations.[92,105] LDA is an integral part of therapy for antiphospholipid antibody syndrome, either primary or associated with SLE. LDA is often used with heparin and prednisone.

Intravenous gammaglobulin[106,107] has been used in pregnancy and is considered safe, but evidence of efficacy has not been established. Concerns about allergic reactions and blood-borne pathogens should limit the use of intravenous gammaglobulin to conditions in which efficacy has been established by appropriate clinical trials. Nonsteroidal antiinflammatory drugs (NSAID) are relatively contraindicated in pregnancy, especially during the second and third trimester, because of studies demonstrating premature closure of the patent ductus arterosus,[108,109] oligohydramnios,[110,111] fetal renal dysfunction,[112,113] necrotizing enterocolitis,[114] and effects on cerebral blood flow.[115]

Antimalarial medications are commonly used in the treatment of SLE. There is evidence that chloroquine, used in doses for treatment of SLE, may cause abnormalities of the eye and ear.[116,117] No evidence of teratogenicity has been demonstrated with the lower doses of chloroquine used in antimalarial therapy.[118] Hydroxychloroquine is thought to be safer than chloroquine.[119,120] Many rheumatologists and obstetricians in the USA will attempt to discontinue antimalarials prior to conception. Currently, there is a large body of evidence attesting to the safety of antimalarials in pregnancy. Discontinuation of these medications has been demonstrated to increase the incidence of SLE exacerbation. Continuation of antimalarial medication during pregnancy is now accepted as relatively safe and effective therapy.[121,122]

Effect of SLE on the fetus

The effects of SLE on the fetus and pregnancy outcome is related to the following:

End organ disease

1 The most common organ system involved is the kidney, with resultant lupus nephritis, renal insufficiency, and often hypertension. Patients with renal disease are divided into three broad categories:
   (a) Those without significant hypertension or renal impairment will have successful pregnancies over 90% of the time.[123,124]
   (b) Patients with renal disease and significant hypertension have a higher incidence of fetal loss, intrauterine growth retardation, and superimposed preeclampsia.[86,87,125]
   (c) Patients with significant renal impairment are subject to the same complications as patients with significant hypertension, but also run the risk of irreversible renal compromise.[125]
2 CNS and pulmonary involvement are less common than renal disease, but when present are potentially extremely serious.
   (a) Patients with CNS involvement or pulmonary manifestations of SLE are at greater risk of serious maternal morbidity.
   (b) Premature delivery in SLE is often indicated for maternal indications.

Lupus activity at time of conception

1 Patients with significant lupus activity at time of conception have a higher incidence of fetal loss.[82,84,86]

Presence of antiphospholipid antibodies and SS-A (Ro) and SS-B (La) antibodies.

1 The presence of autoantibodies is one of the more important predictors of fetal and neonatal outcome in SLE pregnancy.
2 Antiphospholipid (aPL) antibody syndrome occurs in about 25% of patients with SLE. Antiphospholipid antibodies consist of anticardiolipin antibody (ACLA) and lupus anticoagulant (LAC).

The following summary represents reasonable conclusions based on the available literature regarding aPL and pregnancy outcome:

(a) The presence of LAC or ACLA is a marker of fetal outcome.
(b) Prior fetal loss is an independent predictor of future fetal death.
(c) High-titer ACLA (greater than 40 immunoglobulin IgG binding units (GPL)) combined with prior loss increases the risk of fetal death in the index pregnancy.
(d) Decreasing titers of aPL during pregnancy do not correlate with improved fetal prognosis.
(e) aPL correlates with an increased incidence of intrauterine growth retardation.
(f) aPL correlates with an increased incidence of maternal complications, including preeclampsia,[126] postpartum complications,[127] arterial and venous thrombosis and, rarely, catastrophic occlusion syndrome.[128,129]

3 Neonatal lupus erythematosus (NLE) is strongly correlated with the presence of SSA (anti-Ro) and SSB (anti-La) autoantibodies, which can cross the placenta. Complete congenital heart block is the most serious, but least common, manifestation of NLE and may lead to fetal death or require pacemaker placement in the neonatal period.[130,131] More often, NLE manifests as a transient rash and thrombocytopenia, which resolve in 4–6 weeks.

Management of pregnancy complicated by SLE

Close cooperation between the rheumatologist, internist, and obstetrician is essential for optimal outcome in SLE in pregnancy. Neonatologists and pediatricians should be involved when decisions about delivery at early gestational ages are contemplated. The optimal time to deal with the issues surrounding SLE and pregnancy is prior to the patient becoming pregnant. The patient should be advised to defer pregnancy until she has been in remission for at least 6 months. Renal function must be evaluated, particularly if the patient has a history of lupus nephritis. The presence or absence of aPL antibodies, SS-A, and SS-B should be determined. If aPL antibodies are not detected prior to pregnancy, repeat titers should be evaluated in the late first or early second trimester, as the presence of positive titers after pregnancy confirmation has been reported to occur. Attempts should be made to maintain remission on glucocorticoids, azathioprine, or antimalarials. Cyclophosphamide and methotrexate are contraindicated during pregnancy.

Patient in remission, without renal disease and without aPL antibodies or SS-A, SS-B antibodies

Pregnancy should be attempted while in remission. Routine obstetrical follow-up is appropriate with a second-trimester sonogram and sonograms every 4–6 weeks thereafter to follow fetal growth. Fetal monitoring should begin in the third trimester with nonstress tests, contraction stress tests, biophysical profile,[132] and umbilical artery velocimetry.[133]

Patient in remission with SS-A or SS-B antibodies

Patients should be counseled about neonatal lupus. The risk is greatest if the mother has human leukocyte antigen (HLA)-DR3 and both anti-Ro and anti-La.[130] Serial fetal echocardiograms from 16 weeks' gestation can detect the fetus at risk. Incomplete forms of heart block, if detected early, may be treatable.[134–136] Empiric therapy of SS-A and/or SS-B antibody-positive patients in an attempt to prevent congenital heart block is not justified given the low prevalence of the condition. Intensive fetal surveillance from 16 weeks' gestation and treatment of the fetus with evidence of early cardiac involvement are recommended.[136] Serial sonography every 2–4 weeks should be performed if heart block is detected. If early fetal hydrops (pleural pericardial effusions and ascites) is detected, prompt delivery may be necessary, even at an early gestational age. If hydrops does not develop and biophysical testing is normal, the pregnancy should be allowed to continue. Spontaneous onset of labor should be anticipated. Involvement of pediatric cardiology should occur as soon as the condition is diagnosed or suspected.

Patient with renal disease, normotensive or mildly hypertensive, no autoantibodies

These patients should continue on antihypertensive medications and immunosuppressive therapy as required. Baseline renal function should be determined prior to pregnancy, and every trimester. Monthly sonograms for fetal growth and fetal monitoring from 26 to 28 weeks should be instituted. Frequent blood pressure and urine monitoring (for proteinuria) should be done to detect the onset of preeclampsia.

Patients with severe hypertension or severely compromised renal function (creatinine clearance <50 ml/min, serum creatinine greater than 1.2 mg/dl)

These patients should be discouraged from becoming pregnant because of the risk of irreversible renal deterioration and possible need for dialysis and/or transplantation.

Patients with aPL antibodies, no history of fetal loss, no history of thromboembolic disease

If the antibody titer is low (ACLA<40 GPL), low-dose aspirin (81 mg/day) is added to their immunosuppressive medications. If the antibody titer is high, LDA and low dose subcutaneous heparin should be used.[137,138] Early and intensive fetal monitoring is indicated.

Patients with aPL antibodies and history of fetal loss

These patients should be started on LDA and low-dose subcutaneous heparin. Early and intensive fetal monitoring is indicated.

Patients with aPL antibodies and prior history of thromboembolism, venous or arterial

In addition to LDA, these patients should be fully anticoagulated with heparin during pregnancy and continue lifelong anticoagulation following pregnancy.[139,140] Intensive fetal monitoring is recommended.

Patients with prior fetal loss and immunoglobulin M and aCL antibodies only

LDA only and intensive fetal monitoring is indicated. A recent study on the outcome of treated pregnancies in women with antiphospholipid syndrome and pregnancy concluded that pregnancy outcome in women with aPL appears to be improved by treatment but fetal loss may still occur, despite treatment.[141] Therefore, all patients should have repeat aCL titers done in late first or early second trimester if initial pregnancy titers were negative or low-titer. If high-titer immunoglobulin G aCL is detected, addition of low-dose heparin should be considered.

Patients with SLE and autoimmune disorders will often have unremarkable pregnancies. Routine obstetrical evaluation and laboratory tests should be performed, as these patients may have obstetrical problems unrelated to their autoimmune disorders. The patients should be seen every 2–4 weeks by both the obstetrician and rheumatologist or internist. Patients with SLE can often have normal spontaneous vaginal deliveries. Cesarean section should be reserved for routine obstetrical indications. There must be no reluctance to treat serious medical complications in these patients simply because they are pregnant. Maternal health is of paramount importance. Maternal mortality is rare and the majority of patients with autoimmune disorders can have successful pregnancies.

Summary

In summary, a wide range of maternal disorders may affect the development of the fetus. Some genetic diseases result in early pregnancy loss, congenital malformations, or developmental derangements that are evident at birth, whereas other genetic diseases affect postnatal and childhood development. In fact, a wide range of human disease may result from even more subtle genetic programming. Other inherited or acquired maternal disease may result in a suboptimal environment for fetal development. Treatment for maternal disease must take into account potential fetal teratogenicity and direct neurotoxicity.

REFERENCES

1 Seckol JR. Physiologic programming of the fetus. *Clin Perinatol* 1998; 25: 939–962.

2 Rizzo TA, Metxger BE, Dooly SA, Cho NH. Early malnutrition and neurobehavioral development: insights from the study of the children of diabetic mothers. *Child Dev* 1997; 68: 26–38.

3 Jones KL and Smith DW. *Smith's Recognizable Patterns of Human Malformation*, 5th edn. Philadelphia, PA: Saunders, 1997: 683.

4 Towner D, Kjos SL, Leung B et al. Congenital malformations in pregnancies complicated by NIDDM. *Diabetes Care* 1995; 18: 1446–1451.

5 Greene MF. Prevention and diagnosis of congenital anomalies in diabetic pregnancies. *Clin Perinatol* 1993; 20: 533–547.

6 Simpson JL, Elias S, Martin AO et al. Diabetes in pregnancy. Northwestern University Series (1977–1981) I. Prospective study of anomalies in offspring of mothers with diabetes mellitus. *Am J Obstet Gynecol* 1983; 146: 263–270.

7 Becerra JE, Khoury MJ, Cordero JF, Erikson JD. Diabetes mellitus and pregnancy and the risk of specific birth defects: a population based, case-control study. *Pediatrics* 1990; 85: 1–9.

8 Freinkel N. Diabetic embryopathy and fuel-mediated teratogenesis: lessons from animal models. *Horm Metab Res* 1988; 20: 463–475.

9 Eriksson U. The pathogenesis of congenital malformations in the diabetic pregnancy. *Diabetes Metab Rev* 1995; 11:63–82.

10 Pinter E, Reece EA, Leranth CZ et al. Arachadonic acid prevents hyperglycemia-associated yolk sac damage and embryopathy. *Am J Obstet Gynecol* 1986; 166: 691–702.

11 Goldman AS, Baker L, Piddington R et al. Hyperglycemia induced teratogenesis is mediated by a functional deficiency of arachadonic acid. *Proc Natl Acad Sci* 1985; 82: 8227–8231.

12 Eriksson NJ and Borg LA. Protection by free oxygen scavenging enzymes against glucose-induced embryonic malformations in vitro. *Diabetologia* 1991; 34: 325–331.

13 Rosenn B, Miodovnik M, Combs CA, Khoury J, Siddiqi TA. Glycemic thresholds for spontaneous abortions and congenital malformations in insulin dependent diabetes mellitus. *Obstet Gynecol* 1994; 84: 515–520.

14 Schefer UM, Songster G, Xiang A et al. Congenital malformations in offspring of women with hyperglycemia first detected during pregnancy. *Am J Obstet Gynecol* 1997; 177; 1165–1171.

15 Mills J, Simpson JL, Driscol SG et al. Incidence of spontaneous abortion among normal and insulin dependent diabetic women whose pregnancies were recognized within 21 days of conception. *N Engl J Med* 1988; 319: 1617–1623.

16 Pederson J. Weight and length of infants of diabetic mothers. *Acta Endocrinol* 1954; 16: 330–342.

17 Kitzmiller JL. Macrosomia in infants of diabetic mothers: characteristics, causes, prevention. In Jovanovic L, Peterson CM, Furhmann K (eds) *Diabetes and Pregnancy: Teratology, Toxicology and Treatment.* New York: Praeger, 1986: 85–120.

18 Widness JA, Cowett RM, Coustan DR et al. Neonatal morbidities in infants of mothers with glucose intolerance in pregnancy. *Diabetes* 1985; 61(suppl. 2): 65.

19 Rich-Edwards JW, Colditz GA, Stampfer MJ et al. Birth weight and the risk for type 2 diabetes mellitus in adult women. *Ann Intern Med* 1999; 130: 278–284.

20 Kuhl C, Anderson GE, Brandt NJ et al. Metabolic events in infants of diabetic mothers during the first 24 hours after birth. *Acta Paediatr Scand* 1982; 71: 19–25

21 Bourbon JR and Farrell PM. Fetal lung development in the diabetic pregnancy. *Pediatr Res* 1985; 19: 253.

22 Smith BT, Giroud CJP, Robert M et al. Insulin antagonism of cortisol action on lecithin synthesis by cultures of fetal lung cells. *J Pediatr* 1975; 87: 953–955.

23 Rizzo T, Metzger BE, Burns WJ, Burns K. Correlations between antepartum maternal metabolism and intelligence of offspring. *N Engl J Med* 1991; 325: 911–916.

24 Rizzo TA, Dooley SL, Metzger BE et al. Prenatal and perinatal influences on long-term psychomotor development in offspring of diabetic mothers. *Am J Obstet Gynecol* 1995; 173: 1753–1758,

25 Vulsma T, Gons MH, de Vijlder JJM. Maternal–fetal transfer of thyroxine in congenital hypothyroidism due to a total organification defect or thyroid agenesis. *N Engl J Med* 1989; 321: 13–16.

26 Pop VJ, Kuijpens JL, van Baar AL et al. Low maternal free thyroxine concentrations during early pregnancy are associated with impaired psychomotor development in infancy. *Clin Endocrinol (Oxf)* 1999; 50: 149–155.

27 Man EB, Brown JF, Serunian SA. Maternal hypothyroxinemia: psychoneurological deficits of progeny. *Ann Clin Lab Sci* 1991; 21: 227–239.

28 Haddow JE, Palomaki GE, Allan WC et al. Maternal thyroid deficiency during pregnancy and subsequent neuropsychological development of the child. *N Engl J Med* 1999; 341: 549–555.

29 Volpe JJ. Neuronal proliferation, migration, organization and myelination. In Volpe JJ (ed.). *Neurology of the Newborn*, 3rd edn. Philadelphia: W.B. Saunders, 1995: 43–92.

30 Badawi N, Kurinczuk JJ, Mackenzie CL et al. Maternal thyroid disease: a risk factor for newborn encephalopathy in term infants. *Br J Obstet Gynaecol* 2000; 107: 798–801.

31 Momotani N, Ito K, Hamada N et al. Maternal hyperthyroidism and congenital malformations in the offspring. *Clin Endocrinol* 1984; 20: 695–700.

32 Page DV, Brady K, Mitchell LJ et al. The pathology of intrauterine thyrotoxicosis: two case reports. *Obstet Gynecol* 1988; 72: 479–481.

33 Therrell B, Berenbaum SA, Manter-Kapanke V et al. Results of screening 1.9 million Texas newborns for 21-hydroxylase deficient congenital adrenal hyperplasia. *Pediatrics* 1998; 101: 583–590.

34 White PC, New MI. Genetic basis of endocrine disease: 2 Congenital adrenal hyperplasia due to 21-hydroxylase deficiency. *J Clin Endocrinol Metab* 1992; 74: 6–11.

35 Kuhnle U, Bullinger M, Schwarz HP, Knorr D. Partnership and sexuality in adult female patients with congenital adrenal hyperplasia. First results of a cross sectional study. *J Steroid Biochem Mol Biol* 1993; 45: 123–126.

36 Zucker KJ, Bradley SJ, Oliver G et al. Psychosexual development of women with congenital adrenal hyperplasia. *Horm Behav* 1996; 30: 300–318.

37 Meyer-Bahlburg HF, Gruen RS, New M et al. Gender changes from female to male in classical congenital adrenal hyperplasia. *Horm Behav* 1996; 30: 319–332.

38 Forest MG. Prenatal diagnosis, treatment and outcome in infants with congenital adrenal hyperplasia. *Curr Opin Endocrinol Diabet* 1997; 4: 209–217.

39 Forest MG, Morel Y, David M. Prenatal treatment of congenital adrenal hyperplasia. *Trends Endocrinol Metab* 1998; 9: 284–289.

40 Mercado AB, Wilson C, Cheng KC, Wei JQ, New MI. Extensive personal experience: prenatal diagnosis and treatment of congenital adrenal hyperplasia owing to steroid 21-hydroxylase deficiency. *J Clin Endocrinol Metab* 1995; 80: 2014–2020.

41 Speiser PW, New MI. Prenatal diagnosis and treatment of congenital adrenal hyperplasia. *J Pediatr Endocrinol* 1994; 7: 183–191.

42 Quercia N, Chitayat D, Babul-Hirji R, New MI, Daneman D. Normal external genitalia in a female with classic adrenal hyperplasia who was not treated during embryogenesis. *Prenat Diagn* 1998; 18: 83–85.

43 Miller WL. Dexamethasone treatment of congenital adrenal hyperplasia in utero: an experimental therapy of unproven safety. *J Urol* 1999; 162: 537–540.

44 Pang S, Clark AT, Freeman LC et al. Maternal side effects of prenatal dexamethasone therapy for fetal congenital adrenal hyperplasia. *J Clin Endocrinol Metab* 1992; 75: 249–253.

45 Celsi G, Kistner A, Aizman R et al. Prenatal dexamethasone causes oligonephria, sodium retention, and higher blood pressure in the offspring. *Pediatr Res* 1998; 44: 317–322.

46 Lajic S, Wendell A, Bui T-H, Ritzen E, Holst M. Long term somatic follow up of prenatally treated children with congenital adrenal hyperplasia. *J Clin Endocrinol Metab* 1998; 83: 3872–3880

47 Lo JC, Schwitzgebel VM, Tyrrell JB et al. Normal female infants born to women with classic congenital adrenal hyperplasia due to 21-hydroxylase deficiency. *J Clin Endocrinol Metab* 1999; 84: 930–936.

48 ElSayed YY. Obstetric and gynecologic care of women with epilepsy. *Epilepsia* 1998; 39: S17–S25.

49 Annegers JF, Hauser WA, Elveback LR et al. Seizure disorders in offspring of parents with a history of seizures: a maternal–paternal difference? *Epilepsia* 1976; 17: 1–9.

50 Fairgrieve SD, Jackson M, Jonas P et al. Population based, prospective study of the care of women with epilepsy in pregnancy. *Br Med J* 2000; 321: 674–675.

51 Hanson JW, Myrianthopoulos NC, Harvey MAS, Smith DW. Risks to the offspring of women treated with hydantoin anti-convulsants, with emphasis on the fetal hydantoin syndrome. *J Pediatr* 1976; 89: 662–668.

52 Rodriguez-Pinilla E, Arroyo I, Fondevilla J, Garcia MJ, Martinez-Frias ML. Prenatal exposure to acid during pregnancy and limb deficiencies: a case control study. *Am J Med Genet* 2000; 28: 376–381.

53 Samren EB, van Duijn CM, Christiaens GC, Hofman A, Lindhout D. Antiepileptic drug regimens and major congenital abnormalities in the offspring. *Ann Neurol* 1999; 46: 739–746.

54 Dasky LV, Rosenblatt DS, Anderman E. Mechanism of teratogenesis: folic acid and anti-epileptic therapy. *Neurology* 1992; 42: S32–S42.

55 Craig J, Morrison P, Morrow J, Patterson V. Failure of folic acid to prevent a neural tube defect in the offspring of a mother taking sodium valproate. *Seizure* 1999; 8: 253–254.

56 Yerby MS. Pregnancy and epilepsy. *Epilepsia* 1991; 32: S51–S59.

57 Aube M. Migraine in pregnancy. *Neurology* 1999; 53: S26–S28.

58 Wisner KL, Peindl KP, Hanusa BH. Relationship of psychiatric illness to childbearing status: a hospital based epidemiologic study. *J Affect Disord* 1993; 28: 39–50.

59 Wisner KL, Gelenberg AJ, Leonard H, Zarin D, Frank E. Pharmacologic treatment of depression during pregnancy. *JAMA* 1999; 282: 1264–1269.

60 Altshculer L, Cohen L, Szuba MP et al. Pharmacologic management of psychiatric illness in pregnancy: dilemmas and guidelines. *Am J Psychiatry* 1996; 153: 592–606.

61 Pastuszal A, Schick-Boschetto B, Zuber C. Pregnancy outcome following first trimester exposure to fluoxetine (Prozac). *JAMA* 1993; 269: 2246–2248.

62 Kulin NA, Pastuszak A, Sage SR et al. Pregnancy outcome following the new selective serotonin reuptake inhibitors. *JAMA* 1998; 279: 609–610.

63 Chambers CD, Johnson KA, Dick LN, Felix RJ, Jones KL. Birth outcomes in women taking fluoxetine. *N Engl J Med* 1996; 335: 1010–1015.

64 Nulman I, Rovet J, Stewart DE et al. Neurodevelopment of children exposed in utero to antidepressant drugs. *N Engl J Med* 1997; 336: 258–262.

65 Wisner KL, Stowe ZN. Psychobiology of postpartum mood disorders. *Semin Reprod Endocrinol* 1997; 15: 77–90.

66 Cohen LS, Friedman JM, Jefferson JW, Johnson EM, Weiner ML. A re-evaluation of risk of in utero exposure to lithium. *JAMA* 1994; 271: 146–150.

67 Sloane D, Suskind V, Heinonen OP et al. Antenatal exposure to phenothiazines in relation to congenital malformations, perinatal mortality rate, birth weight and intelligence quotient score. *Am J Obstet Gynecol* 1977; 128: 486–488.

68 Kris EB. Children of mothers maintained on pharmacotherapy during pregnancy and post partum. *Curr Ther Res Clin Exp* 1965; 7: 785–789.

69 Abel EL, Sokol RJ. Fetal alcohol syndrome is now the leading cause of mental retardation. *Lancet* 1986; 2: 222.

70 Abel EL, Sokol RJ. A revised conservative estimate of the incidence of FAS and its economic impact. *Alcohol Clin Exp Res* 1991; 15: 514.

71 Committee on Drugs, American Academy of Pediatrics. Use of psychoactive medication during pregnancy and possible effects on the fetus and newborn. *Pediatrics* 2000; 105: 880–887.

72 Kelly SJ, Day N, Streissguth AP. Effects of prenatal alcohol exposure on social behavior in humans and other species. *Neurotoxicol Teratol* 2000; 22: 143–149.

73 Johnson JJ, Leff M. Children of substance abusers: overview of research findings. *Pediatrics* 1999; 103: 1085–1099.

74 Lynch BC, Pitt DB, Maddison TG et al. Maternal phenylketonuria: successful outcome in four pregnancies treated prior to conception. *Eur J Pediatr* 1988; 148: 72–75.

75 Lenke RR and Levy HL. Maternal phenylketonuria and hyperphenylalaniuria: an international survey of the outcome of untreated and treated pregnancies. *N Engl J Med* 1980; 303: 1202–1208.

76 Waisbren SE, Hanley W, Levy HL et al. Outcome at 4 years in offspring of women with maternal phenylketonuria: the maternal PKU collaborative study. *JAMA* 2000; 283: 756–762.

77 Spohr HL, Williams J, Steinhausen HC. Prenatal alcohol exposure and long-term developmental consequences. *Lancet* 1993; 341: 907–910.

78 Rogers BB, Bloom SL, Buchanan GR. Autosomally inherited Diamond–Blackfan anemia resulting in non-immune hydrops. *Obstet Gynecol* 1997; 89: 805–807.

79 Vogel F. Clinical consequences of heterozygosity for autosomal-recessive diseases. *Clin Genet* 1984; 25: 381–415.

80 Brown WT. The fragile X syndrome. *Neurol Clin* 1989; 7: 107–121.

81 Kallinen J, Heinonen S, Mannermaa A, Ryynanen M. Prenatal diagnosis of fragile X syndrome and the risk of expansion of a permutation. *Clin Genet* 2000; 58: 111–115.

82 Mintz G, Niz J, Guiterrez C et al. Prospective study of pregnancy in systemic lupus erythematosus: results of a multidisciplinary approach. *J Rheumatol* 1986; 13: 732–739.

83 Estes D and Larson DL. Systemic lupus erythematosus and pregnancy. *Clin Obstet Gynecol* 1965; 8: 307–321.

84 Hayslett JP and Lynn RI. Effect of pregnancy in patients with lupus nephropathy. *Kidney Int* 1980; 18: 207–220.

85 Tozman EC, Urowitz MB, Gladman DD. Systemic lupus erythematosus and pregnancy. *J Rheumatol* 1980; 7: 624–632.

86 Jungers P, Dougados M, Pelissier C et al. Lupus nephropathy and pregnancy: report of 104 cases in 36 patients. *Arch Intern Med* 1982; 142: 771–776.

87 Packham DK, Lam SS, Nicholls K et al. Lupus nephritis and pregnancy. *Q J Med* 1992; 83: 315–324.

88 Imbasciati E, Surian M, Bottino S et al. Lupus nephropathy and pregnancy: a study of 26 pregnancies in patients with systemic lupus erythematosus and nephritis. *Nephron* 1984; 36: 46–51.

89 Druzin ML. Pregnancy induced hypertension and preeclampsia: the fetus and the neonate. In Rubin PD (ed.) *Handbook of Hypertension*, vol. 10: *Hypertension in Pregnancy*. Amsterdam: Elsevier, 1988: 267–289.

90 Buyon JP, Cronstein BN, Morris M et al. Serum complement values (C3 and C4) to differentiate between systemic lupus activity and preeclampsia. *Am J Med* 1986; 81: 194–200.

91 Sharon E, Jones J, Diamond H et al. Pregnancy and azathioprine in systemic lupus erythematosus. *Am J Obstet Gynecol* 1974; 118: 25–28.

92 Roubenooff R, Hoyt M, Petri M et al. Effects of anti-inflammatory and immunosuppressive drugs on pregnancy and fertility. *Semin Arthritis Rheum* 1988; 18: 88–110.

93 Reinisch JM, Simon NG, Karow WG et al. Prenatal exposure to prednisone in humans and animals retards intrauterine growth. *Science* 1978; 202: 436–438.

94 Scott J. Fetal growth retardation associated with maternal administration of immunosuppressive drugs. *Am J Obstet Gynecol* 1977; 128: 668–676.

95 Lockshin MD, Druzin ML, Qamar T. Prednisone does not prevent recurrent fetal death in women with antiphospholipid antibody. *Am J Obstet Gynecol* 1989; 160: 439–443.

96 Cowchock FS, Reece EA, Balaban D et al. Repeated fetal losses associated with antiphospholipid antibodies: a collaborative randomized trial comparing prednisone with low-dose heparin treatment. *Am J Obstet Gynecol* 1992; 166: 1318–1323.

97 Arias F and Zamora J. Antihypertensive treatment and pregnancy outcome in patients with mild chronic hypertension. *Obstet Gynecol* 1979; 53: 489–494.

98 Blake S and MacDonald D. The prevention of the maternal manifestation of preeclampsia by intensive and antihypertensive treatment. *Br J Obstet Gynaecol* 1991; 98: 244–248.

99 Phippard AF, Fischer WE, Horvath JS et al. Early blood pressure control improves pregnancy outcome in primigravid women with mild hypertension. *Med J Aust* 1991; 154: 378–382.

100 Constantine G, Beevers DG, Reynolds AL et al. Nifedipine as a second-line antihypertensive drug in pregnancy. *Br J Obstet Gynaecol* 1987; 94: 1136–1142.

101 Ulmsten U. Treatment of normotensive and hypertensive patients with preterm labor using oral nifedipine, a calcium antagonist. *Arch Gynecol* 1984; 236: 69–72.

102 Schubiger G, Flurry G, Nussberger J. Enalapril for pregnancy-induced hypertension: acute renal failure in a neonate. *Ann Intern Med* 1988; 149: 2233–2236.

103 Hall JAG, Pauli RM, Wilson KM. Maternal and fetal sequelae of anticoagulation during pregnancy. *Am J Med* 1980; 68: 122–140.

104 Melissari E, Das S, Kanthou C et al. The use of LMW heparin in treating thromboembolism during pregnancy and prevention of osteoporosis (abstract). *Thromb Haemost* 1991; 65: 926a.

105 Nelson M and Forfar J. Associations between drugs administered during pregnancy and congenital abnormalities of the fetus. *Br Med J* 1971; 1: 523–525.

106 Kaaja R, Julkunen H, Ammala P et al. Intravenous immunoglobulin treatment of pregnant patients with recurrent pregnancy losses associated with antiphospholipid antibodies. *Acta Obstet Gynecol Scand* 1993; 72: 63–66.

107 Parke A. The role of IVIG in the management of patients with antiphospholipid antibodies and recurrent pregnancy losses. *Clin Rev Allergy* 1992; 10: 105–118.

108 Goudie B, Dossetor J. Effect on the fetus of indomethacin given to suppress labour. *Lancet* 1979; 2: 1187–1188.

109 Levin D, Fixler D, Morriss F et al. Morphologic analysis of the pulmonary vascular bed in infants exposed in utero to prostaglandin synthetase inhibitors. *J Pediatr* 1978; 92: 478–483.

110 Dewit W, Van Monrik I, Wisenhaan PE. Prolonged maternal indomethacin therapy associated with oligohydramnios. Case reports. *Br J Obstet Gynaecol* 1988; 95: 303–305.

111 Goldenberg RL, Davis RO, Baker RC. Indomethacin-induced oligohydramnios. *Am J Obstet Gynecol* 1989; 160: 1196–1197.

112 Kirshon B, Moise KJ, Wassertrum N et al. Influence of short-term indomethacin therapy on fetal urine output. *Obstet Gynecol* 1988; 72: 51–53.

113 Simeoni V, Messer J, Weisburd P et al. Neonatal renal dysfunction and intrauterine exposure to prostaglandin synthesis inhibitors. *Eur J Pediatr* 1989; 148: 371–373.

114 Major CA, Lewis DF, Harding JA et al. Does tocolysis with indomethacin increase the incidence of necrotizing enterocolitis in the low birth weight neonates? *Am J Obstet Gynecol* 1992; 166: 381.

115 Wennmalm A, Eriksson S, Wahren J. Effect of indomethacin on basal and carbon dioxide stimulated cerebral blood flow in man. *Clin Physiol* 1983; 1: 227–232.

116 Parke AL. Antimalarial drugs, systemic lupus erythematosus and pregnancy. *J Rheumatol* 1988; 15: 607–610.

117 Lindquist N and Ullberg S. The melanin affinity of chloroquine and chlorpromazine studied by whole body auto radiography. *Acta Pharmacol Toxicol* 1972; 31 (suppl. 2): 1–32.

118 Wolfe M and Cordero J. Safety of chloroquine in chemosuppression of malaria during pregnancy. *Br Med J* 1985; 290: 1446–1447.

119 Kitridou RC and Mintz G. The mother in systemic lupus erythematosus. In Wallace DJ, Hahn BH (eds) *Dubouis' Lupus Erythematosus.* Philadelphia: Lea & Febiger 1993; 487–507.

120 Levy M, Buskila D, Gladman DD et al. Pregnancy outcome

following first trimester exposure to chloroquine. *Am J Perinatol* 1991; 8: 174–178.
121 Buchanan NM, Toubi E, Khamashta MA et al. Hydroxychloroquine and lupus pregnancy: review of a series of 36 cases. *Ann Rheum Dis* 1996; 55:486–488.
122 Parke A and West B. Hydroxychloroquine in pregnant patients with systemic lupus erythematosus. *J Rheum* 1996; 23: 1715–1718.
123 Ferris TF. *Renal Disease*. Philadelphia: WB Saunders, 1975: 1.
124 Strauch BS and Hayslett JP. Kidney disease and pregnancy. *Br Med J* 1974; 4: 578–581.
125 Imbasciati E, Surian M, Botino S et al. Lupus nephropathy and pregnancy: a study of 26 pregnancies in patients with systemic lupus erythematosus and nephritis. *Nephron* 1984; 36: 46–51.
126 Branch DW, Andres R, Digre KB et al. The association of antiphospholipid antibodies with severe preeclampsia. *Obstet Gynecol* 1989; 73: 541–545.
127 Kochenour NK, Branch DW, Rote NS et al. A new postpartum syndrome associated with antiphospholipid antibodies. *Obstet Gynecol* 1987; 69: 460–468.
128 Greisman SG, Thayaparan R-S, Godwin TA et al. Occlusive vasculopathy in systemic lupus erythematosus: association with anti-cardiolipin antibody. *Arch Intern Med* 1991; 151: 389–392.
129 Hochfeld M, Druzin ML, Maia D et al. Pregnancy complicated by primary antiphospholipid antibody syndrome. *Obstet Gynecol* 1994; 83: 804–805.
130 Buyon JP. Neonatal lupus syndromes. *Am J Reprod Immunol* 1992; 28: 259–263.
131 Lockshin MD, Bonfa E, Elkon K et al. Neonatal lupus risk to newborns of mothers with systemic lupus erythematosus. *Am J Reprod Immunol* 1992; 31: 697–701.
132 Adams D, Druzin MD, Edersheim T et al. Condition specific antepartum testing. Systemic lupus erythematosus and associated serologic abnormalities. *Am J Reprod Immunol* 1992; 28: 159–163.
133 Kerslake S, Morton KE, Versi E et al. Early Doppler studies in lupus pregnancy. *Am J Reprod Immunol* 1992; 28: 172–175.
134 Buyon JP, Swersky SH, Fox HE et al. Intrauterine therapy for presumptive fetal myocarditis with acquired heart block due to systemic lupus erythematosus. Experience in a mother with a predominance of SS-B (La) antibodies. *Arthritis Rheum* 1987; 30: 44–49.
135 Friedman DM. Fetal echocardiography in the assessment of lupus pregnancies. *Am J Reprod Immunol* 1992; 28: 164–167.
136 Rosenthal D, Druzin ML, Chin C et al. A new therapeutic approach to the fetus with congenital complete heart block: preemptive, targeted therapy with dexamethasone. *Obstet Gynecol* 1998; 92: 689–691.
137 Cowchock FS, Wapner RJ, Needleman L et al. A comparison of pregnancy outcomes after two treatments for antibodies to cardiolipin (ACA). *Clin Exp Rheumatol* 1988; 6: 200.
138 Kalunian KC, Peter JB, Middlekauff HR et al. Clinical significance of a single test for anti-cardiolipin antibodies in patients with systemic lupus erythematosus. *Am J Med* 1988; 85: 602–608.
139 Rosove MH, Brewer PMC. Antiphospholipid thrombosis: clinical course after the first thrombotic event in 70 patients. *Ann Intern Med* 1992; 117: 303–308.
140 Derksen RHWM, De Groot PhG, Kater L et al. Patients with antiphospholipid antibodies and venous thrombosis should receive life-long anticoagulant treatment. *Clin Exp Rheumatol* 1992; 10: 662.
141 Branch DW, Silver RM, Blackwell JL et al. Outcome of treated pregnancies in women with antiphospholipid syndrome: an update of the Utah experience. *Am J Obstet Gynecol* 1992; 80: 614–620.

10

Antepartum evaluation of fetal well-being

Deirdre J. Lyell and Maurice L. Druzin

Stanford University Medical Center, Stanford, CA, USA

In the USA, nearly 50% of all perinatal death occurs prior to birth.[1] While fetal death from acute events such as cord accidents cannot be predicted, identifying, testing, and intervening for the fetus at risk for chronic in utero compromise may prevent neonatal and infant morbidity. This chapter discusses the antenatal assessment of fetal well-being.

An antepartum fetal test should reduce perinatal morbidity and mortality, and reassure parents. The test of choice depends on gestational age. When a fetus at risk for acidosis and asphyxia has reached viability, one of several tests may be employed for screening, including the nonstress test (NST), the contraction stress test (CST), fetal movement monitoring, the biophysical profile (BPP), and Doppler ultrasound. The specificity of these tests is generally high, while the sensitivity is highly variable. Diagnostic ultrasound and prenatal diagnostic procedures such as chorionic villus sampling (CVS) or amniocentesis are the most common tests performed during the early stages of pregnancy to identify chromosomal or major fetal anomalies.

The purpose of this chapter is to discuss common antepartum screening tests, including a description of each test, its indication, and its accuracy.

Perinatal mortality

Since 1965, the perinatal mortality rate (PMR) in the USA has fallen steadily, and the pattern of perinatal death has changed considerably. Improved techniques of antepartum fetal evaluation likely contribute to the decreasing PMR.

The PMR is defined in several ways. According to the National Center for Health Statistics (NCHS), the PMR is the number of late fetal deaths (28 weeks' gestation or more) plus early neonatal deaths per 1000 live births.[2] The World Health Organization (WHO) defines the PMR as the number of deaths of fetuses and live births weighing at least 500 g per 1000 live births. If the weight is unavailable, a fetus is counted if the gestational age is 22 weeks or greater, or the crown-to-heel length is 25 cm or more in a newborn that dies before day 7 of life, per 1000 live births. The American College of Obstetricians and Gynecologists (ACOG) has recommended including in PMR statistics only fetuses and neonates weighing 500 g or more.[3] For international comparisons, ACOG recommends counting fetuses and neonates weighing 1000 g or more at delivery.

Using the NCHS definition, the PMR reported in 1991 was 8.7/1000, of which 5.6/1000 was due to neonatal death, and 3.1/1000 was due to fetal death.[4] In 1997, the PMR decreased to 7.3/1000. It was divided nearly evenly between fetal and neonatal mortality, with rates of 3.5/1000 and 3.8/1000, respectively. A racial difference exists. The PMR for blacks was nearly double that of whites in 1991 and 1997, at 15.7/1000 vs 7.4/1000 in 1991, and 13.2/1000 v 6.3/1000 in 1997, respectively. This increased PMR among blacks includes higher rates of both fetal and neonatal deaths.

The decline in the fetal death rate may be attributed to improved methods of antepartum fetal surveillance, the prevention of Rh sensitization, improved ultrasound detection of intrauterine growth restriction (IUGR) and fetal anomalies, and improved care of maternal diabetes mellitus and preeclampsia. In Canada, Fretts and colleagues[5,6] analyzed the cause of fetal death among 94 346 total deliveries weighing at least 500 g at the Royal Victoria Hospital in Montreal from 1961 to 1993. Overall, the fetal death rate declined by 70%, from 11.5/1000 in the 1960s to 3.2/1000 from 1990 to 1993. Fetal deaths fell from 13.1 to 1.2/1000 for intrapartum asphyxia, and from 4.3 to 0.7/1000 for Rh disease. Deaths due to lethal anomalies declined by 50%, from 10.8 to 5.4/1000, primarily because of improved detection and early termination of pregnancy. Fetal mortality from IUGR fell 60%, from 17.9 to 7.0/1000 births. However, the growth-restricted fetus had a greater than 10-fold increased risk for fetal death compared to an appropriately grown fetus.

Infant mortality during the past 20 years can be attributed most frequently to birth defects. In 1995, malformations were responsible for 22% of all infant deaths, one-third of which were caused by cardiac anomalies; chromosomal, respiratory, and nervous system defects were responsible for approximately 15% each.[7]

The pattern of perinatal death in the USA has changed during the past 30 years. According to data collected between 1959 and 1966 by the Collaborative Perinatal Project, 30% of perinatal deaths were attributed to complications of the cord and placenta.[8] Other major causes of perinatal death were unknown (21%), maternal and fetal infection (17%), prematurity (10%), congenital anomalies (8%), and erythroblastosis fetalis (4%). Lammer and colleagues[9] reviewed the causes of 574 fetal deaths in Massachusetts in 1982. For the first time in that state, the fetal mortality rate exceeded the neonatal mortality rate. Overall, 30% of fetal death was attributed to maternal disease such as hypertension and diabetes, 28% to hypoxia, 12% to congenital anomalies, and 4% to infection. Ten percent of fetal death occurred in multiple gestations, giving a fetal mortality rate of 50 per 1000. This was seven times the rate of women with singleton pregnancies. Fetal death was higher among women who were older than age 34, younger than age 20, unmarried, black, of parity of five or greater, and received no prenatal care or care in the third trimester only. Data from Denmark also confirmed that the highest fetal death rate was found in teenagers and women over age 35.[10,11]

Most fetal deaths occur before 32 weeks' gestation. However, as pregnancy progresses, the risk of intrauterine fetal demise increases among high-risk patients. To plan a strategy for antepartum fetal testing, one must examine the risk of fetal death in a population of women still pregnant at that point in pregnancy.[12,13] When this approach is taken, one finds that fetuses at 40–41 weeks are at a threefold greater risk of intrauterine death than are fetuses at 28–31 weeks, and fetuses at 42 weeks or more are at a 12-fold greater risk.[13]

Sensitivity, specificity, positive and negative predictive value

Any test of fetal well-being should ideally meet several criteria:

1 The test reliably predicts the fetus at risk for hypoxia.
2 The test reduces the risk of fetal death.
3 A false-positive test does not materially increase the risk of poor outcome to the patient or the fetus.
4 If an abnormality is detected, treatment options are available.
5 The test provides information not already apparent from the patient's clinical status.
6 The information is helpful to patient management.

Screening tests are applied broadly to healthy patients. The small screen-positive group subsequently undergoes more costly, potentially more invasive, confirmatory testing. In obstetrics, the sensitivity of most tests is limited by a low prevalence of conditions which lead to intrauterine fetal death, and by the variability of the normal fetal neurologic state.

The prevalence of an abnormal condition is directly proportional to the predictive value of its screening test. When fetal tests are applied widely to populations with low disease prevalence, the tests' sensitivity is generally low. Because a missed diagnosis of fetal hypoxia may result in lifelong neurologic problems, most obstetricians accept tests of low sensitivity in clinical practice. While tests of high sensitivity are ideal, the low prevalence of the most worrisome obstetric conditions, coupled with the need to identify all fetuses at risk, has created acceptance of tests which have a high false-positive rate, a low sensitivity, and a low positive predictive value. When interpreting the results of studies of antepartum testing, the obstetrician must consider the application of that test to his or her own population. If the population is at greater risk of poor fetal outcomes, the likelihood is greater that an abnormal test will be associated with an abnormal fetus. If the population is generally low-risk, an abnormal test will more likely be associated with a false-positive diagnosis.

Given the frequency of false-positive tests in obstetrics, to act upon a single test could result in iatrogenic prematurity. In this setting, multiple tests may be helpful. Multiple normal tests tend to exclude disease, while additional abnormal tests support the diagnosis of disease and may merit intervention.

The fetal neurologic state

During the third trimester, the normal fetal neurologic state varies markedly,[14,15] and limits the sensitivity of fetal testing. The fetus may spend up to 25% of its time in quiet sleep, a condition during which fetal testing may appear nonreassuring. During quiet, non-rapid eye movement (REM), sleep, the fetal heart rate slows and heart rate variability is reduced. Breathing and startle movements may be infrequent. Electrocortical activity recordings reveal high-voltage, low-frequency waves. Near term, periods of quiet sleep may last 20 min, and those of active sleep approximately 40 min.[15] The mechanisms that control these periods of rest and activity in the fetus are not well established. Active sleep, in which the fetus spends approximately 60–70% of its time, is associated with REM. The fetus exhibits regular breathing movements, intermittent abrupt movements of its head, limbs, and trunk, increased variability of its heart rate and frequent accelerations with movement, all of which are reassuring, as discussed below.

Biophysical techniques of fetal evaluation

During the 1970s and early 1980s biochemical tests such as human placental lactogen and estriol were considered the optimal methods of fetal evaluation. These tests have since fallen out of favor, replaced by more sensitive and less cumbersome biophysical surveillance techniques. The most commonly used tests are the CST, the NST, maternal perception of fetal movement, and the BPP.

Antenatal tests are limited in their scope. They can often identify chronic events such as progressive metabolic acidosis, though the point at which a fetus experiences long- or short-term negative sequelae from mild acidemia is unknown. Antenatal tests may not predict acute events such as umbilical cord accidents or placental abruption. The tests may be influenced by prematurity, maternal medication exposure, fetal sleep–wake cycle, and fetal anomalies.

Contraction stress test

The first widely adopted test of fetal well-being was the CST, also called the oxytocin challenge test. The CST mimics the first stage of labor with uterine contractions, and thus indirectly assesses fetal–placental reserve. Uterine contractions reduce blood to the intervillous space, causing transient fetal hypoxia. The fetus at risk for uteroplacental insufficiency will demonstrate an abnormal response to contractions, forming the basis for this test. If fetal and placental reserve is poor, the fetus will often develop evidence of hypoxia that is not physiologic and may manifest late decelerations. A well-oxygenated fetus with good reserve should tolerate contractions without evidence of pathological hypoxia. The CST is performed during the antepartum period.

The CST should take place in the labor and delivery suite, or in an adjacent area with easy access to labor and delivery. The patient is placed in the semi-Fowler's position at a 30–45° angle, with a slight left tilt in order to avoid supine hypotension. Baseline fetal heart rate and uterine tone are simultaneously recorded for at least 10 min. Following this, the fetal heart rate is observed during three contractions of at least 40 s duration within 10 min. If there are no spontaneous uterine contractions, oxytocin is administered by an infusion pump at a rate of 0.5 mIU/min. The infusion rate is doubled every 20 min until adequate contractions have been achieved.[16] Nipple stimulation may be used to initiate or augment contractions, and may reduce testing time by half when used with oxytocin.[17] In one technique, the patient is instructed to rub one nipple through her clothing for 2 min, or until a contraction appears. If a contraction does not appear she should stop for 5 min and then repeat the process.

Although the CST has never been shown to cause premature labor,[18] it is contraindicated when preterm labor is a significant risk, such as in the setting of premature rupture of the membranes, cervical incompetence, or multiple gestation. The CST should also be avoided when labor is contraindicated, such as among patients with a prior classical cesarean section, placenta previa, or extensive uterine surgery.

How to interpret the test

The contraction stress test is interpreted as follows:[19]

Negative (normal): no late or significant variable decelerations

Positive: late decelerations following 50% or more contractions (regardless of contraction frequency)

Unsatisfactory: fewer than three contractions in 10 min, or a tracing that cannot be interpreted

Equivocal suspicious: intermittent late decelerations or suspicious variable decelerations

Equivocal hyperstimulatory: fetal heart rate decelerations in the presence of contractions lasting more than 90 s or more frequent than every 2 min

A negative (normal) CST is associated with good fetal outcome, permitting the obstetrician to prolong a high-risk pregnancy safely. The incidence of perinatal death within 1 week of a negative test is less than 1/1000.[20,21] A suspicious or equivocal CST should be repeated within 24 h. A positive CST merits further evaluation and possibly delivery, as it may indicate uteroplacental insufficiency. Variable decelerations seen during the CST suggest cord compression, often associated with oligohydramnios. In such cases, ultrasonography should be performed to assess amniotic fluid volume. Low amniotic fluid may reflect chronic stress, as fetal blood is shunted preferentially to the brain and away from the kidneys. A positive CST has been associated with an increased incidence of intrauterine death, late decelerations in labor, low 5-min Apgar scores, IUGR, and meconium-stained amniotic fluid.[21]

The CST is limited by a high false-positive rate. Supine hypotension decreases uterine perfusion and may cause transient fetal heart rate abnormalities, heart rate tracings may be misinterpreted, oxytocin or nipple stimulation may cause uterine hyperstimulation, or the fetal condition may improve after the CST has been performed.

In addition to high-risk pregnancies, the CST has also been used to assess low-risk postterm pregnancies. There were no perinatal deaths among 679 prolonged pregnancies evaluated primarily with the CST.[22] When both the NST and the nipple stimulation CST were used to determine the need for delivery, there were no antepartum deaths in a series of 819 patients tested at 40 weeks or more.[23]

Druzin et al. found the CST to be most beneficial as a test to follow up a nonreactive NST.[23] Otherwise, the CST provided no information that significantly improved antepartum or intrapartum outcome. Merrill et al.[24] evaluated all nonreactive NSTs with a CST and found that if the CST were negative and a biophysical profile (to be discussed later) were six or greater, the pregnancy could be prolonged for up to 13 days. This approach should be used only when prematurity is an issue and when careful follow-up with daily assessment can be performed reliably.

The CST obtained between 28 and 33 weeks' gestation appears as accurate as a test performed at a greater gestational age.

The nonstress test

Fetal heart rate monitoring, or cardiotocography, was developed during the 1960s as a means of evaluating the fetus in labor. The concept of fetal monitoring was eventually extrapolated to the developing fetus with the NST, CST, and BPP. The antenatal use of the NST in the assessment of fetal well-being has become an integral part of obstetric care.[16]

The NST is based on the observation that fetal heart rate accelerations reflect fetal well-being.[25] A "reactive" test is defined as the occurrence of two accelerations of 15 beats/min above the fetal heart rate baseline, lasting at least 15 s, during any 20-min period. A "nonreactive" test is one that does not meet the afore-mentioned criteria. A reactive NST suggests the absence of fetal hypoxia or asphyxia. The incidence of stillbirth within 1 week of a normal test, corrected for lethal congenital anomalies and unpredictable causes of in utero demise such as cord accidents or placental abruption, is approximately 1.9 per 1000.[21]

The basis for the NST

The premise behind the NST is that the well-oxygenated nonacidotic, nonimpaired fetus will temporarily accelerate its heart rate in response to movement. Regulation of the fetal heart rate and variability is complex and not entirely understood. The fetal heart rate is modulated by the vagal nerve and the sympathetic nervous system. Like the adult, the fetal heart has intrinsic pacemakers, including the sinoatrial (SA) and atrioventricular (AV) nodes. Both nodes are normally under continuous influence of the vagus nerve, which prevents the fetal heart from beating at its more rapid intrinsic rate. The interplay between the sympathetic and parasympathetic nervous systems results in beat-to-beat variability of the fetal heart rate, an important clinical predictor of fetal well-being.

In sheep, vagal influence increases fourfold during acute hypoxia,[26] while the influence of the sympathetic nervous system increases to a lesser degree. In sum, vagal influence over the fetal heart dominates sympathetic influence during hypoxia. Baroreceptors located in the aortic arch and carotid sinus immediately signal the vagus or glossopharyngeal nerve, increasing vagal influence and slowing the heart rate. Fetal hypoxia results in a compensatory bradycardia with hypertension. The fetus also has functioning chemoreceptors in the medulla oblongata and carotid and aortic bodies. Interaction between the fetal chemoreceptors is poorly understood.[26]

Uterine contractions reduce blood flow to the intervillous space, causing transient hypoxia. Using a sheep model, Parer[26] demonstrated that the abrupt cessation of uterine blood flow for 20 s in normally oxygenated sheep resulted in a delayed deceleration in the fetal heart rate, known now as a late deceleration. Pretreatment with atropine abolished any change in the fetal heart rate. The author concluded that chemoreceptors signal the vagus nerve to slow the heart during hypoxemic conditions, resulting in a deceleration of the heart rate following the contraction peak. Repetitive late decelerations suggest fetal hypoxemia.

When under hypoxic conditions, the fetus redistributes blood to its vital organs: the brain, heart, and adrenal glands. Blood is shunted away from the gut, spleen, and kidneys, leading to oligohydramnios. This, along with compensatory mechanisms such as decreased total oxygen consumption and anaerobic glycolysis, allows the fetus to survive for periods of up to 30 min in conditions of decreased oxygen.

Loss of reactivity is associated most commonly with a fetal sleep cycle, but may result from any cause of central nervous system depression, the most ominous being fetal acidosis.

When to perform the NST

The NST, or cardiotocography, can identify the suboptimally oxygenated fetus, and provides the opportunity for intervention before progressive metabolic acidosis results in morbidity or death. Patients with risk factors for uteroplacental insufficiency should undergo NST. In general, this includes maternal disease such as diabetes, hypertensive disorders, Rh-sensitization, antiphospholipid syndrome, poorly controlled hyperthyroidism, hemoglobinopathies, chronic renal disease, systemic lupus erythematosus, and pulmonary disease, also fetal–placental conditions such as IUGR, decreased movement, oligo- or polyhydramnios, and finally other situations of increased risk such as multiple gestation, pregnancies past their due date, poor obstetric history, and bleeding.

Identifying the appropriate time to initiate fetal testing depends on several factors, including the prognosis for neonatal survival, the risk of intrauterine fetal death, the degree of maternal disease, and the potential for a false-positive test leading to iatrogenic prematurity. Most high-risk patients begin NSTs between 32 and 34 weeks, and are tested weekly.

The NST is generally not recommended prior to 26 weeks.[19] An NST should be performed only after viability, when intervention for a nonreassuring test is an option. The limit of viability is poorly defined. Recent survival rates of neonates born at 22 and 23 weeks have been reported at 21% and 30%, respectively.[27] However, given the significant morbidity associated with birth at these gestational ages, testing and intervention prior to 24 weeks' gestation are controversial and should be evaluated on a case-by-case basis only.

How to perform the test

The fetal heart rate is monitored using a Doppler ultrasound transducer attached with a belt to the maternal abdomen. At the same time, a tocodynameter is applied to the maternal abdomen to monitor for uterine contractions or fetal movement. Signals from the Doppler transducer and tocodynameter are then relayed to tracing paper. Ideally, the patient should not have smoked cigarettes recently, as this has been shown to interfere with the NST.[28]

How to interpret the test

Using the most common definition, a normal or "reactive" test is when the fetal heart rate accelerates 15 beats/min from the baseline, for 15 s, twice during a 20-min period.[29] A nonreactive NST is one that lacks these accelerations during 40 min of testing.

A reactive NST is associated with fetal survival for at least 1 week in more than 99% of patients.[30] In the largest series of NSTs, the stillbirth rate among 5861 tests was 1.9 per 1000, when corrected for lethal anomalies and unpredictable causes of demise.[31] The negative predictive value of the NST is 99.8%.[21] The low false-negative rate depends on the appropriate follow-up of significant changes in maternal status or perception of fetal movement. The false-positive rate of the nonreactive NST is quite high. A nonreactive NST must be evaluated further, unless the fetus is extremely premature.

The fetal ability to generate a reactive heart rate tracing depends on gestational age, as it likely reflects the maturation of the parasympathetic and sympathetic nervous systems. Druzin et al. demonstrated that, among women who delivered infants with normal Apgar scores, 73% had nonreactive NSTs between 20 and 24 weeks' gestation, 50% were nonreactive between 24 and 32 weeks, and 88% became reactive by 30 weeks. Between 32 and 36 weeks, 98% were reactive.[32]

The high incidence of the false-positive nonreactive NST is primarily due to the normal quiet fetal sleep state. The near-term fetus has four neurologic states, described as 1F, 2F, 3F, and 4F. State 1F is a period of quiet sleep in which the fetus spends approximately 25% of its time. This state may last up to 70 min. During this time the fetal heart rate has few accelerations and reduced variability, and the fetus demonstrates only occasional gross body movements. The fetus spends 60–70% of its time in state 2F, or active sleep. During this time, heart rate variability and accelerations are increased, as are body and eye movements. During state 3F, eye and body movements are common, but accelerations are diminished. State 4F is characterized by continuous movement, and constant fetal heart rate accelerations and variability are seen. While a nonreactive NST may reflect sleep state 1F, it alternatively might indicate fetal compromise and must be evaluated further.

Fetal bradycardia during routine antepartum testing is potentially ominous, and merits further evaluation or delivery. Bradycardia, defined in some studies as a slowing of the fetal heart rate of 40–90 beats/min lasting for at least 60s, has been associated with stillbirth,[33] significant cord compression, meconium passage, congenital abnormalities, and abnormal heart rate patterns in labor.[34] In a study of 121 cases of antepartum fetal bradycardia managed by active intervention and delivery, there were no fetal deaths.[34]

Efficacy

To date there are no prospective, double-blinded, randomized controlled trials of the use of the NST to reduce perinatal morbidity or mortality. The NST was widely adopted without demonstration of benefit among well-conducted trials. Observational studies have shown a correlation between abnormal NSTs and poor fetal outcome.[35]

Four randomized controlled trials of NST among intermediate- and high-risk patients failed to show reduction in perinatal morbidity or mortality due to asphyxia.[36–39] The study populations ranged from 300 to 550 patients, and lacked sufficient power to assess low-prevalence events such as perinatal mortality. A metaanalysis of these four trials also lacked the power to demonstrate a difference.[40] The metaanalysis demonstrated a trend toward increased perinatal morbidity among the tested group, although most of the deaths in the tested group were considered unavoidable, and reflect a weakness of the studies. NST did not lead to early delivery when compared to controls. The authors of the metaanalysis acknowledge that these trials are old, dating from the introduction and widespread use of NST, were not double-blinded, and vary in quality. Practice styles and interpretation of the tests may have since changed.

Given the current medical–legal climate, a randomized, double-blinded controlled trial is unlikely to be performed as use of the NST has become the standard of care. Further, given the fact that adverse outcomes such as fetal death are uncommon even among high-risk populations, any investigation would require enormous patient enrollment.[41]

Several retrospective studies have suggested that the NST decreases perinatal mortality in the tested, high-risk population. Schneider et al.[42] reviewed their experience with antenatal testing from 1974 to 1983, before antenatal testing was widespread. The authors utilized the contraction stress test for the first 2 years of study period, and the NST for the remaining 7 years. They found that perinatal mortality was 2.24% in the nontested population and 0.12% in the high-risk tested population. Studies such as these fueled the widespread adaptation of the NST as a means of fetal assessment.

Vibroacoustic stimulation

To differentiate whether a nonreactive NST is due to the quiet fetal sleep state or to fetal compromise, vibroacoustic stimulation (VAS) is performed. VAS, the application of a vibratory stimulus to the patient's abdomen above the fetal vertex, increases the NST's sensitivity without adversely affecting perinatal outcome.[43–45] VAS creates a startle response in the noncompromised fetus, resulting in fetal heart accelerations.[46] The stimulus should be applied for at least 3 s.

VAS increases the NST's positive predictive value. Smith et al. found the PPV for fetal well-being of a VAS-induced reactive NST to be 99%, compared with 87–99% for a spontaneously reactive NST.[43] The incidence of fetal death within 7 days of a VAS-induced reactive NST was similar to that of a spontaneously reactive NST (1.9 v 1.6/1000 fetuses). There were no significant differences in Apgar scores, operative intervention, or meconium staining between groups.

The fetal response to VAS relies on an intact and mature auditory system. Anencephalic fetuses do not manifest heart rate accelerations in response to VAS.[47] The blink–startle response to VAS does not occur prior to 24 weeks, and is seen consistently only after 28–31 weeks.[48,49] The incidence of reactivity after VAS increases significantly after 26 weeks.[50]

The intensity and duration of the stimulus are

important. A stimulus lasting for 3–5 s significantly increases fetal heart rate accelerations, while no difference is seen with a 1-s VAS.[51]

If VAS fails to achieve a reactive NST, a BPP should be performed, as described later in this text.

Maternal perception of fetal movement

Maternal perception of fetal movement, or fetal "kick counts," is an inexpensive, easily implemented, reliable test of fetal well-being and may be ideal for routine antepartum fetal surveillance.

The normal fetus is active. Studies using real-time ultrasound show that, during the third trimester, the fetus generates gross body movements 10% of the time, making 30 such movements each hour.[52] Most women can perceive 70–80% of gross body movements. The fetus also makes fine body movements, more difficult to perceive, such as limb flexion and extension, sucking, and hand grasping. Fine body movements probably reflect more coordinated central nervous function. Decreased maternal perception of fetal movement often precedes fetal death, sometimes by several days.[53] Cessation of fetal movement has been correlated with a mean umbilical venous pH of 7.16.[54] Several studies have shown that maternal awareness of changes in fetal activity can prevent unexplained fetal death.

There are several protocols for monitoring fetal movement. Using Cardiff Count-to-Ten, a woman starts counting fetal movements in the morning and records the time needed to reach 10 movements. The optimal number of fetal movements has not been established. However, there were at least 10 movements per 12-h period in 97.5% of movement periods recorded by women who delivered healthy babies.[53] The ACOG recommends having the patient count movements while lying on her side. Her perception of 10 movements within 2 h is considered acceptable.[19]

Fetal movement-counting protocols have been shown to decrease fetal demise. In a prospective, randomized trial, 1562 women counted movements three times a week, 2h after their largest meal, starting after 32 weeks' gestation. Fewer than three fetal movements each hour prompted further evaluation with a NST and ultrasound. One stillbirth occurred in the monitored group, while 10 occurred in a comparable control group of 1549 women ($P<0.05$).[55] In a cohort study, Moore and Piacquadio[56] demonstrated a substantial reduction in fetal death using the Cardiff Count-to-Ten approach. Women were asked to monitor fetal movements in the evening, typically a time of increased activity. On average, women observed 10 movements by 21 min. Patients who failed to perceive 10 movements within 2 hours were told to report immediately to the hospital for further evaluation. Compliance was greater than 90%. As a control, the authors used a 7-month period preceding the study when no instructions were given regarding fetal movement counting. The fetal death rate during the study period was 2.1/1000, substantially lower than 8.7/1000 among 2519 patients during the control period. Of the 290 patients who presented with decreased fetal movement in the Cardiff Count-to-Ten group, only one presented after fetal death had occurred. Antepartum testing to assess patients with decreased fetal activity increased 13% during the study period. During the control period, 247 women presented to the hospital with decreased fetal movement, 11 of whom had already suffered an intrauterine fetal death.[56] The study of intensive maternal surveillance was expanded to include almost 6000 patients. A fetal death rate of 3.6/1000 was achieved – less than half the rate observed during the control period.[57]

The only other prospective, randomized trial in the literature suggests that there is no benefit to increased surveillance of fetal activity. Grant and coworkers[58] randomized 68 000 European women to fetal movement counting using the Cardiff Count-to-Ten method, or to standard care. Women counted movements for nearly 3 h per day. Approximately 7% of patients experienced at least one episode of decreased movement. The antepartum death rate for normal, singleton fetuses was equal in both groups (2.9/1000 among the study group versus

2.7/1000 among controls). This study contains serious flaws and should be interpreted with caution. Compliance for reporting decreased fetal movement among the study group was low – only 46%. Compliance was even lower among study patients who suffered a fetal death. Of the 17 study patients who later experienced an intrauterine fetal demise, none received emergency intervention when she presented to the hospital complaining of decreased fetal movement. Why? Grant et al. ascribed the lack of intervention to errors of clinical judgment and to falsely reassuring follow-up testing. One might conclude that this large prospective study disproves the benefit of fetal kick counts. To the contrary, the study clearly demonstrates the need for appropriate interventions, and follow-up of patients who present complaining of decreased fetal activity.

Maternal perception of fetal movement is influenced by several factors. An anterior placenta, polyhydramnios, and maternal obesity can decrease perception of fetal movement.[59] Movements lasting 20–60 s are more likely to be felt by the mother.[60] Fetal anomalies, sometimes associated with polyhydramnios, were linked in one study with decreased movement perception in 26% of cases, as compared with 4% of normal controls.[61]

Fetal activity does not increase in response to food or glucose administration, despite popular belief.[62,63] Hypoglycemia is associated with increased fetal movement.[64] Normal fetal activity ranges widely, and each mother and fetus serve as their own control. Fetal movements tend to peak between 9 p.m. and 1 a.m., when maternal glucose levels are falling.[65]

Intensive maternal surveillance of fetal activity helps to identify fetuses at risk for death due to chronic insult. "Kick counts" are unlikely to prevent an acute event such as fetal death caused by cord prolapse. Charting fetal movement may increase anxiety for some,[66,67] but generally reassures most women and may enhance maternal–fetal attachment. When educated and encouraged, women are more likely to present early if they experience decreased fetal movement.

The biophysical profile

The discovery that decreased fetal activity is associated with hypoxia, combined with the 1970's development of B-mode ultrasound which allowed for real-time observation of the fetus, led to the creation of the BPP. Hypoxic animals reduce activity in order to conserve oxygen. By decreasing movement and employing other protective mechanisms, the hypoxic fetus can reduce oxygen consumption by up to 19% minutes into a hypoxic event.[68] Observation of such reduction in movement can provide clues into the fetus's acid–base status.

The BPP is based upon a 10-point score. The fetus receives two points for the presence of each of the following:

1 Reactive NST
2 Fetal breathing movement
3 Gross body movement
4 Fetal tone
5 Amniotic fluid volume

The lower the BPP, the greater the risk of fetal asphyxia.

A BPP is typically performed to evaluate a nonreactive or nonreassuring NST. It may be used for other indications, such as the evaluation of a fetus with an abnormal cardiac rhythm. Given the variation in the normal fetal neurologic state, an abnormal test should be evaluated by extending the testing time or repeating the test shortly thereafter in order to distinguish quiet sleep from asphyxia. VAS during the BPP can change the fetal behavioral state and improve the score without increasing the false-negative rate.[69]

The BPP has been shown to have 90% sensitivity, 96% specificity, 82% positive predictive value, and 98% negative predictive value for cord arterial pH of less than 7.20.[70] The incidence of intrauterine fetal demise within 7 days of a normal BPP ranges from 0.411 to 1.01 per 1000.[71] Manning[72] recently discovered a significant relationship between the risk of cerebral palsy and a decreased BPP. While controlling for gestational age, birth weight, and timing of injury, the incidence of cerebral palsy was 0.7 per 1000 live births for a normal BPP score, 13.1 per 1000 live births for a score of 6, and 333 per 1000 live births for a score of 0.

The BPP correlates well with acid–base status. By performing BPPs immediately prior to cordocentesis, Manning et al. demonstrated that a nonreactive NST and an otherwise normal BPP correlated with a mean umbilical vein pH of 7.28 (±0.11).[54] Fetuses with abnormal movement had an umbilical vein pH of 7.16 (±0.08) Vintzileos et al.[70] evaluated 124 patients undergoing cesarean section prior to labor. All patients underwent a BPP prior to surgery, followed by cord pH at delivery. Reasons for delivery included severe preeclampsia, growth restriction, placenta previa, breech presentation, fetal macrosomia, and elective repeat cesarean section. Acidosis was defined as a cord pH less than 7.20. The earliest biophysical signs of acidosis were a nonreactive NST and loss of fetal breathing movements. Among patients with a BPP of eight or more, the mean arterial pH was 7.28. Two of 102 fetuses were acidotic. Nine fetuses with scores of four or less had a mean arterial pH of 6.99. These data suggest that the NST is the most sensitive of the biophysical tests, followed by fetal breathing movements. Fetal movement is the least sensitive, ceasing at the lowest pH. The NST may be omitted from the BPP without fetal compromise if the other four components are normal.[73] Manning et al. postulate that the graded biophysical response to hypoxia is due to variation in sensitivity of the central nervous system regulatory centers.

Fetal adaptation to chronic hypoxemia may occur eventually, lowering the pH threshold of the biophysical response. This might explain why a chronically stressed fetus can die shortly after a reactive NST, and why oligohydramnios, which may reflect chronic hypoxia and reshunting of blood from the kidneys to the brain, is associated with increased morbidity and mortality regardless of other test results. The lowered threshold likely results from a shift in the hemoglobin dissociation curve, improved fetal extraction of maternal oxygen, and an increase in fetal hemoglobin. Manning postulates that resetting of the central nervous system threshold may occur in part because some biophysical activity is necessary, especially for limb and lung development.[71]

Recent studies suggest that antenatal corticosteriods may adversely affect the BPP, decreasing the score. Antenatal steroids are administered most commonly between 24 and 34 weeks, when premature delivery is anticipated. Kelly et al.[74] reported that among one-third of fetuses who received steroids between 28 and 34 weeks, BPP scores were decreased. The effect was seen within 48 h of corticosteroid administration. Repeat BPPs performed within 24–48 h were normal in cases where the BPP score had decreased by 4 points. Neonatal outcome was not affected. Similarly, Deren et al.[75] reported transient suppression of heart rate reactivity, breathing movements, and movement when corticosteroids were administered at less than 34 weeks' gestation. These changes were transient and returned to normal by 48–96 h. This effect must be considered at institutions where BPPs are used to evaluate the fetus.

A modified BPP, which uses only the NST and amniotic fluid index, may be used in lieu of the full biophysical profile to identify the at-risk fetus.[76] The amniotic fluid index is an ultrasound measurement, calculated by adding the length of the largest vertical fluid pockets free of umbilical cord in the four quadrants of the gravid uterus. If either the NST is nonreactive or the amniotic fluid index is less than 5.0, further evaluation is mandated. Delivery is indicated if the fetus is full-term.

Doppler

Doppler ultrasound is used primarily to assess placental insufficiency and IUGR.[77,78]

Blood flow through arteries supplying low-impedance vascular beds, such as the placenta, normally flow forward during systole and diastole. Diastolic forward flow in the umbilical artery is high during a normal pregnancy, and increases more than systolic flow. As gestation advances, placental resistance normally decreases, and the systolic to diastolic (S/D) ratio should decrease.[79] An increased S/D ratio suggests an increase in placental resistance.[80,81]

If the placenta is compromised, diastolic flow may be absent or reversed. This eventually leads to IUGR. Absent end-diastolic flow is associated with increased perinatal morbidity and mortality. Reversed end-diastolic flow is even more predictive of poor perinatal outcome. Farine et al. summarized data from 31 studies of 904 fetuses demonstrating absent or reversed end-diastolic velocities.[82] Perinatal mortality was 36%. Eighty percent of the fetuses weighed less than the 10th percentile for gestational age. Abnormal karyotypes were found in 6%, and malformations in 11%. Absent or reversed end-diastolic flow in the umbilical artery, while not an indication for immediate delivery, is considered an indication for intensive ongoing fetal surveillance. Delivery is usually based on results of fetal heart rate monitoring or of the BPP, depending on maternal condition and gestational age.

Studies support the use of Doppler to assess high-risk pregnancies. A metaanalysis of six published randomized controlled clinical trials of 2102 fetuses followed with Doppler compared to 2133 controls demonstrated a reduction in perinatal morality with Doppler.[83] An analysis of 12 published and unpublished randomized controlled clinical trials in 7474 high-risk patients revealed fewer antenatal admissions, inductions of labor, cesarean deliveries for fetal distress, and a lower perinatal mortality among high-risk pregnancies monitored with Doppler.[84] A recent report by Neilson and Alfirevic confirmed these findings.[85] Doppler ultrasound appears to reduce perinatal mortality without increasing maternal or neonatal morbidity among patients with high-risk pregnancies.[86] Studies of the use of Doppler ultrasound in low-risk pregnancies have not shown a benefit.[87]

Investigators have reported Doppler investigation of several different arteries, such as the middle cerebral and splenic arteries. However, the umbilical arteries are most commonly used because their large size, lack of branches, and length make them easy to identify and study. Doppler studies are commonly conducted later in pregnancy. Prior to 15 weeks' gestation one cannot consistently identify diastolic flow in the umbilical artery.[88]

Fetuses with congenital malformations and chromosomal abnormalities may demonstrate markedly abnormal Doppler studies.

Summary

Antepartum testing of fetal well-being should reduce perinatal morbidity and mortality. The prevalence of an abnormal condition significantly impacts the predictive value of antepartum fetal tests. When any test is applied widely to a low-prevalence population, the sensitivity of the test is reduced. Obstetrical intervention based on false-positive fetal evaluation is justified based on the severe consequences of a missed diagnosis. The complete clinical situation should be considered when decisions are made to intervene in a pregnancy based on results of fetal evaluation techniques.

The incidence of stillbirth within 1 week of a negative CST test is less than 1/1000, and for a reactive NST, 1.9/1000.

The high false-positive rate of antepartum fetal tests is due in part to the fact that the near-term fetus spends approximately 25% of its time in a quiet sleep state. To design a strategy to reduce perinatal morbidity and mortality, maneuvers such as VAS, serial testing, and careful selection of patients tested should be employed given the high false-positive rates and low prevalence of the most serious conditions.

REFERENCES

1 Centers for Disease Control and Prevention, NCHS, National Vital Statistics System. (2000) *Vital statistics of the United States*, vol. II, *Mortality*, Part A; *Infant Mortality Rates, Fetal Mortality Rates, and Perinatal Mortality Rates, According to Race: United States, Selected Years 1950–1998.* Public Health Service. Washington: US Government Printing Office.

2 Fried A, Rochat R. (1985) Maternal mortality and perinatal mortality: definitions, data, and epidemiology. In Sachs B (ed.) *Obstetric Epidemiology*, p. 35. Littleton, MA: PSG.

3 American College of Obstetricians and Gynecologists. (1995) *Perinatal and Infant Mortality Statistics.* Committee Opinion 167. Washington, DC: ACOG.

4 US Department of Health and Human Services. (1995) *ChildHealth USA '94*. Washington, DC: US Government Printing Office.

5 Fretts RC, Boyd ME, Usher RH et al. (1992) The changing pattern of fetal death, 1961–1988. *Obstet Gynecol* 79:35–39.

6 Fretts RC, Schmittdiel J, McLean FH et al. (1995) Increased maternal age and the risk of fetal death. *N Engl J Med* 333:953–957.

7 Morbidity and Mortality Weekly Report. (2000) Trends in infant mortality attributable to birth defects – United States, 1980–1995. Massachusetts Medical Society.

8 Naeye RL. (1977) Causes of perinatal mortality in the United States Collaborative Perinatal Project. *JAMA* 238:228–229.

9 Lammer EJ, Brown LE, Anderka MR et al. (1989) Classification and analysis of fetal deaths in Massachussetts. *JAMA* 261:1757–1762.

10 Nybo Andersen AM, Wohlfahrt J, Christens P et al. (2000) Maternal age and fetal loss: population based register linkage study. *Br Med J* 320:1708–1712.

11 Stein Z, Susser M. (2000) The risks of having children later in life. *Br Med J* 320:1681–1682.

12 Grant A, Elbourne D. (1989) Fetal movement counting to assess fetal well-being. In Chalmers I, Enkin M, Keirse MJNC (eds) *Effective Care in Pregnancy and Childbirth*, p. 440. Oxford: Oxford University Press.

13 Cotzias CS, Paterson-Brown S, Fisk NM. (1999) Prospective risk of unexplained stillbirth in singleton pregnancies at term: population based analysis. *Br Med J* 319:282–288.

14 Manning FA. (1985) Assessment of fetal condition and risk: analysis of single and combined biophysical variable monitoring. *Semin Perinatol* 9:168–183.

15 Van Woerden EE, VanGeijn HP. (1992) Heart-rate patterns and fetal movements. In Nijhuis J (ed.) *Fetal Behaviour*, p. 41. New York: Oxford University Press.

16 Antepartum fetal surveillance. (1994) *Am Coll Obstet Gynecol Tech Bull* 188.

17 Huddleston JF, Sutliff G, Robinson D. (1984) Contraction stress test by intermittent nipple stimulation. *Obstet Gynecol* 63:669–673.

18 Braly P, Freeman R, Garite T et al. (1981) Incidence of premature delivery following the oxytocin challenge test. *Am J Obstet Gynecol* 141:5–8.

19 ACOG Practice Bulletin. (1999) Antepartum fetal surveillance. Number 9.

20 Nageotte MP, Towers CV, Asrat T et al. (1994) The value of a negative antepartum test: contraction stress test and modified biophysical profile. *Obstet Gynecol* 84:231–234.

21 Freeman R, Anderson G, Dorchester W. (1982) A prospective multi-institutional study of antepartum fetal heart rate monitoring. I. Risk of perinatal mortality and morbidity according to antepartum fetal heart rate test results. *Am J Obstet Gynecol* 143:771–777.

22 Freeman R, Garite T, Mondanlou H et al. (1981) Postdate pregnancy: utilization of contraction stress testing for primary fetal surveillance. *Am J Obstet Gynecol* 140:128–135.

23 Druzin ML, Karver ML, Wagner W et al. (1992) Prospective evaluation of the contraction stress test and non stress tests in the management of post-term pregnancy. *Surg Gynecol Obstet* 174:507–512.

24 Merrill PM, Porto M, Lovett SM et al. (1995) Evaluation of the non-reactive positive contraction stress test prior to 32 weeks: the role of the biophysical profile. *Am J Perinatol* 12:229–237.

25 Hammacher K. (1969) The clinical significance of cardiotocography. In Huntingford P, Huter K, Saling E (eds) *Perinatal Medicine*, p. 80. 1st European Congress, Berlin. San Diego: Academic Press.

26 Parer JT. (1994) Fetal heart rate. In Creasy RK and Resnick R (eds) *Maternal–Fetal Medicine: Principles and Practice*, 3rd edn. W.B. Saunders.

27 Lemons JA, Bauer CR, Oh W. (2001) Very low birth weight outcomes of the National Institute of Child Health and Human Development Neonatal Research Network, January 1995 through December 1996. *Pediatrics* 107:1.

28 Graca LM, Cardoso CG, Clode N et al. (1991) Acute effects of maternal cigarette smoking on fetal heart rate and fetal body movements felt by the mother. *J Perinat Med* 19:385–390.

29 Lavery J. (1982) Nonstress fetal heart rate testing. *Clin Obstet Gynecol* 25:689–705.

30 Schifrin B, Foye G, Amato J et al. (1979) Routine fetal heart rate monitoring in the antepartum period. *Obstet Gynecol* 54:21–25.

31 Miller DA, Rabello YA, Paul RH. (1996) The modified biophysical profile: antepartum testing in the 1990s. *Am J Obstet Gynecol* 174:812–817.

32 Druzin ML, Fox A, Kogut E et al. (1985) The relationship of the nonstress test to gestational age. *Am J Obstet Gynecol* 153:386–389.

33 Dashow EE, Read JA. (1984) Significant fetal bradycardia during antepartum heart rate testing. *Am J Obstet Gynecol* 148:187–190.

34 Druzin ML. (1989) Fetal bradycardia during antepartum testing. *J Reprod Med* 34:1.

35 Phelan JP. (1981) The nonstress test: a review of 3000 tests. *Am J Obstet Gynecol* 139:7–10.

36 Brown VA, Sawers RS, Parsons RJ et al. (1982) The value of antenatal cardiotocography in the management of high risk

pregnancy: a randomised controlled trial. *Br J Obstet Gynaecol* 89:716–722.
37 Flynn A, Kelly J, Mansfield H et al. (1982) A randomized controlled trial of non-stress antepartum cardiotocography. *Br J Obstet Gynaecol* 89:427–433.
38 Kidd L, Patel N, Smith R. (1985) Non-stress antenatal cardiotocography-a prospective randomized clinical trial. *Br J Obstet Gynaecol* 92:1156–1159.
39 Lumley J, Lester A, Anderson I et al. (1993) A randomised trial of weekly cardiotocography in high risk obstetric patients. *Br J Obstet Gynaecol* 90:1018–1026.
40 Pattison N, McCowan L. (2000) Cardiotocography for antepartum fetal assessment. Cochrane Database of Systematic Reviews (Issue 4).
41 Thornton JG, Lilford RJ. (1993) Do we need randomised trials of antenatal tests of fetal wellbeing? *Br J Obstet Gynaecol* 100:197–200.
42 Schneider EP, Hutson JM, Petrie RH. (1988) An assessment of the first decade's experience with antepartum fetal heart rate testing. *Am J Perinatol* 5:134.
43 Smith CV, Phelan JP, Broussard PM et al. (1988) Fetal acoustic stimulation testing III. Prediction value of a reactive test. *J Reprod Med* 33:217–218.
44 Sarno AP, Bruner JP. (1990) Fetal acoustic stimulation as a possible adjunct to diagnostic ultrasound: a preliminary report. *Obstet Gynecol* 76:668–690.
45 Serafini P, Lindsay MBJ, Nagey DA et al. (1984) Antepartum fetal heart rate response to sound stimulation, the acoustic stimulation test. *Am J Obstet Gynecol* 148:41–45.
46 Divon MY, Platt LD, Cantrell CJ. (1985) Evoked fetal startle response: a possible intrauterine neurological examination. *Am J Obstet Gynecol* 153:454–456.
47 Ohel G, Simon A, Linder N et al. (1986) Anencephaly and the nature of fetal response to vibroacoustic stimulation. *Am J Perinatol* 3:345–346.
48 Birnholz JC, Benacerraf BR. (1983) The development of fetal hearing. *Science* 148:41–45.
49 Crade M, Lovett S. (1988) Fetal response to sound stimulation: preliminary report exploring use of sound stimulation in routine obstetrical ultrasound examination. *J Ultrasound Med* 7:499–503.
50 Druzin ML, Edersheim TG, Hutson JM. (1989) The effect of vibroacoustic stimulation on the nonstress test at gestational ages of thirty-two weeks or less. *Am J Obstet Gynecol* 1661:1476–1478.
51 Pietrantoni M, Angel JL, Parsons MT et al. (1991) Human fetal response to vibroacoustic stimulation as a function of stimulus duration. *Obstet Gynecol* 78:807–911.
52 Patrick J, Campbell K, Carmichael L et al. (1982) Patterns of gross fetal body movements over 24-hour observation intervals during the last 10 weeks of pregnancy. *Am J Obstet Gynecol* 142:363–371.
53 Pearson JF, Weaver JB. (1976) Fetal activity and fetal wellbeing: an evaluation. *Br Med J* 1:1305–1307.
54 Manning FA, Snijders R, Harman CR et al. (1993) Fetal biophysical profile score. VI. Correlation with antepartum umbilical venous pH. *Am J Obstet Gynecol* 169:755–763.
55 Neldam S. (1983) Fetal movements as an indicator of fetal well being. *Dan Med Bull* 30:274–278.
56 Moore TR, Piacquadio K. (1989) A prospective evaluation of fetal movement screening to reduce the incidence of antepartum fetal death. *Am J Obstet Gynecol* 160:1075–1080.
57 Elbourne D, Grant A. (1990) Study results vary in count-to-10 method of fetal movement screening. *Am J Obstet Gynecol* 163:264–265.
58 Grant A, Valentin L, Elbourne D. (1989) Routine formal fetal movement counting and risk of antepartum late death in normally formed singletons. *Lancet* 2:345–349.
59 Sorokin Y, Kierker L. (1982) Fetal movement. *Clin Obstet Gynecol* 25:719–734.
60 Johnson TR, Jordan ET, Paine LL. (1990) Doppler recordings of fetal movement: II. Comparison with maternal perception. *Obstet Gynecol* 76:42–43.
61 Rayburn W, Barr M. (1982) Activity patterns in malformed fetuses. *Am J Obstet Gynecol* 142:1045–1048.
62 Phelan JP, Kester R, Labudovich ML. (1982) Nonstress test and maternal glucose determinations. *Obstet Gynecol* 60:437–439.
63 Druzin ML, Foodim J. (1982) Effect of maternal glucose ingestion compared with maternal water ingestion on the nonstress test. *Obstet Gynecol* 67:425–426.
64 Holden K, Jovanovic L, Druzin M et al. (1984) Increased fetal activity with low maternal blood glucose levels in pregnancies complicated by diabetes. *Am J Perinatol* 1:161–164.
65 Schwartz RM, Luby AM, Scanlon JW et al. (1994) Effect of surfactant on morbidity, mortality and resource use in newborn infants weighing 500–1500 grams. *N Engl J Med* 330:1476–1480.
66 Draper J, Field S, Thomas H. (1986) Women's views on keeping fetal movement charts. *Br J Obstet Gynaecol* 93:334–338.
67 Mikhail MS, Freda MC, Merkatz RB et al. (1991) The effect of fetal movement counting on maternal attachment to fetus. *Am J Obstet Gynecol* 165:988–991.
68 Rurak DW, Gruber NC. (1983) Effect of neuromuscular blockade on oxygen consumption and blood gases. *Am J Obstet Gynecol* 145:258–262.
69 Inglis SR, Druzin ML, Wagner WE et al. (1993) The use of vi-

broacoustic stimulation during the abnormal or equivocal biophysical profile. *Obstet Gynecol* 82:371–374.

70 Vintzileos AM, Gaffrey SE, Salinger IM et al. (1987) The relationship between fetal biophysical profile score and cord pH in patients undergoing cesarean section before the onset of labour. *Obstet Gynecol* 70:196–201.

71 Manning F. (1999) Fetal assessment by evaluation of biophysical variables: fetal biophysical profile score. In Creasy R and Resnik R (eds) *Maternal–Fetal Medicine*. Philadelphia, PA: W.B. Saunders.

72 Manning FA. (1999) Fetal biophysical profile. *Obstet Gynecol Clin North Am* 26:557–577.

73 Manning FA, Morrison I, Lange IR et al. (1987) Fetal biophysical profile scoring: selective use of the nonstress test. *Am J Obstet Gynecol* 156:709–712.

74 Kelly MK, Schneider EP, Petrikovsky BM et al. (2000) Effect of antenatal steroid administration on the fetal biophysical profile. *J Clin Ultrasound* 28:224–226.

75 Deren O, Karaer C, Onderoglu L et al. (2000) The effect of steroids on the biophysical profile of the healthy preterm fetus and its relationship with time. *Am J Obstet Gynecol* 182 (1, part 2):S108.

76 Nageotte MP, Towers CV, Asrat T et al. (1994) Perinatal outcome with the modified biophysical profile. *Am J Obstet Gynecol* 170:1672–1676.

77 McCowan LME, Harding JE, Stewart AW et al. (2000) Umbilical artery Doppler studies in small for gestational age babies reflect disease severity. *Br J Obstet Gynaecol* 107:916–925.

78 Pollack RN, Divon MY. (1995) Intrauterine growth retardation: diagnosis. In Copel JA and Reed KL (eds) *Doppler Ultrasound in Obstetrics and Gynecology*, p. 171. New York: Raven Press.

79 Itskovitz J. (1987) Maternal–fetal hemodynamics. In Maulik D and McNellis D (eds) *Reproductive and Perinatal Medicine* (VIII). *Doppler Ultrasound Measurement of Maternal–Fetal Hemodynamics*, p. 13. Perinatology Press.

80 Morrow R, Ritchie K. (1989) Doppler ultrasound fetal velocimetry and its role in obstetrics. *Clin Perinatol* 16:771.

81 Copel JA, Schlafer D, Wentworth R et al. (1990) Does the umbilical artery systolic/diastolic ratio reflect flow or acidosis? *Am J Obstet Gynecol* 163:751.

82 Farine D, Kelly EN, Ryan G et al. (1995) Absent and reversed umbilical artery end-diastolic velocity. In Copel JA, Reed KL (eds) *Doppler Ultrasound in Obstetrics and Gynecology*, p. 187. New York: Raven Press.

83 Giles WB, Bisets A. (1993) Clinical use of Doppler in pregnancy: information from six randomized trials. *Fetal Diagn Ther* 8:247–255.

84 Alfirevic Z, Neilson JP. (1995) Doppler ultrasonography in high-risk pregnancies: systematic review with meta-analysis. *Am J Obstet Gynecol* 172:1379.

85 Neilson JP, Alfirevic Z. (1999) Doppler ultrasound in high-risk pregnancies (Cochrane Review). In The Cochrane Library, Issue 4. Oxford, Update Software.

86 Divon MY, Ferber A. (2000) Evidence-based antepartum fetal testing. *Perinatal Neonatal Med* 5:3–86.

87 Goffinet F, Paris-Llado J, Nisand I et al. (1997) Umbilical after Doppler velocimetry in unselected and low risk pregnancies: a review of randomized controlled trials. *Br J Obstet Gynaecol* 104:425.

88 Rizzo G, Arduini D, Romanini C. (1995) p. 105. First trimester fetal and uterine Doppler. In Copel JA, Reed KL (eds) *Doppler Ultrasound in Obstetrics and Gynecology*, p. 105. New York: Raven Press.

11

Intrapartum evaluation of the fetus

Julian T. Parer and Tekoa King

University of California Health Sciences Center, San Francisco, CA, USA

Introduction

Fetal heart rate (FHR) monitoring during labor was introduced into clinical practice in the 1970s. At the time, obstetric providers and researchers in fetal physiology believed electronic fetal monitoring (EFM) would identify changes in the FHR and/or rhythm that reflect fetal acidosis. Second, it was presumed that detection would be early enough to allow clinical intervention that would prevent perinatal asphyxia. Despite 20 years of widespread use and multiple randomized clinical trials, FHR monitoring has not been shown to decrease perinatal mortality.[1] The relationship between intrapartum FHR monitoring and fetal acidosis is complex. Both of the suppositions stated above were problematic. This chapter reviews the physiology underlying FHR patterns, the reasons why randomized trials of EFM have failed to demonstrate efficacy, and the current knowledge that guides interpretation of EFM in the intrapartum period.

The history of EFM

The discovery of fetal heart tones in 1821 marked the beginning of modern obstetric practice.[2,3] Jean Alexandre Lejumeau, Vicomte de Kergaradec, correctly identified the FHR when using a stethoscope, hoping to hear the noise of the water in the uterus. FHR detection was rapidly used to improve obstetrical care. The ability to determine life or death of the fetus supported the decision to do a postmortem cesarean section (albeit a rare occurrence), helped determine fetal position, diagnosed multiple pregnancies, and quickly became the definitive positive sign of pregnancy.

During the mid 1800s several FHR patterns became evident and observations of a relationship between FHR changes and fetal asphyxia set the stage for scientific pursuit. In 1833 the British obstetrician Kennedy published the first descriptions of "fetal distress" by describing a late deceleration and associating it with poor prognosis.[4] By the late 1800s the occurrence of fetal bradycardias was well described.[3] The presence of bradycardia (<120 beats/min) or tachycardia (>160 beats/min) was used clinically as an indication for forceps delivery. In 1893, Von Winkel published criteria for fetal distress that were used through the mid twentieth century.[3,5]

In 1906 Cramer produced the first electrocardiographic (ECG) recording of the fetal heart beat.[6] Research using abdominal leads to obtain the fetal electrocardiogram continued but remained impractical for clinical use until the mid-1960s when techniques capable of excluding the maternal ECG became available.

Knowledge of the physiology of the FHR progressed in tandem with human observations and animal research. As early as 1947, Barcroft discovered the cardiovascular changes in fetal rabbits and sheep when subjected to umbilical cord occlusion and proposed vagal stimulation as the etiology.[7] Myers provided data on the development of brainstem lesions and cerebral palsy-type disorders following cerebral anoxia in monkeys.[8]

These works supported the beliefs of the time that cerebral palsy was a consequence of intrapartum asphyxia and that umbilical cord occlusion was the most common cause of oxygen deprivation in the fetus. Thus, when EFM improved to the point that it was clinically technically feasible, FHR monitoring was rapidly incorporated into routine use. Unfortunately, clinical practice proceeded before controlled trials could establish a true cause-and-effect relationship between specific FHR patterns and fetal acidemia.

Early studies of EFM

The first randomized controlled trial (RCT) of continuous electronic FHR monitoring compared to intermittent auscultation was published in 1976,[9] and found no improvement in newborn outcome with FHR monitoring, but a several-fold increase in cesarean sections in the group of women who were monitored during labor. Several randomized trials were conducted and published in the 1980s with similar results.[10–17] Women monitored during labor with EFM had higher operative delivery rates compared to women monitored with intermittent auscultation without a significant reduction in perinatal mortality or decrease in the incidence of cerebral palsy.

A decade after the Dublin report,[15] a metaanalysis by Thacker et al.[1] and the secondary analysis of trials[18] provided the beginnings of insight into why EFM had not proven to be efficacious in randomized trials. Thacker et al.[1] reviewed the results of 12 randomized trials with greater than 18 000 patients and found that newborn seizures occurred with a relative risk of 0.5 in the group monitored electronically, compared to a randomized group of patients managed by auscultation during labor. Approximately 1.1% of the fetuses in the auscultated group experienced seizures in the newborn period, whereas 0.8% of the newborns in the monitored group had seizures in the same time period. An important caveat to these findings is that in some studies long-term follow-up of the newborns with seizures failed to reveal significant neurologic sequelae. In fact, the majority of newborns in some of these trials who developed cerebral palsy were not in the group of those fetuses who had FHR tracings that were considered ominous.[18,19]

The results of these two studies raised two questions: first, do the abnormal FHR patterns thought to be indicative of fetal asphyxia in labor reflect acidosis severe enough to cause brain damage to the fetus? Second, is fetal acidosis during labor the cause of cerebral palsy? Both questions challenged the beliefs underlying clinical use of EFM and rephrased the questions recent research in FHR monitoring has investigated. Today it is understood that several of the FHR patterns presumed "abnormal" do not reflect fetal acidosis and, although cerebral palsy is a result of hypoxemic–ischemic injury, only about 10% of the children with cerebral palsy had an asphyxial event during labor.[20]

Despite the apparent lack of efficacy with regard to perinatal mortality that emerged from the randomized trials and metaanalysis, the use of EFM during labor has continued to grow in hospital settings and interpretation is being refined as knowledge of fetal physiology grows. Before summarizing how EFM is used today, a review of what is known about the physiology of the FHR and the factors that influence it is pertinent.

Physiology of the fetal heart rate

Fetal oxygenation

The transfer of oxygen and carbon dioxide between the fetal and maternal circulations depends upon the structure and adequate function of the uterine vasculature, the intervillous space, the fetal placenta, and the umbilical cord. The fetal umbilical vein blood, which carries oxygenated blood from the placenta to the fetus, has about the same partial pressure of oxygen (Po_2) as that in the maternal uterine vein blood – approximately 35 mmHg. Although the system of gas exchange across the placenta is efficient, the Po_2 in fetal oxygenated blood is poor relative to arterial values in adults.[21]

There are several physiologic mechanisms that

enable the fetus to maintain normal metabolism in an environment with a lower Po_2:

1 Fetal blood has more hemoglobin than adult blood. The extra "carrying capacity" allows the fetus to extract maximal amounts of oxygen.
2 Fetal hemoglobin has increased oxygen affinity relative to adult hemoglobin.
3 The pattern of blood flow in the fetus allows overperfusion of some organs with higher oxygen requirements, i.e., cerebral blood flow.[22]
4 The fetus has an increased cardiac output and heart rate, which results in a rapid circulation or turnover time.[21,23]
5 Finally, the fetus has more capillaries per unit of tissue than do adults.

The most common etiologies of interruption of oxygen delivery to the fetus during labor are acute decreases in uterine blood flow secondary to uterine contractions or decrease in umbilical blood flow secondary to cord occlusion. The fetus is able to maintain normal aerobic metabolism during transient decreases in blood flow to the uterus. Certain FHR patterns, namely variable decelerations, have been ascribed to transient umbilical cord compression in the fetus during labor, and manipulation of maternal position either to the lateral or Trendelenburg position can sometimes abolish these patterns. Under normal conditions, the fetus compensates for short-term transient decreases in Po_2 without altering normal metabolic function.

Role of the autonomic nervous system

The heart is innervated by both parasympathetic (primarily vagus) and sympathetic fibers. Parasympathetic nerve activity results in a decrease in the heart rate, because it decreases the rate of firing of the sinoatrial node, and slows the rate of transmission of impulses from atrium to ventricle. Stimulation of the sympathetic nerves to the heart releases norepinephrine, resulting in an increase in heart rate and an increase in cardiac contractility, a combination that results in an increase in cardiac output (Figure 11.1).

A number of factors can increase or decrease either parasympathetic or sympathetic activity. Variation or changes in the FHR from beat to beat, as well as longer-term changes over periods of less than a minute, are the result of the interplay of various inputs from the cerebral cortex and the cardioregulatory centers in the brainstem. These short-term changes in rate are visible as a jagged line on Doppler or ECG recordings and are termed "variability." Variability is of great prognostic importance clinically and valuable empiric predictions can be made from evaluation of its characteristics.

Chemoreceptors, baroreceptors, and cardiac output

Chemoreceptors are found in the carotid and aortic bodies of the aorta and the carotid sinus. In the adult, when the central chemoreceptors perceive a decrease in circulating oxygen, a reflex tachycardia is initiated, presumably to circulate more blood. The fetus, in contrast, responds to hypoxia with a decrease in heart rate. The cardiovascular responses to hypoxia in the fetus are instituted rapidly and are mediated by neural and hormonal mechanisms.[24] Baroreceptors in the aortic arch and carotid sinus are small stretch receptors sensitive to changes in blood pressure (Figure 11.2). When blood pressure rises, impulses from the baroreceptors are sent to the brainstem via afferent fibers in the vagus and impulses returned via vagal efferent fibers, rapidly resulting in a slowing of the FHR.

Cardiac output depends on heart rate, preload, afterload, and intrinsic contractility.[25,26] Each of these four determinants interacts dynamically to modulate the fetal cardiac output during physiologic conditions. The Frank–Starling mechanism is probably not well developed in the fetal heart.[27] Because the fetal cardiac muscle is less developed than that of the adult, increases or decreases in preload do not initiate compensatory changes in stroke volume. In addition, the fetal heart function appears to be highly sensitive to changes in the afterload, represented by the fetal arterial blood pressure. Increases in afterload elicit a dramatic reduction in the stroke volume or cardiac output. In clinical

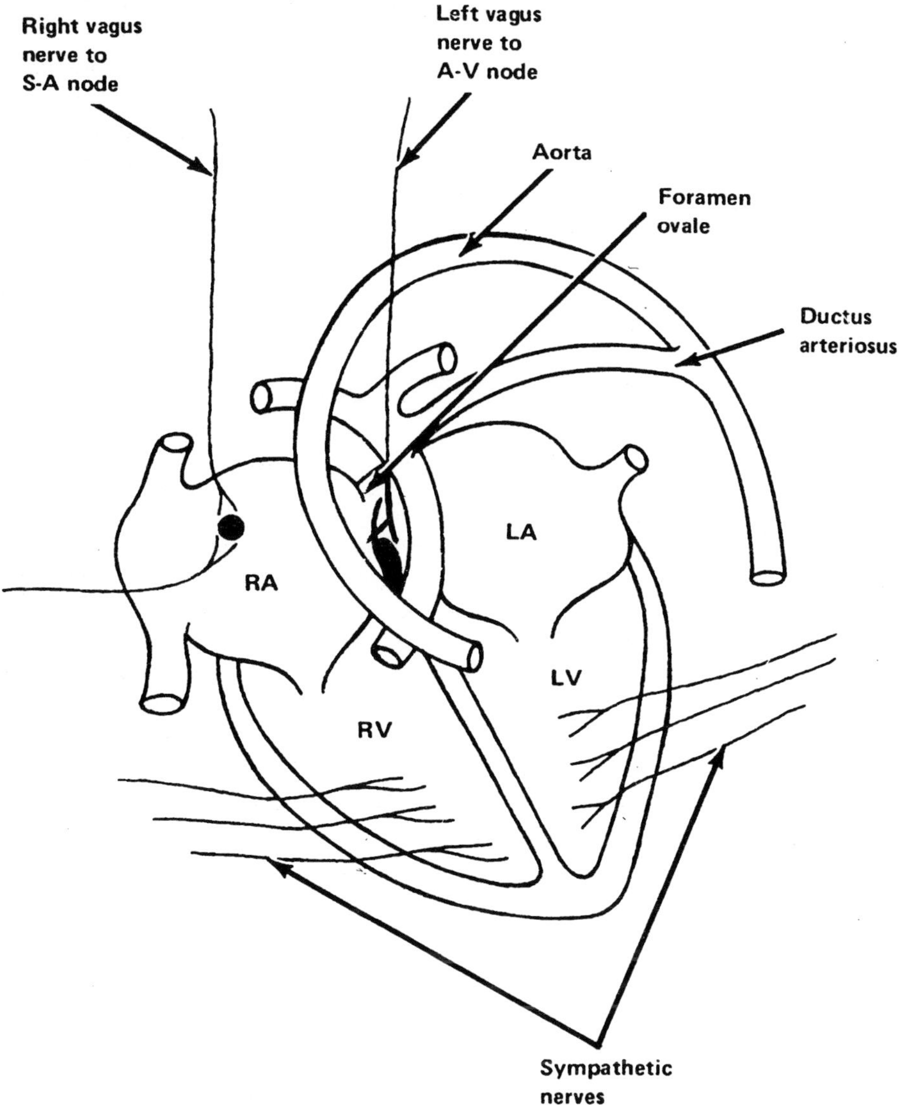

Figure 11.1 The fetal heart and its connections. RA and LA, right and left atria; RV and LV, right and left ventricle; S-A, sinoatrial; A-V, atrioventricular. From Parer JT. Physiological regulation of fetal heart rate. *J Obstet Gynecol Neonatal Nurs*, 1976; 5: 265–295 with permission.

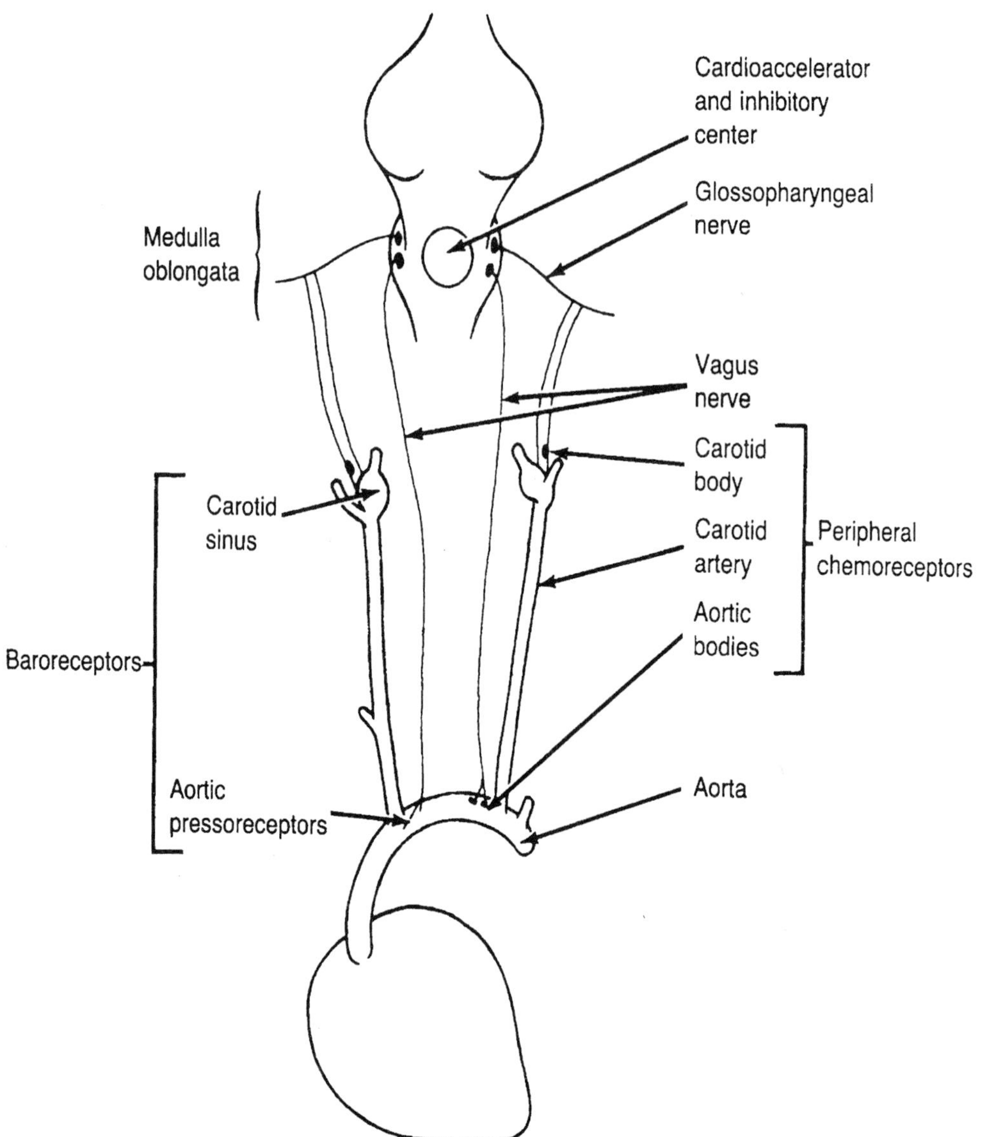

Figure 11.2 The peripheral chemo- and baroreceptors and their input to the cardiac integrating center in the medulla oblongata. From Parer JT. Physiologic regulation of fetal heart rate. *J Obstet Gynecol Neonatal Nurs*, 1976; 5: 265–295 with permission.

practice it is reasonable to assume that at small variations of heart rate, there are relatively small effects on the cardiac output in the fetus. However, at extremes (for example, a tachycardia above 240 beats/min or a bradycardia below 60 beats/min), cardiac output and umbilical blood flow are likely to be substantially decreased.

Other factors which either directly or indirectly alter FHR and the fetal circulation include central nervous system activity (sleep and awake cycles change the FHR variability), hormones, and blood volume shifts. The primary hormones involved in regulation of FHR, cardiac contractility, and distribution of blood flow in the fetus include epinephrine, norepinephrine, the renin–angiotensin system, arginine vasopressin, prostaglandins, melanocyte-stimulating hormone, atrial natriuretic hormone, neuropeptide Y, and thyrotropin-releasing hormone. In addition, nitric oxide and adenosine can affect the fetal circulation

Characteristics of the normal fetal heart rate

The characteristics of the FHR and common FHR patterns are classified as baseline or periodic/episodic.[28,29] The baseline features, heart rate and variability, are those recorded between uterine contractions. Periodic changes occur in association with uterine contractions, and episodic changes are those not obviously associated with uterine contractions. Periodic and episodic changes can be a response to decreases in oxygenation but may not be reflective of clinically significant hypoxia in the fetus. Before reviewing variant FHR patterns, a brief review of baseline FHR characteristics and the fetal response to hypoxia is in order.

The baseline features of the FHR, that is, those predominant characteristics which can be recognized between uterine contractions, consist of the following:

Baseline rate

The baseline FHR is the approximate mean FHR rounded to 5 beats/min during a 10-min segment, excluding:

- Periodic or episodic changes
- Periods of marked FHR variability
- Segments of the baseline which differ by >25 beats/min

In any 10-min window the minimum baseline duration must be at least 2 min, otherwise the baseline for that period is indeterminate, in which case one may need to refer to the previous 10-min segment(s). The normal baseline FHR is considered to be between 110 and 160 beats/min. Values below 110 beats/min are termed bradycardia and those above 160 beats/min are termed tachycardia.[29]

Variability

Variability refers to the irregularity in the line one sees when examining an FHR monitor tracing. The FHR variability represents a slight difference in time interval between each beat as counted and recorded by the monitor. If all intervals between heart beats were identical, the line would be regular or smooth. Baseline variability is defined as fluctuations in the baseline FHR of 2 cycles per minute or greater.[29] These fluctuations are somewhat akin to sine waves, but they are irregular in amplitude and frequency. The sinusoidal pattern (see below) differs from variability in that it has a smooth sine wave-like pattern of regular frequency and amplitude, and is excluded from the definition of FHR variability. As stated above, variability is a critical determinant of adequate perfusion and/or function in the central nervous system.

Accelerations

An acceleration is a visually apparent abrupt increase (defined as onset of acceleration to peak in <30 s) in FHR above the baseline. The increase is calculated from the most recently determined portion of the baseline. The acme is ≥15 beats/min above the baseline, and the acceleration lasts ≥15 s and <2 min from the onset to return to baseline.[29] Before 32 weeks of gestation, accelerations are defined as having an acme ≥10 beats/min above the baseline and duration of ≥10 s. A prolonged acceleration is

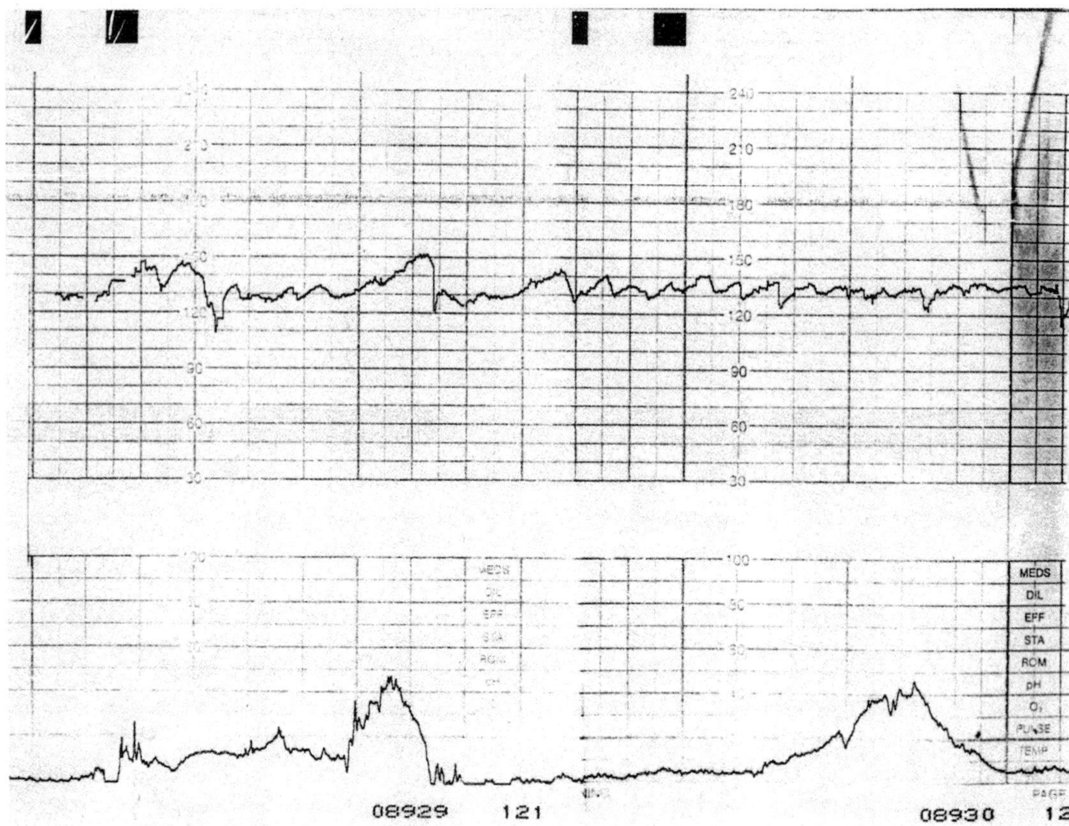

Figure 11.3 Normal fetal heart rate (FHR) pattern with normal rate (approximately 135 beats/min) and normal short-term and long-term variability (amplitude range approximately 20 beats/min) and absence of periodic changes. This pattern represents a normally oxygenated fetus without evidence of asphyxial stress.

≥2 min and <10 min in duration. There is a close association between the presence of accelerations and normal FHR variability and both accelerations and normal variability have the same positive prognostic significance of normal fetal oxygenation (Figure 11.3).

Fetal response to hypoxia/asphyxia

The tonic influence of the autonomic nervous system on the heart rate, blood pressure, and umbilical circulation in the well-oxygenated fetus is quantitatively minor. This is in marked contrast to autonomic activity during hypoxia. Studies of chronically prepared animals have shown that a number of responses occur during acute hypoxia or asphyxia. Parasympathetic activity is augmented three to five times and beta-adrenergic activity doubles when measured by heart rate response during a hypoxic episode.[30] The net result of these changes is vagal dominance and a decrease in FHR during hypoxia.

Augmented beta-adrenergic activity may be important in maintaining cardiac output and umbilical blood flow during hypoxia, by increasing the inotropic effect on the heart. Alpha-adrenergic activity is important in determining regional distribution of blood flow in the hypoxic fetus by selective vasoconstriction.[31]

The initial response to hypoxia includes a decrease in fetal oxygen consumption to values as low as 60% of control.[32] This decrease is rapidly instituted, stable for periods up to 45 min, proportional to the degree of hypoxia, and rapidly reversible on cessation of maternal hypoxia. It is accompanied by a fetal bradycardia of about 30 beats/min below control and an increase in fetal arterial blood pressure. If hypoxia persists, metabolic acidosis develops. This is due to lactic acid accumulation as a result of anaerobic metabolism primarily in those partially vasoconstricted beds where oxygenation is inadequate for normal basic needs.[33]

It has been shown in experimental animals that a fetus's ability to tolerate asphyxial stress depends on cardiac carbohydrate reserves. Whether this also applies to a human fetus is unknown, but clinical observations support the view that carbohydrate-depleted fetuses with intrauterine growth restriction succumb more readily than those with normal reserves. Such nutritionally growth-restricted fetuses are also more susceptible to intrauterine asphyxia and depression than a normal fetus.[34] The prime aim of compensatory responses during hypoxia is maintenance of the circulation, and maintenance of the integrity of cardiac function is paramount in this regard. It is likely that carbohydrate availability is critical in supplying substrates for glycolysis at more severe degrees of hypoxia.

In summary, the fetus responds to hypoxia with a redistribution of blood flow favoring certain vital organs – namely, heart, brain, and adrenal glands – and a decrease in blood flow to the gut, spleen, kidneys, and carcass. In addition there is bradycardia, decreased total oxygen consumption, and anaerobic glycolysis.[35] These compensatory mechanisms enable a fetus to survive moderately long periods (e.g., 30–60 min) of limited oxygen supply, without damage to vital organs. The response of blood flow to oxygen availability achieves a constancy of oxygen delivery in the fetal cerebral circulation[36] and in the fetal myocardium.[37]

During more severe asphyxia or sustained hypoxemia, the responses described above are no longer maintained, and decreases in cardiac output, arterial blood pressure, and blood flow to the brain and heart have been described.[38]

Fetal oxygenation can be impaired by a decrease in umbilical vessel perfusion, a decrease in maternal placental perfusion, an increase in fetal need for oxygen (e.g., fetal infection or anemia) or, rarely, a decrease in maternal arterial oxygen content (e.g., maternal anemia or cardiopulmonary disease.[39] In addition, the fetal outcome is dependent upon both the magnitude and duration of the insult.

Variant fetal heart rate patterns

Periodic patterns: late, early, and variable decelerations

Periodic patterns are the alterations in FHR that are associated with uterine contractions. The three characteristic periodic patterns seen are late decelerations, early decelerations, and variable decelerations. Prolonged decelerations are a subcategory of variable or late decelerations. Episodic decelerations are similar to periodic patterns, but do not have the same constant association with contractions.

Late deceleration of the FHR is a visually apparent gradual decrease (defined as onset of deceleration to nadir ≥30 s) and return to baseline FHR associated with a uterine contraction.[29] It is delayed in timing, with the nadir of the deceleration late in relation to the peak of the contraction. In most cases the onset, nadir, and recovery are all late in relation to the beginning, peak, and ending of the contraction respectively.

Originally, all late decelerations were thought to represent the fetal response to decreased oxygenation in the presence of significant uteroplacental insufficiency. More recent research has identified two different mechanisms: late decelerations that have retained variability are neurogenic in origin.[24] When a well-oxygenated fetus has an acute reduction in oxygenation during a contraction, chemoreceptors detect the hypoxemia and initiate the vagal bradycardiac response. It takes a short time for hypoxemia to develop in this setting, thus the chemoreceptor reflex occurs as the hypoxemia is detected. The FHR baseline has a slower decline and the nadir of the deceleration is "late" relative to the peak of the contraction. Because the fetus is centrally well oxygenated and not acidemic (i.e., the heart and central nervous system), variability is retained (Figure 11.4).[40]

Late decelerations with decreased or absent variability are possibly asphyxial. Late decelerations with absent variability occur when there is insufficient oxygen for myocardial metabolism and/or normal cerebral function. These are likely to occur in the fetus with chronic and prolonged placental insufficiency.

Early deceleration of the FHR is a visually apparent gradual decrease (defined as onset of deceleration to nadir (≥30 s) and return to baseline FHR associated with a uterine contraction.[29] The nadir of the deceleration is coincident to the peak of the contraction. In most cases the onset, nadir, and recovery are all coincident to the beginning, peak, and ending of the contraction respectively. They are not associated with significant fetal acidemia.

Variable decelerations are visually apparent abrupt decreases (defined as onset of deceleration to beginning of nadir <30 s) in FHR from the baseline. The decrease in FHR below the baseline is at least 15 beats/min, lasting (from baseline to baseline) at least 15 s, and <2 min.[29] When variable decelerations are associated with uterine contractions, their onset, depth, and duration commonly vary with successive uterine contractions (Figure 11.5).

Variable decelerations are secondary to either head compression that causes vagal stimulation or umbilical cord compression that causes baroreceptor stimulation.[41] During rapid fetal descent, sudden increases in pressure on the fetal cranium result in molding that accommodates different pelvic diameters. Umbilical cord compression causes an increase in blood pressure secondary to umbilical artery occlusion. The sudden increase in blood pressure stimulates baroreceptors in the aortic arch. The baroreceptor reflex through the vagus to the medulla oblongata and back to the pacemaker of the heart is extremely fast and the bradycardial response is quick, thus the abrupt descent of the fetal heart rate. If variable decelerations are persistent and/or severe, one may see the development of tachycardia, late return to baseline with progressive decelerations, and/or decreased variability. The evolution of moderate variables to variables with or absent variability reflects developing fetal acidemia.[42]

Episodic decelerations: prolonged deceleration

A prolonged deceleration is a subcategory of the variable deceleration. The decrease in FHR below the baseline is at least 15 beats/min, lasting ≥2 min, but <10 min. The definition changes to a change in baseline rate (e.g., bradycardia) if the prolonged deceleration is ≥10 min in duration.[29] Prolonged decelerations can lead to hypoxia. These patterns may reflect a stepwise decrease in fetal oxygenation secondary to an acute asphyxial insult.[24] The stimulus may be anything that causes a sudden drop in blood flow to the intervillous space (e.g., maternal hypotension or tetanic contractions).

Changes in baseline rate: tachycardia and bradycardia

Nonasphyxial causes of fetal tachycardia include the administration of some drugs such as beta-sympathomimetics or atropine. Nonasphyxial causes that may develop into asphyxia include maternal fever, fetal infection, and fetal cardiac tachyarrhythmia. Tachycardia signifying a fetal acidemia is most frequently seen with absent variability, recurrent late decelerations, recurrent variable decelerations, or a combination of the above patterns.[43] Mild tachycardia with normal variability and no periodic changes is not associated with fetal acidemia.[44–47] Tachycardia can also be seen transiently when the fetus recovers from an acute hypoxial stress. This tachycardia is considered a physiologic response secondary to adrenal stimulation with release of catecholamines.

By definition, bradycardia refers to a baseline rate

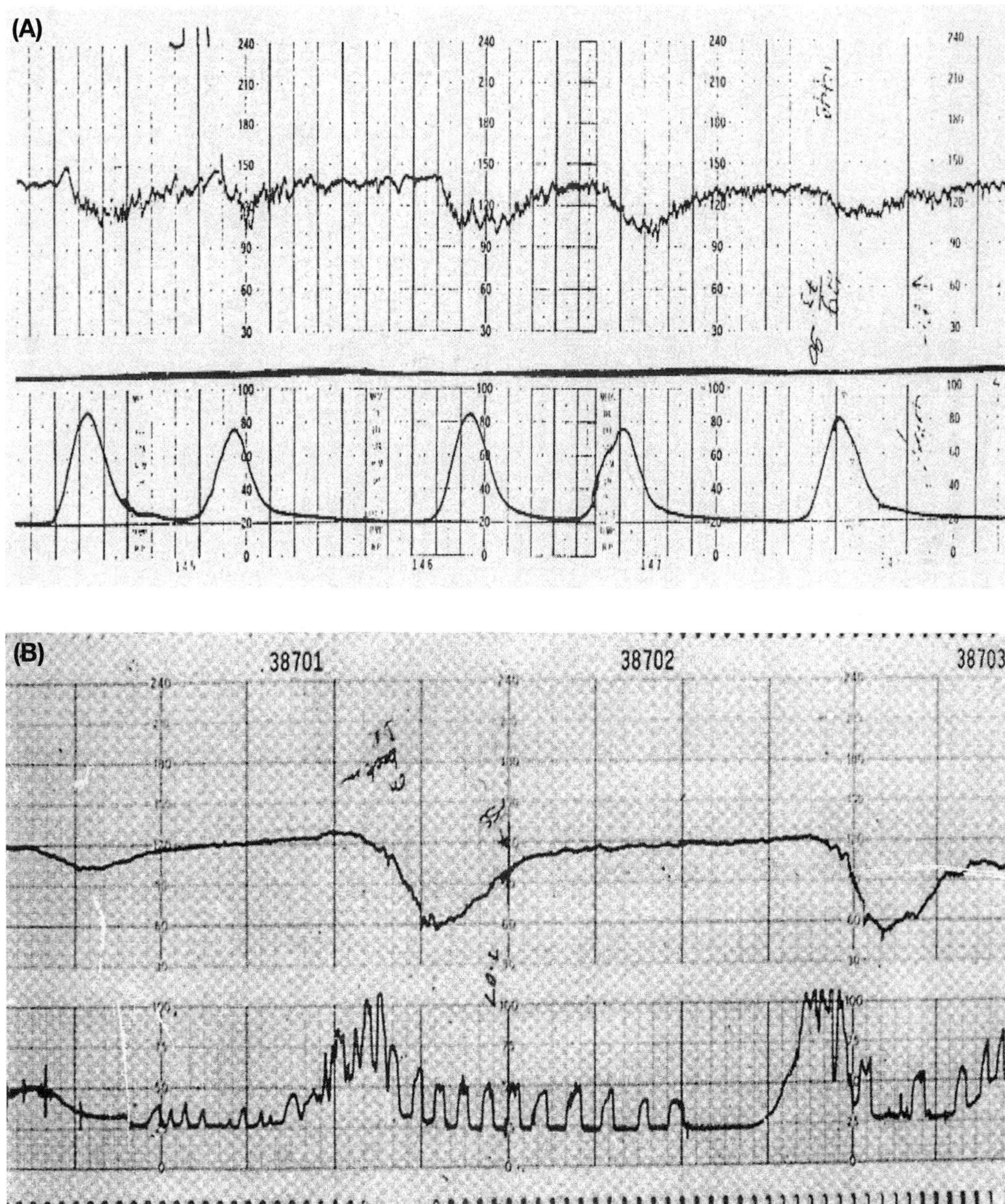

Figure 11.4 (A) Reflex late decelerations with normal fetal heart rate (FHR) variability. (B) Late decelerations with virtually absent FHR variability. These findings represent transient asphyxial myocardial failure as well as intermittent vagal decreases in heart rate. The lack of FHR variability also signifies a decreased cerebral oxygenation. Note the acidosis in fetal scalp blood (7.07). A 3340-g girl with Apgar scores of 3 (1 min) and 4 (5 min) was delivered soon after this tracing was made. Cesarean section was considered to be contraindicated because of severe preeclamptic coagulopathy.

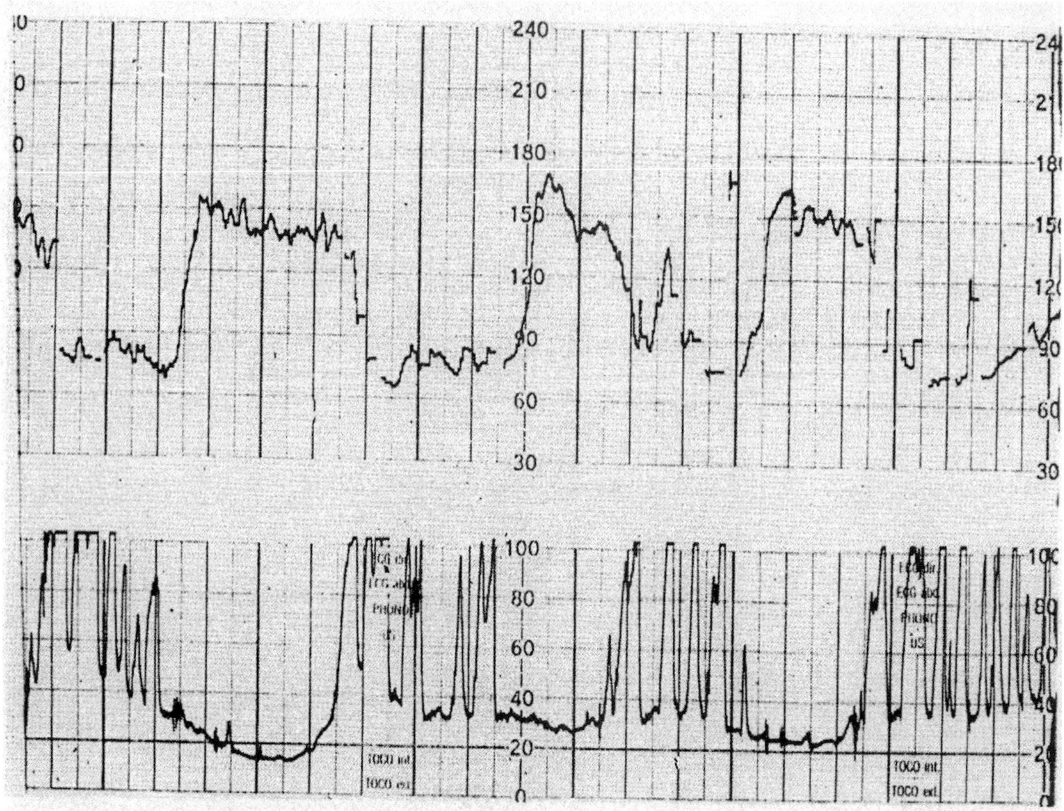

Figure 11.5 Variable decelerations. Intrapartum recording using fetal scalp electrode and tocodynamometer. The spikes in the uterine activity channel represent maternal pushing efforts in the second stage of labor. Note normal baseline variability between contractions, signifying normal central oxygenation despite the intermittent asphyxial stress represented by the severe variable decelerations.

of <110 beats/min.[29] Uncomplicated bradycardias of >80 beats/min with retained variability are not associated with fetal acidemia.[43,44,46,48] Nonasphyxial causes of bradycardia include complete heart block and treatment with significant doses of β-adrenergic blockers. Occasionally a fetus will have a baseline below 110 beats/min without pathologic implications.

Like the patterns described above, bradycardial episodes in the fetus may cause hypoxia or they may be the cause of hypoxia. Bradycardias that occur during the final moments of the second stage (end-stage bradycardias) are an example of an FHR pattern that can lead to hypoxia if sufficiently prolonged and severe. These bradycardias can be secondary to head compression and vagal stimulation or secondary to acute umbilical cord occlusion. The fetus can tolerate end-stage bradycardias as long as the baseline remains above 80 beats/min and the variability is retained.[49,50]

If a bradycardia becomes severe, oxygen and carbon dioxide transfer will become impaired, a metabolic acidosis will develop, and variability will diminish. Bradycardias that result from severe hypoxia do not return to baseline and have decreased or absent variability.[46,51] The progressive flat-line bradycardia can be seen following a period of severe late or variable decelerations (Figure 11.6). This evolution from severe periodic changes to the progressive bradycardia with minimal or absent variability is associated with metabolic acidemia and eventually fetal hypotension. It may be seen in uterine rupture, extensive placental abruption, or just prior to fetal death.

Sinusoidal patterns

The sinusoidal pattern was first described in a group of severely affected Rh-isoimmunized fetuses,[52] but has subsequently been noted in association with fetuses that are anemic for other reasons, such as fetal–maternal bleeding, and in severely asphyxiated infants. This pattern appears as a regular, smooth sine wave-like baseline, with a frequency of approximately 3–6 per min and an amplitude range of up to 30 beats/min. The regularity of the waves distinguishes it from long-term variability complexes, which are more crudely shaped and irregular. In addition, sinusoidal patterns exhibit an absence of beat-to-beat or short-term variability. The essential characteristic of a true sinusoidal pattern is extreme regularity and smoothness.[42]

Sinusoidal patterns have also been described in cases of normal infants born without depression or acid–base abnormalities, although in these cases there is dispute about whether the patterns are truly sinusoidal or whether, because of the moderately irregular pattern, they are variants of long-term variability. Such patterns, called pseudosinusoidal, are sometimes seen after administration of narcotics to the mother.

The presence of a sinusoidal pattern in an Rh-sensitized patient suggests fetal anemia, generally with a hematocrit below 25%. In cases of fetal–maternal bleeding, the appearance of a striking sinusoidal pattern has given rise to the belief that the pattern is caused by acute anemia, rather than a slow development of anemia, as seen usually with erythroblastosis fetalis.[42] However, there may be a less striking blunted variant in Rh-affected babies. As yet there is little evidence for this, although the association of the acute anemia in fetal arginine vasopression levels is consistent with the theory.[53] If the pattern is irregularly sinusoidal or pseudosinusoidal, intermittently present, and not associated with intervening periodic decelerations, it is unlikely to indicate fetal compromise.[42]

Absent or minimal variability

Minimal variability can be secondary to fetal sleep, medication, or early hypoxia. Minimal variability without decelerations is almost always nonasphyxial.[54] Absent variability can be asphyxial or nonasphyxial as well. Examples of nonasphyxial causes include central nervous system depressants, anencephaly, defective cardiac conduction system, and congenital neurologic abnormalities (Figure 11.7). Conversely, absent variability is seen when the fetus has cerebral asphyxia with accompanying loss of either fine-tuning within the cardioregulatory center in the brain and/or direct myocardial depression. Loss of variability, especially in the presence of other periodic patterns during labor, is the most sensitive indicator of metabolic acidemia in a fetus.[44,47,55–57]

In summary, when assessing periodic or episodic FHR patterns, variability is the key reflection of intact cerebral oxygenation. Periodic FHR patterns have specific physiologic mechanisms but, because such variant patterns are common during labor, the degree of hypoxia or asphyxia experienced by an individual fetus is not well predicted by them.

Role of EFM in predicting perinatal asphyxia

It is believed that the evolution of the FHR from a normal baseline with moderate variability to recurrent decelerations and absent variability parallels the evolution from acidemia to serious asphyxia. However, the link between the FHR pattern and the actual acid–base status of the fetus is not well demarcated. Thirty-nine percent of the intrapartum FHR tracings obtained during labor display periodic

(A)

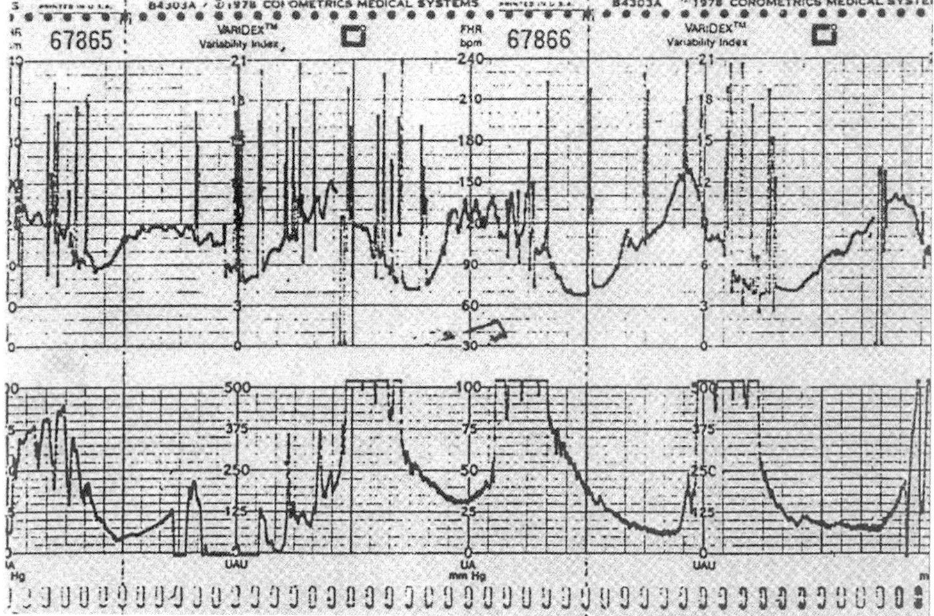

(B)

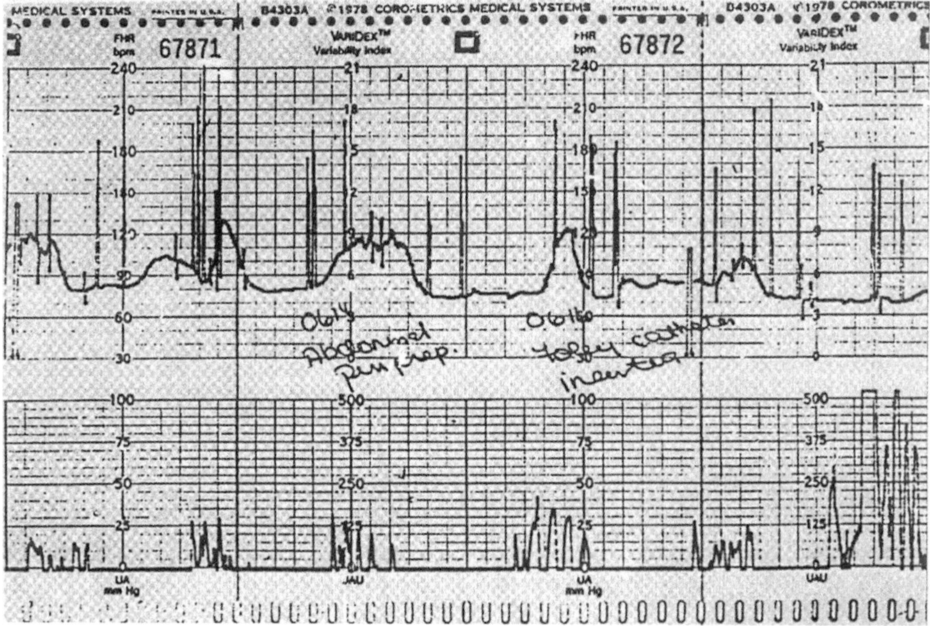

Figure 11.6 (A and B). A case of fetal cardiorespiratory decompensation showing the evolution of the smooth baseline over 30 min. In this case the asphyxial stress is manifested as late decelerations. Death occurred in utero about 20 min later.

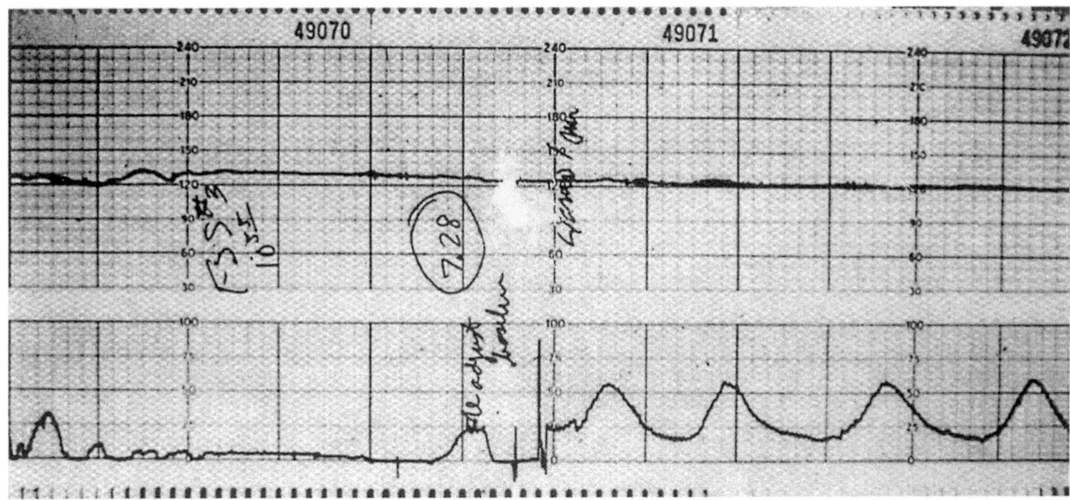

Figure 11.7 No variability of fetal heart rate (FHR). The patient was a severe preeclamptic receiving magnesium sulfate and narcotics. The normal scalp blood pH (7.28) assures one that the absence of variability is nonasphyxic in origin and that the fetus is not chronically asphyxiated and decompensated. The uterine activity channel has an inaccurate trace in the first half.

FHR patterns, yet only 2% of all newborns have evidence of metabolic acidemia (pH <7.1 with base excess <12 mmol/l).[43,58]

The original outcome measures used in early studies of FHR monitoring were intrapartum stillbirth and cerebral palsy. FHR monitoring has been associated with a virtual disappearance of intrapartum stillbirth. Prior to the introduction of FHR monitoring, approximately one-third of all stillbirths or 3 per 1000 births occurred in the intrapartum period.[59] Currently, the overall incidence of intrapartum stillbirth is at most 0.5/1000 births. The hope that EFM during labor would abolish cerebral palsy through the diagnosis of "fetal distress" and early intervention has proven to be an unrealistic goal because the majority of children with cerebral palsy develop the disorder prior to labor.[18–20,60] In fact, the incidence of cerebral palsy due to intrapartum asphyxia is of the order of 0.025%, i.e., more than 1000-fold less than the incidence of variant FHR patterns during labor.

Other outcome measures of potential significance are Apgar scores, newborn seizures, and acidemia at birth. Normal FHR tracings predict normal Apgar scores 96% of the time and 83% of newborns with low 5-min Apgar scores are presaged by variant FHR patterns.[61] However, this concordance is unhelpful because Apgar scores do not predict neonatal morbidity well.

Seizures that first occur in the newborn period are predictive of long-term neurologic abnormality[62] and neonatal seizures that occur secondary to perinatal asphyxia generally manifest within the first day of life.[63] Several authors have evaluated the relationship between various variant FHR patterns and markers of neonatal encephalopathy, including seizures, intraventricular hemorrhage, and cerebral palsy.[64] The sensitivity for specific variant FHR patterns ranges from 23 to 100%. The positive predictive value is worse (0.3–30%). Neonatal seizures are a low-prevalence outcome, yet the frequency of variant FHR patterns is high.

Fetal acidemia precedes metabolic acidosis and is therefore the precursor to the level of asphyxia one hopes to avoid through interpretation of EFM. A pH value of less than 7.0, which occurs in about 3 per 1000 births, is associated with (but not predictive of) neurologic and other organ damage.[65–68] Recent evidence is accumulating that some morbidity (though rarely permanent) is seen in fetuses with an umbilical arterial pH between 7.0 and 7.1. It is important to note that umbilical cord gases provide a quantitative measure of acidemia but the degree of asphyxia cannot be accurately determined via umbilical cord sampling because the values obtained from a sample taken immediately after birth do not reliably reflect the duration of the insult or the fetal (or neonatal) response.[62] Thus, the outcome variables used in studies of FHR monitoring have some limitations. The above notwithstanding, umbilical cord gas analysis is probably the best outcome measure of intrapartum fetal acid–base status that we have to date.

The independent variables, i.e., "abnormal" FHR patterns, are also problematic. Approximately 30% of fetuses have some sort of pattern which is variant from normal[43] which could be interpreted as suspicious or ominous. If one narrows the definition of suspicious to those variant patterns with reduced or absent FHR variability, the prevalence drops to 3%. Even this rate is 10-fold higher than the incidence of an umbilical arterial pH of <7.0, although it is similar to the incidence of newborns born with a pH ≤7.1.

"Fetal stress/distress" is a continuum that ranges from normal compensatory mechanisms to decompensation and deep central asphyxia. In any individual fetus, the impact of an asphyxial event will be the result of interplay between the severity and duration of the insult, and the reserve of the fetus. As the wide variation in fetal response to oxygen deprivation has become evident, the term "distress," which is nonspecific, has become inappropriate as a diagnosis that incites intervention.[54,69]

The published studies comparing the incidence of periodic FHR patterns to newborn acidemia have been retrospective case-control studies of asphyxiated newborns[47,48,70,71] or prospective studies comparing specific FHR patterns to fetal scalp sample pH or umbilical cord blood pH values at birth.[44–46,72,73] Case-control and prospective observational designs can demonstrate a statistically significant association but cannot prove that the association elucidated is actually a cause-and-effect relationship. Despite this limitation, the remarkable consistency across this literature supports the application of these findings in clinical management. Normal baseline rate, moderate variability, accelerations, and absence of periodic patterns are highly predictive of the absence of fetal acidemia. Second, in the presence of absent variability, severe bradycardia, late decelerations (mild or severe), and/or severe variable decelerations are predictive of newborn acidemia (Table 11.1).

Table 11.1. Fetal heart rate patterns associated with risk for acidemia

Absent or minimal variability and:
Recurrent late decelerations
Recurrent severe variable decelerations
Bradycardia (<80 beats/min)
Sinusoidal pattern

Source: Adapted from: [40, 43, 44, 46, 49, 50, 57]

In summary, attempts to date to compare FHR patterns to subsequent neonatal morbidity have been imprecise. Cerebral palsy and neonatal seizures are extremely rare events and variant heart rate patterns are common. Apgar scores do correlate well with FHR patterns but they do not correlate well with long-term outcome or with concomitant newborn acidemia. Although there are no specific FHR patterns or group of patterns that reliably predict brain damage, there is a growing literature that suggests there is a correlation between absent variability with severe periodic decelerations or bradycardia and progressive metabolic acidemia in the fetus. The degree of acidemia that reliably predicts newborn complications is as yet undetermined.

Methods for detecting fetal acidemia

There are two ancillary methods of assessing fetal acidemia that, when used in conjunction with FHR monitoring, can help identify nonacidemic fetuses. Fetal blood sampling from the fetal scalp after adequate dilatation of the cervix[74] was developed at about the same time as continuous electronic FHR monitoring, and, in fact, for a time was a competitor to FHR monitoring for primary screening of fetal condition during labor. Later, a combination of the two techniques, with FHR monitoring as the screening tool and fetal blood sampling as a follow-up in cases of uncertainty, was recommended by a number of investigators.[44] Such an approach was utilized with great enthusiasm by tertiary institutions, but the technique of fetal blood sampling never penetrated to any great extent to community hospitals, where the vast majority of North America's 4 million births per year are carried out.

Stimulation testing has largely taken the place of scalp sampling. The presence of an acceleration in FHR in response to tactile or vibroacoustic stimulation virtually assures a fetal pH above 7.2.[57] Scalp stimulation can be a useful adjunct when delivery is remote and the FHR tracing is nonreassuring but not clearly indicative of fetal acidemia.

Current recommendations

The fetus lives in a state of decreased oxygen tension relative to the adult yet has similar metabolic needs. The physiologic mechanisms that enhance oxygen delivery to fetal tissue are intricate and able to accommodate varying degrees of lowered Po_2 without pathologic sequelae. The biochemical events that herald irreversible asphyxial injury have not been determined in terms of acid–base indices and, because there is wide variability in physiologic responses from fetus to fetus, acid–base status at birth may never be a perfect predictor. To date, there are no clinical markers or specific FHR patterns that reliably predict intrapartum asphyxia. Neither are there any single neonatal indices, such as Apgar scores, umbilical cord gases, or neonatal seizures, that reliably correlate to intrapartum asphyxia severe enough to cause brain injury. The combination of a mixed acidemia, 5-min Apgar score of <3, seizures within 24 h of birth, and multiorgan dysfunction as a constellation are the indicators most associated with intrapartum asphyxia.[65]

Given these complexities, the goal of clinical FHR monitoring is the detection of those patterns that herald a significant risk of acidemia at a value well before irreversible damage occurs. Absent or minimal variability, especially in the presence of late or severe variable decelerations, and bradycardias are the patterns most associated with severe fetal acidemia.

REFERENCES

1 Thacker SB, Stroup DF and Peterson HB. (1995). Efficacy and safety of intrapartum electronic fetal monitoring: an update. *Obstet Gynecol*, **86**, 613–620.

2 Sureau C. (1996). Historical perspectives: forgotten past, unpredictable future. *Baillieres Clin Obstet Gynecol*, **10**, 167–184.

3 Goodlin RC. (1979). History of fetal monitoring. *Am J Obstet Gynecol*, **133**, 323–352.

4 Kennedy E. (1833). *Observations of Obstetrical Auscultation*, p. 311. Dublin: Hodges and Smith.

5 Freeman RK and Garite TL. (1981). *Fetal Heart Rate Monitoring*. Baltimore: Williams and Wilkins.

6 Cramer MV. (1906). Ueber die dierkte Ableitung der Akionsstrome des menschlichen Herzens vom Oesophagus und uber das Elektrokardiogramm des Fotus. *Munch Med Wschr*, **53**, 811–813.

7 Barcroft J. (1947). *Researches on Prenatal Life*. Springfield, IL: Charles C Thomas.

8 Myers RE. (1972). Two patterns of perinatal brain damage and their conditions of occurrence. *Am J Obstet Gynecol*, **112**, 246–276.

9 Havercamp AD, Thompson HE, McFee JG et al. (1976). The evaluation of continuous fetal heart rate monitoring in high-risk pregnancy. *Am J Obstet Gynecol*, **125**, 310–320.

10 Renou P, Chang A, Anderson I et al. (1976). Controlled trial of fetal intensive care. *Am J Obstet Gynecol*, **126**, 470–475.

11 Kelso IM, Parsons RJ, Lawrence GF et al. (1978). An assessment of continuous fetal heart rate monitoring in labor. *Am J Obstet Gynecol*, **131**, 526–532.

12 Havercamp AD, Orleans M, Langerdoerfer S et al. (1979). A controlled trial of differential effects of intrapartum fetal monitoring. *Am J Obstet Gynecol*, **134**, 399–408.

13 Wood C, Renou P, Oats J et al. (1981). A controlled trial of fetal heart rate monitoring in a low risk obstetric population. *Am J Obstet Gynecol*, **141**, 527–534.

14 Neldam S, Osler M, Hansen PK et al. (1986). Intrapartum

fetal heart rate monitoring in a combined low-and high-risk population: a controlled trial. *Eur J Obstet Gynecol Reprod Biol*, **23**, 1–11.

15 MacDonald D, Grant A, Sheridan-Pereira M et al. (1985). The Dublin randomized controlled trial of intrapartum fetal heart rate monitoring. *Am J Obstet Gynecol*, **152**, 524–539.

16 Leveno J, Cunningham FG, Nelson S et al. (1986). A prospective comparison of selective and universal electronic fetal monitoring in 34995 pregnancies. *N Engl J Med*, **315**, 615–641.

17 Luthy DA, Shy KK, van Belle G et al. (1987). A randomized trial of electronic monitoring in labor. *Obstet Gynecol*, **69**, 687–695.

18 Shy NE, Luthy DA, Bennett FC et al. (1990). Effects of electronic fetal heart rate monitoring as compared with periodic auscultation on the neurologic development of premature infants. *N Engl J Med*, **322**, 588–593.

19 Grant S, O'Brien N, Joy MT et al. (1989). Cerebral palsy among children born during the Dublin randomized trial of intrapartum monitoring. *Lancet*, **2**, 1233–1235.

20 Nelson KB. (1988). What proportion of cerebral palsy is related to birth asphyxia? *J Pediatr*, **112**, 572–574.

21 Martin CB Jr and Gingerich B. (1976). Uteroplacental physiology. *J Obstet Gynecol Neonatal Nurs*, **5** (suppl. 5), 16s–25s.

22 Richardson BS. (1989). Fetal adaptive responses to asphyxia. *Clin Perinatol*, **16**, 595–611.

23 Jepson JH. (1974). Factors influencing oxygenation in mother and fetus. *Obstet Gynecol*, **44**, 906–914.

24 Parer JT. (1997). *Handbook of Fetal Heart Rate Monitoring*, 2nd edn, p. 286. Philadelphia: Saunders.

25 Anderson PAW, Glick KL, Killam AP et al. (1986). The effect of heart rate on in utero left ventricular output in the fetal sheep. *J Physiol*, **372**, 557–573.

26 Anderson PAW, Killam AP, Mainwaring RD et al. (1987). In utero right ventricular output in the fetal lamb: the effect of heart rate. *J Physiol*, **387**, 297–316.

27 Rudolph AM and Heymann MA. (1973). Control of the foetal circulation. In *Fetal and Neonatal Physiology.* Proceedings of the Barcroft Centenary Symposium, ed. Comline KS, Cross KW, Dawes GS et al., pp. 89–111. Cambridge: Cambridge University Press.

28 Hon EH and Quilligan EJ. (1967). The classification of fetal heart rate. *Conn Med*, **31**, 779–784.

29 National Institute of Child Health and Human Development Research Planning Workshop. (1997). Electronic fetal heart rate monitoring; research guidelines for interpretation. *Am J Obstet Gynecol*, **17**, 1385–1390; *J Obstet Gynecol Neonatal Nurs*, **26**, 635–640.

30 Court DJ and Parer JT. (1985). Experimental studies in fetal asphyxia and fetal heart rate interpretation. In *Research in Perinatal Medicine*, vol. 1, eds. Nathanielsz PW, Parer JT, pp.114–164. Ithaca, NY: Perinatology Press.

31 Reuss ML, Parer JT, Harris JL et al. (1982). Hemodynamic effects of alpha adrenergic blockade during hypoxia in fetal sheep. *Am J Obstet Gynecol*, **142**, 410–415.

32 Parer JT, Krueger TR and Harris JL. (1980). Fetal oxygen consumption and mechanisms of heart rate response during artificially produced late decelerations of fetal heart rate in sheep. *Am J Obstet Gynecol*, **136**, 478–482.

33 Mann LI. (1970). Effects in sheep of hypoxia on levels of lactate, pyruvate, and glucose in blood of mothers and fetus. *Pediatr Res*, **4**, 46–54.

34 Mann LI, Tejani NA and Weiss RR. (1974). Antenatal diagnosis and management of the small gestational age fetus. *Am J Obstet Gynecol*, **120**, 995–1004.

35 Cohn HE, Sacks EJ, Heymann MA et al. (1974). Cardiovascular responses to hypoxemia and acidemia in fetal lambs. *Am J Obstet Gynecol*, **120**, 817–824.

36 Jones MD, Sheldon RE, Peeters LL et al. (1977). Fetal cerebral oxygen consumption at different levels of oxygenation. *J Appl Physiol*, **43**, 1080–1084.

37 Fisher DS, Heymann MA and Rudolph AM. (1982). Fetal myocardial oxygen and carbohydrate consumption during acutely induced hypoxemia. *Am J Physiol*, **242**, H657–H661.

38 Yaffe H, Parer JT, Block BS et al. (1987). Cardiorespiratory responses to graded reductions of uterine blood flow in the sheep fetus. *J Dev Physiol*, **9**, 325–336.

39 Carter BS, Havercamp AD and Merenstein GB. (1993). The definition of acute perinatal asphyxia. *Clin Perinatol*, **20**, 287–304.

40 Paul RH, Suidan AK, Yeh S et al. (1975). Clinical fetal monitoring: VII. The evaluation and significance of intrapartum baseline FHR variability. *Am J Obstet Gynecol*, **123**, 206–210.

41 Ball RH and Parer JT. (1992). The physiological mechanisms of variable decelerations. *Am J Obstet Gynecol*, **166**, 1683–1689.

42 Parer JT and King TL. (1999). Whither fetal heart rate monitoring? *Obstet Gynecol Fertility*, **22**, 149–192.

43 Krebs HB, Petres RE, Dunn LJ et al. (1979). Intrapartum fetal heart rate monitoring. I. Classification and prognosis of fetal heart rate patterns. *Am J Obstet Gynecol*, **133**, 762–772.

44 Beard RW, Filshiw GM, Knight CA et al. (1971). The significance of the changes in the continuous fetal heart rate in the first stage of labor. *J Obstet Gynecol Br Commonwealth*, **78**, 865–881.

45 Tejani N, Mann LI, Bhakthavathsalan A et al. (1975). Correlation of fetal heart rate and uterine contraction patterns with fetal scalp blood pH. *Obstet Gynecol*, **46**, 392–396.

46 Berkus MD, Langer O, Samueloff A et al. (1998). Electronic fetal monitoring: what's reassuring? *Acta Obstet Gynecol Scand*, **78**, 15–21.

47 Low JA, Victory R and Derrick EJ. (1999). Predictive value of electronic fetal monitoring for intrapartum fetal asphyxia with metabolic acidosis. *Obstet Gynecol*, **93**, 285–291.

48 Low JA, Cox MJ, Karchmar EJ et al. (1981). The prediction of intrapartum fetal metabolic acidosis by fetal heart rate monitoring. *Am J Obstet Gynecol*, **139**, 229–305.

49 Gilstrap LC, Hauth JC, Hankins GD et al. (1987). Second stage fetal heart rate abnormalities and type of neonatal acidemia. *Obstet Gynecol*, **70**, 191–195.

50 Gull H, Jaffa AJ, Oren M et al. (1996). Acid accumulation during end stage bradycardia in term fetuses: how long is too long? *Br J Obstet Gynaecol*, **103**, 1096–1101.

51 Dellinger EH, Boehm FH and Crane MM. (2000). Electronic fetal heart rate monitoring: early neonatal outcomes associated with normal rate, fetal stress and fetal distress. *Am J Obstet Gynecol*, **182**, 14–20.

52 Rochard F, Schifrin BS, Goupil F et al. (1976). Non-stressed fetal heart rate monitoring in the antepartum period. *Am J Obstet Gynecol*, **126**, 699–706.

53 Murata Y, Miyake Y, Yamamoto T et al. (1985). Experimentally produced sinusoidal fetal heart rate patterns in choronically instrumental fetal lamb. *Am J Obstet Gynecol*, **153**, 693–702.

54 Parer JT and Livingston EG. (1990). What is fetal distress? *Am J Obstet Gynecol*, **162**, 1421–1427.

55 Wood C, Ferguson R, Leeton J et al. (1967). Fetal heart rate and acid–base status in the assessment of fetal hypoxia. *Am J Obstet Gynecol*, **98**, 62–70.

56 Paul RH, Suidan AK, Yeh S et al. (1975). Clinical fetal monitoring. VII. The evaluation and significance of intrapartum baseline FHR variability. *Am J Obstet Gynecol*, **123**, 206–210.

57 Clark SL, Gimovsky ML and Miller FC. (1984). The scalp stimulation test: a clinical alternative to fetal scalp blood sampling. *Am J Obstet Gynecol*, **148**, 274–277.

58 Helwig JT, Parer JT, Kilpatrick SJ et al. (1996). Umbilical cord blood acid base state: what is normal? *Am J Obstet Gynecol*, **174**, 1807–1812.

59 Lilien AA. (1970). Term intrapartum fetal death. *Am J Obstet Gynecol*, **107**, 595–603.

60 Paneth N and Kiely J. (1984). The frequency of cerebral palsy: a review of population studies in industrial nations since 1950. In *The Epidemiology of the Cerebral Palsies*, ed. Stanley FJ and Alberman E, pp. 46–56. Philadelphia: JB Lippincott.

61 Shiffrin BS and Dame L. (1972). Fetal heart rate patterns: prediction of Apgar Score. *JAMA*, **219**, 1322–1325.

62 Low JA, Galbraith RS, Muir DW et al. (1988). Motor and cognitive defects after intrapartum asphyxia in the mature fetus. *Am J Obstet Gynecol*, **158**, 356–361.

63 Minchom P, Niswander K, Chalmers I et al. (1987). Antecedents and outcome of very early neonatal seizures in infants born at or after term. *Br J Obstet Gynecol*, **94**, 431–439.

64 Rosen MG and Dickinson JC. (1993). The paradox of electronic fetal monitoring: more data may not enable us to predict or prevent neurologic morbidity. *Am J Obstet Gynecol*, **168**, 745–751.

65 Gilstrap LC, Leveno KJ, Burris J et al. (1989). Diagnosis of birth asphyxia on the basis of fetal pH, Apgar score, and newborn cerebral dysfunction. *Am J Obstet Gynecol*, **161**, 825–830.

66 Winkler Cl, Hauth JC, Tucker MJ et al. (1991). Neonatal complications at term as related to the degree of umbilical artery acidemia. *Am J Obstet Gynecol*, **164**, 637–641.

67 Goldaber KG, Gilstrap LC, Leveno KJ et al. (1991). Pathologic fetal acidemia. *Obstet Gynecol*, **78**, 1103–1108.

68 Low JA, Panagiopoulos C and Derrick EJ. (1994). Newborn complications after intrapartum asphyxia with metabolic acidosis in the term fetus. *Am J Obstet Gynecol*, **170**, 1081–1087.

69 American College of Obstetricians and Gynecologists. (1998). *Inappropriate Use of the Terms Fetal Distress and Birth Asphyxia*. Committee Opinion #197. Washington, DC: American College of Obstetricians and Gynecologists.

70 Phelan JP and Ahn MO. (1994). Perinatal observations in forty-eight neurologically impaired term infants. *Am J Obstet Gynecol*, **171**, 424–431.

71 Ellison PH, Foster M, Sheridan-Pereira M et al. (1991). Electronic fetal heart monitoring, auscultation and neonatal outcome. *Am J Obstet Gynecol*, **164**, 1281–1288.

72 Kubli FW, Hon EH, Khazin AF et al. (1969). Observations on heart rate and pH in the human fetus during labor. *Am J Obstet Gynecol*, **104**, 1190–1206.

73 Fleischer A, Schulman H, Jagani N et al. (1982). The development of fetal acidosis in the presence of an abnormal fetal heart tracing. *Am J Obstet Gynecol*, **142**, 55–60.

74 Saling E and Schneider D. (1967). Biochemical supervision of the foetus during labor. *J Obstet Gynaecol Br Commonwealth*, **74**, 799–811.

12

Obstetrical conditions and practices that affect the fetus and newborn

Section I

Reinaldo Acosta and Yasser Y. El-Sayed

Stanford University Medical Center, Stanford, CA, USA

Placenta previa

The implantation of the placenta over the cervical os or very near to it is known as placenta previa. It may be total, when the internal cervical os is completely covered by placenta; partial, when the internal os is partially covered by placenta; marginal, when the edge of the placenta is at the margin of the internal os; and low-lying, when the placental edge does not reach the internal os but is in close proximity to it.[1]

Incidence

The incidence of placenta previa is about 3–6 per 1000 singleton pregnancies.[2,3] This condition in an unscarred uterus has been reported to be 0.26%, and it increases almost linearly with the number of prior cesarean sections up to 10% in patients with four or more.[4] In a study from the state of New Jersey evaluating almost 550 000 deliveries where the diagnosis of placenta previa was confirmed only in pregnancies delivered by cesarean section, the incidence was 5 per 1000 births.[5]

Etiology and risk factors

The likelihood of placenta previa rises with multiparity,[6] advancing maternal age, especially in women older than 35 years old,[7] and a history of prior cesarean deliveries.[8] Smoking during pregnancy can double the risk of this condition,[9,10] and women of Asian origin have been reported to have an increased risk of a delivery complicated by placenta previa compared to caucasian women.[11]

Clinical presentation and diagnosis

The classic symptom of placenta previa is painless bright-red vaginal bleeding in the second or third trimester of pregnancy. In fact, almost three-fourths of all women with placenta previa experience at least one episode of painless antepartum bleeding, which usually presents without warning. In most situations, the initial episode resolves spontaneously.[12] The anteparum diagnosis of placenta previa is primarily based on the ultrasonographic visualization of the placental location and its relationship to the internal cervical os. Transvaginal sonography is more accurate than transabdominal sonography in making the diagnosis.[13,14] Transperineal[15] and translabial ultrasonography[16] may also provide good resolution of the internal os. Placenta previa has been diagnosed in 5% of patients undergoing ultrasound examination between 16 and 18 weeks; however 90% of these placentas are no longer identified as previas in the third trimester. This phenomena has been called placental migration. In these patients extra care is not required unless the diagnosis persists beyond 30 weeks of gestation or if the patient becomes symptomatic before that time. In general the earlier in pregnancy the initial episode of bleeding occurs, the worse is the outcome of the pregnancy.[17]

Management

Management of placenta previa varies according to the clinical situation. In preterm pregnancies with no active bleeding, expectant management is the general rule. Strict bedrest, providing the mother with blood transfusions if required, administration of corticosteroids to reduce the rate and severity of respiratory distress syndrome, as well as the occasional use of tocolytic agents for inhibition of premature labor in the presence of vaginal bleeding are appropriate in the conservative aggressive management of this condition.[18–20] One of the most controversial issues is whether the mother should be kept hospitalized after she has been stabilized. D' Angelo and Irwin reported an improved outcome in neonatal morbidity in these patients maintained in hospital,[21] but Wing and coworkers noted that, in selected patients, outpatient management may be safe and appropriate.[22] Anti-D immunoglobulin (RhoGAM) should be given after a bleeding episode if the patient is Rh-negative. It is advisable to perform an elective cesarean section after determination of fetal pulmonary maturity; this approach significantly reduces overall neonatal morbidity and mortality.[18] However, expeditious cesarean delivery, after the mother is adequately stabilized, is warranted in cases of persistent hemorrhage, failed tocolysis, fetal distress, or coagulopathy.

Complications

Major complications are related to massive bleeding leading to hemorrhagic shock. Following placental removal, hemorrhage at the site of implantation may occur. Almost 7% of placenta previas have an abnormal placental attachment to the myometrium (placenta accreta).[3] If uterotonic medication, hemostatic sutures, and other conservative methods fail to control the hemorrhage, hysterectomy may become necessary.

Some investigators have reported a high incidence of fetal growth restriction with previa.[23] Others have not found this association after controlling for gestational age.[2,5,24] Despite tocolysis and transfusions to delay delivery, nearly two-thirds of the patients are delivered before 36 weeks and account for at least 10–15% of all premature births.[5] The perinatal mortality due to placenta previa has decreased significantly since the early 1970s from 37%[25] to as low as 4–8% in the 1980s.[26] Crane et al., in a population-based retrospective cohort study of over 92000 births in Nova Scotia, identified 305 cases of placenta previa.[2] The perinatal mortality rate in their patients was 2.3% as compared to 0.78% in controls. These investigators also noted no differences in birth weights after controlling for gestational age in the patients and controls. After controlling for potential confounders, neonatal complications, which are associated with placenta previa, include major congenital anomalies, respiratory distress syndrome, and anemia.[2] There is a significant correlation between antepartum maternal hemorrhage and the need for neonatal transfusion, and between the neonatal anemia and the amount of intrapartum maternal blood loss.[17]

Summary

Placenta previa is a life-threatening condition for the mother and the fetus. Prompt diagnosis, mainly by ultrasound, and treatment with strict bedrest, tocolysis, and blood transfusions are mainstays of care. An elective delivery as close to term as feasible and with documented fetal maturity is optimal. However emergency preterm delivery is frequently necessary.

Placental abruption

The premature separation of the normally implanted placenta is known as placental abruption. Usually this phenomena is accompanied by painful uterine contractions and a variable amount of vaginal bleeding. Bleeding may also be concealed behind the detached placenta.

Incidence

The incidence of placental abruption is between 5 and 7 per 1000 births.[27,28] Ananth and Wilcox, evaluating 7508655 singleton births in the USA in the years 1995 and 1996, found that abruption was encountered in 6.5 per 1000 live births.[29] A perinatal mortality rate of 119 per 1000 live births has been reported,[29] and up to 14% of the fetuses that survive may have significant neurological deficits.[30]

Etiology and risk factors

Although the precise cause of placental abruption remains unknown, various risk factors have been identified. Many reports suggest that the incidence increases with advancing maternal age and parity,[31,32] however other studies have been unable to confirm this association.[33,34] It has also been reported to be more common in African-American women than Caucasians and less frequent in Hispanic women.[31] There is a strong association of this condition with hypertension, either preexisting or pregnancy-associated;[28,35–37] in fact, there is a threefold increased incidence of abruption with chronic hypertension and a fourfold increase with severe preeclampsia.[38] Women who smoke during their pregnancies also have an increased risk of abruption.[39] If one adds the effects of smoking and hypertension during pregnancy, the risk is increased even greater.[28] There is also an increased incidence of abruption with premature rupture of membranes,[36] especially in patients who have recurrent bleeding episodes during the period of expectant management.[40,41] Studies have consistently documented placental abruption as a maternal reproductive risk associated with cocaine use.[42–44] Recent reports have also found an increased frequency of genetic thrombophilias in patients with placental abruption.[45,46] Placental abruption may also be present even in cases of minor trauma and may not be a clinically immediately evident condition.[47,48] Uterine leiomyomas may predispose to abruption, especially if they are located behind the placental implantation site.[49] A history of placental abruption may increase the risk of occurrence up to 10-fold in subsequent pregnancies.[27] Other risk factors that have been associated with this condition include severe fetal growth restriction, chorioamnionitis, polyhydramnios, a short umbilical cord, sudden uterine decompression, external version, and diabetes.[32,33,50]

Clinical presentation and diagnosis

Because of the wide variety of signs and symptoms associated with this clinical condition, it is necessary to have a high index of suspicion in order to make an accurate diagnosis. The spectrum ranges from asymptomatic states in which the diagnosis is made only after delivery upon the evaluation of the placenta, to cases with fetal demise, hypovolemic shock, and severe coagulopathy. However, the most common presentation is an acute onset of vaginal bleeding accompanied by intermittent cramping or constant abdominal pain. Other findings that may be present are fetal distress, frequent and intense contractions, preterm labor, and intrauterine fetal demise.[51] Ultrasound visualization of a clot occurs in only about 25% of the cases, and appears to have little or no impact on course or management. The absence of these findings should not preclude the diagnosis. However ultrasound assessment as well as clinical inspection are essential in order to rule out placenta previa and other causes of bleeding. In assessing a woman with placental abruption, the possibility of physical abuse or the use of cocaine must not be disregarded. Unless specific questions about these issues are asked, the precipitating cause of the abruption may not be identified.[50]

Management

Once the diagnosis of placental abruption has been made, intravenous access, blood product availability, and maternal hemodynamic stability must be secured. The next step in management will depend upon gestational age and maternal and fetal status.

In preterm pregnancies without evidence of maternal–fetal compromise expectant management may be considered. Tocolysis in this clinical situation is a matter of controversy.[51–53] Administration of steroids should be considered, in the hope of reducing the risk of respiratory distress syndrome.

Expectant management generally is not a choice for the majority of patients and delivery is indicated because of maternal or fetal deterioration or both. Delivery is also indicated in viable, mature fetuses. If vaginal delivery is not imminent, cesarean section is the best approach. However, if the fetus has died, labor can be pursued provided that the mother does not continue to have deterioration of her clinical status. Cesarean section in this case must be reserved for maternal indications alone.[20] Rh-negative mothers with placental abruptio require anti-D immunoglobulin (RhoGAM) to avoid Rh-isoimmunization.

Complications

Most of the serious maternal complications are related to hypovolemia secondary to maternal hemorrhage, which may lead to acute renal and other organ failure. Almost 40% of cases of renal failure in pregnancy are secondary to placental abruption.[54] Abruption is also the most frequent cause of disseminated intravascular coagulation (DIC) in pregnancy. DIC may aggravate hemorrhagic problems, is found in about 30% of women with abruption, and is severe enough to cause fetal demise.[55] In some cases extravasation of blood into the myometrium may create a blue-purple discoloration of the uterus known as a Couvelaire uterus, which has been associated with uterine atony and postpartum hemorrhage. With respect to the fetus, most of the complications result from prematurity and hypoxia. Low-birth-weight infants delivered after abruptio placentae tend to have low Apgar scores, and are at increased risk of death, having intraventricular hemorrhage, and developing cerebral palsy.[56]

Summary

Abruptio placentae is an extremely dangerous condition for both the mother and the fetus, and carries significant morbidity and mortality for both. The diagnosis requires a high index of suspicion as well as prompt assessment of the fetal–maternal status. Expectant management or expeditious delivery depends upon the severity of the condition and the gestational age at the time of diagnosis. The route of delivery is dictated by the severity of the condition and the viability of the fetus.

Vasa previa

Vasa previa is a rare condition in which the fetal blood vessels, unsupported by either the umbilical cord or placental tissue, traverse the fetal membranes of the lower segment of the uterus below the presenting part.[57]

Incidence

It is difficult to estimate the true incidence of this condition, as vasa previa is likely to be underreported. It has been estimated to occur in about 1 in 2000 to 1 in 3000 deliveries. Thus, a relatively active obstetric service may expect one case per year.[58]

Etiology and risk factors

Vasa previa has been associated with in vitro fertilization, multiple pregnancies, low-lying placentas, multilobed, and succenturiated lobed placentas.[59–61]

Clinical presentation and diagnosis

Usually the clinical presentation of this condition is vaginal bleeding after either spontaneous or artificial rupture of membranes, leading to the rupture of the velamentous vessels, and fetal death from exsanguination. However, vessel rupture may occur independently of membrane rupture; therefore, this condition should be suspected in any patient with antepartum or intrapartum hemorrhage.[62] Occasionally, progressive severe variable decelerations and bradycardia, secondary to compression of the velamentous vessels by the presenting part or a sinusoidal pattern due to fetal anemia, may be the only manifestations of vasa previa.[63,64]

Transvaginal ultrasound with color Doppler is the current method used for the antenatal diagnosis of vasa previa.[57,65–68] Also three-dimensional ultrasound has been reported as a useful diagnostic tool for this condition.[69] Some authors have proposed the use of amnioscopy[57,64] and low intrauterine transcervical endoscopy (LITE)[70] before amniotomy in those cases identified by ultrasound as being suspicious for vasa previa. This diagnosis should be suspected in any case of bleeding in the second half of the pregnancy; therefore it is crucial to determine whether the bleeding is of maternal or fetal origin. The Ogita may be helpful in this regard.[71]

Management

If the diagnosis has been made antenatally and there is no evidence of fetal compromise, the safest form of delivery would be by elective cesarean when the fetus is mature. This approach mitigates the risk of membrane rupture and fetal exsanguinations. Immediate delivery is mandatory in a viable pregnancy. The infant has a total blood volume of approximately 250 ml at term, and so is very intolerant to blood loss. If the cervix is fully dilated and vaginal delivery can be accomplished rapidly, this becomes the route of choice.[58] Vaginal delivery is also indicated when the fetus is too immature to survive or fetal demise has already occurred. An emergency cesarean section provides the most favorable outcome if performed immediately upon recognition of the condition. Optimizing neonatal outcome requires rapid and aggressive neonatal resuscitative techniques. These include immediate basic and advanced life support measures, and establishment of vascular access for fluids, blood, and blood component therapy.[72] Rh-negative patients should receive anti-D immunoglobulin when indicated.

Complications

Vasa previa is mainly a risk to the fetus. The fetal mortality rate ranges from 33 to 100%.[57] Fortunately, there is little, if any, increase in maternal complications.[58]

Summary

Vasa previa is an obstetric condition that may have catastrophic consequences for the fetus. Ultrasound and color Doppler studies may help identify this condition in patients at risk. If hemorrhage is present, immediate delivery and aggressive resuscitation of the newborn are mandatory.

Vaginal birth after previous cesarean section (VBAC)

At present, a trial of labor after previous cesarean delivery is an accepted form of therapy in the attempt to decrease the overall cesarean delivery rate. Elective repeat cesarean births account for one-third of all cesarean deliveries.[73–78] By 1996, 28% of women with prior cesarean section had vaginal deliveries, which represented a 50% increase in VBAC since 1989.[79] Although there is strong consensus that trial of labor is appropriate for most women who have had a previous low transverse cesarean delivery, increased experience with VBAC shows that there are many potential problems associated with a small but significant risk of uterine rupture.[80–85]

Candidate selection

The American College of Obstetricians and Gynecologists has issued the following recommendations for selection of candidates for VBAC:[80]

- One or two prior low transverse cesarean deliveries
- Clinically adequate pelvis
- No other uterine scars or previous rupture
- Physician immediately available throughout active labor capable of monitoring labor and performing emergency cesarean delivery
- Availability of anesthesia and personnel for emergency cesarean delivery

There has been a trend to extend the clinical situations in which VBAC may be attempted including an unknown uterine scar,[86] breech presentation,[87,88] twin gestation,[89,90] postterm pregnancy,[91,92] suspected macrosomia,[93,94] and multiple previous cesarean deliveries.[95,96] However, uterine rupture has been reported to be three to five times more common in women who had a trial of labor after two or more previous cesareans.[78,97] It is still debatable if VBAC option should be offered with these clinical situations and a history of a previous low vertical uterine incision.[98–101]

The VBAC success rate is in the range of 60–80%.[75,102] Patients with nonrecurring indications have a higher probability of success than women with recurring indications.[103,104] Women with a previous vaginal delivery either before or after a cesarean birth have a significantly higher rate of success in a subsequent trial of labor.[105–107]

Limited data suggest that external cephalic version is a reasonable option in patients with a prior low transverse uterine scar;[108,109] however the safety and efficacy of this procedure in this clinical situation must be examined further.[110]

Counseling patients

Every patient with a prior cesarean delivery should be thoroughly counseled regarding the benefits and risks of a trial of labor. Neither repeat cesarean delivery nor trial of labor is riskfree. A successful trial of labor is associated with fewer postpartum transfusions, postpartum infections, and a decreased length of hospital stay, when compared with elective repeat cesarean deliveries.[75,77] However a significant increase in maternal morbidity has been noted among patients whose trial of labor resulted in a repeat cesarean section.[73,111–114] There is also an increased rate of infection among infants who are delivered after a failed trial of labor.[115]

Risks of uterine rupture

Rupture of the uterine scar is the most significant and worrisome risk in a patient undergoing a trial of labor after a cesarean section. The risk of uterine rupture with one prior low transverse uterine incision is about 0.5–1.0%.[77,78,101] This risk has been reported to be almost the same in patients who had a previous low vertical incision,[98,100,101] but can be as high as 12% in classical incisions.[75] In patients who have had a prior lower segment uterine rupture the risk of a repeat rupture is 6%. In those whose prior rupture was in the upper uterus, the recurrence risk was 32%.[116,117]

Managing labor in patients undergoing VBAC

A number of issues have been raised regarding the management of patients with prior cesarean section who opt for a trial of labor. Some of these include:

1. Anesthesia. The use of epidural anesthesia was once felt to be contraindicated in women undergoing a trial of labor, due to the fear that this technique could mask the pain of uterine rupture. However, pain and bleeding are unlikely findings in uterine scar separation as these are infrequently encountered.[118] The literature strongly suggests that epidural anesthesia is safe even when oxytocin is used for augmentation of labor.[119–121] More important than the type of anesthesia is the immediate availability of anesthesia coverage should an emergency suddenly develop.
2. Intrapartum management. Continuous electronic fetal monitoring is of paramount importance during a trial of labor, in view that prolonged fetal heart rate decelerations are the most common manifestation of a scar separation, and these may be the only indication that uterine rupture has occurred.[76,118] An intrauterine pressure catheter is probably not helpful since a change in intrauterine pressure is not a useful indicator of uterine rupture.[122] Every patient should have an intravenous access, and have type and screen drawn.
3. Induction and augmentation of labor. Spontaneous labor is preferred over induction of women who have experienced previous cesarean deliveries.[123] Although there have been many reports to indicate that prostaglandins and/or oxytocin may be used safely in patients with prior low segment cesarean sections,[75,124–129] most recent studies have documented that induction of labor, with either of these agents, is associated with a risk of uterine rupture that is five times

greater than if labor occurs spontaneously.[111,130–132] The American College of Obstetricians and Gynecologists recommends close patient monitoring when oxytocin or prostaglandin gel is used in women undergoing a trial of labor.[80]

4. Examining the scar. The routine exploration of the uterine segment after a successful VBAC is a matter of controversy. Most asymptomatic scar dehiscences heal well and surgical correction is necessary only if significant bleeding is found. Asymptomatic separations do not generally require exploratory laparotomy and repair.
5. Elective sterilization. Desire for permanent sterilization in a woman with a prior cesarean section is not an indication for a repeat operation, because the morbidity of vaginal birth and postpartum tubal ligation is considerably less than that of a repeat cesarean.

Complications of uterine rupture

Maternal

Maternal deaths from uterine rupture are rarely encountered, but unfortunately do occur.[84,85,132,133] Major puerperal infection, severe posthemorrhagic anemia, bladder injury, and paralytic ileus are well-recognized complications. Hysterectomy may be required following uterine rupture, and the incidence of this complication ranges from as low as 0.12%[77,131] to as great as 17%.[133] The length of hospital stay is also increased following uterine rupture,[132] although in some situations it may be the same as that following cesarean delivery.[134]

Fetal

The primary danger of uterine rupture is the adverse effect on the fetus. Even if the uterine rupture is partial, and the fetus is not extruded into the mother's peritoneal cavity, perinatal asphyxia and subsequent neurological damage can occur. The ability to provide immediate operative management for a woman with a ruptured uterus is the key to enhancing optimal outcome for the fetus. In a recent study from San Francisco in which 21 patients with uterine rupture were managed, only two neonatal deaths occurred.[134] One was a fetus of 23 weeks' gestation, and the other was a 25-week fetus with Potter's syndrome. Although four infants had umbilical cord pH recorded below 7.0, none of the infants was found to have suffered neurological sequelae at the time of discharge from the hospital. Unfortunately, the long-term evaluation of these infants has not been reported, but the authors have demonstrated that, with excellent inhouse personnel and equipment, these infants can be rescued appropriately.

Porter et al. reported on 23 patients with uterine rupture who were attempting VBAC at the time.[135] Six of the infants (23%) either died or suffered adverse neurological sequelae. Interestingly, poor neurological outcome was found in 31% of the infants delivered within 30 min of either severe variable decelerations or bradycardia and in 33% of infants delivered within 20 min of the event.

The studies of Leung et al. are the most widely quoted as to the timing of delivery of the fetus following overt signs of uterine rupture.[133] If delivery could be accomplished within 17 min of prolonged deceleration, the infants survived and no significant abnormalities were noted at the time of discharge. If, however, the prolonged deceleration was preceded by severe late decelerations, perinatal asphyxia occurred as early as 10 min from the onset of the prolonged deceleration and delivery. Unfortunately, the long-term evaluation of these survivors has not been reported.

Summary

VBAC remains an acceptable option for appropriately selected patients. The ideal candidate is the patient with one prior low transverse uterine incision following a cesarean section for a nonrecurring indication who presents in spontaneous labor to a hospital with inhouse obstetrics and anesthesia. The decision to proceed with the trial of labor after a previous cesarean section must only be made after thorough counseling between the patient and her physician that balances the risk and benefits of the procedure, especially the potential of adverse affects on the fetus should uterine rupture occur.[136]

REFERENCES

1 Cunningham FG, Gant NF, Leveno KJ, et al. (2001). *Williams Obstetrics*, 21st edn, pp. 630–635. New York: McGraw-Hill.

2 Crane JM, van den Hof MC, Dodds L, et al. (1999). Neonatal outcomes with placenta previa. *Obstet Gynecol*, **93**, 541–544.

3 Frederiksen MC, Glassenberg R and Stika CS. (1999). Placenta previa: a 22-year analysis. *Am J Obstet Gynecol*, **180**, 1432–1437.

4 Clark SL, Koonings PP and Phelan JP. (1985). Placenta previa/accreta and prior cesarean sections. *Obstet Gynecol*, **66**, 89–92.

5 Ananth CV, Demissie K, Smulian JC, et al. (2001). Relationship among placenta previa, fetal growth restriction and preterm delivery: a population-based study. *Obstet Gynecol*, **98**, 299–306.

6 Babinszki A, Kerenyi T, Torok O, et al. (1999). Perinatal outcome in grand and great grand multiparity: effects of parity on obstetric risk factors. *Am J Obstet Gynecol*, **181**, 669–674.

7 Iyasu S, Saftlas AK, Rowley DL, et al. (1987). The epidemiology of placenta previa in the United States, 1979 through 1987. *Am Obstet Gynecol*, **168**, 1424–1429.

8 Ananth CV, Smulian JC and Vintzileos AM. (1997). The association of placenta previa with history of cesarean delivery and abortion: a meta-analysis. *Am J Obstet Gynecol*, **177**, 1071–1078.

9 Williams MA, Mittendorf R, Lieberman E, et al. (1991). Cigarette smoking during pregnancy in relation to placenta previa. *Am J Obstet Gynecol*, **165**, 28–32.

10 Handler AS, Mason ED, Rosenberg DL, et al. (1994). The relationship between exposure during pregnancy to cigarette smoking and cocaine use and placenta previa. *Am J Obstet Gynecol*, **170**, 884–889.

11 Taylor VM, Peacock S, Kramer MD, et al. (1995). Increased risk of placenta previa among women of Asian origin. *Obstet Gynecol*, **86**, 805–808.

12 Love CD and Wallace EM. (1996). Pregnancies complicated by placenta previa: what is appropriate management? *Br J Obstet Gynaecol*, **103**, 864–867.

13 Farine D, Fox HE, Jakobson S, et al. (1989). It is really a placenta previa? *Eur Obstet Gynecol Reprod Biol*, **31**, 103–108.

14 Smith RS, Lauria MR, Comstock CH, et al. (1997). Transvaginal ultrasonography for all placentas that appear to be low lying or over the internal cervical os. *Ultrasound Obstet Gynecol*, **9**, 22–24.

15 Hertzberg BS, Bowie JD, Carroll BA, et al. (1992). Diagnosis of placenta previa during the third trimester: role of transperineal sonography. *Am J Roetgenol*, **159**, 83–87.

16 Dawson WB, Dumas MD, Romano WM, et al. (1996). Translabial ultrasonography and placenta previa: does measurement of the os-placenta distance predict outcome? *Ultrasound Med*, **15**, 441–446.

17 McShane PM, Heyl PS and Epstein MF. (1985). Maternal and perinatal morbidity resulting from placenta previa. *Obstet Gynecol*, **65**, 176–182.

18 Cotton DB, Read JA, Paul RH, et al. (1980). The conservative aggressive management of placenta previa. *Am J Obstet Gynecol*, **137**, 687–695.

19 Besinger RE, Moniak CW, Paskiweicz LS, et al. (1995). The effect of tocolytic use in the management of symptomatic placenta previa. *Am J Obstet Gynecol*, **172**, 1770–1775.

20 Chamberlain G and Steer P. (1999). ABC of labour care: obstetric emergencies. *Br Med J*, **318**, 1342–1345.

21 D' Angelo LJ and Irwin LF. (1984). Conservation management of placenta previa: a cost benefit analysis. *Am J Obstet Gynecol*, **149**, 320–326.

22 Wing DA, Paul RH and Millar LK. (1996). Management of the symptomatic placenta previa: a randomized, controlled trial of inpatient versus outpatient expectant management. *Am J Obstet Gynecol*, **175**, 806–811.

23 Brar HS, Platt LD, De Vore GR, et al. (1988). Fetal umbilical velocimetry for the surveillance of pregnancies complicated by placenta previa. *Reprod Med*, **33**, 741–744.

24 Wolf EJ, Mallozi A, Rodis JF, et al. (1991). Placenta previa is not an independent risk factor for a small for gestational age infant. *Obstet Gynecol*, **77**, 707–709.

25 Crenshaw C Jr, Jones DED and Parker RT. (1973). Placenta previa: a survey of twenty years experience with improved perinatal survival by expectant therapy and cesarean delivery. *Obstet Gynecol Surv*, **28**, 461–470.

26 Silver R, Depp R, Sabbagha RE, et al. (1984). Placenta previa: aggressive expectant management. *Am J Obstet Gynecol*, **150**, 15–22.

27 Karegard M and Genneser G. (1986). Incidence and recurrence rate of abruption placentae in Sweden. *Obstet Gynecol*, **67**, 523–528.

28 Ananth CV, Smulian JC and Vintzileos AM. (1999). Incidence of placental abruption in relation to cigarette

smoking and hypertensive disorders during pregnancy: a meta-analysis of observational studies. *Obstet Gynecol*, **93**, 622–628.

29 Ananth CV and Wilcox AJ. (2001). Placental abruption and perinatal mortality in the United States. *Am J Epidemiol*, **153**, 332–337.

30 Abdella TN, Sibai BM, Hays JM Jr, et al. (1984). Perinatal outcome in abruptio placentae. *Obstet Gynecol*, **63**, 365–370.

31 Pritchard JA, Cunningham FG, Pritchard SA, et al. (1991). On reducing the frequency of severe abruption placentae. *Am J Obstet Gynecol*, **165**, 1345–1351.

32 Kramer MS, Usher RH, Pollack R, et al. (1997). Etiologic determinants of abruption placentae. *Obstet Gynecol*, **89**, 221–226.

33 Krohn M, Voig L, McKnight B, et al. (1987). Correlates of placental abruption. *Br J Obstet Gynaecol*, **94**, 333–340.

34 Toohey JS, Keegan KA Jr, Morgan MA, et al. (1995). *Am J Obstet Gynecol*, **172**, 683–686.

35 Ananth CV, Savitz DA and Williams MA. (1996). Placental abruption and its association with hypertension and prolonged rupture of membranes: a methodologic review and meta-analysis. *Obstet Gynecol*, **88**, 309–318.

36 Ananth CV, Savitz DA, Bowes WA Jr, et al. (1997). Influence of hypertensive disorders and cigarette smoking on placental abruption and uterine bleeding during pregnancy. B*r J Obstet Gynaecol*, **104**, 572–578.

37 Sibai BM, Lindheimer M, Hauth J, et al. (1998). Risk factors for preeclampsia, abruption placentae and adverse neonatal outcomes among women with chronic hypertension. National Institute of Child Health and Human Development network of maternal–fetal medicine units. *N Engl J Med*, **339**, 667–671.

38 Ananth CV, Berkowitz GS, Savitz DA, et al. (1999b). Placental abruption and adverse perinatal outcomes. *JAMA*, **282**, 1646–1651.

39 Misra DP and Ananth CV. (1999). Risk factor profiles of placental abruption in first and second pregnancies: heterogeneous etiologies. *J Clin Epidemiol*, **52**, 453–461.

40 Gonen R, Hannah ME and Milligan JE. (1989). Does prolonged premature rupture of the membranes predispose to abruptio placentae? *Obstet Gynecol*, **74**, 347–350.

41 Major CA, de Veciana M, Lewis DF, et al. (1995). Preterm premature rupture of membranes and abruption placentae: is there an association between these pregnancy complications? *Am J Obstet Gynecol*, **172**, 672–676.

42 Bingol N, Fuchs M, Diaz V, et al. (1987). Teratogenicity of cocaine in humans. *J Pediatr*, **110**, 93–96.

43 Hoskins IA, Friedman DM, Frieden FJ, et al. (1991). Relationship between antepartum cocaine abuse, abnormal umbilical artery Doppler velocimetry, and placental abruption. *Obstet Gynecol*, **78**, 279–282.

44 Slutsker L. (1992) Risks associated with cocaine use during pregnancy. *Obstet Gynecol*, **79**, 778–789.

45 Kupferminc MJ, Eldor A, Steinman N, et al. (1999). Increased frequency of genetic thrombophilia in women with complications of pregnancy. *N Engl J Med*, **340**, 50–52.

46 Gherman RB and Goodwin TM. (2000). Obstetric implications of activated protein C resistance and factor V Leiden mutation. *Obstet Gynecol*, **55**, 117–122.

47 Kettel LM, Branch DW and Scott JR. (1988) Occult placental abruption after maternal trauma. *Obstet Gynecol*, **71**, 449–453.

48 Stafford PA, Biddinger PW and Zumwalt RE. (1988). Lethal intrauterine fetal trauma. *Am J Obstet Gynecol*, **159**, 485–489.

49 Rice JP, Kay HH and Mahony BS. (1989). The clinical significance of uterine leiomyomas in pregnancy. *Am J Obstet Gynecol*, **160**, 1212–1216.

50 Nimrod CA and Oppenheimer LW. (1999). *Medicine of the Fetus and Mother*, 2nd edn, pp. 1498–1501. Philadelphia: Lippincott-Raven.

51 Hurd WW, Miodovnik M, Hertzberg V, et al. (1983). Selective management of abruptio placentae: a prospective study. *Obstet Gynecol*, **61**, 467–473.

52 Combs CA, Nyberg DA, Mack LA, et al. (1992). Expectant management after sonographic diagnosis of placental abruption. *Am J Perinatol*, **9**, 170–174.

53 Towers CV, Pircon RA and Heppard M. (1999). Is tocolysis safe in the management of third trimester bleeding? *Am J Obstet Gynecol*, **180**, 1572–1578.

54 Grunfeld JP and Pertuiset N. (1987). Acute renal failure in pregnancy: 1987. *Am J Kidney Dis*, **9**, 359–362.

55 Shaw KJ. (1994). Abruptio placentae In *Management of Common Problems in Obstetrics and Gynecology*, 3rd edn, ed. Mishell DR and Brenner PF, pp. 211–215. Boston: Blackwell Scientific Publications.

56 Spinillo A, Fazzi E, Stronati I, et al. (1994). Early morbidity and neurodevelopmental outcome in low birth weight infants born after third trimester bleeding. *Am J Perinatol*, **11**, 85–90.

57 Oyelese KO, Turner M, Lees C, et al. (1999). Vasa previa: an avoidable obstetric tragedy. *Obstet Gynecol Surv*, **54**, 138–145.

58 Pent D. (1979). Vasa previa. *Am J Obstet Gynecol*, **134**, 151–155.

59 Englert Y, Imbert MC, Van Rosendael E, et al. (1987). Morphological anomalies in the placentae of IVF pregnan-

cies: preliminary report of a multicentric study. *Hum Reprod*, **2**, 155–157.
60 Burton G and Saunders DM. (1988). Vasa praevia: another cause of concern in in vitro fertilization pregnancies. *Aust NZ J Obstet Gynaecol*, **28**, 180–181.
61 Oyelese KO, Schwarzler P, Coates S, et al. (1998). A strategy for reducing the mortality rate from vasa previa using transvaginal sonography with color Doppler. *Ultrasound Obstet Gynecol*, **12**, 377–379.
62 Carp HJ, Mashiach S and Serr DM. (1979). Vasa previa: a major complication and its management. *Obstet Gynecol*, **53**, 273–275.
63 Cordero DR, Helfgoftt AW, Landy HJ, et al. (1993). A nonhemorrhagic manifestation of vasa previa: a clinico-pathologic case report. *Obstet Gynecol*, **82**, 698–700.
64 Antoine C, Young BK, Silverma, F, et al. (1982). Sinusoidal fetal heart rate pattern with vasa previa in twin pregnancy. *J Reprod Med*, **27**, 295–300.
65 Harding JA, Lewis DF, Major CA, et al. (1990). Color flow Doppler – a useful instrument in the diagnosis of vasa previa. *Am J Obstet Gynecol*, **163**, 1566–1568.
66 Meyer WJ, Blumenthal L, Cadkin A, et al. (1993). Vasa previa: prenatal diagnosis with transvaginal color Doppler flow imaging. *Am J Obstet Gynecol*, **169**, 1627–1629.
67 Hata K, Hata T, Fujiwaki R, et al. (1994). An accurate antenatal diagnosis of vasa previa with transvaginal color Doppler ultrasonography. *Am J Obstet Gynecol*, **171**, 265–267.
68 Clerici G, Burnelli L, Lauro V, et al. (1996). Prenatal diagnosis of vasa previa presenting as amniotic band. "A not so innocent amniotic band." *Ultrasound Obstet Gynecol*, **7**, 61–63.
69 Lee W, Kirk JS, Comstock CH, et al. (2000). Vasa previa: prenatal detection by three-dimensional ultrasonography. *Ultrasound Obstet Gynecol*, **16**, 384–387.
70 Young M, Yule N and Barham K. (1991). The role of light and sound technologies in the detection of vasa previa. *Reprod Fertil Dev*, **3**, 439–445.
71 Odunsi K, Bullough CH, Henzel J, et al. (1996). Evaluation of chemical tests for fetal bleeding from vasa previa. *Int J Gynaecol Obstet*, **55**, 207–212.
72 Schellpfeffer MA. (1995) Improved neonatal outcome of vasa previa with aggressive intrapartum management: a report of two cases. *J Reprod Med*, **40**, 327–332.
73 Merril BS and Gibbs CE. (1978). Planned vaginal delivery following cesarean section. *Obstet Gynecol*, **52**, 50–52.
74 Flamm BL, Newma, LA, Thomas SJ, et al. (1990). Vaginal birth after cesarean delivery: results of a 5-year multicenter collaborative study. *Obstet Gynecol*, **76**, 750–754.
75 Rosen MG, Dickinson JC and Westhoff CL. (1991). Vaginal birth after cesarean: a meta-analysis of morbidity and mortality. *Obstet Gynecol*, **77**, 465–470.
76 Cowan RK, Kinch RA, Ellis B, et al. (1994). Trial of labor following cesarean delivery. *Obstet Gynecol*, **83**, 933–936.
77 Flamm BL, Goings JR, Liu,Y, et al. (1994). Elective repeat cesarean delivery versus a trial of labor: a prospective multicenter study. *Obstet Gynecol*, **83**, 927–932.
78 Miller DA, Diaz FG and Paul RH. (1994). Vaginal birth after cesarean: a 10-year experience. *Obstet Gynecol*, **84**, 255–258.
79 Leveno KJ. (1999). Controversies in Ob/gyn: should we rethink the criteria for VBAC? *Contemp Ob-Gyn*, **44**, 57–65.
80 American College of Obstetricians and Gynecologists. (1999). Vaginal birth after previous cesarean delivery. *ACOG Practice Bulletin*, 5.
81 Scott JR. (1991). Mandatory trial of labor after cesarean delivery: an alternative viewpoint. *Obstet Gynecol*, **77**, 811–814.
82 Jones RO, Nagashima AW, Hartnett-Goodman MM, et al. (1991). Rupture of low transverse cesarean scars during trial of labor. *Obstet Gynecol*, **77**, 817–817.
83 Leung AS, Farmer RM, Leung EK, et al. (1993). Risk factors associated with uterine rupture during trial of labor after cesarean delivery: a case control study. *Am J Obstet Gynecol*, **168**, 1358–1363.
84 Rageth JC, Juzi C and Grossenbacher H. (1999). Delivery after previous cesarean: a risk evaluation. *Obstet Gynecol*, **93**, 332–337.
85 Mozurkewich EL and Hutton EK. (2000). Elective repeat cesarean delivery versus trial of labor: a meta-analysis of the literature from 1989 to 1999. *Am J Obstet Gynecol*, **183**, 1187–1197.
86 Beall M, Eglinton EE, Clark SL, et al. (1984). Vaginal delivery after cesarean section in women with unknown types of uterine scar. *J Reprod Med*, **29**, 31–35.
87 Ophir E, Oettinger M, Yagoda A, et al. (1989). Breech presentation after cesarean section: always a section? *Am J Obstet Gynecol*, **161**, 25–28.
88 Sarno AP Jr, Phelan JP, Ahn MO, et al. (1989). Vaginal birth after cesarean delivery. Trial of labor in women with breech presentation. *J Reprod Med*, **34**, 831–833.
89 Strong TH Jr, Phelan JP, Ahn MO, et al. (1989). Vaginal birth after cesarean delivery in the twin gestation. *Am J Obstet Gynecol*, **161**, 29–32.
90 Miller DA, Mullin P, Hou D, et al. (1996). Vaginal birth after cesarean section in twin gestation. *Am J Obstet Gynecol*, **175**, 194–198.
91 Yeh S, Huang X and Phelan JP. (1984). Postterm pregnancy after a previous cesarean section. *J Reprod Med*, **29**, 41–44.

92 Callahan C, Chescheir N and Steiner BD. (1999). Safety and efficacy of attempted vaginal birth after cesarean section beyond the estimated date of delivery. *J Reprod Med*, **44**, 606–610.

93 Phelan JP, Eglinton GS, Horenstein JM, et al. (1984). Previous cesarean birth. Trial of labor in women with macrosomic infants. *J Reprod Med*, **29**, 36–40.

94 Flamm BL and Goings JR. (1989). Vaginal birth after cesarean section: is suspected fetal macrosomia a contraindication? *Obstet Gynecol*, **74**, 694–697.

95 Pruett KM, Kirshon B, Cotton DB, et al. (1988). Is vaginal birth after two or more cesarean sections safe? *Obstet Gynecol*, **72**, 163–165.

96 Granovski-Grisaru S, Shaya M and Diamant YZ. (1994). The management of labor in women with more than one uterine scar: is a repeat cesarean section really the only "safe" option? *J Perinat Med*, **22**, 13–17.

97 Caughey AB, Shipp TD, Repke JT, et al. (1999). Rate of uterine rupture during a trial of labor in women with one or two prior cesarean deliveries. *Am J Obstet Gynecol*, **181**, 872–876.

98 Naef RW 3rd, Ray MA, Chauhan SP, et al. (1995). Trial of labor after cesarean delivery with a lower-segment, vertical uterine incision: is it safe? *Am J Obstet Gynecol*, **172**, 1666–1673.

99 Adir CD, Sanchez-Ramos L, Whitaker D, et al. (1996). Trial of labor in patients with a previous lower uterine vertical cesarean section. *Am J Obstet Gynecol*, **174**, 966–970.

100 Martin JN Jr, Perry KG Jr, Roberts WE, et al. (1997). The case for trial of labor in the patient with a prior low-segment vertical cesarean incision. *Am J Obstet Gynecol*, **177**, 144–148.

101 Shipp TD, Zelop CM, Repke JT, et al. (1999). Intrapartum uterine rupture and dehiscense in patients with prior low uterine segment vertical and transverse incisions. *Obstet Gynecol*, **94**, 735–740.

102 Pridjian G. (1992). Labor after prior cesarean section. *Clin Obstet Gynecol*, **35**, 445–456.

103 Demianczuk NN, Hunter DJ and Taylor DW. (1982). Trial of labor after previous cesarean section: prognostic indicators of outcome. *Am J Obstet Gynecol*, **142**, 640–642.

104 Hoskins IA and Gomez JL. (1997). Correlation between maximum cervical dilatation at cesarean delivery and subsequent vaginal birth after cesarean delivery. *Obstet Gynecol*, **89**, 591–593.

105 Bedoya C, Bartha JL, Rodriguez I, et al. (1992). A trial of labor after cesarean section in patients with or without a prior vaginal delivery. *Int J Gynaecol Obstet*, **39**, 285–289.

106 Flamm BL and Geiger AM. (1997). Vaginal birth after cesarean delivery: an admission scoring system. *Obstet Gynecol*, **90**, 907–910.

107 Caughey AB, Shipp TD, Repke TJ, et al. (1998). Trial of labor after cesarean delivery: the effect of previous vaginal delivery. *Am J Obstet Gynecol*, **179**, 938–941.

108 Flamm BL, Frie MW, Lonky NM, et al. (1991). External cephalic version after previous cesarean section. *Am J Obstet Gynecol*, **165**, 370–372.

109 De Meeus JB, Ellia F and Magnin G. (1998). External cephalic version after previous cesarean section: a series of 38 cases. *Eur J Obstet Gynecol Reprod Biol*, **81**, 65–68.

110 Schachter M, Kogan S and Blickstein I. (1994). External cephalic version after previous cesarean section – a clinical dilemma. *Int J Gynaecol Obstet*, **45**, 17–20.

111 Blanchette H, Blanchette M, Mc Cabe J, et al. (2001). Is vaginal birth after cesarean safe? Experience at a community hospital. *Am J Obstet Gynecol*, **184**, 1478–1487.

112 Mootbar H, Dwyer JF, Surur F, et al. (1984). Vaginal delivery following previous cesarean section in 1983. *Int J Obstet Gynaecol*, **22**, 155–160.

113 Yetman TJ and Nolan TE. (1989). Vaginal birth after cesarean section: a reappraisal of risk. *Am J Obstet Gynecol*, **161**, 1119–1123.

114 McMahon MJ, Luther ER, Bowes WA Jr, et al. (1996). Comparison of a trial of labor with an elective second cesarean section. *N Engl J Med*, **335**, 689–695.

115 Hook B, Kiwi R, Amini SB, et al. (1997). Neonatal morbidity after elective repeat cesarean section and trial of labor. *Pediatrics*, **100**, 348–353.

116 Richie EH. (1971). Pregnancy after rupture of pregnant uterus. A report of 36 pregnancies and a study of cases reported since 1932. *J Obstet Gynaecol Br Commonwealth*, **78**, 642–648.

117 Reyes-Ceja L, Cabreara R, Insfran E, et al. (1969). Pregnancy following previous uterine rupture. Study of 19 patients. *Obstet Gynecol*, **34**, 387–389.

118 Farmer RM, Kirschbaum T, Potter D, et al. (1991). Uterine rupture during trial of labor after previous cesarean section. *Am J Obstet Gynecol*, **165**, 996–1001.

119 Stovall TG, Shaver DC, Solomon SK, et al. (1987). Trial of labor in previous cesarean section patients, excluding classical cesarean sections. *Obstet Gynecol*, **70**, 713–717.

120 Sakala EP, Kaye S, Murray RD, et al. (1990). Epidural analgesia. Effect on the likelihood of a successful trial of labor after cesarean section. *J Reprod Med*, **35**, 886–890.

121 Johnson C and Oriol N. (1990). The role of epidural anesthesia in trial of labor. *Reg Anesthes*, **15**, 304–308.

122 Rodriguez MH, Masaki DI, Phelan JP, et al. (1989). Uterine rupture: are intrauterine pressure catheters useful in the diagnosis? *Am J Obstet Gynecol*, **161**, 666–669.

123 Kobelin CG. (2001). Intrapartum management of vaginal birth after cesarean section. *Clin Obstet Gynecol*, **44**, 588–593.

124 Horenstein JM and Phelan JP. (1985). Previous cesarean section: the risks and benefits of oxytocin usage in a trial of labor. *Am J Obstet Gynecol*, **151**, 564–569.

125 Flamm BL, Goings JR, Fuelberth NJ, et al. (1987). Oxytocin during labor after previous cesarean section: results of a multicenter study. *Obstet Gynecol*, **70**, 709–712.

126 Chelmow D and Laros RK Jr. (1992). Maternal and neonatal outcomes after oxytocin augmentation in patients undergoing a trial of labor after prior cesarean delivery. *Obstet Gynecol*, **80**, 966–971.

127 Blanco JD, Collins M, Willis D, et al. (1992). Prostaglandin E_2 gel induction of patients with a low transverse cesarean section. *Am J Perinatol*, **9**, 80–83.

128 Stone JL, Lockwood CJ, Berkowitz G, et al. (1994). Use of cervical prostaglandin E_2 gel in patients with previous cesarean section. *Am J Perinatol*, **11**, 309–312.

129 Flamm BL, Anton D, Goings JR, et al. (1997). Prostaglandin E_2 for cervical ripening: a multicenter study of patients with prior cesarean delivery. *Am J Perinatol*, **14**, 157–160.

130 Turner MJ. (1997). Delivery after one previous cesarean section. *Am J Obstet Gynecol*, **176**, 741–744.

131 Zelop CM, Shipp TD, Repke JT, et al. (1999). Uterine rupture during induced or augmented labor in gravid women with one prior cesarean delivery. *Am J Obstet Gynecol*, **181**, 882–886.

132 Lyndon-Rochelle M, Holt VL, Easterling TR, et al. (2001). Risk of uterine rupture during labor among women with a prior cesarean delivery. *N Engl J Med*, **345**, 3–8.

133 Leung AS, Leung EK and Paul RH. (1993). Uterine rupture after previous cesarean delivery. Maternal and fetal consequences. *Am J Obstet Gynecol*, **169**, 945–950.

134 Yap OW, Kim ES and Laros RK Jr. (2001). Maternal and neonatal outcomes after uterine rupture in labor. *Am J Obstet Gynecol*, **184**, 1576–1581.

135 Porter TF, Clark SL, Esplin MS, et al. (1998). Timing of delivery and neonatal outcome in patients with clinically overt uterine rupture during VCAC. *Am J Obstet Gynecol*, **178**, 531.

136 Phelan JP. (1998). Point/counterpoint. II The VBAC "con" game. *Obstet Gynecol Surv*, **53**, 662–663.

Section II

Maurice L. Druzin, Susan R. Hintz, David K. Stevenson, and Philip Sunshine

Stanford University Medical Center, Stanford, CA, USA

Preeclampsia and HELLP syndrome

Introduction

Hypertensive disorders during pregnancy are not uncommon, but can be complex entities both in terms of diagnosis and therapy. Accurate classification of the particular hypertensive disorder is essential since important differences in management and outcome exist for both mother and fetus depending on the diagnosis. Historically, hypertension during pregnancy has been classified in four general groups: preeclampsia/eclampsia; chronic hypertension; chronic hypertension complicated by preeclampsia; and transient hypertension of late pregnancy.[1,2] Because some of the distinctions within this scheme relate to previous medical history, timely and appropriate diagnosis of a specific disorder may be challenging for the clinician, especially if no prior medical information can be obtained. Similarly, debate regarding the definitions of these hypertensive disorders exists and modifications of the scheme continue.[3,4] However, these difficulties should not deter the practitioner from pursuing a complete and correct diagnosis when hypertension is encountered during pregnancy; the approach to the level of maternal and fetal surveillance may be dramatically altered. Standard initial laboratory evaluation of women who develop hypertension during pregnancy, especially after 20 weeks' gestation, should assist the clinician in differentiating types of hypertensive disorders (Table 12.1).

Preeclampsia

Definition

The American College of Obstetricians and Gynecologists (ACOG) has defined preeclampsia as blood pressure greater than 140 mmHg systolic or 90 mmHg diastolic or a rise of 30 mmHg over normal systolic or 15 mmHg over diastolic blood pressure, along with other signs such as edema and proteinuria after 20 weeks' gestation.[4] This definition is further refined as mild or severe on the basis of blood pressure and other maternal and fetal characteristics (Table 12.2). As the severity of preeclampsia may worsen suddenly, management of mild preeclampsia usually includes modified bedrest, careful blood pressure and fetal monitoring, and serial laboratory evaluation. Depending upon the status of the fetus and mother, this close observation may be undertaken in the hospital. Severe preeclampsia and hemolysis, elevated liver enzymes, and low platelet count (HELLP) syndrome (see below) are considered to be imminent medical crises; prompt delivery is indicated if eclampsia or multiorgan involvement is threatened, or if fetal distress is noted.

Etiology and pathophysiology

Epidemiology

Preeclampsia occurs in 3–7% of human pregnancies and is a leading cause of maternal and perinatal

Table 12.1. Laboratory evaluation of women with hypertension after 20 weeks' gestation

Hemoglobin and hematocrit
Blood smear
Platelet count
Urinalysis
Serum BUN and creatinine levels
Serum uric acid level
Liver enzyme panel, including SGOT, SGPT, LDH
Serum albumin

Notes:
BUN, blood urea nitrogen; SGOT, serum glutamic oxaloacetic transaminase; SGPT, serum glutamic pyruvic transaminase; LDH, lactate dehydrogenase.
Source: Modified from August P (1999): Hypertensive disorders in pregnancy. In Burrow GN and Duffy TP (eds), *Medical Complications in Pregnancy*, 5th edn, pp. 53–77. Philadelphia, PA: WB Saunders.

Table 12.2. Clinical characteristics of severe pregnancy-induced hypertension

Blood pressure more than 160–180 mmHg systolic or more than 110 mmHg diastolic
Significant renal failure as evidenced by severe proteinuria (>5 g/24 h), elevated serum creatinine, or oliguria
Seizures or coma (eclampsia)
Microangiopathic hemolysis
Thrombocytopenia
Hepatocellular dysfunction
Fetal growth retardation or oligohydramnios

Source: Modified from American College of Obstetricians and Gynecologists (1996). *Hypertension in Pregnancy.* Technical bulletin 219 (replaces 91, February 1986). Washington, DC: ACOG.

morbidity and mortality.[5,6] There are a number of risk factors associated with preeclampsia.[7,8] Preeclampsia is more common among nulliparous women; those younger than 18 or older than 35; women with a family history of preeclampsia; those carrying multiple gestations; those with diabetes; and in women who have had a previous pregnancy complicated by hypertension or preeclampsia.

Pathophysiology

The placenta is of central importance to the pathophysiologic consideration of preeclampsia. Animal models, blood flow, and histopathologic examination of placentas suggest that failed spiral artery remodeling leads to increased resistance to uteroplacental blood flow and subsequent ischemia.[9–11] In normal pregnancies, spiral ateries are replaced by low-resistance, thin-walled vessels through the process of trophoblastic invasion that occurs from the 10th to the 18th week of gestation.[12] This process appears to be incomplete in the pregnancies of women destined to develop preeclampsia. Atherotic changes have been detected in the placental bed as early as the first trimester, suggesting pathologic evidence of preeclampsia long before clinical presentation of the disease.[13] However, the factors or signaling mechanisms associated with these placental changes may be of greater importance for prediction and therapy of preeclampsia, and are the basis for ongoing research.

A genetic basis for preeclampsia?

As epidemiologic studies have confirmed a familial predilection for preeclampsia, and due to the suggested role of the renin–angiotensin system in the development of hypertension in preeclampsia, focus has turned to variants of the angiotensinogen (AGT) gene which may be associated with the disease. Linkage study and molecular analysis data from several laboratories support the connection of AGT with the development of preeclampsia.[14–16] Specifically, the variant T235, a common allele in the caucasian population, may be associated with the development of preeclampsia in women homozygous for this allele compared with the apparently "protective" M235 allele.[17] In addition, a mutation in the AGT promoter region, which is in very tight linkage disequilibrium with T235, appears to cause elevated AGT expression.[18,19] Elevated local AGT expression may lead to increased local angiotensin II levels and subsequent abnormal remodeling of the spiral arteries. However, other studies have not demonstrated an association with this allele and clinical preeclampsia, leading to the suggestion that this genetic finding may be correlated with hypertension rather than preeclampsia.[20] The factor V Leiden mutation and 5,10-methylenetetrahydrofolate reductase (MTHFR) C677T polymorphism have also been implicated as potential correlates with preeclampsia. Although it appears that women with preeclampsia are significantly more likely to be heterozygous for the G1691A Leiden mutation than normotensive pregnant women,[21,22] the specific pathophysiologic mechanism and implications for this finding have yet to be elucidated.

Neonatal outcome

Although significant improvements have been made in recent years, maternal morbidity and mortality are still major problems in hypertensive disorders of pregnancy. Because the ultimate "cure" for these disorders is termination of the pregnancy, neonatal morbidity is greatly impacted by the degree of interventional prematurity in cases of severe preeclampsia.[23] Improvements in neonatal intensive care therapy appear to have improved the outcomes of infants born to mothers with severe preeclampsia. Early studies of conservative management of severe preeclampsia from 1985 reported greater than 50% neonatal mortality at approximately 28 weeks' gestational age.[24] A study undertaken almost 10 years later by the same group comparing aggressive with expectant management reported no fetal or neonatal deaths.[25] Gestational age at delivery was approximately 30.8 weeks in the aggressively managed group and 32.9 weeks in the conservatively managed group. In addition to the improved therapies available for premature infants available during the more recent study period, it is also crucial to emphasize that meticulous obstetrical monitoring and fetal surveillance were employed in the management of the conservatively treated patients.[26]

It has also been suggested that fetuses of preeclamptic mothers actually have improved short-term outcomes due to the "stress" to which they are subjected in utero. A gestational age-matched cohort study by Friedman et al.[27] found no difference in neonatal death rate, respiratory distress syndrome incidence, rates of grade 3 or 4 intraventricular hemorrhage, necrotizing enterocolitis, or sepsis between preeclamptic and control infants. Not surprisingly, mean birth weight in the preeclampsia group was significantly lower than that of the control group (1515 vs 1875 g, $P=0.0001$). Spinello et al.[28] examined longer-term outcomes of premature infants born to mothers with preeclampsia, comparing them with gestational age-matched controls. The authors found that rates of cerebral palsy at 2 years corrected age were the same, but that rates of minor neurodevelopmental impairment were increased in the groups whose mothers had severe preeclampsia.

HELLP

Definition

HELLP syndrome is a relatively rare but extremely serious variant of pregnancy-induced hypertension which can be associated with pulmonary edema, acute kidney failure, DIC, placental abruption, and hepatic rupture.[4] Thrombocytopenia has generally been defined as $<100\,000/\mu l$. Clinical features of HELLP may include right upper quadrant or midepigastric pain, nausea, and vomiting, and may present postpartum. This syndrome has been reported to occur in 4–12% of women with preeclampsia, up to 20% of women with severe preeclampsia, and 10% of women with eclampsia.[29–31] Unfortunately, because HELLP syndrome may have very little, if any, hypertension or proteinuria, it can be difficult to diagnose, and may be initially misinterpreted as another platelet disorder of pregnancy or microangiopathic syndrome. Ascertaining the correct diagnosis is critical, as entities such as hemolytic–uremic syndrome or thrombotic thrombocytopenic purpura may require therapies such as plasmapheresis, whereas delivery might be the approach to HELLP syndrome.[32]

Etiology and pathophysiology

Epidemiology

HELLP is viewed as a subset of preeclampsia. However, it is important to recognize that women of all productive ages, both primagravida and multiparous, and of all ethnic groups have been afflicted with HELLP. Reportedly, approximately 19% of women with HELLP have preexisting chronic hypertension.[31]

Pathophysiology

As with preeclampsia, the etiology of HELLP is not clear. Theoretical considerations suggest that placental ischemia leads to release of circulating chemical mediators and subsequent endothelial injury. This injury is then thought to contribute to capillary leakage, leading to proteinuria and edema, and platelet aggregation with DIC. This tendency toward activation of fibrinolysis and consumption of coagulation factors was demonstrated by Paternoster and colleagues, who showed significantly increased plasma fibronectin and D-dimer levels and decreased antithrombin III levels in patients with HELLP compared with non-HELLP preeclamptic patients.[33] As with preeclampsia, research into the etiology of HELLP has also explored prothrombotic tendencies. Remote postpartum testing in patients who had HELLP has revealed abnormalities in activated protein C, protein S deficiency, anticardiolipin antibodies, and hyperhomocysteinemia.[34] Although some studies have suggested that hyperhomocysteinemia is associated with preeclampsia[35] and therefore a potential genetic risk factor and basis for screening in the C677T MTHFR mutation, others have failed to confirm these findings.[36] Finally, there are similarities, both histologic and clinical, of HELLP syndrome with acute fatty liver of pregnancy (AFLP). Although some have suggested that these entities are part of a diagnostic spectrum,[37] there are characteristic distinctions between the diagnoses, including differences in specific fatty infiltration location.[38]

Neonatal outcome

Delivery

Because birth weight and gestational age appear to be the most important factors in neonatal outcome from pregnancies complicated by HELLP syndrome,[39] efforts to temporize delivery have been studied. Higher perinatal mortality rates, up to 19.6%, have been reported in studies of expectant management;[40,41] most deaths were attributable to stillbirths. Conversely, delivery after 48 h of antenatal steroid therapy has been advocated,[42] and immediate delivery with cesarean section has been reported to be associated with much lower perinatal mortality rates.[43] It has therefore been considered prudent that, if the diagnosis of HELLP has been made and there is a reasonable chance of neonatal survival, expeditious delivery be undertaken at a facility equipped to provide intensive care to both mother and infant.

Outcome studies

Several studies have attempted to describe the short- and long-term outcome of infants born to mothers with HELLP, and to differentiate them from the outcomes of infants born to mothers with uncomplicated preeclampsia. In an early retrospective report, Eeltink and colleagues reported on the outcome of 87 pregnancies complicated by HELLP and found that 9.9% of the infants were stillborn, 44% were small-for-gestational-age (SGA), and mechanical ventilation was necessary in 47% of survivors.[44] Thrombocytopenia was noted in over 30% of the infants. An additional nine infants died within the first week of life. Harms et al.[43] reported on 89 infants born to mothers with HELLP and found them to be SGA in 39% of cases, with high rates of thrombocytopenia and leukopenia. Infection appeared to be correlated with neutropenia. The authors compared HELLP infants of <1500 g with all very-low-birth-weight (VLBW) infants born during the study period, and found that the mortality and pulmonary morbidity rates were statistically similar. The incidence of intraventricular hemorrhage was 12.5% compared with 18.2% in the non-HELLP VLBW infants. Dotsch et al.[45] also suggested increased neonatal morbidity in a retrospective review in which infants born to mothers with HELLP were compared to infants born to mothers with uncomplicated hypertension in pregnancy (HIP) and control infants matched for gestational age, sex and birth date. HELLP infants less than 32 weeks' estimated gestational age (EGA) were more likely than either HIP or control infants to be SGA. Cardiovascular instability requiring volume resuscitation was significantly more frequent among HELLP infants. Although platelet counts were lower among HELLP and HIP infants compared with controls, incidence of neutropenia, infection, or intraventricular hemorrhage was not mentioned. Raval et al. conducted a comparative chart review[46] and found that there were no significant differences in gestational age, birth weight, head circumference, hematocrit, or platelet counts between infants born to mothers with HELLP versus those born to mothers with preeclampsia. Infants of mothers with HELLP were, however, significantly more likely to require resuscitation at delivery, have a 1-min Apgar score of <5, require assisted ventilation, and present with hypotension on admission. Cerebral complications, such as intraventricular hemorrhage, were not reported.

Other reports have suggested that factors other than the presence of HELLP in the mother, such as gestational age, are more critical indicators for neonatal outcome. Kandler and colleagues reported on the outcome of infants born to mothers with HELLP compared with a complete age group from the same neonatal intensive care unit.[47] Gestational age and birth weight were significantly lower in the HELLP group, but there were no significant differences in the incidences of leukopenia, thrombocytopenia, or intraventricular hemorrhage. Mortality differences did not reach significance, nor did incidence of respiratory distress syndrome. Although normal or only minor disabilities were reported in 90.3% of HELLP infants undergoing neurodevelopmental follow-up, only 58% of the original group were actually examined. Abramovici et al. examined and compared infant outcomes from pregnancies complicated by HELLP, partial HELLP, or severe preeclampsia without signs of HELLP.[48] Gestational age and birth weight were significantly lower among the HELLP and partial HELLP infants, and the incidence of 5-min Apgar score of <6 was higher. However, after controlling for gestational age, no statistically significant differences were found in mortality rate, respiratory distress syndrome, requirement for mechanical ventilation, or incidence of intraventricular hemorrhage grade 3 or 4, necrotizing enterocolitis or bronchopulmonary dysplasia. Murray et al. reported on 20 cases over a 5-year period (1995–9) of infants born to mothers with HELLP,[49] and concluded that, although neonatal morbidity was high, it was more closely related to gestational age than severity of maternal disease.

Fetal effect of disorders of ß-oxidation of fatty acids on maternal health

There is now convincing evidence that a fetal–maternal interaction leading to development of maternal HELLP syndrome or AFLP can occur when a fetus is afflicted with long-chain 3-hydroxyacyl-coenzyme A (CoA) dehydrogenase (LCHAD) deficiency, an autosomal recessive condition. LCHAD is an inner membrane-bound mitochondrial enzyme which dehydrogenates 3-hydroxyacyl CoA compounds of 12–18 carbon length, and along with long-chain enoyl-CoA hydratase and long-chain ketoacyl-CoA thiolase makes up the mitochondrial trifunctional protein complex, or TFP. These enzymes are essential to the process of ß-oxidation of fatty acids. This fetal–maternal relationship was first reported in 1991,[50] and has been expanded upon since that time with further cases and extensive molecular testing.[51–53] The mechanism by which the fetal deficiency causes maternal disease has not been fully elucidated. It has been suggested[52] that, due to the genetic nature of the disease, there may be maternal reduction in fatty acid ß-oxidation capability complicating the already increased fatty acid levels and decreased mitochondrial fatty acid metabolism normally present in later pregnancy.

Ibdah and colleagues[53] reported on the pregnancy history and molecular analysis of 24 families in which one child had clinical features consistent with LCHAD or TFP deficiency. Nineteen of the children were found to have isolated LCHAD deficiency; eight of those were homozygous for the E474Q mutation, while the other 11 were compound heterozygotes with the E474Q mutation on one allele and a different mutation on the other allele. Seventy-nine percent of the heterozygous mothers had HELLP or AFLP syndrome while carrying a fetus with the E474Q mutation. The other five children had TFP deficiency, did not carry the specific E474Q mutation, and their mothers did not experience HELLP or AFLP. This would suggest that at least one copy of the E474Q mutation in the fetus is consistent with a tendency toward liver disease of pregnancy, and that fetal TFP deficiency does not result in HELLP or AFLP. A recent case series disputes this theory, suggesting that significant hepatic dysfunction can occur in women carrying fetuses with TFP deficiency in the absence of the E474Q mutation.[54] In any case, implications for the evaluation of infants born to mothers with AFLP or HELLP, as well as for the parents and other offspring, are clear. Early diagnosis of these fatty acid oxidation disorders with subsequent appropriate dietary intervention offers the best chance for survival and good outcome.[53] Recommendations for biochemical and detailed molecular analysis for the E474Q and other mutations have been made by Strauss et al.[52] (Table 12.3).

Table 12.3. Recommended evaluation of families with maternal liver disease of pregnancy

In the setting of maternal AFLP in the current pregnancy:

- Prenatal E474Q mutation screening of both parents
- At delivery, cord blood should be sent for acylcarnitine profile, acylglycine analysis, and E474Q mutation screening
- Rigorous avoidance of fasting and vigilant monitoring of any symptoms of illness are recommended for the infant born to a mother with AFLP until results of cord blood analysis have returned

In the setting of AFLP in a previous pregnancy:

- Molecular mutation analysis for all family members
- Metabolic testing (acylcarnitine profile; total, free, and esterified carnitine; acylglycine analysis) of AFLP pregnancy offspring

In the setting of HELLP syndrome:

- Consider prenatal molecular testing of parents
- Consider molecular and metabolic screening of infant

In families with proven LCHAD deficiency:

- Expanded molecular mutation analysis
- Genetic counseling
- First-trimester molecular analysis

Notes:
AFLP, acute fatty liver of pregnancy; HELLP, hemolysis, elevated liver enzymes, and low platelet count; LCHAD, long-chain 3-hydroxyacyl-coenzyme A dehydrogenase.
Source: Modified from Strauss AW, Bennett MJ, Rinaldo P et al. (1999). Inherited long-chain 3-hydroxyacyl coenzyme A dehydrogenase deficiency and a fetal–maternal interaction cause maternal liver disease and other pregnancy complications. *Semin Perinatol* 23:100–112.

Amniotic fluid embolism

One of the most acute and devastating complications of pregnancy is amniotic fluid embolism (AFE). It usually presents suddenly and will often be rapidly fatal. AFE is a very rare condition, but is one of the leading causes of peripartum deaths in developed countries.[55]

The incidence of AFE has been stated to range between 1 in 8000 to 1 in 80 000 pregnancies.[56,57] With such a wide variation, and with the infrequency of recognition by any single practitioner or group, the true incidence is not known. Also the various manners with which the entity presents may make the diagnosis difficult, and it may only be thought of retrospectively or discovered at postmortem examination.

AFE tends to occur primarily during labor or in the immediate postpartum period, but it has been described during cesarean sections, during second-trimester termination, and even in the absence of labor.[56,58] It has also been reported following amnioinfusion in the getting of meconium staining of amniotic fluid.

The etiology and pathogenesis are incompletely understood, and the mechanism by which the amniotic fluid gains access to the mother's circulation is speculative at best. For many years, the traditional view was that debris from the amniotic fluid gained access to the mother's circulation and led to obstruction of the pulmonary vasculature by embolic phenomenon.[59] This has been encountered in a few, but not most patients.[60,61] Clark, who has been a leading influence in the study of patients with AFE, has suggested a biphasic hemodynamic model to explain the pathophysiology of the disorder.[55,57] Initially, acute pulmonary hypertension and vasospasm occur in response to the amniotic fluid in the mother's circulation. This period, which has also been documented in laboratory animals by Hankins et al.,[62] lasts about 30 min and is then replaced by the development of left ventricular failure.[57] Since this symptomatology is similar to that seen in patients with anaphylaxis or sepsis, Clark et al. have suggested that AFE be renamed anaphylactoid syndrome of pregnancy.[57] This response to a foreign substance entering the maternal circulation results in the release of various cytokines and other mediators, especially endothelin, which produce the pathophysiology seen in these patients.

Clinical manifestation

Because AFE is uncommonly encountered, Clark and his coworkers established a national registry in 1988.[57] After reporting on the data accumulated in 1995, the registry was subsequently abandoned. However, important data were presented, including clinical manifestation, morbidity, and mortality. A total of 46 patients were reported, and Table 12.4 lists the most common findings encountered. All patients developed hypotension and 40 patients had cardiac arrest. Four additional patients had a serious dysrhythmia without frank arrest. The types of dysrhythmias included electromechanical dissociation, bradycardia, ventricular tachycardia, or fibrillation and asystole.

Table 12.4. Signs and symptoms noted in patients with amniotic fluid embolism

Signs or symptoms	Incidence
Hypotension	100%
Pulmonary edema or adult respiratory distress syndrome	93%
Cardiorespiratory arrest	87%
Coagulopathy	48%

Source: Modified from Clark et al.[57]

Table 12.5. Presenting signs and symptoms of intrapartum amniotic fluid embolism (30 patients)

Seizures or seizure-like activity
Dyspnea
Hypotension
Fetal heart rate abnormalities

Source: Modified from Clark et al.[57]

Coagulopathy was encountered frequently. Of all patients, eight expired before the coagulation status could be evaluated; four additional patients had clinical evidence of a coagulopathy, but died before laboratory confirmation could be ascertained. Thus, 83% of the patients had evidence of a coagulopathy. This type of presentation has been documented in other reports as well.[58,63]

Table 12.5 lists the most common presenting factors among the women who had AFE before they delivered their babies. Seizure activity, dyspnea, and hypotension were the most common presenting symptoms. Clark et al.[57] also noted that, in all of the undelivered patients at the time of the embolism, fetal bradycardia or the abrupt onset of severe variable deceleration leading within minutes to bradycardia was noted.

Risk factors

In the reviews of Morgan[56] and Clark et al.[57] there were no identifiable maternal risk factors for AFE, other than multiparity. Clark et al. reported no relationships "between oxytocin or antecedent hyperstimulation and AFE." They also noted that AFE was much more common in women carrying a male fetus.[57] Certainly, when the amniotic fluid is meconium-stained, the severity of the disease is intensified.[57] This was clearly demonstrated in the pregnant goat model as well.[62]

Differential diagnosis

Often the diagnosis is one of exclusion,[58] but any devastating entity such as an acute myocardial infarction, air embolism, any thromboembolic episode, or an anaphylaxis reaction must be considered in the differential diagnosis[58,64–66] (Table 12.6). In most situations, entities that cause severe abdominal pain such as uterine rupture or abruptio placentae are not considered in the differential diagnosis, unless the pain is masked by anesthesia, such as an epidural.

Management of the mother and fetus

The management of AFE is to maintain adequate oxygenation and cardiac output in a critically ill patient. Appropriate techniques using ventilation and the enhancement of cardiac output with pressors and fluids are paramount to improving outcome. Correction of coagulopathies with fresh frozen plasma, platelet concentrations, and even cryoprecipitate may be of benefit in these patients.[67] The use of nitric oxide, aerosolized prostacycline, and/or high doses of corticosteroids has been encouraging.[57,58]

While it is recommended that a cesarean section be performed as rapidly as possible, it may not be possible in a patient who is in cardiovascular collapse and who is also coagulopathic. In such situations, intensive care of the mother is a priority. However, cardiopulmonary resuscitation is unlikely to be successful unless the uterus is emptied.

Obviously, in a situation when the mother's condition is not dire or is rapidly stabilized, it would be appropriate to deliver the fetus by cesarean section as rapidly as possible.

Table 12.6. Differential diagnosis of amniotic fluid embolism[58,65]

Acute myocardial infarction
Thromboemolic phenomenon (especially pulmonary embolism)
Air embolus
Anaphylaxis reaction
Hemorrhagic shock
Cerebral hemorrhage or infarction
Massive aspiration
Toxic reaction to anesthetic agents
Transfusion reaction

Source: Modified from Davies[58] and Locksmith.[65]

Outcome

In Morgan's review, published in 1979, the mortality rate was 86%.[56] The registry reported a mortality rate of 61%, but only 15% of the survivors were neurologically intact.[57] Clark et al. also noted that, of the 28 fetuses that were alive in utero at the time of the AFE, 22 survived, but only 11 (50%) were neurologically normal.[57] Obviously, the more rapidly the fetus was delivered in the mothers where AFE was recognized, the greater was the infant survival, albeit with significant neurological sequelae.

Summary

AFE continues to be a devastating problem with a high rate of mortality and morbidity. Rapid approach to recognition and response is clearly indicated, but may still not be sufficient to prevent damage to the mother or infant. Whether the development of international registries would be of help in improving the understanding or foster research endeavors remains speculative.

Shoulder dystocia

Shoulder dystocia is an obstetrical emergency, and if an adverse outcome is encountered, litigation is certain to be initiated against the treating physician and other care givers.[68] Because the problem is often unanticipated, many teaching centers initiate educational programs, including, "shoulder dystocia drills," during the first week of postgraduate training in order to prepare the house officers and midwives regarding the anticipation, recognition, and management of the problem.[69,70] However, even if optimal care is provided, the neonate as well as the mother may suffer injury during the peripartum period.

Table 12.7. Incidence of shoulder dystocia in infants weighing greater than 3500 g delivered in acute care hospitals in California in 1992

	Incidence of shoulder dystocia (%)			
	Nondiabetic		Diabetic	
Weight (g)	Unassisted	Assisted	Unassisted	Assisted
4000–4250	5.2	8.6	8.4	12.2
4250–4500	9.1	12.9	12.3	16.7
4500–4750	14.3	23	19.9	27.3
4750–5000	21.1	29	23.5	34.8

Source: Data from Nesbitt et al.[74]

Definition and diagnosis

Although there is a lack of a standard definition of shoulder dystocia, it is generally understood to indicate difficulty in the prompt delivery of the infant's anterior shoulder when gentle downward traction on the fetal head is utilized.[70,71] The difficulty encountered in a vertex delivery is when the infant's anterior shoulder is impacted behind the mother's symphysis pubis. Since uniform definitions are often not utilized, and incomplete documentation of the event may occur, the true incidence of the problem may vary from center to center. The usual incidence ranges from 0.2% to 3% of deliveries depending upon the types of patients enumerated.[70–73] In a retrospective review of 175 886 vaginal births in California in 1992 of infants weighing greater than 3500 g, the incidence was 3%.[74] The incidence increased significantly with increasing fetal weight, with pregnancies complicated by diabetes, and with forceps and/or vacuum-assisted deliveries (Table 12.7). In other reports the incidence was much lower, but infants of all weights were included, not just those weighing greater than 3500 g and delivered vaginally.[69,73,75]

The diagnosis may be suspected prior to delivery when the care taker recognizes excessive molding of the fetal head, a prolonged second stage of labor, or when there is retraction of the fetal chin after delivery of the head – the "turtle sign."[71]

Table 12.8. Risk factors for predicting fetal macrosomia

Maternal diabetes
Previous infant with macrosomia and/or shoulder dystocia
Excessive maternal weight gain (>20 kg)
Maternal obesity
Postdates pregnancy
Increased maternal age

Risk factors

The major risk factor in shoulder dystocia is fetal macrosomia. The incidence of infants weighing greater than 4000 g at birth appears to be increasing.[76] The factors for predicting macrosomia are listed in Table 12.8. Some authors have stated that fetal macrosomia can be predicted and perhaps prevented to a reasonable degree if risk factors are identified early in pregnancy, frequent ultrasonographic evaluations are carried out, and induction of labor or cesarean sections are utilized at or before 40 weeks' gestation.[68] The use of ultrasonographic measurements comparing ratios or differences in head circumference, biparietal diameters, abdominal circumference, and femur length have been utilized to predict macrosomia and the risks of shoulder dystocia.[69–73,75,77,78] Modanlou and coworkers have suggested that, when an ultrasonographic measurement demonstrated a difference between chest circumference and head circumference of greater than 1.6 cm or a shoulder to head circumference difference of 4.8 cm or more, a significant risk of shoulder dystocia exists.[79] Other investigators have not confirmed that ultrasonographic studies are very accurate in predicting which patients will be at risk for shoulder dystocia. As fetal weight increases, there is decreasing accuracy in estimating fetal weight.[72,73,75,77,78]

After performing a detailed Medline search, Sacks and Chen noted that, in published reports, 15–81% (median 67%) of babies predicted to be macrosomic were confirmed to be so at birth; as few as 50% to as many as 100% of macrosomic infants were successfully predicted by ultrasound evaluations.[80] Even when shoulder widths of infants were measured in the neonatal period, there was a poor prediction that shoulder dystocia would have occurred.[81] One of the major problems in predicting fetal macrosomia and shoulder dystocia is that in most situations all macrosomic infants are evaluated in the same manner. Infants of diabetic pregnancies tend to have asymmetric growth with a disproportionate increase in chest, shoulder, and probably abdominal growth in comparison to head growth.[82] While the head can be delivered readily in these infants, the delivery of the shoulder may create a problem. This type of asymmetric growth may not be applicable to macrosomic infants whose mothers are not diabetic and who are large for other reasons.

Despite the numerous studies and theories published, the two most prominent factors that predict shoulder dystocia are diabetic pregnancies and a history of a previous infant with shoulder dystocia.[70,80,83]

The ACOG Practice Patterns published in 1997 on shoulder dystocia noted that most cases of shoulder dystocia could not be predicted or prevented; that ultrasonographic measurements to detect macrosomia have limited accuracy; and that planned cesarean delivery on the basis of suspected macrosomia in the general population was not reasonable, but planned cesarean birth was reasonable for pregnancies complicated by diabetes when the estimated fetal weight exceeded 4250–4500 g.[72] In the *ACOG Practice Bulletin* published in 2000 many of these recommendations were reiterated and it was noted that the diagnosis of fetal macrosomia is imprecise; that suspected fetal macrosomia is not an indication for induction of labor; that labor and vaginal delivery are not contraindicated for women with estimated fetal weight up to 5000 g in the absence of maternal diabetes; with an estimated fetal weight of greater than 4500 g, a prolonged second stage of labor or arrest of descent in the second stage is an indication for cesarean delivery; that prophylactic cesarean section may be considered for suspected macrosomia with estimated fetal weight greater than 5000 g in women without diabetes and greater than 4500 g in women with diabetes.[77] It was also stated that suspected fetal macrosomia is not a contraindication to attempt vaginal birth after a previous cesarean section.[77]

Management of shoulder dystocia

The management of these infants is well outlined in numerous publications in the obstetrical literature.[69–71,75,76,80,83] Since it is an obstetrical emergency, and often unanticipated, one must call for assistance quickly and have personnel present who can resuscitate the infant appropriately. One also requires assistance in performing the McRoberts maneuver with or without suprapubic pressure to dislodge the anterior shoulder and facilitate delivery. The mother should also be instructed to stop pushing as suprafundal pressure may worsen the situation. The all-fours position or the Gaskin maneuver, the Woods screw maneuver, the Rubin technique, and other techniques to facilitate delivery of the posterior shoulder, are other approaches used to manage the dystocia. The Zavanelli maneuver, or cephalic replacement followed by cesarean section, hysterotomy with abdominal rescue and symphysiotomy are techniques utilized when the previous maneuvers fail.

Complications of shoulder dystocia

Injuries to both the mother and infant can result from complications encountered with shoulder

Table 12.9. Maternal complications of shoulder dystocia

Perineal lacerations
Bladder injury
Hemorrhage
Uterine atony
Uterine rupture
Infection
Fistula formation

Table 12.10. Neonatal complications of shoulder dystocia

Fractures
Clavicle
Humerus
Dislocation of the shoulder
Brachial plexus palsy
Birth asphyxia
Intracranial hemorrhage
Diaphragmatic paralysis
Horner's syndrome
Tracheal tear
Spinal cord injuries
Facial nerve injury

dystocia. Maternal complications are listed in Table 12.9, and include trauma to the birth canal with third- and fourth-degree lacerations, hemorrhage, infection, and even uterine rupture. In the rare cases where symphysiotomy is required, healing will usually occur, but it is often associated with a great deal of pain.[70,71]

Neonatal complications are more severe, may result in permanent damage, and are found in 15–30% cases with shoulder dystocia[83–86] (Table 12.10). The most severe and least frequently encountered is intrapartum asphyxia with delay in delivery of the infant. This can result in the death of the infant or produce neurological injury of varying severity. Fortunately, these occur rarely in modern obstetrics. Fractures of the clavicle and humerus resolve without long-term sequelae. Brachial plexus palsy, which is reported to occur in approximately 2–2.5 per 1000 live full-term births, is another dreaded complication of shoulder dystocia.[84] The severity of the problem depends upon the type of injury, with avulsion of the roots from the spinal cord being the most serious, often resulting in permanent neurological damage. More commonly, hemorrhage and edema to either or both the nerve sheaths and axons occur and the outcome is much more favorable. Intermediate types of injuries have variable prognosis; but if the nerve sheath is intact even if the axons are torn, the likelihood of recovery is good.[86]

In neonates, over 90% of the patients with brachial plexus injury have Erb's palsy, with cervical segments 5 and 6 being involved in half of the patients and 5, 6, and 7 in the other 50%. Diaphragmatic paralysis can accompany these injuries when C3–C5 are injured. Total brachial plexus palsy involving C8 and T1 in addition to C5–C7 occur in less than 10% of patients. In these latter infants, Horner's syndrome is also frequently encountered.[86]

Although brachial plexus palsy had been thought to be a result of deliveries associated only with shoulder dystocia, recent studies have shown that Erb's palsy occurs in the absence of shoulder dystocia.[85,87] Erb's has been encountered in infants delivered by cesarean section without undue traction placed on the head or neck, and it can also affect the posterior shoulder without affecting the anterior shoulder.[85,87–90] Thus, there are a number of infants with in utero-acquired Erb's palsy and the etiology of this is often unknown. Interestingly, the infants with brachial plexus palsy not associated with shoulder dystocia usually have a worse prognosis than those associated with shoulder dystocia.[88,90]

In most of the series reported, there is excellent recovery with brachial plexus palsies. In the follow-up of the National Collaborative Perinatal Study, 92% of affected infants were normal at 12 months of age and only 7% were abnormal at 4 years of age.[91] Overall, excellent outcome has been reported in as few as 50% to as many as 90% of the infants affected. Most infants will have complete recovery by 6 months of age, but if the impairment persists to 18 months of age, it is usually permanent.[86] Those individuals who provide surgical repair for these infants, and who would see the most severely affected patients, offer a more dismal picture as far as outcome is concerned.[92]

Spinal cord injuries can result from shoulder dystocia but this is a very rare occurrence. When excessive pressure is used to depress the head, tracheal tears have been encountered. These are often difficult to recognize, and the initial finding may be the development of subcutaneous emphysema. Intubation may be very difficult in these infants, but they may be able to be managed with bag-and-mask ventilation. If these infants can be successfully intubated and resuscitated, the trachea will usually heal without surgical correction.[93]

Summary

Shoulder dystocia is an obstetrical emergency and is unanticipated in about 50% of patients. Measures to predict the birth of these infants are not precise and may be misleading. Routine cesarean sections for most macrosomic infants is not warranted and would result in an inordinate number being performed with little decrease in complications in the infants.

Operative intervention

Obstetric interventions, such as forceps delivery and vacuum extraction, are important instrumental procedures to assist vaginal delivery and avoid cesarean section, especially among nulliparous pregnant women.[94–96] While forceps have been used in obstetrics for nearly two centuries, vacuum extraction is a twentieth-century phenomenon, with usage increasing over the last 15 years. Concomitant with the recent increase in vacuum extraction has been a decrease in the number of forceps-assisted deliveries.[97] The latter circumstance probably complicates any analysis comparing the maternal and neonatal outcomes of forceps to vacuum instrumental deliveries, because the skill of the instrument user is likely to vary indirectly with the frequency of the use. Moreover, it could be interpreted as suggesting that less skilled users of forceps would contribute to higher rates of maternal and neonatal injuries, but the ease of vacuum application could also tempt less skilled, inexperienced users to try this alternative instrumental procedure. Although technical skill is necessary to minimize the risk of complications, it is not sufficient.

Table 12.11. Indications and contraindications for vacuum extraction

Indications
Prolonged second stage
Overly dense epidural analgesia/anesthesia
Maternal paralysis
Shortening of the second stage (indicated)
Nonreassuring fetal status (presumed fetal jeopardy)
Abnormal fetal scalp/umbilical cord pH readings
Abruptio placentae/maternal hemorrhage
Cord prolapse
Maternal exhaustion
Contraindications
Operator inexperience
Inability to achieve proper application
Malpresentations
Incomplete cervical dilatation
Prophylactic procedures
Relative contraindications
Prematurity (<36 weeks)
Teaching/resident instruction

Source: Reproduced with permission from O'Grady JP, Pope CS and Patel SS (2000). Vacuum extraction in modern obstetric practice: a review and critique. *Curr Opin in Obstet and Gynecol*, **12**, 475.

Knowing when an instrumental delivery is indicated is also critical to success. The indications for instrumental delivery are similar for birth procedures (Table 12.11).[98] In general, failure rates are higher with vacuum extraction compared to forceps, and there is little advantage to flexible cups compared to rigid cups besides less fetal cosmetic injury, probably because of their inability to sustain

Table 12.12. Adjusted odds ratios (OR) and 95% confidence intervals (CI) for the effects of the instruments (vacuum or forceps) on major adverse maternal and infant outcomes obtained from multiple logistic regression analysis, Quebec, Canada, 1991/1992–1995/1996

	Vacuum vs unassisted		Forceps vs unassisted		Vacuum vs forceps	
Adverse outcomes	OR	95% CI	OR	95% CI	OR	95% CI
Third-/fourth-degree perineal laceration	3.9	3.8,4.1	8.4	8.0,8.7	0.5	0.5, 0.5
Intracranial hemorrhage	4.5	3.0, 6.6	5.0	3.3, 7.7	1.3	0.7, 2.3
Subdural or cerebral	4.6	2.6, 8.4	8.5	4.9, 14.7	1.0	0.5, 1.9
Intraventricular	1.6	0.5, 5.6	2.1	0.6, 7.5	1.0	0.2, 6.0
Subarachnoid	5.3	2.9, 9.6	3.0	1.3, 6.8	5.4	1.3, 23.4
Cephalhematoma	9.9	9.4, 10.5	5.9	5.5, 6.3	2.0	1.9, 2.2
Facial nerve injury	2.3	1.6, 3.4	9.8	7.3, 13.1	0.2	0.2, 0.4
Brachial plexus injury	1.6	1.3, 2.2	1.6	1.1, 2.1	1.1	0.8, 1.6
Convulsions	1.8	1.3, 2.4	2.0	1.4, 2.7	0.9	0.6, 1.4
Central nervous system depression	1.7	0.8, 3.8	0.8	0.3, 2.3	1.7	0.5, 5.4
Feeding difficulty	1.3	1.1, 1.5	1.2	1.0, 1.5	1.1	0.9, 1.4
Neonatal in-hospital death	0.9	0.4, 2.1	1.0	0.4, 2.3	0.9	0.3, 2.7

Source: Reproduced with permission from Wen SW, Liu S, Kramer MS, et al. (2001). Comparison on maternal and infant outcomes between vacuum extraction and forceps deliveries. *Am J Epidemiol*, **153**, 106.

comparable traction. The latter factor contributes to an even greater failure rate compared to rigid cups, metal, or plastic.[99,100] Inaccurate placement of the cups, off mid saggital position, centrally located over the cranial pivot or flexion point, is a major contributing cause of failure.[101] Knowing when to stop and accept failure is also important – four to five tractions, or two to three cup detachments maximum, with advances of the presenting part on initial traction and total procedure duration of 20 min or less.[99–110] There is some evidence that vacuum extraction after failed forceps may be associated with an increased risk of intracranial hemorrhage,[96] but it is also possible that the underlying circumstance, such as cephalopelvic disproportion, which has not been recognized, is the real danger in the context of attempted instrumental delivery, whether singular or in series.

Of course, there are advantages and disadvantages to both instrumental procedures, which may vary with the clinical circumstances, operator experience, and expertise. None the less, the weight of the published evidence suggests that forceps have lower failure rates and result in fewer scalp injuries. On the other hand, vacuum extraction causes less maternal perineal injury and neonatal facial nerve injury, but intracranial hemorrhage, especially subarachnoid hemorrhage, is more likely (Table 12.12).[111] Another retrospective study added another interpretive wrinkle to the debate. Notably, the common factor associated with intracranial hemorrhage is abnormal labor, which tracks with vacuum extraction, forceps, and cesarean section with labor compared with cesarean section before labor (Table 12.13).[96]

Finally, it is important to point out that the occurrence of intracranial hemorrhage is not always associated with adverse long-term neurodevelopmental outcome.[112] The large study by Seidman et al.[94] suggests no increased risk for physical or cognitive impairment at 17 years of age for either instrumental procedure. Other small studies affirm this

Table 12.13. Incidence of major neonatal morbidity and risk associated with operative procedures as compared with spontaneous delivery

(a) Spontaneous

	Spontaneous incidence	Vacuum (n=59354)		Forceps (n=15945)		Vacuum and forceps (n=2817)	
	(n=387–799)	Incidence	Odds ratio	Incidence	Odds ratio	Incidence	Odds ratio
Subdural or cerebral hemorrhage	2.9	8.0	2.7 (1.9–3.9)	9.8	3.4 (1.9–5.9)	21.3	7.3 (2.9–17.2)
Intraventricular hemorrhage	1.1	1.5	1.4 (0.7–3.0)	2.6	2.5 (0.9–6.9)	3.7	3.5 (1.5–25.5)
Subarachnoid hemorrhage	1.3	2.2	1.7 (0.9–3.2)	3.3	2.5 (0.9–6.6)	10.7	8.2 (2.1–27.4)
Facial nerve injury	3.3	4.6	1.7 (0.9–2.1)	45.4	13.6 (10.0–18.4)	28.5	8.5 (3.9–18.0)
Brachial plexus injury	7.7	17.6	2.3 (1.8–2.9)	25.0	3.2 (2.3–4.6)	46.4	6.0 (3.3–10.7)
Convulsions	6.4	11.7	1.8 (1.4–2.4)	9.8	1.6 (0.9–2.7)	24.9	3.9 (1.7–8.6)
Central nervous system depression	3.1	9.2	2.9 (2.9–4.1)	5.2	1.4 (0.6–2.8)	21.3	6.9 (2.7–16.2)
Feeding difficulty	68.5	72.1	1.1 (1.0–1.2)	74.6	1.1 (0.9–1.3)	60.7	0.9 (0.5–1.5)
Mechanical ventilation	25.8	39.1	1.5 (1.3–1.8)	45.4	1.8 (1.4–2.3)	50.0	1.9 (1.1–3.4)

(b) Cesarean

	Total (n=117425)		During labour (n=84417)		During labor, failed vaginal delivery (n=2342)†		During labour, no attempt at vaginal delivery (n=82075)†		No labor (n=33008)	
	Incidence	Odds ratio	Incidence	Odds ratio	Incidence	Odds ratio	Incidence	Odds ratio	Incidence	Odds ratio
Subdural or cerebral hemorrhage	6.7	2.3 (1.7–3.1)	7.4	2.5 (1.8–3.4)	25.7	8.8 (3.9–19.9)	6.8	2.3 (1.7–3.2)	4.1	1.4 (0.8–2.6)
Intraventricular hemorrhage	2.1	2.0 (1.2–3.3)	2.5	2.3 (1.4–4.0)	0.0	0.0 (0.0–1.1)	2.6	2.4 (1.4–4.1)	0.8	0.6 (0.1–2.5)
Subarachnoid hemorrhage	0.9	0.7 (0.4–1.4)	1.2	0.9 (0.4–1.9)	4.3	3.3 (0.5–23.9)	1.1	0.9 (0.4–1.7)	0.0	0.0 (0.0–19.7)
Facial nerve injury	3.5	1.1 (0.7–1.5)	3.1	0.9 (0.6–1.4)	12.8	3.8 (1.2–12.1)	2.8	0.8 (0.5–1.3)	4.9	1.5 (0.8–2.6)
Brachial plexus injury	3.0	0.4 (0.3–0.5)	1.8	0.2 (0.1–0.4)	8.6	1.1 (0.3–4.4)	1.6	0.2 (0.1–0.4)	4.1	0.5 (0.3–1.0)
Convulsions	18.7	2.9 (2.4–3.6)	21.3	3.3 (2.8–4.1)	68.8	10.8 (6.5–17.8)	19.9	3.1 (2.6–3.8)	8.6	1.4 (0.9–2.1)
Central nervous system depression	8.9	2.9 (2.2–3.7)	9.6	3.1 (2.3–4.1)	17.1	5.5 (1.7–15.5)	9.4	3.0 (2.3–4.0)	67.6	2.2 (1.3–3.6)
Feeding difficulty	114.7	1.7 (1.6–1.8)	117.2	1.7 (1.6–1.8)	94.8	1.4 (0.9–2.1)	117.9	1.7 (1.6–1.8)	106.3	1.6 (1.4–1.8)
Mechanical ventilation	96.0	3.7 (3.4–4.1)	103.2	4.0(3.6–4.3)	156.1	6.0 (4.3–8.3)	101.7	2.6 (2.2–3.0)	71.3	2.8 (2.4–3.3)

Source: Reproduced with permission from Towner D, Castro MA, Eby-Wilkens E and Gilbert WM (1999). Effect of mode of delivery in nulliparous women on neonatal intracranial injury. *N Engl J Med*, **341**, 1711.

finding.[113,114] Another important point is that none of the published studies has addressed the issue of subgaleal hemorrhage, although there is some rationale for suspecting its association with vacuum extraction because of the increased incidence of scalp injuries. This kind of scalp bleeding is life-threatening and a cause of significant morbidity in the neonate. Whether the incidence of subgaleal hemorrhage has increased is an important question that deserves systematic analysis.

REFERENCES

1 FA Davis (1972). *Obstetric–Gynecologic Terminology*, ed. Hughes EC, pp. 422–423. Philadelphia, PA: FA Davis.

2 August P. (1999). Hypertensive disorders in pregnancy. In *Medical Complications in Pregnancy*, 5th edn, ed. Burrow GN and Duffy TP, pp. 53–77. Philadelphia, PA: WB Saunders.

3 Brown MA and Buddle ML. (1997). What's in a name? Problems with the classification of hypertension in pregnancy. *J Hypertens*, **15**, 1049.

4 American College of Obstetricians and Gynecologists. (1996). *Hypertension in Pregnancy*. Technical bulletin 219 (replaces 91, February 1986). Washington, DC: ACOG.

5 Kaunitz A, Hughes J, Grimes D, et al. (1990). Causes of maternal mortality in the United States 1979–1986. *Am J Obstet Gynecol*, **163**, 460–465.

6 Working Group on High Blood Pressure in Pregnancy. (1990). National High Blood Pressure Education Program Working Group report on high blood pressure in pregnancy: consensus report. *Am J Obstet Gynecol*, **163**, 1689–1712.

7 Sibai BM, Ewell M, Levine RJ, et al. (1997). Risk factors associated with preeclampsia in healthy nulliparous women. *Am J Obstet Gynecol*, **177**,1003.

8 Ness RB and Roberts JM. (1996). Heterogeneous causes constituting the single syndrome of pre-eclampsia: a hypothesis and its implications. *Am J Obstet Gynecol*, **175**,1365.

9 Combs C, Katz M, Kitzmiller J, et al. (1993). Experimental preeclampsia produced by chronic constriction of the lower aorta: validation with longitudinal blood pressure measurements in conscious rhesus monkeys. *Am J Obstet Gynecol*, **169**, 215–223.

10 Lunell NO, et al. (1984). Uteroplacental blood flow in pregnancy-induced hypertension. *Scand J Clin Lab Invest*, **169**, 28.

11 Pijnenborg R, et al. (1991). Placental bed spiral arteries in the hypertensive disorders of pregnancy. *Br J Obstet Gynaecol*, **98**, 648.

12 Pijnenborg R, et al. (1980). Trophoblastic invasion of human decidua from 8 to 18 weeks of pregnancy. *Placenta*, **1**, 3.

13 Ghidini A, Salafia CM and Pezzullo JC. (1997). Placental vascular lesions and likelihood of diagnosis of pre-eclampsia. *Obstet Gynecol*, **90**, 542.

14 Ward K, Hata A, Jeunemaitre X, et al. (1993). A molecular variant of angiotensinogen associated with preeclampsia. *Nat Genet*, **4**, 59–61.

15 Arngrimsson R, Purandare S, Conner M, et al. (1993). Angiotensinogen: a candidate gene involved in preeclampsia? *Nat Genet*, **4**, 114–115.

16 Takimoto E, Ishida J, Sugiyama F, et al. (1996). Hypertension induced in pregnant mice by placental renin and maternal angiotensinogen. *Science*, **274**, 995–997.

17 Jeunemaitre X, Soubrier F, Kotelevtsev Y, et al. (1992). Molecular basis of human hypertension: role of angiotensinogen. *Cell*, **71**, 169–180.

18 Inoue I, Nakajima T, Williams C, et al. (1997). A nucleotide substitution in the promoter of human angiotensinogen transcription. *J Clin Invest*, **99**, 1786–1797.

19 Morgan T, Craven C, Nelson L, et al. (1997). Angiotensinogen T235 expression is elevated in decidual spiral arteries. *J Clin Invest*, **100**, 1406–1415.

20 Wilton AN, Kaye JA, Guo G, et al. (1995). Is angiotensinogen a good candidate gene for preeclampsia? *Hypertens Pregnancy*, **14**, 251–260.

21 Dizon-Townson D, Nelson L, Easton K, et al. (1996). The factor V Leiden mutation may predispose women to severe preeclampsia. *Am J Obstet Gynecol*, **175**, 902–905.

22 Rigo J Jr, Nagy B, Fintor L, et al. (2000). Maternal and neonatal outcome of preeclamptic pregnancies: the potential roles of factor V Leiden mutation and 5,10 methylenetetrahydrofolate reductase. *Hypertens Pregnancy*, **19**, 163–172.

23 Shah DM and Reed G. (1996). Parameters associated with adverse perinatal outcome in hypertensive pregnancies. *J Hum Hypertens*, **10**, 511.

24 Sibai BM, Taslimi MM, Abdella TN, et al. (1985). Maternal and perinatal outcome of conservative management of severe preeclampsia in midtrimester. *Am J Obstet Gynecol*, **152**, 32–37.

25 Sibai BM, Mercere BM, Schiff E, et al. (1994). Aggressive versus expectant management of severe preeclampsia at 28 to 32 weeks gestation: a randomized controlled trial. *Am J Obstet Gynecol*, **171**, 818–822.

26 Chari RS, Friedman SA, O'Brien JM, et al., (1995). Daily

antenatal testing in women with severe preeclampsia. *Am J Obstet Gynecol*, **173**, 1207–1210.

27 Friedman SA, Schiff E, Kao L, Sibai BM. (1995). Neonatal outcome after preterm delivery for preeclampsia. *Am J Obstet Gynecol*, **172**, 1785–1792.

28 Spinello A, Iasci A, Capuzzo E, et al. (1994). Two-year infant neurodevelopmental outcome after expectant management and indicated preterm delivery in hypertensive pregnancies. *Acta Obstet Gynecol Scand*, **73**, 625–629.

29 Sibai BM, Taslimi MM and El-Nazer A. (1986). Maternal-perinatal outcome associated with the syndrome of hemolysis, elevated liver enzymes, and low platelets in severe preeclampsia–eclampsia. *Am J Obstet Gynecol*, **155**, 501–509.

30 Mackenna J, Dover NL and Brame RG. (1982). Preeclampsia associated with hemolysis, elevated liver enzymes, and low platelets: an obstetrical emergency? *Obstet Gynecol*, **62**, 751–754.

31 Sibai BM, Ramadan MK, Usta I, et al. (1993). Maternal morbidity and mortality in 442 pregnancies with hemolysis, elevated liver enzymes, and low platelets. *Am J Obstet Gynecol*, **169**, 1000–1006.

32 Sibai BM, Kustermann L and Velasco J. (1994). Current understanding of severe preeclampsia, pregnancy-associated hemolytic uremic syndrome, thrombotic thrombocytopenic purpura, hemolysis, elevated liver enzymes and low platelet syndrome, and postpartum acute renal failure: different clinical syndromes or just different names? *Curr Opin Nephrol Hypertens*, **3**, 436.

33 Paternoster DM, Stella A, Simioni P, et al. (1995). Coagulation and plasma fibronectin parameters in HELLP syndrome. *Int J Gynecol Obstet*, **50**, 263–268.

34 Dekker GA, deVries JIP, Doelitsch PM, et al. (1995). Underlying disorders associated with severe early-onset preeclampsia. *Am J Obstet Gynecol*, **173**, 1042–1048.

35 Rajkovic A, Catalano PM and Malinow MR. (1997). Elevated homocysteine levels with preeclampsia. *Obstet Gynecol*, **90**, 168–171.

36 Raijmakers MTM, Zusterzeel PLM, Steegers EAP, et al. (2001). Hyperhomocysteinaemia: a risk factor for preeclampsia? *Eur J Obstet Gynecol Reprod Biol*, **95**, 226–228.

37 Dani R, Mendes GS, de Laurentys Medeiros J, et al. (1996). Study of the liver changes occurring in preeclampsia and their possible pathogenetic connection with acute fatty liver of pregnancy. *Am J Gastroenterol*, **91**, 292–294.

38 Barton J, Riely C, Ademec T, et al. (1992). Hepatic histopathologic condition does not correlate with laboratory abnormalities in HELLP syndrome. *Am J Obstet Gynecol*, **167**, 1538.

39 Magann EF, Perry KG, Chauhan SP, et al. (1994). Neonatal salvage by weeks gestation in pregnancies complicated by HELLP syndrome. *J Soc Gynecol Invest*, **1**, 206–209.

40 Visser W and Wallenburg HCS. (1995). Temporising management of severe pre-eclampsia with and without the HELLP syndrome. *Br J Obstet Gynaecol*, **102**, 111–117.

41 Van Pampus MG, Wolf H, Westerberg SM, et al. (1998). Maternal and perinatal outcome after expectant management of the HELLP syndrome compared with preeclampsia without HELLP syndrome. *Eur J Obstet Gynecol Reprod Biol*, **76**, 31–36.

42 Sibai BM. (1990). The HELLP syndrome: much ado about nothing? *Am J Obstet Gynecol*, **162**, 311–316.

43 Harms K, Rath W, Herting E, et al. (1995). Maternal hemolysis, elevated liver enzymes, low platelet count, and neonatal outcome. *Am J Perinatol*, **12**, 1–7.

44 Eeltink CM, van Lingen RA, Aarnoudse JG, et al. (1993). Maternal haemolysis, elevated liver enzymes, and low platelets syndrome: specific problems in the newborn. *Eur J Pediatr*, **152**, 160–163.

45 Dotsch J, Hohmann M and Kuhl PG. (1997). Neonatal morbidity and mortality associated with maternal haemolysis, elevated liver enzymes and low platelets syndrome. *Eur J Pediatr*, **156**, 389–391.

46 Raval ES, Co S, Reid MA, et al. (1997). Maternal and neonatal outcome of pregnancies complicated with maternal HELLP syndrome. *J Perinatol*, **17**, 266–269.

47 Kandler C, Kevekordes B, Zenker M, et al. (1998). Prognosis of children born to mothers with HELLP-syndrome. *J Perinat Med*, **26**, 486–490.

48 Abramovici D, Friedman SA, Mercer BM, et al. (1999). Neonatal outcome in severe preeclampsia at 24 to 36 weeks' gestation: does the HELLP syndrome matter? *Am J Obstet Gynecol*, **180**, 221–225.

49 Murray D, O'Riordan MO, Geary M, et al. (2000). The HELLP syndrome: maternal and perinatal outcome. *Ir Med J*, **94**, 16–18.

50 Schoeman MN, Batey RG and Wilcken B. (1991). Recurrent acute fatty liver of pregnancy associated with a fatty-acid oxidation defect in the offspring. *Gastroenterology*, **100**, 544–548.

51 Treem W, Shoup ME, Hale DE, et al. (1996). Acute fatty liver of pregnancy, hemolysis, elevated liver enzymes and low platelets syndrome and long-chain 3-hydroxyacyl coenzyme A dehydrogenase deficiency. *Am J Gastroenterol*, **91**, 2293–2300.

52 Strauss AW, Bennett MJ, Rinaldo P, et al. (1999). Inherited long-chain 3-hydroxyacyl coenzyme A dehydrogenase deficiency and a fetal–maternal interaction cause maternal

liver disease and other pregnancy complications. *Semin Perinatol*, **23**, 100–112.

53 Ibdah JA, Bennett MJ, Rinaldo P, et al. (1999). A fetal fatty-acid oxidation disorder as a cause of liver disease in pregnant women. *N Engl J Med*, **340**, 1723–1731.

54 Chakrapani A, Olpin S, Cleary M, et al. (2000). Trifunctional protein deficiency: three families with significant maternal hepatic dysfunction in pregnancy not associated with E474Q mutation. *J Inherit Metab Dis*, **23**, 826–834.

55 Clark SL. (1990). New concepts of amniotic fluid embolism: a review. *Obstet Gynecol Surv*, **45**, 360–368.

56 Morgan M. (1979). Amniotic fluid embolism. *Anesthesia*, **341**, 20–32.

57 Clark SL, Hankins GDV, Dudley DA, et al. (1995). Amniotic fluid embolism: analysis of the national registry. *Am J Obstet Gynecol*, **172**, 1158–1169.

58 Davies S. (2001). Amniotic fluid embolus: a review of the literature. *Can J Anaesth*, **48**, 88–98.

59 Steiner PE and Lushbaugh CC. (1986). Maternal pulmonary embolism by amniotic fluid as a cause of obstetric shock and unexpected deaths in obstetrics. *JAMA*, **255**, 2187–2203.

60 Esposito RA, Gross EA, Coppa G, et al. (1990). Successful treatment of postpartum shock caused by amniotic fluid embolism with cardiopulmonary bypass and pulmonary artery thromboembolectomy. *Am J Obstet Gynecol*, **163**, 572–574.

61 Bauer P, Lelarge P, Hennequin L, et al. (1995). Thromboembolism during amniotic fluid embolism. *Intensive Care Med*, **21**, 384.

62 Hankins GDV, Snyder RR, Clark SL, et al. (1993). Acute hemodynamic and respiratory effects of amniotic fluid embolism in the pregnant goat model. *Am J Obstet Gynecol*, **163**, 1113–1130.

63 Awad IT and Shorten GD. (2001). Amniotic fluid embolism and isolated coagulopathy: atypical presentation of amniotic fluid embolism. *Eur J Anaesthesiol*, **18**, 410–413.

64 Martin RW. (1996). Amniotic fluid embolism. *Clin Obstet Gynecol*, **39**, 101–106.

65 Locksmith GJ. (1999). Amniotic fluid embolism. *Obstet Gynecol Clin North Am*, **26**, 435–444.

66 St Amand J. (1993). Mediocolegal nightmare: a tragic case, a needless trial. *Can Med Assoc J*, **148**, 806–809.

67 Rodgers GP and Heymach GJ III. (1984). Cryoprecipitate therapy in amniotic fluid embolization. *Am J Med*, **76**, 916–920.

68 O'Leary JA and Leonetti HB. (1990). Shoulder dystocia: prevention and treatment. *Am J Obstet Gynecol*, **162**, 5–9.

69 Kees S, Margalet V, Schiff E, et al. (2001). Features of shoulder dystocia in a busy obstetric unit. *J Reprod Med*, **46**, 583–588.

70 Wagner RK, Nielsen PE and Gonik B. (1999). Shoulder dystocia. *Obstet Gynecol Clin North Am*, **26**, 371–383.

71 Bennett BB. (1999). Shoulder dystocia: an obstetrical emergency. *Obstet Gynecol Clin North Am*, **26**, 445–458.

72 ACOG Practice Patterns. (1997). In *Shoulder Dystocia*, pp. 1137–1143. Washington: American College of Obstetrics and Gynecology.

73 Nocon JJ, McKenzie DK, Thomas LJ, et al. (1993). Shoulder dystocia: an analysis of risks and obstetric maneuvers. *Am J Obstet Gynecol*, **168**, 1732–1739.

74 Nesbitt TS, Gilbert WM and Herrchen B. (1998). Shoulder dystocia and associated risk factors with macrosomic infants born in California. *Am J Obstet Gynecol*, **179**, 476–480.

75 Morrison JC, Sanders JR, Magann EF, et al. (1992). The diagnosis and management of dystocia of the shoulder. *Surg Gynecol Obstet*, **175**, 515–522.

76 Geary M, McParland P, Johnson H, et al. (1995). Shoulder dystocia – is it predictable? *Eur J Obstet Gynecol*, **62**, 15–18.

77 ACOG Practice Bulletin. (2000). *Fetal macrosomia*, pp. 929–939. Washington: American College of Obstetrics and Gynecology.

78 Weeks JW, Pitman T and Spinnato JA II. (1995). Fetal macrosomia: does antenatal prediction affect delivery route and birth outcome? *Am J Obstet Gynecol*, **173**, 1215–1219.

79 Modanlou HD, Komatsu G, Dorchester W, et al. (1982). Large-for-gestational age neonates: anthropomorphic reasons for shoulder dystocia. *Obstet Gynecol*, **60**, 417–423.

80 Sacks DA and Chen W. (2000). Estimating fetal weight in the management of macrosomia. *Obstet Gynecol Surv*, **55**, 229–239.

81 Verspyck E, Goffinet F, Hellot MF, et al. (1999). Newborn shoulder width: a prospective study of 2222 consecutive measurements. *Br J Obstet Gynaecol*, **106**, 589–593.

82 Bahar AM. (1996). Risk factors and fetal outcome in cases of shoulder dystocia compared with normal deliveries of a similar birthweight. *Br J Obstet Gynaecol*, **103**, 868–872.

83 Ginsberg NA and Moisidis C. (2001). How to predict recurrent shoulder dystocia. *Am J Obstet Gynecol*, **184**, 1427–1430.

84 Levine MG, Holroyde J, Woods JR Jr, et al. (1984). Birth trauma: incidence and predisposing factors. *Obstet Gynecol*, **63**, 792–795.

85 Gilbert WM, Nesbitt TS and Danielsen B. (1999). Associated factors in 1611 cases of brachial plexus injury. *Obstet Gynecol*, **93**, 536–540.

86 Volpe JJ. (2001). *Neurology of the Newborn*, 3rd edn, pp. 825–829. Philadelphia: Saunders.

87 Sandmire HF and De Mott RK. (2001). Erb's palsy: concepts of causation. *Obstet Gynecol*, **95**, 940–942.
88 Gherman RB, Goodwin TM, Ouzounian JG, et al. (1997). Brachial plexus palsy associated with cesarean section: an in utero injury? *Am J Obstet Gynecol*, **177**, 1162–1164.
89 Gherman RB, Ouzounian JG and Goodwin TM. (1999). Brachial plexus palsy: an in utero injury. *Am J Obstet Gynecol*, **180**, 1303–1307.
90 Ouzounian JG, Korst LM and Phelan JP. (1998). Permanent Erb's palsy: a lack of a relationship with obstetrical risk factors. *Am J Perinatol*, **15**, 221–223.
91 Gordon M, Rich H, Deutschberger J, et al. (1973). The immediate and long-term outcome of obstetric birth trauma. I. Brachial plexus paralysis. *Am J Obstet Gynecol*, **117**, 51–57.
92 Adler JB and Patterson RL Jr. (1967). Erb's palsy. Long-term results of treatment in eighty-eight cases. *J Bone Joint Surg Am*, **49**, 1052–1064.
93 DeBree R, Van Nieuwkerk EBJ, Vos A, et al. (1999). Ruptuur van de larynx of de trachea als geboortetrauma. *Ned Tijdschr Geneeskd*, **143**, 1564–1568.
94 Seidman DS, Laor A, Gale R, et al. (1991). Long-term effects of vacuum and forceps deliveries. *Lancet*, **337**, 1583–1585.
95 Drife JO. (1996). Choice and instrumental delivery. *Br J Obstet Gynaecol*, **103**, 608–611.
96 Towner D, Castro MA, Eby-Wilkens E, et al. (1999). Effect of mode of delivery in nulliparous women on neonatal intracranial injury. *N Engl J Med*, **341**, 1709–1714.
97 Ventura SJ, Martin JA, Taffel SM, et al. (1994). Advance report of final natality statistics. *Mon Vital Stat Rep*, **43** (suppl.), 20.
98 O'Grady JP, Pope CS and Patel SS. (2000). Vacuum extraction in modern obstetric practice: a review and critique. *Curr Opin Obstet Gynecol*, **12**, 475–480.
99 Johanson RB and Menon BVK. (2001). Vacuum extraction versus forceps for assisted vaginal delivery. *Cochrane Database Syst Rev*, **2**, 1–5.
100 Johanson R and Menon V. (1999). Soft versus rigid vacuum extractor cups for vaginal assisted delivery. *Cochrane Database Syst Rev*, **1**, 44.
101 Vacca A. (1992). *Handbook of Vacuum Extraction in Obstetrical Practice*. London: Edward Arnold.
102 Bofill JA, Rust OA, Schorr SJ, et al. (1996). A randomized prospective trial of the obstetric forceps versus the M-cup vacuum extractor. *Am J Obstet Gynecol*, **175**, 1325–1330.
103 Bofill JA, Rust OA, Schorr SJ, et al. (1997). A randomized trial of two vacuum extraction techniques. *Obstet Gynecol*, **89**, 758–762.
104 Vacca A, Grant A, Wyatt G, et al. (1983). Portsmouth operative delivery trial: a comparison of vacuum extraction and forceps delivery. *Br J Obstet Gynaecol*, **90**, 1107–1112.
105 Sjostedt JE. (1967). The vacuum extractor and forceps in obstetrics. A clinical study. *Acta Obstet Gynecol Scand*, **46** (suppl. 10), 1–208.
106 O'Grady JP. (2000). Instrumental delivery: a critique of current practice. In *Gynecologic, Obstetric and Related Surgery*, ed. Nichols D and Clarke-Pearson D, pp. 1081–1105. St Louis: Mosby.
107 Berkus MD, Ramamurthy RS, O'Connor PS, et al. (1985). Cohort study of Silastic obstetric vacuum cup deliveries: I. Safety of the instrument. *Obstet Gynecol*, **66**, 503–509.
108 Berkus MD, Ramamurthy RS, O'Connor PS, et al. (1986). Cohort study of Silastic obstetric vacuum cup deliveries: II. Unsuccessful vacuum extraction. *Obstet Gynecol*, **68**, 662–666.
109 Johanson R, Pusey J, Livera N, et al. (1989). North Stafordshire/Wigan assisted delivery trial. *Br J Obstet Gynaecol*, **96**, 537–544.
110 Johanson RB, Heycock E, Carter J, et al. (1999). Maternal and child health after assisted vaginal delivery: five-year follow-up of a randomized controlled study comparing forceps and ventouse. *Br J Obstet Gynaecol*, **106**, 544–549.
111 Wen SW, Liu S, Kramer MS, et al. (2001). Comparison on maternal and infant outcomes between vacuum extraction and forceps deliveries. *Am J Epidemiol*, **153**, 103–107.
112 Schmidt B, Davis P, Moddeman D, et al. (2001). Long-term effects of indomethacin prophylaxis in extremely-low-birth-weight infants. *N Engl J Med*, **344**, 1966–1972.
113 Ngan H, Miu P, Ko L, et al. (1990). Long-term neurological sequelae following vacuum extractor delivery. *Aust NZ J Obstet Gynecol*, **30**, 111–114.
114 Carmody F, Grant A, Mutch L, et al. (1986). Follow up of babies delivered in a randomized controlled comparison of vacuum extraction and forceps delivery. *Acta Obstet Gynecol Scand*, **65**, 763–766.

13

Fetal and neonatal injury as a consequence of maternal substance abuse

Louis P. Halamek

Stanford University Medical Center, Palo Alto, CA, USA

Introduction

Substance abuse is widely prevalent in our society and women in their child-bearing years are not immune to this epidemic. In addition to the many problems substance abuse causes for these women it also places the children they are carrying at risk for lifelong sequelae. Virtually all pregnant women are exposed to drugs in some form (such as acetaminophen, iron, multivitamins, and antimicrobials) and it is estimated that approximately 10% are exposed to illicit substances.[1] The purpose of this chapter will be to describe the fetal and neonatal effects of various sensorium-altering licit and illicit substances ingested by pregnant women.

Drug distribution in pregnancy

Before discussing the various substances that may be ingested, it is important to understand general principles of drug distribution during pregnancy, including the roles of the placenta and breast in biotransformation and secretion. Drugs that are abused are capable of easily and rapidly entering the nervous system. The characteristics that favor transport of a drug across the lipoprotein barriers between the circulation and the central and peripheral nervous systems include high lipid solubility, minimal ionization at physiologic pH, low protein-binding, and low molecular weight. High lipid solubility may result in storage of such substances in maternal body fat with subsequent release and transfer into fetal lipid stores during pregnancy. These same characteristics also enable drugs to cross the placenta readily and enter the fetal circulation. The placenta harbors many enzyme systems that play roles in drug metabolism: such roles may consist of breaking down toxic substances to innocuous waste products or converting such substances into more active (and harmful) metabolites.[2] Deposition and retention of drugs in placental tissue, while limiting acute fetal exposure during maternal binges, may result in chronic long-term exposure to low levels of the same substance or its metabolites. Because the levels and activities of certain fetal hepatic enzyme systems critical in drug metabolism are suboptimal, the potential exists for concentrations of such substances to be higher in the fetus than in the mother. Fetal organs such as the kidney may also be relatively inefficient in drug excretion, producing higher serum levels. Fetal urine composes an increasing fraction of amniotic fluid as gestation progresses; fetal swallowing of amniotic fluid contaminated with active drugs and metabolites results in continued exposure. The umbilical cord and its vessels along with the vessels present on the surface of the placenta provide yet another potential route of absorption of drugs and metabolites present in amniotic fluid.[3] The cutting of the umbilical cord at birth does not fully protect the newborn from maternal substance abuse. Drugs stored in fetal fat can be released over time, resulting in continued exposure of the neonate over the first hours, days, weeks, or months of life. High lipophilicity enables these same substances to pass into breast milk, resulting in continued neonatal exposure and potential overdose. Certain substances such as tobacco smoke found in the environment are capable of producing serious consequences for mothers, fetuses, and newborns indirectly exposed to them. Finally it is only now being realized that adverse fetal consequences are not limited solely to maternal exposure to substances of abuse; the effects of various drugs on paternal sperm are now being delineated.

General effects of substance abuse during pregnancy

Substance-abusing women often do not seek or lack access to health care and are at high risk for serious sequelae, including withdrawal, malnutrition, iron and folate deficiency, anemia, and parenterally transmitted diseases such as bacterial endocarditis, human immunodeficiency virus, and hepatitis B virus. Pregnancy further increases the risks to health faced by these women.

Fetal effects of maternal substance abuse depend on multiple variables. The specific substance used by the mother may have profound effects on the fetus readily apparent during pregnancy or shortly after birth, subtle influences manifested during the school-age years, or no detectable consequences. The dose of the substance ingested and the duration of exposure also play an important role. Heavy use of any drug over a long period of time places the fetus at greater risk than light use over a similar time frame. Binge use, i.e., high intake of a drug over a relatively short period of time, even when infrequent, is also potentially very toxic to the fetus. Similarly, the timing of ingestion during pregnancy determines the fetal and neonatal effects. Use early in gestation during the period critical for organogenesis may result in malformations of these organs. Use in later trimesters may unduly influence processes occurring late in gestation, such as synapse formation in the central nervous system, that may produce neurobehavioral abnormalities or result in the neonatal abstinence syndrome. The genetic constitution of both mother and fetus is likewise important, in that drug metabolism by enzyme systems is under genetic control and inherited enzymatic defects may greatly potentiate the deleterious effects of various ingested substances. Variability in placental metabolic capacity also plays a role in the differential fetal effects of maternal substance abuse.[4]

Exposure to substances of abuse in utero may carry lifelong consequences. Serious teratologic influences will present in the neonatal period; these may be incompatible with long-term survival. Other more subtle alterations in morphogenesis may present months or even years after birth, in the form of neurodevelopmental delay or similar abnormalities. Clamping of the umbilical cord produces an abrupt cessation of drug administration and may result in withdrawal as newborn blood levels fall. Continuing exposure of the neonate to substances of abuse, as through breast-feeding, may produce a state of prolonged intoxication.

Methodologic limitations

Many methodologic problems exist with studies performed on substance-abusing women and their children. Because many women abuse more than a single substance (polydrug abuse) during pregnancy, simple identification of a population of women and neonates exposed to a single substance is difficult at best. Small selective sample sizes and the lack of suitable control groups are problems which plague many clinical investigations. Such small sample sizes are not representative of the entire spectrum of pregnant women who abuse a particular substance; rather they tend to focus on those with the most intense exposures who are most likely to exhibit detectable effects. Studies based on these small patient populations lack the power to achieve statistical significance. Concomitant use of multiple drugs may produce an additive harmful effect when compared to use of a single substance. Investigators are faced with an inherent inability to document the frequency and dose of drug exposure.

Illicit drugs are not regulated for purity and are often adulterated or "cut" with other substances, making dose ascertainment problematic, even in those who apparently have limited their exposure to a single drug. While elicitation of a drug use history is a vital component of any obstetric or neonatal examination, it has been shown in multiple studies that patient historical recall alone grossly underestimates prenatal substance abuse. Therefore historical data must be accompanied by analysis of maternal and neonatal body fluids or tissues. Analysis of urine is capable of detecting only relatively recent (hours to days) exposure. Neonatal meconium analysis, while more sensitive than urine analysis, is useless in the detection of drug exposure very early in gestation as meconium is formed beginning at approximately 16 weeks' gestation. It therefore is uninformative for exposures occurring during the crucial first trimester. Maternal hair analysis may provide the best information regarding timing of exposure, dose ingested, and duration of exposure but requires the cooperation of the mother. Neonatal hair may be lacking in sufficient quantity to allow study and also is not present early in gestation (fetal hair begins to appear at approximately 9 weeks' gestation). Selection of only the most severely affected cases for presentation in the medical literature (publication bias) and ignorance of negative studies (studies finding no apparent effect of the drug) are common. The presence of numerous confounding variables such as poor nutrition, poverty, previous obstetric history, and lack of access to prenatal and pediatric care greatly complicates any study of the effects of maternal substance abuse. That in utero exposure and subsequent biologic predisposition or vulnerability are complicated by environmental influences is reflected in the multihit model of neurologic handicap.[5] Follow-up studies are hampered by high attrition rates. The most dysfunctional families (arguably those with the most severely impaired children) fail to return for follow-up; this results in bias in favor of those performing relatively well. Little experimental evidence exists for the many clinical observations of potential effects of transplacental acquisition of various substances of abuse. Thus, while many of these substances are associated with adverse maternal, fetal, and neonatal outcome, it is impossible to state that a cause-and-effect relationship exists for most of the drugs ingested by pregnant women.

Substances of abuse

Ethanol

Ethanol is a drug which alters the sensorium. The production and distribution of ethanol is regulated by the US government. Its consumption is also regulated in the sense that sales of alcoholic beverages to minors is illegal; however, irresponsible consumption by both minors and adults is a major societal problem. Ethanol consumption is common in the population at large and various studies indicate that approximately one-half of women in their childbearing years drink. The incidence of ethanol ingestion by pregnant women steadily declines as pregnancy advances; by the third month only 10–15% of women continue to ingest ethanol.[6] Many women are unaware they are pregnant until they reach the second or third month; therefore their fetuses are exposed to ethanol and its metabolites during the critical period of organogenesis.

Signs and symptoms of ethanol intoxication vary directly with blood levels. Acute intoxication in the adult is characterized by incoordination and mood changes when levels are relatively low (approximately 5 mmol/l) and nystagmus, diplopia, ataxia, dysarthria, hypotension, and confusion at higher (20 mmol/l) levels. Coma, respiratory depression, and death may follow as blood levels rise. The effects of chronic exposure to ethanol include malnutrition (ethanol is a source of nonnutritive calories), Wernicke's encephalopathy (encephalopathy, ophthalmoplegia, ataxia) secondary to thiamine deficiency, Korsakoff's syndrome (selective memory deficits and apathy), cerebellar degeneration, central pontine myelinolysis, myoneuropathies, and dementia. Ethanol withdrawal has been well described in the adult literature.

The mechanism of action of ethanol is complex

and not fully understood. Ethanol is not thought to interact with specific receptors in a manner similar to the opioids; rather it dissolves into the plasma membrane of cells in the central nervous system, producing alterations in the structure and function of membrane lipids and proteins.[7] Ethanol may interact in a manner similar to barbiturates and benzodiazepines with the receptor for gamma-aminobutyric acid (GABA), functioning as an inhibitory neurotransmitter.[8]

The level of glucuronyl transferase and alcohol dehydrogenase activity is decreased in the fetus as compared to maternal levels.[9] Catabolism is delayed, resulting in higher fetal than maternal ethanol concentrations. It has long been recognized that maternal ethanol consumption during pregnancy produces a range of effects in the fetus and neonate: such effects may be subtle, expressing themselves in mild neurodevelopmental abnormalities, or profound, with characteristic phenotypic manifestations and mental retardation.[10,11] This variability in phenotype has historically been designated as fetal alcohol effects (mildly affected) and fetal alcohol syndrome (severely involved). The diagnosis of fetal alcohol syndrome is dependent upon a positive history of maternal ethanol use during gestation, characteristic facial dysmorphology, mental retardation, and growth deficiency of pre- or postnatal onset. Because of the imprecision of the designation "fetal alcohol effects," the potential for indiscriminate labeling of children whose problems may only partially be secondary to prenatal ethanol exposure, and the maternal and neonatal stigma associated with it, it is recommended that use of this term be avoided.[12] Just as the intoxicating effects of ethanol on adults vary directly with blood levels, the effects seen in the newborn undoubtedly reflect the variability in dose, timing of exposure during gestation, frequency of exposure, and the genotype of mother and fetus. Fetal alcohol syndrome is the most common identifiable cause of mental retardation in the USA, affecting 0.1–0.5% of all live births.

Both ethanol and its primary metabolite acetaldehyde are teratogenic to numerous organ systems. Affected neonates are readily recognized by characteristic facies. Specific facial abnormalities include short palpebral fissures, hypoplasia of the upper lip, thin vermillion, diminished philtrum, upturned nose, and maxillary hypoplasia.[13] Central nervous system abnormalities, especially involving midline structures, are a prominent component of fetal alcohol syndrome.[14] Structural malformations include microcephaly, cerebellar dysplasia, heterotopias, agenesis of the corpus callosum, and anomalies secondary to the interruption of neuronal and glial migration.[15]

The exact mechanism(s) by which ethanol and its metabolites impair normal development is unknown. Events such as neuronal migration depend upon the developmentally regulated expression and function of cell adhesion molecules (CAMs); CAMs are also expressed in osteoblasts and appear to play a role in bone formation. Ethanol has been shown to alter the migration of neurons into the cortex in animal models and suppress the expression of CAMs in tissue culture in a dose-dependent fashion.[16,17] Alteration of CAM expression may be one of the teratogenetic mechanisms by which ethanol alters brain and craniofacial development. Ethanol alters the levels of endogenous retinoids and the expression of retinoic acid receptors in rats, producing cardiac anomalies similar to those seen in vitamin A teratogenesis.[18]

Some studies have revealed that ethanol inhibits cell division and protein synthesis. Quantitative decreases in brain DNA and delays in the appearance of messenger RNA for various developmentally regulated central nervous system proteins have been detected in rat pups.[19] Delayed neuronal migration and proliferation have been documented in rats exposed to ethanol in utero.[20] The incidence of central nervous system (germinal matrix and intraventricular) hemorrhage is increased in ethanol-exposed premature human neonates.[21] This may be indicative of an ethanol-induced alteration in the developmental biology of the germinal matrix, the site of both neuroblastogenesis and glioblastogenesis. Evidence also exists that ethanol may in certain circumstances stimulate cell proliferation and thereby inhibit terminal neuronal differentiation and synapse formation.[22] These studies indicate that ethanol is capable of impairing gene expression at the transcriptional level, disrupting the temporal and spatial patterns of differential gene expression, potentially having a profound impact on eventual structure and function.

Functional abnormalities such as mental retardation, hypotonia, irritability, and poor coordination are seen in patients with fetal alcohol syndrome. Exposure to ethanol in utero has been shown quantitatively and temporally to alter the development of numerous neurotransmitters, including the serotonergic, cholinergic, dopaminergic, and glutamatergic systems, as well as alter the activity of membrane-bound receptors for various neurotransmitters.[23,24]

Prenatal ethanol exposure is associated with amblyopia, astigmatism, and other visual defects in humans. Animal studies in rats indicate that ethanol produces both macroscopic and microscopic changes in the optic nerves, including a gross decrease in cross-sectional diameter; cytostructural maldevelopment of glial cells, neurons, and myelin; and abnormalities in various organelles.[25] External ear anomalies and sensorineural hearing loss have also been described.[26]

Associated cardiovascular abnormalities include atrial septal defect, ventricular septal defect, and anomalies of the great vessels. Myocardial ultrastructural changes, including decreased myofibrillar density and dysplasia, have been produced in rats exposed to ethanol prenatally.[27] The genitourinary system may also be involved and hydronephrosis is a common finding. Murine embryos exposed to ethanol show excessive cell death in the region of the mesonephric duct proximal to the cloaca and in neural crest cells proximal to the posterior neuropore.[28] This is followed by abnormalities in the location of the ureterovesicle junction, leading to ureteral obstruction and hydronephrosis. Other common anomalies include hirsutism, cleft lip and palate, nail hypoplasia, pectus excavatum, diastasis recti, hypospadius, and camptodactyly.

Prenatal and postnatal growth deficiency are manifested as decreased weight, length and head circumference.[29] Animal data indicate that prenatal ethanol exposure reduces fetal concentrations of insulin-like growth factor-1 (IGF-1) as well as the concentration of IGF-binding proteins later in life.[30] Ethanol has also been shown to reduce the secretion of IGF-2 from explanted fetal rat organs.[31] Such studies indicate that this may be but one mechanism by which prenatal ethanol exposure results in both short- and long-term alterations in growth and development. Lactase activity in the small intestine of rat pups exposed to transplacental ethanol is decreased in comparison to controls and may represent another factor contributing to the growth retardation seen in this syndrome.[32]

Women giving birth to babies with fetal alcohol syndrome typically use more ethanol and use it earlier in gestation. While it is clear that daily consumption of more than approximately 1.5 oz (42 g) of absolute ethanol (the equivalent of three beers) greatly increases the risk of alcohol-induced teratogenicity, there is no uniform fetal response to a particular dose of ethanol: therefore there is no amount of alcohol that can be considered entirely safe for the pregnant woman to consume. The American Medical Association, the American Academy of Pediatrics, the American College of Obstetricians and Gynecologists, and the Surgeon General recommend that women who are attempting to conceive or who are already pregnant should not drink ethanol in any amount.

In addition to its teratogenic effects on the fetus, chronic ethanol abuse is associated with an increase in the risk of spontaneous abortion and abruptio placentae.

Ethanol withdrawal has been described in neonates born to chronically intoxicated mothers. Given the potent teratogenic effects of ethanol, it may be difficult to determine whether such manifestations represent true withdrawal or are manifestations of the central nervous system effects of fetal alcohol syndrome.

Maternal ethanol abuse complicates breastfeeding in several ways.[33] Lactation is impaired and the let-down reflex is inhibited by ethanol. Ethanol is readily secreted in breast milk and acute neonatal intoxication can result. The motor development of infants regularly exposed to ethanol in breast milk as measured by the Psychomotor Development Index has been shown to be significantly lower in a dose–response fashion at 1 year of age.[34] It is interesting to note that in this study mental development was not affected.

Investigators have shown that the facial characteristics and other stigmata of fetal alcohol syndrome persist beyond the neonatal and infancy periods. It has also become apparent that children with a history of prenatal exposure but lacking the typical stigmata at birth may develop signs and symptoms over time. Longitudinal follow-up of neonates with prenatal ethanol exposure is necessary.[35]

The neurodevelopmental deficits seen in the fetal alcohol syndrome persist into adulthood. They manifest an inability to stay on task, poor memory, and are at increased risk for attention deficit disorder with hyperactivity.[36] Their comprehension, judgment, and reasoning are also impaired, making it difficult for them to anticipate the consequences of their actions. Because of mood lability, social interaction is impaired; this may accentuate feelings of withdrawal and depression.[37]

Tobacco

Tobacco leaves when burned liberate thousands of compounds including toxins (such as carbon monoxide and hydrogen cyanide), trace elements (lead, nickel, and cadmium) and carcinogens. While the prevalence of smoking has declined in the general population, it has become and remains a significant problem among women, especially those of child-bearing age. Though smoking may be a form of rebellion or a response to societal pressures to "grow up," it is the addicting nature of nicotine which undoubtedly plays the major role in its widespread use.

Carbon monoxide avidly binds to hemoglobin, competitively inhibiting oxygen from being taken up in the pulmonary capillaries. At atmospheric partial pressures this results in essentially irreversible displacement of oxygen. Carboxyhemoglobin levels in pregnant women who smoke are many times those of nonsmokers.[38] Increased maternal carboxyhemoglobin implies increased fetal carboxyhemoglobin, impaired oxygen content and delivery, and fetal hypoxemia.[39] Neonates born to mothers who smoke tobacco have elevated levels of erythropoietin in umbilical cord blood and increased numbers of nucleated red blood cells in peripheral circulation; both of these results indicate a response to hypoxemia.[40] Cyanide acts in a similar manner by binding to the iron moiety of both hemoglobin and mitochondrial cytochrome oxidase, inhibiting oxygen uptake and delivery as well as cellular respiration. Cyanide is also capable of inhibiting carbonic anhydrase, resulting in decreased carbon dioxide excretion. Chronic fetal hypoxemia results in intrauterine growth retardation and a small-for-gestational-age neonate. Newborns so affected are at risk for sequelae such as hypoxic–ischemic encephalopathy, polycythemia, and pulmonary hypertension.

The onset of action of nicotine is rapid and the effects sustained for minutes to hours. Nicotine is primarily excreted by the kidneys, although the lungs and liver are also sites of metabolism. Nicotine intoxication produces enhancement of memory and attention, suppression of appetite, relaxation of skeletal muscle, and generalized stimulation of the peripheral and central nervous systems. Higher doses can result in tachycardia, vasoconstriction, hypertension, and dysrhythmias. Withdrawal from nicotine is characterized by signs such as headache, memory and attention difficulties, nausea, constipation or diarrhea, generalized fatigue, and insomnia.

Nicotine crosses the placenta and accumulates in the amniotic fluid and fetus to the extent that fetal levels exceed those seen in the mother.[41–43]

It is commonly known among pregnant adolescents that smoking will allow for an easier (quicker and less painful) vaginal delivery. Indeed studies have shown that mothers who smoke deliver neonates weighing 200–300 g less than gestational age-matched controls; this appears to be due to a difference in fat-free mass.[9,44] Some studies have indicated a dose–response relationship between weight and length at birth and prenatal exposure to tobacco.[45] Another series revealed less severe growth restriction in neonates born to mothers who quit smoking during pregnancy compared with women who continued to smoke.[46] The pathophysiology of the intrauterine growth retardation seen in offspring of smoking mothers is multifactorial. Uterine artery vasoconstriction and decreased substrate delivery to the fetus may play a role.[47] Cigarette smoking may also alter the bioavailability of certain nutrients such as folate, zinc, and vitamins, producing relative maternal and fetal deficiencies. While gross placental size is not affected by smoking, structural changes in the cytoarchitecture at the placental–lacunar interface have been described.[48,49] Epidermal growth factor plays an important role in implantation, placental growth and endocrine function, and other aspects of fetoplacental development. Alterations in epidermal growth factor receptor autophosphorylation have been described and may represent another mechanism by which smoking may impair fetal growth.[50] It is also possible that embryonic and fetal cell number and size are diminished by premature termination of cell division, abnormal differentiation, alterations in neuronal synapse formation, or an as yet undetermined mechanism.[51]

The existence of a tobacco embryopathy is unclear. The association of smoking with cleft lip and cleft lip/palate remains controversial.[52,53]

Placenta previa is an abnormality in placentation resulting in the placenta being located close to or extending over the cervical os. Onset of labor with cervical effacement and dilatation produces hemorrhage as the placenta, fixed at one pole, separates from the cervix. Maternal and neonatal morbidity and mortality are high if this condition is undiagnosed and the woman begins to labor. Smoking during pregnancy increases the risk of placenta previa.[54] In addition, a dose–response relationship exists between cigarette smoking and placenta previa.[55] Pregnant women smoking more than 20 cigarettes per day have been shown to be at more than twice the risk of nonsmokers for developing placenta previa.

Intrauterine exposure to tobacco may have serious consequences for the fetus and neonate that extend beyond the immediate newborn period. Alterations in cerebral blood flow have been documented in animal models.[56] Prenatal exposure to tobacco decreases arousal to auditory stimuli and appears to increase the risk of obstructive sleep apnea.[57,58] Maternal smoking during pregnancy is a risk factor for sudden infant death syndrome.[59–61] Brainstem gliosis has been found in a number of autopsies of victims of sudden infant death syndrome; this histologic finding is consistent with repetitive hypoxemia, possibly secondary to abnormalities in the control of respiration.[62,63] In addition, maternal smoking appears to have an adverse effect on early intellectual function.[64–66]

Nicotine, cotinine, and other substances found in tobacco are secreted in breast milk. Levels in the neonate correlate with those seen in the mother. Nicotine has been shown to impair lactation and decrease the supply of breast milk. Nicotine is secreted in breast milk and has been associated with neonatal emesis, respiratory problems such as frequent upper respiratory tract infections, and reactive airway disease, and an increased risk of childhood cancer.[67,68] The effects on the newborn of the many other substances found in tobacco and secreted in breast milk are currently unknown. This is especially concerning as many women who quit smoking during pregnancy are likely to start again after delivery, feeling that the danger to their newborn no longer exists. All mothers should be counseled as to the potential risks presented by tobacco products secreted in breast milk and those found in environmental smoke.[69]

The consumption of smokeless tobacco ("chew," "chaw," "dip"), while primarily a male activity in the population at large, is more common in females in certain ethnic groups, such as native Americans. Animal studies indicate that ingestion of this form of tobacco increases the risk of intrauterine growth retardation, decreased bone ossification, and embryonic demise.[70,71]

The maternal effects of tobacco ingestion are multiple and well documented: chronic obstructive pulmonary disease, myocardial infarction, and cancer are just a few of the serious consequences. The dangers of environmental tobacco smoke ("second-hand smoke," "passive" or "involuntary" smoking) are only now coming to light. Environmental tobacco smoke refers to smoke which is exhaled by smokers or released from burning cigarettes ("sidestream" smoke) which can then be inhaled by nonsmokers. Estimates of the percentage of nonsmoking pregnant women exposed to environmental smoke range as high as 50%. It appears that fetal exposure to nicotine and its metabolites is significant even in cases of passive maternal exposure to smoke, as similar levels of cotinine and *trans*-3′-hydroxycotinine have been found in neonates born to nonsmoking passively exposed mothers and mothers identified as light (less than one pack per day) active smokers.[72] Fetal exposure to environmental smoke appears to increase the risk of poor developmental outcome. Children between the ages of 6 and 9 years who were exposed to environmental smoke in utero were found to perform at a level inferior to those born to nonsmoking mothers but superior to those born to smoking mothers.[73] Paternal smoking with subsequent maternal passive inhalation of "sidestream" smoke has also been associated with intrauterine growth retardation.[74,75] An increased risk of respiratory tract disease (recurrent infection, reactive airway disease), impaired pulmonary development, otitis media, and lung cancer in later life has been associated with the inhalation of environmental tobacco smoke; however most of these studies are retrospective in nature and prospective, well-controlled analyses are lacking. One of the most alarming findings to date is that passive smoking in the same room as the infant increases the risk of sudden infant death syndrome in a dose-dependent fashion.[76]

Marijuana

Δ-9-tetrahydrocannabinol (Δ-9–THC) is the major active metabolite derived from the plant *Cannabis sativa* (over 60 similar cannabinoid compounds are present). Marijuana is the term applied to the dried leaves, stems, and seeds of this plant. It is the most frequently abused of all illicit drugs in the USA and its use by women in their child-bearing years is extremely common. Despite this, little is known about potential effects on the mother and her fetus. Other derivatives of marijuana include hashish, a resin derived from the seedless flowering tops of the female plant (sinsemilla), and hashish oil. Hashish oil ("hash") is produced by repeated extraction of marijuana which yields a dark liquid containing high concentrations of Δ-9–THC. While oral consumption is possible, smoking is the usual route of ingestion and results in the absorption of a much greater proportion of active drug.[77] Burning or heating marijuana, hashish, and hashish oil allows for the inhalation of smoke containing Δ-9–THC and rapid absorption across the pulmonary epithelium. Marijuana smoke contains more carcinogens, irritants, and particulates than tobacco smoke.[78] Some of the substances present in marijuana smoke include carbon monoxide, toluene, cyanide, and acetone. Carboxyhemoglobin concentration increases several-fold as the user typically inhales deeply and holds her breath to achieve better absorption and a more intense effect. Marijuana cigarettes ("joints") may be adulterated with other substances such as cocaine and phencyclidine (PCP) to produce a more intense high. Intoxication may also be seen in those exposed to second-hand smoke. Δ-9–THC distributes slowly from the plasma to the tissue compartment over approximately 30 min; it is readily taken up by the brain, liver, and other tissues with high lipid contents. Effects may last for hours as chronic use results in deposition and slow release from fatty tissues; reabsorption by the enterohepatic route also plays a role. Δ-9–THC is metabolized by hepatic hydroxylases and excreted by the liver and kidneys.

Δ-9–THC produces a state of euphoria and relaxation by complex interactions with various neurotransmitters and receptors within the central nervous system. Users may feel a sense of heightened self and sensory awareness as well as experience hallucinations. This eventually gives way to a state of "temporal disintegration" characterized by deficits in attention and memory as well as generalized lethargy.[79]

Physiologic effects include conjunctival reddening, tachycardia, orthostatic hypotension, and dry mouth. No withdrawal has been described.

Prolonged, arrested labor has been reported with acute marijuana intoxication. While no teratogenic effects have been directly linked to prenatal marijuana, the adulteration of cigarettes with other drugs of abuse may raise the potential risk. Frequent marijuana use during pregnancy has been shown to be associated with a small decrease in birth weight, although this decrease does not reach statistical significance in all studies and in and of itself probably carries little clinical significance.[80–82] The effect of prenatal marijuana exposure on long-term growth is also unclear.[83]

Reported effects on neonatal behavior of in utero marijuana exposure include prolongation of the startle response, tremors, irritability, poor state regulation, and altered visual and auditory responses.[84] Reports of the effects of prenatal exposure to marijuana on neurobehavioral development during childhood is contradictory.[85–89] Continued exposure of the neonate to marijuana after birth is experienced by breast-feeding newborns because Δ-9–THC is excreted in breast milk. Another potential source is environmentally acquired smoke which may lead to intoxication.[90]

Cocaine

Cocaine or benzoylmethylecgonine is one of several alkaloids found in the leaves of *Erythroxylon coca* which grows primarily in Peru, Ecuador, and Bolivia; raw leaves contain approximately 0.5–2% cocaine.[91] Cocaine may also be synthesized from ecgonine by esterification with methanol and benzoic acid. Early South Americans discovered the pleasant effects of chewing coca leaves, slowly releasing small amounts of cocaine. The Spanish brought cocaine to Europe where purified forms became both popular and addictive habits. The major metabolite of cocaine is benzoylecgonine. In addition to its local anesthetic and vasoconstrictor properties, it blocks presynaptic catecholamine reuptake, resulting in catecholamine accumulation at postsynaptic receptors and pronounced central nervous system stimulation. In the central nervous system it blocks the reuptake of dopamine at dopaminergic receptors, producing a feeling of euphoria.

Coca paste is extracted from the leaves after harvesting and contains approximately 80% cocaine. The paste can be converted to a hydrochloride salt that can then be diluted with various adulterants such as lidocaine and talc or other psychotropic drugs such as heroin and amphetamine, resulting in a product of varying purity.[91] As a substance of abuse it exists in two forms – a hydrochloride salt and a free alkaloid. Benzoylmethylecgonine hydrochloride ("coke," "snow," "lady," "gold dust") is a benzoic acid ester of ecgonine obtained by dissolving the alkaloid in hydrochloric acid, producing a water-soluble solid with a melting point of approximately 200°C. It is produced in the form of crystals, granules, and powder. This form is suitable for intravenous use or nasal insufflation. Because of varying purity and absorption, nasal insufflation of cocaine produces relatively low serum levels (and therefore less intense effects) than smoking. Cocaine base ("freebase") is formed by the extraction of cocaine from the hydrochloride salt with the use of alkaline solutions and subsequent recrystallization employing highly flammable solvents; extraction of cocaine base in this manner is a dangerous procedure. Once purified the base is then smoked in a water pipe.

In the 1980s a much simpler and safer method of extraction of cocaine base was discovered: cocaine hydrochloride is mixed with water and sodium bicarbonate, forming a paste which is then hardened in a microwave oven. The free alkaloid form ("crack," "rock") makes cracking sounds as it is burned in pipes. It is soluble in ether, acetone, or alcohol; in addition it has a relatively low melting point (98 °C) and is heat-stable. Smoking takes advantage of these properties of the drug, allowing for rapid diffusion (given the large surface area of the lung) and entry into the blood and central nervous system, producing high serum levels and short, very intense highs. Intoxication is marked by disinhibition and a sense of increased physical and sexual energy, enthusiasm, and power. Other effects, which may not be dose-related, include hypertension, vasospasm, central nervous system hemorrhage, and myocardial infarction. Metabolism occurs via three mechanisms: plasma and hepatic cholinesterases to ecgonine methylester (inactive), nonenzymatic hydrolysis to benzoylecgonine (inactive), and *N*-demethylation via the mixed oxidase system to norcocaine (active). Biotransformation within the brain is slow and levels within the central nervous system may be up to 20 times higher than plasma levels.[92] Because cholinesterase activity is low in pregnancy as well as in the fetal and neonatal periods, pregnant women and their newborns may be exposed to high levels of cocaine for protracted periods of time. The placenta binds cocaine and its metabolites and thus may effectively serve as a depot for drug release during pregnancy.[93] Excretion of the water-soluble metabolites (benzoylecgonine and ecgonine methyl ester) is accomplished by the kidney.

A cocaine abstinence syndrome has been described in adults as consisting of three phases. After a binge the user experiences a period of agitation and anxiety with an intense craving for the drug. This is followed by a "crash" marked by hypersomnolence punctuated with episodes of hyperphagia lasting for days. Following the crash, withdrawal symptoms consisting of depression, lack of energy, and disinterest in surroundings occur and are accompanied by drug-seeking behavior. Addicts may continue to suffer strong cravings which gradually diminish over months or years. Extinction finally occurs with persistent abstinence.[94]

The number of individuals in the USA who have tried cocaine is estimated at 30 million; 5 million of these are regular users and 750 000 are women aged 18–34.[95] In women of child-bearing age, cocaine has replaced heroin as the second most commonly abused illicit substance after marijuana.

The perinatal literature is replete with case reports of fetal and neonatal problems involving essentially every organ system attributed to prenatal cocaine exposure. The common pathogenetic mechanism underlying these many and varied effects is suspected to be a disruption of blood flow, either globally to the uteroplacental unit or locally within specific fetal organs.[96] Thus cocaine exerts its teratogenic potential primarily through its ability to produce vasoconstriction, producing disruptions of normally formed tissues, rather than inducing primary malformations.

Global disruption of blood flow to the fetoplacental unit produces generalized rather than focal effects on the fetus. Uterine arterial vasospasm as a result of cocaine ingestion impairs fetal substrate delivery, predisposing the fetus to intrauterine growth retardation.[97,98] Prostaglandin production is altered in placental explants incubated in the presence of cocaine: thromboxane A_2 synthesis is increased and prostacyclin production decreased. Thromboxane A_2 induces vasoconstriction and platelet aggregation and may represent one mechanism whereby uteroplacental blood flow is impaired.[99] Although the duration of action of cocaine in producing uterine arterial vasoconstriction is relatively short-lived, even women who are relatively infrequent users of the drug remain at high risk for fetal growth abnormalities.[100] Therefore it is probable that mechanisms other than vasoconstriction play a role in the increased risk of intrauterine growth retardation. One example of such a mechanism is the ability of cocaine to inhibit the in vitro sodium-dependent uptake of alanine by human placental microvillous and basal membrane vesicles.[101] Even though vasoconstriction may be intermittent, other processes such as placental substrate uptake may be altered in a more chronic fashion.

While generalized compromise in blood flow to the uteroplacental unit may produce global fetal and neonatal effects, focal impairment produces a myriad of disruptive events affecting specific organs or organ systems. One of the more dramatic is the fetal disruption sequence or limb–body wall complex.[102] The fetal disruption sequence is characterized by a severe abdominal wall defect which results in exposure of viscera such as the liver, stomach, intestine, and spleen, and is accompanied by absence of the umbilicus and umbilical cord, genitourinary abnormalities, and musculoskeletal defects such as vertebral anomalies. Examples of disruptions secondary to cocaine-induced vasospasm that are more focal in nature include limb reduction defects such as terminal transverse defects of the forearm and amputation of the medial rays of the hands, intestinal atresia and infarction secondary to impaired mesenteric artery flow, and cranial defects such as encephalocele and exencephaly.[103–106] Cardiovascular disruptions are produced in murine embryos exposed to cocaine transplacentally; such disruptions are not seen in embryo cultures incubated with cocaine.[107] That disruptive effects are seen in vivo but not in vitro indicates that the maternal compartment may play a role in teratogenesis. Ischemia–reperfusion injury secondary to cocaine-induced uteroplacental ischemia followed by oxygen free radical toxicity upon reperfusion is another possible mechanism; this is supported by evidence that treatment with antioxidants ameliorates the disruptive effects.[108]

Many authors have described genitourinary tract abnormalities, including hydroureter, hydronephrosis, hypospadius, cryptorchidism, and ectopic kidneys, in neonates born to cocaine-abusing women.[109–112] The urethral obstruction sequence is postulated to be secondary to fetal prostatic vasospasm, resulting in subsequent hypoplasia of the prostatic stroma and urethral obstruction. Urinary tract obstruction ensues, producing dilatation of the bladder, ureters, and kidneys. Urinary ascites and abdominal distension stretch the abdominal skin and thin the abdominal musculature; any degree of decompression creates the wrinkled appearance of the abdomen, responsible for the name "prune belly." Animal models have indicated that transplacental cocaine alters neuronal and glial morphology, density, and distribution in the developing mouse cerebral cortex.[113] Cardiovascular anomalies, including peripheral pulmonic stenosis, atrial septal defects, ventricular septal defects, and patent ductus arteriosus, have been described in case reports.[104,114,115] Studies in mammalian animal models have produced cardiac lesions similar to those in human case reports. A pattern of facial dysmorphology consisting of hypertelorism and midfacial flattening has been reported but little agreement exists among dysmorphologists regarding its incidence.[116]

Cocaine use is associated with premature labor, premature rupture of membranes, advanced cervical dilatation at admission, and a shortened latency period to labor and delivery.[109,117,118] In addition, maternal cocaine ingestion appears to carry an increased risk of placenta previa, abruptio placentae, uterine rupture, and precipitous delivery.[119–122] Cocaine appears to enhance myometrial contractility by various mechanisms: increased thromboxane A_2 synthesis, inhibition of beta-adrenergic receptor binding, and a downregulation of beta-adrenergic receptor number.[99,123,124] The incidence of spontaneous abortion and fetal demise is also higher in the cocaine-exposed population.[109]

The pathophysiologic basis of the effects associated with intrauterine cocaine exposure described in the neonatal period is primarily vascular. Necrotizing enterocolitis is a potentially catastrophic gastrointestinal disease which primarily affects premature newborns. Prenatal cocaine exposure is associated with an increased risk of necrotizing enterocolitis in both premature and term newborns.[103,115,125,126] Pregnant rats injected with cocaine delivered newborns with mesenteric vascular thrombosis and focal areas of inflammation, hemorrhage, and necrosis in their gastrointestinal tract.[127]

The effects of cocaine on the developing central nervous system has been a focus of investigation by many. Various central nervous system manifestations have been described in neonates, infants, and children born to cocaine-abusing women. Discrete anatomic lesions such as cerebral artery infarction have been detected in exposed neonates.[128,129] An increased incidence of intracranial hemorrhage has been described; this is felt to be due at least in part to an increase in mean arterial blood pressure and cerebral blood flow velocity.[130,131] Periventricular leukomalacia, felt to be secondary to in utero cerebral ischemia, has also been associated with prenatal cocaine exposure.[132] However, not all studies reveal an association between prenatal cocaine exposure and structural brain abnormalities.[133]

In addition to anatomic lesions, cocaine has been associated with physiologic abnormalities in the newborn. Seizures have been described in neonates after receiving a transplacental cocaine bolus shortly before birth and after passive inhalation of environmental "crack" smoke.[134] Alterations in both respiratory control and sleep regulation in the fetus and neonate have been described in human and animal studies. Periodic breathing and apnea are common in preterm neonates and felt to be secondary to immaturity in respiratory control mechanisms; such findings are rare in neonates born at term. Cocaine-exposed term newborns have been shown to have increased apnea and periodic breathing in comparison with controls.[135,136] The ability of neonates to make a smooth transition between sleep and awake states has been found to be abnormal in those exposed to cocaine.[137] Direct intravascular administration of cocaine to fetal sheep suppresses low-voltage electrocortical activity and increases catecholamine levels.[138] Fetal sleep state regulation is in part controlled by norepinephrine which normally decreases in active fetal sleep. Transplacentally acquired cocaine elevates norepinephrine levels and decreases active sleep. Tryptophan and serotonin also function as regulators of the sleep–wake cycle; cocaine has been found to interfere with tryptophan uptake and serotonin biosynthesis.[139] The effects of these alterations upon the developmental biology of the central nervous system are unknown. Abnormalities in respiratory control and sleep state regulation increase the risk of sudden infant death syndrome (SIDS). However it is not clear that cocaine-exposed neonates are at an increased risk of SIDS as studies have produced conflicting results.[140,141] Home monitoring is not indicated for the neonate exposed to cocaine in utero.[142]

Numerous developmental studies have been performed on children of varying postnatal ages who were exposed to cocaine prenatally. Studies have shown poor on-task performance, fine motor deficits, impaired habituation, low threshold for overstimulation, inability to self-regulate, and cognitive and motor developmental delay at 1.5–2 years of age based on scores achieved on the Mental Development Index and Psychomotor Development Index.[130,143–145] Other studies indicate a dose–response effect of prenatal cocaine exposure upon assessments of growth and behavior.[146–148] While the growth-retarded cocaine-exposed neonate shows a recovery in weight and length, poor head growth persists through age 2 years.[149] Abnormalities in catecholamines and their metabolites have been documented in neonates exposed in utero to cocaine.[150] Cocaine exposure alters the levels of neurotransmitters such as dihydroxyphenylalanine (the conversion of tyrosine to dihydroxyphenylalanine by tyrosine hydroxylase is the rate-limiting step in catecholamine synthesis) in serum and homovanillic acid (the major metabolite of dopamine) in cerebrospinal fluid.[151–153] The relationship between serum and cerebrospinal fluid levels of molecules capable of neurotransmission is yet to be elucidated. Similarly, the effects of such alterations early in gestation on the subsequent developmental biology of the human nervous system are unknown.

The lay press was quick to sensationalize the cocaine epidemic and the purported effects of this drug on the unborn. Despite limited evidence generated by studies complicated by all of the problems outlined earlier, "crack babies" were labeled as irrecoverably damaged and a burden to society. A more scientific analysis of the available data fails to substantiate the universality and inevitability of these early claims. A metaanalysis published in 2001 stated that there was no convincing evidence that in utero exposure to cocaine and its metabolites results in developmental defects in children aged 6 and younger.[154]

Anecdotal experience indicates that neonates exposed to transplacental cocaine rarely become clinically jaundiced. The ability of cocaine to induce Δ^5-3-ketosteroid isomerase, glutathione-*S*-transferase, and bilirubin uridine diphosphate glucuronosyl transferase, hepatic enzymes important in the transport and metabolism of bilirubin, has been shown in a rat model and offers a possible explanation for the clinical observation of a decreased incidence of jaundice in exposed newborns.[155]

No definitive abstinence syndrome from in utero

cocaine exposure has been described in neonates; it is uncertain whether the signs seen in neonates represent true withdrawal or are secondary to the direct effects of the drug still present in the newborn. These signs typically appear in the first 24–48 h after birth and peak in intensity by 72 h.[156] The most frequently observed findings include tachycardia, tachypnea, hypertension, irritability, exaggerated Moro response, impaired visual tracking, increased tremulousness, abnormal sleep patterns, increased generalized motor tone, and feeding abnormalities, including poor suck and emesis.[157]

Cocaine is excreted in breast milk up to 36 h after the last dose, representing another potential route of neonatal exposure. Cases of neonatal intoxication marked by irritability, vomiting, diarrhea, tachycardia, tachypnea, hypertension, and tremulousness in breast-fed newborns have been described.[158] One case describes an 11-day-old breast-feeding neonate who developed apnea and seizures after ingesting cocaine used as a topical anesthetic for maternal nipple soreness.[159] Intoxication may also result from passive inhalation of smoke from the environment.[160]

Opioids

Opium is the dried milky exudate of the common poppy, *Papaver somniferum* (Latin, *papaver*, poppy, + *somnus*, sleep, + *fero*, to bring). Opiate refers to a drug derived from opium. An opioid is a natural or synthetic substance which produces opium- or morphine-like effects when ingested. Narcotic is the nonspecific term applied to any drug derived from opium or similar compounds that is capable of inducing analgesia, sedation, and sleep and which will cause dependence with repeated use. The most commonly abused opioids act as agonists for specific receptors (mu, kappa, delta, sigma, epsilon) within the central and peripheral nervous systems. Opioids inhibit the activity of pain fibers via two mechanisms: decreasing neurotransmitter release and production of membrane hyperpolarization.[161] Their activity is similar to that of endorphins, enkephalins, and dynorphins, peptides that act as endogenous nonaddicting analgesics. The naturally occurring agonists are morphine, papaverine, codeine, and noscapine; others such as diacetylmorphine (heroin), oxycodone (Percodan), meperidine (Demerol), propoxyphene (Darvon), fentanyl (Sublimaze) and methadone (Dolophine) are wholly or partially synthetic. Designer opioids such as 1-methyl-4-phenyl-4-propionoxy-piperidine (MPPP), 1-methyl-4-phenyl-1,2,3,6-tetrahydropyridine (MPTP) and alpha methyl fentanyl ("China white") are extremely potent "designer" opioids, easily and inexpensively synthesized and having a very rapid onset of action with prolonged euphoric effects. Opioids may be ingested orally or inhaled; they may also be injected intravenously, intramuscularly, and subcutaneously. Onset of action is typically rapid and the duration of effect is prolonged for hours to days. The drug of choice among opioid addicts is heroin; its lipid solubility is greater than morphine, thereby allowing it to enter the central nervous system more rapidly and producing a quicker, more intense "high." Maternal intoxication is marked by euphoria and sedation but may progress to hypotension, respiratory depression, and death. Upon discontinuation of opioid use, intense withdrawal occurs.

Despite the frequency of fetal exposure to opioids, no opioid embryopathy has been described. Endogenous opioid peptides and opioid receptors are expressed transiently in the developing mammalian brain.[162–164] The significance of this developmentally regulated process and the effects that exogenous opioids delivered via the umbilical cord have on this phenomenon are unknown at this time. Surfactant is a complex lipoprotein which is produced and secreted by type II alveolar cells within the fetal lung. In preparation for the transition at birth to an air-filled environment, surfactant production is upregulated late in gestation. Methadone delays pulmonary surfactant synthesis by an unknown mechanism and places the newborn at higher risk of respiratory distress syndrome and the concomitant need for assisted ventilation.[165] Opioids also appear to have some beneficial effects on the fetus. Heroin nonspecifically induces several fetal enzyme systems. Unlike methadone, heroin accelerates pulmonary surfactant synthesis; exposed neonates have a decreased risk of respiratory distress. Heroin also induces uridine diphosphate glucuronyl transferase, the hepatic enzyme which catalyzes the formation of bilirubin monoglucuronide, resulting in a decreased incidence of hyperbilirubinemia.

Maternal withdrawal implies fetal withdrawal. While the addicted mother manifests the typical signs and symptoms of opioid withdrawal, the fetus experiences hypoxia and in response may pass meconium. Meconium aspiration carries a significant risk of pneumonitis, air trapping, and pneumothorax. Chronic fetal hypoxia produces pulmonary vascular remodeling and increased vascular reactivity, predisposing the newborn to pulmonary hypertension after birth when adequate pulmonary perfusion is necessary for gas exchange. Both meconium aspiration and pulmonary hypertension increase neonatal morbidity and mortality. Chronic intrauterine hypoxia also increases the risk of hypoxic–ischemic encephalopathy and fetal demise. Because of the significant maternal, fetal, and neonatal sequelae, withdrawal in pregnancy should be treated promptly and appropriately with enrollment of the mother in a methadone program.

A neonate exposed to opioids in utero is at risk of respiratory depression in the hours after birth. Naloxone (Narcan), an opioid antagonist, may be used to reverse respiratory depression in the newborn secondary to maternal opioid administration within 4 h of delivery in the absence of a maternal history of opioid abuse. Given that first, maternal underreporting of substance abuse has been shown in numerous studies comparing drug use histories with body fluid toxicology screening and second, acute opioid reversal in a newborn chronically exposed in utero may produce withdrawal, naloxone should be used very judiciously on a case-by-case basis. In general, it is preferable to support the neonate's respirations with positive-pressure ventilation and achieve a heart rate above 100 beats/min prior to establishing the need for and administration of naloxone. Any neonate receiving naloxone should be monitored carefully in the hours after birth as the duration of action of many opioids is longer than that of naloxone.

Opioids appear to have effects that extend beyond the immediate newborn period. Neonates born to methadone-using mothers have been shown to have a decreased sensitivity to carbon dioxide during the first days of life in comparison to controls.[166] The risk of SIDS in babies born to opioid-abusing mothers is 5–10 times that of nonexposed newborns (approximately 20–30 per 1000 live births versus two to three per 1000 in the general population).[165] Fetal exposure to opioids may also increase the risk of mild developmental delay in infancy.[167]

Once the umbilical cord is clamped, the newborn is disengaged from all that was once supplied by the mother and placenta; this includes any drugs that may have crossed into the umbilical vein. Neonates born to opioid-addicted mothers are at risk for withdrawal. Withdrawal in the newborn is characterized by central nervous system signs such as yawning, lacrimation, mydriasis, irritability, and seizures. While these effects are transitory, some may produce permanent nervous system injury if not treated appropriately (e.g., untreated seizures). Heroin and methadone are the most common opioids used by pregnant women. Heroin has a relatively short half-life and exposed newborns typically experience withdrawal soon after birth. Methadone is a synthetic opioid used in the treatment of maternal addiction and prevention of withdrawal signs and symptoms. It produces similar analgesic effects but results in less sedation and euphoria than heroin and morphine. The half-life of methadone is approximately 12–24 h, making once-a-day oral dosing an attractive feature of this medication in treating addiction. The majority of neonates exposed to methadone in utero undergo withdrawal, usually manifesting signs within 1–2 days of birth. Withdrawal from methadone is typically more severe and longer in duration in comparison with other prenatally acquired opioids. Given the long half-life of this drug and the fact that methadone is present in low concentrations in breast milk, some neonates may not experience withdrawal until several weeks of age. While the presence of methadone in breast milk in levels approximating those found in serum may prevent or delay neonatal withdrawal, it may also result in intoxication, respiratory depression, and death in the breast-feeding newborn.[168] The American Academy of Pediatrics states that breast-feeding is contraindicated if the maternal dose of methadone exceeds 20 mg/day.[169]

Sedative-hypnotics

The group of drugs known as the sedative-hypnotics includes the benzodiazepines (diazepam, lorazepam, triazolam, chlordiazepoxide, etc.), barbiturates (phenobarbital, pentobarbital, secobarbital, hexobarbital, etc.) and miscellaneous others, including methaqualone, meprobamate, and ethchlorvynol. Many of these drugs act by accentuating the effects of the inhibitory neurotransmitter GABA on the function of other stimulatory neurotransmitters.[170] These substances are used to induce sleep, decrease anxiety, and relax muscles. Higher doses result in retrograde amnesia, headache, vertigo, nausea, coma, respiratory depression, and death. Ethanol potentiates the absorption of these drugs and therefore may lead to overdose if used simultaneously. Because they can be ingested orally they are common substances of abuse. They can also be administered intravenously or intramuscularly. Effects are dependent upon route of administration and may be seen within minutes. As a class of drugs these substances typically have long half-lives and their effects may persist for days. They are metabolized by hepatic glucuronidases and excreted by the kidneys. Withdrawal in the adult from sedative-hypnotics is marked by increasing depression or anxiety which may progress to agitation, delirium, and frank psychosis.

Benzodiazepine levels in fetal blood exceed those in maternal blood.[171] Fetal effects include decreased beat-to-beat variability in heart rate pattern. Dysmorphic characteristics similar to those seen in fetal alcohol syndrome (microcephaly, neurodevelopmental delay, hypotonia, feeding difficulties, genitourinary abnormalities, and abnormal facies) and cleft lip and cleft palate have been reported in neonates exposed to benzodiazepines.[172–175] Reduced head circumference and cognitive deficits have been associated with in utero exposure to anticonvulsant barbiturates.[176,177] However no definitive evidence of a "sedative-hypnotic syndrome" exists.

Withdrawal in the neonate is similar to that seen with opioids: at its most severe, hypothermia, hypotonia, and respiratory depression ensue.[178] Sedative-hypnotics are secreted in breast milk and this route affords another possible route of intoxication.

Sympathomimetics

Sympathomimetics produce physiologic responses similar to endogenous catecholamines, stimulating neurotransmitter release at alpha, beta, dopaminergic, and serotonergic receptors.[179] Unlike catecholamines, these drugs retain their efficacy when ingested orally, readily enter the central nervous system, and are metabolized much more slowly than the endogenous catecholamines with large proportions excreted unchanged in urine. Thus they are capable of producing sustained central nervous system stimulation. Plants such as cola nuts and cacao (caffeine) serve as sources for some of the sympathomimetic drugs. Many others can be obtained in over-the-counter medications, including phenylephrine, ephedrine, pseudoephedrine, and phenylpropanolamine. The most commonly abused sympathomimetics include amphetamine, methamphetamine ("crystal"), and methylphenidate. Some drugs in this class also possess hallucinogenic effects, such as 3,4,5-trimethoxyamphetamine (TMA), dimethoxyamphetamine (DOM/STP), and methylenedioxymethamphetamine (MDMA). The amphetamines are collectively known as "speed;" a "speed run" refers to frequent repeated use of amphetamines over the course of several days during which the user sleeps and eats little. This is followed by a "crash" marked by long periods of sleep, hyperphagia, and dysphoria. Some users ingest "speedballs," combinations of amphetamine with barbiturates (to calm the agitated feelings associated with amphetamine use) or heroin (to enhance the "rush" associated with heroin). Routes of ingestion include oral consumption, nasal insufflation, and inhalation of smoke (smokeable methamphetamine hydrochloride is known as "ice") as well as intravenous and subcutaneous injection ("skin popping"). Onset of action and duration of effect vary with the route of ingestion. Effects are usually noticeable within 30–60 min and last for hours. Metabolism occurs in the liver and excretion is renal.

Sympathomimetic intoxication in the adult is characterized by an ability to remain awake for extended periods (days) with decreased total and rapid eye movement sleep, appetite suppression, mood elevation, a sense of greater awareness of one's surroundings and thoughts, and better adherence to task.[179] Pleasurable hallucinations may also be experienced. Toxic effects are dose-dependent. Relatively low doses result in stimulation of peripheral alpha- and beta-receptors producing hypertension and reflex bradycardia; higher doses are capable of inducing tachydysrhythmias, including sinus and ventricular tachycardia. Profound hypertension can result in intracerebral hemorrhage.[180–182] Other signs and symptoms of sympathomimetic toxicity in adults include urinary obstruction, constipation, agitation, anxiety, seizures, choreoathetosis, dystonia, rhabdomyolysis, hyperthermia, respiratory depression and arrest, and death. Amphetamines with hallucinogenic properties are capable of destroying dopaminergic and serotonergic neurons in the central nervous system.[183,184]

As with cocaine, the sympathomimetics may produce potent vasoconstriction and limit blood flow to various organs. Uterine artery constriction results in relative placental insufficiency, decreased substrate delivery to the fetus, and risk of intrauterine growth retardation.[185] A slight reduction in birth weight but no differences in length or head circumference have been reported in studies of antepartum methamphetamine use.[186,187] While pregnant rats given MDMA showed dose-dependent decreases in serotonin and 5-hydroxyindoleacteic acid, their pups did not suffer depletion of these neurotransmitters.[188] Animal studies reveal that prenatal amphetamine exposure is associated with structural and functional alterations in brain development.[189–193] Methamphetamine use in late gestation has been associated with neonatal intracranial lesions, including white-matter cavitary lesions and intraventricular, subarachnoid, and subependymal hemorrhage.[194] Because the fetus has little central nervous system blood flow autoregulatory capacity, it is possible that the sympathomimetic-induced alterations in uterine and placental blood flow produce both uncompensated hypertensive spikes and hypotensive nadirs in the fetal circulation, predisposing the fetus to ischemic damage and reperfusion injury.

Sympathomimetic use during pregnancy has been associated with premature labor, preterm delivery, abruptio placentae, and postpartum hemorrhage.[195,196]

While tolerance to sympathomimetics develops readily, true physical dependence has not been conclusively proven. Abrupt cessation of use in adults produces jitteriness, poor coordination, and excessive rapid eye movement sleep which lasts for days to weeks. Tremors, feeding difficulties, and irritability followed by prolonged periods of lethargy have been described in the first days of life in neonates exposed to methamphetamine in utero. Since methamphetamine persists for days in the neonate after clamping of the umbilical cord it is possible that these signs represent drug toxicity rather than withdrawal.[197]

PCP

PCP (1-(1-phenylcyclohexyl)piperidene hydrochloride) was formerly used as an anesthetic agent until a high incidence of side-effects, including hallucinations and violent behavior, resulted in its removal from legal use in humans.[198] Because of its psychotropic effects and relative ease of manufacture, it has found a place as a substance of abuse. It exists in a liquid and a powder form (PCP, "angel dust"). Cigarettes are dipped into liquid PCP or the marijuana or tobacco leaves are coated with the powdered form of the drug; smoking allows for rapid absorption from the extensive surface area of the lungs. It may also be insufflated, injected intravenously, ingested orally, or absorbed percutaneously.

Effects are seen within minutes of exposure and may persist for hours to days. Because of its high lipid solubility, PCP is deposited in adipocytes and therefore may be slowly released over time from this tissue depot. Hepatic metabolism and renal excretion account for elimination of the drug.

Intoxication in adults produces a variable constellation of signs and symptoms. Common findings include hypertension, nystagmus, tachycardia, and wild swings in mental status, ranging from disorientation, agitation, and violent behavior to catatonia and coma.[199] Serious medical complications reported in adults include seizures, hyperthermia, intracranial hemorrhage, rhabdomyolysis, apnea, cardiac arrest, and death.[200–202] Because of the analgesic properties of PCP, users are capable of sustaining substantial trauma while intoxicated without recognition of the extent of their injury.

PCP readily crosses the placenta and enters the fetal circulation. Reports of microcephaly and dysmorphic facies associated with maternal PCP ingestion are found in the literature but no conclusive evidence of a PCP embryopathy exists.[203,204] Studies using human cerebral cortical tissue culture indicate that PCP has the potential to suppress axonal outgrowth and induce neuronal necrosis, possibly via an inhibitory effect on potassium channels.[205] However, no in vivo correlation of these findings has been made.

Neonates exposed to PCP in utero may manifest jitteriness, irritability, and rapid swings in levels of consciousness, as seen in adults with acute PCP intoxication.[203,206–208] As with many other substances of abuse, signs manifested in the neonatal period most likely reflect continued exposure to the active drug rather than true withdrawal.[209] PCP is secreted in breast milk and the potential exists for neonatal chronic exposure and intoxication.[210]

LSD

LSD ("acid") is a synthetic diethylamide derivative of lysergic acid. It is classified as a psychedelic (a substance capable of producing a distorted perception of reality) rather than a hallucinogen (a substance which produces a vision with no basis in reality). While LSD may be insufflated, inhaled, injected intravenously or subcutaneously, and instilled into the conjunctival sac, it is most commonly taken orally. Sugar cubes, gelatin ("window panes"), paper ("blotter acid"), and tablets ("microdots") can be coated or impregnated with the drug and ingested. Onset of action is within minutes and the effect is prolonged for hours. Metabolism is primarily hepatic and excretion is both renal and hepatic.

Initial effects are not pleasant and consist of chills, flushing, nausea, piloerection, and tachycardia. Later, however, a sense of well-being and "communion with creation" may be had; reality is distorted and users describe sensations such as the slowing of time. Other effects include the ability to hear light or feel colors (synesthesia). More serious signs and symptoms such as hypertension, hyperthermia, seizures, and cardiorespiratory arrest may follow. While acute withdrawal has not been described, some users of LSD do report "flashbacks:" psychedelic experiences which occur in the absence of recent ingestion of the drug. Such flashbacks may occur months or years after one has last taken LSD. The mechanism of action of LSD appears to lie in its ability to inhibit serotonin and dopamine activity in the central nervous system. This likely results in "disinhibition" of higher cortical function, producing alterations in perception and thought.[211,212]

LSD has been associated with chromosomal breakage in offspring of mothers abusing the drug. While several reports of cardiac, ophthalmologic and other malformations exist, no causal link has been shown.[213–219] Whether neonates delivered to using mothers experience psychedelic effects is unknown. Withdrawal has not been reported. The extent of excretion into breast milk is also unknown.

Volatile substances of abuse

Any gas or liquid with a low boiling point which is psychoactive but minimally irritating to the airways can be inhaled to produce intoxication. These volatile substances of abuse are primarily hydrocarbon derivatives: aromatic and aliphatic hydrocarbons such as those found in paint solvents, adhesives, and fuels; alkyl halides and nitrites present in aerosol propellants, refrigerant, and cleaning fluids, and fuels; and ether and ketone components of fuels, solvents, oils, sealants, and plastics. Such substances are ubiquitous in modern society, found in products such as lighter fluids, nail polish remover, and typewriter correction fluid. Because they may be obtained so readily (and legally) they are common substances of abuse, especially among those unable to afford the more expensive illicit drugs such as cocaine.

The route of ingestion is inhalation and various methods are employed to accomplish this.[220] Sniffing refers to the inhalation of vapors emanating from a container filled with or a surface freshly coated with the substance. Bagging – breathing into and out of a bag filled with the substance tightly applied to the face – increases the exposure to the substance by reducing that lost to the atmosphere with sniffing. Placing a cloth soaked with a volatile substance of abuse over the nose and mouth is known as huffing. Substances with boiling points above room temperature can be liberated by heating over an open flame, although this carries a risk of ignition. Regardless of the method used, the onset of action is rapid, with effects felt within seconds to minutes; duration of effect is fairly short-lived, persisting for minutes to possibly an hour or more after exposure has ceased. Metabolism is primarily carried out in the liver and metabolites are excreted in bile, urine, and exhaled gas.

Although this category of chemicals contains many different substances with potentially a multitude of effects, intoxication generally produces feelings of euphoria and an increased sense of energy. Other reported psychoactive effects include hallucinations and paranoid ideation. More serious side-effects occur with higher doses and include nystagmus, ataxia, and dysrhythmias, potentially leading to cardiac arrest. Some of these compounds are metabolized to even more toxic products, such as carbon monoxide. The risk of permanent hematologic, hepatic, and renal damage is significant. No withdrawal has been described for the volatile substances of abuse.

The teratogenic potential of many of the chemicals abused in this manner is high, especially in view of the fact that it is impossible to control the amount ingested.[221] Teratogenicity is dependent upon the particular substance abused and is described in the literature regarding the industrial use of these substances. Toluene embryopathy serves as an example. Toluene, an aromatic hydrocarbon found in paints and adhesives, is normally converted to hippuric acid then excreted in the adult, although a large fraction is not metabolized. Toluene readily crosses the placenta; however the fetus appears unable to metabolize toluene adequately.[222,223] Animal studies indicate that prenatal exposure to toluene results in intrauterine growth retardation and neurologic, cardiovascular, skeletal, and craniofacial abnormalities.[224–230] Case reports in humans describe microcephaly, narrow bifrontal diameter, midface hypoplasia, developmental delay, and craniofacial abnormalities, including micrognathia, short palpebral fissures, ear anomalies, unusual scalp hair patterning, thin upper lip, and smooth philtrum.[231,232,233] Much phenotypic similarity exists in patients exposed in utero to toluene and those diagnosed with fetal alcohol syndrome. This has raised the possibility of a common mechanism of craniofacial teratogenesis.

Adulterants, substitutes, and contaminants

Ethanol, while legally sold and purchased in the USA, is commonly used in excess of socially accepted levels of intake. Tobacco, also legal, contains numerous toxic substances and is fatal to many users via a number of different mechanisms, including carcinogenesis and induction of chronic obstructive pulmonary disease. The production of the other substances described in this chapter is not regulated and therefore quality control regarding purity is nonexistent. In order to increase the bulk quantity of illicit drug and maximize profits, drugs are commonly diluted with other substances before being sold.[234] Adulterants are substances that appear similar to the illicit drug in color, structure, and consistency. Common adulterants include talc, sugar, starch, and cellulose. Adulterants are inert and do not possess psychotropic potential; the major complication associated with their incorporation into illicit drugs lies in their ability to embolize. Substitutes, like adulterants, increase the apparent volume of illicit drug by dilution. Substitutes, however, do possess intrinsic psychotropic activity similar to that of the illicit drug. Ephedrine, phenylpropanolamine, and caffeine produce a stimulant effect when added to illicit drugs. Procaine, lidocaine, and other local anesthetics are difficult to distinguish from cocaine. Contaminants are substances used in the preparation of illicit drugs that are not completely removed in the production and purification processes and therefore remain in the final formulation. Contaminants may or may not possess psychotropic or other potentially harmful effects in the user. The presence of adulterants, substitutes, and contaminants in the manufacture of illicit drugs adds further complexity to the determination of potential maternal, fetal, and neonatal toxicities.

The medical prescription of controlled substances during pregnancy has been reported in an attempt to avoid exposure to the unknown and potentially lethal substances which may be used as adulterants and substitutes in street drugs.[235] Dextroamphetamine was prescribed for a pregnant woman seropositive for human immunodeficiency virus and hepatitis B virus who was addicted to methamphetamines, chronically depressed, and felt to be at risk for suicide. The patient experienced normalization of her sleep–wake cycle, maintained her job, and weaned herself from the medication within several weeks. She remained drug-free during her last 2 months of pregnancy and delivered a healthy baby at term.

Screening

A maternal drug history is a mandatory part of any obstetric or neonatal history and physical. The history should be obtained in a nonthreatening manner and should review the use of over-the-counter medications, prescription drugs, tobacco, ethanol, and illicit drugs. When the concern of substance abuse is raised by the history or the examination of the mother, fetus, or neonate, the mother should be informed in a nonjudgmental manner. The physician should always be cognizant of the potential for spouse abuse when contemplating the manner in which this information is communicated to the father. Ideally this is accomplished after obtaining maternal permission and with the support of social workers trained in substance abuse. Maternal self-reporting of substance abuse uniformly underestimates the actual frequency of in utero exposure.[236] In addition it is recognized that drug use cuts across racial and socioeconomic boundaries.[237] Suspected substance abuse should be confirmed not only by elicitation on history but also by appropriate screening of selected maternal, fetal, and neonatal body fluids or tissues. Hospital policies vary, although permission of the mother is generally required for maternal screening, whereas neonatal testing is often considered implied when general consent to treat is provided upon newborn admission.

Urine is the body fluid most frequently tested for substances of abuse. Urine collection is noninvasive and large volumes can be rapidly and easily obtained in either mother or newborn. The kidney acts to concentrate drugs and their metabolites, producing higher concentrations in urine than in serum. Because of the lack of proteins and other cellular constituents which can interfere with the equipment used in assays, urine is relatively easy to analyze. Finally, urine offers the benefit of long-term stability if specimens are frozen. Screening tests commonly used include the fluorescence polarization immunoassay and the enzyme multiplication immunoassay technique. False-positive results depend on the extent of cross-reactivity with other substances. Positive results should be confirmed by more definitive methods such as gas chromatography–mass spectrometry. The most serious drawback in using urine to screen for intrauterine substance exposure lies in the fact that, because of the efficiency of the renal system, drugs and their metabolites are excreted quite quickly, usually within hours to several days after maternal ingestion. Therefore the ability of a urine drug screen to detect any exposure occurring more than 48–72 h preceding sampling is minimal. Other reasons for false-negative results include concentrations below the detectable limits of the assay and alterations in urinary pH affecting drug solubility.[238]

Meconium is the first stool passed by the newborn. It is composed of swallowed amniotic fluid and secretions such as bile, vernix caseosa, and epithelial cells and other debris shed into the lumen of the fetal gastrointestinal tract starting early in the second trimester. Because of its appearance early in gestation it functions as a reservoir for drugs delivered to the fetus via the umbilical cord and amniotic fluid and therefore provides a much better chronologic record of intrauterine drug exposure than does urine. Large quantities can easily be obtained in a noninvasive manner. However it is a tenaciously thick fluid with abundant particulate matter which requires extensive processing before conventional screening methods can be employed. Whereas most hospitals in the USA offer urine toxicologic testing, fewer centers are currently testing meconium on a routine basis. In addition, the number of drugs capable of being detected in meconium is limited in comparison with urine. Nevertheless, its utility in increasing the yield of positive exposures for cocaine and other selected drugs is well documented.[239]

Fetal hair appears at approximately 8 weeks of gestation, appearing first on the face, spreading to the scalp, and covering the rest of the body as development progresses. As epidermal cells surrounding the dermal papillae divide, the hair shaft grows; drugs and metabolites in the intrauterine environment are incorporated into the developing hair shafts. Like meconium, hair acts as a depot for drugs of abuse and provides a source for detection of drugs used early in gestation. The timing of exposure during gestation can be approximated by measuring the length of the hairs in the sample, incorporating the average rate of hair growth (1.3 ± 0.2 cm/month in adult women) and preserving the proximal–distal orientation of the hair strands.[240] Obviously, the longer the strands of hair obtained, the better the historical assessment of substance exposure will be; therefore it is best to obtain full-length hair. A core of hair approximately the same circumference as the eraser on a pencil is required. Because of the quantity of hair required the mother is usually a much better source than the neonate. The hair is then decontaminated (washed) and any drugs extracted.[241] Quantitative analysis is then carried out by radioimmunoassay with a specific antibody or gas chromatography–mass spectrometry. While it is an extremely useful tool in the determination of prenatal drug exposure, hair analysis is not completely foolproof as various hair treatments may limit the amount of drug which can be extracted.[241,242]

Serum may also be used for drug screening, although its use entails all of the limitations of urine testing, including the inability to establish distant or chronic exposures. In addition it is more difficult to obtain as it requires an invasive procedure, thus resulting in higher costs.

Summary

With the exception of ethanol (fetal alcohol syndrome), toluene (toluene embryopathy), and cocaine (fetal disruption sequence), little is definitively known about the potential fetal and neonatal consequences of intrauterine drug exposure. While the many case reports and abundant anecdotal experience allow for the listing of numerous associations of the substances of abuse with various malformations, disruptions, and neurodevelopmental disabilities, few well-designed, controlled, prospective clinical studies with appropriate follow-up have been carried out. The further elucidation of embryopathic effects will require expansion of the concept of teratogenesis beyond gross morphologic abnormalities. A lack of gross structural anomalies does not imply normal molecular structure nor normal physiologic function. Direct damage to DNA is but one mechanism by which drugs may affect the fetus. The cytoplasm is truly "where action is" and it is in this dynamic milieu that drugs may exert their effects on transcription, mRNA stability, and other processes vital to normal cellular function. This is an especially important concept in view of the many neurobehavioral problems purportedly associated with prenatal substance abuse that occur in the absence of gross nervous system malformations. Further clinical studies coupled with bench research at the molecular level should provide a better understanding of the impact of prenatal drug use on the fetus.

The fetal and neonatal brain exhibits remarkable resilience. Although prenatal drug exposure may create vulnerability, it is clear that the majority of children, given appropriate care, stimulation, and follow-up can overcome such potential insults. It is also clear that the quality of the postnatal environment may be just as important as, if not more important than, the intrauterine environment in determining long-term outcome. Although children with drug exposure have been shown to attain a performance level equal to nonexposed peer groups, it is also true that such peer groups function at levels below the national norm. This illustrates the profound effect other factors such as poverty and malnutrition can have on child development. It also illustrates how elimination of these other factors can positively impact the development of our youth.

The transition to an extrauterine existence is a difficult task. A baby must learn what actions elicit the desired responses from its parents. Caring for a newborn is a tremendous challenge and parents must learn to interpret their baby's wants and needs and be able to respond appropriately. A neonate exposed to drugs in utero may be lethargic or irritable and thus unable to process stimuli from the outside world. Substance-abusing parents may be unable to care for themselves adequately, let alone their newborn. The potential for frustration, under- or overstimulation, neglect, and abuse is great. The importance of family support, beyond that provided by substance abuse programs, cannot be underestimated. Multidisciplinary assessment and intervention programs must be easily accessible to those most in need of their services. Intrauterine drug exposure, unlike many other hazards faced by the fetus and neonate, is potentially a preventable problem.

Finally, criminalization of drug use and legitimization of the concept of "fetal abuse" in regard to prenatal drug use is not the means to achieve adequate care for a mother and her unborn child. For physicians who have not experienced, either personally or professionally, a dependency disorder, it is difficult to understand how a woman can knowingly risk potential harm to her unborn child. We can only understand when we realize that these women, plagued by a society that not only reinforces their feelings of inadequacy but also convinces them that inadequacy is their fault, are ridden with guilt and self-deprecation and therefore easily succumb to the temporary but nevertheless real reprieve offered by illicit drugs.

REFERENCES

1 Committee on Substance Abuse, American Academy of Pediatrics. (1995). Drug-exposed infants. *Pediatrics*, **96**, 364–367.

2 Little BB and VanBeveren TT. (1996). Placental transfer of selected substances of abuse. *Semin Perinatol*, **20**, 147–153.

3 Mahone PR, Scott K, Sleggs G, et al. (1994). Cocaine and metabolites in amniotic fluid may prolong fetal drug exposure. *Am J Obstet Gynecol*, **171**, 465–469.

4 Potter S, Klein J, Valiante G, et al. (1994). Maternal cocaine use without evidence of fetal exposure. *J Pediatr*, **125**, 652–654.

5 Snodgrass SR. (1994). Cocaine babies: a result of multiple teratogenic influences. *J Child Neurol*, **9**, 227–233.

6 Day NL and Richardson GA. (1991). Prenatal alcohol exposure: a continuum of effects. *Semin Perinatol*, **15**, 271–279.

7 Charness ME, Simon RP, Greenberg DA. (1989). Ethanol and the nervous system. *N Engl J Med*, **321**, 442–454.

8 Greenberg DA, Cooper EC, Gordon A, Diamond I. (1984). Ethanol and the gamma-aminobutyric acid-benzodiazepine receptor complex. *J Neurochem*, **42**, 1062–1068.

9 Jacobson JL, Jacobson SW, Sokol RJ, et al. (1994). Effects of alcohol use, smoking, and illicit drug use on fetal growth in black infants. *J Pediatr*, **124**, 757–764.

10 Jones KL, Smith DW, Ulleland CW, et al. (1973). Pattern of malformation in offspring of alcoholic mothers. *Lancet*, **1**, 1267–1271.

11 Clarren SK and Smith DW. (1978). The fetal alcohol syndrome. *N Engl J Med*, **298**, 1063–1067.

12 Aase JM, Jones KL, Clarren SK. (1995). Do we need the term "FAE"? *Pediatrics,* **95**, 428–430.

13 Sulik KK and Johnston MC. (1983). Sequence of developmental alterations following acute ethanol exposure in mice: craniofacial features of the fetal alcohol syndrome. *Am J Anat,* **166**, 257–269.

14 Swayze VW, Johnson VP, Hanson JW, et al. (1997). Magnetic resonance imaging of brain anomalies in fetal alcohol syndrome. *Pediatrics,* **99**, 232–240.

15 Clarren SK, Alvord EC, Sumi SM, et al. (1978). Brain malformations related to prenatal exposure to ethanol. *J Pediatr,* **92**, 64–67.

16 Miller M. (1993). Migration of cortical neurons is altered by gestational exposure to ethanol. *Alcohol Clin Exp Res,* **17**, 304–314.

17 Charness ME, Safran RM, Perides G. (1994). Ethanol inhibits neural cell-cell adhesion. *J Biol Chem,* **269**, 9304–9309.

18 DeJonge MH and Zachman RD. (1995). The effect of maternal ethanol ingestion on fetal rat heart vitamin A: a model for fetal alcohol syndrome. *Pediatr Res,* **37**, 418–423.

19 Naus CCG and Bechberger JF. (1991). Effect of prenatal ethanol exposure on postnatal neural gene expression in the rat. *Dev Genet,* **12**, 293–298.

20 Miller MW. (1990). Prenatal exposure to ethanol delays the schedule and rate of migration of neurons to rat somatosensory cortex. In *Fifth Congress of the International Society for Biomedical Research on Alcoholism.* Toronto, Canada.

21 Holzman C, Paneth N, Little R, et al. (1995). Perinatal brain injury in premature infants born to mothers using alcohol in pregnancy. *Pediatrics,* **95**, 66–73.

22 Armant DR and Saunders DE. (1996). Exposure of embryonic cells to alcohol: contrasting effects during preimplantation and postimplantation development. *Semin Perinatol,* **20**, 127–139.

23 Druse MJ, Kuo A, Tajuddin N. (1991). Effects of in utero ethanol exposure on the developing serotonergic system. *Alcohol Clin Exp Res,* **15**, 678–684.

24 Nio E, Kogure K, Yae T, et al. (1991). The effects of maternal ethanol exposure on neurotransmission and second messenger systems: a quantitative autoradiographic study in the rat brain. *Exp Brain Res,* **62**, 51–60.

25 Pinazo-Duran MD, Renau-Piqueras J, Guerri C. (1993). Developmental changes in the optic nerve related to ethanol consumption in pregnant rats: analysis of the ethanol-exposed optic nerve. *Teratology,* **48**, 305–322.

26 Church MW and Gerkin KP. (1988). Hearing disorders in children with fetal alcohol syndrome: findings from case reports. *Pediatrics,* **82**, 147–154.

27 Syslak PH, Nathaniel EJH, Novak C, et al. (1994). Fetal alcohol effects on the postnatal development of the rat myocardium: an ultrastructural and morphometric analysis. *Exp Mol Pathol,* **60**, 158–172.

28 Gage JC and Sulik KK. (1991). Pathogenesis of ethanol-induced hydronephrosis and hydroureter as demonstrated following in vivo exposure of mouse embryos. *Teratology,* **44**, 299–312.

29 Day NL, Richardson G, Robles N, et al. (1990). Effect of prenatal alcohol exposure on growth and morphology of offspring at 8 months of age. *Pediatrics,* **85**, 748–752.

30 Breese CR, D'Costa A, Ingram RL, et al. (1993). Long-term suppression of insulin-like growth factor-1 in rats after in utero ethanol exposure: relationship to somatic growth. *J Pharmacol Exp Ther,* **264**, 448–457.

31 Mauceri HJ, Lee W, Conway S. (1994). Effect of ethanol on insulin-like growth factor-II release from fetal organs. *Alcohol Clin Exp Res,* **18**, 35–41.

32 Guo W, Gregg JP, Fonkalsrud EW. (1994). Effect of maternal ethanol intake on fetal rabbit gastrointestinal development. *J Pediatr Surg,* **29**, 1030–1034.

33 American College of Obstetricians and Gynecologists Educational Bulletin Number 258. (2000). Breastfeeding: maternal and infant aspects. *Obstet Gynecol,* **96** (suppl.) 1–13.

34 Little RE, Anderson KW, Ervin CH, et al. (1989). Maternal alcohol use during breast-feeding and infant mental and motor development at one year. *N Engl J Med,* **321**, 425–430.

35 Graham JM, Hanson JW, Darby BL, et al. (1988). Independent dysmorphology evaluations at birth and 4 years of age for children exposed to varying amounts of alcohol in utero. *Pediatrics,* **81**, 772–778.

36 Streissguth AP. (1986). The behavioral teratology of alcohol: performance, behavioral, and intellectual deficits in prenatally exposed children. In: *Alcohol and Brain Development,* West JR (ed.), pp. 3–44. New York, NY: Oxford University Press.

37 Streissguth AP, Aase JM, Clarren SK, et al. (1991). Fetal alcohol syndrome in adolescents and adults. *JAMA,* **265**, 1961–1967.

38 Secker-Walker RH, Vacek PM, Flynn BS, et al. (1997). Smoking in pregnancy, exhaled carbon monoxide, and birth weight. *Obstet Gynecol,* **89**, 648–653.

39 Visnjevac V and Mikov M. (1986). Smoking and carboxyhemoglobin concentrations in mothers and their newborn infants. *Toxicology,* **5**, 175–177.

40 Jazayeri A, Tsibris JCM, Spellacy WN. (1998). Umbilical cord plasma erythropoietin levels in pregnancies complicated by maternal smoking. *Am J Obstet Gynecol,* **178**, 433–435.

41 Luck W and Nau H. (1984). Exposure of the fetus, neonate and nursed infant to nicotine and cotinine from maternal smoking. *N Engl J Med*, **311**, 672.
42 Etzel RA, Greenberg RA, Haley NJ, et al. (1985). Urine cotinine excretion in neonates exposed to tobacco smoke products in utero. *J Pediatr*, **107**, 146–148.
43 Jordanov JS. (1990). Cotinine concentrations in amniotic fluid and urine of smoking, passive smoking and non-smoking pregnant women at term and in the urine of their neonates on the 1st day of life. *Eur J Pediatr*, **149**, 734–737.
44 Bernstein IM, Plocienik K, Stahle S, et al. (2000). Impact of maternal cigarette smoking on fetal growth and body composition. *Am J Obstet Gynecol*, **183**, 883–886.
45 Bardy AH, Seppälä T, Lillsunde P, et al. (1993). Objectively measured tobacco exposure during pregnancy: neonatal effects and relation to maternal smoking. *Br J Obstet Gynaecol*, **100**, 721–726.
46 Cliver SP, Goldenberg RL, Cutter GR, et al. (1995). The effect of cigarette smoking on neonatal anthropometric measurements. *Obstet Gynecol*, **85**, 625–630.
47 Resnik R, Brink GW, Wilkes M. (1979). Catecholamine-mediated reduction in uterine blood flow after nicotine infusion in the pregnant ewe. *J Clin Invest*, **63**, 1133–1136.
48 Van der Velde WJ and Treffers PE. (1985). Smoking in pregnancy: the influence on percentile birthweight, mean birthweight, placental weight, menstrual age, perinatal mortality and maternal diastolic blood pressure. *Gynaecol Obstet Invest*, **19**, 57–63.
49 Burton GJ, Palmer ME, and Dalton KJ. (1989). Morphometric differences between the placental vasculature of non-smokers, smokers and ex-smokers. *Br J Obstet Gynecol*, **96**, 907–915.
50 Gabrial R, Alsat E, and Evain-Brion D. (1994). Alteration of epidermal growth factor receptor in placental membranes of smokers: relationship with intrauterine growth retardation. *Am J Obstet Gynecol*, **170**, 1238–1243.
51 Slotkin TA, McCook EC, Lappi SE, et al. (1992). Altered development of basal and forskolin-stimulated adenylate cyclase activity in brain regions of rats exposed to nicotine prenatally. *Dev Brain Res*, **68**, 233–239.
52 Shiono PH, Klebanoff MA, and Berendes HW. (1986). Congenital malformations and smoking during pregnancy. *Teratology*, **34**, 65–71.
53 Khoury MJ, Gomez-Frias M, and Mulinare J. (1989). Does maternal cigarette smoking during pregnancy cause cleft lip and palate in offspring? *Am J Dis Child*, **143**, 333–337.
54 Williams M, Mittendorf R, Lieberman E, et al. (1991). Cigarette smoking during pregnancy in relation to placenta previa. *Am J Obstet Gynecol*, **165**, 28–32.
55 Handler AS, Mason ED, Rosenberg DL, et al. (1994). The relationship between exposure during pregnancy to cigarette smoking and cocaine use and placenta previa. *Am J Obstet Gynecol*, **170**, 884–889.
56 Arbeille P, Bosc M, Vaillant MC, et al. (1992). Nicotine-induced changes in the cerebral circulation in ovine fetuses. *Am J Perinatol*, **79**, 645–648.
57 Franco P, Groswasser J, Hassid S, et al. (1999). Prenatal exposure to cigarette smoking is associated with a decrease in arousal in infants. *J Pediatr*, **135**, 34–38.
58 Kahn A, Groswasser J, Sottiaux M, et al. (1994). Prenatal exposure to cigarettes in infants with obstructive sleep apneas. *Pediatrics*, **93**, 778–783.
59 Hoffman HF, Damus K, Hillman L, et al. (1988). Risk factors for SIDS: results of the National Institute of Child Health and Human Development Cooperative Epidemiological Study. *Ann NY Acad Sci*, **533**, 13–30.
60 Mitchell EA, Ford RPK, Stewart AW, et al. (1993). Smoking and the sudden infant death syndrome. *Pediatrics*, **91**, 893–896.
61 Hoffman HJ and Hillman LS. (1992). Epidemiology of the sudden infant death syndrome: maternal, neonatal, and postneonatal risk factors. *Clin Perinatol*, **19**, 717–737.
62 Takashima S, Armstrong D, Becker LE, et al. (1978). Cerebral white matter lesions in sudden infant death syndrome. *Pediatrics*, **62**, 155–159.
63 Takashima S, Armstrong D, Becker LE, et al. (1978). Cerebral hypoperfusion in the sudden infant death syndrome, brainstem gliosis and vasculature. *Ann Neurol*, **4**, 257–262.
64 Drews CD, Murphy CC, Yeargin-Allsop M, et al. (1996). The relationship between idiopathic mental retardation and maternal smoking during pregnancy. *Pediatrics*, **97**, 547–553.
65 Olds DL, Henderson CR, Tatelbaum R. (1994). Intellectual impairment in children of women who smoke cigarettes during pregnancy. *Pediatrics*, **93**, 221–227.
66 Lichtensteiger W, Ribary U, Schlumpl M, et al. (1988). Prenatal adverse effects of nicotine on the developing brain. *Prog Brain Res*, **73**, 137–157.
67 John EM, Savitz DA, Sandler DP. (1991). Prenatal exposure to parents' smoking and childhood cancer. *Am J Epidemiol*, **133**, 123–132.
68 Stjernfeldt M, Berglund K, Lindsten J, et al. (1986). Maternal smoking during pregnancy and risk of childhood cancer. *Lancet*, **1**, 1350–1352.
69 Charlton A. (1994). Children and passive smoking: a review. *J Fam Pract*, **38**, 267–277.
70 Paulson RB, Shanfeld J, Prause L, et al. (1991). Pre- and

post-conceptional tobacco effects on the CD-1 mouse fetus. *J Craniofac Genet Dev Biol*, **11**, 48–57.
71 Paulson RB, Shanfeld J, Mullet D, et al. (1994). Prenatal smokeless tobacco effects on the rat fetus. *J Craniofac Genet Dev Biol*, **14**, 16–25.
72 Ostrea EM, Knapp DK, Romera A, et al. (1994). Meconium analysis to assess fetal exposure to nicotine by active and passive maternal smoking. *J Pediatr*, **124**, 471–476.
73 Makin J, Fried PA, and Watkinson B. (1991). A comparison of active and passive smoking during pregnancy: long-term effects. *Neurotoxicol Teratol*, **13**, 5–12.
74 Witschi H, Lundgaard SM, Rajini P, et al. (1994). Effects of exposure to nicotine and to sidestream smoke on pregnancy outcome in rats. *Toxicol Lett*, **71**, 279–286.
75 Davis DL. (1991). Paternal smoking and fetal health. *Lancet*, **337**, 123.
76 Klonoff-Cohen HS, Edelstein SL, Lefkowitz ES, et al. (1995). The effect of passive smoking and tobacco exposure through breast milk on sudden infant death syndrome. *JAMA*, **273**, 795–798.
77 Selden BS, Clark RF, and Curry SC. (1990). Marijuana. *Emerg Med Clin North Am*, **8**, 8527–8539.
78 Wu T-C, Tashkin DP, Djahed B, et al. (1988). Pulmonary hazards of smoking marijuana as compared with tobacco. *N Engl J Med*, **318**, 347–351.
79 Melges FT, Tinklenberg JR, Hollister LE, et al. (1970). Temporal disintegration and depersonalization during marijuana intoxication. *Arch Gen Psychiatry*, **23**, 204–210.
80 English DR, Hulse GK, Milne E, et al. (1997). Maternal cannabis use and birth weight: a meta-analysis. *Addiction*, **92**, 1553–1560.
81 Cornelius MD, Taylor PM, Geva D, et al. (1995). Prenatal tobacco and marijuana use among adolescents: effects on offspring gestational age, growth, and morphology. *Pediatrics*, **95**, 738–743.
82 Zuckerman B, Frank DA, Hingson R, et al. (1989). Effects of maternal marijuana and cocaine use on fetal growth. *N Engl J Med*, **320**, 762–768.
83 Fried PA, Watkinson B, and Gray R. (1999). Growth from birth to early adolescence in offspring prenatally exposed to cigarettes and marijuana. *Neurotoxicol Teratol*, **21**, 513–525.
84 Fried PA and Makin JE. (1987). Neonatal behavioral correlates of prenatal exposure to marijuana, cigarettes and alcohol in a low risk population. *Neurotoxicol Teratol*, **9**, 1–7.
85 Dahl RE, Scher MS, Williamson DE, et al. (1995). A longitudinal study of prenatal marijuana use. Effects on sleep and arousal at age 3 years. *Arch Pediatr Adolesc Med*, **149**, 145–150.
86 Fried PA. (1995). Prenatal exposure to marijuana and tobacco during infancy, early and middle childhood: effects and an attempt at synthesis. *Arch Toxicol Suppl*, **17**, 233–260.
87 Fried PA. (1995). The Ottawa Prenatal Prospective Study (OPPS): methodologic issues and findings – it's easy to throw the baby out with the bathwater. *Life Sci*, **56**, 2159–2168.
88 Coles CD, Platzman KA, Smith I, et al. (1992). Effects of cocaine, alcohol, and other drug use in pregnancy on neonatal growth and neurobehavioral status. *Neurotoxicol Teratol*, **14**, 22–33.
89 Dreher MC, Nugent K, and Hudgins R. (1994). Prenatal marijuana exposure and neonatal outcomes in Jamaica: an ethnographic study. *Pediatrics*, **93**, 254–260.
90 Schwartz RH. (1989). Passive inhalation of marijuana, phencyclidene, and freebase cocaine ('crack') by infants. *Am J Dis Child*, **143**, 644.
91 Farrar HC and Kearns GL. (1989). Cocaine: clinical pharmacology and toxicology. *J Pediatr*, **115**, 665–675.
92 Ellenhorn M and Barceloux D. (1988). *Medical Toxicology: Diagnosis and Treatment of Human Poisoning*, pp. 644–661. New York: Elsevier Science.
93 Bailey DN. (1997). Cocaine and cocaethylene binding to human placenta in vitro. *Am J Obstet Gynecol*, **177**, 527–531.
94 Gawin FH and Kleber HD. (1986). Abstinence symptomatology and psychiatric diagnosis in cocaine abusers. *Arch Gen Psychiatry*, **43**, 107–113.
95 Rosenak D, Diamont YZ, Yaffe H, et al. (1990). Cocaine: maternal use during pregnancy and its effect on the mother, the fetus, and the infant. *Obstet Gynecol Surv*, **45**, 3483–3459.
96 Jones KL. (1991). Developmental pathogenesis of defects associated with prenatal cocaine exposure: fetal vascular disruption. *Clin Perinatol*, **18**, 139–146.
97 Woods JR, Plessinger MA, Clark KE. (1987). Effects of cocaine on uterine blood flow and fetal oxygenation. *JAMA*, **257**, 957–961.
98 Arbeille P, Maulik D, Salihagic A, et al. (1997). Effect of long-term cocaine administration to pregnant ewes on fetal hemodynamics, oxygenation, and growth. *Obstet Gynecol*, **90**, 795–802.
99 Monga M, Chmielowiec S, Andres RL, et al. (1994). Cocaine alters placental production of thromboxane and prostacyclin. *Am J Obstet Gynecol*, **171**, 965–969.
100 Burkett G, Yasin SY, Palow D, et al. (1994). Patterns of cocaine binging: effect on pregnancy. *Am J Obstet Gynecol*, **171**, 372–379.

101 Dicke JM, Verges DK, and Polakoski KL. (1994). The effects of cocaine on neutral amino acid uptake by human placental basal membrane vesicles. *Am J Obstet Gynecol*, **171**, 485–491.

102 Viscarello RR, Ferguson DD, Nores J, et al. (1992). Limb–body wall complex associated with cocaine abuse: further evidence of cocaine's teratogenicity. *Obstet Gynecol*, **80**, 523–526.

103 Hoyme HE, Jones KL, Dixon SD, et al. (1990). Prenatal cocaine exposure and fetal vascular disruption. *Pediatrics*, **85**, 743–747.

104 Bingol N, Fuchs M, Diaz V, et al. (1987). Teratogenicity of cocaine in humans. *J Pediatr*, **110**, 93–96.

105 Dixon SD and Bejar R. (1988). Brain lesions in cocaine and methamphetamine exposed neonates. *Pediatr Res*, **23**, 405A.

106 Dominguez R, Vila-Coro AA, Slopis JM, et al. (1991). Brain and ocular abnormalities in infants with in utero exposure to cocaine and other street drugs. *Am J Dis Child*, **145**, 688–695.

107 Fisher JE, Potturi RB, Collins M, et al. (1994). Cocaine-induced embryonic cardiovascular disruption in mice. *Teratology*, **49**, 182–191.

108 Zimmerman EF, Potturi RB, Resnick E, et al. (1994). Role of oxygen free radicals in cocaine-induced vascular disruption in mice. *Teratology*, **49**, 192–201.

109 Chasnoff IJ, Burns WJ, Schnoll SH, et al. (1985). Cocaine use in pregnancy. *N Engl J Med*, **313**, 666–669.

110 Chasnoff IJ, Chisum GM, and Kaplan WE. (1988). Maternal cocaine use and genitourinary tract malformations. *Teratology*, **37**, 201–204.

111 Chavez GF, Mulinare J, and Cordero JF. (1989). Maternal cocaine use during early pregnancy as a risk factor for congenital urogenital anomalies. *JAMA*, **262**, 795–798.

112 Lezcano L, Antia DE, Sahdev S, et al. (1994). Crossed renal ectopia associated with maternal alkaloid cocaine abuse: a case report. *J Perinatol*, **14**, 230–233.

113 Kosofsky BE, Wilkins AS, Gressens P, et al. (1994). Transplacental cocaine exposure: a mouse model demonstrating neuroanatomic and behavioral abnormalities. *J Child Neurol*, **9**, 234–241.

114 Kain ZN, Kain TS, and Scarpelli EM. (1992). Cocaine exposure in utero: perinatal development and neonatal manifestations – review. *Clin Toxicol*, **30**, 607–636.

115 Bays J. (1991). Fetal vascular disruption with prenatal exposure to cocaine and methamphetamines. *Pediatrics*, **87**, 416–418.

116 Astley SJ, Clarren SK, Little RE, et al. (1992). Analysis of facial shape in children gestationally exposed to marijuana, alcohol, and/or cocaine. *Pediatrics*, **89**, 67–77.

117 Dinsmoor MJ, Irons SJ, and Christmas JT. (1994). Preterm rupture of the membranes associated with recent cocaine use. *Am J Obstet Gynecol*, **171**, 305–309.

118 Kliegman RM, Madura D, Kiwi R, et al. (1994). Relation of maternal cocaine use to the risks of prematurity and low birth weight. *J Pediatr*, **124**, 751–756.

119 Iriye BK, Bristow RE, Hsu CD, et al. (1994). Uterine rupture associated with recent antepartum cocaine abuse. *Obstet Gynecol*, **83**, 840–841.

120 Gonsoulin W, Borge D, and Moise KJ. (1990). Rupture of the unscarred uterus in primigravid woman in association with cocaine abuse. *Am J Obstet Gynecol*, **163**, 526–527.

121 Hsu CD, Chen S, Feng TI, et al. (1992). Rupture of uterine scar with extensive bladder laceration after cocaine abuse. *Am J Obstet Gynecol*, **197**, 129–130.

122 Macones GA, Sehdev HM, Parry S, et al. (1997). The association between maternal cocaine use and placenta previa. *Am J Obstet Gynecol*, **177**, 1097–1100.

123 Hurd WW, Gauvin JM, Dombrowski MP, et al. (1993). Cocaine selectively inhibits beta-adrenergic receptor binding in pregnant human myometrium. *Am J Obstet Gynecol*, **169**, 644–649.

124 Smith YR, Dombrowski MP, Leach KC, et al. (1995). Decrease in myometrial beta-adrenergic receptors with prenatal cocaine use. *Obstet Gynecol*, **85**, 357–360.

125 Telsey AM, Merrit TA, and Dixon SD. (1988). Cocaine exposure in a term neonate: necrotizing enterocolitis as a complication. *Clin Pediatr*, **27**, 547–550.

126 Czyrko C, Del Pin CA, O'Neill JA, et al. (1991). Maternal cocaine abuse and necrotizing enterocolitis: outcome and survival. *J Pediatr Surg*, **26**, 414–418.

127 Büyükünal C, Kiliç N, Dervisoglu S, et al. (1994). Maternal cocaine abuse resulting in necrotizing enterocolitis – an experimental study in a rat model. *Acta Paediatr, Suppl*, **396**, 91–93.

128 Chasnoff IJ, Bussey ME, Savich R, et al. (1986). Perinatal cerebral infarction and maternal cocaine use. *J Pediatr*, **108**, 456–459.

129 Tenorio GM, Nazvi M, Bickers GH, et al. (1988). Intrauterine stroke and maternal polydrug abuse. *Clin Pediatr*, **27**, 565–567.

130 Singer LT, Yamashita TS, Hawkins S, et al. (1994). Increased incidence of intraventricular hemorrhage and developmental delay in cocaine-exposed, very low birth weight infants. *J Pediatr*, **124**, 765–771.

131 van de Bor M, Walther FJ, Sims ME. (1990). Increased cerebral blood flow velocity in infants of mothers who abuse cocaine. *Pediatrics*, **85**, 733–736.

132 Sims ME and Walther FJ. (1989). Antenatal brain injury and maternal cocaine use. *J Perinatol*, **9**, 349–350.

133 Behnke M, Eyler FD, Conlon M, et al. (1998). Incidence and description of structural brain abnormalities in newborns exposed to cocaine. *J Pediatr*, **132**, 291–294.

134 Mott SH, Packer RJ, Soldin SJ. (1994). Neurologic manifestations of cocaine exposure in childhood. *Pediatrics*, **93**, 557–560.

135 Chasnoff IJ, Hunt CE, Kletter R, et al. (1989). Prenatal cocaine exposure is associated with respiratory pattern abnormalities. *Am J Dis Child*, **143**, 583–587.

136 Chen C, Duara S, Neto GS, et al. (1991). Respiratory instability in neonates with in utero exposure to cocaine. *J Pediatr*, **119**, 111–113.

137 Tronick EZ, Frank DA, Cabral H, et al. (1996). Late dose–response effects of prenatal cocaine exposure on newborn neurobehavioral performance. *Pediatrics*, **98**, 76–83.

138 Chan K, Dodd PA, Day L, et al. (1992). Fetal catecholamine, cardiovascular, and neurobehavioral responses to cocaine. *Am J Obstet Gynecol*, **167**, 1616–1623.

139 Knapp S and Mandell AJ. (1972). Narcotic drugs: effect on the serotonin biosynthetic systems of the brain. *Science*, **177**, 1209–1211.

140 Durand DJ, Espinoza AM, and Nickerson BG. (1990). Association between prenatal cocaine exposure and sudden infant death syndrome. *J Pediatr*, **117**, 909–911.

141 Bauchner H, Zuckerman B, McClain M, et al. (1988). Risk of sudden infant death syndrome among infants with in utero exposure to cocaine. *J Pediatr*, **113**, 831–834.

142 Bauchner H and Zuckerman B. (1990). Cocaine, sudden infant death syndrome, and home monitoring. *J Pediatr*, **117**, 904–906.

143 Freier MC, Griffith DR, Chasnoff IJ. (1991). In utero drug exposure: developmental followup and maternal–infant interaction. *Semin Perinatol*, **15**, 310–316.

144 Mayes LC, Granger RH, Frank MA, et al. (1993). Neurobehavioral profiles of neonates exposed to cocaine prenatally. *Pediatrics*, **91**, 778–783.

145 Eisen LN, Field TM, Bandstra ES, et al. (1991). Perinatal cocaine effects on neonatal stress behavior and performance on the Brazelton scale. *Pediatrics*, **88**, 477–480.

146 Eyler FD, Behnke M, Conlon M, et al. (1998). Birth outcome from a prospective, matched study of prenatal crack/cocaine use: I. Interactive and dose effects on health and growth. *Pediatrics*, **101**, 229–237.

147 Eyler FD, Behnke M, Conlon M, et al. (1998). Birth outcome from a prospective, matched study of prenatal crack/cocaine use: II. Interactive and dose effects on neurobehavioral assessment. *Pediatrics*, **101**, 237–241.

148 Delaney-Black V, Covington C, Ostrea E, et al. (1996). Prenatal cocaine and neonatal outcome: evaluation of dose–response relationship. *Pediatrics*, **98**, 735–740.

149 Chasnoff IJ, Griffith DR, Freier C, et al. (1992). Cocaine/polydrug use in pregnancy: two-year follow-up. *Pediatrics*, **89**, 284–289.

150 Scafadi FA, Field TM, Wheedon A, et al. (1996). Cocaine-exposed preterm neonates show behavioral and hormonal differences. *Pediatrics*, **97**, 851–855.

151 Mirochnick M, Meyer J, Cole J, et al. (1991). Circulating catecholamine concentrations in cocaine-exposed neonates: a pilot study. *Pediatrics*, **88**, 481–485.

152 Ward S, Schuetz S, Wachsman L, et al. (1991). Elevated plasma norepinephrine levels in infants of substance-abusing mothers. *Am J Dis Child*, **145**, 44–48.

153 Needlman R, Zuckerman BS, Anderson G, et al. (1993). CSF monoamine precursors and metabolites in human neonates following in utero cocaine exposure. *Pediatrics*, **92**, 55–60.

154 Frank DA, Augustyn M, Knight WG, et al. (2001). Growth, development, and behavior in early childhood following prenatal cocaine exposure: a systematic review. *JAMA*, **285**, 1613–1625.

155 Wennberg RP, Yin J, Miller M, et al. (1994). Fetal cocaine exposure and neonatal bilirubinemia. *J Pediatr*, **125**, 613–616.

156 Roland EH and Volpe JJ. (1989). Effect of maternal cocaine use on the fetus and newborn: review of the literature. *Pediatr Neurosci*, **15**, 88–94.

157 Oro A and Dixon S. (1987). Perinatal cocaine and methamphetamine exposure: maternal and neonatal correlates. *J Pediatr*, **111**, 571–578.

158 Chasnoff IJ, Lewis DE, and Squires L. (1987). Cocaine intoxication in a breast-fed infant. *Pediatrics*, **80**, 836–838.

159 Chaney NE, Franke J, and Waddington WB. (1988). Cocaine convulsions in a breast-feeding baby. *J Pediatr*, **112**, 134–135.

160 Bateman DA and Heagarty MC. (1989). Passive free-base cocaine ("crack") inhalation by infants and toddlers. *Am J Dis Child*, **143**, 25–27.

161 Ford M, Hoffman RS, and Goldfrank LR. (1990). Opioids and designer drugs. *Emerg Clin North Am*, **8**, 495–511.

162 Rius RA, Barg J, Bem WT, et al. (1991). The prenatal developmental profile of expression of opioid peptides and receptors in the mouse brain. *Dev Brain Res*, **58**, 237–241.

163 Barg J, Rius A, Bem WT, et al. (1992). Differential development of β-endorphin and μ opioid binding sites in mouse brain. *Dev Brain Res*, **66**, 71–76.

164 Barg J and Simantov R. (1991). Transient expression of opioid receptors in defined regions of developing brain: are

embryonic receptors selective? *J Neurochem*, **57**, 1978–1984.
165 Suguihara C and Bancalari E. (1991). Substance abuse during pregnancy: effects on respiratory function in the infant. *Semin Perinatol*, **15**, 302–309.
166 Olson GD and Lees MH. (1980). Ventilatory response to carbon dioxide of infants following chronic prenatal methadone exposure. *J Pediatr*, **96**, 983–989.
167 Bunikowski R, Grimmer I, Heiser A, et al. (1998). Neurodevelopmental outcome after prenatal exposure to opiates. *Eur J Pediatr*, **157**, 724–730.
168 Smialek JE, Monforte JR, Aronow R, et al. (1977). Methadone deaths in children – a continuing problem. *JAMA*, **238**, 2516–2517.
169 Committee on Drugs, American Academy of Pediatrics. (1989). Transfer of drugs and other chemicals into human milk. *Pediatrics*, **84**, 924–936.
170 Haefely W. (1984). Benzodiazepine interactions with GABA-receptors. *Neurosci Lett*, **47**, 201–206.
171 Idänpäan-Heikkilä JE, Jouppila PI, Puolakka JO, et al. (1971). Placental transfer and fetal metabolism of diazepam in early pregnancy. *Am J Obstet Gynecol*, **109**, 1011–1016.
172 Laegreid L, Olegärd R, Walström J, et al. (1989). Teratogenic effects of benzodiazepine use during pregnancy. *J Pediatr*, **114**, 126–131.
173 Aarskog D. (1975). Associations between maternal intake of diazepam and oral clefts. *Lancet*, **2**, 921.
174 Saxen I. (1975). Associations between oral clefts and drugs taken during pregnancy. *Int J Epidemiol*, **4**, 37–44.
175 Safra MJ and Oakley GP. (1975). Association between cleft lip with or without cleft palate and prenatal exposure to diazepam. *Lancet*, **2**, 478–481.
176 Dessens AB, Cohen-Kettenis PT, Mellenbergh GJ, et al. (2000). Association of prenatal phenobarbital and phenytoin exposure with small head size at birth and with learning problems. *Acta Paediatr*, **89**, 533–541.
177 Reinisch JM, Sanders SA, Mortensen EL, et al. (1995). In utero exposure to phenobarbital and intelligence deficits in adult men. *JAMA*, **274**, 1518–1525.
178 Rementeria JL and Bhatt K. (1977). Withdrawal symptoms in neonates from intrauterine exposure to diazepam. *J Pediatr*, **90**, 123–126.
179 Aaron CK. (1990). Sympathomimetics. *Emerg Med Clin North Am*, **8**, 513–526.
180 Delaney P and Estes M. (1980). Intracranial hemorrhage with amphetamine abuse. *Neurology*, **30**, 1125–1128.
181 Rothrock JF, Rubenstein B, Lyden PD. (1988). Ischemic stroke associated with methamphetamine inhalation. *Neurology*, **38**, 589–592.
182 Harrington H, Heller HA, Dawson D, et al. (1983). Intracerebral hemorrhage and oral amphetamine. *Arch Neurol*, **40**, 503–507.
183 Battaglia G, Yeh SY, deSouza EB. (1988). MDMA-induced neurotoxicity: parameters of degeneration and recovery of brain serotonin neurons. *Pharmacol Biochem Behav*, **29**, 269–274.
184 Pan ZZ and Williams JT. (1989). Differential actions of cocaine and amphetamine on dorsal raphe neurons in vitro. *J Pharmacol Exp Ther*, **251**, 56–62.
185 Stek AM, Baker RS, Fisher BK, et al. (1995). Fetal responses to maternal and fetal methamphetamine administration in sheep. *Am J Obstet Gynecol*, **173**, 1592–1598.
186 Little BB, Snell LM, and Gilstrap LC. (1988). Methamphetamine abuse during pregnancy: outcome and fetal effects. *Obstet Gynecol*, **72**, 541–544.
187 Ramin SM, Little BB, Trimmer KJ, et al. (1994). Peripartum methamphetamine use in a large urban population. *J Maternal–Fetal Med*, **3**, 101–103.
188 St. Omer VE, Ali SF, Holson RR, et al. (1991). Behavioral and neurochemical effects of prenatal methylenedioxymethamphetamine (MDMA) exposure in rats. *Neurotoxicol Teratol*, **13**, 13–20.
189 Nasif FJ, Cuadra GR, and Ramirez OA. (1999). Permanent alteration of cerebral noradrenergic system by prenatally administered amphetamine. *Brain Res Dev Brain Res*, **112**, 181–188.
190 Tavares MA and Silva MC. (1996). Differential effects of prenatal exposure to cocaine and amphetamine on growth parameters and morphometry of the prefrontal cortex in the rat. *Ann N Y Acad Sci*, **801**, 256–273.
191 Tavares MA, Silva MC, Silva-Araujo A, et al. (1996). Effects of prenatal exposure to amphetamine in the medial prefrontal cortex of the rat. *Int J Dev Neurosci*, **14**, 585–596.
192 Acuff-Smith KD, Schilling MA, Fisher JE, et al. (1996). Stage-specific effects of prenatal *d*-methamphetamine exposure on behavioral and eye development in rats. *Neurotoxicol Teratol*, **18**, 199–215.
193 Weissman AD and Caldecott-Hazard S. (1995). Developmental neurotoxicity to methamphetamines. *Clin Exp Pharmacol Physiol*, **22**, 372–374.
194 Dixon SD and Bejar R. (1989). Echoencephalographic findings in neonates associated with maternal cocaine and methamphetamine use: incidence and clinical correlates. *J Pediatr*, **115**, 770–778.
195 Ericksson M, Larsson C, Windblath B, et al. (1978). The influence of amphetamine addiction on pregnancy and the newborn infant. *Acta Paediatr Scand*, **67**, 95–99.
196 Ericksson M, Larsson C, and Zetterström R. (1981).

Amphetamine addiction and pregnancy. *Acta Obstet Gynecol Scand*, **60**, 253–259.
197 Oro AS and Dixon SP. (1987). Perinatal cocaine and methamphetamine exposure: maternal and neonatal correlates. *J Pediatr*, **111**, 571–578.
198 Baldridge EB and Bessen HA. (1990). Phencyclidine. *Emerg Med Clin North Am*, **8**, 541–550.
199 McCarron MM, Schulze BW, Thompson GA, et al. (1981). Acute phencyclidene intoxication: incidence of clinical findings in 1000 cases. *Ann Emerg Med*, **10**, 237–242.
200 Armen R, Kanel G, and Reynolds T. (1984). Phencyclidene-induced malignant hyperthermia causing submassive liver necrosis. *Am J Med*, **77**, 167–172.
201 Bessen HA. (1982). Intracranial hemorrhage associated with phencyclidene abuse. *JAMA*, **248**, 585–586.
202 Patel R and Connor G. (1985–6). A review of thirty cases of rhabdomyolysis-associated acute renal failure among phencyclidene users. *Clin Toxicol*, **23**, 547–556.
203 Strauss AA, Modanlou HD, and Bosu SK. (1981). Neonatal manifestations of maternal phencyclidene (PCP) abuse. *Pediatrics*, **68**, 550–552.
204 Golden NL, Sokol RJ, and Rubin IL. (1980). Angel dust: possible effects on the fetus. *Pediatrics*, **65**, 18–20.
205 Mattson MP, Rychlik B, and Cheng B. (1992). Degenerative and axon outgrowth-altering effects of phencyclidine in human fetal cerebral cortical cells. *J Pharmacol*, **31**, 279–291.
206 Wachsman L, Schuetz S, Chan LS, et al. (1989). What happens to babies exposed to phencyclidene (PCP) in utero? *Am J Drug Alcohol Abuse*, **15**, 31–39.
207 Golden NL, Kuhnert BR, Sokol RJ, et al. (1987). Neonatal manifestations of maternal phencyclidene exposure. *J Perinat Med*, **15**, 185–191.
208 Chasnoff IJ, Burns WJ, Hatcher RP, et al. (1983). Phencyclidene: effects on the fetus and neonate. *Dev Pharmacol Ther*, **6**, 404–408.
209 Rahbar F, Fomufod A, White D, et al. (1993). Impact of intrauterine exposure to phencyclidene (PCP) and cocaine on neonates. *J Natl Med Assoc*, **85**, 349–352.
210 Kaufman KR, Petrucha RA, Pitts FN, et al. (1983). PCP in amniotic fluid and breast milk: case report. *J Clin Psychiatry*, **44**, 269–270.
211 Strassman RJ. (1984). Adverse reactions to psychadelic drugs – a review of the literature. *J Nerv Ment Dis*, **172**, 577–592.
212 DaPrada M, Saner A, Burkard WP, et al. (1975). Lysergic acid diethylamide: evidence for stimulation of cerebral dopamine receptors. *Brain Res*, **94**, 67–73.
213 Eller JL and Morton JA. (1970). Bizarre deformities in offspring of users of lysergic acid diethylamide. *N Engl J Med*, **283**, 395–397.
214 Pilapil V, Harp R, Ehrhardt O. (1973). LSD and cyanotic congenital heart disease. *J Am Med Women's Assoc*, **28**, 131–132.
215 Hecht F, Beals RK, Lees MH, et al. (1968). Lysergic-acid-diethylamide and cannabis as possible teratogens in man. *Lancet*, **2**, 1087.
216 Carakushansky G, Neu RL, and Gardner LI. (1969). Lysergide and cannabis as possible teratogens in man. *Lancet*, **1**, 150–151.
217 Bogdanoff B, Rorke LV, Yanoff M, et al. (1972). Brain and eye abnormalities: possible sequelae to prenatal use of multiple drugs including LSD. *Am J Dis Child*, **123**, 145–148.
218 Jacobson CB and Berlin CM. (1972). Possible reproductive detriments in LSD users. *JAMA*, **222**, 1367–1373.
219 Geleherter D. (1970). Lysergic acid diethylamide (LSD) and exstrophy of the bladder. *J Pediatr*, **77**, 1065–1066.
220 Linden CH. (1990). Volatile substances of abuse. *Emerg Med Clin North Am*, **8**, 559–578.
221 Jones HE and Balster RL. (1998). Inhalant abuse in pregnancy. *Obstet Gynecol Clin North Am*, **25**, 153–167.
222 Ghantous H and Danielsson BRG. (1986). Placental transfer and distribution of toluene, xylene, and benzene and their metabolites during gestation in mice. *Biol Res Pregnancy*, **7**, 98–105.
223 Goodwin TH. (1988). Toluene abuse and renal tubular acidosis in pregnancy. *Obstet Gynecol*, **71**, 715–718.
224 da Silva VA and Malheiros LR. (1990). Developmental toxicity of in utero exposure to toluene on malnourished and well nourished rats. *Toxicology*, **64**, 155–168.
225 Stoltenbeurg-Didinger G, Altenkirch H, and Wagner M. (1990). Neurotoxicity of organic solvent mixtures: embryotoxicity and fetotoxicity. *Neurotoxicol Teratol*, **12**, 585–589.
226 Kostas J and Hotchin J. (1981). Behavioral effects of low-level perinatal exposure to toluene in mice. *Neurobehav Toxicol Teratol*, **3**, 467–469.
227 Gospe SM and Zhou SS. (2000). Prenatal exposure to toluene results in abnormal neurogenesis and migration in rat somatosensory cortex. *Pediatr Res*, **47**, 362–368.
228 Hougaard KS, Hass U, Lund SP, et al. (1999). Effects of prenatal exposure to toluene on postnatal development and behavior in rats. *Neurotoxicol Teratol*, **21**, 241–250.
229 Gospe SM and Zhou SS. (1998). Toluene abuse embryopathy: longitudinal neurodevelopmental effects of prenatal exposure to toluene in rats. *Reprod Toxicol*, **12**, 119–126.
230 Gospe SM, Zhou SS, Saeed DB, et al. (1996). Development of a rat model of toluene-abuse embryopathy. *Pediatr Res*, **40**, 82–87.

231 Toutant C and Lippman S. (1979). Fetal solvents syndrome. *Lancet*, **1**, 1356.

232 Pearson MA, Hoyme HE, Seaver LH, et al. (1994). Toluene embryopathy: delineation of the phenotype and comparison with fetal alcohol syndrome. *Pediatrics*, **93**, 211–215.

233 Arnold GL, Kirby RS, Langendoerfer S, et al. (1994). Toluene embryopathy: clinical delineation and developmental followup. *Pediatrics*, **93**, 216–220.

234 Schauben JL. (1990). Adulterants and substitutes. *Emerg Med Clin North Am*, **8**, 595–611.

235 Joffe GM and Kasnic T. (1994). Medical prescription of dextroamphetamine during pregnancy. *J Perinatol*, **14**, 301–303.

236 Schutzman DL, Frankenfield-Chernicoff M, Clatterbaugh HE, et al. (1991). Incidence of intrauterine cocaine exposure in a suburban setting. *Pediatrics*, **88**, 825–827.

237 Chasnoff IJ, Landres HJ, and Barrett ME. (1990). The prevalence of illicit-drug or alcohol use during pregnancy and discrepancies in mandatory reporting in Pinellas County, Florida. *N Engl J Med*, **322**, 1202–1206.

238 Farrar HC and Kearns GL. (1989). Cocaine: clinical pharmacology and toxicology. *J Pediatr*, **115**, 665–675.

239 Ryan RM, Wagner CL, Schultz JM, et al. (1994). Meconium analysis for improved identification of infants exposed to cocaine in utero. *J Pediatr*, **125**, 435–440.

240 Saitoh M, Uzuka M, and Sakamoto M. (1969). Rate of hair growth. *Adv Biol Skin*, **9**, 183–201.

241 Baumgartner WA, Hill VA, and Bland WH. (1989). Hair analysis for drug abuse. *J Forensic Sci*, **34**, 1433–1453.

242 Marques PR, Tippetts AS, and Branch DG. (1993). Cocaine in the hair of mother–infant pairs: quantitative analysis and correlations with urine measurements and self report. *Am J Drug Alcohol Abuse*, **19**, 159–175.

14

Chorioamnionitis and its possible relation to subsequent cerebral palsy

Boaz Weisz and Daniel S. Seidman

Department of Obstetrics and Gynecology, Sheba Medical Center, Tel-Hashomer, and Sackler Faculty of Medicine, Tel-Aviv University, Israel

Clinical chorioamnionitis is a primary infection that involves the chorioamniotic membranes and the intraamniotic cavity.[1] Microscopically, clinical chorioamnionitis is defined by bacteria and leukocytes that are found between the chorion and the amnion, and by isolation of bacteria from the amniotic fluid. Other terms used in the literature are intraamniotic infection, amnionitis, amniotic fluid infection, intrauterine infection, and intrapartum infection.[2] However, clinical chorioamnionitis is distinct from histological chorioamnionitis, which is defined by the infiltration of polymorphonuclear cells into the placenta and choriamniotic membranes.[3]

Clinical manifestations

The clinical manifestations of chorioamnionitis include fever, maternal and fetal tachycardia, uterine tenderness, foul odor of the amniotic fluid, and leukocytosis. Although a combination of these signs may be present in most women with chorioamnionitis, they are by no means universal. Recent studies are usually based on the clinical criteria defined by Gibbs and Duff[3,4] which include maternal fever of 37.8°C or greater as a mandatory sign, plus two or more minor signs (maternal tachycardia >100 beats/min, fetal tachycardia >160 beats/min, uterine tenderness, foul odor of the amniotic fluid and leukocytosis >15 000/mm^3).

Fever accompanies virtually all cases of clinical chorioamnionitis. The criteria that define maternal and fetal tachycardia exceed the 90th percentile and are discovered in a wide range (20–80%) of patients with intraamniotic infection. Leukocytosis can be a normal finding in women during labor without obvious signs of infection. The mean intrapartum white blood cell count is 12 500 ± 3900/mm^3 and increases in linear fashion with an extending duration of labor.[5] Leukocytosis greater than 15 000/mm^3 is seen in 63% of cases of intraamniotic infection vs 21% of matched controls.[6] Leukocyte counts greater than 20 000/mm^3 (which is above the 95th percentile for asymptomatic women) should be considered abnormal and infection must be searched for and excluded.

Laboratory investigation

Several other laboratory studies are associated with chorioamnionitis. C-reactive protein (CRP) is an acute-phase reactant that increases in conjunction with various inflammatory states.[7] It has been suggested that an elevated CRP in women with premature ruptured membranes might be indicative of intraamniotic infection. However, due to high false-positive and false-negative results,[8] this test adds little to the clinical diagnosis of chorioamnionitis. Other laboratory tests require the aspiration of amniotic fluids for the assay of markers of intraamniotic infection. These include Gram stain and measurement of leukocyte esterase activity, glucose,

Table 14.1. Clinical and laboratory studies suggestive of chorioamnionitis

	Test	Pathologic values
Maternal blood	Body temperature	>37.8
	Leukocytosis	>15000 mm^3
	C-reactive protein	>2 mg/dl
	Interleukin-8	
Amniotic fluid	Leukocyte esterase	Positive
	Interleukin-1	
	Interleukin-6	
	Glucose concentration	<15 mg/dl
	Gram staining	Positive
	Culture	Positive

various cytokines, ceramide lactoside, and fetal fibronectin. Many of these tests require special equipment; however, Gram stain, glucose, and leukocyte esterase activity assays are performed easily in most laboratories. Gram stain and culture of amniotic fluid are of value in confirming the diagnosis of chorioamnionitis and will be discussed later.

The assay of leukocyte esterase activity identifies the esterase enzyme (found in polymorphonuclear cells) in the amniotic fluid. This assay is easily measured and provides sensitivity, specificity, and positive and negative predicted values of 91–95%.[9] The presence of more than six leukocytes (on 20 high-powered field (HPF) microscopic examination) in a clean aspirate is abnormal. A relatively simple assay is the measurement of glucose level in the amniotic fluid. Positive cultures are associated with decreased glucose levels and any level less than 15 mg/dl is highly suggestive of intraamniotic infection[2] (Table 14.1).

Ultrasonographic imaging

An ultrasound scan can be used to support the diagnosis of infection in patients with ruptured membranes. Some reports have shown a correlation between low biophysical profile (BPP) score and the risk of infection.[10,11] A nonreassuring (<7/10) BPP score performed within 24 h before labor was initiated was associated with a >90% incidence of infection. However, others have reported little correlation between fetal activity and the risk of infection.[12,13] Low amniotic fluid volumes (after rupture of membranes) defined either as a pocket less than 1 × 1 cm[14,15] or an amniotic fluid index (AFI) <5 cm[16] were also related to increased risk of chorioamnionitis (perhaps as a result of decreased urine production in the inflammatory states).

Incidence

The incidence of chorioamnionitis varies widely among centers. In previous retrospective studies the overall incidence varied from 0.5 to 2%.[17–20] However, two recent prospective studies reported a substantially higher incidence of 4% and 10.5%.[21,22] This variation might be a methodology-based variation (i.e., improved diagnosis of chorioamnionitis in prospective studies); however, it might also represent a true increased rate of intraamniotic infection due to changes in obstetric practice (such as conservative management of preterm premature rupture of membranes (PPROM) and increased use of invasive techniques during labor). Other factors are associated with increased risk for chorioamnionitis, including women younger than 21 years, nulliparity, women of lower socioeconomic class, nutritional disorders (obesity and starvation), drug abuse, chronic disease such as diabetes, autoimmune disorders, and infection with human immunodeficiency virus and drugs (e.g., steroids, cancer chemotherapy). Preterm labor at 36 weeks or less is the most significant predictor of intrapartum fever (odds ratio 9.1; range 7.5–13.7).[23] Independent predictors of PPROM (which might lead to intrapartum fever) include antepartum bleeding and previous preterm delivery. Chorioamnionitis in a previous pregnancy does not increase the risk of subsequent intraamniotic infection.[24]

The histologic appearance of chorioamnionitis includes an initial inflammatory and exudative reaction that involves the chorionic plate with progressive spread to the amnion, decidua, and the amniotic fluid.[17] Most cases of chorioamnionitis are the result of ascending infection caused by cervicovaginal pathogens after rupture of membranes. The incidence of intraamniotic infection correlates negatively with gestational age at rupture of membranes. While the rate of clinical chorioamnionitis is 0.5–2% at term PROM, this rate increases to approximately 15% at 32 weeks and 40% at 24 weeks.[2] Interestingly, histological chorioamnionitis is also less common with increasing gestational age.[25] When membranes rupture, the risk of clinical chorioamnionitis increases with more intensive obstetric manipulations, including repeated vaginal exams and prolonged use of internal monitoring during labor.[21]

Microbiologic pathogens

Another mechanism for the development of chorioamnionitis is introduction of bacteria during an invasive procedure. The risk of intraamniotic infection is specific for each procedure. While the risk of infection after diagnostic amniocentesis is low (about 0.1%), this risk increases to approximately 5% after invasive procedures such as intrauterine infusions.[26] Other procedures that do not involve the amniotic cavity might cause infection as well. The placement of a cervical cerclage, for example, is associated with a risk of about 1% for chorioamnionitis. This risk increases significantly to approximately 25% when the procedure is performed after cervical dilatation and prolapsed membranes.[27] In rare cases of maternal bacteremia (*Listeria monocytogenes*, *Streptococcus* group A, or *Campylobacter* species) hematogenous spread was reported to cause intraamniotic infection.[28,29]

The microbiologic composition of amniotic fluid in patients with intraamniotic infection consists primarily of pathogens that are indigenous to the lower genital tract. Women with clinical chorioamnionitis are more likely to have greater than 100 colony-forming units (71%) when compared to matched controls with ruptured membranes, but without signs of infection (8%).[6] The predominant organisms in cases of intraamniotic infection are *Ureaplasma urealyticum* (47%), *Mycoplasma hominis* (31%), *Bacteroides bivius* (29%), and *Gardnerella vaginalis* (24%). Interestingly, the rate of *U. urealyticum* is the same as in patients without signs of infection. Group B streptococci and *Escherichia coli* were found in 15% and 8% of patients, respectively.[30] Since the bacteriologic composition of the amniotic fluid was polymicrobial, interesting associations were found. Anaerobes *G. vaginalis* and associations of *M. hominis* and anaerobes appeared to interact with each other.[31] These associations of pathogens might suggest that the organisms arise concurrently from bacterial vaginosis rather than independently from the vagina, but there is also a causal relationship between bacterial vaginosis and clinical chorioamnionitis. Other studies have also shown that bacterial vaginosis is significantly related to both clinical and histological chorioamnionitis.[32] Some studies have demonstrated that pregnant women with bacterial vaginosis have an attenuated rate of both preterm deliveries and postpartum endometritis after appropriate antimicrobial therapy.[33] However, others have shown no benefit in treating women with bacterial vaginosis.[34] In addition, common combinations of organisms found in clinical chorioamnionitis include gut-related pathogens such as *E. coli* and aerobic Gram-negative rods.

Although group B streptococcus and *E. coli* are present in the amniotic fluid of only 20% of the patients, they account for about two-thirds of either maternal or neonatal bacteremia and sepsis. Intraamniotic infection with *E. coli* is associated with an 18% risk for neonatal sepsis and a 15% risk for maternal sepsis. Infection with group B streptococci is associated with a 7% risk for neonatal sepsis and a 18% risk for maternal sepsis.[30,31] Other organisms that can cause either maternal or neonatal bacteremia include: *Staphylococcus aureus*, *L. monocytogenes*, *Bacteroides* spp., enterococci, *Pseudomonas aeruginosa*, and *Streptococcus pneumoniae*. Interestingly, no cases of neonatal bacteremia were associated with anaerobic organisms; however, this might be related to culture methodology.

Several studies have described intraamniotic infection in cases complicated by preterm labor with intact membranes. The prevalence of positive amniotic cultures (obtained by amniocentesis) has varied from 0% to 25.8%; however, only about one-eighth of these women had signs of clinical chorioamnionitis.[35] The disparity among different studies is probably attributed to population characteristics, the criteria used for diagnosis of preterm labor, the threshold required for performing amniocentesis, and different techniques of microbiologic isolation. The rate of positive cultures in women proceeding to preterm delivery approximates 20%. A similar rate of histological chorioamnionitis was observed in the pathologic examination of placenta from women delivering preterm infants without PPROM.[36] These observations indicate that almost one-fifth of preterm deliveries with intact membranes are associated with subclinical intraamniotic infection.

Adverse maternal outcome

Previously, chorioamnionitis was a major cause of severe maternal morbidity and mortality. Pregnant women with clinical infection, who were not treated early in their course, had complications such as septic shock, adult respiratory distress syndrome, and coagulopathy and had high rates of mortality. Currently, with immediate availability of intensive medical care and appropriate usage of antibiotics, the prospects of survival without complications are greatly increased.

Clinical chorioamnionitis is associated with labor abnormalities such as dystocia, need for oxytocin augmentation, and increased rates of cesarean section (26–43%).[18,37] Interestingly, the oxytocin initiation to delivery interval is shorter when delivery begins with signs of infection (compared to uninfected controls), while the same interval tends to be significantly longer when signs of infection appear after the initiation of oxytocin.[38] Moreover, patients with positive cultures but without clinical signs of infection required higher doses of oxytocin for augmentation of labor.[39] Women with clinical infection which began after initiation of augmentation had a higher rate of cesarean sections compared to controls (40% vs 10%). Other studies have shown that infections with high-virulence organisms are associated with slower progress of labor despite a maximal dose of oxytocin augmentation.[3] Women with chorioamnionitis are also prone to a greater risk of surgical complications, including longer duration of surgery, increased incidence of blood loss, and wound infection.[4]

Adverse fetal outcome

Chorioamnionitis is associated with adverse fetal outcome in both term and preterm infants. The incidence of neonatal infection after rupture of membranes for greater than 24 h is about 1–3%.[40–42] This risk rises to about 3–16% when signs of clinical chorioamnionitis are present.[40,41] In a multivariate analysis, clinical chorioamnionitis was highly predictive of neonatal infection (odds ratio (OR) 5.89). Other independent predictors were positive group B streptococcal status (OR 3.08), multiple digital examinations, and time elapsed from membrane rupture to active labor.[40]

The major complications in term infants born from an infected environment are sepsis, meningitis, pneumonia, and respiratory distress, which might be an early sign of development of severe pneumonia. The incidence of culture-proved sepsis is about six times greater in infants born of women with chorioamnionitis.[43] The incidence of pneumonia in full-term neonates whose mothers had chorioamnionitis varies between 1.9 and 23%.[19,43] There are several other significant risk factors (such as prolonged second stage, prolonged labor, oxytocin use, and postterm pregnancies) that are related to chorioamnionitis and might be associated with adverse outcome. However, even after adjustment by multivariate analysis, chorioamnionitis is significantly associated with pneumonia, sepsis, and the need for intubation in full-term neonates.[43]

Preterm neonates are prone to higher rates of complications if born to mothers infected with chorioamnionitis. About 4–25% of preterm deliveries with intact membrane have positive amniotic cultures.[35,44,45] These pregnancies are associated with a worse neonatal outcome, including a sixfold ratio of infectious morbidity, a twofold ratio of respiratory distress syndrome, and low Apgar scores at both 1 and 5 min postdelivery.[35] However, since positive amniotic cultures are also related to a significantly lower gestational age at delivery, most of the afore-mentioned adverse outcomes might be related to prematurity and not to the infectious status. Chorioamnionitis after rupture of membranes in preterm infants is associated with a two- to fourfold increased rate of mortality, sepsis, respiratory distress syndrome, and intraventricular hemorrhage, as compared to noninfected preterm infants with PROM, but without signs of chorioamnionitis.[37,46] Infants weighing less than 2500 g at birth are more prone to chorioamnionitis-related sequelae when compared to newborns whose birth weight exceeds 2500 g.[30] Interestingly, Gram-negative anaerobes were more commonly associated with chorioamnionitis in the low-birth-weight group. This might be a possible explanation for the major differences in weight-dependent outcome.

Neonatal asphyxia

Controversy exists regarding the association between chorioamnionitis and neonatal asphyxia at birth. Some experts argue that, similar to the extra-uterine environment, sepsis in utero by itself might lead to metabolic acidemia and birth asphyxia.[47] In contrast, others have found no such association.[10] Since asphyxia implies acidemia to an extent leading to metabolic acidosis, determination of umbilical acid–base balance in infected labors is important. Several studies have shown that chorioamnionitis is not associated with lower mean umbilical artery pH in preterm neonates.[48] Moreover, the same proportion of neonates, infected and noninfected, had metabolic acidemia, defined by pH of less than 7.20. One study demonstrated a slight, though statistically significant, decrease in pH, but only in full-term infants.[49] Apgar scores were significantly lower (without difference between term and preterm infants) in association with chorioamnionitis. Nevertheless, other studies have shown that the lower Apgar scores observed in infected deliveries are partly attributed to prolonged labors, need for oxytocin, and general anesthesia.[43,48]

Chorioamnionitis and cerebral palsy

Cerebral palsy is a complex of symptoms characterized by the aberrant control of movement or posture that appears in early life and can lead to costly lifelong disability.[50] Despite previous expectations, the tremendous improvement in perinatal medicine has not been accompanied by a decrease in the prevalence of cerebral palsy. Moreover, the incidence of cerebral palsy has increased in the last two decades and is 0.06% for term newborns and 4.4–2.1% for neonates born before 32 weeks of gestation.[51,52] The etiology of cerebral palsy is poorly understood. Most cases remain unexplained and are primarily attributed to unknown prenatal factors.[53,54] Contrary to common belief, birth asphyxia plays only a minor role in the development of cerebral palsy.[55] Chorioamnionitis has been implicated as a potential cause of cerebral palsy.[50,56,57] Chorioamnionitis is common and often subclinical. It is postulated that both clinical and subclinical intrauterine infection might either cause or predispose the neonate to severe brain injury and subsequent cerebral palsy. In a 6-year study, beginning in 1959 and including approximately 54 000 pregnancies, chorioamnionitis was associated with a 4.8-fold increased risk for cerebral palsy.[58] However, the last four decades have yielded a substantial improvement in both fetal monitoring and preterm neonatal survival. During this time interval, numerous articles have been published trying to clarify the association between chorioamnionitis and cerebral palsy in term and preterm infants. A metaanalysis of relevant studies was performed by Wu and Colford,[59] evaluating the risk of cystic periventricular leukomalacia (cPVL) and subsequent cerebral palsy in infants born of women with either histologic or clinical chorioamnionitis. Based on this recent metaanalysis, chorioamnionitis appears to be associated with an increased incidence of both cerebral palsy and cPVL (Table 14.2).

In experimentally induced chorioamnionitis using an animal model, ascending infection was

Table 14.2. Chorioamnionitis and relative risk of subsequent cerebral palsy

	Term	No. of studies	Preterm	No. of studies
Histologic chorioamnionitis	RR 8.9 (CI 1.9–40.0)	1	RR 1.6 (CI 0.9–2.7)	5
Clinical chorioamnionitis	RR 4.7 (CI 1.3–16.2)	2	RR 1.9 (CI 1.4–2.5)	17

Note:
RR, relative risk; CI, confidence interval.
Source: Adapted from Wu and Colford.[59]

associated with fetal brain matter lesions.[60] Other studies have demonstrated elevated cytokine production after experimental induction of intrauterine infection.[61] The cytokine hypothesis states that the elevated blood and brain cytokine levels resulting from maternal infection are associated with brain damage and subsequent cerebral palsy.[62]

Prematurity is the leading identifiable cause of cerebral palsy.[63,64] Subclinical and overt chorioamnionitis are associated with approximately 25% of preterm deliveries.[65] Both preterm parturition and chorioamnionitis are associated with elevation of certain plasma cytokines[66] when dried blood samples that were taken routinely after birth for hypothyroidism screening demonstrated significantly higher concentrations of interleukin-1, -6, -8, and -9 and tumor necrosis factor-α in samples obtained from neonates diagnosed later as suffering from cerebral palsy.[67] Another study that focused on preterm deliveries demonstrated that amniotic fluid concentrations of interleukin-6 and -8, and amniotic fluid white blood cell counts, were significantly higher in fetuses with subsequent development of cerebral palsy when compared to those who did not develop cerebral palsy (OR = 5.6, confidence interval (CI) = 1.0–30.7). Yet, the higher level of certain cytokines among children with cerebral palsy does not imply that cerebral palsy originates from the same etiology in all infants.

Cytokine production is influenced by a variety of factors, including infection, autoimmune states, trauma, and ischemia. Furthermore, cytokine expression (translation) is influenced by genetic variables (as polymorphism), which might predispose a cluster of neonates to the development of cerebral palsy. Therefore, the elevation of certain cytokines in these children may mark a common pathway linking a number of different causes with adverse neurological outcome.

Cerebral palsy has also been associated with several placental lesions in preterm infants. These lesions, namely chorionic plate thrombi and diffuse villous edema, were associated with histologic chorioamnionitis. The number of lesions was related to the risk of subsequently developing cerebral palsy.[68] Furthermore, funisitis, which is a marker of the fetal inflammatory response, was associated with both the development of white-matter lesions and the occurrence of cerebral palsy (OR = 6.6, CI = 1.4–31.8) at the age of 3 years.[69] Of note, the relationship between histologic chorioamnionitis and brain damage is not clearly established. Some studies document a significant relationship between histologic chorioamnionitis and brain damage, increased periventricular echodensity, echolucency, intraventricular hemorrhage grade III–IV, and ventriculomegaly by ultrasound.[70] However, others[68,69,71,72] have found no association between histologic subclinical chorioamnionitis, acute inflammatory changes on examination of a membrane roll and chorionic plate, and white-matter damage when controlled for gestational age. As reported elsewhere,[68] the fetal inflammatory response and vasculitis, rather than the maternal inflammation, are associated with the subsequent pathological brain lesions. Other factors, such as gestational age and maternal disease (e.g., pre-eclampsia or diabetes), may interact with chorioamnionitis in the pathogenesis of cerebral palsy. Some neonates might be genetically predisposed to inflammatory brain injury by cytokine functional polymorphism.[73] Such genetic factors may in part determine the extent of fetal inflammation that occurs in the face of maternal infection.

Cerebral palsy is also associated with chorioamnionitis in infants born at term.[50,58] Chorioamnionitis is associated with both short- (e.g., low Apgar score, need for resuscitation, seizures) and long-term (e.g., cerebral palsy and neurologic morbidity) adverse neonatal outcome. Maternal fever in labor is a risk factor for neonatal encephalopathy in term infants.[74] Furthermore, the major cause of mortality for term neonates with low Apgar score is maternal infection,[75] and intrauterine exposure to infection apparently endangers the brains of infants of normal birth weight. Future investigations will be required to explicate further the exact mechanism of injury. Lastly, preterm infants have a markedly increased incidence of chronic lung disease (bronchopulmonary dysplasia) if chorioamnionitis is present. While the incidence and severity of respiratory distress syndrome are decreased in these infants, they often have more significant bronchopulmonary dysplasia.[76]

Treatment

Patients with acute intraamniotic infection are usually treated by prenatal antibiotic therapy and labor is induced. Previously it was recommended that antibiotic therapy be withheld until after delivery in order to culture the neonate accurately. Currently, most agree that treatment should start as soon as clinical signs of infection are recognized. While intrapartum therapy is associated with a 0–2.8% risk of neonatal sepsis, postponing therapy raises the risk to an excessive rate, estimated at 6–21%.[20,77,78] Moreover, maternal outcome, consisting of postpartum hospital stay, febrile illness, and sequelae, was improved in patients who received antibiotic therapy before and during labor.

The most commonly recommended antibiotic regimen includes penicillin or ampicillin plus an aminoglycoside. This combination covers the most common organisms associated with early neonatal sepsis (group B streptococci and Enterobacteriaceae), that are also found in intraamniotic infections. In light of the increasing incidence of anaerobic organisms identified, it may be appropriate to broaden the antibiotic coverage. Therefore, combination therapy using clindamycin and aminoglycosides is advised, especially after cesarean delivery.[79] Another approach is the use of broad-spectrum single-agent therapy, such as second- or third-generation cephalosporins and extended-spectrum penicillins. These agents are usually less toxic, easily administered, and are efficacious in 80–90% of patients.[1]

Prevention of chorioamnionitis is advocated in situations that involve a higher risk for infection. It is well established that prophylactic antibiotics should be given to patients undergoing cesarean section in order to reduce the postpartum febrile morbidity. Recently, prophylactic antibiotic therapy has been recommended during expectant management of PPROM. Antibiotic treatment was advocated in these situations in order to prolong the latency period until delivery and to reduce fetal, and possibly maternal, morbidity. A metaanalysis of seven randomized clinical trials has demonstrated a significant reduction in relative risk of neonatal sepsis (68% reduction) and intraventricular hemorrhage (50% reduction). Respiratory distress syndrome, necrotizing enterocolitis, and overall neonatal mortality were not significantly affected by such treatment.[80–86]

Another randomized controlled trial has demonstrated that ampicillin and erythromycin also reduce the rate of respiratory distress and necrotizing enterocolitis. The reduction in fetal morbidity was more significant for group B beta-hemolytic streptcoccus-negative patients.[87] Treated patients also had a lower incidence of clinical amnionitis. Therefore, it is recommended that woman with PPROM, who are expectantly managed remote from term, should receive antibiotics in order to reduce the associated morbidity.

Once the diagnosis of clinical chorioamnionitis is established, many obstetricians feel that the fetus should be removed as soon as possible from the infected environment. The average interval between the diagnosis of chorioamnionitis and delivery is 3–7 h. The critical time interval beyond which maternal and neonatal complications increase has never been determined.[78,88] However, it seems from clinical experience that in most situations vaginal delivery is superior. Intrapartum antibiotic therapy should cover the fetus with appropriate bactericidal concentrations within less than an hour. Furthermore, in most cases, when the progress of labor is within normal limits, the time interval from the presentation of the clinical signs of infection to delivery is not as long as to endanger the neonate.[78] It is also reasonable to suggest that a fetus compromised due to infection will develop a nonreassuring fetal heart rate, which may lead to an operative delivery. Cesarean delivery should be reserved for cases of intraamniotic infection with additional standard obstetric indications for abdominal delivery. Therefore, due to a higher rate of dystocia and nonreassuring fetal conditions, the rate of cesarean delivery is often increased to 35–40%.[76]

REFERENCES

1 Casey BM and Cox SM. (1997). Chorioamnionitis and endometritis. *Infect Dis North Am*, **11**, 203–222.

2 Newton ER. (1993). Chorioamnionitis and intraamniotic infection. *Clin Obstet Gynecol*, **36**, 795–808.

3 Gibbs RS and Duff P. (1991). Progress in pathogenesis and management of clinical intraamniotic infection. *Am J Obstet Gynecol*, **164**, 1317–1326.

4 Gilstrap LC and Cox SM. (1989). Acute chorioamnionitis. *Obstet Gynecol Clin North Am*, **16**, 373–379.

5 Newton ER, Prihoda TJ and Gibbs RS. (1989). Logistic regression analysis of risk factors for intraamniotic infection. *Obstet Gynecol*, **73**, 571–575.

6 Gibbs RS, Blanco JD, Clair PJ, et al. (1982). Quantitative bacteriology of amniotic fluid from patients with clinical intraamniotic infection at term. *J Infect Dis*, **145**, 1–8.

7 Morley JJ and Kushner I. (1982). Serum C-reactive protein levels in disease. *Ann NY Acad Sci*, **389**, 406–411.

8 Fisk NM, Fysh J, Child AG, et al. (1987). Is C-reactive protein really useful in preterm premature rupture of the membranes? *Br J Obstet Gynaecol*, **94**, 1159–1164.

9 Hoskins IA, Johnson TRB and Winkel CA. (1987). Leukocyte esterase activity in human amniotic fluid for the rapid detection of chorioamnionitis. *Am J Obstet Gynecol*, **157**, 730–732.

10 Vintzileos AM, Campbell WA, Nochimson DJ, et al. (1985). The fetal biophysical profile in patients with premature rupture of membranes – an early predictor of fetal infection. *Am J Obstet Gynecol*, **152**, 510–516.

11 Roussis P, Rosemond RL, Glass C, et al. (1991). Preterm premature rupture of membranes: detection of infection. *Am J Obstet Gynecol*, **165**, 1099–1104.

12 Del Valee GO, Joffe GM, Izquierdo LA, et al. (1992). The biophysical profile and the non-stress test: poor predictors of chorioamnionitis and fetal infection in prolonged preterm premature rupture of membranes. *Obstet Gynecol*, **80**, 106–110.

13 Miller JM Jr, Kho MS, Brown HL, et al. (1990). Clinical chorioamnionitis is not predicted by an ultrasonic biophysical profile in patients with premature rupture of membranes. *Obstet Gynecol*, **76**, 1051–1054.

14 Gonik B, Bottoms SF and Cotton DB. (1985). Amniotic fluid volume as a risk factor in preterm premature rupture of membranes. *Obstet Gynecol*, **65**, 456–459.

15 Vintzileos AM, Campbell WA, Nochimson DJ, et al. (1986). Qualitative amniotic fluid volume versus amniocentesis in predicting infection in preterm premature rupture of membranes. *Obstet Gynecol*, **67**, 579–583.

16 Vermillion ST, Kooba AM and Soper DE. (2000). Amniotic fluid index values after preterm premature rupture of membranes and subsequent perinatal infection. *Am J Obstet Gynecol*, **183**, 271–276.

17 Gibbs RS, Castillo MS and Rodjers PJ. (1980). Management of acute chorioamnionitis. *Am J Obstet Gynecol*, **180**, 709–715.

18 Koh KS, Chan FH, Monfared AH, et al. (1979). The changing perinatal and maternal outcome in chorioamnionitis. *Obstet Gynecol*, **53**, 730–734.

19 Yoder PR, Gibbs RS, Blanco JD, et al. (1983). A prospective controlled study of maternal and perinatal outcome after intraamniotic infection at term. *Am J Obstet Gynecol*, **145**, 695–701.

20 Gilstrap LC, Leveno KJ, Cox SM, et al. (1988). Intrapartum treatment of acute chorioamnionitis: impact on neonatal sepsis. *Am J Obstet Gynecol*, **159**, 579–583.

21 Newton ER, Prihoda TJ and Gibbs RS. (1989). Logistic regression analysis of risk factors for intraamniotic infection. *Obstet Gynecol*, **73**, 571–575.

22 Soper DE, Mayhall CG and Dalton HP. (1989). Risk factors for intraamniotic infection: a prospective epidemiologic study.

Am J Obstet Gynecol, **161**, 562–568.

23 Sturchler D, Menegoz F and Daling J. (1986). Reproductive history and intrapartum fever. *Gynecol Obstet Invest*, **21**, 182–186.

24 Harger JH, Hsing AW, Tuomala RE, et al. (1990). Risk factors for preterm premature rupture of fetal membranes: a multicenter case-control study. *Am J Obstet Gynecol*, **163**, 130–137.

25 Hillier S, Krohn MA, Kiviat NB, et al. (1991). Microbilogic causes and neonatal outcomes associated with chorioamnion infection. *Am J Obstet Gynecol*, **165**, 955–961.

26 Queenan JT. (1977). *Modern Management of the Rh Problem*, 2nd edn, p. 180. Hagerstown, Maryland: Harper & Row.

27 Charles D and Edwards WR. (1981). Infectious complications of cervical cerclage. *Am J Obstet Gynecol*, **141**, 1065–1070.

28 Halliday HL and Hirata T. Perinatal listeriosis: a review of twelve patients. *Am J Obstet Gynecol*, **133**, 405–410.

29 Monif GR. (1975). Antenatal group A streptococcal infection. *Am J Obstet Gynecol*, **123**, 213–214.

30 Sperling RS, Newton E and Gibbs RS. (1988). Intraamniotic infection in low-birth weight infants. *J Infect Dis*, **157**, 113–117.

31 Silver HM, Sperling RS, Clair PJ, et al. (1989). Evidence relating bacterial vaginosis to intraamniotic infection. *Am J Obstet Gynecol*, **161**, 808–812.

32 Gibbs RS. (1993). Chorioamnionitis and bacterial vaginosis. *Am J Obstet Gynecol*, **169**, 460–462.

33 Steele RW. (1996). Reduced incidence of preterm delivery with metronidazole and erythromycin in women with bacterial vaginosis. *Clin Pediatr*, **35**, 378–379.

34 Kekki M, Pelkonen J, Kurkinen-Raty M, et al. (2001). Vaginal clindamycin in preventing preterm birth and peripartal infections in asymptomatic women with bacterial vaginosis: a randomized controlled trial. *Obstet Gynecol*, **94**, 643–648.

35 Romero R, Sirtori M, Oyarzun E, et al. (1989). Prevalence, microbiology and clinical significance of intraamniotic infection in women with preterm labor and intact membranes. *Am J Obstet Gynecol*, **161**, 817–824.

36 Guzick DS and Winn K. (1985). The association of chorioamnionitis with preterm delivery. *Obstet Gynecol*, **65**, 11–16.

37 Ferguson MG, Rhodes PG, Morrison JC, et al. (1985). Clinical amniotic fluid infection and its effect on the neonate. *Am J Obstet Gynecol*, **151**, 1058–1061.

38 Satin AJ, Maberry MC, Leveno KJ, et al. (1992). Chorioamnionitis: a harbinger of dystocia. *Obstet Gynecol*, **79**, 913–915.

39 Silver RS, Gibbs RS, Castillo M, et al. (1986). Effect of amniotic fluid bacteria on the course of labor in nulliparous women at term. *Obstet Gynecol*, **68**, 587–592.

40 Seaward PGS, Hannah ME, Myhr TL, et al. (1998). International multicenter term PROM study: evaluation of predictors of neonatal infection in infants born to patients with premature rupture of membranes at term. *Am J Obstet Gynecol*, **179**, 635–639.

41 Gerdes JS. (1991). Clinicopathologic approach to the diagnosis of neonatal sepsis. *Clin Perinatol*, **18**, 361–379.

42 Haque KN. (1993). Indications for antimicrobial therapy in babies after PROM: the Saudi Arabian experience. *Post Grad Doctor*, **16**, 342–347.

43 Alexander JM, McIntire DM and Leveno KJ. (1999). Chorioamnionitis and the prognosis for term infants. *Obstet Gynecol*, **94**, 274–278.

44 Wallace RL and Herrick CN. (1981). Amniocentesis in the evaluation of premature labor. *Obstet Gynecol*, **57**, 483–486.

45 Gravett MG, Hummel D, Eschenbach DA, et al. (1986). Preterm labor associated with subclinical amniotic fluid infection and with bacterial vaginosis. *Obstet Gynecol*, **67**, 229–237.

46 Morales WJ. (1987). The effect of chorioamnionitis on the developmental outcome of preterm infants at one year. *Obstet Gynecol*, **70**, 183–186.

47 Peevey KJ and Chalhub EG. (1983). Occult group B streptococcal infection: an important cause of intrauterine asphyxia. *Am J Obstet Gynecol*, **146**, 989–990.

48 Maberry MC, Ramin SM, Gilstrap LC, et al. (1990). Intrapartum asphyxia in pregnancies complicated by intraamniotic infection. *Obstet Gynecol*, **76**, 351–354.

49 Meyer BA, Dickinson JE, Chambers C. (1992). The effect of fetal sepsis on umbilical cord blood gases. *Am J Obstet Gynecol*, **166**, 612–617.

50 Grether JK and Nelson KB. (1997). Maternal infection and cerebral palsy in infants of normal birth weight. *JAMA*, **278**, 207–211.

51 Bhushan V, Paneth N and Kiely JL. (1993). Impact of improved survival of very low birth weight infants on recent secular trends in the prevalence of cerebral palsy. *Pediatrics*, **91**, 1094–1100.

52 Cummins SK, Nelson KB, Grether JK, et al. (1993). Cerebral palsy in four northern California counties; births 1983 through 1985. *J Pediatr*, **123**, 230–237.

53 Nelson KB and Ellenberg JH. (1986). Antecedents of cerebral palsy: multivariate analysis of risk. *N Engl J Med*, **315**, 81–86.

54 Blair E and Stanley FG. (1988). Intrapartum asphyxia: a rare cause of cerebral palsy. *J Pediatr*, **112**, 515–519.

55 Perlman JM. (1997). Intrapartum hypoxic–ischemic

cerebral injury and subsequent cerebral palsy: medicolegal issues. *Pediatrics*, **99**, 851–859.

56 Dammann O and Leviton A. (1997). Maternal intrauterine infection, cytokines and brain damage in the preterm newborn. *Pediatr Res*, **42**, 1–8.

57 Adinolfi M. (1993). Infectious diseases in pregnancy, cytokines and neurological impairment: an hypothesis. *Dev Med Child Neurol*, **35**, 549–553.

58 Nelson KB and Ellenberg JH. (1985). Antecedents of cerebral palsy. Univariate analysis of risks. *Am J Dis Child*, **139**, 1031–1038.

59 Wu YW and Colford JM. (2000). Chorioamnionitis as a risk factor for cerebral palsy. A meta-analysis. *JAMA*, **284**, 1417–1424.

60 Yoon BH, Kim CJ, Romero R, et al. (1997). Experimentally induced intrauterine infection causes fetal brain white matter lesions in rabbits. *Am J Obstet Gynecol*, **177**, 797–802.

61 Cai Z, Pan Z, Pang Y, et al. (2000). Cytokine induction in fetal rat brains and brain injury in neonatal rats after maternal lipopolysaccharide administration. *Pediatr Res*, **47**, 64–72.

62 Dammann O and Leviton A. (1998). Infection remote from the brain, neonatal white matter damage and cerebral palsy in the preterm infant. *Semin Pediatr Neurol*, **5**, 190–201.

63 Kuban KCK and Leviton A. (1994). Cerebral palsy. *N Engl J. Med*, **330**, 188–195.

64 Evans PM, Evans SJW and Alberman E. (1990). Cerebral palsy: why we must plan for survival. *Arch Dis Child*, **65**, 1329–1333.

65 Yoon BH, Jun JK, Romero R, et al. (1997). Amniotic fluid inflammatory cytokines (IL-6, IL-1β and TNF-α), neonatal brain white matter lesions and cerebral palsy. *Am J Obstet Gynecol*, **177**, 19–26.

66 Romero R, Mazor M, Munoz H, et al. (1994). The preterm labor syndrome. *Ann NY Acad Sci*, **734**, 414–429.

67 Nelson KB, Dambrosia JM, Grether JK, et al. (1998). Neonatal cytokines and coagulation factors in children with cerebral palsy. *Ann Neurol*, **44**, 665–675.

68 Redline RW, Wilson-Costello D, Borawski E, et al. (1998). Placental lesions associated with neurologic impairment and cerebral palsy in very low-birth-weight infants. *Arch Pathol Lab Med*, **122**, 1091–1098.

69 Yoon BH, Romero R, Park JS, et al. (2000). Fetal exposure to an intraamniotic inflammation and the development of cerebral palsy at the age of three years. *Am J Obstet Gynecol*, **182**, 675–681.

70 De Felice C, Toti P, Laurini R, et al. (2001). Early neonatal brain injury in histologic chorioamnionitis. *J Pediatr*, **138**, 101–104.

71 Dammann O and Leviton A. (2000). Role of the fetus in perinatal infection and neonatal brain damage. *Curr Opin Pediatr*, **12**, 99–104.

72 O'Shea TM, Klinepeter KL, Meis PJ, et al. (1998). Intrauterine infection and the risk of cerebral palsy in very low birth weight infants. *Paediatr Perinat Epidemiol*, **12**, 72–83.

73 Dammann O, Durum SK and Leviton A. (1999). Modification of the infection-associated risks of preterm birth and white matter damage in the preterm newborn by polymorphisms in the tumor-necrosis-factor locus. *Pathogenesis*, **1**, 171–177.

74 Adamson J, Alessandri LM, Badawi N, et al. (1995). Predictors of neonatal encephalopathy in full term infants. *Br Med J*, **311**, 598–602.

75 Naeye RL. (1979). Underlying disorders responsible for the neonatal deaths associated with low Apgar scores. *Biol Neonate*, **35**, 150–155.

76 Watterberg KL, Demers LM, Scott SM, et al. (1996). Chorioamnionitis and early lung inflammation in infants in which bronchopulmonary dysplasia develops. *Pediatrics*, **97**, 210–215.

77 Sperling RS, Ramamurthy RS and Gibbs RS. (1987). A comparison of intrapartum versus immediate postpartum treatment of intraamniotic infection. *Obstet Gynecol*, **70**, 861–865.

78 Gibbs RS, Dinsmoor MJ, Newton ER, et al. (1988). A randomized trial of intrapartum versus immediate post-partum treatment of women with intra amniotic infection. *Obstet Gynecol*, **72**, 823–828.

79 Gibbs RS, Blanco JD, Castaneda YS, et al. (1982). A double-blind randomized comparison of clindamycin-gentamicin versus cefamandole for treatment of post-cesarean endomyometritis. *Am J Obstet Gynecol*, **144**, 261–266.

80 Egarter C, Leitich H, Karas H, et al. (1996). Antibiotic treatment in preterm premature rupture of membranes and neonatal morbidity: a metaanalysis. *Am J Obstet Gynecol*, **174**, 589–597.

81 Kirschbaum T. (1993). Antibiotics in the treatment of preterm labor. *Am J Obstet Gynecol*, **168**, 1239–1246.

82 Ernest JM and Givner LB. (1994). A prospective randomized, placebo-controlled trial of penicillin in premature rupture of membranes. *Am J Obstet Gynecol*, **170**, 516–521.

83 Johnson MM, Sanchez-Ramos L, Vaughn AJ, et al. (1990). Antibiotic therapy in preterm premature rupture of membranes: a randomized, prospective, double-blind trial. *Am J Obstet Gynecol*, **163**, 743–747.

84 McCaul JF, Perry KG, Moore JL, et al. (1992). Adjunctive antibiotic treatment of women with preterm rupture of membranes or preterm labor. *Int J Gynecol Obstet*, **38**, 19–24.

85 McGregor JA, French JI and Seo K. (1991). Antimicrobial

therapy in preterm premature rupture of membranes: results of a prospective , double-blind, placebo-controlled trial of erythromycin. *Am J Obstet Gynecol*, **165**, 632–640.

86 Morales WJ, Angel JL, O'Brien WF, et al. (1989). Use of ampicillin and corticosteroids in premature rupture of membranes: a randomized study. *Obstet Gynecol*, **73**, 721–726.

87 Mercer BM, Miodovnik M, Thurnau GR, et al. (1997). Antibiotic therapy for reduction of infant morbidity after preterm premature rupture of the membranes. *JAMA*, **278**, 989–995.

88 Hauth JC, Gilstrap LC, Hankins GDV, et al. (1985). Term maternal and neonatal complications of acute chorioamnionitis. *Obstet Gynecol*, **55**, 59–64.

15

Bacterial sepsis in the neonate

Hayley A. Gans

Stanford University Medical Center, Stanford, CA, USA

Introduction

Bacterial sepsis of the neonate is defined as systemic signs of infection with bacteremia, occurring in the first 30 days of life. Meningitis accompanies sepsis in approximately one-quarter of cases of neonatal disease, but the two processes share a common etiology and pathogenesis. This chapter will cover only bacterial sepsis of the term infant; meningitis is covered elsewhere. Prematurity and residence in an intensive care unit are independent risk factors for bacterial sepsis that differ from sepsis in the term infant. In addition, the emphasis of this chapter will be on early-onset neonatal disease, with less of a concentration on late-onset sepsis.

Epidemiology

Although the ability to diagnose bacterial sepsis has improved, septicemia remains a frequent cause of neonatal morbidity and mortality. The first records of positive blood cultures were reported from Yale in 1928.[1] Since this time there has been a changing prevalence of prominent bacterial organisms that cause sepsis in the neonate, requiring an ever-vigilant approach to this disease,[1,2] and it is likely that changes will continue to occur with the use of intrapartum antibiotics.[3]

Two distinct patterns of neonatal sepsis have been described, differentiated by time of disease onset, predominant organism, and associated risk factors.[1,4] Early-onset disease is defined as occurring ≤7 days postnatally with a strong association with obstetrical complications or risk factors. Therefore, disease is caused by microorganisms that colonize the maternal genital tract.[4,5] Some authors argue for a further stratification of this early septic group into "very-early" onset, within 48 h, since the pathophysiology may be different. It is believed that this group acquires infection in utero at a particularly susceptible stage, accounting for the very high mortality in these infants who are symptomatic at the time of delivery or shortly after birth. The early-onset group in the later model would acquire the infecting organism at the time of delivery, and this group has a lower case-fatality rate than the very-early-onset group.[5,6]

Late-onset disease presents >7 days of life,[7] in infants lacking a history of obstetrical risk factors, and involves organisms that could be acquired perinatally as well as postnatally. Focal infections, such as meningitis, are more commonly seen in late-onset disease,[4] and pose a unique set of prognostic factors (see Chapter 16).

The incidence of neonatal sepsis has remained unchanged, despite advances in prevention practices, and occurs in 1–10 per 1000 live term births in developed countries.[2,9] Early-onset disease has an annual incidence of 2.2–3.9/1000 live births and late-onset 2.5/1000 live births.[1,6] The incidence rates for the major individual organisms are described below.

Risk factors

A neonate's susceptibility to infection is well documented and thought to be multifactorial. Unique to the neonatal host is deficiencies of various arms of the immune system and circumstances where exposure to a large number of organisms occurs. Susceptibility to infections in the neonate also arises when there are interruptions in the natural barriers of the body, which occur frequently in the birthing process, such as breaks in the skin with monitoring devices.

Immunologic limitations have been documented in both the innate immunity, including cellular defenses (such as eosinophils, neutrophils, platelets, and monocytes) and adaptive immunity involving both cell-mediated immunity and humoral responses.[8,9] Antigen presentation by dendritic cells and activity of natural killer cells have also been shown to be deficient in the neonate and in neonatal sepsis in particular.[10] The lack of opsonizing antibody to encapsulated bacteria confers a susceptibility to many of the bacteria in the maternal genital tract to which the neonate is exposed.[11,12]

Obstetrical risk factors for the term infant include prolonged rupture of membranes ≥18 h, maternal fever, with the height of fever reflecting strongly on risk to the infant.[6] Additional risk factors for group B streptococcus (GBS) infection include a pregnancy complicated by GBS bacteriuria and history of an infant with invasive GBS disease.[13] The determination of these risk factors is vitally important because intensive focus in this area has decreased the incidence and thus mortality rates from GBS substantially (see below).

Etiology

Overall there are only a small group of organisms accounting for the majority of neonatal sepsis, with a very large and varied group of organisms accounting for the minority of cases.[6] Before the introduction of antibiotics the predominant organisms were Gram-positive, with group A β-hemolytic streptococcus (*Streptococcus pyogenes*) the major etiologic entity. This was replaced by the intestinal Gram-negative bacilli, particularly *Escherichia coli* (*E. coli*) after the introduction of sulfonamides in the early 1940s.[1] *Staphylococcus aureus* was observed to be a major pathogen from 1950–63, but for reasons that are not clear has diminished in importance since this time.[1,2] Even in the early reports, GBS held its place as a major contributor to neonatal sepsis, and was a leader in early fulminant disease. Over time, the predominance of GBS has risen to assume the leading cause of Gram-positive septicemia in early-onset neonatal disease. GBS accounts for 25–35% of sepsis overall, with 80% occurring in the first 48 h of life, resulting in 55% of early-onset disease. This is in contrast to *E. coli* which causes 27% of sepsis overall, only 13% of early-onset sepsis, but 31% of late-onset disease.[1,2] *Klebsiella pneumoniae* and *Enterobacter cloacae* are seen in about 15% of cases of septicemia, with other organisms being reported less frequently, such as *Listeria monocytogenes, Haemophilus* spp., *Pseudomonas* spp., *Streptococcus pneumoniae, viridans streptococcus,* enterococcal group D streptococcus (enterococcus), and *staphylococcus* spp. Some of the latter organisms have a strong association with prematurity or an underlying condition or procedure. The important individual organisms are discussed separately below.

Clinical presentation

The spectrum of clinical signs in neonates that develop sepsis is varied and symptoms are nonspecific. During delivery, signs of fetal distress, such as tachycardia,[14] and low Apgar scores[15] have been associated with sepsis, but both lack specificity.

Subtle signs of infection include poor feeding, decreased responsiveness, and more prominent symptoms include temperature instability, apnea, respiratory distress, jaundice, lethargy, vomiting, and diarrhea.[16] Though a serious bacterial infection is rare in asymptomatic neonates,[17] infants who are bacteremic may have no symptoms initially, but deteriorate rapidly,[18] and develop multiorgan failure. Due to the nonspecific and subtle presenting clinical signs of septic neonates, clinical symptoms cannot be used alone to identify high-risk infants.

Diagnosis

The optimal workup of a newborn with suspected sepsis is not well defined. Presenting clinical symptoms are often nonspecific and thus differentiating truly infected infants from infants symptomatic as a result of noninfectious causes is challenging. The importance of initiating prompt antimicrobial therapy to reduce the high mortality rate attributed to neonatal sepsis makes identifying the septic infant essential. Standard culturing procedures do not offer a timely method to differentiate between these infant groups, and further cultures may not prove helpful if intrapartum antibiotics were used.

Given this inherent difficulty in determining which infants are at risk for developing sepsis, infants with symptoms consistent with sepsis of any pattern historically have received therapy to reduce the potential morbidity and mortality. It is estimated that 11–23 infants are treated for every documented case of neonatal sepsis,[19] accounting for the treatment of 4.4–10.5% of all infants born in the USA.[20,21] This overutilization of antibiotics in all clinically symptomatic infants results in most infants receiving antibiotics unnecessarily, putting these infants at risk for complications of therapy and contributing to the development of multiple drug-resistant bacteria.

Many researchers are turning their efforts to the evaluation of rapid diagnostic methods for the early detection of those infants who will progress to sepsis, and identifying those infants who are symptomatic for noninfectious reasons. In the latter group the goal is safely to allow for the discontinuation of antibiotics but ideally aiming for the development of a rapid test that would aid in guiding the initiation of therapy on only those infants where it is necessary.[19,22] Thus, in addition to the standard culturing methods used for diagnosis, adjunctive tests have been evaluated. These include markers such as C-reactive protein (CRP), interleukin-6 (IL-6), interleukin-8 (IL-8), neutrophil CD-11b, granulocyte colony-stimulating factor (G-CSF), and hematologic abnormalities such as immature-to-mature neutrophil ratio.

Cultures are the gold standard for the definitive diagnosis of neonatal sepsis. All infants suspected of sepsis should have a blood culture drawn prior to the initiation of antibiotics. Venous puncture is the preferred method for obtaining blood for culture.[23] The number of optimal blood cultures is under debate. Extrapolating from recommendations for older children and adults, some authors have suggested obtaining blood from two sites in order to increase the yield of a positive result, especially when a small bacterial load is expected, as in the case of infants born to mothers who received intrapartum antibiotics.[24] In addition, it is argued that this may help clarify when a contaminating organism is isolated. There are obvious limitations to this in a neonate; among them is the desire to limit the amount of blood taken from small infants to reduce the potential need for blood transfusion. Additionally, the density of bacteria may be higher in neonates and the bacteremia more continuous compared with older patients and thus a single blood culture may be adequate.[25]

Studies looking at the time to positivity of blood culture isolates in neonates have shown that approximately 92% of true pathogens are easily isolated from blood culture within 48 h,[26,27] and 99% of cultures will be positive by day 4.[28] Therefore, some authors would suggest that this high bacterial isolation rate – 92% by day two of life – would support the discontinuation of antibiotics in the asymptomatic term neonate who is undergoing a suspected sepsis rule-out. It will be important to determine if this remains the case in the era of increased use of intrapartum antibiotics.

The utility of cultures from sterile sites other than blood, such as the cerebrospinal fluid and urine, has been debated. The necessity of doing a lumbar puncture in a neonate suspected of sepsis is covered elsewhere. Urine cultures have been shown to be important in late-onset neonatal disease,[29] but the data are variable for early-onset disease. Given that neonatal urine tract infections are thought to be a result of hematogenous spread of the organism and not direct inoculum into the urinary tract, the low yield of urine cultures in the evaluation of infants with suspected sepsis – about 0.1–1% – would warrant eliminating urine cultures from the workup in the first 24 h of life.[30–32] There does not appear to be any additional information obtained from the culturing of nonsterile surface sites.[33]

In an attempt to develop a rapid diagnostic test to distinguish between infants suspected of and infants with sepsis, many researchers have looked to blood test assays other than cultures. One study evaluated multiple rapid tests and their utility in diagnosing neonatal bacteremia in cases of suspected sepsis.[34] The results showed the nonspecific nature of an elevated white blood cell count (WBC) since it was positive in 71% of culture-proven bacteremia but also 42% of infants with negative blood cultures. Immature-to-total neutrophil ratios were not elevated in the majority of infants with negative blood cultures, but it was also <0.2 in 29% of infants with positive blood cultures.

CRP, an acute-phase reaction to inflammation or tissue necrosis, has also received a lot of attention and use in neonatal units. CRP is thought to be a good predictor of bacterial sepsis in the neonate,[35] with its predictability peaking at 24–48 h after presentation with infection and thus the recommendation for serial levels.[36] The majority of the highest titers have been documented in response to bacterial illnesses, with moderate elevations tending to be more nonspecific. Levels decline rapidly once the ongoing process resolves and thus serial titers are a helpful measure of disease activity.[37] In particular, authors have shown that the negative predictive value of a negative CRP after 24 h is approximately 99% predictive of not having a bacterial process[19,36,38] and thus would warrant the discontinuation of antibiotics. Unfortunately the positive predictive value is low, approximately 89% in proven early-onset neonatal disease,[36] given that other processes, such as the stresses of delivery (prolonged rupture of membranes, low Apgars) correlate with a nonspecific rise of CRP for approximately 3 days.[37,39] Thus CRP cannot be used to guide the initiation of therapy to only infants who are truly infected and in the early stages of sepsis, but has value in discontinuing therapy in neonates undergoing a sepsis evaluation if levels remain low.

The poor positive predictive value of CRP has led to evaluations of other cytokines, independently or in combination with CRP, to increase the sensitivity of rapid determination of infants at risk for sepsis, since many of these cytokines may become abnormal prior to elevations in CRP. IL-6, the major inducer of CRP, has been one prime target of investigation.[39] Early studies are promising in distinguishing those infants that are not infected, but a clearer understanding of levels in infants that have sepsis compared with those that do not is needed before its role as a predictor of bacterial sepsis can be determined. IL-8 has also been studied in combination with CRP[22] since it is an early proinflammatory marker. Franz et al. showed that using high thresholds for both IL-8 and CRP (≥70 pg ml and ≥10 mg/l, respectively) achieved a sensitivity of 96–100%, but a positive predictive value of only 65–77% for determining neonatal bacterial sepsis over the study period. By restricting therapy to only infants in this group, there was a 60% reduction in antimicrobial use and only 23% of infants were treated unnecessarily. Once again there was a good negative predictive value of having two negative tests 24 h apart.[22] This same study has not been evaluated for early-onset neonatal disease in a large cohort of term infants.

Neutrophil CD11b is a surface marker activated early in the host's innate immune response to invading microbes. It shows promise in the very early detection of neonatal sepsis because it is positive upon first evaluation of the symptomatic neonate and thus does not have the delay seen with CRP. Neutrophil CD11b is elevated in infants with proven and suspected sepsis,[40,41] and remains low in infants with symptoms caused by noninfectious disorders.[41] Once again, if CD11b is determined to be helpful in the diagnosis of neonatal bacterial sepsis, it will most likely be in concert with the other markers described above, especially CRP. Weirich et al. showed that, while CD11b was elevated in infants with proven viral illnesses and symptoms indistinguishable from bacterial sepsis, the CRP never rose in these infants,[40] and Nupponen et al. showed that, used in combination with IL-8, most proven and suspected bacterial illnesses were determined very early in the workup of symptomatic neonates.[41]

Both G-CSF and intercellular adhesion molecule-1 (ICAM-1) have been studied and shown to have some promise for the early detection of neonatal sepsis. They lack reliable positive predictive values and sensitivity but again report good negative predictive values.[42,43]

Though newer diagnostic tests are sought, none of the studied methods has improved upon the positive predictive value of using risk factors and clinical signs consistent with infection, low absolute neutrophil count, and immature-to-total neutrophil ratio $\geq$0.25 to determine infants with sepsis, even in the age of intrapartum antibiotics, as revealed by a large outcome study of 2785 infants.[17] In this study, the majority of infants that had either culture-proven or suspected sepsis were identified as "at risk for infection" using obstetrical risk factors including maternal chorioamnionitis, prolonged rupture of membranes (>18 h), maternal fever (>100.4), GBS carriage, foul-smelling amniotic fluid, and prematurity. The rest of the infants were picked up through screening, complete blood count (CBC), and clinical presentations. Eighty percent of these infants were symptomatic within 12 h of birth. All of the infants, including the 20% that were asymptomatic at the time of evaluation, had significantly lower absolute neutrophil counts than the infants without sepsis and all received antibiotics by 12 h of age. The infants whose mothers had received intrapartum antibiotics were more likely to be asymptomatic, less likely to be critically ill or to be infected, and had better outcomes compared with infants whose mothers did not receive intrapartum treatment.

Treatment

Empiric treatment with broad-spectrum antibiotics guided by the knowledge of etiologic organisms and their susceptibility patterns is the standard of care in neonatal sepsis. The goal of any antibiotic therapy is the elimination of the bacteria from the blood as quickly as possible to reduce the source for the host inflammatory process that is responsible for the symptoms related to sepsis. In addition, it is important to avoid hematogenous dissemination of the infecting organism to secondary sites. Ampicillin is most commonly chosen for its coverage of GBS, group D nonenterococcal streptococci, *L. monocytogenes*, enterococcus, and other anaerobes. In addition, an aminoglycoside is added for appropriate coverage of Gram-negative organisms[44] and for synergy with ampicillin for treatment of enterococcus, GBS,[45] and *L. monocytogenes*. The choice of initial antibiotic therapy will require close monitoring in the growing age of intrapartum antibiotics and the potential for emerging microbial resistance. Antibiotic treatment can be narrowed in culture-proven sepsis once susceptibility of the organism is known.

Despite the use of appropriate antibiotic treatment, the mortality rate for neonates remains high. Therefore there is interest in determining if adjunctive therapy, targeted at areas of immune immaturity in the neonate, would be effective. Given the success of intravenous immune globulin (IVIG) in the prevention of bacterial infections in primary agammaglobulinemia, studies have been tried as adjunctive therapy in neonatal sepsis. In a meta-analysis, Jenson and Pollock[46] reviewed three studies all of which showed a six-fold decrease in acute mortality in the infants treated with one dose of 500–750 mg/kg of IVIG, but long-term mortality and morbidity must still be evaluated.

The use of granulocyte–macrophage colony-stimulating factor (GM-CSF) has been evaluated to target neonatal neutropenia, which is associated with increased morbidity and mortality when present during bacterial sepsis.[47] Studies have documented the safety of both G-CSF[48] and GM-CSF[49] in neonates and a recent randomized controlled trial[50] showed a significant increase in neutrophil count in the GM-CSF-treated infants compared with the conventionally treated septic neonates. In addition, the mortality rate in this study was decreased by 20% in the infants treated with GM-CSF. Though promising for improving outcome of neonatal sepsis, there is concern about the long-term toxicity on the developing bone marrow of the neonate, and further efficacy studies in larger cohorts are still required before GM-CSF is used as standard adjunctive therapy for neonatal sepsis.

Outcome

There is a clear association between sepsis and mortality, with a less defined causal relationship with long-term morbidity. Mortality from sepsis accounts for approximately 16% of neonatal deaths, but reports on early-onset mortality rates attributable to sepsis range from 15 to 50%.[6,9] Mortality in the first couple of days after birth was highest and is not dependent on the causative agent.[6] Late-onset disease carries a much lower case-mortality rate of approximately 17–22%, and is more dependent on the etiologic organism, with *E. coli* carrying the highest rates of mortality, followed by *Staphylococcus aureus* and GBS.[6]

Over time a dramatic decrease in mortality has been demonstrated, most closely associated with changes in mortality due to GBS sepsis. In the 1930s mortality rates as high as 80% were demonstrated, with a continued decline to present levels, which appears to have plateaued.[9] Mortality from GBS sepsis peaked at 47% in 1974, reaching a nadir in 1978 of 18%. Mortality from other entities remained appreciably unchanged during the same period despite the use of appropriate antimicrobial therapy.[1] The cases of GBS reported in the later series also document a falling rate of fulminant disease. The decline in neonatal mortality secondary to sepsis is multifactorial, related to prevention, early detection, advanced supportive care, and antimicrobial therapy.[2]

Sequelae resulting from neonatal septicemia have not been well studied. With declining mortality rates, and more survivors of neonatal sepsis, defining what morbidity exists in these survivors is becoming increasingly more important. Most of the documented adverse outcomes, particularly neurologic deficits, are seen in neonates that had meningitis as part of their sepsis,[51] and there are clear orthopedic deformities as a result of neonatal osteomyelitis.[52] These infants though are neurologically intact. Bennet et al.[53] reviewed the outcomes of survivors of neonatal sepsis over the 15-year period 1969–83, including premature and term neonates. In their study approximately 8% of septic neonates that survive and have neither meningitis nor osteomyelitis will have long-term sequelae. These infants account for 40% of the infants that developed sequelae and include 50% with severe developmental delay. Other outcomes were shown to be deafness, hydrocephalus, and mild developmental delay. The hearing impairment observed was associated with Gram-negative sepsis, but it could not be determined if it was as a result of treatment with an aminoglycoside, sepsis alone, or both. All of the infants that developed sequelae were those with obstetrical and neonatal risk factors, and thus identifying these infants and utilizing preventive measures should impact not only survival, but long-term outcome in these septic neonates. Unfortunately the same does not hold true for meningitis. Alfven et al.[54] studied 90 infants with neonatal sepsis and also reported that most survivors of sepsis without meningitis that developed long-term sequelae had other underlying conditions, such as prematurity, and maternal preconditions such as diabetes. Most other survivors were noted to have normal growth and development at the time of follow-up 2–6 years later.

The role of bacterial sepsis as an independent factor in the poor outcomes and long-term morbidity in infants with other neonatal complications, such as perinatal asphyxia[55] preterm labor, and prematurity cannot be easily determined and has not been reported. Therefore the reader is referred to the chapters that deal directly with these confounding abnormalities.

Prevention

Prevention measures have been targeted almost exclusively at GBS sepsis and are covered below.

Specific organisms

The major organisms associated with bacterial sepsis will be covered in more detail, but an exhaustive review of all etiologic agents of neonatal sepsis is beyond the scope of this chapter. Given the importance of GBS in neonatal sepsis and mortality, it will be discussed in more detail than other organisms, which will be reviewed for the qualities that are unique to them and deserve mention beyond the general discussion above.

Group B streptococcus

The organism

GBS emerged as a leading cause of neonatal infections and mortality in the 1970s[56] and remains an important cause of disease in the term and preterm infant.[57] The organism is a Gram-positive coccus and is found as a colonizer of the female genital and rectal areas. The organism gains access to these secondary sites of colonization from the gastrointestinal tract, which serves as the most likely human reservoir.[58] Approximately 10–35% of women are asymptomatic carriers of GBS. The colonization rate of infants exposed to maternal sources of GBS is high – about 50% – but the majority – around 98% – of these infants are asymptomatic. Eighty percent of the remaining 1–2% of exposed infants will develop early-onset disease presenting as sepsis, pneumonia, or meningitis.[57,58] The majority of these infants are symptomatic within 2 days of birth with the rest presenting within the first week.

Approximately nine serotypes of GBS have been identified, with serotype III causing approximately 36% of early-onset disease, 90% of early-onset meningitis, and 71% of late-onset disease (regardless of site of infection), despite a smaller representation in maternal colonization rates.[59–61] Recently serotype V has been increasing as an important isolate in neonatal disease, accounting for about 14% of early-onset GBS disease.[62] In early-onset disease without meningitis the non-III GBS serotypes are evenly distributed, with nontypable strains accounting for approximately 2–10% of disease.[61]

The capsular polysaccharide (CPS) antigens are recognized as major virulence factors of GBS and immunity is known to be a type-specific anticapsular antibody that promotes opsonization of homologous GBS strains in concert with the complement system. The concentration of CPS-specific antibody that is protective is not known and may depend on serotype and bacterial inoculum, as well as the maturity of the immune system.[63] In a large cohort study, women colonized with type III GBS had lower CPS-specific immunoglobulin G levels compared with women colonized with other serotypes.[61] The lack of passive antibodies at protective levels may partially explain the virulence of GBS serotype III in early-onset neonatal disease with meningitis and late-onset disease.

Epidemiology

The exact incidence of GBS disease is hard to determine. Published reports are variable, reflecting reporting practices based on high-risk groups and single institutions, and may not correctly reflect disease incidence in a larger population. Studies looking at a 10-year period from 1989 to 1999 in the USA report an incidence for early-onset disease of 1.4–3.2/1000 births and 0.24–0.5/1000 births for late-onset disease.[64–66] Early-onset disease results in approximately 2200 infections annually in the USA.[67] Reports from the Centers for Disease Control and Prevention (CDC) surveillance from a very large population, but in only four geographic areas of the country, showed a decline in the incidence of early-onset GBS disease by 43% in some sites from the years 1993–95, but no changes were found at other locations. There was a decline from 1.4 to 0.8 cases per 1000 births in the areas that showed a decline. In this evaluation there were clear differences in rates when race was considered, with African-American rates the highest,[68] and this has been substantiated in other studies.[69] During the same period the incidence for late-onset disease remained unchanged. This trend, therefore, most likely represents practices that interrupt intrapartum transmission of GBS, including practice guidelines, and enhanced detection techniques and not decreasing GBS carriage rates. Recurrent disease appears to occur in only a small percentage (0.4–0.9%) of appropriately treated infants that survive their initial GBS infection.[70,71] Though GBS is strongly associated with disease in preterm infants, the majority of cases (up to 82%) in institutions are still seen in term infants.[13]

Pathogenesis

The pathogenesis of very-early-onset GBS disease is thought to occur through ascending spread of the organism into amniotic fluid from which the fetus aspirates.[58] This is thought to present a larger inoculum of organisms than could be achieved through other routes. GBS has been shown to cross intact membranes.[72] As noted above, the early-onset syndrome presenting at 3–7 days of life is thought to represent acquisition of the organism at the time of delivery. Late-onset sepsis is less well understood, with only a portion of cases reflecting colonization at the time of delivery. Only 50% of infants with late-onset disease are born to mothers with positive cultures for GBS,[73] with nosocomial[74] and community[75] acquisition thought to account as the source of the remainder of disease.

Risk factors

The major risk factors associated with early-onset invasive GBS disease have to do with infant exposure to a high inoculum of organisms and a relatively immunocompromised host. Disease of all serotypes has been documented in early-onset disease, reflecting the colonizing strains found in women, but there is a strong representation of serotype III in invasive neonatal disease, especially when meningitis is present. Invasive disease is more likely to develop in an infant who lacks anticapsular antibodies to the specific serotype that is present in the birth canal. This occurs if maternal levels are low or the baby is born prior to significant antibody transfer.[58] There is also evidence that immunologic protection provided by maternal antibodies is not sufficient to protect the neonate from GBS disease, as incidence is highest in the first weeks of life, when titers of passive antibodies are expected to be the highest. While deficiencies in a neonate's complement pathways creates a particular susceptibility to encapsulated organisms, such as GBS,[76] there remains a unique susceptibility to GBS that differs from other encapsulated organisms.[77]

An infant will be at an increased risk for colonization with GBS if the mother is heavily colonized, or if obstetrical manipulations allow for bacterial replication.[78] Obstetrical manipulations also increase the risk for invasive disease by allowing ascension of the organism and increase the inoculum to which the fetus is exposed.[79] African-American women have higher rates of heavy colonization with GBS that may account for the higher rates of neonatal disease.[80] Bacteriuria in the mother signals heavy colonization with GBS, and thus is defined as an individual risk factor for disease in the neonate.[81] Prolonged rupture of membranes, also considered an individual risk factor, will increase the inoculum of organisms presented to the fetus. Multiple pregnancies and congenital malformations are known to predispose to prematurity and prematurity is also a risk factor for early-onset GBS disease.[60] With the goal to identify infants at high risk for invasive GBS disease the CDC, American College of Obstetricians and Gynecologists (ACOG), and American Academy of Pediatrics (AAP) have focused on the above risk factors when creating the prevention strategies outlined below.[3,82,83]

Clinical presentation

The clinical presentations of GBS disease are nonspecific and include sepsis, meningitis, pneumonia and less frequently cellulitis, omphalitis, osteomyelitis, and septic arthritis. Bacteremia with or without pneumonia accounts for 89% of disease in infants $\leq$90 days, with meningitis only complicating 10% of these cases.[60,68] Septicemia (signs of sepsis in bacteremic infants without a focus) accounts for 25–40% of presentations, and pneumonia 35–55%.[7,71]

Infants presenting with sepsis represent the full range of the spectrum of disease, including multiorgan failure, acidemia, and hypotension requiring full life support measures, as well as interventions to correct metabolic abnormalities. Respiratory findings were prominent in the majority of early-onset disease (80%), but poor feeding, lethargy, hypothermia or fever, abdominal distension, pallor, tachycardia, and jaundice have all been described.[7]

Diagnosis

The only definitive diagnostic test for GBS sepsis is a positive culture. Culture results are obviously not available at the time of presentation, and all symptomatic neonates require a full septic evaluation and initiation of broad-spectrum antibiotics, usually with ampicillin and an aminoglycoside. These can be narrowed once culture results and sensitivities of the organism are determined (see below).

The evaluation and management of high-risk infants born to women with risk factors, particularly if they have received intrapartum antibiotics, present particular difficulties and are very controversial. This is particularly true if the infant is asymptomatic, as some infants that are bacteremic may be asymptomatic at birth and partial treatment afforded by antibiotics given to the mother may mask early symptoms.[84] Guidelines have been created in some institutions that include obtaining a blood culture and CBC in infants that have one or more risk factors for sepsis. Empiric antibiotics are initiated if the CBC had a total WBC count $<5000/\text{mm}^3$ or of >0.2 ratio of immature to total neutrophils (I/T ratio). These are discontinued at 48 h if blood cultures remain negative.[66] Some of the rapid diagnostic methods mentioned above may aid in guiding therapy for this group of infants.

Treatment

Antibiotics are the hallmark of treatment for all forms of GBS sepsis, with the drug of choice being penicillin at 2000000 units/kg per day. There have been no clinical isolates of GBS that have been resistant to penicillin, and the microbiologic inhibitory concentration (MIC) remains very low. Isolates are also routinely sensitive to ampicillin, though this antibiotic has a slightly broader spectrum and thus, when GBS has been confirmed, it is often recommended that penicillin be used when possible. These organisms are also sensitive to cephalosporins, vancomycin, and semisynthetic penicillins at variable activities. Erythromycin resistance has been reported in 7–21% of isolates, and resistance to clindamycin in 4–15% of isolates.[85,86] There is evidence of synergy with an aminoglycoside, as stated previously. The duration of treatment of bacteremia without meningitis is 10–14 days.

Outcome

Initial reports of GBS sepsis in the neonate documented mortality rates of approximately 50%,[5] but this dropped quickly in the 1980s to 15% and further to present levels of about 4–6% with improved recognition, prompt treatment, and better supportive care.[64,68]

Morbidity has been more difficult to define, but reports from the 1970s showed profound neurologic sequelae if meningitis was documented,[5] and more recently, reports of infants treated with extracorporeal membrane oxygenation (ECMO) have shown some long-term neurologic impairments.[74] It is difficult to differentiate between the individual effects of ECMO and those of sepsis on these outcomes, as the most severe infants are placed on ECMO. In addition, newer evaluations are needed for infants that survive GBS sepsis in the age of intensive supportive care of these infants.

Prevention

With the increase in GBS incidence and the decline in mortality due to better treatment modalities, efforts have now turned to prevention. The strategies for the prevention of GBS transmission from mother to fetus have evolved over the past 20 years, but it was not until the CDC, ACOG, and AAP reached a consensus that prevention made sense and was economically affordable, that practices started changing.[3,82,83] ACOG first published guidelines in 1992, and supported a risk-based strategy to prevention. In the same year the AAP published a screening-based approach to GBS prevention. Confusion persisted for a number of years as to the best strategy to use, and in 1996–7 all three bodies – the CDC, ACOG, and AAP – reissued consensus statements. Currently, all institutions that offer obstetrical services must either adapt a screening-based or a risk-based approach to GBS prevention.

Screening-based approaches provide intrapartum antibiotics to all women with positive cultures for GBS performed late in gestation and all women without cultures that are delivering <37 weeks' gestation. Risk-based approaches provide intrapartum antibiotics to women with the following risk factors; delivery <37 weeks' gestation, prolonged rupture of membranes >18 h, intrapartum temperature ≥38°C. Both strategies provide intrapartum antibiotics to women with GBS bacteriuria and to women who previously delivered an infant with GBS disease (both markers of heavy genital tract colonization).

The screening-based approach allows for the potential use of antibiotics early in delivery (as opposed to the alternative of waiting 18 h after ruptured membranes or until a fever develops in the mother), and in mothers who may still colonize their infants despite the lack of symptoms. Reviews of maternal and infant records of infants with early-onset disease show that 50–70% of these infants were born to mothers who lack risk factors.[13,87] One of these studies reported that up to 79% of early-onset disease could be prevented by the screening-based approach.[87]

There is also evidence to suggest that at least 4 h of intrapartum antibiotics is better than shorter courses; up to 40% of infants born to colonized mothers were still colonized if antibiotics were given within 1 h of delivery, but only 1% of infants were colonized if the mothers received ampicillin ≥4 h before delivery.[88]

The screening-based strategy is more cumbersome since it depends on the collection of prenatal cultures that need to be performed correctly and processed appropriately, as well as the information being available at time of delivery. It is also unclear who to screen, and because data based on large populations showed no reliable information to predict which populations to screen, this strategy must be applied universally.[80]

Correct culturing techniques are vital to the success of the screening-based protocol. It has been shown that cervical cultures have low predictive value of GBS colonization and that ideally both vaginal and rectal cultures should be performed,[89] although this appears to be practiced only 83% of the time.[69] Processing of these cultures on nonselective media will miss up to 50% of GBS carriers from the overgrowth of other bacteria.[69] Thus there must be good communication between the practitioner and the laboratories that the samples are GBS screens and need selective media. In a study evaluating the implementation of the prevention strategies, only 12% of specimens were cultured on selective media.[69] Further, studies have shown that cultures are most accurate when collected within 5 weeks of delivery,[79] thus it is recommended to collect prenatal cultures at 35–37 weeks' gestation.[82,83]

The risk-based strategy has the ease of implementation. The risk factors should be easily recognizable, and the only issues would be around educating the delivery staff. Though this strategy may be appropriate for institutions that have low rates of carrier states or with a large proportion of women delivering without prenatal care, it can only be expected to prevent less than 40% of early-onset disease.[87] Even if risk factors were reevaluated to include more women whose infants have been shown to have early-onset disease, there is usually less than 4 h between the presentation of a risk factor and delivery – too short a time for the effective use of intrapartum antibiotics.[13,58] It does appear that using a risk-based prevention approach may be more appropriate for preterm labor since more infected preterm neonates were born to mothers with symptoms that were defined in the prevention guidelines.[13]

More recent recommendations are concentrating on a combination strategy, selective intrapartum chemoprophylaxis (SIC), using chemoprophylaxis on women with risk factors that are culture-positive for GBS.[90–92] The goal is to prevent the majority of GBS cases (approximately 60%) and restrict the exposure of antibiotics to <5% of women. Infected neonates born to women who are culture-negative on examination carry lower rates of mortality and morbidity, and thus the remainder of cases (40%) would have a better prognosis. The risk factors used were prolonged rupture of membranes (>12 h) and prematurity.

This combined strategy has obvious limitations, and institutions have documented failures,[93,94] but decreased incidence of GBS early-onset disease has also been reported.[95,96] The obvious problems are with women lacking prenatal care, the predictive value of cultures, the inability to prevent intrauterine infection, the elimination of chorioamnionitis as a risk factor, and the protection of infants with early-onset disease born to women who are asymptomatic.

Some of the issues raised above are addressed by combining this strategy with the use of intramuscular penicillin in neonates of colonized mothers without risk factors (selective neonatal chemoprophylaxis). The use of penicillin in neonates has been shown to reduce the rate of GBS early-onset disease without an increase in incidence of late-onset disease.[97,98] Adverse reactions to antimicrobials in this population are much smaller than in adults. Further, the incidence of producing resistance has not been documented.[97]

Gotoff and Boyer proposed combining SIC with selective neonatal chemoprophylaxis (SNC).[91,92] In their proposal all prenatal cultures would be obtained at 35 weeks' gestation, and risk factors extended to include all women without prenatal care and delivering prematurely. In addition, any woman with a febrile course consistent with chorioamnionitis would receive full treatment with ampicillin and an aminoglycoside, and not just prophylaxis. Further, all asymptomatic infants born to GBS-colonized women would be given penicillin. This approach would be expected to protect those infants born to colonized mothers that are symptomatic at time of delivery and thus bacteremic at birth. SIC has been shown to be effective in this group of infants. Infants more likely to be infected with GBS at the time of delivery are more likely to be born to colonized mothers without risk factors and therefore should be protected by SNC. This would be expected to decrease the incidence of GBS early-onset disease by approximately 75–90% and limit the exposure to penicillin to <10%. There is still concern about the use of this strategy, particularly with the postpartum use of penicillin in neonates[99] and vigilance of mortality rates, incidence of late-onset disease, and emergence of resistance must continue.

It is clear that the use of prevention strategies reduces the incidence of early-onset disease. Despite successes, only a minority (35%) of institutions surveyed as of 1994 followed any prevention strategy, and most of these (48%) offered intrapartum antimicrobial prophylaxis to women with risk factors. Of the institutions having some prevention strategy, most did not follow the prevention strategies as they were outlined by the recommending bodies, but adapted some part of the protocol.[69]

The CDC through active Bacterial Core Surveillance System surveyed hospitals in eight states, and reported that the proportion of hospitals with formal intrapartum GBS prevention policies increased to 59% in 1997,[68] but remained unchanged in 1999.[67] Of institutions surveyed with guidelines, 53% used screening-based approaches, 31% risk-based, and 14% utilized a combined approach. Of these institutions, 80% used penicillin as the chemoprophylatic agent in 1999. It has been shown that even limited compliance with any prevention strategy that reduces the risk of early-onset GBS neonatal disease is cost-effective.[100,101]

Chemoprophylaxis

Chemoprophylaxis during pregnancy, prior to onset of labor, has been studied as a way of preventing neonatal GBS disease. Most studies show that there is no impact on maternal carriage and that colonization rates revert to baseline by the time of delivery.[102,103] Some success has been demonstrated if antibiotics are given late in the third trimester, at which time the maternal colonization can be reduced or eradicated with one dose of penicillin.[104]

The use of penicillin as intramuscular injections postnatally in infants has also been studied. This strategy showed a reduction in the incidence of early-onset disease, but there was no significant impact on mortality of infected neonates, and the protection of term infants against disease was not as clear as with premature neonates.[98,105] Further, this method could not be expected to prevent the very early-onset cases that are already established at the time of birth.[105]

The use of intrapartum chemoprophylaxis carries the highest likelihood for success and has been shown in studies to reduce the colonization of neonates and invasive GBS disease, but is linked to the flaws of the prevention strategies, as outlined above.[106,107] The administration of antepartum chemoprophylaxis to all GBS carriers has potential risks for adverse events.[108] Given the population that would require treatment, there is the potential for approximately 10 deaths annually from anaphylaxis,[109] and a proportion of women and fetuses suffering less severe reactions.[110] In addition, the use of antepartum chemoprophylaxis challenges the pediatrician to understand how to treat the neonates born to mothers who have been treated with antibiotics.[96]

The use of intrapartum antibiotics is also plagued with the potential emergence of resistant microbes, including non-GBS organisms. Towers et al.[110] showed that, while the incidence of GBS in their institution declined over an 8-year study period as a result of increasing intrapartum ampicillin use, there was also a coincident rise in early-onset neonatal disease caused by non-GBS organisms. The majority of these cases were in infants whose mothers had been given intrapartum ampicillin and 87% of the bacteria were ampicillin-resistant. The conclusion was drawn that the use of penicillin with a more narrow spectrum would be more prudent in this setting. These findings have been supported by other authors.[111] Further, there has been an association with increased mortality in infants infected with ampicillin-resistant *E. coli* compared with sensitive strains.[112]

Immunoprophylaxis

Even though the prevention strategies outlined above and the use of intrapartum antibiotics are expected to reduce the incidence of GBS sepsis, there are concerns about the frequent use of antibiotics and the emergence of resistant strains of GBS and other organisms. In addition, the prevention strategies are not expected to prevent late-onset disease, GBS-related stillbirths, or prematurity, and so recent developments are focusing on vaccines. Vaccines are expected to be effective, by providing a boost in the maternal anticapsular antibody titers so that higher levels are transferred transplacentally to the neonate. The hope is to overcome the neonatal susceptibility to GBS disease that is believed to arise from deficiencies in protective levels of maternal anticapsular antibodies, particularly to serotype III.[61]

The initial attempts at producing an effective vaccine concentrated on GBS serotype III, but it was not until the polysaccharide was conjugated to tetanus toxoid that promising results were observed.[113] In addition the initial target populations for these vaccines were pregnant women in their second trimester, but this proved to be very controversial. Therefore the focus for vaccine-induced immunity to GBS has shifted to women in the child-bearing age prior to pregnancies, and to childhood. The immunity for a conjugate vaccine is expected to be lasting and thus vaccinating the latter two populations would offer protection even to newborns born years after effective immunization.

One obvious goal of GBS vaccination would be to achieve decreases in mucosal colonization as well as protective antibody titers, as has been seen with the *Haemophilus influenzae* vaccines[114] which are also conjugate vaccines and serve as a model for GBS vaccine development. One obvious difference is that, unlike *H. influenzae*, where one serotype is responsible for invasive disease, several serotypes of GBS have been implicated in invasive disease. Thus a multivalent vaccine will be the only viable strategy to potential disease elimination, although great accomplishments can be expected using vaccines targeted at GBS serotype III since it is the major cause of early-onset disease associated with meningitis and late-onset sepsis.

Escherichia coli

Escherichia coli is the second most important pathogen in neonatal sepsis, and the primary Gram-negative coliform causing disease.[1,6,115] The antigenic structure of *E. coli* is very complex, and a great genetic diversity exists in the strains that colonize humans. Despite the large number of different colonizing strains, there is a strikingly small number of strains that cause disease.[116] One of the capsular antigens of *E. coli*, the K1 antigen, is related to invasive disease and is uniquely associated with neonatal meningitis. Approximately 80% of *E. coli* meningitis in neonates is caused by K1 strains, and though this association is not as strong with bacteremia, it has been cultured from the blood of infants with sepsis without meningitis.[117] There is also a higher rate of morbidity and mortality associated with sepsis and meningitis caused by the K1 strains compared with disease caused by non-K1 strains. The increased morbidity and mortality are related to the concentration and persistence of the capsular polysaccharides of these K1 strains in blood and cerebrospinal fluid.[118]

Pili on the surface of *E. coli* K1 strains are important for mucosal colonization, but a shift to a nonpiliated form where the capsular protein becomes important is the form of the bacteria that is found in the blood stream of animal models. The importance of these phase shifts in the *E. coli* K1 strain's ability to avoid immune recognition by the host defenses is speculated[119] and considered an important virulence factor.

The pathogenesis of fetal colonization is similar to that of GBS and other organisms that are acquired from the maternal birth canal either prior to or at the time of delivery (see above). Though *E. coli* only causes approximately 13% of early-onset disease, it is responsible for 31% of late-onset disease for reasons that are not clearly understood.[1,2] McCracken et al.[117,118] have shown that in the acquisition of K1 strains of *E. coli* there is also a role for postnatal transmission of the organism. They demonstrated high rates of carriage in hospital personnel and subsequent acquisition of identical strains in the neonates they cared for. In addition, there was acquisition of these strains in neonates born to mothers that were not colonized with these strains.

Treatment for *E. coli* bacteremia without meningitis is dictated by the susceptibility to antibiotics of the isolate. Treatment with ampicillin in susceptible strains alone or in combination with an aminoglycoside is appropriate therapy. The use of broader regimens, particularly cephalosporins, should be carefully considered and used only if deemed necessary since there is concern for the emergence of cephalosporin-resistant strains of *Enterobacter cloacae*, *Klebsiella* species, and *Serratia* species in the institutions where these infants reside. The duration of therapy for uncomplicated disease is usually 10–14 days.

Streptococcus pyogenes (group A beta-hemolytic streptococcus)

Streptococcus pyogenes has been a historically important cause of neonatal sepsis from the sixteenth century and the predominant organism causing disease from 1930–40,[1] but incidence dropped off markedly in the antibiotic era.[120]

S. pyogenes has been cultured from the anus and vagina of pregnant women, the umbilical stumps of neonates, and the hands and nasopharynx of neonates, mothers, and nursery personnel. Transmission is thought to be at the time of delivery and potentially postnatally. Most colonized infants are asymptomatic, but rare cases of invasive disease, such as sepsis and meningitis, have been documented.[121] In the past, most disease presented as indolent omphalitis.[120,121] This is in contrast to more recent reports of neonates with a severe early-onset sepsis associated with high mortality rates, pointing to the possibility of a resurgence of disease with a more aggressive course similar to early-onset GBS disease.[122,123] If there appears to be a true increased incidence of such disease then preventive measures such as those utilized to decrease the incidence of GBS may become increasingly more important.

No strains of *S. pyogenes* have emerged that are resistant to penicillin, and this remains the drug of choice for treatment.[124,125] In the era of new more invasive neonatal sepsis caused by *S. pyogenes*, adjunctive therapies with clindamycin[126] and IVIG[127] may be warranted, but studies in neonates are lacking at the present time.

Enterococcal group D streptococci

The incidence of enterococcal group D streptococci (enterococcus) as a cause of neonatal sepsis has risen over the last decade from approximately 0.12/1000 live births to 0.8/1000 live births in one study[128] and threefold in another.[129] Eliminating prematurity as a risk factor, early-onset disease was not associated with obstetrical complications, and very few term infants were noted to have late-onset disease, and these were associated with complicated postnatal courses with invasive procedures. Further, the increased incidence was not a result of the use of broader-spectrum antibiotics, which are not in common use at the reporting institutions. Since the increased cases are late, occurring in hospitalized neonates, they are thought to represent longer survival of mostly preterm infants in invasive intensive care units.[128,129]

The organism is a Gram-positive, catalase-negative cocci, and has been known as a human pathogen for approximately 100 years.[130] The two important species that cause disease in humans are *Enterococcus faecalis* and *E. faecium*.[129]

The clinical symptoms again are often subtle and nonspecific, but the major signs of enterococcal sepsis include respiratory distress and apnea,[128,129] but rarely are chest roentgenograms positive.[128] Temperature instability and hypothermia are also present in 15–60% of infants.[129] Diarrhea was the second most frequent symptom encountered in early-onset disease, and rarely does meningitis complicate early-onset disease. About 40% of infants with early-onset disease can be expected to be asymptomatic at birth and are often screened only because of maternal risk factors.[128]

Enterococci are moderately resistant to ampicillin and penicillin and highly resistant to all cephalosporins. Optimal therapy includes both a penicillin and an aminoglycoside for synergy, or vancomycin. There are concerns that neonatal enterococcal infections will continue to rise and be more difficult to treat given the appearance of strains that are vancomycin-resistant in the USA. The hospital survival rates in infants with vancomycin-resistant enterococcus (VRE) are significantly worse compared to infants with susceptible strains.[129]

Outcomes for enteroccocus sepsis appear to be good, with quick clinical improvements, but long-term studies are lacking. Case-fatality rates are low – approximately 5.5–10% – and appear to relate to underlying conditions.[128,129]

Summary

The changing prevalence of organisms responsible for neonatal sepsis and emerging resistance in these organisms underscores the necessity for close vigilance and surveillance of this disease. Many advances have been made in the prevention and treatment of neonatal bacterial sepsis, but mortality and morbidity remain high. By adapting more stringent prevention guidelines and developing better diagnostic and treatment strategies, there is hope that dramatic improvement will occur in both the mortality rates and the incidence of morbidity in the survivors of sepsis from all etiologic organisms.

REFERENCES

1 Freedman RM, Ingram DL, Gross I, et al. (1981). A half century of neonatal sepsis at Yale: 1928 to 1978. *Am J Dis Child*, **135**, 140–144.

2 Gladstone IM, Ehrenkranz RA, Edberg SC, et al. (1990). A ten-year review of neonatal sepsis and comparison with the previous fifty-year experience. *Pediatr Infect Dis J*, **9**, 819–825.

3 Centers for Disease Control and Prevention. (1996). Prevention of perinatal group B streptococcal disease: a public health perspective. *MMWR*, **45**, 1–24.

4 Eichenwald EC. (1997) Perinatally transmitted neonatal bacterial infections. *Infect Dis Clin North Am*, **11**, 223–239.

5 Baker CJ. (1978). Early onset group B streptococcal disease. *J Pediatr*, **93**, 124–125.

6 Vesikari T, Janas M, Gronroos P, et al. (1985). Neonatal septicaemia. *Arch Dis Child*, **60**, 542–546.

7 Baker CJ and Edwards MS. (1988). Group B streptococcal infections. Perinatal impact and prevention methods. *Ann NY Acad Sci*, **549**, 193–202.

8 Lewis D and Wilson C. (1995). Developmental immunology and role of the host defenses in neonatal susceptibility to

infection. In *Infectious Diseases of the Fetus and Newborn Infant,* ed. Remington J and Klein J, pp. 20–98. Philadelphia: W.B. Saunders.

9 Arachaisri T and Ballow M. (1999). Developmental immunology of the newborn. *Immunol Allergy Clin North Am,* **19**, 253–279.

10 Georgeson GD, Szony BJ, Streitman K, et al. (2001). Natural killer cell cytotoxicity is deficient in newborns with sepsis and recurrent infections. *Eur J Pediatr,* **160**, 478–482.

11 Wilson CB. (1986). Immunologic basis for increased susceptibility of the neonate to infection. *J Pediatr,* **108**, 1–12.

12 Baker CJ, Edwards MS, Kasper DL. (1981). Role of antibody to native type III polysaccharide of group B streptococcus in infant infection. *Pediatrics,* **68**, 544–549.

13 Towers CV, Suriano K, Asrat T. (1999). The capture rate of at-risk term newborns for early-onset group B streptococcal sepsis determined by a risk factor approach. *Am J Obstet Gynecol,* **181**, 1243–1249.

14 Schiano MA, Hauth JC, Gilstrap LC 3rd. (1984). Second-stage fetal tachycardia and neonatal infection. *Am J Obstet Gynecol,* **148**, 779–781.

15 Soman M, Green B, Daling J. (1985). Risk factors for early neonatal sepsis. *Am J Epidemiol,* **121**, 712–719.

16 Powell KR. (1990). Evaluation and management of febrile infants younger than 60 days of age. *Pediatr Infect Dis J,* **9**, 153–157.

17 Escobar GJ, Li DK, Armstrong MA, et al. (2000). Neonatal sepsis workups in infants >/=2000 grams at birth: a population-based study. *Pediatrics,* **106**, 256–263.

18 Baker CJ. (1997). Group B streptococcal infections. *Clin Perinatol,* **24**, 59–70.

19 Bomela HN, Ballot DE, Cory BJ, et al. (2000). Use of C-reactive protein to guide duration of empiric antibiotic therapy in suspected early neonatal sepsis. *Pediatr Infect Dis J,* **19**, 531–535.

20 Townsend TR, Shapiro M, Rosner B, et al. (1979). Use of antimicrobial drugs in general hospitals: IV. Infants and children. *Pediatrics,* **64**, 573–578.

21 Hammerschlag MR, Klein JO, Herschel M, et al. (1977). Patterns of use of antibiotics in two newborn nurseries. *N Engl J Med,* **296**, 1268–1269.

22 Franz AR, Steinbach G, Kron M, et al. (1999). Reduction of unnecessary antibiotic therapy in newborn infants using interleukin-8 and C-reactive protein as markers of bacterial infections. *Pediatrics,* **104**, 447–453.

23 Paerregaard A, Bruun B, Andersen GE, et al. (1989). No advantage of capillary blood compared with venous blood for culture in neonates. *Pediatr Infect Dis J,* **8**, 659–660.

24 Wiswell TE and Hachey WE. (1991). Multiple site blood cultures in the initial evaluation for neonatal sepsis during the first week of life. *Pediatr Infect Dis J,* **10**, 365–369.

25 Franciosi RA and Favara BE. (1972). A single blood culture for confirmation of the diagnosis of neonatal septicemia. *Am J Clin Pathol,* **57**, 215–219.

26 Rowley AH and Wald ER. (1986). Incubation period necessary to detect bacteremia in neonates. *Pediatr Infect Dis,* **5**, 590–591.

27 Pichichero ME and Todd JK. (1979). Detection of neonatal bacteremia. *J Pediatr,* **94**, 958–960.

28 Kurlat I, Stoll BJ, McGowan JE Jr. (1989). Time to positivity for detection of bacteremia in neonates. *J Clin Microbiol,* **27**, 1068–1071.

29 Visser VE and Hall RT. (1979). Urine culture in the evaluation of suspected neonatal sepsis. *J Pediatr,* **94**, 635–638.

30 Abbott GD. (1972). Neonatal bacteriuria: a prospective study in 1460 infants. *Br Med J,* **1**, 267–269.

31 Littlewood JM, Kite P, Kite BA. (1969). Incidence of neonatal urinary tract infection. *Arch Dis Child,* **44**, 617–620.

32 DiGeronimo RJ. (1992). Lack of efficacy of the urine culture as part of the initial workup of suspected neonatal sepsis. *Pediatr Infect Dis J,* **11**, 764–766.

33 Evans ME, Schaffner W, Federspiel CF, et al. (1988). Sensitivity, specificity, and predictive value of body surface cultures in a neonatal intensive care unit. *JAMA,* **259**, 248–252.

34 Kite P, Millar MR, Gorham P, et al. (1988). Comparison of five tests used in diagnosis of neonatal bacteraemia. *Arch Dis Child,* **63**, 639–643.

35 Schouten-Van Meeteren NY, Rietveld A, Moolenaar AJ, et al. (1992). Influence of perinatal conditions on C-reactive protein production. *J Pediatr,* **120**, 621–624.

36 Benitz WE, Han MY, Madan A, et al. (1998). Serial serum C-reactive protein levels in the diagnosis of neonatal infection. *Pediatrics,* **102**, E41.

37 Jaye DL, and Waites KB. (1997). Clinical applications of C-reactive protein in pediatrics. *Pediatr Infect Dis J,* **16**, 735–747.

38 Ehl S, Gering B, Bartmann P, et al. (1997). C-reactive protein is a useful marker for guiding duration of antibiotic therapy in suspected neonatal bacterial infection. *Pediatrics,* **99**, 216–221.

39 Chiesa C, Signore F, Assumma M, et al. (2001). Serial measurements of C-reactive protein and interleukin-6 in the immediate postnatal period: reference intervals and analysis of maternal and perinatal confounders. *Clin Chem,* **47**, 1016–1022.

40 Weirich E, Rabin RL, Maldonado Y, et al. (1998). Neutrophil CD11b expression as a diagnostic marker for early-onset neonatal infection. *J Pediatr*, **132**, 445–451.

41 Nupponen I, Andersson S, Jarvenpaa AL, et al. (2001)Neutrophil cd11b expression and circulating interleukin-8 as diagnostic markers for early-onset neonatal sepsis. *Pediatrics*, **108**, E12.

42 Kennon C, Overturf G, Bessman S, et al. (1996). Granulocyte colony-stimulating factor as a marker for bacterial infection in neonates. *J Pediatr*, **128**, 765–759.

43 Edgar JD, Wilson DC, McMillan SA, et al. (1994). Predictive value of soluble immunological mediators in neonatal infection. *Clin Sci (Colch)*, **87**, 165–171.

44 Starr SE. (1985). Antimicrobial therapy of bacterial sepsis in the newborn infant. *J Pediatr*, **106**, 1043–1048.

45 Backes RJ, Rouse MS, Henry NK, et al. (1986). Activity of penicillin combined with an aminoglycoside against group B streptococci in vitro and in experimental endocarditis. *J Antimicrob Chemother*, **18**, 491–498.

46 Jenson HB and Pollock BH. (1997). Meta-analyses of the effectiveness of intravenous immune globulin for prevention and treatment of neonatal sepsis. *Pediatrics*, **99**, E2.

47 Manroe BL, Rosenfeld CR, Weinberg AG, et al. (1977). The differential leukocyte count in the assessment and outcome of early-onset neonatal group B streptococcal disease. *J Pediatr*, **91**, 632–637.

48 Schibler KR, Osborne KA, Leung LY, et al. (1998). A randomized, placebo-controlled trial of granulocyte colony-stimulating factor administration to newborn infants with neutropenia and clinical signs of early-onset sepsis. *Pediatrics*, **102**, 6–13.

49 Gillan ER, Christensen RD, Suen Y, et al. (1994). A randomized, placebo-controlled trial of recombinant human granulocyte colony-stimulating factor administration in newborn infants with presumed sepsis: significant induction of peripheral and bone marrow neutrophilia. *Blood*, **84**, 1427–1433.

50 Bilgin K, Yaramis A, Haspolat K, et al. (2001). A randomized trial of granulocyte–macrophage colony-stimulating factor in neonates with sepsis and neutropenia. *Pediatrics*, **107**, 36–41.

51 Bennet R, Eriksson M, Zetterstrom R. (1987). Neonatal septicemia: comparison of onset and risk factors during three consecutive 5-year periods. *Acta Paediatr Scand*, **76**, 361–362.

52 Mok PM, Reilly BJ, Ash JM. (1982). Osteomyelitis in the neonate. Clinical aspects and the role of radiography and scintigraphy in diagnosis and management. *Radiology*, **145**, 677–682.

53 Bennet R, Bergdahl S, Eriksson M, et al. (1989). The outcome of neonatal septicemia during fifteen years. *Acta Paediatr Scand*, **78**, 40–43.

54 Alfven G, Bergqvist G, Bolme P, et al. (1978). Longterm follow-up of neonatal septicemia. *Acta Paediatr Scand*, **67**, 769–773.

55 Sehdev HM, Stamilio DM, Macones GA, et al. (1997). Predictive factors for neonatal morbidity in neonates with an umbilical arterial cord pH less than 7.00. *Am J Obstet Gynecol*, **177**, 1030–1034.

56 Baker CJ and Barrett FF. (1973). Transmission of group B streptococci among parturient women and their neonates. *J Pediatr*, **83**, 919–925.

57 Schuchat A. (2001). Group b streptococcal disease: from trials and tribulations to triumph and trepidation. *Clin Infect Dis*, **33**, 751–756.

58 Schuchat A. (1998). Epidemiology of group B streptococcal disease in the United States: shifting paradigms. *Clin Microbiol Rev*, **11**, 497–513.

59 Baker CJ and Barrett FF. (1974). Group B streptococcal infections in infants. The importance of the various serotypes. *JAMA*, **230**, 1158–1160.

60 Yagupsky P, Menegus MA, Powell KR. (1991). The changing spectrum of group B streptococcal disease in infants: an eleven-year experience in a tertiary care hospital. *Pediatr Infect Dis J*, **10**, 801–808.

61 Davies HD, Adair C, McGeer A, et al. (2001). Antibodies to capsular polysaccharides of group B streptococcus in pregnant Canadian women: relationship to colonization status and infection in the neonate. *J Infect Dis*, **184**, 285–291.

62 Blumberg HM, Stephens DS, Modansky M, et al. (1996). Invasive group B streptococcal disease: the emergence of serotype V. *J Infect Dis*, **173**, 365–373.

63 Klegerman ME, Boyer KM, Papierniak CK, et al. (1983). Estimation of the protective level of human IgG antibody to the type-specific polysaccharide of group B streptococcus type Ia. *J Infect Dis*, **148**, 648–655.

64 Zangwill KM, Schuchat A, Wenger JD. (1992). Group B streptococcal disease in the United States, 1990: report from a multistate active surveillance system. *MMWR CDC Surveill Summ*, **41**, 25–32.

65 Weisman LE, Stoll BJ, Cruess DF, et al. (1992). Early-onset group B streptococcal sepsis: a current assessment. *J Pediatr*, **121**, 428–433.

66 Schuchat A, Deaver-Robinson K, Plikaytis BD, et al. (1994). Multistate case-control study of maternal risk factors for

neonatal group B streptococcal disease. The Active Surveillance Study Group. *Pediatr Infect Dis J*, **13**, 623–629.

67 Morbidity and Mortality Weekly Report. Early-onset group B streptococcal disease – United States, 1998–1999. (2000). *MMWR*, **49**, 793–796.

68 Morbidity and Mortality Weekly Report. Decreasing incidence of perinatal group B streptococcal disease – United States, 1993–1995. (1997). *MMWR*, **46**, 473–477.

69 Whitney CG, Plikaytis BD, Gozansky WS, et al. (1997). Prevention practices for perinatal group B streptococcal disease: a multi-state surveillance analysis. Neonatal Group B Streptococcal Disease Study Group. *Obstet Gynecol*, **89**, 28–32.

70 Harrison LH, Ali A, Dwyer DM, et al. (1995). Relapsing invasive group B streptococcal infection in adults. *Ann Intern Med*, **123**, 421–427.

71 Schuchat A, Oxtoby M, Cochi S, et al. (1990). Population-based risk factors for neonatal group B streptococcal disease: results of a cohort study in metropolitan Atlanta. *J Infect Dis*, **162**, 672–677.

72 Katz V and Bowes WA Jr. (1988). Perinatal group B streptococcal infections across intact amniotic membranes. *J Reprod Med*, **33**, 445–449.

73 Dillon HC Jr, Khare S, Gray BM. (1987). Group B streptococcal carriage and disease: a 6-year prospective study. *J Pediatr*, **110**, 31–36.

74 Glass P, Wagner AE, Papero PH, et al. (1995). Neurodevelopmental status at age five years of neonates treated with extracorporeal membrane oxygenation. *J Pediatr*, **127**, 447–457.

75 Trager JD, Martin JM, Barbadora K, et al. (1996). Probable community acquisition of group B streptococcus in an infant with late-onset disease: demonstration using field inversion gel electrophoresis. *Arch Pediatr Adolesc Med*, **150**, 766–768.

76 Davis CA, Vallota EH, Forristal J. (1979). Serum complement levels in infancy: age related changes. *Pediatr Res*, **13**, 1043–1046.

77 Smith CL, Baker CJ, Anderson DC, et al. (1990). Role of complement receptors in opsonophagocytosis of group B streptococci by adult and neonatal neutrophils. *J Infect Dis*, **162**, 489–495.

78 Ancona RJ, Ferrieri P, Williams PP. (1980). Maternal factors that enhance the acquisition of group-B streptococci by newborn infants. *J Med Microbiol*, **13**, 273–280.

79 Yancey MK, Duff P, Kubilis P, et al. (1996). Risk factors for neonatal sepsis. *Obstet Gynecol*, **87**, 188–194.

80 Regan JA, Klebanoff MA, Nugent RP. (1991). The epidemiology of group B streptococcal colonization in pregnancy. Vaginal Infections and Prematurity Study Group. *Obstet Gynecol*, **77**, 604–610.

81 Wood EG and Dillon HC Jr. (1981). A prospective study of group B streptococcal bacteriuria in pregnancy. *Am J Obstet Gynecol*, **140**, 515–520.

82 ACOG committee opinion. (1996). Prevention of early-onset group B streptococcal disease in newborns. Number 173 – June 1996. Committee on Obstetric Practice. American College of Obstetrics and Gynecologists. *Int J Gynaecol Obstet*, **54**, 197–205.

83 American Academy of Pediatrics Committee on Infectious Diseases and Committee on Fetus and Newborn. Revised guidelines for prevention of early-onset group B streptococcal (GBS) infection. (1997). *Pediatrics*, **99**, 489–496.

84 Morbidity and Mortality Weekly Report. Hospital-based policies for prevention of perinatal Group B streptococcal disease – United States, 1999. (2000). *MMWR*, **49**, 936–940.

85 Baker CJ, Webb BJ, Barrett FF. (1976). Antimicrobial susceptibility of group B streptococci isolated from a variety of clinical sources. *Antimicrob Agents Chemother*, **10**, 128–131.

86 Fernandez M, Hickman ME, Baker CJ. (1998). Antimicrobial susceptibilities of group B streptococci isolated between 1992 and 1996 from patients with bacteremia or meningitis. *Antimicrob Agents Chemother*, **42**, 1517–1519.

87 Rosenstein NE and Schuchat A. (1997). Opportunities for prevention of perinatal group B streptococcal disease: a multistate surveillance analysis. The Neonatal Group B Streptococcal Disease Study Group. *Obstet Gynecol*, **90**, 901–906.

88 Cueto M, Sancez M, Sampedro A, et al. (1995). Relationship between timing of intrapartum ampicillin administration and its effectiveness in preventing vertical transmission of group B streptococci. In *Program and Abstracts of the 35th Interscience Conference on Antimicrobial Agents and Chemotherapy*. Washington, DC: American Society for Microbiology.

89 Hillier S and Schuchat A. (1997). Preventing neonatal group B streptococcal disease: the role of the clinical microbiology laboratory. *Clin Microbiol Newslett*, **19**, 113–116.

90 American Academy of Pediatrics Committee on Infectious Diseases and Committee on Fetus and Newborn. (1992). Guidelines for prevention of group B streptococcal (GBS) infection by chemoprophylaxis. *Pediatrics*, **90**, 775–778.

91 Gotoff SP and Boyer KM. (1997). Prevention of early-onset neonatal group B streptococcal disease. *Pediatrics*, **99**, 866–869.

92 Gotoff SP and Boyer K. (1997). Combined, selective chemo-

prophylaxis of early onset neonatal group B streptococcal disease (GBS EOD). *Adv Exp Med Biol*, **418**, 267–268.
93 Ohlsson A and Myhr TL. (1994). Intrapartum chemoprophylaxis of perinatal group B streptococcal infections: a critical review of randomized controlled trials. *Am J Obstet Gynecol*, **170**, 910–917.
94 Rouse DJ, Goldenberg RL, Cliver SP, et al. (1994). Strategies for the prevention of early-onset neonatal group B streptococcal sepsis: a decision analysis. *Obstet Gynecol*, **83**, 483–494.
95 Garland SM and Fliegner JR. (1991). Group B streptococcus (GBS) and neonatal infections: the case for intrapartum chemoprophylaxis. *Aust NZ J Obstet Gynaecol*, **31**, 119–122.
96 Pylipow M, Gaddis M, Kinney JS. (1994). Selective intrapartum prophylaxis for group B streptococcus colonization: management and outcome of newborns. *Pediatrics*, **93**, 631–635.
97 Siegel JD and Cushion NB. (1996). Prevention of early-onset group B streptococcal disease: another look at single-dose penicillin at birth. *Obstet Gynecol*, **87**, 692–698.
98 Siegel JD, McCracken GH Jr, Threlkeld N, et al. (1980). Single-dose penicillin prophylaxis against neonatal group B streptococcal infections. A controlled trial in 18738 newborn infants. *N Engl J Med*, **303**, 769–775.
99 Benitz WE. (1998). The neonatal group B streptococcal debate. *Pediatrics*, **101**, 494–496.
100 Boyer KM and Gotoff SP. (1986). Prevention of early-onset neonatal group B streptococcal disease with selective intrapartum chemoprophylaxis. *N Engl J Med*, **314**, 1665–1669.
101 Gibbs RS, McDuffie RS Jr, McNabb F, et al. (1994). Neonatal group B streptococcal sepsis during 2 years of a universal screening program. *Obstet Gynecol*, **84**, 496–500.
102 Gardner SE, Yow MD, Leeds LJ, et al. (1979). Failure of penicillin to eradicate group B streptococcal colonization in the pregnant woman. A couple study. *Am J Obstet Gynecol*, **135**, 1062–1065.
103 Hall RT, Barnes W, Krishnan L, et al. (1976). Antibiotic treatment of parturient women colonized with group B streptococci. *Am J Obstet Gynecol*, **124**, 630–634.
104 Bland ML, Vermillion ST, Soper DE. (2000). Late third-trimester treatment of rectovaginal group B streptococci with benzathine penicillin G. *Am J Obstet Gynecol*, **183**, 372–376.
105 Pyati SP, Pildes RS, Jacobs NM, et al. (1983). Penicillin in infants weighing two kilograms or less with early-onset Group B streptococcal disease. *N Engl J Med*, **308**, 1383–1389.
106 Yow MD, Mason EO, Leeds LJ, et al. (1979). Ampicillin prevents intrapartum transmission of group B streptococcus. *JAMA*, **241**, 1245–1247.
107 Lim DV, Morales WJ, Walsh AF, et al. (1986). Reduction of morbidity and mortality rates for neonatal group B streptococcal disease through early diagnosis and chemoprophylaxis. *J Clin Microbiol*, **23**, 489–492.
108 Schwartz B, Schuchat A, Oxtoby MJ, et al. (1991). Invasive group B streptococcal disease in adults. A population-based study in metropolitan Atlanta. *JAMA*, **266**, 1112–1114.
109 Heim K, Alge A, Marth C. (1991). Anaphylactic reaction to ampicillin and severe complication in the fetus. *Lancet*, **337**, 859–860.
110 Towers CV, Carr MH, Padilla G, et al. (1998). Potential consequences of widespread antepartal use of ampicillin. *Am J Obstet Gynecol*, **179**, 879–883.
111 Mercer BM, Carr TL, Beazley DD, et al. (1999). Antibiotic use in pregnancy and drug-resistant infant sepsis. *Am J Obstet Gynecol*, **181**, 816–821.
112 Schuchat A, Zywicki SS, Dinsmoor MJ, et al. (2000). Risk factors and opportunities for prevention of early-onset neonatal sepsis: a multicenter case-control study. *Pediatrics*, **105**, 21–26.
113 Kasper DL, Paoletti LC, Wessels MR, et al. (1996). Immune response to type III group B streptococcal polysaccharide-tetanus toxoid conjugate vaccine. *J Clin Invest*, **98**, 2308–2314.
114 Mohle-Boetani JC, Ajello G, Breneman E, et al. (1993). Carriage of *Haemophilus influenzae* type b in children after widespread vaccination with conjugate *Haemophilus influenzae* type b vaccines. *Pediatr Infect Dis J*, **12**, 589–593.
115 Robbins JB, McCracken GH Jr, Gotschlich EC, et al. (1974). *Escherichia coli* K1 capsular polysaccharide associated with neonatal meningitis. *N Engl J Med*, **290**, 1216–1220.
116 Bingen E, Picard B, Brahimi N, et al. (1998). Phylogenetic analysis of *Escherichia coli* strains causing neonatal meningitis suggests horizontal gene transfer from a predominant pool of highly virulent B_2 group strains. *J Infect Dis*, **177**, 642–650.
117 Sarff LD, McCracken GH, Schiffer MS, et al. (1975). Epidemiology of *Escherichia coli* K1 in healthy and diseased newborns. *Lancet*, **1**, 1099–1104.
118 McCracken GH Jr, Sarff LD, Glode MP, et al. (1974). Relation between *Escherichia coli* K1 capsular polysaccharide antigen and clinical outcome in neonatal meningitis. *Lancet*, **2**, 246–250.
119 Guerina NG, Kessler TW, Guerina VJ, et al. (1983). The role of pili and capsule in the pathogenesis of neonatal infection with *Escherichia coli* K1. *J Infect Dis*, **148**, 395–405.
120 Charles D and Larsen B. (1986). Streptococcal puerperal

sepsis and obstetric infections: a historical perspective. *Rev Infect Dis*, **8**, 411–422.

121 Stevens DL, Tanner MH, Winship J, et al. (1989). Severe group A streptococcal infections associated with a toxic shock-like syndrome and scarlet fever toxin A. *N Engl J Med*, **321**, 1–7.

122 Panaro NR, Lutwick LI and Chapnick EK. (1993). Intrapartum transmission of group A streptococcus. *Clin Infect Dis*, **17**, 79–81.

123 Greenberg D, Leibovitz E, Shinnwell ES, et al. (1999). Neonatal sepsis caused by *Streptococcus pyogenes*: resurgence of an old etiology? *Pediatr Infect Dis J*, **18**, 479–481.

124 Macris MH, Hartman N, Murray B, et al. (1998). Studies of the continuing susceptibility of group A streptococcal strains to penicillin during eight decades. *Pediatr Infect Dis J*, **17**, 377–381.

125 Kaplan EL, Johnson DR, Del Rosario MC, et al. (1999). Susceptibility of group A beta-hemolytic streptococci to thirteen antibiotics: examination of 301 strains isolated in the United States between 1994 and 1997. *Pediatr Infect Dis J*, **18**, 1069–1072.

126 Zimbelman J, Palmer A, Todd J. (1999). Improved outcome of clindamycin compared with beta-lactam antibiotic treatment for invasive *Streptococcus pyogenes* infection. *Pediatr Infect Dis J*, **18**, 1096–1100.

127 Norrby-Teglund A, Ihendyane N, Kansal R, et al. (2000). Relative neutralizing activity in polyspecific IgM, IgA, and IgG preparations against group A streptococcal superantigens. *Clin Infect Dis*, **31**, 1175–1182.

128 Dobson SR and Baker CJ. (1990). Enterococcal sepsis in neonates: features by age at onset and occurrence of focal infection. *Pediatrics*, **85**, 165–171.

129 McNeeley DF, Saint-Louis F, Noel GJ. (1996). Neonatal enterococcal bacteremia: an increasingly frequent event with potentially untreatable pathogens. *Pediatr Infect Dis J*, **15**, 800–805.

130 Murray BE. (1990). The life and times of the *Enterococcus*. *Clin Microbiol Rev*, **3**, 46–65.

16

Neonatal bacterial meningitis

Alistair G. S. Philip

Stanford University Medical Center, Stanford, CA, USA

Introduction

The term "meningitis" refers to inflammation of the leptomeninges covering the brain. Bacterial infection of the meninges usually produces a suppurative process or "purulent meningitis." However, it is probably more correct in the newborn infant to consider the condition as bacterial meningoencephalitis, since it is common to have involvement of the cerebral hemispheres as well as involvement of the meninges.

From the clinician's perspective it has been traditional to think of neonatal sepsis (septicemia) and meningitis together, because the clinical manifestations may be indistinguishable. For many years, the proportion of cases of neonatal sepsis that also had documented meningitis was considered to be one-quarter to one-third. For instance, in 1986 it was estimated that one case of neonatal meningitis occurs for every four cases of sepsis.[1] Indeed, this was my personal experience in Vermont between 1975 and 1980, when 12 of 41 cases (29%) with neonatal sepsis in the first week after birth had associated meningitis.[2] However, in recent years the proportion of cases seems to be decreasing to as low as 5%.[3–5] This may be less true in other countries, with 32 of 229 (14%) noted in Israel,[6] and 107 of 577 (18.5%) in Panama.[7]

Incidence

The incidence of neonatal bacterial meningitis will vary from one center to the next, but national studies have shown the incidence to be quite similar (Table 16.1). In the Netherlands,[8] the incidence in 1976–82 was 0.23 per 1000 live births and in England and Wales[9] the incidence in 1985–87 was 0.32 per 1000 live births. The lowest incidence of 0.16–0.17 per 1000 live births was reported from Australia.[5,12] In Sweden, the national incidence fell between 1976 and 1983.[11] More recently, this was true in Australia, with falling rates of sepsis and meningitis in the 1990s.[5] Estimates from earlier years (1960s and 1970s) suggest somewhat higher numbers – 0.46 per 1000 live births in the Collaborative Perinatal Research Project[12] and 0.49 and 0.5 per 1000 live births in two different time periods in Göttingen, Germany.[13] The incidence of sepsis and meningitis is higher in neonates of low birth weight (<2500 g)[12,14,15] and especially very low birth weight (VLBW: <1500 g).[15,16] There is also a slight male preponderance in most reports.

Need for lumbar puncture

It is unusual to encounter meningitis in the first 24 h after delivery[4,17] and because of this, many clinicians elect not to perform a lumbar puncture at that time, particularly when evaluation for sepsis/meningitis is being performed only for risk factors (e.g., prolonged rupture of membranes, maternal fever, etc.).

This issue remains controversial,[17,18] with a paper by Wiswell et al.[19] stimulating a good deal of discussion.[20–23] While there are differences of opinion about the best approach to adopt in the term infant, there is also no uniformity of opinion regarding the VLBW infant.[17] This is because the procedure itself

Table 16.1. Incidence of neonatal bacterial meningitis

Authors	Country	Years	Rate[a]
Overall 1970[12]	USA	1959–66	0.46
Speer et al. 1985[13]	Germany	1962–74	0.49
		1975–82	0.50
Tessin et al. 1990[15]	Sweden	1975–86	0.40
Bennhagen et al. 1987[11]	Sweden	1976	0.36
		1983	0.19
Mulder and Zanen 1984[8]	The Netherlands	1976–82	0.23
De Louvois et al. 1991[9]	England and Wales	1985–87	0.32
Francis and Gilbert 1992[10]	Australia	1987–89	0.17
Hristeva et al. 1993[174]	England	1984–91	0.25
Greenberg et al. 1997[6]	Southern Israel	1986–94	0.45
Isaacs et al. 1999[5]	Australia	1991–97	0.16

Notes:
[a] per 1000 live births.

may cause disruption of normal physiology, may produce a "traumatic tap,"[17] or may be unsuccessful.[24]

Some authors[25–27] have documented an extremely low yield from cerebrospinal fluid (CSF) obtained very early, particularly when performed for features of respiratory distress syndrome, and may add little to blood culture alone. For example, Weisman et al.[16] showed that only 11 of 176 neonates with group B-beta-hemolytic streptococcus (GBS) infection in the first week after birth had positive CSF cultures prior to antibiotic therapy. All had positive blood cultures and seven of the 11 were obtained at less than 12 h of age. On the other hand, Visser and Hall[28] reported that 15% of neonates with meningitis did not demonstrate bacteremia; and an even higher percentage was noted in another study.[29] Wiswell et al.[19] documented that 28% of infants (12 of 43) with meningitis had a negative blood culture, including seven of the eight infants whose mothers received prenatal antibiotics. With an increasing number of women receiving prenatal antibiotics to prevent GBS infection,[20] this does raise some concern, but there may be alternative strategies that can be adopted (see Diagnosis, below). A 5-year analysis of neonatal bacterial sepsis also stressed the possible interference of intrapartum maternal antibiotics in obtaining positive blood cultures, but recorded only five cases of bacterial meningitis and 209 cases of septicemia.[30]

Other authors have had a somewhat different experience, with Hendricks-Munôz and Shapiro[26] reporting that the lumbar puncture was omitted from the admission evaluation of sepsis (within 6 h of birth) during a 7-year period. Among 1390 inborn infants <34 weeks' gestation evaluated for sepsis, 32 had sepsis. Fifteen of them died within 24 h; none had meningitis at postmortem evaluation. The 17 survivors of sepsis also did not have meningitis.

At about the same time, MacMahon et al.[17] evaluated the yield from lumbar puncture in a cohort of 62107 live births at three institutions during 1979–85. Lumbar puncture was only performed on babies with signs and symptoms of severe sepsis (i.e., it was not part of the routine preantibiotic screen). There were 1554 lumbar punctures on 1084 babies, with 17 cases of documented bacterial meningitis (five were <1500 g birth weight and 12 >1500 g). Only three cases of meningitis were encountered on the first day after birth, with only one of a total of 773 VLBW (<1500 g) with meningitis on the first day. They considered "routine" lumbar puncture prior to antibiotics to be questionable and believed that a selective approach to lumbar puncture "is not only justified, but correct."

More recently, Johnson et al. (in 1997)[31] looked at 24452 full-term newborns from 1987 to 1993. There were 3423 (14%) evaluated for risk factors who were asymptomatic. Among this group, 17 (0.5%) were bacteremic, but none had meningitis. An additional 1712 (7%) were evaluated for signs of sepsis, 55 of whom (3.2%) were bacteremic, with 11 cases of meningitis (10 of whom had positive blood cultures). They concluded that lumbar puncture is unnecessary in asymptomatic full-term newborns – a position affirmed by Pong and Bradley in a recent review.[32]

I agree with this approach and, even in the presence of signs of sepsis, would recommend a selective policy on the first day, taking specific signs and markedly abnormal laboratory values into consideration (see Diagnosis, below). After the first day, evaluation for sepsis/meningitis should include a lumbar puncture, in most cases. Particularly when neonates with nonspecific illnesses are seen in an outpatient setting, the need to consider meningitis has recently been emphasized.[33]

Case-fatality

Despite a decrease in meningitis relative to sepsis, the case-fatality rate has remained extremely high until recently. In the Netherlands (1976–82), the rate among 280 cases was 27%.[8] The rate in England and Wales (1985–87) among 450 cases was 20%.[9] Case-fatality rates are usually higher in neonates with Gram-negative infections, with a rate of 32% in England and Wales[9] and a threefold increase compared to Gram-positive infections in another study.[34] On the other hand, a more recent report of a 21-year experience in Dallas indicated a case-fatality rate with Gram-negative bacillary meningitis of 17% for the years 1969 through 1989.[35] It should also be noted that 61% of the survivors in Dallas had long-term sequelae. Even with Gram-positive meningitis the outcome frequently involves impairment. For instance, Edwards et al.[36] evaluated 38 survivors of group B streptococcal meningitis at over 3 years of age. Only 50% were functioning normally. In a recent study from Toronto, Canada, the case-fatality rate was 13% in 101 infants with definitive bacterial meningitis born between 1979 and 1998 and an additional 17% had moderate or severe disability at 1 year of age.[37] The best outcome was recently reported from Greece, where 70 of 72 term infants with Gram-negative bacterial meningitis survived to discharge and survivors had a low incidence of neurologic sequelae.[38] Experience in England and Wales[39] also suggests a marked decrease in case-fatality in recent years (8% in 1996–97), but other countries (less well developed) continue to report high case-fatality rates of 30–40% with a high incidence of neurologic sequelae in survivors.[40–42]

Thus, it is clear that neonatal meningitis remains an important cause of mortality and morbidity. Early diagnosis and treatment remain desirable goals, but prevention may be even more desirable. These areas will be discussed later.

Etiology

Prior to the mid-1970s, *Escherichia coli* was the leading cause of neonatal bacterial meningitis in most developed countries. Even in the period 1975–83, *E. coli* was the leading cause of neonatal meningitis in England and Wales,[43] and the same was true in the Netherlands from 1976 to 1982. However, as long ago as the early 1970s, group B streptococci accounted for 31% of 131 cases of neonatal meningitis and *E. coli* for 38% in the Neonatal Meningitis Co-operative Study.[44] Since the late 1970s, GBS, also known as *Streptococcus agalactiae*, has assumed the dominant role in most countries reporting on the causative organisms of neonatal meningitis. This included Sweden,[11,15] England and Wales,[9,43] Australia,[10] Spain,[45] Canada,[37] South Africa,[46] and Taiwan[34] as well as the USA.[29,34,47] However, Gram-negative bacteria (*Klebsiella* spp. and *E. coli*) continue to predominate in some developing countries,[6,7,14,48] although GBS is increasing.[6,42] Experience from Dallas during 1987–94 indicated that GBS accounted for 52% and *E. coli* for only 9% of 74 cases of neonatal bacterial meningitis. (Trujillo and McCracken, personal communication). On the other hand, in Toronto, Canada, between 1979 and 1998 GBS decreased from 59% to 42% and *E. coli* increased from 22% to 27%.[37] Similar figures were noted in Lyons, France, with GBS in 36% and *E. coli* in 28% during the period 1982–97.[49]

Meningitis due to GBS is usually associated with late-onset infection, generally considered to be more than 5 days after birth, in contrast to the clinical picture of sepsis and pneumonia associated with early-onset infection,[50] although cases of early-onset meningitis certainly occur.[16,50] Similarly, babies infected with *Listeria monocytogenes* are more likely to have meningitis as the most frequent clinical manifestation with late-onset infection.[51,52] Although *L. monocytogenes* is not as prevalent in the USA, it has been an important organism in some countries[53] and has been implicated in epidemics in North America.[54] Indeed, in a report from Kuwait, *L. monocytogenes* was the commonest organism isolated in 45 neonates with bacterial meningitis, accounting for 31% of the total, compared to 15% for GBS and 11% for *E. coli*.[55]

Meningitis due to GBS is most frequently due to serotype III, even with early-onset meningitis. In contrast to a broad distribution of serotypes in neonatal early-onset sepsis, Baker[50] documented that over 85% of early-onset (n=46) and late-onset (n=121) meningitis cases were due to serotype III. Rather similar findings were reported by Carstensen et al.[56] when describing a national study from Denmark, when 77% of early-onset (n=13) and 100% of late-onset (n=18) meningitis cases were type III infections. Experience from the Netherlands showed 57% of GBS meningitis to be the result of type III.[8] Cases of neonatal meningitis attributed to *E. coli* are predominantly the result of those carrying the K_1 capsular antigen.[57] Most reports indicate that 75% of strains of *E. coli* causing neonatal meningitis are K_1 strains and Mulder et al.[58] had 88% K_1 strains.

There are many other organisms that have been implicated in neonatal meningitis, most of which are relatively uncommon. (For extensive lists, with references, see Klein and Marcy,[59] Davies and Rudd,[60] and Pong and Bradley.[32]) It should be noted that the fourth commonest organism in England and Wales was *Streptococcus pneumoniae* (or pneumococcus), which was almost as common as *L. monocytogenes*.[9,43] *Neisseria meningitidis*, which is a frequent etiologic agent in older infants and children, is an uncommon cause of neonatal meningitis[9] but cases continue to be reported.[61] *Hemophilus influenzae*, which was a common causative organism of meningitis in infancy until recently,[47] has also been an uncommon etiologic agent in the neonate and is usually nontypable (not type b), even in years prior to the introduction of *H. influenzae* type b vaccine.

Some organisms have a penchant for causing more difficulty than others. Important among them is *Citrobacter diversus*, which seems to predispose to the development of brain abscess (or abscesses),[62–64] for reasons that are not completely clear.

Pathophysiology and pathology

Bacteremia and susceptibility

Although some cases of neonatal meningitis are encountered without accompanying bacteremia, the most likely route of spread is via blood-stream infection. Indeed, it has been suggested that the magnitude of bacteremia is associated with the occurrence of Gram-negative meningitis.[65] Thus, those factors that predispose to neonatal sepsis (septicemia) may also be considered as risk factors for meningitis.

Infection may be acquired from the mother or may be acquired after birth. Bacteria may also possibly gain access to the meninges by direct spread from the oropharynx. Prenatal risk factors include prolonged rupture of the fetal membranes, particularly if there is evidence of chorioamnionitis, and preterm labor without apparent explanation. Much recent research has linked amniotic fluid infection to preterm labor.[66,67] Male infants seem to be more susceptible to infection than female, with a higher incidence in almost every series. VLBW ($<$1500 g) infants are at particularly high risk (see Introduction, above) and an increased risk for GBS infection has been reported in twins,[68] although this may be related to the higher incidence of preterm delivery with multiple pregnancy. An additional high-risk group is infants with galactosemia, who are particularly susceptible to infection with *E. coli*.[69]

The characteristics of some bacteria seem to be associated with an increased propensity to cause neonatal meningitis.[70] The capsular polysaccharide of GBS type III, *E. coli* K_1 and *L. monocytogenes* serotype IVb all contain sialic acid in high concentration.[71] All these organisms have been closely linked to meningitis. The ability of bacteria to interact with neutrophils may also affect virulence. It has been shown that impaired interaction with neutrophils is characteristic of virulent clones of *E. coli*, more likely to produce invasive infection.[72]

The hospital environment can be particularly hostile for VLBW infants, who may require prolonged intubation with endotracheal tubes or prolonged catheterization of major blood vessels. Central venous catheters in particular seem to predispose to bacteremia, with the possibility of meningitis as a consequence. Another association is the presence of meningitis in a small proportion of infants who develop necrotizing enterocolitis, a condition seen most often in VLBW infants.[73]

Anatomical pathology

Because meningitis is now relatively infrequent, it is necessary to rely on older information for a description of the morphological inflammatory response.[74] Initially (during the first week) polymorphonuclear leukocytes (PMNs) aggregate in a meshwork of fibrin over the outer part of the arachnoid membrane. This exudate may occur over the cerebral hemispheres, but is also found at the base of the brain. Later (second and third week) PMNs decrease, while histiocytes and macrophages increase.[74]

Pathologically, changes in blood vessels are very common, with inflammatory infiltrates leading to thromboses of arachnoidal or subependymal veins. There may be severe congestion or hemorrhagic encephalopathy of the brain substance. This may lead to necrosis of nerve cells and leukomalacia. Additional findings that may help to explain the sequelae among survivors of bacterial meningitis are segmental arteritis of meningeal and perforating branches of the carotid artery, compression or collapse of surface veins by purulent meningeal exudate and by cerebral edema, and phlebitis of cortical veins.[75] The major neuropathological features of neonatal bacterial meningitis are summarized in Table 16.2.

Table 16.2. Neuropathological features of neonatal bacterial meningitis

Acute	Chronic
Arachnoiditis	Cerebral cortical atrophy
Cerebral edema	Developmental defects
Encephalopathy	Hydrocephalus
Infarction	Multicystic encephalomalacia
Vasculitis	Organizational defects
Ventriculitis	White-matter atrophy

Source: Adapted from Volpe.[71]

Cytokines

In recent years, there has been an increased awareness that outcome may be related to circulating humoral factors as well as direct bacterial invasion of the meninges. McCracken et al.[76] demonstrated that many neonates have significant increases in the levels of certain cytokines. In particular, interleukin-1β and tumor necrosis factor-α (cachectin) levels were detected in the CSF of most neonates with Gram-negative bacterial meningitis and peak concentrations of interleukin-1β correlated with outcome. While some cytokines may produce adverse effects, others have been shown to have beneficial effects (e.g., interleukin-10) and could prove useful as adjunctive therapy.[77]

Blood-brain barrier

Another factor that normally plays a role in protection against the spread of bacterial infection is the blood–brain barrier. The permeability of the blood–brain barrier has been shown to increase in stressed neonates and those with bacterial meningitis, when compared to "healthy" infants or neonates with aseptic meningitis.[78] The brain is normally protected from undesirable fluctuations of humoral factors by the blood–CSF–brain barrier, which primarily exists at the arachnoid membranes, the choroid plexus, and the endothelial cells of brain capillaries. The endothelial cells produce continuous tight junctions in the walls of capillaries which act as the barrier, but can be disrupted by hyperosmotic solutions.[79]

The ability of lipopolysaccharide derived from *E. coli* O_{111} B_4 to disrupt the blood–brain barrier has been shown in newborn piglets during experimental neonatal meningitis.[80] This was demonstrated by leakage of sodium fluorescein from blood vessels within about 1 hour of intracisternal injection of lipopolysaccharide. *E. coli* was chosen because this organism remains a frequent cause of meningitis in human newborns. The authors postulate that "the products of Gram-negative organisms could adhere to the adventitial surface of cerebral capillaries, resulting directly in separation of the tight junctions between endothelial cells and a marked increase in pinocytotic activity within the endothelium."[80] This model could prove useful for studying both pathogenesis of neonatal meningitis and also its therapy.

Disruption of the blood–brain barrier with exudation of albumin across the leaky junctions may lead to cerebral edema, with increased intracranial pressure and altered cerebral blood flow. These in turn can produce cranial nerve injury, seizures, and hypoxic–ischemic injury.

There is recent evidence to suggest that genetic factors may contribute to bacterial penetration of the blood–brain barrier. This transcellular penetration (transcytosis) has been demonstrated for GBS, *E. coli* K_1, *L. monocytogenes, Citrobacter freundii,* and *Streptococcus pneumoniae.*[81]

Diagnosis

Clinical features

Bell and McGuinness[75] have noted that there were only occasional publications on neonatal bacterial meningitis in the first half of the twentieth century, with authors stressing the rareness of the condition and the difficulty of clinical diagnosis until the advanced stages were reached. As we enter the twenty-first century, the condition is becoming relatively rare, but any of the clinical features which initiate investigation for sepsis continue to be those that should also raise the possibility of meningitis. These clinical manifestations include lethargy, abdominal distension, respiratory distress, temperature instability, irritability, apnea, or cyanotic spells.[29,35,82,83] When these features cannot be explained by other diagnoses, it is important to evaluate the baby for infection, including a lumbar puncture to obtain cerebrospinal fluid. A recent paper from France notes the nonspecific nature of the clinical presentation in neonates beyond 1 week of age, but emphasizes that fever is almost universal.[49]

Late signs of bacterial meningitis are a bulging anterior fontanel and seizures, although in recent reports seizures were surprisingly common.[35,37,38] Nuchal rigidity is almost never seen in the neonate,[38,49] although a report from Thailand had a high incidence.[39] If investigation of meningitis is not performed until these late signs are seen, serious mortality and morbidity are likely to result.[39] Unfortunately, in many cases of later onset, this is the situation that prevails.

Cerebrospinal fluid

In contrast to older infants and children, CSF obtained early in the course of meningitis may not demonstrate specific cellular changes in the neonate. The interpretation of CSF changes is compounded by the presence of up to 25–30 white blood cells per cubic millimeter (WBC/mm^3) in neonates without infection (Table 16.3) and by the difficulties in obtaining CSF uncontaminated with blood. In the study of Visser and Hall,[28] analysis of CSF samples for cell count was possible in 21 samples from 39 neonates with meningitis on CSF culture. Only 12 of 21 had more than 25 WBC/mm^3, illustrating the importance of sending the fluid for culture in every case where lumbar puncture is performed. It also illustrates that, when infection is suspected, antibiotics should be initiated promptly after specimens for culture have been sent. Decisions about discontinuing antibiotics can be made 48–72 h later.

Culture of CSF remains the "gold standard" as far as diagnosis of bacterial meningitis in the neonate is concerned. As mentioned earlier, it is possible to have a lack of pleocytosis, but to have a positive culture (presumably early in the course of the illness). For this reason, CSF should always be sent for culture. A case has also been made for repeating lumbar punctures when bacteremia is documented, since pleocytosis developed in several infants whose

Table 16.3. Findings in the cerebrospinal fluid (CSF) of noninfected neonates

Authors	*n*	WBC/mm^3 mean (range)	Protein (mg/dl) mean (range)	Glucose (mg/dl) mean (range)	Comment
Naidoo[175]	Term 20	3 (0–9)	47 (27–65)	55 (48–62)	Age 7 days
Escobedo et al.[176]	394	6	180	59	1st week preterm
		3	117	(65% of blood)	4th week preterm
Sarff et al.[177]					*CSF/Blood Glucose*
	Term 87	8.2 (0–32)	90 (20–170)	52 (34–119)	81% (44–248%)
	Preterm 30	9 (0–29)	115 (65–150)	50 (24–63)	74% (55–105%)
Pappu et al.[178]	Term 24	11 (1–38)			
	Preterm 22	7 (0–28)			
Bonadio et al.[179]	Term 35	11 (0–35)	84	47	0–4 weeks
Ahmed et al.[180]	Term 108	7.3 (0–130) only 3 > 20	64	51	0–30 days initial evaluation in Emergency Department

Notes:
WBC, white blood cells.

CSF was initially normal.[84] In cases of meningitis which grow Gram-negative organisms, it is common for the CSF to remain culture-positive for several days.[35] This seems to be less true with Gram-positive organisms, but whenever persistently positive cultures occur, it suggests ventriculitis.

The technique of performing a lumbar puncture (or spinal tap) is important. Care needs to be taken to avoid excessive flexion of the trunk or neck, since this may produce hypoxemia.[85] Although intuitively local anesthesia might seem to lessen physiologic instability, this was not observed in a controlled trial.[86] On the other hand, it seems important to use needles with stylets, since needles without stylets carry the risk of introducing epithelial cells into the spinal canal with subsequent development of epidermoid tumors.[87] Short needles for this purpose are available and allow considerable stability during manipulation.

Examination of CSF microscopically may reveal a specific organism more rapidly than waiting for culture.[88] In one large cooperative study, smear with Gram's stain correctly identified 80% of organisms prior to culture results.[89]

Although it was suggested in older children[90] that CSF C-reactive protein (CRP) levels might help to make a rapid diagnosis of bacterial meningitis, CRP in CSF was not shown to be helpful in neonates.[91,92]

It is also possible to detect bacterial antigen in CSF using either countercurrent immunoelectrophoresis or latex particle agglutination (LPA). The latter is quicker and simpler and has proved quite useful in type III GBS meningitis.[93] Although there is an LPA test for *E. coli* K_1 antigen, which cross-reacts with *Neisseria meningitidis* group B, this has not been shown to be particularly reliable or useful.

Other laboratory evaluations

Additional help in evaluating infants with suspected sepsis and/or meningitis comes from leukocyte counts and CRP measurements. As with any severe infection, total leukocyte counts are frequently low (below 5.0×10^9/l) with increased ratios of immature to total neutrophils.[94] Important observations on the usefulness of serum CRP determinations in bacterial meningitis were published over 25 years ago.[95] The most uniform pattern of high serum CRP values in neonates was seen with cases of *E. coli* meningitis. Marked increases in serum CRP were noted in four cases of neonatal meningitis reported by Sabel and Wadsworth,[96] with three cases seen on the first day after delivery. Although serum CRP may not always be elevated at the initial evaluation for suspected sepsis/meningitis,[94,97,98] it increases reliably in cases of meningitis, sometimes to very high levels within 24–48 h.[94] Pourcyrous et al.[98] documented increased levels of CRP in 11 of 13 (85%) neonates with meningitis at initial evaluation. By 12 h later, all 13 had elevated levels. This was also my experience with 18 cases of neonatal bacterial meningitis seen during the decade 1983–92 (unpublished observations). Consequently, CRP determinations may be particularly helpful if a decision had been made to defer performing a lumbar puncture in an unstable infant. If the serum CRP remains normal, meningitis is virtually eliminated, but if it increases substantially (above 4 mg/dl) lumbar puncture should be performed. This number proved useful in infants over 2 months of age, who had been ill for more that 12 hours and had fever.[99] When CRP was less than 2 mg/dl, all had confirmed or probable viral infection, whereas above 4 mg/dl 79% had bacterial infection.[99]

Imaging studies

The most useful technique for imaging the brain in cases of bacterial meningitis is probably ultrasonographic imaging. This is because it can be accomplished at the bedside (through the anterior fontanel) and considerable experience has accumulated with this technique in the last 20 years.[100–103] It seems likely that magnetic resonance imaging will prove valuable for prognostic purposes, but there is little information available in the literature to date. Computed tomography may also provide better delineation than ultrasonography.[32]

One of the earlier reports of cephalic ultrasonography documented echogenic sulci and possible ventriculitis, as well as multicystic parenchymal change later in the course.[100] More recently, in a series of infants from Toronto, a constellation of abnormalities was documented in the great majority (25 of 34) with pyogenic meningitis.[101] Abnormalities included ventriculomegaly, echogenic sulci, subdural effusion, ventriculitis, infarction, cerebritis, cerebral edema, and porencephalic cysts.[101]

As noted earlier, brain abscess (or abscesses) may be seen more commonly in association with meningitis due to *Citrobacter diversus* and imaging studies are particularly valuable in this context.[65,104]

Antibody to common bacteria

Susceptibility to infection is related to the presence (or absence) of antibody. This has been most strikingly demonstrated with regard to group B streptococcal infection. Vogel et al.[105] documented the lack of serospecific antibody in neonates who acquired GBS infection. The increased susceptibility of VLBW infants is probably related (in part) to decreased transfer of antibody from mother to baby, since transfer of immunoglobulin G occurs predominantly after 32 weeks' gestation.[106] Only immunoglobulin G usually traverses the placenta.

Since meningitis is a serious infection, it would be suspected that survivors would have a significant antibody response. It is therefore interesting to learn that the patterns of response in survivors of type III GBS meningitis were quite variable.[107] In five of 10 infants, specific immunoglobulin M antibody failed to develop at a mean of 3.8 weeks after diagnosis, increased after another 4–8 weeks, and declined to baseline again another 2–4 months later. This inability to sustain an antibody response is akin to the comparatively low response of mothers to unconjugated GBS vaccine.[108]

The prominence of *E. coli* has been attributed to the fact that antibody to this and other Gram-negative organisms is predominantly found in the immunoglobulin M fraction, which does not cross the placenta. However, it has been documented that selective transport of anti-*E. coli* antibody in the immunoglobulin G fraction can provide some protection, even in very preterm infants.[109]

Complications

There are several acute complications that have been reported in association with bacterial meningitis in the neonate. The most frequently reported are ventriculitis, hydrocephalus, and cerebral abscess, but more recently cerebral infarction has been noted in infants with meningitis.[110] Although frequently recognized in older infants, very few cases of inappropriate secretion of antidiuretic hormone have been documented in the neonate.[111,112] A recent report of diabetes insipidus was associated with GBS sepsis/meningitis.[113] This was presumed to be related to brain edema, inflammation, and vasculitis leading to infarction.[113] In a few instances, the inflammatory process and ischemic change may lead to liquefaction of the brain. The author has encountered three such cases, one with GBS[94] and one each with *Streptococcus pneumoniae* and *E. coli* (unpublished). In the latter two cases, a "lava lamp" or "wobbly jello" sign was seen with cephalic ultrasound evaluation when the head was moved.

Because ventriculitis was so commonly encountered with Gram-negative organisms, the first Neonatal Meningitis Co-operative Study Group used intrathecal antibiotics[89] and the second used intraventricular gentamicin.[114] The results of these interventions were no better (and possibly worse) than intravenous antibiotics alone, so that intrathecal or intraventricular therapy is not considered necessary or particularly beneficial. It may be possible to detect ventriculitis using cephalic ultrasound.[102,103]

Hydrocephalus seems to be the result of outflow obstruction secondary to high CSF protein levels. Earlier treatment may possibly minimize this problem, but when it develops (possibly in one-third) it usually requires ventriculoperitoneal shunt repair.[63,115]

As noted earlier, cerebral abscesses seem to be particularly common in association with neonatal meningitis caused by *Citrobacter diversus*.[62] In recent years, the diagnosis has become easier to make because of newer imaging techniques. Cranial ultrasonography, in particular, allows the imaging to be performed at the bedside.[103] Another organism which has been associated with neonatal brain abscesses is *Proteus*. In one series, among 30 cases of brain abscess, 27 were caused by *Proteus* species infections.[116] Many of them were enormous and easily detected with ultrasonography or computed tomography scans. In only 20 cases did meningitis precede the brain abscess.

Ment et al.[110] performed cranial computed tomographic scans on all eight neonates with bacterial meningitis admitted during a 36-month period. Six had large areas of infarction related to major arterial vascular distributions. They suggest that computed tomographic scans be done on all neonates with bacterial meningitis, although magnetic resonance imaging might now be considered. Long-term complications (such as deafness) are discussed in the subsection on neurological sequelae in the outcome section, below.

Treatment and management

Although antibiotic therapy is often referred to as "specific treatment," it should be remembered that antibiotics are used to suppress bacterial growth, so that the baby's defense mechanisms have time to respond. There are many instances where appropriate antibiotic therapy is used, with a sensitive organism, but the baby with sepsis and/or meningitis is overwhelmed by the infection and dies.

In addition, as mentioned earlier, there may be other humoral factors that produce undesirable effects (e.g., cytokines). With Gram-negative enteric organisms there is frequently release of endotoxin and with GBS, "endotoxin-like effects" have been described.[117] The presence of endotoxin was found in the CSF of all infants with Gram-negative bacterial meningitis who died, but was also frequently found in those with an abnormal or normal outcome.[118]

Thus, although antibiotic therapy is very important for the eradication of bacteria, other adjunctive measures may be almost as important in determining survival and in minimizing the long-term sequelae. The two major supportive measures that are used are assisted ventilation (for those infants who develop respiratory failure) and cardiovascular support. It is common with severe infections to have shock and the use of volume (colloid or crystalloid) replacement, as well as pressor agents (such as dopamine) to support blood pressure, may be life-saving. It is also important to recognize (and aggressively treat) seizure activity. In this situation, assisted ventilation may be particularly valuable and there may be benefits from moderate hyperventilation which may decrease increased intracranial pressure. Extreme hypocarbia ($P\text{CO}_2$ less than 20 mmHg) may substantially decrease cerebral blood flow[119] and should probably be avoided.

Choice of antibiotics

The recommendations made by an American Academy of Pediatrics Task Force[1] regarding antibiotic therapy for neonatal meningitis still seem to be valid. Initial antibiotic therapy in the first week after birth seems to be fairly well agreed upon in most developed countries and consists of ampicillin and an aminoglycoside (usually gentamicin). This combination has stood the test of time (somewhat remarkably) and seems to be effective for the most common etiologic bacteria, although this may be changing and the combination of ampicillin and cefotaxime has been suggested more recently.[120] In a retrospective review from Sweden, covering the years 1975–86, of the 365 pathogens isolated from blood and/or CSF, 91% were sensitive to either ampicillin or aminoglycosides or both.[121] Treatment failed in six of 34 patients with neonatal meningitis, but the failure was not related to ampicillin or aminoglycoside resistance.[121] Ampicillin resistance occurred most frequently with late-onset infections in VLBW and low-birth-weight infants,[121] but currently, initial antibiotic therapy after the first week usually includes antistaphylococcal coverage in such infants.

It is often stated that aminoglycosides do not penetrate well into CSF, but in the presence of inflamed meninges the penetration may be better. Certainly, intrathecal administration combined with intravenous gentamicin seemed to offer no advantage over intravenous therapy alone.[89] Nevertheless, one disadvantage of aminoglycosides is that levels may need to be monitored to avoid toxicity, although data about nephrotoxicity and ototoxicity in neonates are limited. Much of what is written concerns potentially toxic concentrations rather than documented permanent sequelae.[122,123]

While there seems to be reasonable unanimity of opinion about ampicillin–aminoglycoside in the first week after birth, this is not the case beyond that age. Another Swedish study has documented (in infants up to 1 year) that ampicillin plus gentamicin is inadequate empiric therapy for meningitis.[124] The combination of ampicillin and ceftazidime has proved superior[125] and cefotaxime has also shown more effective coverage.[124] However, when cefotaxime is incorporated into empiric therapy, it has been shown to increase bacterial resistance.[126]

It should perhaps be noted that the only large-scale evaluation of cephalosporins in the treatment of neonatal meningitis involved moxalactam. It was combined with ampicillin and compared to amikacin and ampicillin. There were no significant differences between groups in the case-fatality rates (23% vs 15%) or the duration of positive CSF cultures (3 days in both groups) in infants with Gram-negative enteric bacillary meningitis.[127] Moxalactam has been virtually abandoned, and replaced by other cephalosporins, because it produced a bleeding tendency. In older infants and children, both cefuroxime and ceftriaxone proved efficacious, with ceftriaxone perhaps superior.[128] However, the prolonged excretion time for ceftriaxone makes it difficult to know what should be its dosing frequency in the neonate.

Prior to the introduction of the cephalosporins, another antibiotic that was deemed to be of considerable value was chloramphenicol. Although it fell out of favor for a number of years following reports of a shock-like syndrome (called the "gray baby syndrome") associated with high doses,[129] it was shown more recently to be quite effective in the management of Gram-negative bacillary meningitis.[130] Nevertheless, in contrast to the cephalosporins, use of chloramphenicol necessitates the determination of levels to accomplish therapeutic, but nontoxic, levels.[130,131] This is certainly a disadvantage, but does not exclude chloramphenicol from the therapeutic armamentarium, if sensitivities suggest that it may

Table 16.4. Antibiotics commonly used in neonatal meningitis and their dosage[a]

	<1 week	>1 week	Frequency
Penicillin G	100000 units	200000 units	b.i.d./q.i.d.
Ampicillin	200 mg	300 mg	b.i.d./q.i.d.
Gentamicin[b] [181]	4 mg load, then	3 mg	Daily
Cefotaxime	100 mg	150 mg	b.i.d./t.i.d.
Vancomycin[b]	30 mg	45 mg	b.i.d./t.i.d.
Chloramphenicol[b]	25 mg	50 mg	Daily/b.i.d.
Nafcillin	50 mg	100 mg	b.i.d./q.i.d.

Notes:

[a] All as per kg per day.

[b] Serum levels need to be monitored.

be the antibiotic of choice. In addition, chloramphenicol is comparatively inexpensive, especially when compared to the cephalosporins. Although frequently used in England and Wales in the mid-1980s, chloramphenicol use has decreased from 50% to less than 5% in the late 1990s.[39] The cost factor may make chloramphenicol particularly valuable in developing countries.

With late-onset infection in VLBW infants, there is the strong possibility of staphylococcal infection. There are now many methicillin-resistant strains of *Staphylococcus aureus* and most hospital-acquired strains of *S. epidermidis* are resistant to the penicillins. With these organisms, it may be possible to use nafcillin or oxacillin,[120] but it is frequently necessary to use vancomycin and in the sick infant beyond the first week it is probably wise to initiate antibiotic treatment with vancomycin and a cephalosporin, although few data are available concerning its use in neonatal meningitis.[132] Vancomycin levels need to be monitored.

Since there is considerable variation from one country to another (and even within countries), it is important to keep track locally of the most frequent organisms causing sepsis and meningitis and to know local antibiotic sensitivities. The more frequently used antibiotics are displayed in Table 16.4. Successful treatment of Gram-negative bacterial meningitis in term neonates was recently reported using cefotaxime and amikacin.[38]

Special mention was made earlier of *Citrobacter diversus* and its propensity to lead to brain abscesses. One report describes the poor response to third-generation cephalosporins, aminoglycosides, and trimethoprim-sulfamethoxazole, but the successful treatment of *C. diversus* meningitis complicated by brain abscesses using imipenem-cilastatin.[133] On the other hand, a favorable outcome has been reported with protracted courses of more traditional antibiotics.[134]

Duration of antibiotics

Since there is reasonable consensus regarding which antibiotics to use in the first week, one might imagine that duration of therapy would also be agreed upon. Unfortunately, although many authors have firm opinions about duration of therapy for neonatal bacterial meningitis, there are very few data upon which to base those opinions. In older infants and children there has been recent reevaluation of the duration of therapy for sepsis/meningitis. In particular, the "7–10–14-day rule" has been called in question.[135] To quote Radetsky:[135] "The numerology of infectious disease has never been investigated. Even in the absence of specific data certain numbers have an unaccountable power to satisfy and reassure, and they are the numbers that are preferentially chosen. For the duration of antimicrobial therapy 7, 10, 14 and 21 days have consistently appeared ... The numbers 7, 10, and 14 are enshrined in the treatment recommendations for meningitis in all current textbooks."

In older infants and children, serum CRP levels have been shown to be helpful in following the course of illness. Peltola[136] in Finland documented that, in uncomplicated cases of bacterial meningitis, CRP levels returned to normal within 7 days. Secondary elevations of CRP may indicate complications such as subdural effusion.[136] A very similar experience was also reported more recently from Chile.[137] Further experience from Finland[138] documented the value of CRP in helping to determine the duration of antibiotic therapy. Although the mean duration was 10 days, it varied from 5.5 to 34 days and antibiotic therapy was not discontinued unless CRP values had normalized.[138]

The ability of serum CRP to distinguish complicated cases from uncomplicated cases of bacterial meningitis in infants and children was also reported from France.[139] All patients were observed in hospital for at least 10 days, but antibiotics were stopped when the patient was clinically well and the CRP was normal. They were able to shorten the duration of antibiotic therapy in the majority of these children to 4–5 days for 21 of 24 with meningococcal meningitis and to 7 days for 16 of 22 with *Haemophilus influenzae* meningitis and four of six with pneumococcal meningitis, without an increase in neurological sequelae. Further data from the Philippines showed that CRP was usually above 5 mg/dl in cases of bacterial meningitis on admission.[140] Mild elevation of CRP may be seen with viral meningitis, but CRP less than 1 mg/dl excluded bacterial meningitis.[140]

Data in neonates are quite limited, but in the early experience of Sabel and Hanson,[95] relapse of meningitis was only encountered (in three cases) when the CRP remained elevated at the time of discontinuance of antibiotics. In my reported experience[94] and unpublished observations, serum CRP was elevated in neonatal meningitis for a minimum of 5 days and not infrequently for more than 10 days. It therefore seems reasonable to discontinue antibiotics within 2–3 days of the CRP level returning to normal (less than 1.0 mg/dl or 10 mg/l). Indeed, Saez-Llorens and McCracken[120] have recently supported this position. While acknowledging traditional and commonly recommended durations of therapy (quite prolonged), they recommend that "duration of antibiotics should be individualized, on the basis of clinical, laboratory and bacteriologic responses. Normalization of the acute-phase reaction (i.e. ESR [erythrocyte sedimentation rate] and CRP) can be considered one index for when antimicrobial therapy could be safely stopped."[120]

Peak levels of CRP with neonatal meningitis are frequently in excess of 10 mg/dl (100 mg/l) and almost always greater than 7.0 mg/dl.[94–96] It is not completely clear whether extremely high levels of CRP (e.g., over 20 mg/dl) can predict an adverse neurological outcome, although limited experience suggests this.[94]

Corticosteroids

The role of corticosteroids in the management of neonatal meningitis is not well defined. Even in infants and children, the benefits of dexamethasone are debated. The arguments for and against have been summarized by Prober.[141] It seems reasonably clear that dexamethasone administered before antibiotics are given is beneficial in meningitis due to *Haemophilus influenzae* type b[142] but the picture is not clear with other organisms, particularly when dexamethasone is given after antibiotics have been started.[143] The rationale for use of corticosteroids is to decrease meningeal inflammation and swelling and to decrease concentrations of potentially harmful cytokines.[143] To date, there is limited experience in neonates. Experience from Australia almost 40 years ago suggested an advantage in steroid-treated neonates, with fewer deaths (9/22 (41%) vs 16/22 (73%)), although development of hydrocephalus or subdural effusions did not seem to be influenced.[144] More recently, Daoud et al.[145] in Jordan performed a randomized controlled trial of dexamethasone use in 52 cases of neonatal bacterial meningitis, the majority being due to *Klebsiella pneumoniae*, and showed no benefit. Of 27 in the dexamethasone group, six died and six had permanent neurological deficit. The control group had 25 neonates, with seven deaths and seven neurologically impaired.[145]

Other antiinflammatory therapy

While there are limited data concerning corticosteroids in neonates, even less is known about most other inflammatory agents which could be used in human bacterial meningitis. Various animal studies have dealt with indometacin, anticytokine antibodies or inhibitors, antiendothelium leukocyte adhesion agents, etc.[120]

Outcome

Case-fatality

It was mentioned in the introduction that case-fatality (mortality) rates are high in almost every series dealing with neonatal bacterial meningitis, although very recent experience provides a more optimistic view.[37–39] Even with the availability of the aminoglycoside antibiotics and improved supportive care, the mortality was high. A report from Sydney, Australia, showed a case-fatality rate of 46% in the early 1970s.[146] The authors noted that this was an improvement in survival compared to earlier reports, but at the expense of increased major neurological sequelae in the survivors.

The national studies from the Netherlands,[8] from England and Wales[9] and from Australia[10] had case-fatality rates of 27%, 20%, and 26% respectively and more recent experience from Dallas[35] documented a case-fatality rate of 17%. My own limited experience in Maine, with 18 cases,[4] was associated with a case-fatality rate of 25% within 1 week of diagnosis and 28% if one late death (5 months later following cerebral infarction) was included. Age at diagnosis may also be important, with higher case-fatality at younger ages. Mulder et al.[58] documented case-fatality rates of 77% at 0–2 days, 28% at 3–6 days, and 15% at 7–27 days in cases of neonatal meningitis caused by *E. coli*. Different rates may also be seen with different strains of *E. coli*. The *E. coli* K1 strains produced a 31% case-fatality rate in one study, vs 0% with non-K1 strains.[147] In addition, case-fatality rates are usually higher in VLBW infants and those with a high CSF protein.[45]

More recently, data from England and Wales documented a case-fatality rate in 1996–97 of only 8%.[39] Experience in Toronto, Canada, for 1979–98 revealed a case-fatality rate of 13%[37] and in Athens, Greece, the rate was only 3% for Gram-negative bacterial meningitis during the period 1983–97.[38] These data are summarized in Table 16.5.

Neurological sequelae

The high percentage of major neurological sequelae in survivors was noted by Lewis and Gupta[146] and emphasized in a series of papers in the mid-1980s dealing with GBS meningitis.[36,57,147,148] With case-fatality rates varying between 26% and 38%, major neurological sequelae were found in 15–29% of the survivors (Table 16.6). Edwards et al.[36] summarized the long-term sequelae of several groups reporting on GBS meningitis. Of a total of 218, the case-fatality was 26% and, of the 152 survivors, 17% had major neurodevelopmental sequelae, 16% had mild/moderate sequelae, and 67% were considered normal. More recent experience is not dissimilar.[37,39]

In their review in 1982, Bell and McGuinness[75] noted that sequelae had been reported in 31–56% of survivors in different reports. Almost identical figures were reported from Stockholm, Sweden, for 5-year periods from 1969–83, with sequelae from neonatal meningitis noted in 31–53% of survivors, and case-fatality rates of 23–35%.[149] The highest rate of sequelae accompanied the lowest case-fatality rate.

The most common severe sequelae include "hydrocephalus, seizures, mental retardation, hyperactivity and cranial nerve or long tract signs. Localized deficits include hearing loss, optic atrophy and hypothalamic injury manifested by endocrine

Table 16.5. Case-fatality rate for neonatal meningitis

Author	Country	Years	Number	Case-fatality (%)	Neurological sequelae (%)[a]	Predominant bacteria
Mulder and Zanen 1984[8]	The Netherlands	1976–82	380	27	N/A	*Escherichia coli*
Longe et al. 1984[14]	Nigeria (Benin City)	1974–82	53	38	N/A	*Escherichia coli, Staphylococcus aureus*
Bennet et al. 1989[149]	Sweden (Stockholm)	1969–83	60	28	40	*Staphylococcus aureus*[b]
Bell et al. 1989[182]	N. Ireland (Belfast)	1973–86	41	49	38	*Escherichia coli*
DeLouvois et al. 1991[9]	England and Wales	1985–87	280	25	20	GBS, *Escherichia coli*
Francis and Gilbert 1992[10]	Australia	1987–89	116	26	23	GBS, *Escherichia coli*
Unhanand et al. 1993[35]	USA (Dallas)	1969–89	98	17	61	*Escherichia coli*
Chotpitayasunondh 1994[41]	Thailand (Bangkok)	1980–90	77	45	N/A	*Pseudomonas aeruginosa*
		1987–90		(26)		*Klebsiella pneumoniae*
Daoud et al. 1996[40]	Jordan	1992–94	53	32	39	*Klebsiella pneumoniae*
Gebremariam 1998[48]	Ethiopia (Addis Ababa)	10 years	55	40	21	*Klebsiella pneumoniae, Escherichia coli, Enterobacter* species
Molyneux et al. 1998[42]	Malawi (Blantyre)	1996–97	61	40	N/A	GBS, *Salmonella typhimurium*
Harvey et al. 1999[39]	England and Wales	1996–97	119	8	N/A	GBS
Klinger et al. 2000[37]	Canada (Toronto)	1979–98	101	13	26	GBS
Dellagrammaticas et al. 2000[38]	Greece (Athens)	1983–97	72	3	8	*Escherichia coli*

Notes:

N/A, not available; GBS, group B beta-hemolytic streptococcus.

[a] percent of survivors.

[b] Cases of sepsis, N/A for meningitis.

Table 16.6. Outcome in infants with group B beta-hemolytic streptococcus (GBS) meningitis

Authors	Age at diagnosis	Case-fatality	Number of survivors	Major neurological sequelae	Age at follow-up
Chin and Fitzhardinge[150]	0–7 days	26%	20	3 (15%)[a]	1½–7 years
Carstensen et al.[56]	0–12 weeks	26%	26	6 (23%)	3 months–5 years
Edwards et al.[36]	0–3 months	38%	38	11 (29%)	3.3–9.0 years
Wald et al.[148]	0–6 months	27%	54	9 (17%)	3–18 years
Klinger et al.[37]	1–28 days	13%[b]	50	15(30%)	1–19 years
Harvey et al.[39]	0–28 days	25%	65	12(18%)	5 years

Notes:

[a] Percentages of survivors.

[b] Based on all cases, not just GBS.

deficiencies, diabetes insipidus, precocious puberty or abnormalities of temperature regulation".[75] In addition, spastic paresis (hemiplegia or quadriplegia) is frequently mentioned.[36,146–148,150,151]

In the large experience with Gram-negative enteric bacillary meningitis reported by Unhanand et al.,[35] hydrocephalus, seizure disorder, cerebral palsy, developmental delay, and hearing loss were seen in 28%, 28%, 19%, 25%, and 16% respectively in 32 term infants and 36%, 36%, 45%, 55%, and 18% respectively in 11 preterm infants who survived. On the other hand, more recently, Dellagrammaticas et al.[38] reported both a high survival rate and a low incidence of sequelae, with persisting seizures, spastic paralysis, developmental delay, and hearing deficit in 4%, 3%, 4%, and 6% respectively. Delay in achieving sterile CSF may increase the frequency of sequelae.[38]

Clinical manifestations on admission that were predictive of a poor outcome (death or severe impairment) in the study of Edwards et al.[36] were presence of coma or semicoma, decreased perfusion, total peripheral WBC count $<5.0\times10^9$/l, absolute neutrophil count $<1.0\times10^9$/l or CSF protein >3 g/l. The recent study by Klinger et al.[37] showed that the best predictors of an adverse outcome were quite similar. Both at 12 h and 96 h after admission, seizures, coma, use of inotropes to maintain blood pressure and leukopenia ($<5.0\times10^9$/l) were predictive of a poor outcome. Of 101 infants (born in the years 1979–98)with bacterial meningitis, 13 died and 17 others had moderate-to-severe disability at 1 year of age.[37] Among 50 infants with GBS meningitis, 15 (30%) had an adverse outcome.

As noted earlier, McCracken et al.[76] suggested that peak concentrations of interleukin-1β correlated with outcome. Klein et al.[1] suggested that a cautiously optimistic note be struck with parents when discussing the long-term complications of meningitis, since "there is a tendency for even major neurologic defects to resolve unpredictably with time."

Prevention

Before discussing the potential for preventing specific kinds of meningitis, it should be remembered that general infection control measures (especially careful hand washing) may be particularly important in preventing the spread of infection. Even in recent years, there have been reports of nosocomial spread of meningitis due to unusual organisms such as *Campylobacter jejuni*,[152] *Citrobacter diversus*,[153] and *Serratia marcescens*.[154] These organisms may also produce devastating effects on the brain.

Attempts to prevent neonatal bacterial meningitis have largely dealt with those organisms that are frequently implicated. There are two major strategies that have been employed. The first is chemoprophylaxis and the second is immunoprophylaxis. Both strategies have been used to prevent neonatal sepsis and meningitis, rather than specifically preventing meningitis. In keeping with the important role it plays in many countries, GBS infection has received the most attention.

Neonatal approach

Both chemo- and immunoprophylaxis have been evaluated from the maternal or neonatal approach. While there has been some success using the maternal approach, using only the neonatal approach has been contradictory or disappointing. For instance, prophylactic administration of penicillin to neonates seemed to be beneficial in reducing GBS infection in some centers,[155] but not in others.[156] There was also the possibility that one problem (early-onset GBS infection) might be exchanged for another (late-onset GBS or Gram-negative bacterial infection). Similarly, the use of prophylactic intravenous immunoglobulin in VLBW infants seemed beneficial in one large ($n=588$) study,[157] but not in an even larger ($n=2416$) study.[158] Different preparations were used in the two studies, which may explain the differences. Another large study ($n=753$), using the same preparation as Fanaroff et al.,[158] also failed to find a protective effect in early-onset or late-onset infection.[159,160] It has been documented that considerable variability of availability of specific antibody to the common pathogens occurs within different lots of immunoglobulin.[161] Greater success seems likely if preparations with species-specific antibody can be administered.

Maternal approach

The use of maternal chemoprophylaxis has proved to be much more striking. The study of Yow et al.[162] documented that intravenous ampicillin given to the mother during labor could prevent transmission of GBS to the baby. This was strongly supported by the work of Boyer and Gotoff,[163] with bacteremia in none of 85 babies born to ampicillin-treated women vs five of 79 babies born to untreated mothers. Although this strategy does not prevent transmission of infection in all cases,[164] there seems to be a consensus that women at high risk (rupture of membranes longer than 18 h, preterm labor, or maternal fever possibly caused by choriamnionitis) should be screened and treated.

Since the publication by the CDC in 1996 of new guidelines[165] for the prevention of GBS infection based on this consensus, there has been a substantial change in obstetrical practice in North America with approximately 25% of women receiving intrapartum antibiotics (penicillin or ampicillin).[166] This has led to a marked decrease in the incidence of early-onset GBS infection, with a 65% decrease from 1.7 cases per 1000 live births in 1993 to 0.6 cases per 1000 live births in 1998. Only 6% with early-onset GBS infection had meningitis.[166] This contrasts with a study from Finland, where 17% had meningitis in 1985–94.[167] To date, this increased use of intrapartum antibiotics has not changed antibiotic sensitivity patterns substantially, although it has created some difficulty in deciding which neonates should be treated after delivery.[168]

With regard to maternal immunoprophylaxis, there is variable enthusiasm. While intuitively it would seem that this might be the most effective strategy, there are several possible drawbacks. One significant disadvantage is that, since transfer of antibody from mother to infant occurs primarily after 32 weeks' gestation, the group of infants at greatest risk might not be protected. Another disadvantage (to date) is that the response of women to a polysaccharide vaccine of GBS has been disappointing.[108] Of 35 women with low or unprotected antibody levels before immunization, only 20 (57%) responded to the vaccine in a study published in 1988.[108] This study used type III capsular polysaccharide vaccine. While it is true that this serotype accounts for the majority of cases of neonatal meningitis, it would be preferable to have a polyvalent vaccine with increased immunogenicity.[169,170] The many problems in finding and distributing a suitable vaccine have been discussed.[170] One approach that has shown promise is to increase the immunogenicity of vaccines by conjugating (coupling) them to tetanus toxoid or other agents.[171–173] Polyvalent conjugate vaccines for GBS infection have been tested and may soon be commercially available. With other organisms, particularly *E. coli*, the ability to provide protection by maternal immunization seems a daunting prospect.

Conclusion

Despite the fact that the incidence of neonatal bacterial meningitis may be falling, there is little room for complacency. This is a disease with very high case-fatality rates and morbidity rates. The neurological sequelae can be quite devastating in some cases and a completely normal outcome can be anticipated in only half of the survivors. It is therefore important to consider the possibility of sepsis/meningitis in any sick neonate, so that treatment can be initiated as early as possible. However, prevention is even more desirable and continued efforts in this direction must remain a high priority.

REFERENCES

1 Klein JO, Feigin RD and McCracken GH Jr. (1986). Report on the task force on diagnosis and management of meningitis. *Pediatrics*, **78** (suppl.), 959–982.

2 Philip AGS. (1985). *Neonatal Sepsis and Meningitis*, Appendix. Boston: G.K. Hall.

3 Hack M, Horbar JD, Malloy MH, Tyson JE, Wright E, Wright L. (1991). Very low birth weight outcomes of the National Institutes of Child Health and Human Development Neonatal Network. *Pediatrics*, **87**, 587–597.

4 Philip AGS. (1994). The changing face of neonatal infection: experience at a regional medical center. *Pediatr Infect Dis J*, **13**, 1098–1102.

5 Isaacs D and Royle JA for the Australia Study Group for Neonatal Infections. (1999). Intrapartum antibiotics and early onset neonatal sepsis caused by group B streptococcus and by other organisms in Australia. *Pediatr Infect Dis J*, **18**, 524–528.

6 Greenberg D, Shinwell ES, Yagupsky P, et al. (1997). A prospective study of neonatal sepsis and meningitis in southern Israel. *Pediatr Infect Dis J*, **16**, 768–773.

7 Moreno MT, Vargas S, Poveda R, et al. (1994). Neonatal sepsis and meningitis in a developing Latin American country. *Pediatr Infect Dis J*, **13**, 516–520.

8 Mulder CJJ and Zanen HC. (1984). A study of 280 cases of neonatal meningitis in the Netherlands. *J Infect*, **9**, 177–184.

9 De Louvois J, Blackbourn J, Hurley R, et al. (1991). Infantile meningitis in England and Wales: a two year study. *Arch Dis Child*, **66**, 603–607.

10 Francis BM and Gilbert GL. (1992). Survey of neonatal meningitis in Australia: 1987–1989. *Med J Aust*, **156**, 240–243.

11 Bennhagen R, Svenningsen NW and Békássy AN. (1987). Changing pattern of neonatal meningitis in Sweden: a comparative study 1976 vs 1983. *Scand J Infect Dis*, **19**, 587–593.

12 Overall JC Jr. (1970). Neonatal bacterial meningitis: analysis of predisposing factors and outcome compared with matched control subjects. *J Pediatr*, **76**, 499–511.

13 Speer CP, Hauptmann D, Stubbe P, et al. (1985). Neonatal septicemia and meningitis in Göttingen, West Germany. *Pediatr Infect Dis J*, **4**, 36–41.

14 Longe AC, Omene JA and Okolo AA. (1984). Neonatal meningitis in Nigerian infants. *Acta Paediatr Scand*, **73**, 477–481.

15 Tessin I, Trollfors B and Thiringer K. (1990). Incidence and etiology of neonatal septicemia and meningitis in western Sweden 1975–1986. *Acta Paediatr Scand*, **79**, 1023–1030.

16 Weisman LE, Stoll BJ, Cruess DF, et al. (1992). Early-onset group B streptococcal sepsis: a current assessment. *J Pediatr*, **121**, 428–433.

16 Hristeva L, Booy R, Bowler I, et al. (1993). Prospective surveillance of neonatal meningitis. *Arch Dis Child*, **69**, 14–18.

17 MacMahon P, Jewes L and de Louvois J. (1990). Routine lumbar punctures in the newborn – are they justified? *Eur J Pediatr*, **149**, 797–799.

18 Halliday HL. (1989). When to do a lumbar puncture in a neonate. *Arch Dis Child*, **64**, 313–316.

19 Wiswell TE, Baumgart S, Gannon CM, et al. (1995). No lumbar puncture in the evaluation for early neonatal sepsis: will meningitis be missed? *Pediatrics*, **95**, 803–806.

20 Tierney AJ and Finer NN. (1996). Lumbar puncture in the evaluation for early neonatal sepsis. *Pediatrics*, **97**, 929–930.

21 Beeram M, Oltorf C and Cipriani C.(1996). Lumbar puncture in the evaluation for early neonatal sepsis. *Pediatrics*, **97**, 930.

22 Boyer KM and Gotoff SP. (1996). Lumbar puncture in meningitis? *Pediatrics*, **98**,166.

23 Escobar GJ. (1996). Lumbar puncture in meningitis? *Pediatrics*, **98**, 166–167.

24 Weiss MG, Ionides SP and Anderson CL. (1991). Meningitis in premature infants with respiratory distress: role of admission lumbar puncture. *J Pediatr*, **119**, 973–975.

25 Eldadah M, Frenkel LD, Hiatt IM, et al. (1987). Evaluation of routine lumbar punctures in newborn infants with respiratory distress syndrome. *Pediatr Infect Dis J*, **6**, 243–245.

26 Hendricks-Munôz KD and Shapiro DL. (1990). The role of the lumbar puncture in the admission sepsis evaluation of the premature infant. *J Perinatol*, **10**, 60–64.

27 Schwersenski J, McIntyre L and Bauer CR. (1991). Lumbar puncture frequency and cerebrospinal fluid analysis in the neonate. *Am J Dis Child*, **145**, 54–58.

28 Visser VE and Hall RT. (1980). Lumbar puncture in the evaluation of suspected neonatal sepsis. *J Pediatr*, **96**, 1063–1067.

29 Shattuck KE and Chonmaitree T. (1992). The changing spectrum of neonatal meningitis over a fifteen-year period. *Clin Pediatr*, **31**, 130–136.

30 Sanghvi KP and Tudehope DI. (1996). Neonatal bacterial sepsis in a neonatal intensive care unit: a 5 year analysis. *J Paediatr Child Health*, **32**, 333–338.

31 Johnson CE, Whitwell JK, Pethe K, et al. (1997). Term newborns who are at risk for sepsis: are lumbar punctures necessary? *Pediatrics*, **99**, E10

32 Pong A and Bradley JS. (1999). Bacterial meningitis and the newborn infant. *Infect Dis Clin North Am*, **13**, 711–733.

33 Albanyan EA and Baker CJ. (1998). Is lumbar puncture necessary to exclude meningitis in neonates and young infants: lessons from the group B streptococcus cellulitis–adenitis syndrome. *Pediatrics*, **102**, 985–986.

34 Franco SM, Cornelius VE and Andrews B.F. (1992). Long-term outcome of neonatal meningitis. *Am J Dis Child*, **146**, 567–571.

35 Unhanand M, Mustafa MM, McCracken GH Jr, et al. (1993). Gram-negative enteric bacillary meningitis: a twenty-one-year experience. *J Pediatr*, **122**, 15–21.

36 Edwards MS, Rench MA, Haffar AAM, et al. (1985). Long-term sequelae of group B streptococcal meningitis in infants. *J Pediatr*, **106**, 717–722.

37 Klinger G, Chin C-N, Beyene J, et al. (2000). Predicting the outcome of neonatal bacterial meningitis. *Pediatrics*, **106**, 477–482.

38 Dellagrammaticas HD, Christodoulou C, Megaloyanni E, et al. (2000). Treatment of gram-negative bacterial meningitis in term neonates with third generation cephalosporins plus amikacin. *Biol Neonate*, **77**, 139–146.

39 Harvey D, Holt DE and Bedford H. (1999). Bacterial meningitis in the newborn: a prospective study of mortality and morbidity. *Semin Perinatol*, **23**, 218–225.

40 Daoud AS, al-Sheyyab M, Abu-Ekteish F, et al. (1996). Neonatal meningitis in northern Jordan. *J Trop Pediatr*, **42**, 267–270.

41 Chotpitayasunondh T. (1994). Bacterial meningitis in children: etiology and clinical features, an 11 year review of 618 cases. *SE Asian J Trop Med Pub Health*, **25**, 107–115.

42 Molyneux E, Walsh A, Phiri A, et al. (1998). Acute bacterial meningitis in children admitted to the Queen Elizabeth Central Hospital, Blantyre, Malawi in 1996–97. *Trop Med Int Health*, **3**, 610–618.

43 Synnott MD, Morse DL and Hall SM. (1994). Neonatal meningitis in England and Wales: a review of routine national data. *Arch Dis Child*, **71**, F75–F80.

44 Howard JB and McCracken GH Jr. (1974). The spectrum of group B streptococcal infections in infancy. *Am J Dis Child*, **128**, 815–818.

45 Hervás JA, Alomer A, Salvá F, et al. (1993). Neonatal sepsis and meningitis in Mallorca, Spain, 1977–91. *Clin Infect Dis*, **16**, 719–724.

46 Nel E. (2000). Neonatal meningitis: mortality, cerebrospinal fluid, and microbiological findings. *J Trop Pediatr*, **46**, 237–239.

47 Dawson KG, Emerson JC and Burns JL. (1999). Fifteen years of experience with bacterial meningitis. *Pediatr Infect Dis J*, **18**, 816–822.

48 Gebremariam A. (1998). Neonatal meningitis in Addis Ababa: a 10 year review. *Ann Trop Paediatr*, **18**, 279–283.

49 Zanelli S, Gillet Y, Stamm D, et al. (2000). Bacterial meningitis in infants 1 to 8 weeks old (article in French). *Arch Pediatr*, suppl. 3, 565s-571s.

50 Baker CJ. (1979). Group B streptococcal infections in neonates. *Pediatr Rev*, **1**, 5–15.

51 Annotation. (1980). Perinatal listeriosis. *Lancet*, **i**, 911.

52 Mulder CJJ and Zanen HC. (1986). *Listeria monocytogenes* neonatal meningitis in the Netherlands. *Eur J Pediatr*, **145**, 60–62.

53 Relier JP, Amiel-Tison C, Krauel J, et al. (1977). Listériose néonatale: à propos de 53 cas. *J Gynecol Obstet Biol Reprod*, **6**, 367–381.

54 Linnan MJ, Mascola L, Lou XD, et al. (1988). Epidemic listeriosis associated with Mexican-style cheese. *N Engl J Med*, **319**, 823–828.

55 Zaki M, Daoud AS, al Saleh Q, et al. (1990). Bacterial meningitis in the newborn: a Kuwaiti experience. *J Trop Pediatr*, **36**, 62–65.

56 Carstensen H, Henrichsen J and Jepsen OB. (1985). A national survey of severe group B streptococcal infections in neonates and young infants in Denmark, 1978–83. *Acta Paediatr Scand*, **74**, 934–941.

57 Robbins JB, McCracken GH Jr, Gotschlich EC, et al. (1974). *Escherichia coli* K1 capsular polysaccharide associated with neonatal meningitis. *N Engl J Med*, **290**, 1216–1220.

58 Mulder CJJ, van Alphen L and Zanen HC. (1984). Neonatal meningitis caused by *Escherichia coli* in the Netherlands. *J Infect Dis*, **150**, 935–940.

59 Klein JO and Marcy SM. (1990). Bacterial sepsis and meningitis. In *Infectious Diseases of the Fetus and Newborn Infant*, 3rd edn, eds. Remington JS and Klein JO, pp. 601–656. Philadelphia:W.B. Saunders.

60 Davies PA and Rudd PT. (1994). *Neonatal Meningitis, Clinics in Developmental Medicine* no. 132. London: MacKeith Press.

61 Arango CA and Rathore MH. (1996). Neonatal meningococcal meningitis: case reports and review of literature. *Pediatr Infect Dis J*, **15**, 1134–1136.

62 Graham DR and Band JD. (1981). *Citrobacter diversus* brain abscess and meningitis in neonates. *JAMA*, **245**, 1923–1925.

63 Kairam R and De Vivo DC. (1981). Neurologic manifestations of congenital infection. *Clin Perinatol*, **81**, 445–465.

64 Tse G, Silver M, Whyte H, et al. (1997). Neonatal meningitis and multiple brain abscesses due to *Citrobacter diversus*. *Pediatr Pathol Lab Med*, **17**, 977–982.

65 Dietzman DE, Fischer GW and Schoenknecht FD. (1974). Neonatal *Escherichia coli* septicemia – bacterial counts in blood. *J Pediatr*, **85**, 128–130.

66 Drife J. (1989). Infection and preterm birth. *Br J Obstet Gynecol*, **96**, 1128–1132.

67 Goldenberg RL, Hauth JC and Andrews WW. (2000). Intrauterine infection and preterm delivery. *N Engl J Med*, **342**, 1500–1507.

68 Edwards MS, Jackson CV and Baker CJ. (1981). Increased risk of group B streptococcal disease in twins. *JAMA*, **245**, 2044–2046.

69 Levy HL, Sepe SJ, Shih VE, et al. (1977). Sepsis due to *Escherichia coli* in neonates with galactosemia. *N Engl J Med*, **297**, 823–825.

70 Bingen E, Bonacorsi S, Brahimi N, et al. (1997). Virulence

patterns of *Escherichia coli* K1 strains associated with neonatal meningitis. *J Clin Microbiol*, **35**, 2981–2982.
71 Volpe JJ. (1987). Bacterial meningitis. In *Neurology of the Newborn*, ed. Volpe JJ, pp. 596–623. Philadelphia: W.B. Saunders.
72 Öhman L, Tullus K, Katouli M, et al. (1995). Correlation between susceptibility of infants to infection and interaction with neurotrophils of *Escherichia coli* strains, causing neonatal and infantile septicemia. *J Infect Dis*, **171**, 128–133.
73 Kliegman RM and Walsh MC. (1987). The incidence of meningitis in neonates with necrotizing enterocolitis. *Am J Perinatol*, **4**, 245–248.
74 Berman P and Banker B (1966). Neonatal meningitis: a clinical and pathological study of 29 cases. *Pediatrics*, **38**, 6–24.
75 Bell WE and McGuinness GA. (1982). Suppurative central nervous system infections in the neonate. *Semin Perinatol*, **6**, 1–24.
76 McCracken GH.Jr, Mustafa MM, Ramilo O, et al. (1989). Cerebrospinal fluid interleukin 1-beta and tumor necrosis factor concentrations and outcome from neonatal gram-negative enteric bacillary meningitis. *Pediatr Infect Dis J*, **8**, 155–159.
77 Cairo MS. (1991). Cytokines: a new immunotherapy. *Clin Perinatol*, **18**, 343–359.
78 Anagnostakis D, Messaritakis J, Damianos D, et al. (1992). Blood–brain barrier permeability in "healthy," infected and stressed neonates. *J Pediatr*, **121**, 291–294.
79 Goldstein GW, Robertson P and Betz AL. (1988). Update on the role of the blood–brain barrier in damage to immature brain. *Pediatrics*, **81**, 732–734.
80 Temesvari P, Abraham CS, Speer CP, et al. (1993). *Escherichia coli* O111 B4 lipopolysaccharide given intracisternally induces blood–brain barrier opening during experimental neonatal meningitis in piglets. *Pediatr Res*, **34**, 182–186.
81 Huang S, Stins MF and Kim KS. (2000). Bacterial penetration across the blood–brain barrier during the development of neonatal meningitis. *Microbes Infect*, **2**, 1237–1244.
82 Chang Chien HY, Chiu NC, Li WC, et al. (2000). Characteristics of neonatal bacterial meningitis in a teaching hospital in Taiwan from 1984–1997. *J Microbiol Immunol Infect*, **33**, 100–104.
83 Perlman JM, Rollins N and Sanchez PJ. (1992). Late-onset meningitis in sick, very-low-birth weight infants: clinical and sonographic observations. *Am J Dis Child*, **146**, 1297–1301.
84 Sarman G, Moise AA and Edwards MS. (1995). Meningeal inflammation in neonatal Gram-negative bacteremia. *Pediatr Infect Dis J*, **14**, 701–704.
85 Weisman LE, Merenstein GB and Steenbarger JR. (1983). The effect of lumbar puncture position in sick neonates. *Am J Dis Child*, **137**, 1077–1079.
86 Porter FL, Miller JP, Cole FS, et al. (1991). A controlled clinical trial of local anesthesia for lumbar puncture in newborns. *Pediatrics*, **88**, 663–669.
87 Halcrow SJ, Crawford PJ and Craft AW. (1985). Epidermoid spinal cord tumour after lumbar puncture. *Arch Dis Child*, **60**, 978–979.
88 Marks MI and Welch DF. (1981). Diagnosis of bacterial infections of the newborn infants. *Clin Perinatol*, **8**, 537–558.
89 McCracken GH Jr and Mize SG. (1976). A controlled study of intrathecal antibiotic therapy in gram negative enteric meningitis of infancy: report of the Neonatal Meningitis Co-operative Study Group. *J Pediatr*, **89**, 66–72.
90 Corrall CJ, Pepple JM, Moxon ER, et al. (1981). C-reactive protein in spinal fluid of children with meningitis. *J Pediatr*, **99**, 365–369.
91 Philip AGS and Baker CJ. (1983). Cerebrospinal fluid C-reactive protein in neonatal meningitis. *J Pediatr*, **102**, 715–717.
92 Ben Gershõm E, Briggeman-Mol GJJ and de Zegher F. (1986). Cerebrospinal fluid C-reactive protein in meningitis: diagnostic value and pathophysiology. *Eur J Pediatr*, **145**, 246–249.
93 Edwards MS, Kasper DL and Baker CJ. (1979). Rapid diagnosis of type III group B streptococcal meningitis by latex particle agglutination. *J Pediatr*, **95**, 202–205.
94 Philip AGS. (1985). Response of C-reactive protein in neonatal group B streptococcal infection. *Pediatr Infect Dis J*, **4**, 145–148.
95 Sabel KG and Hanson LA. (1974). The clinical usefulness of C-reactive protein (CRP) determinations in bacterial meningitis and septicemia in infancy. *Acta Paediatr Scand*, **63**, 381–388.
96 Sabel KG and Wadsworth C. (1979). C-reactive protein (CRP) in early diagnosis of neonatal septicemia. *Acta Paediatr Scand*, **68**, 825–831.
97 Mathers NJ and Pohlandt F. (1987). Diagnostic audit of C-reactive protein in neonatal infection. *Eur J Pediatr*, **146**, 147–151.
98 Pourcyrous M, Bada HS, Korones SB, et al. (1993). Significance of serial C-reactive protein responses in neonatal infection and other disorders. *Pediatrics*, **92**, 431–435.
99 Putto A, Ruuskanen O, Meurman O, et al. (1986). C-reactive protein in the evaluation of febrile illness. *Arch Dis Child*, **61**, 24–29.

100 Han BK, Babcock DS and McAdams L. (1985). Bacterial meningitis in infants: sonographic findings. *Radiology*, **154**, 645–650.

101 Raju VSN, Rao MN and Rao VSRM. (1995). Cranial sonography in pyogenic meningitis in neonates and infants. *J Trop Pediatr*, **41**, 68–73.

102 Horbar JD, Philip AGS and Lucey JF. (1980). Ultrasound scan in neonatal ventriculitis. *Lancet*, **i**, 976.

103 Hill A, Shackelford GD and Volpe JJ. (1981). Ventriculitis with neonatal bacterial meningitis: identification by real-time ultrasound. *J Pediatr*, **99**, 133–136.

104 Wilson DA, Nguyen DL and Marshall K. (1988). Sonography of brain abscesses complicating *Citrobacter* neonatal meningitis. *Am J Perinatol*, **5**, 37–39.

105 Vogel LC, Boyer KM, Gadzala CA, et al. (1980). Prevalence of type-specific group B streptococcal antibody in pregnant women. *J Pediatr*, **96**, 1047–1051.

106 Sidiropoulos D, Hermann U, Morell A, et al. (1986). Transplacental passage of intravenous immunoglobulin in the last trimester of pregnancy. *J Pediatr*, **109**, 505–508.

107 Edwards MS, Hall MA, Rench MA, et al. (1990). Patterns of immune response among survivors of group B streptococcal meningitis. *J Infect Dis*, **161**, 65–70.

108 Baker CJ, Rench MA, Edwards MS, et al. (1988). Immunization of pregnant women with a polysaccharide vaccine of group B streptococcus. *N Engl J Med*, **319**, 1180–1185.

109 Sennhauser FH, Balloch A, Mac Donald RA, et al. (1990). Materno-fetal transfer of IgG anti-*Escherichia coli* antibodies with enhanced avidity and opsonic activity in very premature neonates. *Pediatr Res*, **27**, 365–371.

110 Ment LR, Ehrenkranz RA and Duncan CC (1986). Bacterial meningitis as an etiology of perinatal cerebral infarction. *Pediatr Neurol*, **2**, 276–279.

111 Sloane E. (1989). Transient diabetes insipidus following listeria meningitis. *Irish Med J*, **82**, 132–134.

112 MacGilvray SS and Billow M. (1990). Diabetes insipidus as a complication of neonatal group B streptococcal meningitis. *Pediatr Infect Dis J*, **9**, 742–743.

113 Cohen C, Rice EN, Thomas DE, et al. (1998). Diabetes insipidus as a hallmark neuroendocrine complication of neonatal meningitis. *Curr Opin Pediatr*, **10**, 449–452.

114 McCracken GH Jr, Mize SG and Threlkeld N. (1980). Intraventricular gentamicin therapy in gram-negative bacillary meningitis of infancy. Report of the Second Neonatal Meningitis Co-operative Study Group. *Lancet*, **i**, 787–791.

115 Lorber J and Pickering D. (1966). Incidence and treatment of post-meningitic hydrocephalus in the newborn. *Arch Dis Child*, **41**, 44–50.

116 Renier D, Flandin C, Hirsch E, et al. (1988). Brain abscesses in neonates: a study of 30 cases. *J Neurosurg*, **69**, 877–882.

117 Fenton LJ and Strunk RC. (1977). Complement activation and group B streptococcal infection in the newborn: similarities to endotoxin shock. *Pediatrics*, **60**, 901–907.

118 McCracken GH Jr and Sarff LD. (1976). Endotoxin in cerebrospinal fluid: detection in neonates with bacterial meningitis. *JAMA*, **235**, 617–620.

119 Bruce DA. (1984). Effects of hyperventilation on cerebral blood flow and metabolism. *Clin Perinatol*, **11**, 673–680.

120 Saez-Llorens X and McCracken GH Jr. (1999). Antimicrobial and anti-inflammatory treatment of bacterial meningitis. *Infect Dis Clin North Am*, **13**, 619–636.

121 Tessin I, Trollfors B, Thiringer K, et al. (1991). Ampicillin–aminoglycoside combination as initial treatment for neonatal septicaemia or meningitis: a retrospective evaluation of 12 years experience. *Acta Paediatri Scand*, **80**, 911–916.

122 Mulhall A, De Louvois J and Hurley R. (1983). Incidence of potentially toxic concentrations of gentamicin in the neonate. *Arch Dis Child*, **58**, 897–900.

123 Adelman RD, Wirth F and Rubio T. (1987). A controlled study of the nephrotoxicity of mezlocillin and gentamicin plus ampicillin in the neonate. *J Pediatr*, **111**, 888–893.

124 Tullus K, Olsson-Liljequist B, Lundstrom G, et al. (1991). Antibiotic susceptibility of 629 bacterial blood and CSF isolates from Swedish infants and the therapeutic implications. *Acta Paediatr Scand*, **80**, 205–212.

125 De Louvois J, Dagan R and Tessin I. (1992). A comparison of ceftazidime and aminoglycoside based regimens as empirical treatment in 1316 cases of suspected sepsis in the newborn. *Eur J Pediatr*, **151**, 876–884.

126 Quinn JP and Rodvold KA. (2000). Antibiotic policies in neonatal intensive-care units. *Lancet*, **355**, 946–947.

127 McCracken GH Jr, Threlkeld N, Mize S, et al. and the Neonatal Meningitis Co-operative Study Group (1984). Moxalactam therapy for neonatal meningitis due to gram-negative enteric bacilli: a prospective controlled evaluation. *JAMA*, **252**, 1427–1432.

128 Lebel MH, Hoy MJ and McCracken GH Jr. (1989). Comparative efficacy of ceftriaxone and cefuroxime for treatment of bacterial meningitis. *J Pediatr*, **114**, 1049–1054.

129 Weiss CF, Glazko AJ and Weston JK. (1960). Chloramphenicol in the newborn infant: a physiologic explanation of its toxicity when given in excessive doses. *N Engl J Med*, **262**, 787.

130 Mulhall A, De Louvois J and Hurley R. (1983). Efficacy of chloramphenicol in the treatment of neonatal and infantile meningitis: a study of 70 cases. *Lancet*, **i**, 284–287.

131 Black SB, Levine P and Shinefield HR. (1978). The necessity for monitoring chloramphenicol levels when treating neonatal meningitis. *J Pediatr*, **92**, 235–236.

132 Ahmed A, Hickey SM, Ehrett S, et al. (1996). Cerebrospinal fluid values in the term neonate. *Pediatr Infect Dis J*, **15**, 298–303.

133 Haimi-Cohen Y, Amir J, Weinstock A, et al. (1993). The use of imipenem-cilastatin in neonatal meningitis caused by *Citrobacter diversus*. *Acta Paediatr Int J Paediatr*, **82**, 530–532.

134 Leggiadro RJ. (1996). Favorable outcome possible in *Citrobacter* brain abscess. *Pediatr Infect Dis J*, **15**, 557.

135 Radetsky M. (1990). Duration of treatment in bacterial meningitis: a historical inquiry. *Pediatr Infect Dis J*, **9**, 2–9.

136 Peltola HO. (1982). C-reactive protein for rapid monitoring of infectious of the central nervous system. *Lancet*, **i**, 980–982.

137 Roine I, Banfi A, Bosch P, et al. (1991). Serum C-reactive protein in childhood meningitis in countries with limited laboratory resources: a Chilean experience. *Pediatr Infect Dis J*, **10**, 923–928.

138 Peltola H, Luhtala K and Valmari P. (1984). C-reactive protein as a detector of organic complications during recovery from childhood purulent meningitis. *J Pediatr*, **104**, 869–872.

139 Astruc J, Taillebois L, Rodière F, et al. (1990). Raccourcissement du traitment antibiotiques des méningites bactériennes de l'enfant: interêt de la surveillance de la C-réactive protéine. *Arch Franc Pédiatr*, **47**, 637–640.

140 Sutinen J, Sombrero L, Paladin FJ, et al. (1998–99). Etiology of central nervous system infections in the Philippines and the role of serum C-reactive protein in excluding acute bacterial meningitis. *Int J Infect Dis*, **3**, 88–93.

141 Prober CG. (1995). The role of steroids in the management of children with bacterial meningitis. *Pediatrics*, **95**, 29–31.

142 Odio CM, Faingezicht I, Paris M, et al. (1991). The beneficial effects of early dexamethasone administration in infants and children with bacterial meningitis. *N Engl J Med*, **324**, 1525–1531.

143 Wald ER, Kaplan SL, Mason EO, et al. for the Meningitis Study Group (1995). Dexamethasone therapy for children with bacterial meningitis. *Pediatrics*, **95**, 21–28.

144 Yu JS and Grauaug A. (1963). Purulent meningitis in the neonatal period. *Arch Dis Child*, **38**, 391–396.

145 Daoud AS, Batieha A, Al-Sheyyab M, et al. (1999). Lack of effectiveness of dexamethasone in neonatal bacterial meningitis. *Eur J Pediatr*, **158**, 230–233.

146 Lewis BR and Gupta JM. (1977). Present prognosis in neonatal meningitis. *Med J Aust*, **I**, 696–697.

147 McCracken GH Jr, Sarff LD, Glode MP, et al. (1974). Relation between *Escherichia coli* K1 capsular polysaccharide antigen and clinical outcome in neonatal meningitis. *Lancet*, **ii**, 246–250.

148 Wald ER, Bergman I, Taylor HG, et al. (1986). Long-term outcome of group B streptococcal meningitis. *Pediatrics*, **77**, 217–221.

149 Bennet R, Bergdahl S, Eriksson M, et al. (1989). The outcome of neonatal septicemia during fifteen years. *Acta Paediatr Scand*, **78**, 40–43.

150 Chin KC and Fitzhardinge PM. (1985). Sequelae of early-onset group B hemolytic streptococcal neonatal meningitis. *J Pediatr*, **106**, 819–822.

151 Moffett KS and Berkowitz FE. (1997). Quadriplegia complicating *Escherichia coli* meningitis in a newborn infant: case report and review of 22 cases of spinal cord dysfunction in patients with acute bacterial meningitis. *Clin Infect Dis*, **25**, 211–214.

152 Goossens H, Henocque G, Kremp L, et al. (1986). Nosocomial outbreak of *Campylobacter jejuni* meningitis in newborn infants. *Lancet*, **ii**, 146–149.

153 Lin F-YC, Devoe WF, Morrison C, et al. (1987). Outbreak of neonatal *Citrobacter diversus* meningitis in a suburban hospital. *Pediatr Infect Dis J*, **6**, 50–55.

154 Campbell JR, Diacovo T and Baker CJ. (1992). *Serratia marcescens* meningitis in neonates. *Pediatr Infect Dis J*, **11**, 881–886.

155 Siegel JD, McCracken GH Jr, Threlkeld N, et al. (1982). Single-dose penicillin prophylaxis of neonatal group B streptococcal disease: conclusion of a 41 month controlled trial. *Lancet*, **i**, 1426–1430.

156 Pyati SP, Pildes RS, Jacobs NM, et al. (1983). Penicillin in infants weighing two kilograms or less with early-onset group B streptococcal disease. *N Engl J Med*, **308**, 1383–1389.

157 Baker CJ, Melish ME, Hall RT, et al., and the Multicenter Group for the Study of Immune Globulin in Neonates (1992). Intravenous immune globulin for the prevention of nosocomial infection in low-birth weight neonates. *N Engl J Med*, **327**, 213–219.

158 Fanaroff AA, Korones SB, Wright LL, et al. (1994). For the National Institute of Child Health and Human Development Neonatal Research Network: a controlled trial of intravenous immune globulin to reduce nosocomial infections in very-low-birth-weight infants. *N Engl J Med*, **330**, 1107–1113.

159 Weisman LE, Stoll BJ, Kueser TJ, et al. (1992). Intravenous immune globulin therapy for early-onset sepsis in premature neonates. *J Pediatr*, **121**, 434–443.

160 Weisman LE, Stoll BJ, Kueser TJ, et al. (1994). Intravenous immune globulin prophylaxis of late-onset sepsis in premature neonates. *J Pediatr*, **125**, 922–930.

161 Weisman LE, Cruess DF and Fischer GW. (1994). Opsonic activity of commercially available standard intravenous immunoglobulin preparations. *Pediatr Infect Dis J*, **13**, 1122–1125.

162 Yow MD, Mason ED, Leeds LJ, et al. (1979). Ampicillin prevents intrapartum transmission of group B streptococcus. *JAMA*, **241**, 1245–1247.

163 Boyer KM and Gotoff SP. (1986). Prevention of early-onset neonatal group B streptococcal disease with selective intrapartum chemoprophylaxis. *N Engl J Med*, **314**, 1665–1669.

164 Ascher DP, Becker JA, Yoder BA, et al. (1992). Failure of intrapartum antibiotics to prevent culture-proved neonatal group B streptococcal sepsis. *J Perinatol*, **13**, 212–216.

165 Morbidity and Mortality Weekly Report. (1996). Prevention of perinatal group B streptococcal disease: a public health perspective. *MMWR*, **45**, 1–24.

166 Schrag SJ, Zywicki S, Farley MM, et al. (2000). Group B streptococcal disease in the era of intrapartum antibiotic prophylaxis. *N Engl J Med*, **342**, 15–20.

167 Kalliola S, Vuopio-Varkilla J, Takala AK, et al. (1999). Neonatal group B streptococcal disease in Finland: a ten-year nationwide study. *Pediatr Infect Dis J*, **18**, 806–810.

168 Philip AGS and Mills PC. (2000). Use of C-reactive protein in minimizing antibiotic exposure: experience with infants initially admitted to a well-baby nursery. *Pediatrics*, **106**, e4.

169 Insel RA. (1988). Maternal immunization to prevent neonatal infections. *N Engl J Med*, **319**, 1219–1220.

170 Schuchat A. (1999). Group B streptococcus. *Lancet*, **353**, 51–56.

171 Noya FJD and Baker CJ. (1992). Prevention of group B streptococcal infection. *Infect Dis Clin North Am*, **6**, 41–55.

172 Baker CJ, Paoletti LC, Wessels MR, et al. (1999). Safety and immunogenicity of capsular polysaccharide-tetanus toxoid conjugate vaccines for group B streptococcal types Ia and Ib. *J Infect Dis*, **179**, 142–150.

173 Paoletti LC, Pinel J, Kennedy RC, et al. (2000). Maternal antibody transfer in baboons and mice vaccinated with a group B streptococcal polysaccharide conjugate. *J Infect Dis*, **181**, 653–658.

174 Hristeva L, Booy R, Bowler I, et al. (1993). Prospective surveillance of neonatal meningitis. *Arch Dis Child*, **69**, 14–18.

175 Naidoo BT. (1968). The cerebrospinal fluid in the healthy newborn infant. *S Afr Med J*, **42**, 933–936.

176 Escobedo M, Barton LL and Volpe J. (1975). Cerebrospinal fluid studies in an intensive care nursery. *J Perinatol*, **3**, 204–210.

177 Sarff LD, Platt LH and McCracken GH Jr. (1976). Cerebrospinal fluid evaluation in neonates: comparison of high-risk infants with and without meningitis. *J Pediatr*, **88**, 473–477.

178 Pappu LD, Purohit DM, Levkoff AH, et al. (1982). CSF cytology in the neonate. *Am J Dis Child*, **136**, 297–298.

179 Bonadio WA, Stanco L, Bruce R, et al. (1992). Reference values of normal cerebrospinal fluid composition in infants ages 0 to 8 weeks. *Pediatr Infect Dis J*, **11**, 589–591.

180 Ahmed A. (1997). A critical evaluation of vancomycin for treatment of bacterial meningitis. *Pediatr Infect Dis J*, **16**, 895–903.

181 Mickas NA and Benitz WE. (2001). Individualized gentamicin pharmokinetics in the neonate (abstract). *J Invest Med*, **49**, 90A.

182 Bell AH, Brown D, Halliday HL, et al. (1989). Meningitis in the newborn – a 14 year review. *Arch Dis Child*, **64**, 873–874.

17

Neurologic sequelae of congenital perinatal infection

Andrea M. Enright and Charles G. Prober

Stanford University School of Medicine, Department of Pediatrics, Division of Infectious Diseases, Stanford, CA, USA

Introduction

Maternal infections, contracted during pregnancy, may be without fetal consequence or they may have serious adverse effects on the fetus. These adverse effects may include fetal death, stillbirth, intrauterine growth retardation, or congenital infection. Congenitally infected neonates may be symptomatic or asymptomatic at birth. Those who are symptomatic at birth generally have significant long-term sequelae. Those who are asymptomatic at birth may never manifest evidence of damage or they may develop clinically evident sequelae later in life. The overwhelming morbidity attributable to congenital infections is borne by this latter group.

The following chapter will discuss the neurologic consequences of congenital infections. The specific infectious agents that will be discussed are often referred to as the TORCH agents; T represents the parasite *Toxoplasma gondii*; O represents other agents such as varicella-zoster virus (VZV), human immunodeficiency virus (HIV), and *Treponema pallidum* (syphilis); R represents rubella virus; C represents cytomegalovirus (CMV); and H represents herpes simplex virus (HSV). With the exception of HSV, the major clinical impact of these agents results from exposure in utero. Morbidity and mortality attributable to neonatal HSV infection usually result from infection contracted at delivery.

Toxoplasmosis

The etiologic agent of toxoplasmosis, *Toxoplasma gondii*, was first demonstrated in the brain of a newborn infant with encephalomyelitis in 1939.[1] The incidence of congenital toxoplasmosis in the USA is estimated to range from 1:1000 to 1:10 000 live births.[2–5] Among immunocompetent women, transmission to the fetus is limited almost solely to those who contract primary infection during gestation. Most cases of vertical transmission resulting from reactivation of previous maternal infection have occurred in women with immunodeficiency from acquired immune deficiency syndrome (AIDS), neoplasm, or autoimmune disease.[3,4]

The risk of fetal infection increases as pregnancy progresses.[3] Increasing placental blood flow with advancing gestation may explain the increased transplacental transmission.[4] The transmission rate may be as low as 5% if maternal infection occurs before 16 weeks' gestation and as high as 75–80% if maternal infection occurs near term.[3] Fortunately, the severity of neonatal disease decreases with advancing gestational age.[3,4] Thus, although transmission of toxoplasmosis to the fetus is greatest late in pregnancy, manifestations resulting from infection are uncommon.

Several studies suggest that the incidence and severity of neonatal infection may be reduced if mothers who acquire toxoplasmosis during pregnancy receive antiparasitic therapy.[6] In one study of 1240 women with proven toxoplasmosis during pregnancy, fetal transmission was reduced to 7% and 81% of these infected newborns had subclinical disease if mothers were treated with spiramycin or pyrimethamine/sulfadiazine/folinic acid during pregnancy. Thus, treatment appeared to decrease both the incidence and severity of congenital toxoplasmosis. Although a second study failed to demonstrate a decrease in transplacental transmission of *T. gondii* by prenatal treatment, it did confirm that the severity of neonatal illness was significantly decreased by prenatal treatment.[7]

The clinical spectrum of congenital toxoplasmosis is broad.[3,4] Although the majority of infants infected in utero with *T. gondii* are asymptomatic at birth, approximately 90% of infected infants will manifest sequelae at a later age, particularly ophthalmologic and intellectual impairment.[3–8]

Outcome in infants asymptomatic at birth

Congenital toxoplasmosis is not as prevalent as congenital CMV, but it is potentially more dangerous for the individual. Although about 85% of infants with congenital toxoplasmosis appear normal at birth, subclinical infection with *T. gondii* is more frequently associated with impaired intellectual performance and chorioretinitis than subclinical infection with CMV.[2–4,8–10] An estimated 85% of untreated infants with congenital toxoplasmosis will suffer at least one episode of chorioretinitis, developmental delay will be evident in 20–75%, and hearing loss will occur in 10–30%.[2–4,8–10] These sequelae of congenital infection may not become clinically apparent until 6–18 years of age.[3,8]

Outcome in infants symptomatic at birth

Only about 15% of neonates congenitally infected with *T. gondii* are symptomatic at birth.[3] Their infection is rarely fulminant but it is often severe. Symptoms and signs of generalized infection are prominent and signs of central nervous system involvement are invariably present.[3] The "classic triad" in these symptomatic neonates is hydrocephalus, chorioretinitis, and diffuse intracranial calcifications. The most frequent extraneural signs associated with symptomatic congenital toxoplasmosis include: hepatosplenomegaly, fever, anemia, and jaundice.[3] The mortality rate of these infants is 10–15%. Approximately 85% of untreated survivors develop mental retardation, 75% develop convulsions, spasticity, and palsies, and 50% develop severe visual impairment.[2] Deafness, a prominent sequela of congenital viral infections (e.g., CMV and rubella), occurs less frequently after congenital toxoplasmosis. The approximate incidence of hearing loss is 0–30%.[2,4,11,12] Microcephaly, also commonly seen in other congenital infections, is less common in congenital toxoplasmosis, the highest reported incidence being less than 25%.[12] When microcephaly does occur it is a predictor of poor outcome. Other factors associated with poor prognosis in congenital toxoplasmosis include: neonatal hypothermia, apnea, bradycardia, prolonged hypoxemia, cerebrospinal fluid (CSF) protein >1 g/dl, delayed treatment and brain atrophy on computed tomography (CT) scan which persists for months after ventriculoperitoneal shunt placement.[3,12]

Good outcomes have occurred in children with significant central nervous system (CNS) involvement at birth treated with antiparasitic drugs for 1 year. The Chicago Collaborative Treatment Trial was a longitudinal study of 44 children treated for 1 year with pyrimethamine, sulfadiazine, and folinic acid.[12] These children were routinely evaluated at diagnosis, and at frequent intervals thereafter. The mean follow-up for individuals was 3.75 years; the maximum follow-up was 10 years. Signs of active infection resolved within weeks of treatment. Many infected children with significant disease at birth were normal or had only minor disabilities at follow-up. Excluding visual deficits, all infected children without hydrocephalus and 50% of those with hydrocephalus were functioning normally. Focal, motor, and neurologic deficits were found in 20 at birth. Following 1 year of therapy, these deficits had completely resolved in 60%. Disseminated calcifications at birth do not necessarily reflect poor prognosis; following treatment, normal development can occur despite these findings.[3] Twenty-five percent of infants with CNS disease evident at birth continued to have severe handicaps despite treatment. In addition, although the cognitive function of many treated children was within the normal range, preliminary data on a small group of patients suggest that their cognitive function was still significantly below that of their uninfected siblings.

Intracranial calcifications may diminish or completely resolve with 1 year of therapy. In one study intracranial calcifications were demonstrated in 40 of 56 newborns with congenital toxoplasmosis.[13] Following 1 year of therapy with pyrimethamine, sulfadiazine, and leucovorin, 75% had decreased or undetectable calcifications.

Screening and prenatal diagnosis

Since the majority of infants with subclinical congenital toxoplasmosis ultimately develop sequelae, identification and treatment of all infected newborns should decrease long-term morbidity. Massachusetts and New Hampshire have screened newborns for congenital toxoplasmosis since 1986 and 1988, respectively. All 50 infected neonates identified by screening had normal newborn exams.[5] However, on the basis of detailed perinatal evaluations conducted shortly after serologic diagnosis, 19% had ocular disease (4% active chorioretinitis, 15% uninflamed retinal scars), 20% had intracranial calcifications found on CT, 25% had increased protein in CSF, and 2% had ventriculomegaly. All infants were treated for 1 year with pyrimethamine, sulfadiazine and folic acid. Only one of 46 infants had persistent neurologic deficits. None of nine infants with macular lesions at birth had progressive ocular disease. However, 10% developed new ocular lesions. Thus, treatment for 1 year with pyrimethamine, sulfadiazine, and folinic acid seems to benefit both symptomatic and asymptomatic neonates with congenital toxoplasmosis. Currently, 1 year of therapy is recommended.

In order to maximize the benefits of prenatal and postnatal therapy, infected neonates must be identified. In France, where the toxoplasmosis seronegative rate among women of child-bearing age is low, monthly serologic screening is performed for all seronegative pregnant women.[3] If seroconversion is documented, prompt therapy is given to the mother during pregnancy and to the neonate from birth. In the USA there has been much debate over systematic universal screening for toxoplasmosis in pregnant women.[3] The seronegative prevalence in the USA is much higher than in Europe; thus, more US women would need routine screening. In addition, the sensitivity, specificity, positive and negative predictive values vary with each serologic test and are less reliable if run outside of reference laboratories.[3,14]

An alternative to screening pregnant women is to screen neonates at birth for serologic evidence of congenital infection. Due to limitations in the immunoglobulin (IgM) assays, newborn screens employing these assays only diagnose 70–80% of congenital infections.[3,14] The 20–30% false-negative rate of neonatal screens may be unacceptably high. In a European study of various prenatal and postnatal screening tests, the sensitivity of IgM testing of neonatal blood was 43%; IgA testing of neonatal blood was 66% sensitive.[14] Sensitivity increased to 70% if results of IgM and IgA testing on neonatal blood were combined. Moreover, maternal prenatal treatment with antiparasitic drugs significantly decreased the incidence of positive serologic diagnosis. The 85% positive rate for specific IgM in neonatal blood dropped to 25% in those neonates whose mothers were treated prenatally. Fetal infection may be detected through amniocentesis or cordocentesis.[3,14,15] Polymerase chain reaction (PCR) on amniotic fluid is superior to cordocentesis with fetal blood serologic evaluation. PCR of amniotic fluid has a sensitivity of 80–90% and a specificity of 96–100%.[3,14,15]

Recommendations

Infants with congenital *T. gondii* infection must be recognized as being at high risk for the development of ophthalmologic and intellectual impairment.

Serial ophthalmologic and intellectual assessments must be performed until the child is at least 18 years of age because onset of sequelae can be delayed.

Normal developmental, ophthalmologic, and neurologic outcomes have been observed in up to 70% of treated infants, despite the presence of systemic disease, hydrocephalus, microcephaly, multiple intracranial calcifications, and extensive macular involvement evident at birth.[3,4,12] Since delays in diagnosis and therapy are associated with worse outcomes, prompt diagnosis and treatment are important.[3,4,12]

Prevention is possible.[3,4,14] Primary prevention to decrease infection of susceptible pregnant women should focus on hygiene: avoiding consumption of raw meat, avoiding potentially contaminated material (cat feces, litter boxes, soil when gardening), and washing fruits and vegetables before consumption. Secondary prevention involves identifying seroconversion in pregnant women and instituting prenatal therapy to reduce transmission and decrease the severity of infection in the fetus. Tertiary prevention includes neonatal evaluation, antiparasitic treatment, and long-term follow-up of congenitally infected infants. Evaluations should include general physical, neurologic, audiologic, and developmental exams, head CT, serologic tests, complete blood counts, liver function tests, cerebrospinal evaluation, and close monitoring for drug toxicity while on therapy.

Cytomegalovirus

CMV is the most common cause of congenital infection; the incidence ranges from 0.2 to 2% of all live births.[16] Congenital CMV infection may result from maternal primary infection, reactivation of a prior latent infection, or, rarely, from reinfection with a new CMV strain.[16] Since most congenital CMV infections result from maternal reactivated infections it is fortunate that maternal immunity attenuates the severity of neonatal illness. More than 90% of neonates with congenital CMV infection are asymptomatic at birth.[16] Approximately 10–15% of these asymptomatic infants develop late-onset sequelae, including sensorineural hearing loss, learning and behavioral abnormalities.[17–29] In contrast, most congenitally infected neonates who are symptomatic at birth manifest severe developmental deficits and mental retardation.[19,30–34] With a few rare exceptions, most symptomatic congenital CMV infection results from a primary maternal infection.[16,17] Primary infections early in pregnancy (before the 27th week of gestation) are more likely to be associated with a poor outcome than those occurring later in gestation.[16,17,23]

Outcome in infants asymptomatic at birth

The majority of neonates with congenital CMV infections are asymptomatic at birth. These infants are likely to be detected only if routine viral cultures of newborns are performed within the first few weeks of life. Several prospective studies assessing the possible long-term effects of these "silent" congenital CMV infections have been conducted.[18,20,21,24–26,28,29,35–37] The most common sequelae of asymptomatic congenital CMV infection are sensorineural hearing loss and possible intellectual impairment. The incidence of sensorineural hearing loss in older children with asymptomatic congenital CMV ranges from 7 to 15%.[28,35,38,39]

Congenital CMV infection is estimated to be responsible for one-third of all cases of sensorineural hearing loss in children.[28] A large prospective study of 307 asymptomatic congenitally infected children and 277 controls found a 7% incidence of sensorineural hearing loss in infected children and no hearing loss in the matched controls.[28] Of those children with sensorineural hearing loss, 50% had bilateral disease; 23% suffered from profound bilateral sensorineural hearing loss. In this study none of the children with sensorineural hearing loss had other risk factors for hearing impairment. Since CMV hearing impairment often presents after the newborn period, is progressive and can fluctuate, researchers estimate that two-thirds of sensorineural hearing loss from asymptomatic congenital CMV infection may be missed by universal newborn hearing screens.[28,28,39] These researchers argue that in order to identify all those at risk for hearing impairment in childhood, universal newborn hearing screening must be accompanied by universal newborn CMV screening.

Hearing impairment's impact on intellectual development has confounded the evaluation of intellectual function in congenitally infected infants. Several studies have attempted to evaluate the possible intellectual consequences of asymptomatic congenital CMV infection. Interpretation of the results of some of the studies is hampered by relatively short periods of follow-up, lack of appropriately matched controls, and failure to control for hearing loss. One well-designed study evaluated the intellectual development of 18 prospectively followed school-aged children with asymptomatic congenital CMV and normal hearing.[29] The results of testing these children were compared with the results from 18 controls matched for age, sex, race, school grade, and socioeconomic status. All children were evaluated between 6.5 and 12.5 years of age using the Wechsler Intelligence Scale for Children – Revised, the Kaufman Assessment Battery for Children, and the Wide Range Achievement Test. No differences between the infected and uninfected children on intelligence scores or subscales, achievement scores, or incidence of learning disabilities were observed. These researchers concluded that children with asymptomatic CMV infection and normal hearing have normal intellectual development. However, the small sample size of this study prohibits a definite conclusion regarding the independent effects of congenital CMV infection on intellectual impairment.

Expression of adverse consequences of asymptomatic CMV infections appears to be influenced by socioeconomic conditions. One study predicted increased school failure rate in infected children of lower socioeconomic class but not in those infected children from middle and higher socioeconomic classes.[26] Future studies must attempt to control for other relevant factors contributing to intellectual development.

Outcome in infants symptomatic at birth

The vast majority of neonates who are symptomatic at birth as a result of congenital CMV have been infected as a result of a primary maternal gestational infection.[16,40] The clinical abnormalities found most frequently in neonates with symptomatic congenital CMV are listed in Table 17.1.[16] Cerebral abnormalities reported in association with congenital CMV infection include: microcephaly, microgyria, periventricular calcifications, migrational abnormalities, disturbed myelination, spongiosus of the brain, encephalomalacia, calcification of the cerebral arteries, parietal lobe cysts, cerebral cortical immaturity, cerebellar hypoplasia, paraventricular cysts, intraventricular strands, and dolichocephaly.[16,18,19,31–34,41,42] CMV has been isolated from CSF by PCR in six of 10 patients with symptomatic congenital infection.[43] Follow-up was available for five of those patients with a positive CSF CMV PCR; all five had developmental delay. Postmortem examination of brains from infants who have died with severe congenital CMV infection have noted decreased brain weight, subependymal cysts, deformed cerebellum, irregular gyri, thickened leptomeninges, cortical and cerebellar neuronal migration abnormalities, and paraventricular bands of necrosis and calcification.[16,33]

Table 17.1. Clinical manifestations of symptomatic congenital cytomegalovirus infection

Petechia	++++
Thrombocytopenia	++++
Hepatosplenomegaly	+++
Jaundice with direct hyperbilirubinemia	+++
Microcephaly	+++
Small-for-gestational-age	++
Prematurity	++
Inguinal hernia	++
Chorioretinitis	+

Notes:
++++ 75–100% incidence; +++ 50–75%; ++ 25–50%; + 0–25%.
Source: Adapted from:[16,19,30–33]

Fortunately, less than 10% of neonates congenitally infected with CMV manifest overt signs of disease at birth because the long-term prognosis of these infants is usually poor.[30,32–44] CNS sequelae include: microcephaly, mental retardation and developmental delays, learning and behavioral disorders, seizures, neuromuscular disorders including facial asymmetry, spasticity, quadriparesis, diplegia, hemiatrophy, and hemiparesis.[16,45] Defects in hearing and vision are also common after symptomatic congenital CMV infection. The largest prospective study of symptomatic neonates was published in 1980.[32] In that study, 34 patients who had clinically evident disease at birth were followed for a mean duration of 4 years. Twenty-nine percent of the patients died and more than 90% of the survivors developed CNS or auditory handicaps; 70% had microcephaly, 61% mental retardation, 35% neuromuscular disorders, 30% hearing loss, and 22% chorioretinitis or optic atrophy. Although the extent of disease apparent at birth was not entirely predictive of CNS sequelae, all children with IQs <50 or neuromuscular disorders were clearly abnormal by 1 year of age. Other studies have documented similarly poor outcomes. In a long-term follow-up of 17 children with symptomatic congenital CMV followed for a mean of 5.5 years, 75% met criteria for mental retardation.[30] In this study, three children with normal hearing and IQ scores still exhibited deficits in expressive language. It is possible that these young children would manifest more severe deficits at later ages. Although the estimated risk of permanent neurologic sequelae after a symptomatic congenital CMV infection is high, in a given case the development may be more favorable than expected.[44]

Recommendations

Congenital CMV infection should be considered in any newborn with unexplained prematurity, growth retardation, hepatomegaly, splenomegaly, jaundice, microcephaly, chorioretinitis, or petechia. This diagnosis can be confirmed by isolating the virus from a urine or salivary culture obtained during the first 3 weeks of life. CMV isolated after the first few weeks of life with a documented negative culture in the neonatal period represents perinatal CMV infection.

Neuroimaging by CT scan or magnetic resonance imaging (MRI) has been shown to be useful in identifying infants at risk for CNS sequelae of congenital CMV infection.[34,42] In a study of 56 infants with symptomatic congenital CMV, 70% had CT abnormalities.[34] Of those with CT abnormalities, 60% had IQ scores less than 70; half of the IQ scores were below 50. In contrast, none of the 17 symptomatic infants with normal CT scans had severe mental retardation. In this study, clinical and laboratory data were not able to predict the neurologic sequelae. Microcephaly, seizures, lethargy, and poor suck did not predict CT scan abnormality. Intracranial calcification was the most common abnormality found in 77% of abnormal scans. White-matter abnormalities were also identified, with MRI more sensitive than CT in a small number of patients.[42]

Currently, there is no known effective antiviral therapy for infants with congenital CMV infection. Ongoing trials by the National Institute of Allergy and Infectious Diseases Antiviral Treatment Group are evaluating ganciclovir therapy for those unfortunate neonates who are symptomatic at birth. Interim analysis suggests that the rate of hearing deterioration is significantly lower in treated patients and hearing is stabilized more often in the treated group[31] (Kimberlin, personal communication).

Despite the current lack of antiviral therapy for infants with congenital infection, it is important to identify all infants with congenital CMV infection as early as possible. Early identification will permit frequent audiometric and intellectual examinations over the first several years of the child's life. In order to maximize a child's full potential, defects, including those in hearing and language, should be corrected as soon as possible.

Rubella

Rubella is an RNA virus, classified as a togavirus, unrelated to any other human viral pathogen.[46,47] Before the introduction of childhood immunization for rubella in the late 1960s, rubella virus caused major epidemics once or twice every decade in the

USA.[47] During rubella epidemics, many infected individuals were asymptomatic while others had classic infection with diffuse exanthem, low-grade fevers, lymphadenopathy, and arthritis/arthralgia.[47] As most children in the USA are now immunized during the second year of life, widespread epidemics of rubella have disappeared. However, outbreaks of rubella and congenital rubella syndrome have occurred in the USA in the late 1980s and early 1990s.[48–50] Most outbreaks have been attributed to a failure to vaccinate susceptible individuals in colleges, prisons, and religious communities.[48–50] Today, an estimated 6–25% of women of childbearing age are susceptible to rubella.[46–48,51] As these recent outbreaks indicate, the risk of congenital rubella syndrome remains.

The transmission of rubella to the fetus

Rubella produces viremia in the susceptible host during primary infection.[47] In pregnant women, this viremic phase often results in placental infection with or without subsequent infection of the fetus.[47] The risk of fetal infection depends on gestational age at the time of maternal infection.[46,47,52,53] The risk of fetal infection is highest in the first trimester, declines during the second trimester, and then increases again during the end of the third trimester.[46,47,52,53] Specifically, the risk of fetal infection is 80–90% during the first 12 weeks of gestation, drops to 25% by 23–26 weeks and then increases to 60–100% near term.[46,47,52,53]

Clinical manifestations of intrauterine rubella infection and the risk of neurologic sequelae

Isolation of virus from the oropharynx of infants with suspected intrauterine rubella is the most reliable method of proving congenital infection.[46,47] Infants with congenital rubella shed virus from this site for 6 months or longer after birth.[46,47] The virus can also be found in the stool, urine, and CSF.[46,47] Although efforts have been made to develop a rubella-specific IgM antibody assay for the diagnosis of congenital rubella infection, many infants with infection proven by culture do not have detectable rubella-specific IgM antibodies using optimal serologic methodology.[46,47,54] The lack of detectable antibodies in infants with congenital rubella syndrome may reflect infection at a time of fetal immune system immaturity in early gestation.[54] Infection before 20–22 weeks may not produce a detectable humoral response despite active viral replication and infection of fetal tissues.[47]

Fewer than 10% of infants with intrauterine rubella have signs of congenital rubella infection at birth.[46,47] The likelihood of clinical manifestations of intrauterine rubella is inversely related to fetal age at the time of maternal infection.[52,55] The estimated risk of defects is 85% following maternal rubella at 8 weeks, 52% at 9–12 weeks, and 16% at 13–20 weeks' gestation.[56] Maternal infection after 20 weeks' gestation can cause fetal infection but these infants are asymptomatic in the newborn period and the risk of late-onset sequelae is low.[47,52,55] Infants infected with rubella virus at the earliest stages of development are more likely to have cardiac defects (patent ductus arteriosus, pulmonary artery stenosis) in addition to the hearing and ocular abnormalities that are characteristic of later in utero infection.

Neurologic manifestations of congenital rubella syndrome include meningoencephalitis, microcephaly, mental and motor retardation, behavioral difficulties, psychiatric disorders, sensorineural hearing loss and, rarely, late-onset progressive rubella panencephalitis.[46,47,52,53,55,57,58] Meningoencephalitis occurs in 10–20% of infected neonates who are symptomatic at birth.[47] In these cases, CSF analysis reveals elevated protein concentrations with or without a pleocytosis.[47] Extensive meningoencephalitis is one cause of early postnatal death from congenital rubella.

The risk of microcephaly depends on the gestational age at infection. Microcephaly occurs in 60% of fetuses infected before 13 weeks' gestation. In contrast, less than 10% infants infected after 20 weeks' gestation are microcephalic.[52] Infants with congenital rubella who are microcephalic can be expected to have additional neurologic impairment.[58] Acquired microcephaly has also been documented in congenital rubella syndrome. Chang et al. described five neonates with confirmed congenital rubella syndrome.[59] Despite having normal head size at birth, head ultrasonography revealed linear and punctuate hyperechogenicities and occasional subependymal cysts. These nonspecific findings of CNS damage were markers for later neurologic sequelae; by 27 months of age, all five had documented microcephaly and profound global developmental delay. In another study white-matter hyperintensities were noted on MRI scans performed on 11 adults with a history of congenital rubella syndrome and schizophrenia-like symptoms.[60] These hyperintensities were not found in any of 19 controls with schizophrenia who had no evidence of congenital infection.

A few children with congenital rubella developed a syndrome of progressive rubella panencephalitis similar to subacute sclerosing panencephalitis caused by the measles virus.[57,60] These children manifest progressive neurologic deterioration after 10 years of age. Neurologic manifestations have included progressive mental retardation, motor incoordination, and cerebellar signs, including nystagmus, ataxia, and choreoathetoid movements. Elevated rubella-specific IgG was demonstrated in the CSF and rubella virus was recovered from brain biopsy in one case.[57] Autopsies revealed diffuse white-matter involvement, microglial nodules, panencephalitis, reactive gliosis, ventricular enlargement, and brain atrophy.[57,61]

Neurologic sequelae of congenital rubella are often subtle and include hearing deficits, language delays, psychomotor retardation, and behavioral/psychiatric disturbances. The progressive nature of intrauterine rubella infection was demonstrated in a group of nonretarded children who were followed for 9–12 years.[62] With increasing age, an increase in the percentage of the population with hearing loss, motor incoordination, and behavioral disturbances was observed. At last follow-up, 86% of the children had hearing deficits, 52% had learning problems, 48% had behavioral problems, and 61% had poor balance and/or muscle weakness. Fifty-year follow-up of cohorts from congenital rubella epidemics in Australia and the USA have been reported.[63,64] In the Australian cohort of 40 individuals long-term outcomes were considered to be "good."[63] Although 100% had hearing deficits, most of which were profound, and 50% had visual deficits, over 50% were employed. In contrast, in the New York cohort one-third had normal lives, one-third were semiindependent, and one-third were institutionalized.[64]

Behavioral and psychiatric disorders are often found at later ages in children with congenital rubella syndrome. Chess et al. described the psychiatric and behavioral consequences of congenital rubella among 243 preschoolers examined at 2.5–5 years of age; 205 children of this cohort were reexamined at 8–9 years of age.[65] Twenty-five to 40% of the children were mentally retarded, 15–20% had diagnoses of reactive or other behavior disorders, and approximately 6% were autistic. In another psychiatric outcome study, the Diagnostic Interview Schedule for Children was administered to 70 young adults with a history of congenital rubella syndrome and 164 controls.[66] Those with congenital rubella syndrome were 5–16 times more likely than age-matched controls to have nonaffective psychiatric disorders defined as delusions and/or hallucinations.[66] Conclusions from these studies are tentative because the impact of multiple handicaps in hearing, visual, and other neurologic domains have not been clearly separated from the direct impact of viral infection on behavior and psychiatric well-being.

Recommendations

The evaluation of a pregnancy potentially complicated by rubella remains a difficult diagnostic problem. The interval required to isolate the virus limits the utility of tissue culture as a diagnostic method.[46,47] If the pregnant woman has not had a previous rubella titer, it is often impossible to determine whether seroconversion has occurred because rubella antibodies are present within a few days of onset of infection.[46,47] The detection of rubella-specific IgM antibodies can be helpful but the method can yield false-positive results and the absence of an IgM response does not exclude recent rubella infection.[46,47] A high titer of rubella antibodies in a single serum sample does not establish a diagnosis of recent infection since many individuals maintain persistently high rubella titers.[46,47] PCR has been performed on amniotic fluid, chorionic villi samples, and fetal blood for detection of in utero rubella infection. The sensitivity, specificity, and clinical value of this and other newer tests need to be further defined before they can be routinely recommended.[67]

If a pregnant woman is exposed to rubella and her immune status is not known, she should be tested for rubella antibodies immediately.[46,47] A positive rubella titer at the time of exposure eliminates any concern. If the titer is negative, it should be repeated at 2 and 6 weeks after exposure to be certain that subclinical infection has not occurred. [46,47] Transplacental transmission of the virus is possible if seroconversion is demonstrated whether or not the pregnant woman has had symptoms.[46,47]

The risk of congenital rubella can be eliminated by an effective vaccination program.[4,6,13,23] Indeed, the rubella vaccination program has reduced the annual number of cases of rubella by 99% compared to the prevaccine era.[49,51,58,68] However, localized rubella outbreaks continue to occur. Most outbreaks of congenital rubella syndrome can be attributed to multiple missed opportunities to vaccinate susceptible women of child-bearing age.[48–50] Immunization coverage rates of 80–90% are needed to prevent rubella transmission in a community.[49] Susceptible young women should be encouraged to receive rubella vaccine. While pregnancy is a contraindication to rubella immunization, inadvertent rubella vaccination during pregnancy has not been associated with congenital rubella syndrome.[46,47] Long-term medical, neurologic, psychiatric, ophthalmologic, audiologic, and developmental evaluations are required for infants with congenital rubella.

Congenital syphilis

In the USA, the late 1980s and early 1990s were marked by a resurgence in the number of congenital infections caused by *Treponema pallidum*, the etiologic agent of syphilis.[69,70] Factors believed to contribute to this increased frequency of infection include: patterns of substance abuse (especially crack cocaine), HIV infection, and changing patterns of sexual activity.[71] In addition, modification of the Centers for Disease Control and Prevention (CDC) case definition of congenital syphilis facilitated the identification and reporting of cases to the CDC.[72,73] Fortunately, the rate of congenital syphilis in the USA has declined steadily since 1992.[74]

The risk of syphilis transmission to the fetus varies with the stage of maternal illness.[75–77] In early, untreated primary maternal infection, transmission rates range from 70 to 100%. In early latent infection (infection of less than 1 year duration) the risk of fetal infection is 40%. Once a mother has late latent infection, fetal transmission rates drop to 10% due in part to low levels of spirochetemia and treponemal proliferation.

There are substantial problems in the diagnosis of congenital syphilis and the evaluation of neurosyphilis in infants.[78–81] *T. pallidum* cannot be cultured from clinical specimens except by inoculation into rabbits, a process that is time-consuming, costly, and impractical.[75,78,82] In addition, *T. pallidum* is often present in low numbers in clinical specimens. Thus, the value of histologic documentation of infection by dark-field microscopy or antigen detection is limited.[75,78,82] Thus, most cases of congenital syphilis are not established by definitive diagnosis, but rather by presumptive diagnosis based on various clinical and laboratory evaluations.[73,75,77,82] Unfortunately, there is no gold standard for diagnosis. Presumptive diagnosis relies on nontreponemal titers: rapid plasma reagin (RPR) card test or Venereal Disease Research Laboratory (VDRL) titers. However, transplacentally acquired maternal antibodies complicate the serologic evaluation of exposed infants. Moreover, an infected infant may have a titer fourfold higher than his/her mother, a lower titer than his/her mother, or a negative titer despite active infection.[77]

Clinical diagnosis of congenital syphilis is also challenging since approximately two-thirds of infants are asymptomatic at birth.[75,77] Sequelae from these asymptomatic infections frequently develop at later ages. When symptoms appear within the first 2 years of life, they are designated early congenital syphilis; those developing thereafter are designated late congenital syphilis.[75,82] Manifestations of syphilitic infections may include: stillbirth, prematurity, intrauterine growth retardation, hepatosplenomegaly, generalized lymphadenopathy, rhinitis ("snuffles"), dermatologic abnormalities, renal disease, hyperbilirubinemia, and CNS abnormalities.[75,76,83] In order to prevent morbidity from congenital syphilis, it is important to identify and treat both asymptomatic and symptomatic newborns.

Early congenital syphilis

Older literature suggested that greater than 60% of neonates with congenital syphilis had abnormal findings on CSF examinations.[84] However, this high rate of abnormality was based on considering CSF abnormal if it contained 5 or more white blood cells/mm[71] and had a protein content >45 mg/dl. These definitions of abnormal CSF may not be appropriate for newborn infants.[75,85–87] A more recent study of 78 newborn infants born to mothers with serologic evidence of syphilis found only one neonate with a positive CSF VDRL titer.[80] None of the 78 infants had more than 32 white blood cells/mm^3 or a CSF protein greater than 170 mg/dl.[80] Another study evaluated the CSF of 19 infants born to mothers with untreated early syphilis using the rabbit infectivity test, PCR, immunoblot IgM assays in addition to CSF cell count, protein and VDRL titer.[78] Eighty-six percent of symptomatic infants with congenital syphilis in this study had evidence of CNS disease. In contrast, only one of 12 asymptomatic newborns had laboratory evidence of CNS disease. The authors concluded that CNS invasion by *T. pallidum* is common in symptomatic congenital syphilis and uncommon in asymptomatic disease.

Sequelae from neurosyphilis include hydrocephalus, cranial nerve palsies, gradual decline in intelligence quotients, mental retardation, seizures, strokes, deafness, blindness, general paresis, and behavioral/learning difficulties.[75,76] Neurologic manifestations of congenital syphilis that are evident during the first 2 years of life are infrequent.[80] When reported, the most common clinical types of CNS involvement with early congenital syphilis are acute leptomeningitis and chronic meningovascular syphilis.[75] Leptomeningitis usually becomes evident between 3 and 6 months of age. It is clinically indistinguishable from other bacterial causes of meningitis. The CSF typically contains 100–200 mononuclear cells/mm^3, has an increased protein concentration, and a positive serologic test for syphilis. This form of neurosyphilis responds to penicillin therapy.[75,76]

Chronic meningovascular syphilis tends to follow a protracted and progressive course starting late in the first year of life. It usually results in communicating hydrocephalus and cranial nerve palsies.[75] Cerebral infarctions from syphilitic endarteritis may also result in a variety of cerebrovascular syndromes, with paresis and seizures being the most consistent features.[75] Unfortunately, these later forms of neurosyphilis often do not respond to penicillin treatment.[75,76]

Neurologic involvement in late congenital syphilis is infrequent.[80,88,89] Interestingly, deafness, a common sequela of other congenital infections, occurs in only 3% of children with congenital syphilis.[75]

Recommendations

The increasing incidence of congenital syphilis underscores the need to optimize identification of infected mothers and neonates. Serologic screening for gestational infection should be conducted early in pregnancy, during the third trimester (especially for high-risk women), and at delivery.[72,73,75,82,90] Even with adherence to these guidelines, some infants with congenital syphilis may be missed, probably because the maternal infection occurred immediately prior to delivery, providing insufficient time for an antibody response to develop.[75,91] Thus in areas where the infection is prevalent, retesting of infants presenting during the first weeks of life with symptoms or signs compatible with congenital syphilis may be prudent.[75,91] Screening should be with a nontreponemal test: VDRL or RPR. RPR is preferred in pregnancy by some experts.[75] If the nontreponemal test is positive, one of the treponemal-specific tests should be performed to confirm maternal infection; either microhemagglutination *Treponema pallidum* (MHA-TP) or fluorescent treponemal antibody absorption (FTA-ABS) may be used. Maternal treatment history must be examined if both nontreponemal and treponemal tests are positive. In addition, any mother with positive syphilis serology needs HIV testing because 15% of adults with syphilis are coinfected with HIV.[76]

The diagnosis of congenital syphilis should be considered in any neonate born to a mother with a reactive serologic test for syphilis. All infants should have a physical exam and nontreponemal antibody titer obtained.[72,73,75,79,82,83,90,92] For accurate comparison, the nontreponemal test must be the same for the infant and mother. Criteria for further evaluation of neonates are listed in Table 17.2. Evaluation for congenital syphilis should also be considered for stillbirths occurring after 20 weeks' gestation and in neonates with unexplained prematurity or low birth weight, bullous skin lesions, maculopapular rashes, rhinitis, skeletal lesions, jaundice, hepatosplenomegaly, or lymphadenopathy.[72,73,75,79,82,83,90,92]

Complete diagnostic evaluation of infants includes: physical exam, nontreponemal titers, long-bone X-rays, and CSF analysis.[72,73,75,78,79,81–83,87,90,92] X-rays are suggested because 6–20% of asymptomatic infants will have detectable abnormalities.[75,76,83] CSF evaluation is still recommended by most experts, despite the low sensitivity with older CSF tests and debate over normal ranges for neonates.[72,73,75,82,83] If the initial evaluation of the neonate is negative, the CDC recommends the performance of a specific treponemal IgM antibody assay on infant's sera before infection is ruled out.[73] Finally, if possible, the placenta and umbilical cord should undergo histologic examination.[73]

Symptomatic infants may require additional testing, including: liver function tests, complete blood counts with platelets, chest X-rays and ophthalmology exams.[73,75,82] CSF analysis should include cell counts, concentrations of glucose and protein, and a VDRL titer. The CSF VDRL titer is highly specific for neurosyphilis, but has a sensitivity of only 22–69%.[78,92] PCR analysis of the CSF has 90% correlation with the rabbit infectivity test.[78] PCR for *T. pallidum* DNA in the CSF is 75% sensitive and 96–100% specific.[78] Thus, if available, PCR should also be performed on CSF fluid.

Ten to 14 days of parenteral procaine or aqueous penicillin is recommended for the treatment of symptomatic congenital syphilis. Procaine or aqueous penicillin is recommended because they provide adequate treatment for possible neurosyphilis; benzathine penicillin does not. This treatment regimen is considered prudent even if tests for neurosyphilis are negative because these tests may be falsely negative. Treatment is also indicated for asymptomatic infants born to women with untreated syphilis, inadequate treatment, treatment with a nonpenicillin regimen, and inadequate documentation of treatment. In addition, treatment should be given to asymptomatic infants born to women treated within 1 month of delivery even if an appropriate regimen was given.[73,75,82]

Table 17.2. Criteria for evaluation of infants for congenital syphilis[75,77,79,82]

Infants born to seropositive women who meet the following criteria should be thoroughly evaluated:

- Mother with untreated syphilis
- Mother treated for syphilis during pregnancy with a nonpenicillin regimen (e.g., erythromycin)
- Mother treated for syphilis less than 1 month before delivery
- Mother treated for syphilis during pregnancy with the appropriate penicillin regimen but nontreponemal antibody titers did not decrease sufficiently after therapy (fourfold decline) to indicate an adequate response to treatment
- Mother did not have syphilis treatment well documented
- Mother was treated appropriately before pregnancy but did not have adequate serologic follow-up to assure response to therapy and to rule out reinfection

Source: Adapted from:[75,77,79,92]

Treatment of asymptomatic infants born to a mother who received appropriate treatment without adequate titer decline is controversial.[73,75,77,80–84,90] The controversy stems from the inability definitely to exclude neurosyphilis or congenital syphilis in at-risk infants. In addition, in late latent maternal infection, nontreponemal titers decline slowly and may remain stably positive at low titers (≤1:4).[75,77] Thus, in some pregnant women, appropriate treatment may fail to produce a fourfold titer decline.[75,77] Debate continues on how to manage infants in this scenario. Some advocate for close observation and follow-up if the complete evaluation is negative.[75,82] Others would treat these infants with a single dose of benzathine penicillin.[75,77,82,83,93] The CDC currently recommends treatment for 10–14 days for this group of infants since infection cannot be excluded definitely.[73,83] Consultation with local infectious disease experts is recommended.

To date, though serology may be less reliable in HIV-infected women, there is no indication to alter maternal treatment or neonatal evaluation and treatment when caring for HIV-infected pregnant women and their children.[73,75] Recommendations are changing constantly and consultation with local infectious disease experts is recommended.

All infants with suspected or proven congenital syphilis, whether or not CNS involvement is confirmed, must undergo careful long-term evaluations of mental and motor function, hearing, and vision.[73,75,82] In addition, serologic tests should be monitored until they become nonreactive.[73,75,79,82] In the absence of fetal infection, the VDRL titer should be decreasing by 3–4 months of age. VDRL is undetectable in most infants by 6 months.[73,75,79,82] If the infant was congenitally infected, adequate treatment should result in a decreasing VDRL, with disappearance by 6 months of age.[73,75,79,82] Treponemal-specific antibodies (e.g., FTA-ABS) may be detectable for up to 15 months of age in uninfected neonates due to persistence of transplacental antibodies.[73,75,79,82] If antibodies persist beyond these limits, the infant should be reassessed and treated. In 85% of infected individuals treponemal antibodies persist for life; therefore, these tests should not be monitored during follow-up assessments of congenitally infected children.[75,77] If the CSF VDRL was originally positive, it should be repeated at 6 months of age. If it remains positive and CSF abnormalities persist by 2 years, retreatment is indicated.[75,77,79,82]

Varicella-zoster virus

Primary infection with VZV causes varicella (chickenpox) while the reactivation of the latent infection results in herpes zoster (shingles). Although pregnant women occasionally develop varicella, this virus is an unusual cause of intrauterine or perinatal infection because more than 90% of women of childbearing age who live in temperate climates have had varicella in childhood.[94] The current rate of pregnancies complicated by varicella is estimated at 0.5–0.7 per 1000 pregnancies.[94–96]

Congenital varicella syndrome was first described in 1947.[97] Infants with congenital varicella syndrome have characteristic cicatricial cutaneous scars, limb atrophy, rudimentary digits, chorioretinitis, and microcephaly.[95,97–103] In 1987, Alkalay et al. proposed three diagnostic criteria for congenital varicella syndrome which included a documented maternal varicella infection in pregnancy, congenital cutaneous lesions in a dermatomal distribution, and evidence of congenital infection by immunologic proof (VZV-specific IgM at delivery) or zoster in infancy accompanied by a rise in VZV antibody titers[103] (Table 17.3). In their study, 77% of the 22 infants fulfilling the diagnostic criteria for congenital varicella syndrome had neurologic abnormalities that included hypoplasia of upper or lower extremities (80%), limb paresis (65%), hydrocephalus/cortical atrophy (35%), seizures (24%), Horner's syndrome (24%), mental retardation (18%), and auditory palsy (6%). The region of neurologic involvement correlated well with the anatomic distribution of dermatomal disease.

The series of Enders et al. of 1373 pregnant women with varicella during pregnancy is the largest experience to date.[101] Nine cases of congenital varicella and an additional 10 cases of zoster in infancy occurred in offspring of these women. The overall risk of congenital varicella syndrome was 1%. This risk increased to 2% if maternal infection occurred between 13 and 20 weeks' gestation. In previous smaller studies the risk of congenital varicella syndrome ranged from 0 to 9%.[95,98,100,101]

Neurologic damage is an important consequence of congenital varicella syndrome.[95,99–106] Table 17.4 lists the various neurologic abnormalities that have been reported. Varicella is a neurotrophic virus. Autopsies of neonates with congenital varicella syndrome have demonstrated VZV virus in the cerebrum and spinal cord by dot-blot and Southern blot hybridization.[107] Postmortem evaluation of suspected and confirmed congenital varicella syndrome cases report cortical and cerebellar necrosis, severe encephalopathy involving gray and white matter, and spinal cord disease including myelopathy, anterior horn cell loss, and gray-matter gliosis.[95,102,107–109]

Maternal varicella during the few days before and after pregnancy can result in transplacental infection or exposure to the virus during delivery.[110] This perinatal infection is not associated with congenital malformations but can be the cause of severe neonatal morbidity and mortality. Infants whose mothers develop varicella more than a week before delivery can be expected to escape infection or to have an uncomplicated illness, probably because the interval between the onset of maternal infection and birth provides sufficient time for transplacental transmission of VZV antibodies.[111] In contrast, maternal chickenpox developing 5 days before or within 2 days following delivery poses a substantial risk to the newborn. The attack rate for perinatal infection under these circumstances is approximately 20% and the incidence of fatal infection is about 30%. Nosocomial exposure of high-risk infants can also result in neonatal varicella.[112]

Infants who contract perinatal VZV during this high-risk period are typically well for the first 5–10 days of age. Infection is recognized thereafter with the typical cutaneous exanthema. The diagnosis is usually obvious because of the characteristic

Table 17.3. Proposed diagnostic criteria for congenital varicella syndrome

1. Documented maternal varicella infection in pregnancy
2. Congenital cutaneous lesions in a dermatomal distribution
3. Evidence of congenital infection by either:
   a. Immunologic proof of in utero varicella infection (VZV-specific IgM at delivery) or
   b. Zoster in infancy accompanied by a rise in VZV antibody titers

Notes:
VZV, varicella-zoster virus; IgM, immunoglobulin M.
Source: Adapted from Alkalay et al.[103]

Table 17.4. Neurologic abnormalities in congenital varicella syndrome

Limb paresis
Hypoplasia of extremities (usually ipsilateral and distal to cutaneous abnormalities)
Seizures
Horner's syndrome
Mental retardation
Auditory nerve palsy
Hydrocephalus
Microcephaly
Cortical atrophy
Central nervous system structural anomalies (prosencephalic cysts, glial fiber proliferation)
Encephalitis
Autonomic dysfunction
Ocular disease (chorioretinitis, microphthalmia, endophthalmos, optic atrophy, cataracts)
Gastrointestinal dysmotility
Genitourinary dysfunction

Notes:
Adapted from:[95,97–99,101–103,105,116,118,119]

vesicular lesions and the recognition of recent maternal varicella. Progressive cutaneous infection is associated with life-threatening illness due to VZV pneumonia, encephalitis, hepatitis, and bleeding diathesis. Encephalitis is suggested by the occurrence of seizures accompanied by CSF and electroencephalogram abnormalities. Because of the limited number of infants with perinatal VZV infection that have been reported, the risk of neurologic involvement has not been established.

Herpes zoster, due to the reactivation of latent VZV, occurs during pregnancy but has not been associated with the classic features of congenital varicella syndrome. Enders et al. followed 366 women with zoster during pregnancy; none of these women had an affected newborn.[101] Other studies also document the absence of fetal/neonatal sequelae in cases of herpes zoster infection during pregnancy.[94,103] The lack of neonatal disease may be explained by the absence of viremia during herpes zoster infection in otherwise healthy pregnant women. Infants whose mothers develop varicella-zoster late in pregnancy or immediately postpartum are not at risk for serious illness because these infants are protected by transplacentally acquired VZV antibodies.

In March 1995 the Food and Drug Administration approved licensure of a live attenuated vaccine for varicella.[113,114] This vaccine is not approved for pregnant women or women who might conceive within 1–3 months following vaccination. The company manufacturing the vaccine and the CDC have established a Varivax Pregnancy Registry to follow inadvertently vaccinated pregnant women.[115] No cases of live births with congenital varicella syndrome have occurred in the pregnancies reported to this registry to date.

Recommendations

If a pregnant woman is known to be susceptible to VZV infection, she should be offered varicella-zoster immune globulin (VZIG) prophylaxis within 96 h of her exposure in order to modify the severity of her infection.[116] It is possible, although not proven, that VZIG may reduce the risk of congenital varicella infection. In the study by Enders et al. none of the 97 women who received VZIG had an infant with congenital varicella syndrome.[101,117]

VZIG should also be given to all infants born to mothers whose onset of varicella is between 5 days before and 2 days after delivery.[116,117] These infants also should be treated with intravenous aciclovir. Although controlled clinical evaluations of aciclovir treatment of infants with perinatal varicella are lacking, the drug prevents progressive VZV infection among other immunodeficient patients.

No intervention is required for infants who are exposed to maternal varicella-zoster. These infants will have transplacentally acquired VZV antibodies and can be expected to be free of infection or to develop mild varicella.

Women who contract varicella during pregnancy should have ultrasounds performed at 20–22 weeks' gestation to look for abnormalities associated with congenital varicella syndrome (limb hypoplasia, microcephaly, intrauterine growth retardation, etc).[103,107] Studies have examined the potential utility of a variety of VZV-specific immunologic studies from blood obtained by cordocentesis from fetuses exposed in utero to maternal VZV infection.[107,108] The potential value of viral culture and PCR from amniotic fluid of pregnancies complicated by varicella has also been assessed.[101,108] To date, the data do not support the routine use of any of these diagnostic methods.

Herpes simplex virus

Approximately 1 in 3000 to 1 in 5000 live-born infants contract HSV infection, resulting in 1500 to 2200 cases of neonatal herpes in the USA each year.[120] Neonatal herpes has four disease manifestations: disease limited to the skin, eye, and mouth (SEM), isolated CNS disease, disseminated disease, and, rarely, congenital disease due to intrauterine infection.[120,121] Approximately 35% of neonatal infections primarily involve the CNS.[120,121]

Transmission of HSV to the fetus and newborn

Neonatal infection with HSV can be caused by either HSV-1 or HSV-2 but two-thirds of these infections result from HSV-2.[120,121] More than 85% of neonates with HSV infection contract the virus during labor and delivery from infected maternal secretions.[120,121] More than 70% of infected neonates are born to women who are asymptomatic during labor and delivery and have no prior history of genital herpes.[122,123] Intrapartum asymptomatic HSV excretion by the mother may represent a primary infection or reactivation of latent virus from a previous genital HSV infection.[124] In a study of almost 16000 women prospectively cultured for HSV at delivery, 56 (0.35%) were found to have asymptomatic HSV excretion.[124] Based on serologic evaluation, one-third of these women had primary genital infections and two-thirds had recurrent infections. The attack rate among infants born to mothers with primary genital herpes at delivery is estimated to be 33–50%.[121] Fortunately, the attack rate for HSV infection among infants whose mothers are experiencing recurrent HSV at delivery is substantially lower: 0–5%.[121,124] The difference in neonatal infection rates following primary vs recurrent maternal infection are due to many factors, including concentration of virus, site of viral excretion (cervix versus labia), and presence of transplacentally acquired protective antibodies in infants born to mothers with recurrent infection.[120,121,124]

Postnatal exposure to HSV accounts for approximately 10% of neonatal infections.[120,121] These infections result from close contact with individuals who have active HSV-1 infection. These infections may be symptomatic or asymptomatic. Nosocomial transmission of HSV from infant to infant, apparently by personnel or fomites, has also occurred in neonatal nurseries.[120]

Fewer than 5% of neonatal HSV infections are congenital.[120,125] The risk factors for HSV infection before birth have not been determined. Affected infants have been born to mothers with symptomatic and asymptomatic, primary and recurrent HSV infections during pregnancy.[120,125] HSV-2 is responsible for most intrauterine infections.[125]

Clinical manifestations and consequences of perinatal and intrauterine HSV infections

Although the rate and severity of neurologic abnormalities varies, SEM, isolated CNS, disseminated disease, and intrauterine infection have all been associated with neurologic deficits at follow-up.

Approximately 40% of perinatal HSV infections are classified as SEM.[120,121] This mucocutaneous form of infection is characterized by vesicular lesions of the skin and mucosal surfaces with or without ocular disease. It is crucial to identify herpetic mucocutaneous lesions as soon as possible because, without proper identification and treatment, SEM disease will progress to the disseminated or CNS forms of neonatal herpes in more than 75% of cases.[120] In addition, during the preantiviral drug era, neurologic sequelae occurred in more than 25% of infants with localized SEM disease.[120] In contrast, with timely aciclovir treatment, the chance that the infant will escape neurologic sequelae exceeds 90%.[126] None the less, even with appropriate therapy for limited mucocutaneous disease, 5–10% will have evidence of neurologic impairment at follow-up.[126] One predictor of neurologic morbidity appears to be the frequency of mucocutaneous recurrences during the first 6 months of life.[127]

Thirty-five percent of neonatal herpes cases have isolated CNS involvement.[121] Herpes encephalitis usually occurs in infants who are about 2 weeks old (range 1–6 weeks). At presentation, some infants have active or resolving mucocutaneous lesions, but the majority do not. Only 60% of infants with CNS herpes have cutaneous lesions documented at any time during the course of their illness.[120] The signs of neonatal HSV encephalitis include fever or temperature instability, lethargy, poor feeding, bulging fontanel, pyramidal tract signs, tremors, and seizures.[120,121] The seizures often begin as focal, unilateral tonic-clonic movements that become generalized. Apnea is common. The CSF can be normal at the onset of symptoms but usually shows a mild lymphocytic pleocytosis (20–100 cells/mm^3) and elevated protein; the glucose may be normal or slightly low. Serial evaluations of the CSF usually show progressive abnormalities with substantial increase in protein (up to 1 g/dl) and inflammatory cells.[120,121] The electroencephalogram is usually diffusely abnormal. CT brain scans may be normal or show diffuse enhancement. MRI is superior to CT in demonstrating subtle abnormalities early in infection. Cultures of the CSF for HSV have a low yield: less than one-third are positive.[120] PCR of CSF is the preferred method to diagnose HSV meningoencephalitis.[120,121,128] The sensitivity of PCR on the CSF is 75–100%, with a specificity of 70–100%.[128] Although antiviral treatment of infants with herpes encephalitis reduces the mortality rate, very few survivors escape serious neurologic sequelae.[126,127] At follow-up, over 60% have neurologic deficits, including persistent seizures, spasticity, chorioretinitis, blindness, learning disabilities, and developmental delays.[126,127] HSV-1 CNS infection may have a better prognosis than CNS disease caused by HSV-2.[127]

Disseminated disease represents 25% of cases of neonatal HSV infection.[121] Infants with disseminated herpes usually present during the first 2 weeks of life with fever and signs indistinguishable from bacterial sepsis.[120] Disseminated HSV is often fulminant and associated with severe hepatitis, coagulopathy, pneumonitis, and possible concomitant encephalitis.[120] Unfortunately, infants with disseminated disease often lack cutaneous symptoms at presentation; 20% never develop mucocutaneous lesions.[120] Disseminated neonatal herpes has a mortality rate of greater than 80% if untreated.[120] The mortality rate is approximately 30% even with appropriate antiviral therapy.[126] Infants who have had CNS infection in the course of their disseminated disease usually have neurologic sequelae if they survive. Despite the severity of the acute illness, up to 80% of treated survivors are developmentally normal at follow-up.[126]

In utero infection accounts for less than 5% of neonatal HSV.[121] The consequences of in utero infection are devastating. Infants with intrauterine infection have skin vesicles or scars at birth, chorioretinitis in the first week of life, microphthalmia, and abnormal head CT.[125] In 13 infants infected in utero, all had multisystem disease.[125] Four died; six had severe neurologic sequelae, including hydranencephaly, brain atrophy, seizures, and severe developmental delay.[125] Antiviral therapy does not reverse CNS damage sustained in utero.[120,125]

Table 17.5. Predictors of mortality with neonatal herpes simplex virus (HSV) infection based on signs at presentation

Coma or semicomatose state
Disseminated intravascular coagulation
Prematurity
Disseminated disease due to HSV-1[a]

Notes:
Mortality was the same in those with central nervous system disease from HSV-1 and HSV-2.
Source: Adapted from Whitley et al.[127] with permission.

Table 17.6. Predictors of morbidity from neonatal herpes infection

Infection with HSV-2
Seizures
Extent of disease at presentation (disseminated, CNS, or SEM)
For SEM only, ≥3 mucocutaneous recurrences in 6 months after therapy

Notes:
HSV, herpes simplex virus; CNS, central nervous system; SEM, skin, eye, and mouth.
Source: Adapted from Whitley et al.[127] with permission.

Predictors of mortality and morbidity from neonatal HSV infections are outlined in Tables 17.5 and 17.6.[127] Morbidity is defined as developmental delay of greater than 6 months, blindness, microcephaly, spastic quadriplegia, and/or seizures. The presence of seizures prior to the initiation of antiviral therapy significantly influences the incidence of neurologic deficits in survivors. Ninety-three percent of survivors with seizures have neurologic deficits compared with 34% incidence of neurologic impairment in the absence of seizures.[127] The highest morbidity occurs in neonates with CNS disease, followed by those infants with disseminated disease.[127] Only a small percentage of those with SEM have neurologic sequelae.[127]

Recommendations

Prevention

Since most neonatal disease is acquired from maternal genital infection at the time of delivery, the first problem is to identify women with active genital HSV at the onset of labor. If the mother has genital lesions or prodromal symptoms consistent with genital HSV, cesarean delivery is recommended to avoid infant exposure.[129] Although some reports suggest that the benefits of cesarean section are more likely to be realized if cesarean section is performed within 4–6 h of membrane rupture, the American College of Obstetrics and Gynecologists (ACOG) recommends cesarean section regardless of the duration of membrane rupture.[120,121,129]

Approximately 0.5–1% of women with a past history of recurrent genital herpes will have HSV excretion without any lesions at the time of delivery.[120,121,124] Unfortunately, these women cannot be identified by antepartum screening cultures.[130,131] Cesarean delivery for every woman with a past history of genital herpes is not reasonable and not recommended by ACOG.[129] Women who have had symptomatic primary genital herpes late in pregnancy may constitute a special subpopulation at greater risk of high-titer asymptomatic shedding; special consideration for cesarean section in these cases may be necessary.[132]

Since most mothers of infants with neonatal herpes have no history of genital herpes, the infant's risk of HSV exposure will not be known. Maternal history of genital infection caused by HSV may be negative because the prior HSV-2 infection was asymptomatic or because the mother had primary genital HSV late in gestation that was not diagnosed or was asymptomatic.

Table 17.7. Mortality and morbidity in neonatal herpes

Diagnosis	Untreated mortality	Treated mortality	Treated morbidity
Disseminated	80%	50–60%	40%
CNS disease	50%	14%	55–65%
SEM disease		0%	5–10%

Notes:

CNS, central nervous system; SEM, skin, eye, and mouth (mucocutaneous only).

Source: Adapted from:[120,121,127]

Diagnosis and treatment

Direct immunofluorescence, PCR, and viral cultures provide the only means of confirming the diagnosis of HSV in the symptomatic infant.[120,121,128,133,134] Serologic tests are not helpful because the majority of newborn infants have passive HSV antibodies due to transplacental acquisition.[120,121] Furthermore, absence of HSV antibodies does not rule out herpes because the infant may have acquired the infection as a result of primary maternal HSV or from a non-maternal source.[120,121] In addition, some infected neonates have delayed or no serologic response to infection. Currently, there is no reliable method for detection of HSV IgM.

Since the maternal history of herpes is not a reliable clue, infants with neonatal herpes will only be recognized if viral diagnostic procedures are included in the evaluation of infants with suspicious mucocutaneous lesions, nonbacterial sepsis, or unexplained seizures. Timely antiviral therapy may result in increased survival and improved long-term outcome for neonates infected with HSV.[127]

High-dose parenteral aciclovir therapy (60 mg/kg per day) is now recommended for the treatment of neonatal herpes. SEM disease should be treated for 14 days and CNS and disseminated disease for 21 days.[121] Survival appears to be improved with this high-dose regimen. For disseminated disease, survival rates were

39% in low-dose groups compared to 69% with high-dose treatment (National Institute of Allergy and Infectious Diseases Collaborative Antiviral Study Group and Kimberlin, personal communication). For CNS disease, survival was 81% and 94% for low- and high-dose regimens, respectively. Morbidity also appears to be improved with high-dose therapy. Only 60% of survivors of disseminated infection were normal at a year on low-dose regimens, compared to 83% who received high-dose treatment. Morbidity following CNS disease was similar after low- and high-dose treatment.

Any infant who has had neonatal HSV should have continued follow-up through childhood.

REFERENCES

1 Wolf ACD and Paige BH. (1939). Toxoplasmic encephalomyelitis. III. A new case of granulomatous encephalomyelitis due to a protozoa. *Am J Pathol*, **15**, 657–694.

2 Wong SY and Remington JS. (1994). Toxoplasmosis in pregnancy. *Clin Infect Dis*, **18**, 853–862.

3 Remington JS, McLeod R, Thulliez, et al. (2001). Toxoplasmosis. In *Infectious Diseases of the Fetus and Newborn Infant*, 5th edn, Remington JS and Klein JO (eds), pp. 205–346. Phildelphia:WB Saunders.

4 Lynfield R and Guerina NG. (1997). Toxoplasmosis. *Pediatr Rev*, **18**, 75–83.

5 Guerina NG, Hsu HW, Meissner HC, et al. (1994). Neonatal serologic screening and early treatment for congenital *Toxoplasma gondii* infection. The New England Regional *Toxoplasma* Working Group. *N Engl J Med*, **330**, 1858–1863.

6 Hohlfeld P, Daffos F, Thulliez P, et al. (1989). Fetal toxoplasmosis: outcome of pregnancy and infant follow-up after in utero treatment. *J Pediatr*, **115**, 765–769.

7 Foulon W, Villena I, Stray-Pedersen B, et al. (1999). Treatment of toxoplasmosis during pregnancy: a multicenter study of impact on fetal transmission and children's sequelae at age 1 year. *Am J Obstet Gynecol*, **180**, 410–415.

8 Koppe JG, Loewer-Sieger DH and de Roever-Bonnet H. (1986). Results of 20-year follow-up of congenital toxoplasmosis. *Lancet*, **1**, 254–256.

9 Stagno S, Reynolds DW, Amos CS, et al. (1977). Auditory and visual defects resulting from symptomatic and subclinical congenital cytomegaloviral and toxoplasma infections. *Pediatrics*, **59**, 669–678.

10 Wilson CB, Remington JS, Stagno S, et al. (1980). Development of adverse sequelae in children born with subclinical congenital *Toxoplasma* infection. *Pediatrics*, **66**, 767–774.

11 Roizen N, Swisher CN, Stein MA, et al. (1995). Neurologic and developmental outcome in treated congenital toxoplasmosis. *Pediatrics*, **95**, 11–20.

12 McAuley J, Boyer KM, Patel D, et al. (1994). Early and longitudinal evaluations of treated infants and children and untreated historical patients with congenital toxoplasmosis: The Chicago Collaborative Treatment Trial. *Clin Infect Dis*, **18**, 38–72 (published erratum appears in *Clin Infect Dis* 1994; **19**, 820).

13 Patel DV, Holfels EM, Vogel NP, et al. (1996). Resolution of intracranial calcifications in infants with treated congenital toxoplasmosis. *Radiology*, **199**, 433–440.

14 Naessens A, Jenum PA, Pollak A, et al. (1999). Diagnosis of congenital toxoplasmosis in the neonatal period: a multicenter evaluation. *J Pediatr*, **135**, 714–719.

15 Foulon W, Pinon JM, Stray-Pedersen B, et al. (1999). Prenatal diagnosis of congenital toxoplasmosis: a multicenter evaluation of different diagnostic parameters. *Am J Obstet Gynecol*, **181**, 843–847.

16 Sagno S. (2001). Cytomegalovirus. In *Infectious Diseases of the Fetus and Newborn Infant*, Remington JS and Klein JO (eds), pp. 389–424. Philadelphia: WB Saunders.

17 Stagno S, Reynolds DW, Huang ES, et al. (1977). Congenital cytomegalovirus infection. *N Engl J Med*, **296**, 1254–1258.

18 Stagno S, Pass RF and Alford CA. (1981). Perinatal infections and maldevelopment. *Birth Defects Orig Artic Ser*, **17**, 31–50.

19 Saigal S, Lunyk O, Larke RP, et al. (1982). The outcome in children with congenital cytomegalovirus infection. A longitudinal follow-up study. *Am J Dis Child*, **136**, 896–901.

20 Reynolds DW, Stagno S, Stubbs KG, et al. (1974). Inapparent congenital cytomegalovirus infection with elevated cord IgM levels. Casual relation with auditory and mental deficiency. *N Engl J Med*, **290**, 291–296.

21 Preece PM, Pearl KN and Peckham CS. (1984). Congenital cytomegalovirus infection. *Arch Dis Child*, **59**, 1120–1126.

22 Noyola DE, Demmler GJ, Williamson WD, et al. (2000). Cytomegalovirus urinary excretion and long term outcome in children with congenital cytomegalovirus infection. Congenital CMV Longitudinal Study Group. *Pediatr Infect Dis J*, **19**, 505–510.

23 Monif GR, Egan EAD, Held B, et al. (1972). The correlation of maternal cytomegalovirus infection during varying stages in gestation with neonatal involvement. *J Pediatr*, **80**, 17–20.

24 Kumar ML, Nankervis GA and Gold E. (1973). Inapparent congenital cytomegalovirus infection. A follow-up study. *N Engl J Med*, **288**, 1370–1372.

25 Ivarsson SA, Lernmark B and Svanberg L. (1997). Ten-year clinical, developmental, and intellectual follow-up of children with congenital cytomegalovirus infection without neurologic symptoms at one year of age. *Pediatrics*, **99**, 800–803.

26 Hanshaw JB, Scheiner AP, Moxley AW, et al. (1976). School failure and deafness after "silent" congenital cytomegalovirus infection. *N Engl J Med*, **295**, 468–470.

27 Halwachs-Baumann G, Genser B, Danda M, et al. (2000). Screening and diagnosis of congenital cytomegalovirus infection: a 5-year study. *Scand J Infect Dis*, **32**, 137–142.

28 Fowler KB, McCollister FP, Dahle AJ, et al. (1997). Progressive and fluctuating sensorineural hearing loss in children with asymptomatic congenital cytomegalovirus infection. *J Pediatr*, **130**, 624–630.

29 Conboy TJ, Pass RF, Stagno S, et al. (1986). Intellectual development in school-aged children with asymptomatic congenital cytomegalovirus infection. *Pediatrics*, **77**, 801–806.

30 Williamson WD, Desmond MM, LaFevers N, et al. (1982). Symptomatic congenital cytomegalovirus. Disorders of language, learning, and hearing. *Am J Dis Child*, **136**, 902–905.

31 Whitley RJ, Cloud G, Gruber W, et al. (1997). Ganciclovir treatment of symptomatic congenital cytomegalovirus infection: results of a phase II study. National Institute of Allergy and Infectious Diseases Collaborative Antiviral Study Group. *J Infect Dis*, **175**, 1080–1086.

32 Pass RF, Stagno S, Myers GJ, et al. (1980). Outcome of symptomatic congenital cytomegalovirus infection: results of long-term longitudinal follow-up. *Pediatrics*, **66**, 758–762.

33 McCracken GH Jr, Shinefield HMR, Cobb K, et al. (1969). Congenital cytomegalic inclusion disease. A longitudinal study of 20 patients. *Am J Dis Child*, **117**, 522–539.

34 Boppana SB, Fowler KB, Vaid Y, et al. (1997). Neuroradiographic findings in the newborn period and long-term outcome in children with symptomatic congenital cytomegalovirus infection. *Pediatrics*, **99**, 409–414.

35 Williamson WD, Demmler GJ, Percy AK, et al. (1992). Progressive hearing loss in infants with asymptomatic congenital cytomegalovirus infection. *Pediatrics*, **90**, 862–866.

36 Kumar ML, Nankervis GA, Jacobs IB, et al. (1984). Congenital and postnatally acquired cytomegalovirus infections: long- term follow-up. *J Pediatr*, **104**, 674–679.

37 Melish ME and Hanshaw JB. (1973). Congenital cytomegalovirus infection. Developmental progress of infants detected by routine screening. *Am J Dis Child*, **126**, 190–194.

38 Fowler KB, Dahle AJ, Boppana SB, et al. (1999). Newborn hearing screening: will children with hearing loss caused by congenital cytomegalovirus infection be missed? *J Pediatr*, **135**, 60–64.

39 Hicks T, Fowler K, Richardson M, et al. (1993). Congenital cytomegalovirus infection and neonatal auditory screening. *J Pediatr*, **123**, 779–782.

40 Stagno S, Pass RF, Cloud G, et al. (1986). Primary cytomegalovirus infection in pregnancy. Incidence, transmission to fetus, and clinical outcome. *JAMA*, **256**, 1904–1908.

41 Butt W, Mackay RJ, de Crespigny LC, et al. (1984). Intracranial lesions of congenital cytomegalovirus infection detected by ultrasound scanning. *Pediatrics*, **73**, 611–614.

42 Steinlin MI, Nadal D, Eich GF, et al. (1996). Late intrauterine cytomegalovirus infection: clinical and neuroimaging findings. *Pediatr Neurol*, **15**, 249–253.

43 Troendle Atkins J, Demmler GJ, Williamson WD, et al. (1994). Polymerase chain reaction to detect cytomegalovirus DNA in the cerebrospinal fluid of neonates with congenital infection. *J Infect Dis*, **169**, 1334–1337.

44 Ahlfors K, Forsgren M, Ivarsson SA, et al. (1982). Congenital cytomegalovirus infection: on the relation between type and time of maternal infection and infant's symptoms. *Scand J Infect Dis*, **15**, 129–138.

45 Atkins JT, Dimmler CJ, Williamson WD, et al. (1994). Polymerase chain reaction to detect cytomegalovirus DNA in the cerebrospinal fluid of neonates with congenital infection. *J Infect Dis*, **169**, 1334–1337.

46 American Academy of Pediatrics. (2000). Rubella. In *2000 Red Book. Report of the Committee on Infectious Diseases*, 25th edn, Pickering LK (ed.), pp. 495–500. Elk Grove, IL: AAP.

47 Cooper LZ and Ahlford CA. (2001). Rubella. In *Infectious Diseases of the Fetus and Newborn Infant*, 5th edn, Remington JS and Klein JO (eds), pp. 347–388. Philadelphia: WB Saunders.

48 Current trends increase in rubella and congenital rubella syndrome — United States, 1988–1990. (1991). *MMWR*, **40**, 93–99.

49 Measles, rubella and congenital rubella syndrome - United States and Mexico, 1997–1999. (2000). *MMWR*, **49**, 1048–1050.

50 Rubella and congenital rubella syndrome – United States, 1994–1997. (1997). *MMWR*, **46**, 350–354.

51 Banatvala JE. (1998). Rubella – could do better. *Lancet*, **351**, 849–850.

52 Miller E, Cradock-Watson JE and Pollock TM. (1982). Consequences of confirmed maternal rubella at successive stages of pregnancy. *Lancet*, **2**, 781–784.

53 Frey TK. (1997). Neurological aspects of rubella virus infection. *Intervirology*, **40**, 167–175.

54 Meitsch K, Enders G, Wolinsky JS, et al. (1997). The role of rubella-immunoblot and rubella-peptide-EIA for the diagnosis of the congenital rubella syndrome during the prenatal and newborn periods. *J Med Virol*, **51**, 280–283.

55 Ueda K, Nishida Y, Oshima K, et al. (1979). Congenital rubella syndrome: correlation of gestational age at time of maternal rubella with type of defect. *J Pediatr*, **94**, 763–765.

56 Peckham CS. (1972). Clinical and laboratory study of children exposed in utero to maternal rubella. *Arch Dis Child*, **47**, 571–577.

57 Weil ML, Itabashi H, Cremer NE, et al. (1975). Chronic progressive panencephalitis due to rubella virus simulating subacute sclerosing panencephalitis. *N Engl J Med*, **292**, 994–998.

58 Macfarlane DW, Boyd RD, Dodrill CB, et al. (1975). Intrauterine rubella, head size, and intellect. *Pediatrics*, **55**, 797–801.

59 Chang YC, Huang CC and Liu CC. (1996). Frequency of linear hyperechogenicity over the basal ganglia in young infants with congenital rubella syndrome. *Clin Infect Dis*, **22**, 569–571.

60 Lane B, Sullivan EV, Lim KO, et al. (1996). White matter MR hyperintensities in adult patients with congenital rubella. *Am J Neuroradiol*, **17**, 99–103.

61 Townsend JJ, Baringer JR, Wolinsky JS, et al. (1975). Progressive rubella panencephalitis. Late onset after congenital rubella. *N Engl J Med*, **292**, 990–993.

62 Desmond MM, Fisher ES, Vorderman AL, et al. (1978). The longitudinal course of congenital rubella encephalitis in nonretarded children. *J Pediatr*, **93**, 584–591.

63 McIntosh ED and Menser MA. (1992). A fifty-year follow-up of congenital rubella. *Lancet*, **340**, 414–415.

64 Congenital rubella – 50 years on. (1991). *Lancet*, **337**, 668.

65 Chess S, Fernandez P and Korn S. (1978). Behavioral consequences of congenital rubella. *J Pediatr*, **93**, 699–703.

66 Brown AS, Cohen P, Greenwald S, et al. (2000). Nonaffective psychosis after prenatal exposure to rubella. *Am J Psychiatry*, **157**, 438–443.

67 Tanemura M, Suzumori K, Yagami Y, et al. (1996). Diagnosis of fetal rubella infection with reverse transcription and nested polymerase chain reaction: a study of 34 cases diagnosed in fetuses. *Am J Obstet Gynecol*, **174**, 578–582.

68 Bart KJ, Orenstein WA, Preblud SR, et al. (1985). Elimination of rubella and congenital rubella from the United States. *Pediatr Infect Dis*, **4**, 14–21.

69 Klass PE, Brown ER and Pelton SI. (1994). The incidence of prenatal syphilis at the Boston City Hospital: a comparison across four decades. *Pediatrics*, **94**, 24–28.

70 Reyes MP, Hunt N, Ostrea EM Jr, et al. (1993). Maternal/congenital syphilis in a large tertiary-care urban hospital. *Clin Infect Dis*, **17**, 1041–1046.

71 Sison CG, Ostrea EM Jr, Reyes MP, et al. (1997). The resurgence of congenital syphilis: a cocaine-related problem. *J Pediatr*, **130**, 289–292.

72 Case definition for public health surveillance. (1990). *MMWR*, **39**, 36–38.

73 1993 Sexually transmitted diseases treatment guidelines. (1993). *MMWR*, **42**, 1–85.

74 Congenital syphilis – United States, 1998. (1999). *MMWR*, **48**, 757–761.

75 Ingall D and Sanchez PJ. (2001). Syphilis. In *Infectious Diseases of the Fetus and Newborn Infant*, 5th edn, Remington JS and Klein JO (eds), pp. 643–682. Philadelphia: WB Saunders.

76 Sung L and MacDonald NE. (1998). Syphilis: a pediatric perspective. *Pediatr Rev*, **19**, 17–22.

77 Stoll BJ. (1994). Congenital syphilis: evaluation and management of neonates born to mothers with reactive serologic tests for syphilis. *Pediatr Infect Dis J*, **13**, 845–853.

78 Sanchez PJ, Wendel GD Jr, Grimprel E, et al. (1993). Evaluation of molecular methodologies and rabbit infectivity testing for the diagnosis of congenital syphilis and neonatal central nervous system invasion by *Treponema pallidum*. *J Infect Dis*, **167**, 148–157.

79 Sanchez PJ. (1998). Laboratory tests for congenital syphilis. *Pediatr Infect Dis J*, **17**, 70–71.

80 Srinivasan G, Ramamurthy RS, Bharathi A, et al. (1983). Congenital syphilis: a diagnostic and therapeutic dilemma. *Pediatr Infect Dis*, **2**, 436–441.

81 Risser WL and Hwang LY. (1996). Problems in the current case definitions of congenital syphilis. *J Pediatr*, **129**, 499–505.

82 American Academy of Pediatrics. (2000). Syphilis. In *2000 Red Book. Report of the Committee on Infectious Diseases*, 25th edn, Pickering LK (ed.), pp. 547–559. Elk Grove: AAP.

83 Glaser JH. (1996). Centers for Disease Control and Prevention guidelines for congenital syphilis. *J Pediatr*, **129**, 488–490.

84 Platou RV. (1949). Treatment of congenital syphilis. *Adv Pediatr*, **4**, 39–81.

85 Ahmed A, Hickey SM, Ehrett S, et al. (1996). Cerebrospinal fluid values in the term neonate. *Pediatr Infect Dis J*, **15**, 298–303.

86 Saraff LPL and McCracken G. (1966). Cerebrospinal fluid

examinate in high risk neonates without meningitis. *J Pediatr*, **88**, 473–475.

87 Beeram MR, Chopde N, Dawood Y, et al. (1996). Lumbar puncture in the evaluation of possible asymptomatic congenital syphilis in neonates. *J Pediatr*, **128**, 125–129.

88 Lapunzina PD, Altcheh JM, Flichman JC, et al. (1998). Neurosyphilis in an eight-year-old child: usefulness of the SPECT study. *Pediatr Neurol*, **18**, 81–84.

89 Fiumara NJ and Lessell S. (1970). Manifestations of late congenital syphilis. An analysis of 271 patients. *Arch Dermatol*, **102**, 78–83.

90 Zenker PN and Berman SM. (1991). Congenital syphilis: trends and recommendations for evaluation and management. *Pediatr Infect Dis J*, **10**, 516–522.

91 Dorfman DH and Glaser JH. (1990). Congenital syphilis presenting in infants after the newborn period (see comments). *N Engl J Med*, **323**, 1299–1302.

92 Ikeda MK and Jenson HB. (1990). Evaluation and treatment of congenital syphilis. *J Pediatr*, **117**, 843–852.

93 Paryani SG, Vaughn AJ, Crosby M, et al. (1994). Treatment of asymptomatic congenital syphilis: benzathine versus procaine penicillin G therapy. *J Pediatr*, **125**, 471–475.

94 Gershan AA. (2001). Chickenpox, measles and mumps. In *Infectious Diseases of the Fetus and Newborn Infant*, 5th edn, Remington JL and Klein JO (eds), pp. 683–732. Philadelphia: WB Saunders.

95 Pastuszak AL, Levy M, Schick B, et al. (1994). Outcome after maternal varicella infection in the first 20 weeks of pregnancy. *N Engl J Med*, **330**, 901–905.

96 Dufour P, de Bievre P, Vinatier D, et al. (1996). Varicella and pregnancy. *Eur J Obstet Gynecol Reprod Biol*, **66**, 119–123.

97 Laforet L. (1947). Multiple congenital defects following maternal varicella. *N Engl J Med*, **236**, 534–537.

98 Paryani SG and Arvin AM. (1986). Intrauterine infection with varicella-zoster virus after maternal varicella. *N Engl J Med*, **314**, 1542–1546.

99 Kent A and Paes B. (2000). Congenital varicella syndrome: a rare case of central nervous system involvement without dermatological features. *Am J Perinatol*, **17**, 253–256.

100 Jones KL, Johnson KA and Chambers CD. (1994). Offspring of women infected with varicella during pregnancy: a prospective study. *Teratology*, **49**, 29–32.

101 Enders G, Miller E, Cradock-Watson J, et al. (1994). Consequences of varicella and herpes zoster in pregnancy: prospective study of 1739 cases. *Lancet*, **343**, 1548–1551.

102 Da Silva O, Hammerberg O and Chance GW. (1990). Fetal varicella syndrome. *Pediatr Infect Dis J*, **9**, 854–855.

103 Alkalay AL, Pomerance JJ and Rimoin DL. (1987). Fetal varicella syndrome. *J Pediatr*, **111**, 320–323.

104 Higa K, Dan K and Manabe H. (1987). Varicella-zoster virus infections during pregnancy: hypothesis concerning the mechanisms of congenital malformations. *Obstet Gynecol*, **69**, 214–222.

105 Ong CL and Daniel ML. (1998). Antenatal diagnosis of a porencephalic cyst in congenital varicella-zoster virus infection. *Pediatr Radiol*, **28**, 94.

106 Bassett DC. (1994). Varicella infection in pregnancy. *N Engl J Med*, **331**, 482.

107 Scharf A, Scherr O, Enders G, et al. (1990). Virus detection in the fetal tissue of a premature delivery with a congenital varicella syndrome. A case report. *J Perinat Med*, **18**, 317–322.

108 Mouly F, Mirlesse V, Meritet JF, et al. (1997). Prenatal diagnosis of fetal varicella-zoster virus infection with polymerase chain reaction of amniotic fluid in 107 cases. *Am J Obstet Gynecol*, **177**, 894–898.

109 Salzman MB, Sharrar RG, Steinberg S, et al. (1997). Transmission of varicella-vaccine virus from a healthy 12-month-old child to his pregnant mother. *J Pediatr*, **131**, 151–154.

110 Myers J. (1974). Congenital varicella in term infants: risk reconsidered. *J Infect Dis*, **129**, 215–219.

111 Gershon AA, Raker R, Steinberg S, et al. (1976). Antibody to varicella-zoster virus in parturient women and their offspring during the first year of life. *Pediatrics*, **58**, 692–696.

112 Gustafson TL, Shehab Z and Brunell PA. (1984). Outbreak of varicella in a newborn intensive care nursery. *Am J Dis Child*, **138**, 548–550.

113 Varicella vaccine. (1995). *Med Lett*, **37**, 55–57.

114 Prevention of varicella: Recommendations of the Advisory Committee on Immunization Practices (ACIP). (1996). *MMWR*, **45**, 1–25.

115 Notice to Readers Establishment of VARIVAX (Registered) Pregnancy Registry. (1996). *MMWR*, **45**, 239.

116 American Academy of Pediatrics. Committee on Infectious Diseases. (2000). Varicella vaccine update. *Pediatrics*, **105**, 136–141.

117 Miller E, Cradock-Watson JE and Ridehalgh MK. (1989). Outcome in newborn babies given anti-varicella-zoster immunoglobulin after perinatal maternal infection with varicella-zoster virus. *Lancet*, **2**, 371–373.

118 Wheatley R, Morton RE and Nicholson J. (1996). Chickenpox in mid-trimester pregnancy: always innocent? *Dev Med Child Neurol*, **38**, 462–466.

119 Borzyskowski M, Harris RF and Jones RW. (1981). The congenital varicella syndrome. *Eur J Pediatr*, **137**, 335–338.

120 Arvin AM and Whitley RJ. (2001). Herpes simplex virus

infections. In *Infectious Diseases of the Fetus and Newborn Infant,* 5th edn, Remington JS and Klein JO (eds), pp. 425–446. Philadelphia: WB Saunders.

121 American Academy of Pediatrics. (2000). Herpes simplex. In *2000 Red Book. Report of the Committee of Infectious Diseases,* 25th edn., Pickering LK (ed.), pp. 309–318. Elk Grove, IL: American Academy of Pediatrics.

122 Whitley RJ, Corey L, Arvin A, et al. (1988). Changing presentation of herpes simplex virus infection in neonates. *J Infect Dis,* **158**, 109–116.

123 Whitley RJ, Nahmias AJ, Visintine AM, et al. (1980). The natural history of herpes simplex virus infection of mother and newborn. *Pediatrics,* **66**, 489–494.

124 Brown ZA, Benedetti J, Ashley R, et al. (1991). Neonatal herpes simplex virus infection in relation to asymptomatic maternal infection at the time of labor. *N Engl J Med,* **324**, 1247–1252.

125 Hutto C, Arvin A, Jacobs R, et al. (1987). Intrauterine herpes simplex virus infections. *J Pediatr,* **110**, 97–101.

126 Whitley R, Arvin A, Prober C, et al. (1991). A controlled trial comparing vidarabine with acyclovir in neonatal herpes simplex virus infection. Infectious Diseases Collaborative Antiviral Study Group. *N Engl J Med,* **324**, 444–449.

127 Whitley R, Arvin A, Prober C, et al. (1991). Predictors of morbidity and mortality in neonates with herpes simplex virus infections. The National Institute of Allergy and Infectious Diseases Collaborative Antiviral Study Group. *N Engl J Med,* **324**, 450–454.

128 Kimberlin DW, Lakeman FD, Arvin AM, et al. (1996). Application of the polymerase chain reaction to the diagnosis and management of neonatal herpes simplex virus disease. National Institute of Allergy and Infectious Diseases Collaborative Antiviral Study Group. *J Infect Dis,* **174**, 1162–1167.

129 ACOG Practice Bulletin. (2000). Management of herpes in pregnancy. *Int J Gyn Obs,* **68**, 165–174.

130 Prober CG, Hensleigh PA, Boucher FD, et al. (1988). Use of routine viral cultures at delivery to identify neonates exposed to herpes simplex virus. *N Engl J Med,* **318**, 887–891.

131 Arvin AM, Hensleigh PA, Prober CG, et al. (1986). Failure of antepartum maternal cultures to predict the infant's risk of exposure to herpes simplex virus at delivery. *N Engl J Med,* **315**, 796–800.

132 Brown ZA, Vontver LA, Benedetti J, et al. (1987). Effects on infants of a first episode of genital herpes during pregnancy. *N Engl J Med,* **317**, 1246–1251.

133 Coleman RM, Pereira L, Bailey PD, et al. (1983). Determination of herpes simplex virus type-specific antibodies by enzyme-linked immunosorbent assay. *J Clin Microbiol,* **18**, 287–291.

134 Jacobs RF. (1998). Neonatal herpes simplex virus infections. *Semin Perinatol,* **22**, 64–71.

18

Perinatal human immunodeficiency virus infection

Yvonne A. Maldonado and Andrea M. Enright

Stanford University Medical Center, Stanford, CA, USA

Introduction

The acquired immunodeficiency syndrome (AIDS), first described in adult male homosexuals in the USA in 1981,[1–3] is one manifestation of infection with the human immunodeficiency virus (HIV).[4–6] HIV infection produces a wide range of clinical manifestations from asymptomatic infection to marked immunodeficiency. The four recognized routes of virus transmission are sexual contact with an HIV-infected individual; receipt of HIV-infected blood or blood products; parenteral exposure to HIV-contaminated equipment, and vertical transmission from an HIV-infected pregnant woman. The HIV pandemic has had a formidable impact on global maternal and child health and survival, with important public health consequences. As of December 2000, the World Health Organization (WHO) estimated that there are over 16 million women and 1.4 million children with HIV/AIDS worldwide.[7] In the USA, over 400 000 cases of AIDS had been reported by June 2000.[8] HIV-1 infection has become one of the leading causes of morbidity and mortality in children worldwide.[9] In the USA, HIV infection was the seventh leading cause of death in children 1–4 years of age in 1996.[10] The most common AIDS-defining conditions in children are listed in Table 18.1.

Descriptions of cases of AIDS in children began in 1982;[11–13] almost 9000 cases of AIDS in individuals under 13 years of age had been reported in the USA by June 2000. Children under 13 years of age account for 1.2% of the total AIDS cases reported in the USA. In the USA and other developed countries, progress has been made in preventing perinatal HIV-1. In 1994, the Pediatric AIDS Clinical Trials Group Protocol 076 (PACTG 076) report on the use of zidovudine (ZDV) in pregnant women with HIV-1 infection and their infants revolutionized the prevention of perinatal HIV-1 transmission.[14] The rate of perinatal transmission of HIV-1 was reduced by two-thirds, utilizing an extended regimen of ZDV given during pregnancy, labor, and delivery, and to the neonate. In 1995, the United States Public Health Service (USPHS) issued guidelines recommending universal counseling and testing for pregnant women and use of ZDV to reduce perinatal transmission.[15] Since that time, pediatric AIDS cases have fallen substantially, raising the possibility that perinatal HIV-1 infection could be eliminated in the USA. The estimated number of children born with HIV infection in the USA peaked in 1992 at 1000–2000 births; however, following the widespread implementation of prenatal HIV testing and therapy to prevent perinatal HIV transmission instituted in 1994, the number of infants born with perinatal HIV infection is now estimated at 200–300 annually.

The first classification system for pediatric HIV infection, which was broader in scope than the AIDS case definition used in adults, was published by the Centers for Disease Control and Prevention (CDC) in 1987.[16] This pediatric classification system did not stage degree of symptomatology and was revised in 1994[17] (Tables 18.2–18.4).

Table 18.1. Acquired immune deficiency syndrome (AIDS)-defining conditions most commonly reported for children <13 years of age, $n=8.718$, reported through 1999, United States

Condition	Number	Percentage of cases[a]
Pneumocystis carinii pneumonia	2900	33
Lymphoid interstitial pneumonia	2061	24
Recurrent bacterial infections	1794	21
HIV wasting syndrome	1564	18
HIV encephalopathy	1462	17
Candida esophagitis	1372	16
Cytomegalovirus disease	838	10
Mycobacterium avium infection	709	8
Severe herpes simplex infection	422	5
Cryptosporidiosis	418	5
Pulmonary candidiasis	326	4

Notes:
[a] From Centers for Disease Control and Prevention,[124] with permission.
Source: HIV, human immunodeficiency virus.

Transmission

Perinatal transmission

Perinatal transmission is the most common source of HIV infection among infants and children in the USA. Over 90% of children under 13 years of age with AIDS contracted infection in this manner.[8] Pediatric HIV infection is therefore dependent on rates of HIV infection among women of child-bearing age. Almost 125000 cases of AIDS in women were reported to the CDC by June 2000, representing 16% of all cases of AIDS. Almost equal numbers of these women contracted infection through intravenous drug use and through heterosexual contact with HIV-infected partners. Whereas the association of intravenous drug use as a risk factor for HIV infection among women has been relatively constant, women with heterosexual contact as the only risk factor for HIV infection increased from 14% in 1982 to 40% in 2000. It is likely that heterosexual transmission of HIV to women of child-bearing age will continue to account for most perinatal HIV infection in the USA. More than 75% of women with AIDS are in the reproductive age group at the time of diagnosis.

Reported vertical perinatal HIV transmission rates range from 7% to 55%, but most rigorously

Table 18.2. Summary of 1994 revised classification of human immunodeficiency virus (HIV) infection in children under 13 years of age[a,b]

	Clinical categories			
Immunologic categories	N: no signs/ symptoms	A: mild signs/ symptoms	B: moderate signs/ symptoms[c]	C: severe signs/ symptoms[c]
1. No evidence of suppression	N1	A1	B1	C1
2. Evidence of moderate suppression	N2	A2	B2	C2
3. Severe suppression	N3	A3	B3	C3

Notes:
[a] Children whose HIV infection status is not confirmed are classified by using the above grid with a letter E (for perinatally exposed) placed before the appropriate classification code (e.g., EN2).
[b] Immunologic categories based on age-specific CD4+ T-lymphocyte counts and percent of total lymphocytes.
[c] Both category c and lymphoid interstitial pneumonitis in category B are reportable to state and local health departments as acquired immunodeficiency syndrome.
Source: From Centers for Disease Control and Prevention,[17] with permission.

Table 18.3. Immunologic categories based on age-specific CD4+ T-lymphocyte counts and percent of total lymphocytes

	Age of child		
Immunologic category	<12 months μl (%)	1–5 years μl (%)	6–12 years μl (%)
1. No evidence of suppression	>=1500 (>=25)	>=1000 (>=25)	>=500 (>=25)
2. Evidence of moderate suppression	750–1499 (15–24)	500–999 (15–24)	200–499 (15–24)
3. Severe suppression	<750 (<15)	<500 (<15)	<200 (<15)

Source: From Centers for Disease Control and Prevention,[17] with permission.

Table 18.4. Clinical categories for children with human immunodeficiency virus (HIV) infection

Category N: not symptomatic

Children who have no signs or symptoms considered to be the result of HIV infection or who have only one of the conditions listed in category A

Category A: mildly symptomatic

Children with two or more of the conditions listed below but none of the conditions listed in categories B and C:

- Lymphadenopathy (0.5 cm at more than two sites; bilateral, one site)
- Hepatomegaly
- Splenomegaly
- Dermatitis
- Parotitis
- Recurrent or persistent upper respiratory infection, sinusitis, or otitis media

Category B: moderately symptomatic

Children who have symptomatic conditions other than those listed for categories A or C that are attributed to HIV infection; examples of conditions in clinical category B include but are not limited to:

- Anemia (<8 g/dl), neutropenia (<1000/mm^3), or thrombocytopenia (<100 000/mm^3) persisting ⩾30 days
- Bacterial meningitis, pneumonia, or sepsis (single episode)
- Candidiasis, oropharyngeal (thrush), persisting (>2 months) in children >6 months of age
- Cardiomyopathy
- Cytomegalovirus infection, with onset before 1 month of age
- Diarrhea, recurrent or chronic
- Hepatitis
- Herpes simplex virus (HSV) stomatitis, recurrent (more than two episodes within 1 year)
- HSV bronchitis, pneumonitis, or esophagitis with onset before 1 month of age
- Herpes zoster (shingles) involving at least two distinct episodes or more than one dermatome
- Leiomyosarcoma
- Lymphoid interstitial pneumonia (LIP) or pulmonary lymphoid hyperplasia complex
- Nephropathy
- Nocardiosis
- Persistent fever (lasting >1 month)
- Toxoplasmosis, onset before 1 month of age
- Varicella, disseminated (complicated chickenpox)

Table 18.4 (*cont.*)

Category C: severely symptomatic

Children who have any condition listed in the 1987 surveillance case definition for AIDS,[16] with the exception of LIP:

- Serious bacterial infections, multiple or recurrent (i.e., any combination of at least two culture-confirmed infections within a 2-year period), of the following types: septicemia, pneumonia, meningitis, bone or joint infection, or abscess of an internal organ or body cavity (excluding otitis media, superficial skin, or mucosal abscesses, and indwelling catheter-related infections)
- Candidiasis, esophageal or pulmonary (bronchi, trachea, lungs)
- Coccidioidomycosis, disseminated (at site other than or in addition to lungs or cervical or hilar lymph nodes
- Cryptococcosis, extrapulmonary
- Cryptosporidiosis isosporiasis with diarrhea persisting >1 month
- Cytomegalovirus disease with onset of symptoms at age >1 month (at a site other than liver, spleen, or lymph nodes)
- Encephalopathy (at least one of the following progressive findings must be present for at least 2 months in the absence of a concurrent developmental illness other than HIV infection that could explain the findings): (1) failure to attain or loss of developmental milestones or loss of intellectual ability, verified by standard developmental scale or neuropsychological tests; (2) impaired brain growth or acquired microcephaly demonstrated by head circumference measurements or brain atrophy demonstrated by computed tomography or magnetic resonance imaging (serial imaging is required for children <2 years of age); (3) acquired symmetric motor deficits manifested by two or more of the following: paresis, pathologic reflexes, ataxia, or gait disturbance
- Herpes simplex virus infection causing a mucocutaneous ulcer that persists for >1 month; or bronchitis, pneumonitis, or esophagitis for any duration affecting a child >1 month of age
- Histoplasmosis, disseminated (at a site other than or in addition to lungs or cervical or hilar lymph nodes)
- Kaposi sarcoma
- Lymphoma, primary, in brain
- Lymphoma, small, noncleaved cell (Burkitt), or immunoblastic or large-cell lymphoma or B-cell or unknown immunologic phenotype
- *Mycobacterium tuberculosis,* disseminated or extrapulmonary
- *M. avium* complex or *M. kansasii,* disseminated (at site other than or in addition to lungs, skin, or cervical or hilar lymph nodes)
- *Pneumocystis carinii* pneumonia
- Progressive multifocal leukoencephalopathy
- *Salmonella* (nontyphoid) septicemia, recurrent
- Toxoplasmosis of the brain with onset at >1 month of age
- Wasting syndrome in the absence of a concurrent illness other than HIV infection that could explain the following findings:(1) persistent weight loss >10% of baseline; or (2) downward crossing of at least two of the following percentile lines on the weight-for-age chart (e.g., 95th, 75th, 50th, 25th, 5th) in a child 1 year of age; or (3) <5th percentile on weight-for-height chart on two consecutive measurements 30 days apart plus 1) chronic diarrhea (i.e., at least two loose stools a day for 30 days); or 2) documented fever (for 30 days, intermittent or constant)

Notes:

AIDS, acquired immune deficiency syndrome.

Source: From Centers for Disease Control and Prevention,[17] with permission.

conducted prospective studies estimate transmission rates of 13% to 30%.[18–24] Variability in estimated rates likely reflects differences in maternal host factors and viral factors. In addition, geographic differences may exist in the predominant mode of perinatal HIV transmission. There are three routes of HIV transmission from an HIV-infected pregnant woman to her fetus or newborn infant: in utero via transplacental infection; intrapartum by exposure to maternal blood at the time of labor and delivery; and postpartum via HIV-contaminated human milk. In utero transmission has been documented by isolation of HIV from tissue of aborted or miscarried fetuses as early as 8 weeks' gestation.[25–29]

Intrapartum transmission is supported by studies failing to detect HIV in infants born to HIV-infected women in the first month of life, but with subsequent detection of virus in these infants after 1–3 months of age.[30–33] Intrapartum transmission is the most common mode of perinatal HIV infection, although studies conducted among HIV-infected African women indicate that up to 30% of perinatal HIV transmission in that population occurs postpartum, from breast-feeding.[34] Retrospective studies of twins born to HIV-infected women found a higher HIV transmission rate among those born by vaginal delivery compared with those born by cesarean delivery and among first-born compared with second-born twins. These data support exposure to maternal virus during delivery as a likely route of transmission.[35,36] The role of cesarean delivery in reducing the risk of perinatal transmission may be beneficial in certain situations, such as for women who are not on antiretroviral therapy or who have high levels of HIV-1 in their blood at the time of labor and delivery.[37,38]

HIV has been isolated from cell-free extracts of human breast milk from HIV-infected women.[39] Postpartum transmission is documented in individual case reports of HIV-infected infants born to mothers infected with HIV at the time of delivery or shortly afterward, and among HIV-infected infants whose mothers were not HIV-infected but who had HIV-infected wet nurses.[40] A prospective study of 212 maternal–infant pairs at high risk of developing HIV infection in Rwanda found that eight of 16 breast-fed infants whose mothers became HIV-infected in the first year of the infant's life also became infected with HIV. All these infants seroconverted to HIV within 3 months of maternal seroconversion, suggesting that the rate of postnatal transmission was higher during early acute maternal infection.[41] Recent studies among breast-feeding African populations suggest that one-third to one-half of transmission may occur via breast-feeding. The highest risk of such transmission is in the first few months of life.[42–45]

Diagnosis of perinatal HIV infection by antibody detection is hampered by the presence of maternal HIV antibodies for up to 15–18 months.[18–20,46,47] Therefore, methods involving direct detection of virus have been evaluated for early identification of perinatal HIV infection. HIV culture and polymerase chain reaction (PCR) appear sensitive and specific in diagnosing HIV infection within the first 6 months of life (Table 18.5).[48–54] Using these techniques, more than 90% of HIV-infected infants are identified during the first 3–6 months of life, but up to 70% of HIV-infected infants can be both HIV culture- and PCR-negative in the first month of life. These early negatives are interpreted as "true negative" results, representing an incubation period of early HIV infection and replication. Measurement of serum p24 antigen is a specific but insensitive method of diagnosing HIV infection.[55] However, acid dissociation of p24 antigen–antibody complexes in infants born to HIV-infected women increases sensitivity and specificity, even in the first week of life.[56,57] The use of other tests, such as determination of HIV immunoglobulin M (IgM) or IgA,[31,32,58,59] and in vitro HIV antibody production from neonatal lymphocytes,[60–62] may also be reliable early diagnostic markers of perinatal HIV infection but have only been reported in small numbers of infants and are not as widely available as HIV PCR. Absence of HIV antibodies in children older than 18 months of age virtually excludes infection, although a small number of HIV-uninfected children have persistent maternal HIV antibodies beyond that time.[17]

Multiple maternal, perinatal, and viral factors have been evaluated as predictors of perinatal infection. Maternal host factors include CD4 and CD8 counts, concentration of HIV-specific neutralizing antibodies, and clinical status. Perinatal factors include presence of primary infection, rupture of membranes for >4 h, chorioamnionitis, invasive obstetric procedures, gestational age, and mode of delivery. Viral factors include HIV-1 levels in maternal blood, inoculum size, and strain characteristics (e.g., "fetotropic" or syncytial morphology). HIV-infected women with progressive symptoms of AIDS, and those with acute HIV infection during pregnancy, are more likely to transmit HIV to their infants than women with asymptomatic HIV infection.[22,23,63,64] Decreased maternal CD4 count[23,65] and neutralizing antibodies to HIV[66–68] and increased viral burden as measured by quantitative DNA PCR or circulating p24 antigen[69–73] are associated with higher rates of perinatal infection. Premature infants born to HIV-infected women have a higher rate of perinatal HIV infection than full-term infants. Studies evaluating the relative risk of HIV transmission associated with vaginal vs cesarean delivery have demonstrated decreased transmission with cesarean section.[36–38] Increased transmission of HIV strains that are fetotropic is reported; isolation of HIV strains with highly conserved gene sequences from HIV-infected infants has been demonstrated despite the large number of genetically diverse strains isolated from their mothers.[74]

Whereas numerous factors have been associated with risk of perinatal transmission of HIV, the strongest predictor of perinatal transmission is maternal serum HIV-1 RNA level.[75,76] Transmission has rarely been documented among pregnant women with undetectable serum levels of HIV-1 around the time of labor and delivery.

Transfusion-acquired infection

Because of HIV antibody screening of blood and blood products and heat treatment of coagulation factors, hemophiliacs and other recipients of blood or blood products represent a small proportion of the population with HIV infection. There is a small risk of transfusion-associated HIV infection due to "silent" infections among blood donors who have recently been infected with HIV and who are still HIV antibody-negative.

Prevalence and risk factors

Prevalence of maternal HIV

Since perinatal transmission is the most common route of pediatric HIV infection, knowledge of maternal HIV seroprevalence rates is the most reliable and uniform predictor of pediatric HIV infection. The CDC directed multistate, population-based HIV seroprevalence studies in women of child-bearing age from 1988 through 1995. Annual seroprevalence rates among postpartum women were determined by testing neonates for HIV antibodies. The average HIV seroprevalence among women in the USA has been estimated at 1.5–1.7 in 1000 women of child-bearing age.[77,78] Regional HIV seroprevalence rates vary, with the highest rates found among women in Florida, New York, New Jersey, Maryland, and the commonwealth of Puerto Rico. Based on these rates, it is estimated that over 7500 HIV-infected women give birth in the USA each year; with a projected perinatal HIV transmission rate of 13%–30%, an estimated 975–2250 HIV-infected infants would be born each year in the USA if preventive therapy were not offered to HIV-infected women.

Risk of transfusion-acquired infection

The current risk of transfusion-associated HIV infection ranges from 1 in 38000 to 1 in 300000 units of blood.[79–81] Based on mathematical modeling of the period of infectivity of silent HIV infection among blood donors, one study estimated that the window period of potential silent HIV infection lasts an average of 45 days from the onset of infectivity to the development of antibody to HIV.[82]

Natural history and prognosis

Perinatal Infection

Time to AIDS

The onset of clinical symptoms occurs earlier among children with perinatal infection compared with those who have transfusion-acquired infection.[83] The observed period to development of AIDS is estimated to be 12 months for perinatal HIV infection compared with 41 months for children with transfusion-acquired HIV infection.[84] In addition, the type of AIDS-defining condition at AIDS diagnosis varies markedly by age. Most infants diagnosed with AIDS in the first 6 months of life present with *Pneumocystis carinii* pneumonia (PCP) whereas at older ages other AIDS-defining conditions are more prevalent. Statistical modeling of the observed AIDS "incubation period" among children with perinatal HIV infection suggests that there may be two distinct patterns of disease progression, with the first sharp peak at about 4 months of age and a second median onset at about 6 years of age.[85] This model projects a 20% incidence of AIDS in the first year of life followed by an 8% annual incidence thereafter, and a median age at AIDS diagnosis of 4.8 years. Another mathematical model of the period from perinatal infection to AIDS predicted that 14% of HIV-infected infants will develop AIDS in the first year of life, followed by a rate of 11–12% a year thereafter.[86] This model projects an overall AIDS incidence of 80–86% at 84 months of age, which is higher than rates of AIDS found in prospective clinical studies. A major drawback of both models is that they were derived from pediatric AIDS cases reported to a county public health department and not from longitudinal cohort studies. Prospective clinical data also support the hypothesis that perinatal HIV infection manifests in a bimodal fashion with early, severe disease in the group with short-term survival, and mild-to-moderate symptoms and longer survival in the second group.[87,88] Whether these short- and long-term survivors correlate with different pathogenetic mechanisms of perinatal HIV acquisition is currently being investigated. One hypothesis suggests that short-term survivors may represent infants with in utero HIV infection, and long-term survivors may reflect intrapartum HIV transmission.[89]

Neurologic manifestations in the infant

Neurologic disease in children with rapid progression of HIV infection has been commonly recognized as HIV encephalopathy. However, only recently have careful clinical studies documented more pervasive and global neurologic manifestation of HIV infection among infants and children. In the current era of treatment for perinatal HIV infection, the incidence of overt and rapidly progressive HIV encephalopathy seems to have decreased, but may also be associated with more subtle central nervous system manifestations. Neuropathologic evidence of HIV-related central nervous system disease includes decreased brain weight, cortical atrophy, symmetric intracerebral calcifications, white-matter changes, reactive astrocytosis, and subcortical gray-matter abnormalities of the basal ganglia, thalamus, claustrum, caudate, putamen, globus pallidus, and hippocampus.[26,90,91] HIV has been isolated from the brain of aborted fetuses from HIV-infected women, and from the brain and cerebrospinal fluid of HIV-infected children and adults.[26,90] HIV RNA and DNA have been detected in central nervous system tissue.[92] Although virus has been recovered from cerebrospinal fluid of patients at all stages of HIV disease, including asymptomatic individuals, the highest rate of viral recovery is from those with symptomatic HIV infection or neurologic complaints.[93] The cerebrospinal fluid profile is often normal; however, mild pleocytosis and elevated protein concentrations may be present.[91,93]

The impact and neurologic manifestations of HIV infection occurring early in development are different from neurologic sequelae in adults infected at the time of central nervous system maturity. This likely reflects the vulnerability of the developing nervous system to infection. Central nervous system targets of HIV infection may be different in children and adults. In contrast to terminally differentiated cells of the mature nervous system of adults, the immature nervous system of children has mitotically active cells. Current research suggests that HIV infection of the immature nervous system alters new synapse formation.[94] In addition, inflammatory mediators from activated macrophages and microglial cells (tumor necrosis factor-α and platelet-activating factor) and HIV proteins (tet and nef) are felt to be neurotoxic.

Central nervous system manifestations in patients with HIV infection may be due to direct effects of HIV viral infection or to secondary effects of opportunistic diseases of the central nervous system that may occur in advanced stages of HIV/AIDS. Children with HIV infection can suffer from progressive encephalopathy, static encephalopathy, neuropsychiatric disorders, motor impairment, and

Table 18.5. Diagnosis of human immunodeficiency virus (HIV) infection in children[a]

Diagnosis: HIV-infected

(a) A child <18 months of age who is known to be HIV-seropositive or born to an HIV-infected mother and:

- has positive results on two separate determinations (excluding cord blood) from one or more of the following HIV detection tests: HIV culture, HIV polymerase chain reaction, HIV antigen p24, or
- meets criteria for acquired immunodeficiency syndrome (AIDS) diagnosis based on the 1987 AIDS surveillance case definition[16]

(b) A child ⩾18 months of age born to an HIV-infected mother or any child infected by blood, blood products, or other known modes of transmission (e.g., sexual contact) who:

- is HIV-antibody-positive by repeatedly reactive enzyme immunoassay (EIA) and confirmatory test (e.g., Western blot or immunofluorescence assay (IFA), or
- meets any of the criteria in (a) above.

Diagnosis: perinatally exposed (prefix E)

A child who does not meet the criteria above who:

- is HIV-seropositive by EIA and confirmatory test (e.g., Western blot or IFA) and is <18 months of age at the time of test, or
- has unknown antibody status, but was born to a mother known to be infected with HIV

Diagnosis: seroreverter (SR)

A child who is born to an HIV-infected mother and who:

- has been documented as HIV-antibody-negative (i.e., two or more negative EIA tests performed at 6–18 months of age or one negative EIA test after 18 months of age), and
- has had no other laboratory evidence of infection (has not had two positive viral detection tests, if performed); and has not had an AIDS-defining condition

Notes:

[a] This definition of HIV infection replaces the definition published in the 1987 AIDS surveillance case definition.[16]

Source: From Centers for Disease Control and Prevention,[17] with permission.

cognitive decline.[93,95–99] Early in the epidemic more than 50% of children with AIDS had progressive encephalopathy. These affected children typically had severe immunosuppression at the time of presentation. More recently, because of the ability to identify asymptomatic and mildly symptomatic HIV infected children, the prevalence of progressive encephalopathy has dropped to less than 25%.[100] Criteria for the definitive diagnosis of encephalopathy are listed in Table 18.5. Encephalopathy in children with HIV is associated with a 28-fold increase in death, a 22 fold increase in wasting and a 16-fold increase in cardiomyopathy.[97] Thus, the diagnosis of encephalopathy in an HIV-infected child is a marker of poor prognosis.

Children infected with HIV display a range of neuropsychological problems, including learning and attention disorders, emotional and behavioral problems, depression, autistic behavior, and social withdrawal.[96,99,101,102] Using various age-appropriate neuropsychological tests (Bayley Scales of Infant Development, McCarthy Scales of Children's Abilities, and the Wechsler Intelligence Scale for Children – Revised), researchers have demonstrated that the overall level of neuropsychological functioning in HIV patients is below normal. HIV-infected children have mean full-scale intelligence quotients (FIQ) of 85.9, compared with FIQs of 100 in noninfected controls.[101] Neuropsychological abnormalities are not observed in HIV-exposed but uninfected infants.[102,103]

Neurologic consequences of HIV infection vary with the state of infection. For example, asymptomatic patients have infrequent or no neurologic deficits while children with advanced AIDS often have profound and persistent neurologic abnormalities.[95,97,98,101,102] It is important to recognize the difficulty in evaluating the impact of the direct effects of HIV infection on neurodevelopment. Multiple confounding variables impacting neurodevelopment are often present in HIV-infected children. These variables include: prematurity, low birth weight, in utero drug exposure, antiviral drug toxicities, nutritional deficits, endocrine abnormalities, and the social impacts of disease.[95,103] Furthermore, secondary central nervous system complications of infection may be present. Thus, it is often not possible to isolate HIV's direct impact on neurodevelopment from the effects of these other variables.

Secondary central nervous system complications of HIV infection include opportunistic infections, neoplasms, and strokes. Opportunistic infections of the central nervous system are less common in children than in adults with HIV infection.[100] When these infections do occur in children, they are often diagnosed in those over 6 years of age with CD4 counts below 200. Central nervous system opportunistic agents include: *Cryptococcus*, toxoplasmosis, cytomegalovirus, herpes simplex virus, *Candida* spp., JC virus, and syphilis.[100] Primary central nervous system lymphomas, non-Hodgkin's lymphoma with central nervous system metastasis, and strokes are rare in children. Table 18.6 compares HIV infection in children and adults.

Antiviral therapy in children may prevent, reduce, or improve neurologic manifestations of HIV infection. ZDV continuous therapy improved cognitive performance and reduced brain atrophy in a small study of symptomatic HIV-infected children.[104] Combination therapy with ZDV and didanosine was more effective than monotherapy with either agent in improving age-appropriate neurocognitive scores in young children with symptomatic HIV.[99,105] Current studies are evaluating the impact of maternal use of highly active antiretroviral therapy (HAART) during pregnancy on perinatal infection. Furthermore, as HAART therapy is used in children, the potential to modulate central nervous system and systemic effects of HIV infection will be determined. Central nervous system penetration differs substantially among current antiretroviral drugs.[105] Thus, physicians are challenged to find adequate drug combinations to prevent and treat both central nervous system and systemic manifestations of HIV infection.

Table 18.6. Comparison of HIV/AIDS in children and adults

HIV Manifestation	Children	Adults
CNS OI	+	+++
PNS involvement	+	+++
Seizures	+	+++
Brain atrophy	++	++
Motor dysfunction	++	++
Psychiatric diagnoses	++[a]	++[b]
Cognitive decline	++	++
Strokes	+	+++
CNS neoplasm	+	+++

Notes:
+ rare; ++ present; +++ common.
HIV, human immunodeficiency virus; AIDS, acquired immune deficiency syndrome; CNS, central nervous system; OI, opportunistic infection; PNS, peripheral nervous system.
[a] psychiatric diagnosis in children includes: learning disorders, attention deficit hyperactive disorders, depression, and autistic behavior.
[b] psychiatric disorders in adults include: dementia, psychosis, depression, delirium.
Source: Adapted from:[97,98,100]

Prognostic factors

A number of clinical and immunologic factors in perinatal HIV infection have been associated with poor prognosis. As in adults, development of AIDS-defining conditions such as encephalopathy and PCP in perinatal-acquired HIV infection is associated with shortened survival.[87,106,107] Children with onset of symptoms at 6–12 months of life, especially with development of PCP and other AIDS-defining symptoms, die earlier than those whose symptoms begin later.[108] Scott et al.[106] found that PCP occurred at a median age of 5 months, with a median survival of 1 month, and that children with other AIDS indicator diseases had median survival times of greater than 12 months. Development of lymphocytic interstitial pneumonitis (LIP) is associated with longer survival. Scott et al.[106] reported a median survival of 72 months among children with LIP, and Thomas et al.[109] found median survival of 54 months with LIP. Maldonado et al.[107] found that PCP prophylaxis was associated with longer AIDS-free survival in the first 3 years of life, related to a decreased incidence of PCP and an increased incidence of HIV encephalopathy.

Laboratory markers associated with progression of HIV symptoms in children with perinatal HIV infection include p24 antigenemia,[110,111] decreased CD4 count,[69] and increasing β_2-microglobulin levels,[112] neopterin levels,[113] and degree of viral burden.[114,115] Syncytium-inducing HIV strains, which are more cytopathic in vitro than other strains, have been associated with rapid disease progression among HIV-infected adults;[116–118] however, syncytium-inducing strains have not been associated with rapidly progressive disease among HIV-infected infants or children to date.[119] By contrast, rapidly growing HIV strains have been associated with progressive disease compared with slow- or intermediate-growing strains isolated from HIV-infected children.[120]

Survival and antiretroviral therapy

Survival estimates among children with perinatal HIV infection demonstrate median life expectancy of 96 months.[121] Survival may improve as HIV-infected children are identified earlier and followed over longer periods. In a prospective study of 124 children with perinatal HIV infection, the European Collaborative Study found that 23% of the children had developed AIDS in the first year of life and 39% by 4 years of age. Mortality was 10% by 1 year of age and 28% by 5 years of age. Forty-eight percent of children were still alive 2 years after the diagnosis of AIDS.[24] The short-term effects of antiretroviral therapy on progression of HIV disease have been reported in small clinical studies; documented effects of antiretroviral therapy such as ZDV and dideoxyinosine include decreased p24 antigenemia and viral burden, and increased CD4 counts.[122,123] Few data are available regarding the effect of antiretroviral therapy on the long-term outcome of HIV-infected children. Data from the Italian Register for HIV Infection in Children demonstrated improved survival among children with perinatal HIV infection from 1996 through 1998 as a result of availability of combination antiretroviral therapy for these children.[115]

A true picture of the evolution and natural history of perinatal HIV infection will be possible only when sufficient numbers of children, enrolled prospectively, have been followed over long periods of time. Current data suggest that the incidence of AIDS is highest early in life but tapers thereafter to a low but constant rate. Survival is inversely linked to development of AIDS and encephalopathy, and prognosis is worst among children developing AIDS in the first year of life. Data are still insufficient to detect definitive differences in survival based on year of birth, temporal differences in availability of therapeutic interventions, and the effect of therapy and prophylaxis on temporal incidence of AIDS and survival.

Recommendations

Optimal methods to recognize and treat perinatal and pediatric HIV infection are changing constantly. In order to decrease vertical transmission of HIV, all pregnant mothers must be screened for infection early in pregnancy and, for those women at high risk, retesting or HIV-infection near term may be indicated. Once a pregnant woman is identified as HIV-infected, she should be offered the most up-to-date treatment to prevent perinatal transmission. Consultation with local infectious disease experts is recommended. Once born, HIV-exposed neonates must be evaluated for HIV infection. Those unfortunate infants with HIV infection need long-term medical treatment and close follow-up evaluations for medical, neurologic, infectious, and other complications of their disease.

REFERENCES

1 Centers for Disease Control. (1981). *Pneumocystis* pneumonia – Los Angeles. *MMWR*, **30**, 250–252.

2 Centers for Disease Control. (1981). Kaposi's sarcoma and *Pneumocystis carinii* pneumonia among homosexual men in New York City and California. *MMWR*, **30**, 305–308.

3 Gottlieb MS, Schroff R, Schanker HM, et al. (1981). *Pneumocystis carinii* pneumonia and mucosal candidiasis in previously healthy homosexual men: evidence for a new severe acquired cellular immunodeficiency syndrome. *N Engl J Med*, **305**, 1425–1431.

4 Barre-Sinoussi F, Chermann JC, Rey F, et al. (1983). Isolation of a T-lymphotropic retrovirus from a patient at risk for acquired immune deficiency syndrome (AIDS). *Science*, **220**, 868–871.

5 Popovic M, Sarngadharan MG, Reed E, et al. (1984). Detection, isolation, and continuous production of cytopathic retroviruses (HTLV-III) from patients with AIDS and pre-AIDS. *Science*, **224**, 503–505.

6 Levy JA, Hoffman AD, Kramer SM, et al. (1984). Isolation of lymphocytopathic retroviruses from San Francisco patients with AIDS. *Science*, **225**, 840–842.

7 World Health Organization. UNAIDS Joint United Nations Program on HIV/AIDS. (2000). AIDS epidemic update: December 2000. Geneva: UNAIDS.

8 Centers for Disease Control and Prevention. (2000). *HIV/AIDS Surveillance Report*, vol. 12, pp. 1–45. Centers for Disease Control and Prevention.

9 Lindegren ML, Steinberg S, and Byers RH. (2000). Epidemiology of HIV/AIDS in children. *Pediatr Clin North Am*, **47**, 1–20.

10 Ventura SJ, Peters KD, Martin JA, et al. (1997). *Births and Deaths: United States, 1996. Monthly Vital Statistics Report*, pp. 32, 46. Hyattsville, MD: National Center for Health Statistics.

11 Scott GB, Buck BE, Leterman JG, et al. (1984). Acquired immunodeficiency syndrome in infants. *N Engl J Med*, **310**, 76–81.

12 Rubinstein A, Sicklick M, Gupta A, et al. (1983). Acquired immunodeficiency with reversed T4/T8 ratios in infants born to promiscuous and drug-addicted mothers. *JAMA*, **249**, 2350–2356.

13 Centers for Disease Control. (1982). Unexplained immunodeficiency and opportunistic infections in infants: New York, New Jersey, California. *MMWR*, **31**, 665–667.

14 Connor EM, Sperling RS, Gelber R, et al. (1994). Reduction of maternal–infant transmission of human immunodeficiency virus type 1 with zidovudine treatment. *N Engl J Med*, **331**, 1173–1180.

15 Centers for Disease Control and Prevention. (1995). US Public Health Service recommendations for human immunodeficiency virus counseling and voluntary testing for pregnant women. *MMWR*, **44**(RR-7), 1–15.

16 Centers for Disease Control. (1987). Classification system for human immunodeficiency virus (HIV) infection in children under 13 years of age. *MMWR*, **36**, 225–235.

17 Centers for Disease Control and Prevention. (1994). 1994 revised classification system for human immunodeficiency virus infection in children less than 13 years of age; official authorized addenda: human immunodeficiency virus infection codes and official guidelines for coding and reporting ICD-9 CM. *MMWR*, **43**, 1–17.

18 Italian Multicentre Study. (1988). Epidemiology, clinical features, and prognostic factors of paediatric HIV infection. *Lancet*, **2**, 1043–1045.

19 Blanche S, Rouzioux C, Moscato MLG, et al. (1989). A prospective study of infants born to women seropositive for human immunodeficiency virus type 1. *N Engl J Med*, **320**, 1643–1648.

20 European Collaborative Study. (1991). Children born to women with HIV-1 infection: natural history and risk of transmission. *Lancet*, **337**, 253–260.

21 Hutto C, Parks WP, and Lai S. (1991). A hospital-based prospective study of perinatal infection with human immunodeficiency virus type 1. *J Pediatr*, **118**, 347–353.

22 Gabiano C, Tobo PA, de Martino M, et al. (1992). Mother-to-child transmission of human immunodeficiency virus type 1: risk of infection and correlates of transmission. *Pediatrics*, **90**, 369–374.

23 Thomas PA, Weedon J, Krasinski K, et al. (1994). Maternal predictors of perinatal human immunodeficiency virus transmission. *Pediatr Infect Dis J*, **13**, 489–495.

24 The European Collaborative Study. (1994). Natural history of vertically acquired human immunodeficiency virus-1 infection. *Pediatrics*, **94**, 815–819.

25 Lewis SH, Reynolds-Kohler C, Fox HE, et al. (1990). HIV-1 trophoblastic and villous Hofbauer cells, and haematological precursors in eight-week fetuses. *Lancet*, **335**, 565–568.

26 Lyman WD, Kress Y, Kure K, et al. (1990). Detection of HIV in fetal central nervous system tissue. *AIDS*, **4**, 917–920.

27 Jovaisas E, Koch MA, Schafer A, et al. (1985). LAV/HTLV-III in a 20-week fetus. *Lancet*, **2**, 1129.

28 Sprecher S, Soumenkoff G, Puissant F, et al. (1986). Vertical transmission of HIV in 15-week fetus. Lancet, **2**, 288–289.

29 Ehrnst A, Lindgren S, Dictor M, et al. (1991). HIV in pregnant women and their offspring: evidence for late transmission. *Lancet*, **338**, 203–207.

30 Rogers MF, Ou CY, Rayfield M, et al. (1989). Use of the polymerase chain reaction for early detection of the proviral sequences of human immunodeficiency virus in infants born to seropositive mothers. *N Engl J Med*, **320**, 1649–1654.

31 Weiblen BJ, Lee FK, Cooper ER, et al. (1990). Early diagnosis of HIV infection in infants by detection of IgA HIV antibodies. *Lancet*, **335**, 988–990.

32 Quinn TC, Kline RL, Halsey N, et al. (1991). Early diagnosis of perinatal HIV infection by detection of viral-specific IgA antibodies. *JAMA*, **266**, 3439–3542.

33 Krivine A, Firtion G, Cao L, et al. (1992). HIV replication during the first weeks of life. *Lancet*, **339**, 1187–1189.

34 Datta P, Embree JE, Kreiss J, et al. (1994). Mother-to-child transmission of human immunodeficiency virus type 1: report from the Nairobi study. *J Infect Dis*, **170**, 1134–1140.

35 Goedert JJ, Duliege AM, Amos CI, et al. (1991). High risk of HIV-1 infection for first-born twins. *Lancet*, **338**, 1471–1475.

36 The International Perinatal HIV Group. (1999). The mode of delivery and the risk of vertical transmission of human immunodeficiency virus type 1. *N Engl J Med*, **340**, 977–987.

37 The European Mode of Delivery Collaboration. (1999). Elective cesarean section versus vaginal delivery in prevention of vertical HIV-1 transmission: a randomized clinical trial. *Lancet*, **353**, 1035–1039.

38 Women and Infants Transmission Study Investigators. (1999). Trends in mother-to-infant transmission of HIV in the WITS cohort: impact of 076 and HAART therapy. In *Second Conference on Global Strategies for the Prevention of HIV Transmission from Mothers to Infants*. Montreal, abstract 212.

39 Thiry L, Sprecher-Goldberger S, and Jonckheer T. (1985). Isolation of AIDS virus from cell-free breast milk of three healthy virus carriers. *Lancet*, **2**, 891–892.

40 Oxtoby MJ. (1988). Human immunodeficiency virus and other viruses in human milk: placing the issues in broader perspective. *Pediatr Infect Dis J*, **7**,825–835.

41 Van de Perre P, Simonon A, Msellati P, et al. (1991). Postnatal transmission of human immunodeficiency virus type 1 from mother to infant. *N Engl J Med*, **325**, 593–598.

42 Dunn DT, Newell ML, Ades AE, et al. (1992). Risk of human immunodeficiency virus type 1 transmission through breastfeeding. *Lancet*, **340**, 585–588.

43 Miotti PG, Taha TET, Kumwenda NI, et al. (1999). HIV transmission through breastfeeding: a study in Malawi. *JAMA*, **282**, 744–749.

44 Nduati R, John G, Mbori-Ngacha D, et al. (2000). Effect of breastfeeding and formula feeding on transmission of HIV-1: a randomized controlled trial. *JAMA*, **283**, 1167–1174.

45 Wiktor SZ, Ekpini E, and Nduati RW. (1997). Prevention of mother-to-child transmission of HIV-1 in Africa. *AIDS*, **11**(suppl. B), S79–S87.

46 De Rossi A, Ades AE, Mammano F, et al. (1991). Antigen detection, virus culture, polymerase chain reaction, and in vitro antibody production in the diagnosis of vertically transmitted HIV-1 infection. *AIDS*, **5**, 15–20.

47 Rakusan TA, Parrott RH, and Sever JL. (1991). Limitations in the laboratory diagnosis of vertically acquired HIV infection. *J Acquir Immune Defic Syndr*, **4**, 116–121.

48 Edwards JR, Ulrich PP, Weintrub PS, et al. (1989). Polymerase chain reaction compared with concurrent viral cultures for rapid identification of human immunodeficiency virus infection among high-risk infants and children. *J Pediatr*, **115**, 200–203.

49 Borkowsky W, Krasinski K, Pollack H, et al. (1992). Early diagnosis of human immunodeficiency virus infection in children less than 6 months of age: comparison of polymerase chain reaction, culture, and plasma antigen capture techniques. *J Infect Dis*, **166**, 616–619.

50 Luzuriaga K, McQuilken P, Alimenti A, et al. (1993). Early viremia and immune responses in vertical human immunodeficiency virus type 1 infection. *J Infect Dis*, **167**, 1008–1013.

51 Palasanthiran P, Ziegler JB, Dwyer DE, et al. (1994). Early detection of human immunodeficiency virus type 1 infection in Australian infants at risk of perinatal infection and factors affecting transmission. *Pediatr Infect Dis J*, **13**, 1083–1090.

52 McIntosh K, Pitt J, Brambilla D, et al. (1994). Blood culture in the first 6 months of life for the diagnosis of vertically transmitted human immunodeficiency virus infection. *J Infect Dis*, **170**, 996–1000.

53 Burgard M, Mayaux MJ, Blanche S, et al. (1992). The use of viral culture and p24 antigen testing to diagnose human immunodeficiency virus infection in neonates. *N Engl J Med*, **327**, 1192–1197.

54 De Rossi A, Ometto L, Mammano F, et al. (1992). Vertical transmission of HIV-1: lack of detectable virus in peripheral blood cells of infected children at birth. *AIDS*, **6**, 1117–1120.

55 Andiman WA, Silva TJ, Shapiro ED, et al. (1992). Predictive value of the human immunodeficiency virus 1 antigen test in children born to infected mothers. *Pediatr Infect Dis J*, **11**, 436–440.

56 Palomba E, Gay V, de Martino M, et al. (1992). Early diagnosis of human immunodeficiency virus infection in infants

by detection of free and complexed p24 antigen. *J Infect Dis*, **165**, 394–395.

57 Miles SA, Balden E, Magpantay L, et al. (1993). Rapid serologic testing with immune-complex dissociated HIV p24 antigen for early detection of HIV infection in neonates. *N Engl J Med*, **328**, 297–302.

58 Weiblen BJ, Schumacher RT, and Hoff R. (1990). Detection of IgM and IgA antibodies to HIV-1 after removal of IgG with recombinant protein G. *J Immunol Methods*, **126**, 199–204.

59 Martin ML, Levy JA, Legg H, et al. (1991). Detection of infection with human immunodeficiency virus (HIV) type 1 in infants by an anti-HIV immunoglobulin A assay using recombinant proteins. *J Pediatr*, **118**, 354–358.

60 Pahwa S, Chirmule N, Leombruno C, et al. (1989). In vitro syntheses of human immunodeficiency virus-specific antibodies in peripheral blood lymphocytes of infants. *Proc Natl Acad Sci USA*, **86**, 7532–7236.

61 Amadori A, Giaquinto C, Zacchello F, et al. (1990). Diagnosis of human immunodeficiency virus 1 infection in infants: in vitro production of virus-specific antibody in lymphocytes. *Pediatr Infect Dis J*, **9**, 26–30.

62 Palomba E, Gay V, Gabiano C, et al. (1990). In-vitro production of HIV-1-specific antibody for diagnosis of perinatal infection. *Lancet*, **336**, 940–941.

63 Mayers MM, Davenny K, Schoenbaum EE, et al. (1991). A prospective study of infants of human immunodeficiency virus seropositive and seronegative women with a history of intravenous drug use or of intravenous drug-using sex partners, in the Bronx, New York City. *Pediatrics*, **88**, 1248–1256.

64 European Collaborative Study. (1992). Risk factors for mother-to-child transmission of HIV-1. *Lancet*, **339**, 1007–1012.

65 Raszka WV Jr, Meyer GA, Waecker NJ, et al. (1989). Variability of serial absolute and percent CD4+ lymphocyte counts in healthy children born to human immunodeficiency virus 1-infected parents. Military Pediatric HIV Consortium. *Pediatr Infect Dis J*, **13**, 70–72.

66 Rossi P, Moschese V, Broliden PA, et al. (1989). Presence of maternal antibodies to human immunodeficiency virus 1 envelope glycoprotein gp120 epitopes correlates with the uninfected status of children born to seropositive mothers. *Proc Natl Acad Sci USA*, **86**, 8055–8058.

67 Goedert JJ, Mendez H, Drummond JE, et al. (1989). Mother-to-infant transmission of human immunodeficiency virus type 1: association with prematurity or low anti-gp120. *Lancet*, **2**, 1351–1354.

68 Scarlatti G, Albert J, Rossi P, et al. (1993). Mother-to-child transmission of human immunodeficiency virus type 1: correlation with neutralizing antibodies against primary isolates. *J Infect Dis*, **168**, 207–210.

69 Dickover RE, Dillon M, Gillette SG, et al. (1994). Rapid increases in load of human immunodeficiency virus correlate with early disease progression and loss of CD4 cells in vertically infected infants. *J Infect Dis*, **170**, 1279–1284.

70 Scarlatti G, Lombardi V, Plebani A, et al. (1991). Polymerase chain reaction, virus isolation and antigen assay in HIV-1-antibody-positive mothers and their children. *AIDS*, **5**, 1173–1178.

71 St Louis ME, Kamenga M, Brown C, et al. (1993). Risk for perinatal HIV-1 transmission according to maternal immunologic, virologic, and placental factors. *JAMA*, **269**, 2853–2859.

72 Borkowsky W, Krasinski K, Cao Y, et al. (1994). Correlation of perinatal transmission of human immunodeficiency virus type 1 with maternal viremia and lymphocyte phenotypes. *J Pediatr*, **125**, 345–351.

73 Farley JJ, Bauer G, Johnson JP, et al. (1994). Phytohemagglutinin-inducible p24 in peripheral blood mononuclear cells as a predictor of human immunodeficiency virus type 1 vertical transmission and infant clinical status. *Pediatr Infect Dis J*, **13**, 1079–1082.

74 Mofenson LM, Lambert JS, Stiehm ER, et al. (1999). Risk factors for perinatal transmission of human immunodeficiency virus type 1 in women treated with zidovudine. *N Engl J Med*, **341**, 385–393.

75 Garcia P, Kalish LA, Pitt J, et al. (1999). Maternal levels of plasma human immunodeficiency virus type-1 RNA and the risk of perinatal transmission. *N Engl J Med*, **341**, 394–402.

76 Wolinsky SM, Wike CM, Korber BTM, et al. (1992). Selective transmission of human immunodeficiency virus type-1 variants from mothers to infants. *Science*, **255**, 1134–1137.

77 Lindegren ML, Byers RH Jr, and Thomas P. (1999). Trends in perinatal HIV/AIDS in the United States. *JAMA*, **282**, 531–538.

78 Davis SF, Rosen DH, and Steinberg S. (1998). Trends in HIV prevalence among childbearing women in the United States, 1989–1994. *J Acquir Immune Defic Syndr Hum Retrovirol*, **19**, 158–164.

79 Busch MP, Eble BE, Khayam-Bashi H, et al. (1991). Evaluation of screened blood donations for human immunodeficiency virus type 1 infection by culture and DNA amplification of pooled cells. *N Engl J Med*, **325**, 1–5.

80 Ward JW, Holmberg SD, Allen JR, et al. (1988). Transmission of human immunodeficiency virus (HIV) by blood transfusions screened as negative for HIV antibody. *N Engl J Med*, **318**, 473–478.

81 Cumming PD, Wallace EI, Schorr JB, et al. (1989). Exposure of patients to human immunodeficiency virus through the transfusion of blood components that test antibody-negative. *N Engl J Med*, **321**, 941–946.

82 Petersen LR, Satten GA, Dodd R, et al. (1994). Duration of time from onset of human immunodeficiency virus type 1 infectiousness to development of detectable antibody. *Transfusion*, **34**, 283–289.

83 Fredrick T, Mascola L, Eller A, et al. (1994). Progression of human immunodeficiency virus disease among infants and children infected perinatally with human immunodeficiency virus or through neonatal blood transfusion. *Pediatr Infect Dis J*, **13**, 1091–1097.

84 Oxtoby MJ. (1991). Perinatally acquired HIV infection. In *Pediatric AIDS: The Challenge of HIV Infection in Infants, Children and Adolescents*, Pizzo PA and Wilfert CM (eds), pp. 3–21. Baltimore: Williams & Wilkins.

85 Auger I, Thomas P, De Gruttola V, et al. (1988). Incubation periods for paediatric AIDS patients. *Nature*, **336**, 575–577.

86 MaWhinney S, Pagano M, and Thomas P. (1993). Age at AIDS diagnosis for children with perinatally acquired HIV. *J Acquir Immune Defic Syndr*, **6**, 1139–1144.

87 Duliege AM, Messiah A, Blanche S, et al. (1992). Natural history of human immunodeficiency virus type 1 infection in children: prognostic value of laboratory tests on the bimodal progression of the disease. *Pediatr Infect Dis J*, **11**, 630–635.

88 Blanche S, Tardieu M, Duliege AM, et al. (1990). Longitudinal study of 94 symptomatic infants with perinatally acquired human immunodeficiency virus infection. *Am J Dis Child*, **144**, 1210–1215.

89 Bryson YJ, Luzuriaga K, Sullivan JL, et al. (1992). Proposed definition for in utero versus intrapartum transmission of HIV-1. *N Engl J Med*, **327**, 1246–1247.

90 Kozlowski PB, Brudkowska J, Kraszpulski M, et al. (1997).Microencephaly in children congenitally infected with human immunodeficiency virus – a gross-anatomical morphometric study. *Acta Neuropathol (Berl)*, **93**, 136–145.

91 Levy JA, Shimabukuro J, Hollander H, et al. (1985). Isolation of AIDS-associated retroviruses from cerebrospinal fluid and brain of patients with neurological symptoms. *Lancet*, **2**, 586–588.

92 Shaw GM, Harper ME, Hahn BH, et al. (1985). HTLV-III infection in brains of children and adults with AIDS encephalopathy. *Science*, **227**, 177–182.

93 Hollander H and Levy JA. (1987). Neurologic abnormalities and recovery of human immunodeficiency virus from cerebrospinal fluid. *Ann Intern Med*, **106**, 692–695.

94 Epstein LG and Gelbard HA. (1999). HIV-1-induced neuronal injury in the developing brain. *J Leukoc Biol*, **65**, 453–457.

95 Belman AL. (1997). Pediatric neuro-AIDS. Update. *Neuroimaging Clin North Am*, **7**, 593–613.

96 Brouwers P, De Carli C, Civitello L, et al. (1995). Correlation between computed tomographic brain scan abnormalities and neuropsychological function in children with symptomatic human immunodeficiency virus disease. *Arch Neurol*, **52**, 39–44.

97 Cooper ER, Hanson C, Diaz C, et al. (1998). Encephalopathy and progression of human immunodeficiency virus disease in a cohort of children with perinatally acquired human immunodeficiency virus infection. Women and Infants Transmission Study Group. *J Pediatr*, **132**, 808–812.

98 Epstein LG, Sharer LR, Oleske JM, et al. (1986). Nerologic manifestations of human immunodeficiency virus infection in children. *Pediatrics*, **78**, 678–687.

99 Raskino C, Pearson DA, Baker CJ, et al. (1999). Neurologic, neurocognitive and brain growth outcomes in human immunodeficiency virus-infected children receiving different nucleoside antiretroviral regimens. *Pediatrics*, **104**, e32.

100 Mintz M. (1999). Clinical features and treatment interventions for human immunodeficiency virus-associated neurologic disease in children. *Semin Neurol*, **19**, 165–176.

101 Brouwers P, Tudor-Williams G, DeCarli C, et al. (1995). Relation between stage of disease and neurobehavioral measures in children with symptomatic HIV disease. *AIDS*, **9**, 713–720.

102 Nozyce M, Hittelman J, Muenz L, et al. (1994). Effect of perinatally acquired human immunodeficiency virus infection on neurodevelopment in children during the first two years of life. *Pediatrics*, **94**, 883–891.

103 Belman AL, Muenz LR, Marcus JC, et al. (1996). Neurologic status of human immunodeficiency virus 1-infected infants and their controls: a prospective study from birth to 2 years. Mothers and Infants Cohort Study. *Pediatrics*, **98**, 1109–1118.

104 DeCarli C, Fugate L, Falloon J, et al. (1991). Brain growth and cognitive improvement in children with human immunodeficiency virus-induced encephalopathy after 6 months of continuous infusion zidovudine therapy. *J Acquir Immune Defic Syndr*, **4**, 585–592.

105 Portegies P. (1995). HIV-1, the brain, and combination therapy. *Lancet*, **346**, 1244–1245.

106 Scott GB, Hutto C, Makuch RW, et al. (1989). Survival in children with perinatally acquired human immunodeficiency virus type 1 infection. *N Engl J Med*, **321**, 1791–1796.

107 Maldonado YA, Araneta RG, and Hersh A. (1998). *Pneumocystis carinii* pneumonia prophylaxis and early clinical manifestations of severe perinatal human immunodeficiency virus type 1 infection. Northern California Pediatric HIV Consortium. *Pediatr Infect Dis J*, **17**, 398–402.

108 Turner BJ, Denison M, Eppes SC, et al. (1993). Survival experience of 789 children with the acquired immunodeficiency syndrome. *Pediatr Infect Dis J*, **12**, 310–320.

109 Thomas P, Singh T, Williams R, et al. (1992). Trends in survival for children reported with maternally transmitted acquired immunodeficiency syndrome in New York City, 1982 to 1989. *Pediatr Infect Dis J*, **11**, 34–39.

110 Epstein LG, Boucher CAB, Morrison SH, et al. (1988). Persistent human immunodeficiency virus type 1 antigenemia in children correlates with disease progression. *Pediatrics*, **82**, 919–924.

111 Ellaurie M and Rubinstein A. (1991). Correlation of serum antigen and antibody concentration with clinical features in HIV infection. *Arch Dis Child*, **66**, 200–203.

112 Ellaurie M and Rubinstein A. (1990). Beta-2-microglobulin concentrations in pediatric human immunodeficiency virus infection. *Pediatr Infect Dis J*, **9**, 807–809.

113 Ellaurie M, Calvelli T, and Rubinstein A. (1992). Neopterin concentrations in pediatric human immunodeficiency virus infection as predictor of disease activity. *Pediatr Infect Dis J*, **11**, 286–289.

114 de Martino M, Tovo PA, and Balducci M. (2000). Reduction in mortality with availability of antiretroviral therapy for children with perinatal HIV-1 infection. Italian Register for HIV Infection in Children and the Italian National AIDS Registry. *JAMA*, **284**, 190–197.

115 Saag MS, Crain MJ, Decker WD, et al. (1991). High-level viremia in adults and children infected with human immunodeficiency virus: relation to disease stage and CD4+ lymphocyte levels. *J Infect Dis*, **164**, 72–80.

116 Tersmette M, De Goede REY, Al BJM, et al. (1988). Differential syncytium-inducing capacity of human immunodeficiency virus isolates: frequent detection of syncytium-inducing isolates in patients with acquired immunodeficiency syndrome (AIDS) and AIDS-related complex. *J Virol*, **62**, 2026–2032.

117 Cheng-Mayer C, Seto D, Tateno M, et al. (1988). Biologic features of HIV-1 that correlate with virulence in the host. *Science*, **240**, 80–82.

118 Tersmette M, Lange JMA, De Goede REY, et al. (1989). Association between biological properties of human immunodeficiency virus variants and risk for AIDS and AIDS mortality. *Lancet*, **1**, 983–985.

119 Spencer LT, Ogino MT, Dankner WM, et al. (1994). Clinical significance of human immunodeficiency virus type 1 phenotypes in infected children. *J Infect Dis*, **169**, 491–495.

120 De Rossi A, Pasti M, Mammano F, et al. (1991). Perinatal infection by human immunodeficiency virus type 1 (HIV-1): relationship between proviral copy number in vivo, viral properties in vitro, and clinical outcome. *J Med Virol*, **35**, 283–289.

121 Tovo PA, De Martino M, Gabiano C, et al. (1992). Prognostic factors and survival in children with perinatal HIV-1 infection. *Lancet*, **339**, 1249–1253.

122 Butler KM, Husson RN, Lewis LL, et al. (1992). CD4 status and p24 antigenemia. Are they useful predictors of survival in HIV-infected children receiving antiretroviral therapy? *Am J Dis Child*, **146**, 932–936.

123 Srugo I, Brunell PA, and Chelyapov NV. (1991). Virus burden in human immunodeficiency virus type 1-infected children: relationship to disease status and effect of antiviral therapy. *Pediatrics*, **87**, 921–925.

124 Centers for Disease Control and Prevention. (2001). *Pediatric HIV/AIDS Surveillance L262 Slide Series*. Available at http://www.cdc.gov/hiv/graphics/pediatri.htm on 30 May 2001.

19

Inborn errors of metabolism with features of hypoxic–ischemic encephalopathy

Gregory M. Enns

Stanford University School of Medicine, Stanford, CA, USA

Introduction

Inborn errors of metabolism that present in the neonatal period can have clinical, biochemical, and neuroradiologic features similar to those of hypoxic–ischemic encephalopathy (HIE). Both metabolic disorders and HIE are associated with severe neurologic distress, metabolic acidosis, and multiorgan system involvement. In general, the patterns of brain injury are different when HIE and inborn errors of metabolism are compared. However, some metabolic disorders may have neuroradiologic findings similar to those seen in HIE. Although inborn errors are rare individually, as a group they affect approximately 1 in 1000 neonates.[1] It is crucial to consider these disorders in the differential diagnosis of patients who present with nonspecific features suggestive of sepsis or asphyxia. Prompt diagnosis may not only prevent mortality or significant morbidity, but also allows the clinician to provide the family with accurate genetic counseling. In this chapter, patterns of brain injury and systemic complications that occur in HIE and metabolic disorders are reviewed. Specific inborn errors of metabolism with clinical presentations that may be seen in patients with HIE are discussed further. For a more comprehensive review of inborn errors of metabolism, the reader is referred to standard metabolic texts.[2–4]

Patterns of brain injury in HIE and inborn errors of metabolism

Neonatal hypoxic–ischemic brain injury may be caused by localized infarction or a diffuse ischemic insult. Focal ischemic infarction in the neonate typically presents with lethargy, hypotonia, or seizures.[5] Metabolic causes of focal ischemia are listed in Table 19.1, but will not be reviewed in this chapter. Perinatal asphyxia affects 2–4/1000 neonates, with encephalopathy occurring in 25% and death in an additional 30%.[6] Diffuse hypoxic–ischemic brain injury presents differently, depending on the duration and severity of the insult, the gestational age of the infant, and the presence or absence of systemic stress.[7]

Mild-to-moderate cerebral hypotension, with impaired brain vascular autoregulation, results in the shunting of blood from the anterior to posterior circulation, in order to maintain blood flow to the basal ganglia, brainstem, and cerebellum. Brain damage, thus, is restricted to the cerebral hemisphere intervascular boundary zones ("watershed regions").[5] Because the location of the watershed regions changes with brain maturation, different patterns of cerebral damage are encountered in premature and term infants. Mild-to-moderate cerebral hypotension in premature infants results in periventricular white-matter injury, with sparing of the

Table 19.1. Inborn errors of metabolism associated with stroke in childhood

Organic acidurias
Propionic acidemia
Methylmalonic acidemia
Isovaleric acidemia
Glutaric aciduria type I
Multiple acyl-coenzyme A (CoA) dehydrogenase deficiency (glutaric aciduria type II)
3-Methylcrotonyl CoA carboxylase deficiency
3-Hydroxy-3-methylglutaryl CoA lyase deficiency
Aminoacidemias
Homocystinuria
Methylenetetrahydrofolate reductase (MTHFR) deficiency
Sulfite oxidase deficiency
Molybdenum cofactor deficiency
Urea cycle disorders
Ornithine transcarbamylase deficiency
Carbamyl phosphate synthetase deficiency
Mitochondrial disorders
MELAS syndrome
Leigh syndrome
Cytochrome oxidase (complex IV) deficiency
Lysosomal storage disorders
Fabry disease
Cystinosis
Other
Congenital disorders of glycosylation[a]
Phosphoglycerate kinase deficiency
Hyperlipoproteinemia
Menkes disease
Purine nucleoside phosphorylase deficiency

Notes:
MELAS, mitochondrial encephalomyopathy, lactic acidosis, and stroke-like episodes.
[a] Formerly carbohydrate-deficient glycoprotein syndrome.
Source: Adapted from Barkovich AJ (2000). *Pediatric Neuroimaging*, 3rd edn. Philadelphia, PA: Lippincott/Williams & Wilkins.

cerebral cortex and subcortical white matter. By the 34th to 36th weeks of gestation, the watershed areas have shifted peripherally to include the subcortical white matter and cerebral cortex. Therefore, term infants who sustain brain injury as a result of mild-to-moderate hypotension have damage primarily in the cortex and underlying subcortical and periventricular white matter.[5]

Severe cerebral hypotension, with complete or near complete interruption of the cerebral blood supply, results in deep gray matter (especially thalami and basal ganglia) and brainstem damage.[8] In this case, the shunting of blood is not sufficient to prevent deep gray-matter damage. Damage to white matter and the cerebral cortex are later sequelae to profound hypotension. Profound cerebral hypotension also causes different patterns of brain injury depending on brain maturity.[5] In the early third trimester, the thalami and brainstem have the highest metabolic activity and relative blood flow. The thalami, brainstem, basal ganglia, and perirolandic region have the highest metabolic activity from the middle of the third trimester through 40 weeks of gestation. By the end of the first postnatal month, the visual cortex has an increased metabolic activity and is susceptible to damage.[5] The basal ganglia remain highly vulnerable to injury from HIE or other environmental stress factors until approximately age 3 years.[9]

Duration of injury is also important in determining the pattern of brain involvement. In mild-to-moderate hypoperfusion, the areas affected by ischemia are limited to the watershed regions and periventricular white matter. Progression of damage beyond watershed regions does not occur unless the hypoperfusion becomes more severe. In severe hypoperfusion, no damage is present if the duration of circulatory arrest is less than approximately 10 min. Damage to the ventrolateral thalami, globus pallidus, posterior putamen, perirolandic cortex, and hippocampi may be seen in arrest lasting 10–15 min. The superior vermis, optic radiation, and calcarine cortex become involved with increasing duration of arrest. By 25–30 min of arrest, injury is present in nearly all the gray matter.[5]

Table 19.2. Inborn errors of metabolism involving gray matter only

Cortical gray matter
Neuronal ceroid lipofuscinosis
Sialidosis
Deep gray matter
Prolonged striatal T2 signal
Mitochondrial disorders: MELAS, Leigh syndrome
Hypoglycemia[a]
Juvenile Huntington disease
Shortened pallidum T2 signal
Neurodegeneration with brain iron accumulation type 1 (NBIA1)[b]
Prolonged pallidum T2 signal
Methylmalonic acidemia
Carbon monoxide poisoning
Kernicterus

Notes:
MELAS, mitochondrial encephalomyopathy, lactic acidosis, and stroke-like episodes.
[a] In older infants, adolescents, and adults.
[b] Formerly Hallervorden–Spatz disease.
Source: Adapted from Barkovich AJ (2000). *Pediatric Neuroimaging*, 3rd edn. Philadelphia, PA: Lippincott/Williams & Wilkins.

Table 19.3. Inborn errors of metabolism involving white matter only

Subcortical white matter early
Macrocephaly
Alexander disease
Normal head circumference
4-Hydroxybutyric aciduria[a]
Galactosemia
Deep white matter early
Pons/medulla corticospinal tract involvement
Peroxisomal disorders
No specific brainstem tracts involved
Phenylketonuria
Maple syrup urine disease[b]
5,10-Methylenetetrahydrofolate reductase (MTHFR) deficiency
Disorders of cobalamin metabolism
Metachromatic leukodystrophy
Lack of myelination
Pelizaeus–Merzbacher disease
Trichothiodystrophy
Nonspecific white-matter pattern
Nonketotic hyperglycinemia
3-Hydroxy-3-methylglutaryl coenzyme A lyase deficiency
Urea cycle disorders

Notes:
[a] Cerebellar atrophy may also be present.
[b] Cerebellar and cerebral peduncle involvement may also be present.
Source: Adapted from Barkovich AJ (2000). *Pediatric Neuroimaging*, 3rd edn. Philadelphia, PA: Lippincott/Williams & Wilkins.

In contrast to the patterns of brain injury encountered in classic HIE, metabolic disorders typically affect different areas of the brain.[5,9] Whereas head MRI evaluation in HIE often shows hyperintense signal in the putamen (with relative sparing of the anterior putamen) and thalamus, metabolic disorders affect other structures. Metabolic conditions with differential involvement of white and gray matter are listed in Tables 19.2–19.4. Disorders of mitochondrial energy metabolism may present with a wide spectrum of lesions, but abnormal hyperintense signal in the globus pallidus and periatrial white matter of the centrum semiovale are often present.[9] Pyruvate dehydrogenase deficiency, organic acidemias, carbon monoxide or cyanide poisoning, and hypothermic circulatory arrest during cardiac surgery have been associated with similar abnormal signals in the globus pallidus.[5,9] Mitochondrial disorders may also present with isolated white-matter disease, Leigh syndrome, or even normal MRI findings.[5] Different patterns of abnormality may suggest other underlying inborn errors of metabolism. For example, basal ganglia "metabolic strokes" have been associated with methylmalonic and propionic acidemias.[10] It is important to emphasize that normal head imaging does not

Table 19.4. Inborn errors of metabolism involving both gray and white matter

Cortical gray matter only
Cortical dysplasia
Muscle–eye–brain disease
Walker–Warburg syndrome
Fukuyama muscular dystrophy
Other congenital muscular dystrophies
Absent cortical dysplasia
Alpers disease
Menkes disease
Abnormal bones
Mucopolysaccharidoses
Lipid storage disorders
Peroxisomal disorders
Deep gray-matter-involvement
Primary thalamic involvement
GM_1 gangliosidosis
GM_2 gangliosidosis
Krabbe disease
Primary globus pallidus involvement
Canavan disease
Methylmalonic acidemia
L-2-Hydroxyglutaric aciduria
Maple syrup urine disease
Mitochondrial disorders: Kearns–Sayre syndrome
Primary striatal involvement
Organic acidemias: propionic acidemia, biotinidase deficiency, multiple carboxylase deficiency, glutaric aciduria type I, β-ketothiolase deficiency, 3-methylglutaconic aciduria, ethylmalonic acidemia
Tricarboxylic acid cycle disorders: malonic acidemia, α-ketoglutaric aciduria
Molybdenum cofactor deficiency
Mitochondrial disorders: MELAS, Leigh syndrome
Wilson disease

Notes:
MELAS, mitochondrial encephalomyopathy, lactic acidosis, and stroke-like episodes.
Source: Adapted from Barkovich A. J. (2000). *Pediatric Neuroimaging*, 3rd edn. Philadelphia, PA: Lippincott/Williams & Wilkins.

exclude the presence of an inborn error of metabolism.[9]

The mechanisms underlying the differential effects of HIE and metabolic disorders on the brain have been the subject of much study.[6,10–17] Recent theories have focused on the position of different deep gray-matter nuclei within the neurotransmitter-specific circuitry of the basal ganglia motor loop.[6,11] HIE following severe asphyxia results in electroencephalographic and positron emission tomographic patterns suggestive of activity in corticothalamic, thalamocortical, and corticoputaminal excitatory projections with strong glutamate innervations.[11] Such hyperexcitability in these circuits could theoretically cause the characteristic thalamus and putamen lesions seen in HIE via glutamate-mediated toxicity.[12] In asphyxia, areas of the brain with a high concentration of glutamate innervations may be particularly vulnerable to injury, because of damage sustained to nerve terminal glutamate reuptake pumps and subsequent high levels of synaptic glutamate. Glutamate can then bind to post-synaptic *N*-methyl-D-aspartate (NMDA) receptors, causing membrane-bound calcium channels to open and subsequent influx of Ca^{2+} and cell death, mediated in part by mitochondrial damage and augmentation of nitric oxide and carbon monoxide production.[6,13,14] Released nitric oxide combines with superoxide to form peroxynitrite, which, in turn, leads to DNA damage, depletion of cellular energy, and cell death.[14] While the cortex, putamen, and thalamus are activated by such a glutamate excitatory stimulus, the globus pallidus is inhibited, resulting in relative sparing of this structure from damage.[11] This neuronal circuitry hypothesis may explain the selective pattern of involvement of deep gray structures in HIE, despite the close proximity and similar vascular supply of these structures.

In contrast, toxic and metabolic disorders that affect mitochondrial energy metabolism (e.g., kernicterus, pyruvate dehydrogenase deficiency, respiratory chain disorders) cause neuronal injury through different mechanisms, although glutamate release may also play a role. Disorders that cause mitochondrial dysfunction may lead to neuronal injury by diminishing the ability of mitochondria to maintain membrane potentials. Neuronal subacute membrane depolarization could result in subsequent opening of postsynaptic voltage-dependent NMDA and sodium channels with resultant cellular injury.[11,15] The globus pallidus may be particularly vulnerable in metabolic disorders, because of the relatively high baseline firing rate of pallidal neurons.[11] This predisposition to oxidative stress may also be related to the relatively high concentration of brain NMDA receptors in neonates when compared to adults.[16,17] Mitochondrial damage may also lead to decreased expression of hypoxia-inducible factor 1 (HIF-1), a transcription factor that induces genes coding for erythropoietin, vascular endothelial growth factor, glycolytic enzymes, and glucose transporters. HIF-1 appears to be important in an adaptive response to hypoxia, because of its role in stimulating cellular glucose uptake, increasing glycolytic capacity, and enhancing tissue O_2 delivery.[18]

Clinical features of HIE and inborn errors of metabolism

Neonates progress through distinctive stages of neurologic impairment following asphyxia severe enough to cause HIE.[7] Seizures occur in 50–70% of acutely asphyxiated neonates and tend to start between 30 min and 24 h after birth, with an earlier occurrence signifying a more severe asphyxial insult.[7] In addition to central nervous system (CNS) complications seen in perinatal asphyxia, systemic involvement of multiple organs, including heart, liver, and kidneys, may also occur (Table 19.5). Such damage to other organs may contribute to the severity of brain injury. Asphyxia in the immediate perinatal period is associated with low Apgar scores (typically 3 or less at 1 min and 6 or less at 5 min); bradycardia, pallor, cyanosis, decreased or absent respirations, and diminished or absent reflex activity may be present. A combined metabolic and respiratory acidosis is characteristic. Other metabolic findings include hypoglycemia, hypocalcemia, hyponatremia (secondary to the syndrome of inappropriate antidiuretic hormone secretion (SIADH)), and multiple electrolyte abnormalities from renal dysfunction. Hyperammonemia may also be present, depending on the severity of hepatic dysfunction.[7,19]

Table 19.5. Systemic complications of hypoxic–ischemic encephalopathy

Cardiomyopathy
Hepatic necrosis
Acute tubular necrosis
Adrenal insufficiency
Necrotizing enterocolitis
Meconium aspiration syndrome
Persistent fetal circulation
Thrombocytopenia
Hypoglycemia
Hypocalcemia
Hyperammonemia
SIADH

Note:
SIADH, Syndrome of inappropriate antidiuretic hormone secretion.

Inborn errors of metabolism may also present with severe neurologic illness and the involvement of multiple organ systems. A high index of suspicion and specific laboratory investigations are necessary to diagnose a metabolic disorder presenting with symptoms and signs suggestive of HIE (Table 19.6). The onset of symptoms of metabolic disease is typically postnatal, appearing after an interval period of apparent good health, and following a normal pregnancy. This interval may be as short as a few hours, or last several days or even longer. Because an asphyxial insult may occur at any time in the prenatal period, the absence of a significant obstetric event does not exclude HIE as a cause of neonatal distress, but may raise the suspicion of an underlying metabolic condition. In general, if the degree of neonatal metabolic distress seems out of proportion to known obstetric or environmental factors, an inborn error of metabolism should be considered. The persistence of markers of metabolic disease

Table 19.6. Laboratory investigations in neonates with a suspected inborn error of metabolism

Routine investigations
Complete blood count + differential
Urinalysis
Electrolytes, blood urea nitrogen, creatinine, calcium, phosphorus, magnesium
Liver enzymes
Creatine kinase
Blood gases
CSF glucose, protein, erythrocytes, and leukocytes
Cultures of blood, urine, and CSF
Basic metabolic investigations
Ammonia
Lactate, pyruvate
Quantitative serum amino acids
Quantitative urine organic acids
Carnitine levels (total, free, and esterified carnitine)
Acylcarnitine profile
Further metabolic investigations[a]
Blood ketone bodies
CSF lactate, glycine, 4-aminobutyric acid levels[b]
Very-long-chain fatty acid analysis
Plasma guanidinoacetate
Urine *S*-sulfocysteine
Urine for homocitrulline
Cultured fibroblasts for specific enzymology[c]
Muscle biopsy for histochemistry, mitochondrial respiratory chain activities
DNA analysis[d]

Notes:
CSF, cerebrospinal fluid.
[a] These investigations are performed on an individual basis depending on the presentation.
[b] Simultaneous serum glycine should be obtained for the investigation of nonketotic hyperglycinemia.
[c] Fibroblast analysis is often used for assay of fatty acid oxidation disorders, some mitochondrial disorders, and disorders of pyruvate metabolism. Other tissues (e.g., liver, muscle) may also be useful for enzyme analysis.
[d] DNA analysis may be routinely available for certain metabolic disorders, including some mitochondrial disorders, but often is only available on a research basis.

(e.g., lactic acid and ammonia) despite vigorous therapy may also point to an underlying metabolic problem. Because most inborn errors of metabolism are characterized by autosomal recessive or maternal inheritance, obtaining a detailed family history is crucial. Parental consanguinity, or a history of a previously affected child, increase the likelihood that neonatal distress is secondary to an underlying inborn error of metabolism.

Other indicators of metabolic imbalance include an anion gap acidosis, lactic acidosis, hyperammonemia, and hypoglycemia, but these markers are not invariably present (Table 19.7). It is apparent that it may be difficult to distinguish HIE from metabolic disorders on clinical presentation, because similar features may occur in both conditions. Furthermore, these conditions are not mutually exclusive. An asphyxial insult may constitute the initial environmental stress that unmasks an underlying inborn error of metabolism. The following sections summarize specific metabolic diseases and their typical presentations in the neonatal period. These clinical classifications are guidelines only, because metabolic disorders may present in atypical ways.

Isolated seizures

Seizures may occur in up to 9% of infants admitted to neonatal intensive care units.[20] The most common causes of neonatal seizures are asphyxia, hypoglycemia, electrolyte abnormalities, infection, CNS malformations, drug exposure and withdrawal, and inborn errors of metabolism.[21] Metabolic disorders that may present with isolated neonatal seizures, without other obvious laboratory or clinical markers of an underlying inborn error of metabolism, are relatively rare and include nonketotic hyperglycinemia (NKH), sulfite oxidase deficiency (either isolated or as part of molybdenum cofactor deficiency), pyridoxine-responsive seizures, folinic-acid responsive seizures, 4-aminobutyrate aminotransferase (GABA transaminase) deficiency, guanidinoacetate methyltransferase (GAMT) deficiency, and glucose transporter (GLUT-1) deficiency.[2,3,4,21–27] Peroxisomal disorders, mitochondrial

Table 19.7. Inborn errors of metabolism with features of hypoxic–ischemic encephalopathy

Isolated seizures	*Severe ketoacidosis*
Nonketotic hyperglycinemia	Propionic acidemia
Sulfite oxidase (molybdenum cofactor) deficiency	Methylmalonic acidemia
Pyridoxine-responsive seizures	Isovaleric acidemia
Folinic acid-responsive seizures	Multiple acyl coenzyme A dehydrogenase deficiency (glutaric aciduria type II)[e]
4-Aminobutyrate aminotransferase (GABA transaminase) deficiency	Holocarboxylase synthetase deficiency (multiple carboxylase deficiency)[d]
Glucose transporter defect (GLUT1 deficiency syndrome)	3-Hydroxyisobutyric aciduria[e]
Peroxisomal disorders[a]	*Lethargy without metabolic acidosis*
Mitochondrial disorders[a]	Maple syrup urine disease[d]
Organic acidemias[a,b]	Mevalonic acidemia[e]
Lactic acidosis, hypotonia, and systemic involvement	*Lethargy with hyperammonemia*
Pyruvate dehydrogenase deficiency[b]	Urea cycle defects
Pyruvate carboxylase deficiency[b]	HHH (hyperammonemia, hyperornithinemia, homocitrullinuria) syndrome
Fatty acid oxidation defects[b,c]	Lysinuric protein intolerance
Mitochondrial disorders	*Other disorders*
3–Methylglutaconic aciduria	Fructose 1,6-diphosphatase deficiency[f,g]
α-Ketoglutarate dehydrogenase deficiency	Glycogen storage disorders types I, II, III, VIII[f,g]
Fumaric aciduria[e]	

Notes:

[a] These conditions commonly have other systemic manifestations (see text).

[b] Hyperammonemia may also be present.

[c] Lactic acidosis is usually not prominent, except in long-chain 3-hydroxyacyl coenzyme A dehydrogenase deficiency and trifunctional protein deficiency, or if there is systemic hypoperfusion.

[d] Metabolic acidosis may occur later in the course of disease.

[e] Dysmorphic features and head magnetic resonance imaging abnormalities are commonly present.

[f] Lactic acidosis may be severe.

[g] Hypoglycemia with hepatomegaly are commonly present. An enlarged heart is present in glycogen storage disorder type II and may be present in glycogen storage disorder type VIII.

disorders, organic acidemias, and urea cycle defects may also have seizures as part of a neonatal presentation, but other organ systems are usually involved. In addition, clues to diagnosis of these conditions are typically present in routine and more specialized metabolic labs.[2,3,4,28] Disorders with an isolated seizure presentation, in contrast, may not have concomitant acidosis, hypoglycemia, or electrolyte abnormalities. Routine metabolic studies are also normal; specific investigations on blood, cerebrospinal fluid (CSF), or urine are required to make a diagnosis.[29]

Nonketotic hyperglycinemia

NKH is an autosomal recessive condition caused by a defect in one of the four components (P protein, H protein, T protein, or L protein) that constitute the glycine cleavage system.[2–4] NKH is characterized by the accumulation of large amounts of glycine in body fluids. Symptoms include lethargy, apnea, profound hypotonia, feeding difficulty, hiccups, and seizures. Approximately two-thirds of patients will have symptoms appear within 48 h of delivery, but symptoms as early as 6 h of life have been described.[2] Routine laboratory evaluations and organic acid analysis are normal. The only consistent abnormality is elevated glycine concentration in urine, plasma, and CSF. A CSF-to-plasma glycine ratio >0.08 is diagnostic of NKH. It is important to obtain CSF and blood samples for glycine analysis as near to simultaneously as possible to allow for an accurate calculation of the glycine ratio. Elevated CSF glycine has also been reported in HIE, but a normal CSF-to-plasma glycine ratio would be expected in this case.[30] Definitive diagnosis is by enzymatic analysis of liver glycine cleavage system activity. The electroencephalogram (EEG) is characterized by a burst-suppression pattern in the first 2 weeks of life. Head computed tomography (CT) evaluation may show cerebral and cerebellar volume loss with hypoattenuation of the periventricular white matter. Head MRI studies show delayed myelination early. Progressive cerebral atrophy, agenesis of the corpus callosum, and atrophic basal ganglia have also been reported.[5] Treatment with sodium benzoate and dextromethorphan (a noncompetitive NMDA receptor antagonist) may improve symptoms, but are not curative. Survivors often display minimal cognitive development and may have seizures recalcitrant to therapy.

Sulfite oxidase deficiency

Sulfite oxidase deficiency may occur in isolation or combined with xanthine oxidase deficiency (molybdenum cofactor deficiency). Inheritance is autosomal recessive. Patients typically present with drug-resistant seizures in the first few days of life. Routine laboratory evaluations and urine organic acid analysis are normal, although a low uric acid level may be noted in molybdenum cofactor deficiency. Elevated *S*-sulfocysteine in plasma or urine is diagnostic.[2–4] (N.B.: *S*-sulfocysteine content is not routinely reported on serum or urine amino acid analyses; a specific assay must be performed). EEG shows a bust-suppression pattern. In the neonatal period, head MRI shows T2 prolongation of the white matter and caudate nuclei, consistent with edema. In the subacute phase, the basal ganglia may have abnormalities similar to those seen in acute asphyxia.[5] There is no current therapy for sulfite oxidase deficiency and most cases are fatal.

Pyridoxine-dependent seizures

Pyridoxine-dependent seizures are caused, at least in part, by glutamic acid decarboxylase deficiency, an autosomal recessive condition with an incidence of approximately 1/160 000.[22] Patients may present on the first day of life with flaccidity, abnormal eye movements, and irritability. Shock, hypothermia, hepatomegaly, and abdominal distension suggestive of intestinal obstruction may also be present.[23] EEG shows intermittent or continuous generalized slow-wave activity. Focal or multifocal spike or spike and wave activity may occur. Patients may have structural brain abnormalities, including cerebellar hypoplasia, generalized brain atrophy, and a thin corpus callosum. Approximately 10% of neonatal cases have features suggestive of HIE.[31] The diagnosis is clinical, with documented response of seizures to intravenous pyridoxine.

Folinic acid-responsive seizures

This is a newly described entity of unknown etiology in which seizures may occur as early as 2 h after birth.[21,27] Routine laboratory studies and metabolic tests are normal. EEG shows a diffuse discontinuous pattern with excessive spikes. Head imaging in two patients between 1 and 2 months of age showed dilated ventricles, cerebellar atrophy, and abnormal signal in frontal and parietal lobe white matter. High-pressure liquid chromatography analysis of CSF shows the presence of a characteristic compound, whose chemical structure has not yet been elucidated. Patients respond to folinic acid supplementation (5–20 mg/day in divided doses).[21]

GABA transaminase deficiency

GABA transaminase catalyzes the first step in the conversion of GABA, a CNS-inhibitory neurotransmitter, to succinic acid. Clinical features of GABA transaminase deficiency include neonatal seizures, lethargy, hypotonia, hyperreflexia, and a high-pitched cry. MRI findings include agenesis of the corpus callosum and cerebellar hypoplasia. Only two patients with this recently identified disorder have been reported, but diagnosis will be missed unless GABA is measured in plasma or CSF.[24]

GAMT deficiency

GAMT deficiency is a recently identified disorder of creatine metabolism characterized by low plasma creatine levels and elevated guanidinoacetate. Patients typically present in infancy with seizures, developmental delay, unusual behavior, and extrapyramidal signs, but this condition has also been diagnosed in neonates. Guanidinoacetate may be assayed in plasma by tandem-mass spectrometry. Treatment with creatine monohydrate has proven efficacy.[25]

GLUT-1 deficiency syndrome

Glut-1 protein is the major glucose transporter in the blood–brain barrier. Mutations in the *GLUT1* gene result in haploinsufficiency of this hexose carrier and severe clinical symptoms, including seizures, acquired microcephaly, and developmental delay. Patients have presented as early as the third week of life, but only a few cases have been reported in the literature. The GLUT-1 deficiency syndrome is an autosomal dominant condition. Characteristic diagnostic findings are a reduced CSF glucose concentration (hypoglycorrhachia) and reduced erythrocyte glucose transporter activity. Peripheral blood glucose and other routine metabolic evaluations are normal. Seizures may stop and children may show a dramatic recovery with the institution of a ketogenic diet.[26]

Peroxisomal disorders

Peroxisomal disorders that may present with neonatal seizures include neonatal adrenoleukodystrophy, Zellweger syndrome, and infantile Refsum disease.[28] Most are inherited in an autosomal recessive fashion, although X-linked adrenoleukodystrophy (which presents in childhood) and rhizomelic chondrodysplasia punctata are X-linked. Clinical features in the neonatal period include severe hypotonia and seizures refractory to therapy. Seizures may be grand mal or myoclonic and EEG typically shows multifocal spike discharges.[3,28] Head imaging in Zellweger syndrome may show subependymal cysts reminiscent of those found in HIE, as well as profound hypomyelination, and cerebral cortex malformations.[5,32] Anterior frontal and temporal lobe microgyri or perisylvian and perirolandic cortex pachygyria may be present. A spectrum of similar brain abnormalities may occur in other peroxisomal disorders, although head imaging may also appear normal in these conditions.[3,5] Patients with peroxisomal disorders may also have prominent ophthalmologic and systemic findings, including large fontanel, cataracts, retinitis pigmentosa, dysmorphic features, hepatomegaly, hepatic fibrosis, and renal cysts. Plasma elevation of very-long-chain fatty acids, bile acid intermediates, and phytanic acid, and decreased erythrocyte plasmalogens are biochemical markers for these conditions. No effective therapy is currently available.[2–4]

Mitochondrial disorders

These conditions may rarely present with neonatal seizures, but more commonly feature hypotonia and lactic acidosis.[33–38] Mitochondrial disorders are discussed further below.

Organic acidemias and urea cycle disorders

Seizures may occur in neonates with classic organic acidemias and urea cycle defects, but are not the major manifestation of these disorders. Overwhelming ketoacidosis, hyperammonemic coma, and characteristic serum amino acids and urine organic acids are usually present. Combined D-2– and L-2-hydroxyglutaric aciduria is a newly described condition that presents with neonatal-onset encephalopathy and intractable seizures.[39] Mevalonic aciduria may present with severe neurologic involvement and seizures, without a metabolic acidosis. However, other findings, including dysmorphic features, hepatosplenomegaly, recurrent fevers, and anemia are more typical.[40,41]

Lactic acidosis, hypotonia, and systemic involvement

Disorders of pyruvate metabolism, tricarboxylic acid cycle disorders, fatty acid oxidation defects, and mitochondrial disease may present in the neonatal period with neuromuscular abnormalities, lactic acidosis, and other systemic manifestations, including cardiomyopathy, liver disease, and renal tubular defects. Anomalies may be present on head imaging, including thinning or agenesis of the corpus callosum and basal ganglia lesions, but the classic findings of HIE are typically absent.[5,11]

Disorders of pyruvate metabolism

Pyruvate dehydrogenase (PDH) deficiency is the most common defect in oxidative metabolism that features persistent lactic acidosis.[3,42,43] Most often a defect in the $E_{1\alpha}$ component of the multimeric pyruvate dehydrogenase complex (PDHC) is the underlying cause of this disorder. $E_{1\alpha}$ deficiency is X-linked. Defects in the E_2, protein X, E_3, and PDH phosphatase components of the PDHC are rare autosomal recessive conditions. Although PDH deficiency often presents later in infancy, a neonatal form exists characterized by lactic acidosis and severe neurologic compromise with hypotonia. Subtle dysmorphic features may be present. In contrast to the acidosis associated with tissue hypoxia, ketosis is often present in primary lactic acidemias. Hyperammonemia has also been reported in some patients.[42,43] Head MRI shows findings typical of Leigh syndrome in about 50% of patients.[5] Cerebral and cerebellar atrophy, delayed myelination, and agenesis of the corpus callosum can be seen.[5] Patients may respond to a diet low in carbohydrate and high in fat. Dichloroacetate reduces lactate in most patients, but is not standard therapy. Some variants have also shown a response to high-dose thiamine administration.[2–4]

The complex form of pyruvate carboxylase deficiency presents with severe neonatal lactic acidosis, hyperammonemia, citrullinemia, and hyperlysinemia. This disorder has been described in patients of European, Egyptian, and Saudi Arabian descent. Most patients with the severe form die by age 3 months. A simple (American Indian) form presents with developmental delay or lactic acidosis in infancy. Both forms are autosomal recessive. No effective treatment is available.[42]

Tricarboxylic acid cycle defects

Alpha-ketoglutarate dehydrogenase deficiency may present with lactic acidemia, hypotonia, hepatomegaly, and elevated creatine kinase immediately after birth. Patients have elevated α-ketoglutaric acid in the urine and a low-normal plasma β-hydroxybutyrate-to-acetoacetate ratio.[44] A combined deficiency of α-ketoglutarate dehydrogenase and pyruvate dehydrogenase has also been described in neonates with lactic acidosis, hypoglycemia, and neurologic abnormalities, including seizures. The combined defects were postulated to be caused by lipoamide dehydrogenase deficiency, because this enzyme is integral to both α-ketoglutarate dehydrogenase and PDHC.[45] Patients with fumaric aciduria may have lactic acidosis, dysmorphic features, and congenital brain malformations, including polymicrogyria, decreased white-matter volume, ventriculomegaly, open operculum, angulation of the frontal horns, and brainstem hypoplasia.[46] Treatment of these conditions is supportive.

Fatty acid oxidation defects

Although the most common defect of fatty acid β-oxidation, medium-chain acyl coenzyme A (CoA) dehydrogenase (MCAD) deficiency, typically presents later in infancy or childhood with a Reye syndrome-like illness, other fatty acid oxidation disorders present in the neonatal or early infantile periods with greater frequency. Short-chain 3-hydroxyacyl CoA dehydrogenase (SCHAD) deficiency, long-chain 3-hydroxyacyl CoA dehydrogenase (LCHAD) deficiency, very long-chain acyl CoA dehydrogenase (VLCAD) deficiency, carnitine palmitoyl transferase II (CPT II) deficiency, and carnitine-acylcarnitine translocase (CAT) deficiency have been described in neonates.[2–4,47–49] These conditions are autosomal recessive. Systemic manifestations include cardiomyopathy, hepatopathy, Reye syndrome-like illness, and muscle weakness and hypotonia. The creatine kinase level may be very elevated and prominent myoglobinuria may lead to renal tubular dysfunction and renal failure. A "salt-and-pepper" retinopathy has been reported in LCHAD deficiency, but usually appears in later childhood. Acute fatty liver of pregnancy and hemolysis, elevated liver enzymes, low platelets (HELLP) syndrome may be present in a heterozygous mother carrying a fetus with LCHAD deficiency.[3,50] Lactic acidosis is often present in LCHAD deficiency and trifunctional protein deficiency, but is usually not a prominent feature in most fatty acid oxidation disorders unless present as part of terminal illness. Patients typically have hypoketotic or nonketotic hypoglycemia, although increased production of ketone bodies may be seen in SCHAD deficiency. Severe hyperammonemia is atypical, but has been described in CAT deficiency.[47] Urine organic acid analysis may show elevated dicarboxylic acids. Plasma total carnitine levels are typically low, but there tends to be an elevation in the esterified carnitine fraction, with elevated esterified-to-free carnitine ratio. An acylcarnitine profile may detect pathognomonic compounds characteristic of specific fatty acid oxidation disorders. However, enzymology on fibroblasts and/or DNA mutation analysis are necessary to establish the diagnosis with certainty. Treatment includes avoidance of fasting, low-fat diet, and carnitine supplementation in patients who survive the neonatal period. Medium-chain triglycerides may be useful in long-chain defects.[3,49]

Mitochondrial disease

The mitochondrial electron transport chain is coded for by the coordinated action of both nuclear and mitochondrial genomes. Thus, these conditions may exhibit either Mendelian (autosomal recessive, autosomal dominant, X-linked) or maternal (mitochondrial) inheritance.[38] Mitochondrial disorders can cause dysfunction of any organ system, either alone or in combination. However, neuromuscular signs and symptoms occur most commonly.[35] Both nuclear and mitochondrial DNA disorders have presented in the neonatal period.[33–37,51–55] Neonates may have hypotonia, lethargy, deafness, dystonia, or seizures. Cataracts and retinal pigmentary abnormalities may also be present. Systemic features include cardiomyopathy, bone marrow suppression, hepatic disease, and renal dysfunction. Fatal mitochondrial disease with presentation soon after birth has been reported in patients with multiple deficiencies of mitochondrial enzymes secondary to deficiency of a nuclear-encoded mitochondrial matrix protein (heat shock protein 60) involved in the folding and assembly of mitochondrial enzymes[53,54] Neonatal lactic acidosis, weakness, lethargy, and feeding difficulties have also been described in patients with multiple mitochondrial enzyme defects secondary to an as yet unidentified nuclear gene mapped to chromosomes 2p14–2p13.[55]

Although some patients with mitochondrial disease may only have nonspecific white-matter abnormalities or delayed myelination, gray-matter involvement is relatively common, especially affecting the dorsal midbrain, thalami, and globi pallidi.[5,11] Mitochondrial disorders may also cause Leigh syndrome (subacute necrotizing encephalomyopathy), but patients tend to present after the neonatal period. The clinician must maintain a high index of suspicion, because these disorders are often difficult to diagnose. For example, a patient initially diagnosed with HIE after presenting with fetal distress, metabolic acidosis, and seizures at 4 h of age was later documented to have complex IV (cytochrome oxidase) deficiency.[36] Elevated lactate-to-pyruvate ratio (>25), β-hydroxybutyrate-to-acetoacetate ratio (>1.0), and urine organic acids with tricarboxylic acid cycle intermediates and other compounds suggestive of mitochondrial dysfunction offer clues to diagnosis.[2,4] Although a muscle biopsy may show changes suggestive of mitochondrial disease (e.g., ragged-red fibers), histopathology may appear normal or have nonspecific findings. Definitive diagnosis is made by mitochondrial respiratory chain analysis in muscle and/or mitochondrial DNA analysis. Various vitamin "cocktails" have been attempted, but there is no proven effective therapy for these conditions.

Severe ketoacidosis

Classic organic acidemias often present in the neonatal period or infancy with overwhelming illness and severe anion gap ketoacidosis. Prominent lactic acidosis is uncommon, but mild-to-moderate elevations may occur, especially if there is superimposed tissue hypoperfusion. Diagnosis of these disorders is relatively straightforward and is based on detection of characteristic metabolites in serum amino acids and urine organic acids.[2–4]

Organic acidemias

Methylmalonic acidemia (MMA), propionic acidemia (PA), isovaleric acidemia (IVA), glutaric aciduria, type II (multiple acyl CoA dehydrogenase deficiency (MADD)), and holocarboxylase synthetase deficiency (multiple carboxylase deficiency (MCD)) are autosomal recessive conditions that may present in neonates with lethargy, vomiting, and severe ketoacidosis.[2–4] Neonatal seizures have also been reported, but are not common. Renal cysts and dysmorphic features are common in MADD with neonatal presentation. An odor of "sweaty feet" may also be noted in patients with MADD or IVA. Routine labs often show neutropenia, hypoglycemia, and a metabolic acidosis. Lactic acidosis is usually not a prominent feature, although high lactate levels may be seen in MCD. Head MRI may show abnormal T2 prolongation in the periventricular white matter and lesions in the basal ganglia, especially the globus pallidus (MMA) or putamen and caudate nucleus (PA).[3,5] Diagnosis is by detection of characteristic organic acids in urine, with confirmation of decreased enzyme activity in leukocytes, fibroblasts, or hepatocytes.

Patients with 3-hydroxyisobutyric aciduria may also present in the neonatal period with overwhelming ketoacidosis. In addition, patients may have lactic acidosis, dysmorphic features, and congenital brain malformations, including intracerebral calcifications, lissencephaly, pachygyria, polymicrogyria, agenesis of the corpus callosum, and an indistinct gray- and white-matter interface.[56] Patients with glutaric aciduria type I may also have severe brain anomalies, including frontotemporal atrophy, delayed myelination, and basal ganglia changes, but this disorder tends to present later in infancy.[5]

Therapy of these disorders consists of dietary restriction of specific amino acids in some conditions and the prompt treatment of acute episodes of ketoacidosis. Carnitine and specific cofactors (e.g., vitamin B_{12} in some forms of MMA or biotin in MCD) are important therapeutic interventions.

Lethargy without metabolic acidosis or hyperammonemia

Maple syrup urine disease

Patients with maple syrup urine disease (MSUD) typically present in the first few days to weeks of life, after appearing normal at birth. Feeding difficulty and vomiting may be the initial symptoms. By the end of the first week, lethargy and progressive neurologic deterioration occur unless appropriate treatment is started. A markedly hypertonic infant with opisthotonus is typical.[3] The characteristic odor is present by the time neurologic symptoms develop, but not all patients have a "maple syrup" smell. Metabolic acidosis is uncommon until later in the course of disease. Neuroimaging is normal in the first few days of life. Characteristic head MRI findings develop with time, including profound localized edema in the deep cerebellar white matter, dorsal brainstem, cerebral peduncles, posterior limb of the internal capsule, perirolandic white matter, and globi pallidi.[5] Generalized cerebral hemisphere edema may also be present. Delayed, or abnormal, myelination is common.[3] Emergency management includes measures to decrease the levels of branched-chain amino acids (BCAA) rapidly (e.g., hemodialysis, BCAA-free parenteral nutrition, and the prevention of catabolism). Restricting intake of branched-chain amino acids, while providing adequate nutrition, and prompt treatment of intercurrent illnesses are the cornerstones of chronic management. One form of MSUD is also thiamine-responsive.

Mevalonic aciduria

Mevalonic aciduria is an autosomal recessive disorder of cholesterol biosynthesis that may present in the neonatal period with lethargy, hypotonia, or other signs of neurologic dysfunction, without a metabolic acidosis. Patients may have dysmorphic features, cataracts, hepatosplenomegaly, recurrent fevers without identifiable infectious agents, and anemia.[40,41]

Lethargy with hyperammonemia

Neonatal hyperammonemia is the predominant laboratory finding in urea cycle disorders, although other inborn errors of metabolism cause hyperammonemia by a secondary inhibition of urea cycle function. Pyruvate carboxylase deficiency, organic acidemias, carnitine-acylcarnitine translocase deficiency, lysinuric protein intolerance, and the HHH (hyperammonemia, hyperornithinemia, homocitrullinuria) syndrome may be associated with neonatal hyperammonemia.[2–4] Prominent hyperammonemia (ammonia 302–960 μg/dl, normal range 38–162 μg/dl) has also been reported in patients with perinatal asphyxia, likely secondary to hepatic dysfunction. However, these patients also had severe fetal bradycardia and low Apgar scores, and required prolonged resuscitation at birth.[19] In contrast, patients with inborn errors of metabolism, including urea cycle disorders, are often normal at birth, without a history of perinatal distress.

Urea cycle disorders

Patients with urea cycle disorders (*N*-acetylglutamate synthetase deficiency, carbamyl phosphate synthetase deficiency, ornithine transcarbamylase deficiency, argininosuccinic acid synthetase deficiency (citrullinemia), and argininosuccinic acid lyase deficiency) typically present with lethargy or poor feeding in the first few days of life.[2–4] Sepsis is often initially suspected, and, unless an ammonia level is checked, these infants may die of unknown cause early in the neonatal period. Aside from the X-linked ornithine transcarbamylase deficiency, these are autosomal recessive conditions. Hyperpnea with respiratory alkalosis may occur. Progression to deep coma supervenes, necessitating intubation and mechanical ventilation. Head imaging is nonspecific in these disorders, but may show cerebral edema. Head MRI in the subacute phase (day of life 3–7) may resemble HIE, with edema in both gray and white matter and gray-matter T1 shortening. Damage to the cortex and underlying white matter, similar to ischemic injury, may be present in the chronic phase.[5] Diagnosis is based on characteristic serum amino acid patterns and urine orotic acid concentration. Enzymology on fibroblasts or hepatocytes may be needed to confirm the diagnosis. DNA analysis has limited availability. Initial emergency treatment consists of hemodialysis, protein restriction, provision of adequate fluids and calories to prevent catabolism, intravenous ammonia-scavenging medications (sodium benzoate and sodium phenylacetate), and intravenous arginine hydrochloride. Chronic therapy includes protein restriction, oral sodium phenylbutyrate and/or sodium benzoate, and arginine or citrulline supplementation.[2–4]

HHH syndrome

This autosomal recessive condition is caused by defective transport of ornithine into mitochondria, resulting in a secondary inhibition of the urea cycle. Most patients present in infancy with lethargy, intermittent hyperammonemia, failure to thrive, developmental delay, and ataxia. Diagnosis is made by detecting characteristic metabolites in blood and urine. Treatment is by protein restriction.[2–4]

Lysinuric protein intolerance

Defective transport of basic amino acids across the basilateral membrane of epithelial cells is the fundamental defect in lysinuric protein intolerance. Patients typically present in infancy with hyperammonemia, vomiting, diarrhea, and failure to thrive. Inheritance is autosomal recessive. Serum concentrations of ornithine, lysine, and arginine are low, while citrulline, glutamine, and alanine tend to be elevated. There is increased urinary excretion of lysine, ornithine, and arginine. Moderate protein restriction and citrulline supplementation are the primary therapies.[2–4]

Other disorders

Glycogen storage disorders (GSD) and disorders of gluconeogenesis may present in neonates with hypoglycemia and lactic acidosis. However, differentiation from HIE and other inborn errors of metabolism should be relatively straightforward.

Glycogen storage disorders

GSD type I patients may have hepatomegaly at birth and symptomatic hypoglycemia, but most patients present in infancy. GSD type III (debrancher enzyme deficiency) tends to be a more mild condition, but may present in neonates. GSD type 0 (glycogen synthetase deficiency) may present with ketotic hypoglycemia and lactic acidosis, without prominent hepatomegaly. GSD type VIII (phosphorylase kinase deficiency) may be inherited as an autosomal recessive or X-linked condition. Clinical features include hepatomegaly, myopathy, and a fatal infantile variant with cardiomyopathy. Pompe disease (GSD type II, α-glucosidase deficiency) may also present with neonatal cardiomyopathy and marked hypotonia secondary to a skeletal myopathy.[57]

Disorders of gluconeogenesis

Fructose 1,6-bisphosphatase deficiency may present with severe neonatal metabolic acidosis. Routine labs show hypoglycemia and lactic acidosis. Patients typically respond well to intravenous fluids containing dextrose and bicarbonate. Avoidance of fasting is the mainstay of therapy for gluconeogenesis disorders.[57]

Other neonatal myopathies and encephalomyopathies

Patients with inherited myopathies (e.g., centronuclear myopathy) may also present with neonatal distress, hypotonia, and signs suggestive of HIE.[58] Boys with Rett syndrome have been described with a nonspecific neonatal encephalopathy and periventricular leukomalacia.[59] Molecular testing for Rett syndrome should be considered in patients with unexplained encephalopathy and normal metabolic investigations.

Summary

Inborn errors of metabolism may present in neonates with features of HIE. In contrast to children with HIE, neonates with metabolic disorders often have an unremarkable delivery and an apparent normal period lasting hours to days. On the other hand, a traumatic delivery or prematurity may constitute environmental stress factors that unmask an underlying inborn error of metabolism; the absence of a normal period, therefore, does not exclude these disorders from consideration. Although patients with metabolic disorders and HIE, in general, have different obstetric histories and head-imaging findings, in practice it may be difficult to distinguish these conditions, because they also share many clinical and laboratory features. There is a tendency to evaluate neonates for a possible underlying metabolic disorder only after more common conditions have been excluded. It is crucial for the clinician to consider metabolic disorders in all neonates with nonspecific features suggestive of sepsis or asphyxia upon initial presentation. Rapid diagnosis and management may prevent death or significant morbidity. By obtaining appropriate laboratory investigations, the clinician can provide the family with the best chance of arriving at a diagnosis for their child during an extremely stressful time. Establishing a diagnosis permits not only optimal management of the child, but also accurate genetic counseling. Tandem-mass spectrometry testing for a wide variety of aminoacidemias, organic acidemias, and fatty acid oxidation defects is currently being integrated into newborn screening programs throughout the world. Such technology provides new hope for the early diagnosis and treatment of inborn errors of metabolism, which collectively account for significant neonatal morbidity and mortality.

REFERENCES

1 Greene, C.L. and Goodman, S.I. (1997). Catastrophic metabolic encephalopathies in the newborn period: evaluation and management. *Clin Perinatol*, **24**, 773–788.

2 Scriver, C.R., Beaudet, A.L., Sly, W.S. and Valle, D., eds. (2001). *The Metabolic and Molecular Bases of Inherited Disease*, 8th edn. New York, NY: McGraw-Hill.

3 Nyhan, W.L. and Ozand, P.T. (1998). *Atlas of Metabolic Diseases*, 1st edn. London: Chapman & Hall Medical.

4 Blau, N., Duran, M. and Blaskovics, M.E., eds. (1996). *Physician's Guide to the Laboratory Diagnosis of Metabolic Diseases*, 1st edn. London: Chapman & Hall Medical.

5 Barkovich, A.J. (2000). *Pediatric Neuroimaging*, 3rd edn, pp. 71–156, 162–205. Philadelphia, PA: Lippincott/Williams & Wilkins.

6 Biagas, K. (1999). Hypoxic–ischemic brain injury: advancements in the understanding of mechanisms and potential avenues for therapy. *Curr Opin Pediatr*, **11**, 223–228.

7 Vannucci, R.C. (2000). Hypoxic–ischemic encephalopathy. *Am J Perinatol*, **17**, 113–120.

8 Roland, E.H., Poskitt, K., Rodriguez, E., Lupton, B.A. and Hill, A. (1998). Perinatal hypoxic–ischemic thalamic injury: clinical features and neuroimaging. *Ann Neurol*, **44**, 161–166.

9 Hoon, A.H., Reinhardt, E.M., Kelley, R.I. et al. (1997). Brain magnetic resonance imaging in suspected extrapyramidal cerebral palsy: observations in distinguishing genetic-metabolic from acquired cases. *J Pediatr*, **131**, 240–245.

10 Haas, R.H., Marsden, D.L., Capistrano-Estrada, S. (1995). Acute basal ganglia infarction in propionic acidemia. *J Child Neurol*, **10**, 18–22.

11 Johnston, M.V. and Hoon, A.H. (2000). Possible mechanisms in infants for selective basal ganglia damage from asphyxia, kernicterus, or mitochondrial encephalopathies. *J Child Neurol*, **15**, 588–591.

12 Ankarcrona, M., Dypbukt, J.M., Bonfoco, E. et al. (1995). Glutamate-induced neuronal death: a succession of necrosis or apoptosis depending on mitochondrial function. *Neuron*, **15**, 961–973.

13 Shi, Y., Pan, F., Li, H. et al. (2000). Role of carbon monoxide and nitric oxide in newborn infants with postasphyxial hypoxic–ischemic encephalopathy. *Pediatrics*, **106**, 1447–1451.

14 Eliasson, M.J.L., Sampei, K., Mandir, A.S. et al. (1997). Poly (ADP-ribose) polymerase gene disruption renders mice resistant to cerebral ischemia. *Nat Med*, **3**, 1089–1095.

15 Penn, A.A., Enzman, D.R., Hahn, J.S. and Stevenson, D.K. (1994). Kernicterus in a full term infant. *Pediatrics*, **93**, 1003–1006.

16 Greenamyre, T., Penney, J.B., Young, A.B. et al. (1987). Evidence of a transient perinatal glutamatergic innervation of globus pallidus. *J Neurosci*, **7**, 1022–1030.

17 Johnston, M.V. (1997). Hypoxic and ischemic disorders of infants and children. Lecture for 38th meeting of Japanese Society of Child Neurology, Tokyo, Japan, July 1996. *Brain Dev*, **19**, 235–239.

18 Agani, F.H., Pichiule, P., Chavez, J.C. and LaManna, J.C. (2000). The role of mitochondria in the regulation of hypoxia-inducible factor 1 expression during hypoxia. *J Biol Chem*, **275**, 35863–35867.

19 Goldberg, R.N., Cabal, L.A., Sinatra, F., Plajstek, C.E. and Hodgman, J.E. (1979). Hyperammonemia associated with perinatal asphyxia. *Pediatrics*, **64**, 336–341.

20 Sheth, R.D., Hobbs, G.R. and Mullett, M. (1999). Neonatal seizures: incidence, onset, and etiology by gestational age. *J Perinatol*, **19**, 40–43.

21 Torres, O.A., Miller, V.S., Buist, N.M.R. and Hyland, K. (1999). Folinic acid-responsive neonatal seizures. *J Child Neurol*, **14**, 529–532.

22 Baxter, P. (1999). Epidemiology of pyridoxine dependent and pyridoxine responsive seizures in the UK. *Arch Dis Child*, **81**, 431–433.

23 Baxter, P., Griffiths, P., Kelly, T. and Gardner-Medwin, D. (1996). Pyridoxine-dependent seizures: demographic, clinical, MRI, and psychometric features, and effect of dose on intelligence quotient. *Dev Med Child Neurol*, **38**, 998–1006.

24 Medina-Kauwe, L.K., Tobin, A.J., De Meirleir, L. et al. (1999). 4-Aminobutyrate aminotransferase (GABA-transaminase) deficiency. *J Inher Metab Dis*, **22**, 414–427.

25 Stöckler, S., Isbrandt, D., Hanefeld, F., Schmidt, B. and von Figura, K. (1996). Guanidinoacetate methyltransferase deficiency: the first inborn error of creatine metabolism in man. *Am J Hum Genet*, **58**, 914–922.

26 De Vivo, D.C., Trifiletti, R.R., Jacobson, R.I. et al. (1991). Defective glucose transport across the blood–brain barrier as a cause of persistent hypoglycorrhachia, seizures, and developmental delay. *N. Engl J Med*, **325**, 703–709.

27 Hyland K., Buist, N.M.R., Powell, B.R. et al. (1995). Folinic acid responsive seizures: a new syndrome? *J Inher Metab Dis*, **18**, 1–5.

28 Takahashi, Y., Suzuki, Y., Kumazaki, K. et al. (1997). Epilepsy in peroxisomal disorders. *Epilepsia*, **38**, 182–188.

29 Hoffmann, G.F., Surtees, R.A.H. and Wevers, R.A. (1998). Cerebrospinal fluid investigations for neurometabolic disorders. *Neuropediatr*, **29**, 61–71.

30 Roldán, A., Figueras-Aloy, J., Deulofeu, R. and Jiménez, R. (1999). Glycine and other neurotransmitter amino acids in cerebrospinal fluid in perinatal asphyxia and neonatal hypoxic–ischemic encephalopathy. *Acta Paediatr*, **88**, 1137–1141.

31 Haenggeli, C-A., Girardin, E. and Paunier L. (1991). Pyridoxine-dependent seizures, clinical and therapeutic aspects. *Eur J Pediatr*, **150**, 452–455.

32 Norman, M.G., McGillivray, B.C., Kalousek, D.K., Hill, A. and Poskitt, K.J. (1995) Perinatal hemorrhagic and hypoxic–ischemic lesions. In Norman, M.G. (ed.) *Congenital Malformations of the Brain: Pathological, Embryological, Clinical, Radiological and Genetic Aspects*, 1st edn, pp. 419–423. Oxford: Oxford University Press.

33 von Döbeln, U., Wibom, R., Åhlman, H. et al. (1993). Fatal neonatal lactic acidosis with respiratory insufficiency due to complex I and IV deficiency. *Acta Paediatr*, **82**, 1079–1081.

34 Muraki, K., Goto, Y., Nishino, I. et al. (1997). Severe lactic acidosis and neonatal death in Pearson syndrome. *J Inher Metab Dis*. **20**, 43–48.

35 Birch-Machin, M.A., Shepherd, I.M., Watmough, N.J. et al. (1989). Fatal lactic acidosis in infancy with a defect of complex III of the respiratory chain. *Pediatr Res*, **25**, 553–559.

36 Willis, T.A., Davidson, J., Gray, R.G.F. et al. (2000). Cytochrome oxidase deficiency presenting as birth asphyxia. *Dev Med Child Neurol*, **42**, 414–417.

37 Procaccio, V., Mousson, B., Beugnot, R. et al. (1999). Nuclear DNA origin of mitochondrial complex I deficiency in fatal infantile lactic acidosis evidenced by transnuclear complementation of fibroblasts. *J Clin Invest*, **104**, 83–92.

38 Zeviani M., Bertagnolia, B. and Uziel, G. (1996). Neurological presentations of mitochondrial diseases. *J Inher Metab Dis*, **19**, 504–520.

39 Muntau, A.C., Röschinger, W., Merkenschlager, A. et al. (2000). Combined D-2- and L-2-hydroxglutaric aciduria with neonatal onset encephalopathy: a third biochemical variant of 2-hydroxyglutaric aciduria? *Neuropediatrics*, **31**, 137–140.

40 Burlina, A.B., Bonalfé, L. and Zacchello, F. (1999). Clinical and biochemical approach to the neonate with a suspected inborn error of amino acid and organic acid metabolism. *Semin Perinatol*, **23**, 162–173.

41 Hoffmann, G.F., Charpentier, C., Mayatepek, E. et al. (1993). Clinical and biochemical phenotype in 11 patients with mevalonic aciduria. *Pediatrics*, **91**, 915–921.

42 Robinson, B.H., MacKay, N., Chun, K. and Ling, M. (1996). Disorders of pyruvate carboxylase and the pyruvate dehydrogenase complex. *J Inher Metab Dis*, **19**, 452–462.

43 Byrd, D.J., Krohn, H.-P., Winkler, L. et al. (1989). Neonatal pyruvate dehydrogenase deficiency with lipoate responsive lactic acidemia and hyperammonemia. *Eur J Pediatr*, **148**, 543–547.

44 Bonnefont, J.-P., Chretien, D., Rustin, P. et al. (1992). Alpha-ketoglutarate dehydrogenase deficiency presenting as congenital lactic acidosis. *J Pediatr*, **121**, 255–258.

45 Haworth, J.C., Perry, T.L., Blass, J.P., Hansen, S. and Urquhart, N. (1976). Lactic acidosis in three sibs due to defects in both pyruvate dehydrogenase and α-ketoglutarate dehydrogenase complexes. *Pediatrics*, **58**, 564–572.

46 Kerrigan, J.F., Aleck, K.A., Tarby, T.J., Bird, C.R. and Heidenreich, R. (2000). Fumaric aciduria: clinical and imaging features. *Ann Neurol*, **47**, 583–588.

47 Stanley, C.A., Hale, D.E., Berry, G.T. et al. (1992). Brief report: a deficiency of carnitine-acylcarnitine translocase in the inner mitochondrial membrane. *N Engl J Med*, **327**, 19–22.

48 Bertrand, C., Largilliere, C., Zabot, M.T., Mathieu, M. and Vianes-Saban, C. (1993). Very long chain acyl-CoA dehydrogenase deficiency: identification of a new inborn error of mitochondrial fatty acid oxidation in fibroblasts. *Biochim Biophys Acta*, **1180**, 327–329.

49 Duran, M., Wanders, R.J.A., de Jaguar, J.P. et al. (1991). 3-Hydroxydicarboxylic aciduria due to long chain 3-hydroxyacyl coenzyme A deficiency associated with sudden neonatal death: protective effect of medium-chain triglyceride treatment. *Eur J Pediatr*, **150**, 190–195.

50 Ibdah, J.A., Yang, Z. and Bennett, M.J. (2000). Liver disease in pregnancy and fetal fatty acid oxidation defects. *Mol Genet Metab*, **71**, 182–189.

51 Valnot, I., Osmond, S., Gigarel, N. et al. (2000). Mutations in the *SCO1* gene in mitochondrial cytochrome *c* oxidase deficiency with neonatal-onset hepatic failure and encephalopathy. *Am J Hum Genet*, **67**, 1104–1109.

52 Poggi, G.M., Lamantea, E., Ciani, F. et al. (2000). Fatal neonatal outcome in a case of muscular mitochondrial DNA depletion. *J Inher Metab Dis*, **23**, 755–757.

53 Agsteribbe, E., Huckriede, A., Veenhuis, M. et al. (1993). A fatal, systemic mitochondrial disease with decreased mitochondrial enzyme activities, abnormal ultrastructure of mitochondria and deficiency of heat shock protein 60. *Biochem Biophys Res Commun*, **193**, 146–154.

54 Briones, P., Vilaseca, M.A., Ribes, A. et al. (1997). A new case of multiple mitochondrial enzyme deficiencies with decreased amount of heat shock protein 60. *J Inher Metab Dis*, **20**, 569–577.

55 Seyda, A., Newbold, R.F., Hudson, T.J. et al. (2001). A novel syndrome affecting multiple mitochondrial functions, located by microcell-mediated transfer to chromosome 2p14–2p13. *Am J Hum Genet*, **68**, 386–396.

56 Chitayat, D., Meagher-Villemure, M., Mamer, O.A. et al. (1992). Brain dysgenesis and congenital intracerebral calcification associated with 3-hydroxyisobutyric aciduria. *J Pediatr*, **121**, 86–89.

57 Tein, I. (1999). Neonatal metabolic myopathies. *Semin Perinatol*, **23**, 125–151.

58 Bruyland, M., Liebaers, I., Sacre, L. et al. (1984). Neonatal myotubular myopathy with a probable X-linked inheritance: observations on a new family with a review of the literature. *J Neurol*, **231**, 220–222.

59 Schanen, N.C., Kurczynski, T.W., Brunelle, D. et al. (1998). Neonatal encephalopathy in two boys in families with recurrent Rett syndrome. *J Child Neurol*, **13**, 229–231.

PART III

Diagnosis of the Infant with Asphyxia

20

Clinical manifestations of hypoxic–ischemic encephalopathy

Jin S. Hahn

Stanford University School of Medicine, Stanford, CA, USA

Hypoxic–ischemic encephalopathy is a well-recognized clinical syndrome and the most common cause of acute neurological impairment and seizures in the neonatal period.[1–5] Hypoxic–ischemic brain injury secondary to birth asphyxia can result in the development of "cerebral palsy," but recent literature has shown that only a small percentage of children with cerebral palsy had intrapartum asphyxia as a possible etiology.[6–8] More emphasis has been placed on antenatal events as having a greater association with cerebral palsy.[9] Nevertheless, severe hypoxic or ischemic injury during the perinatal period can lead to a neurological syndrome in the newborn period, i.e., hypoxic–ischemic encephalopathy, and subsequent neurological sequelae in the survivors.[10] Therefore, recognizing and understanding hypoxic–ischemic encephalopathy are important. The clinical features, the management, and the clinicopathologic syndromes of hypoxic–ischemic encephalopathy are presented in this chapter.

Clinical features and management

The clinical features in the infant with hypoxic–ischemic encephalopathy are presented here by first describing a general approach to the evaluation. Then the specific clinical features, diagnostic studies, prognosis, and management of these infants are described.

General evaluation

The initial assessment of the infant with suspected hypoxic–ischemic encephalopathy relies on obtaining a thorough history and carrying out a careful physical examination. The history should be directed toward determining whether there were any specific antenatal factors that might account for the disorder. Review of the maternal history, fetal monitoring studies, fetal ultrasonographic findings, and fetal acid–base measurements is essential. Information regarding examination of the placenta should also be obtained. Special attention should be paid to possible history of maternal infection and chorioamnionitis.

A general physical examination is required to establish the infant's gestational age, cardiopulmonary status, presence of congenital anomalies, and growth parameters. A carefully performed neurologic examination is essential to obtain information about the infant's current status. This information is used to determine the supplementary evaluations that are indicated and is critical in establishing a prognosis. Many studies have shown that the neonatal neurologic examination is a valuable predictor of outcome.[2,11] A detailed neurologic examination provides the most information in regard to the localization and severity of the encephalopathy, but a clinical staging examination, used in several studies of asphyxiated newborns, should be performed initially.[11]

Table 20.1. Clinical staging and outcome of hypoxic–ischemic encephalopathy

Severity of encephalopathy	Mild	Moderate	Severe
Level of consciousness	Alert	Lethargy	Coma
Tone	Normal or hypertonia	Hypotonia	Flaccidity
Tendon reflexes	Increased	Increased	Depressed or absent
Primitive reflexes	Uninhibited	Depressed	Absent
Autonomic function	Sympathetic overactivity		Autonomic dysfunction
Others	Irritability, jitteriness	Brainstem dysfunction	± Elevated intracranial pressure
Seizures	Absent		± Frequent, often refractory to anticonvulsants
Electroencephalographic background	Normal	Low voltage, periodic or paroxysmal	Periodic or isolectric
Outcome	Normal	20–40% abnormal	Death or 100% abnormal

Sources: Based on Sarnat and Sarnat[12] and Roland and Hill.[4]

Neurologic assessment in hypoxic–ischemic encephalopathy

If the degree of hypoxic–ischemic insult at or shortly before delivery is of sufficient magnitude to cause long-term neurological sequelae, newborns will manifest signs of neurological dysfunction shortly after birth, often within hours. Conversely, the absence of significant neonatal encephalopathy during the newborn period implies the absence of significant hypoxic–ischemic insult during the intrapartum period.

Neurological dysfunctions due to hypoxic–ischemic insult include altered level of consciousness and reactivity, altered tone, and seizures. There is a correlation between the severity and duration of the hypoxic–ischemic insult and the severity of the encephalopathy. Careful documentation of the neurologic examination and staging of the encephalopathy will help determine the severity of the hypoxic–ischemic insult and ultimate outcome.

Several scales have been developed to assess the severity of the hypoxic–ischemic encephalopathy. One of the more widely used scales is the staging system by Sarnat and Sarnat[12] in which the clinical stages of hypoxic–ischemic encephalopathy are divided into three levels. The major clinical features that are used in the assessment are the infant's level of consciousness, cranial nerve findings, muscle tone, deep tendon reflexes, neonatal reflexes, spontaneous motor activity, and autonomic function (Table 20.1).

Infants with a mild degree of encephalopathy (stage I) often have variable levels of consciousness in which periods of lethargy alternate with periods of irritability and "hyperalertness." They often feed poorly, have disturbed sleep–wake cycles with a preponderance of active sleep, and are described as "jittery." Jitteriness is best described as a spontaneous or stimulus-induced myoclonus (nonepileptic). Findings on the cranial nerve examination are normal. Muscle tone is normal or increased and the deep tendon reflexes are hyperactive. The Moro reflex is often exaggerated, but other neonatal reflexes are normal. Pupillary dilation and tachycardia are frequently observed. Mild encephalopathy usually lasts for less than 24 h and is generally associated with a favorable prognosis.[12,13]

Within the first day, the newborn term infant may progress to moderate encephalopathy (stage II) with altered level of consciousness (lethargy or stupor), hypotonia, hyporeflexia, and seizures.[14,15] Infants with a moderate degree of encephalopathy are lethargic and can be aroused with auditory and tactile stimuli. Feeding is extremely poor. Muscle tone is decreased, with a prominent head lag, a positive scarf sign, and a poor response to the Landau maneuver. Exaggerated deep tendon reflexes with clonus are elicited, and clonus of the jaw may be observed. The results of cranial nerve examination are normal except for a decreased gag reflex. Spontaneous motor activity is decreased, and the observed movements may include spontaneous myoclonus or show signs of extrapyramidal dysfunction. Pupils are often constricted, and periodic breathing associated with bradycardia may be present. Seizures may occur and must be differentiated from other abnormal movements and behavior. The duration of moderate encephalopathy is usually 2–14 days. Recovery is heralded by disappearance of myoclonus, increased alertness, and improved suck. Neurologic sequelae occur in approximately 20–40% of infants with moderate encephalopathy, especially if the abnormal neurologic signs persist for one week.[14,16]

Infants who are profoundly affected display severe encephalopathy (stage III) characterized by coma, flaccidity, and unresponsiveness to noxious stimuli.[12] They also have episodic decerebrate posturing and poor brainstem function. Deep tendon and neonatal reflexes are absent. The pupils are poorly reactive or fixed, and the oculocephalic reflex is absent. Seizures are very common. The infant often has bradycardia, systemic hypotension, irregular respirations, periodic breathing, and apnea. The duration of this stage ranges from hours to weeks. If the infant recovers, a period of extensor hypertonia and brainstem dysfunction (abnormal swallowing, sucking movements) may occur. Nearly all of the survivors will develop neurologic sequelae.

Asphyxiated newborns may transition from one stage to another. Most infants who go through stage I also pass through stage II before recovering.[12] More severely asphyxiated infants begin in stage II and progress to stage III. Often the clinical manifestations of stage III may not be apparent until day 2 or 3 after birth, when cerebral edema is at its maximum. Clinically, when severe cerebral edema is present, the anterior fontanel may be bulging or tense and the cranial sutures splayed. If infants remain in moderate or severe encephalopathic states for more than 7 days, there is a high incidence of long-term neurological sequelae.[12]

Laboratory evaluations

Laboratory investigations of the asphyxiated infant should include measurements of cord blood gases, arterial blood gas and pH levels, serum electrolyte levels (including calcium and magnesium), and serum glucose, blood urea nitrogen, creatinine levels, and hepatic enzyme levels. Measurements of several other metabolic indicators of the degree of insult can be carried out, including cerebrospinal fluid (CSF) lactate and serum catecholamine levels.[17,18] The abnormalities found in the majority of these parameters reflect the severity of the systemic asphyxial insult rather than the severity of the insult to the brain. A lumbar puncture with measurement of CSF opening pressure, cell count, and protein and glucose level should be performed.

Concentration of creatine kinase brain isoenzyme (CK-BB) in either blood or CSF shows particular promise for both diagnostic and prognostic measures of brain injury.[19–21] Concentrations of CSF CK-BB were found to be markedly higher in newborns with documented neurologic disorder (intraventricular hemorrhage, asphyxial encephalopathy, central nervous system (CNS) infection, or persistent periventricular intraparenchymal echodensities) when compared to that in normal newborns or those with subarachnoid hemorrhage.[19] CK-BB concentration, particularly in CSF appears to be a sensitive and specific indicator for detection of acquired perinatal brain injury. Further studies are required to determine the usefulness of this and the other metabolic parameters.

Electroencephalography

The electroencephalogram (EEG) is a valuable measure of cerebral function that can be performed at the bedside. It complements the clinical examination in establishing the severity of the encephalopathy and in determining the prognosis.[22] The diagnosis of seizures in this age group is dependent on this study, since a significant number of abnormal behavior patterns thought to represent seizures actually represent other phenomena.[3,23] Furthermore, the clinical seizure type in these infants may often be subtle and fragmentary or masked by anticonvulsant therapy, making the EEG essential for the diagnosis of seizures. The EEG is also helpful in assessing the degree of cerebral dysfunction and providing information about neurological prognosis. Severely depressed backgrounds, such as suppression-burst pattern or isoelectric pattern, indicate severe cerebral dysfunction and usually portend a poor prognosis. The presence of status epilepticus on the EEG also carries an unfavorable prognosis. EEG patterns with less severe background disturbance that revert to normal after the first week usually indicate a more favorable prognosis. The application of EEG in the evaluation of the encephalopathic newborn is described in detail in Chapter 25.

Other neurophysiologic measures of nervous system function, such as somatosensory, brainstem, and visual evoked responses, have only recently been applied to evaluating the asphyxiated newborn and are not routinely recommended as part of the general evaluation.[24–27] Recently amplitude-integrated EEG has been used to monitor neonates with hypoxic–ischemic encephalopathy. This method, which simplifies bedside interpretation of the EEG background, has been found to be useful for identifying infants with more severe encephalopathy and worse outcomes.[28]

Neuroimaging studies

Neuroimaging studies are an essential component of the assessment of the newborn with hypoxic–ischemic encephalopathy. It is helpful for determining the nature, severity, and extent of the hypoxic–ischemic brain injury.

Cranial ultrasonography has proven to be a valuable technique in the diagnosis of intraventricular hemorrhage (IVH) and periventricular leukomalacia (PVL). This study can be readily carried out at the bedside in all newborns with evidence of encephalopathy. However, since IVH and PVL tend to affect premature infants primarily, it may not be as useful in term infants with hypoxic–ischemic insults.

Computed tomography (CT) is widely used to assess the nature and extent of cerebral injury, especially in term infants. It is more useful in assessing cortical and hemorrhagic injury. It can be obtained rapidly, often without need for sedation. CT scans in asphyxiated newborns may show focal or multifocal areas of decreased attenuation in the cerebral gray or white matter. These abnormal areas likely represent areas of ischemia or cerebral edema. Diffuse cerebral edema can manifest as loss of gray-white-matter differentiation, effacement of sulcal spaces, and slit-like ventricles.

Magnetic resonance imaging (MRI) has become the method of choice to assess the newborn brain. MRI has been used to document in the neonate various clinicopathologic syndromes of hypoxic–ischemic brain injury described by Volpe, including basal ganglia injury, parasagittal cerebral injury, PVL, focal ischemic lesions, and selective neuronal necrosis.[29–31] Newer MRI techniques, including diffusion-weighted images and magnetic resonance spectroscopy, have also been developed recently to assess the extent of cerebral injury and to provide prognostic information.[32,33] The disadvantages of MRI include the prolonged scanning time and impaired ability to monitor the mechanically ventilated sick newborns. These considerations limit its use in the early stages of hypoxic–ischemic encephalopathy, when the newborn may be too unstable to undergo MRI. Further details about the use of neuroimaging studies in the newborn are discussed in Chapter 22.

Management of hypoxic–ischemic encephalopathy

The most important aspect of managing the infant with hypoxic–ischemic encephalopathy is supportive care. In the asphyxiated newborn there is involvement of multiple organ systems, all of which require intervention.

Maintenance of adequate ventilation is a critical component of the infant's care. Prevention of further episodes of hypoxemia and hypercarbia may play an important role in determining the ultimate neurological outcome. Hyperoxemia may also be deleterious to the nervous system.[34] Maintenance of adequate cerebral perfusion is also critical; this is best achieved by maintaining normal systemic arterial pressure and avoiding excessive fluctuations. The fluid and electrolyte status requires close observation, since the asphyxiated infant often develops renal failure, resulting in hypocalcemia, hyponatremia, and fluid overload.

Treatment directed toward the control of cerebral edema is controversial. Cerebral edema in a neonate with hypoxic–ischemic encephalopathy may manifest with a bulging fontanel, splayed cranial sutures, and a rapidly enlarging head size. Most pathologic studies suggest that in newborns cerebral edema rarely develops to the extent that herniation is observed at autopsy.[35] The role of brain edema in causing further brain injury is unknown. Various therapies have been used in attempts to reduce cerebral edema, including the use of hyperventilation, corticosteroids, high-dose barbiturates, osmotic agents (mannitol), and hypothermia. There have been no studies that demonstrate that the drugs used to decrease edema diminish the degree of neuronal injury. None of these modalities have proved to be effective in reducing morbidity or mortality in neonatal hypoxic–ischemic encephalopathy. Nevertheless, it is important to avoid fluid overload, realizing that the asphyxiated infant is at higher risk for developing the syndrome of inappropriate antidiuretic hormone secretion and may also have compromised renal function. At present, the available clinical and experimental evidence does not support the use of corticosteroids or osmotic diuretics in neonatal hypoxic–ischemic encephalopathy.[36,37]

High-dose barbiturate therapy has been studied in neonates for hypoxic–ischemic encephalopathy.[38–41] Only one study showed a benefit in outcome.[41] These drugs often cause further systemic complications, such as exacerbating a preexisting cardiovascular instability.[39]

Neonatal seizures associated with hypoxic–ischemic encephalopathies are routinely treated with anticonvulsants such as phenobarbital, phenytoin, and benzodiazepines. To date, it has not been clearly established that frequent seizures *per se* are detrimental to the newborn brain. Nevertheless, neonatal seizures are treated to minimize cardiovascular and metabolic derangements that are associated with seizures. Unfortunately, seizures associated with severe hypoxic–ischemic encephalopathy are often difficult to control, even with high doses of anticonvulsants.[42] Phenobarbital or phenytoin, when given alone, controls seizures in fewer than half of the neonates, but the combination of the two may achieve control in approximately 60% of the neonates.[43] Further management of neonatal seizures is discussed in Chapter 37.

Neuroprotection

As a result of advances in the understanding of mechanisms of hypoxic–ischemic brain injury after a hypoxic–ischemic insult, several neuroprotective agents have been proposed as potential therapy. Many agents have undergone extensive investigation in experimental animal models and in adult humans. They include excitatory amino acid antagonists, oxygen-free radical inhibitors, calcium channel blockers, and inhibitors of nitric oxide production.[44] While these newer agents appear promising, extensive clinical testing in human neonates has not been performed.

Another form of neuroprotection that has been investigated is hypothermia (selective head or systemic cooling). Recently, infants with hypoxic–ischemic encephalopathy have been treated with head cooling and mild hypothermia.[45] This method appears to be safe, but the efficacy in improvement of neurodevelopmental outcome is still being investigated in large controlled studies. It is unlikely that a single "magic bullet" will be effective in blocking the cascade of events that lead to neuronal and white-matter injury, but rather a combination therapy will need to be used in the future.

Clinicopathologic syndromes

The neuropathologic lesions resulting from a hypoxic–ischemic insult have been reviewed extensively.[46–48] The global cerebral insult from perinatal asphyxia results in specific patterns of regional injury, the topography of which is maturation-dependent. The specific type of lesions also varies with the characteristics of the primary insult and the subsequent management. Recent neuroimaging studies with MRI have correlated the specific patterns of neuroradiologic alterations with the specific clinicopathologic syndromes. Recognition of these disorders provides an understanding of the mechanisms leading to their development and allows prediction of possible neurologic disabilities. The neuropathologic changes can be divided into lesions that are the result of primary damage to specific types of cells and structures and those due to hemorrhage.

The pathologic changes observed in the term infant are different from that seen in the premature infant (Table 20.2). The term infant most commonly is observed to have neuropathologic changes involving primarily the gray matter and specific neuroanatomic structures in both the cortical and subcortical regions. IVH occurs in the term infant, but the pathogenic mechanisms are different from those in the preterm infant. On the contrary, periventricular or IVH is the most common neuropathologic finding in the premature infant. Pathologic changes in the white matter are the next most common disorder, followed by lesions involving selected neuronal populations.

The patterns of brain injury observed in the term newborn can be categorized into lesions involving four major areas of the CNS: the cortex, deep gray-matter nuclei, brainstem, and cerebellum. There is often an overlap of these pathologic processes, but primary involvement of one of these regions results in specific clinical characteristics both acutely and over the long term. The clinicopathologic correlates of the major types of hypoxic–ischemic brain injury are presented here.

Table 20.2. Neuropathologic lesions associated with neonatal hypoxic–ischemic encephalopathy

Full-term newborn	Preterm newborn
Focal brain injury	*Periventricular or intraventricular hemorrhage*
Arterial occlusion	
Venous occlusion	*White-matter disease*
"Watershed" lesions	
Necrosis of deep gray nuclei	*Necrosis of deep gray nuclei*
Basal ganglia	Basal ganglia
Thalamus	Thalamus
Diencephalon	Diencephalon
Brainstem necrosis	*Brainstem necrosis*
Pontosubicular necrosis	Pontosubicular necrosis
Selective nuclei	Selective nuclei
Cerebellar necrosis	*Cerebellar necrosis*
Intraventricular hemorrhage	*Cortical infarctions*
White-matter disease	

Parasagittal border-zone injury

This form of cortical injury, resulting from a general decrease in the cerebral blood flow (ischemia), is referred to as the watershed infarction, since the disorder involves the border zones of the three major arterial supply zones. The injury is bilateral, and usually symmetrical. Ulegyria, a term describing cortical gyri that are atrophic, particularly at the depth of sulci, is the chronic lesion resulting from this particular brain injury (Figure 20.1). In one autopsy series of neurologically handicapped children, 30 of 153 subjects had this lesion in the parasagittal watershed region.[49] This type of injury almost invariably affects the term infant and appears to be due to subacute, partial hypoxia–ischemia occurring in the peripartum period. More prolonged partial hypoxic–ischemic insult may lead to a more diffuse neuronal necrosis, with relative sparing of the deep gray matter.

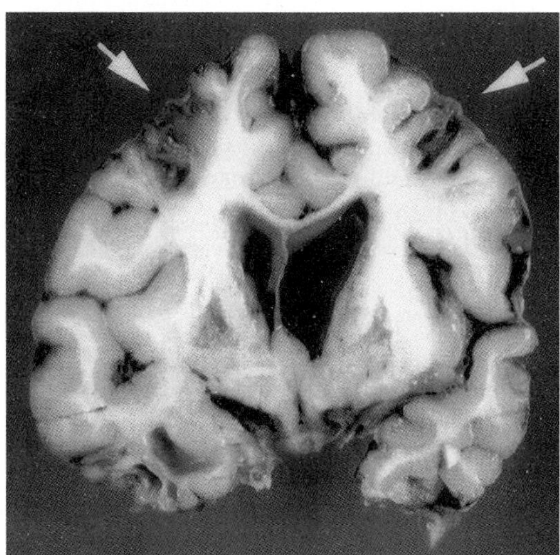

Figure 20.1 Coronal section of a 13-year-old boy who had spastic quadriplegia and mental retardation as a result of perinatal brain injury shows bilateral parasagittal (watershed) atrophy and necrosis (arrows). The cortex in these regions shows thinning (ulegyria) and laminar necrosis that are consistent with remote anoxic/ischemic injury. Courtesy of Jeffrey Twiss, M.D., Ph.D.

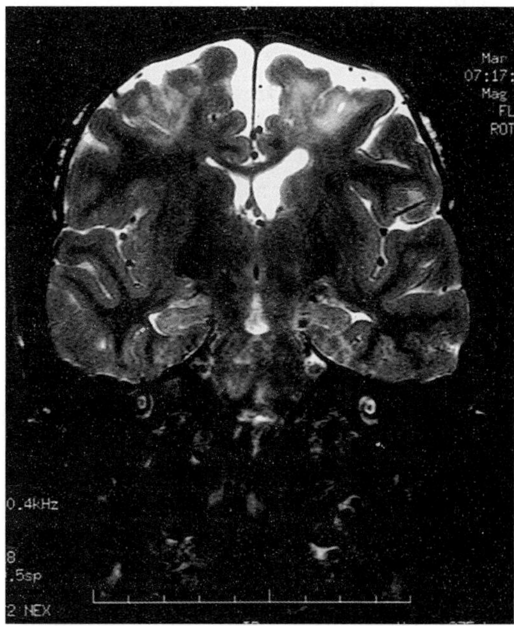

Figure 20.2 Coronal T2-weighted MRI (TE 93/Ef, TR6000) of a 12-year-old girl who had a history of neonatal hypoxic–ischemic encephalopathy and seizures shows bilateral parasagittal signal hyperintensities consistent with border-zone ischemia.

Cortical infarcts in the watershed regions are difficult to diagnose in the neonatal period. This is most likely because CT and ultrasound techniques do not visualize this region well. Radioisotope studies and positron emission tomography have identified infants with decreased cerebral blood flow in the parasagittal cortex.[50,51] MRI is useful in identifying these infants earlier in the course, especially when coronal images are obtained (Figure 20.2).

These newborns often have a moderate encephalopathy in the neonatal period and may show evidence of weakness of the shoulder girdles and the proximal extremities. Seizures can be observed, especially in more severely affected infants. The neurologic sequelae often include a spastic quadriparesis with varying degrees of intellectual impairment. The latter is frequently noted, since this pattern of injury often affects the parietal, posterior temporal, and occipital cortexes. This topographic localization may also account for the frequent occurrence of language and visuospatial disabilities.

Deep gray nuclei, brainstem, and cerebellum

Deep gray nuclei

Lesions in the deep gray nuclei (thalamus, basal ganglia, and diencephalon) have been described for more than a century in children with presumed birth injury who exhibited choreoathetosis and dystonia.[46] Recently infants with this pathologic lesion have been identified in the neonatal period by neuroimaging studies (Figure 20.3).[52] Early in the course there is often hemorrhage and infarction in these structures. Eventually cystic changes develop, particularly in the neostriatum. The neurons and penetrating vessels become calcified.

Recent studies show that acute near-total

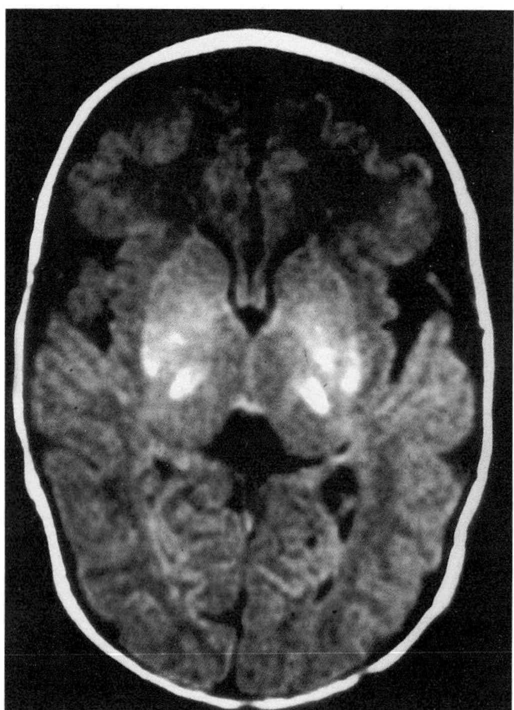

Figure 20.3 Axial T1-weighted MRI (TE 16 ms, TR 600 ms) of a 7-day-old term infant who had an unexplained cardiorespiratory arrest at 12 h of age shows bilateral, symmetric areas of high signal intensity in the basal ganglia and thalami. These areas were low in signal intensity on T2-weighted images. At 1 year of age this child manifested hypotonia, ataxia, and bulbar dysfunction.

asphyxia can lead to specific symmetric lesions of the putamen and the thalamus with sparing of the globus pallidus.[53] This type of injury may occur in setting of severe umbilical cord prolapse, uterine rupture, or severe placental abruption. Affected newborns often manifest evidence of brainstem dysfunction, such as facial diplegia and abnormal eye movements due to concomitant brainstem injury (see below). Children with this type of injury later often develop extrapyramidal cerebral palsy manifested by dystonia, rigidity, axial hypotonia, dysphagia, and abnormal vocalization.

The basal ganglia and thalamus develop a chronic pathologic lesion termed "status marmoratus." This lesion, characterized by neuronal loss, gliosis, and hypermyelination, was observed in 173 of 198 cases of presumed perinatal birth injury in one report.[54] The lesions are probably the result of both impairment of blood flow through the deep penetrating arteries and the high level of metabolic activity of this structure.

These children usually have a poor long-term outcome. Infants with status marmoratus of the basal ganglia develop choreoathetosis, dystonia, tremor, and intellectual deficits. The movement disorder has a delayed onset and may deteriorate over a 1–2-year period.

Brainstem

Pathologic changes of the brainstem are rarely isolated, and other structures, especially the thalamus, are also involved. Brainstem injury usually occurs in the setting of acute hypotension.[55] One particular brainstem lesion, termed *pontosubicular necrosis* by Friede,[56] involves necrosis of neurons in the pons and subiculum of the hippocampus. Friede suggested that these neurons were particularly vulnerable to anoxia, but more recently hyperoxemia was noted to be associated with this lesion.[34] Selective necrosis of specific brainstem nuclei has been observed, and the nuclei adjacent to the floor of the fourth ventricle are more often affected. These nuclei include the inferior colliculi, fifth and seventh cranial nerve nuclei, and nucleus ambiguous (ninth and 10th cranial nerves).

Cerebellum

The cerebellum is especially vulnerable to hypoxic–ischemic insult, and the Purkinje cells are the most vulnerable type of cell. The cerebellum is often affected by bilateral lesions at the boundaries of the superior and inferior cerebellar arterial zones or by lesions of the foliar cortex. White-matter edema and small hemorrhages accompany the neuronal loss. Chronic lesions are referred to as cerebellar sclerosis. In this condition there is a loss of Purkinje cells and an increase in Bergmann's astrocytes. The folia are narrowed and there is an increased space between them.

Cerebellar involvement is often observed concurrently with deep gray nuclei and brainstem lesions. Impairment of the posterior circulation due to hyperextension of the neck at the time of delivery has been suggested as being a factor in the pathogenesis of this lesion.[57] Hypotonia and ataxia are observed as sequelae of cerebellar involvement. Intellectual impairment is common and may be severe.

Infants with disease involving the deep gray-matter nuclei, brainstem, and cerebellum usually have moderate-to-severe encephalopathy in the neonatal period. A history of an acute process that causes near-total asphyxia, such as severe umbilical cord prolapse, uterine rupture, or significant placenta abruption, is often found. Acutely, bifacial weakness, gaze abnormalities, and tongue fasciculations have been described in an infant with brainstem involvement due to "acute" near-total asphyxia.[58–60] Infants with more extensive brainstem involvement may require prolonged ventilatory support. Infants with brainstem involvement have bulbar dysfunction associated with poor feeding, failure to thrive, and recurrent aspiration. Interestingly, in this pattern of injury there may be complete or relative sparing of the cortex and white matter. Also, since the hypoxic–ischemic insult occurs acutely, there is little time for shunting of blood away from extracerebral organs. Hence, there is less evidence of multiorgan dysfunction.

Although there seems to be different topographic distribution of injury caused by chronic partial asphyxia (parasagittal border-zone injury) and acute near-total asphyxia (deep gray nuclei and brainstem), there is often an overlap between the two pathophysiologic syndromes. Hence, when the nature of the injury is widespread, the clinical findings in the neonatal period are diverse. Neurologic examination reveals encephalopathy, brainstem dysfunction, flaccid quadriparesis, and respiration abnormalities. The majority of infants require mechanical ventilation. As the encephalopathy evolves, the infants are described as having clinical seizures, the brainstem signs persist, and temperature instability may be observed. Ultrasonography may be adequate to diagnose thalamic disease, but MRI allows better definition of basal ganglia, thalamic and brainstem involvement.

Focal brain injury

Cortical injury may result from occlusion of an artery, resulting in necrosis of all cellular elements in the distribution of a single vessel. Arterial occlusions occur most often in the term infant and have been observed in 5–9% of autopsy series.[61,62] The middle cerebral artery is most frequently involved. Most are thought to be due to embolic or thrombotic processes. Although the actual etiology is infrequently found, coagulopathy, congenital heart disease, and trauma are common associated disorders. As the infarction evolves, there is dissolution of brain parenchyma and formation of a cavity (porencephalic cyst). If multiple vessels are involved, multicystic encephalomalacia or hydranencephaly may result.

Although the exact incidence of various clinical features in this population is unknown, several clinical features have been observed frequently. The infants may have variable degrees of encephalopathy. Seizures are frequently described in infants with this disorder.[63,64] Focal clonic seizures are often exhibited, and these seizures can be readily diagnosed by clinical criteria.[3] Focal findings may be noted on neurologic examination, but are often subtle. The EEG usually demonstrates lateralized abnormalities and allows assessment of the severity of the encephalopathy in other cortical regions. CT and MRI show a wedge-shaped area of abnormal signal that is in the distribution of a single artery. The neuroimaging findings of infarction may be missed if scans are performed too early in the course. However, the recent MRI technique using diffusion-weighted images may provide a sensitive way of detecting infarcts early in the course.

Infants may develop spastic hemiparesis as long-term sequelae. Because of the frequent involvement of the middle cerebral artery distribution, the upper extremities are more impaired. The extent and location of the pathologic lesion are important factors in determining whether intellectual impairment and epilepsy will also develop.[65]

Focal cerebral injury may also occur with venous occlusions. Venous occlusions often involve the sinuses or major veins, leading to superficial cortical infarcts, which are frequently hemorrhagic. MRI has been particularly useful for diagnosing venous sinus thrombosis and focal injury due to venous occlusions.[66] Venous sinus thrombosis may also cause secondary intraventricular (choroid plexus) hemorrhages in the term newborn. A more severe encephalopathy is noted with venous occlusion because of frequently associated hemorrhage. Seizures are also common.[66,67]

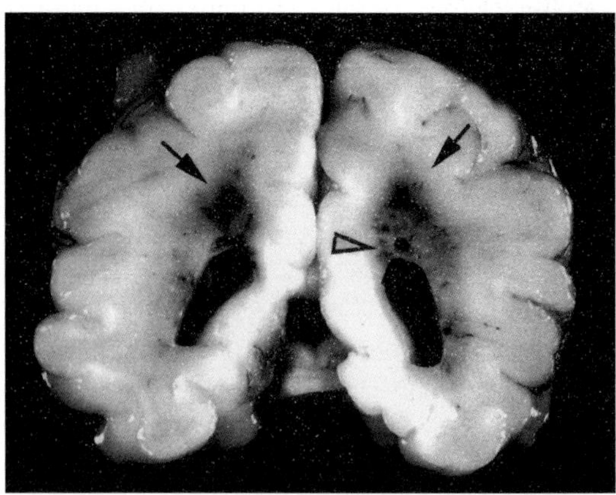

Figure 20.4 Coronal section of a 1-week-old infant (gestational age, 34 weeks) shows periventricular leukomalacia with bilateral areas of congestion and hemorrhage (arrows) in the white matter and a periventricular cyst (arrowhead). The pregnancy was complicated by nonimmune hydrops and an ultrasound study on the first day after birth revealed extensive bilateral periventricular cysts. Courtesy of Raul Bejar, M.D.

White-matter injury

Preterm infants have a predilection for white-matter injury as a result of hypoxic–ischemic insult. There are three types of white-matter lesions observed most commonly in the preterm infant. The first, referred to as glial fatty metamorphosis by Leech and Alvord,[68] is due to deposition of lipid in the white matter. These authors regard this as an abnormal response of immature glia to hypoxia. Others regard this as a normal feature in myelin formation.[46]

The second lesion, characterized by increased reactive astrocytes within the white matter, has also been referred to as perinatal telencephalic leukoencephalopathy.[69] This lesion has been observed in 15–40% of autopsy cases and ultimately may lead to retardation of myelin development.[57,69] Many other factors, such as infectious diseases, hyperbilirubinemia, and nutritional deficiencies, are thought to play a role in the development of this disorder.

The third lesion, characterized by necrosis of the white matter, may include hemorrhage. Periventricular leukomalacia is the term frequently used to describe this disorder.[70] The lesion is readily identified by ultrasonography, and prospective studies have determined that the incidence is 4–26% in low-birth-weight infants.[71–73] Grossly, the acute lesions are characterized by white or white-yellow spots in the periventricular white matter, which occasionally show hemorrhagic infiltration. Microscopically, focal coagulative necrosis is observed. Petechial hemorrhages may also be seen within these lesions. These areas often develop into cystic lesions and later contract into gliotic scars (Figure 20.4). The lesions are observed most frequently in the corona radiata, occipital and temporal horns of the lateral ventricles, and just anterior to the anterior horn of the lateral ventricles. In the term infant the lesions are usually hemorrhagic and are associated with a coagulopathy or congenital heart disease.

The clinical characteristics of infants with necrotic white-matter lesions have only recently been described, but the spectrum of the clinical features during the acute phase still requires further definition.[74] Neonates are usually described as having evidence of decreased tone in the lower extremities associated with increased neck extensor tone. Apnea, pseudobulbar palsy with poor feeding, and irritability have been described. Clinical seizures without EEG confirmation have been reported in 10–30% of the infants. EEGs have been described as having variable degrees of background abnormalities with a high correlation with positive rolandic sharp waves.[75] The diagnosis can be made by ultrasonography, but MRI in later infancy better defines the extent of the disease and the associated abnormalities of myelination.[76] Spastic diplegia with varying degrees of intellectual impairment, especially visuomotor dysfunction, is the usual sequela.

Periventricular/intraventricular hemorrhages

Periventricular or IVH is the most common neuropathologic change observed in the premature infant. It is observed in 31–43% of low-birth-weight infants in prospective neuroimaging studies.[77,78] The hemorrhage arises from the germinal matrix at the ventromedial angle of the lateral ventricle. Cerebral hypoxic–ischemia leads to impaired autoregulation of cerebral blood flow and injury to the germinal matrix and capillary endothelium, which have a high level of oxidative metabolism. Changes in the systemic blood pressure, platelet and coagulation disturbances, and increased cerebral venous pressure also contribute to the pathogenesis of this lesion.

The pathologic findings include subarachnoid hemorrhage with blood in the basal and pontine cisterns and cisterna magna. The hemorrhage may range from a small area of bleeding in the subependymal matrix zone to massive distension of the ventricular system associated with extension of blood into the centrum semiovale. Hydrocephalus may be a complication in infants with this disorder. The hydrocephalus is often secondary to an obstruction at the aqueduct or the foramina exiting from the fourth ventricle or may be due to impairment of reabsorption of CSF over the convexities.

IVH in the term infant often arises from the choroid plexus, and trauma and "hypoxia" are thought to be an important pathogenic factor.[79,80] In 25% of term infants with this disorder there is no identifiable cause for the hemorrhage.[80]

Periventricular or IVH are often clinically silent in the preterm neonate. Severe hemorrhage may present with an acute syndrome, characterized by rapid deterioration of the level of consciousness, brainstem dysfunction, decerebrate posturing, and clinical tonic seizures. The latter events are unlikely to be epileptic seizures, since recent EEG-video monitoring studies have demonstrated that fewer than 10% of these events are accompanied by an electrographic seizure.[3] A subacute presentation is more common, with intermittent neurologic symptoms superimposed on slowly progressive encephalopathy. The newborn may have episodes of abnormal eye movements, hypotonia, and decreased spontaneous motor activity. A fall in the hematocrit level is often an important sign. Ultrasonography is the diagnostic procedure of choice.

The prognosis is extremely variable and many infants have no sequelae. The prognosis is most closely correlated with the degree of parenchymal involvement rather than the extent of the hemorrhage. The EEG has been demonstrated to be a valuable prognostic indicator in this population.[81]

Conclusion and future prospects

The management of the asphyxiated newborn requires early identification, assessment, and stabilization of the cardiopulmonary status and a detailed neurologic evaluation. The identification of infants with specific clinicopathologic syndromes allows prediction of both acute and long-term problems. It is important to identify newborns with these various syndromes early in the course when considering various treatment protocols. Newer neuroimaging techniques and electrophysiologic and biological markers may help in identifying at-risk infants early in the neonatal period. Newer modalities of therapy directed specifically against hypoxic–ischemic injury may soon be available.[44] Further insight into the pathophysiology of hypoxic–ischemic encephalopathy will undoubtedly be obtained through novel application of MRI and spectroscopy and near-infrared spectrophotometry in the human neonate.

REFERENCES

1 Finer NN, Robertson CM, Peters KL, et al. (1983). Factors affecting outcome in hypoxic–ischemic encephalopathy in term infants. *American Journal of Diseases of Children*, **137**, 21–25.

2 Finer NN, Robertson CM, Richards RT, et al. (1981). hypoxic–ischemic encephalopathy in term neonates: perinatal factors and outcome. *Journal of Pediatrics*, **98**, 112–117.

3 Mizrahi EM and Kellaway P. (1987). Characterization and classification of neonatal seizures. *Neurology*, **37**, 1837–1844.

4 Roland EH and Hill A. (1995). Clinical aspects of perinatal hypoxic–ischemic brain injury. *Seminars in Pediatric Neurology*, **2**, 57–71.

5 Vannucci R. (2000). Hypoxic–ischemic encephalopathy. *American Journal of Perinatology*, **17**, 113–120.

6 Blair E and Stanley FJ. (1988). Intrapartum asphyxia: a rare cause of cerebral palsy. *Journal of Pediatrics*, **112**, 515–519.

7 Nelson KB and Ellenberg JH. (1986). Antecedents of cerebral palsy: multivariate analysis of risk. *New England Journal of Medicine*, **315**, 81–86.

8 Nelson KB. (1988). What proportion of cerebral palsy is related to birth asphyxia? *Journal of Pediatrics*, **112**, 572–574.

9 Naeye RL and Peters EC. (1987). Antenatal hypoxia and low IQ values. *American Journal of Diseases of Childhood*, **141**, 50–54.

10 Allan WC and Riviello JJ Jr. (1992). Perinatal cerebrovascular disease in the neonate. *Pediatric Clinics of North America*, **39**, 621–650.

11 Levene MI, Grindulis H, Sands C, et al. (1986). Comparison of two methods of predicting outcome in perinatal asphyxia. *Lancet*, **1**, 67–69.

12 Sarnat HB and Sarnat MS. (1976). Neonatal encephalopathy following fetal distress: a clinical and electroencephalographic study. *Archives of Neurology*, **33**, 696–705.

13 Hill A and Volpe JJ. (1989). Perinatal asphyxia: clinical aspects. *Clinics in Perinatology*, **16**, 435–457.

14 Robertson C and Finer N. (1985). Term infants with hypoxic–ischemic encephalopathy: outcome at 3.5 years. *Developmental Medicine and Child Neurology*, **27**, 473–484.

15 Ishikawa T, Ogawa Y, Kanayama M, et al. (1987). Long-term prognosis of asphyxiated full-term neonates with CNS complications. *Brain and Development*, **9**, 48–53.

16 Hill A. (1991). Current concepts of hypoxic–ischemic cerebral injury in the term newborn. *Pediatric Neurology*, **7**, 317–325.

17 Fernandez F, Verdu A, Quero J, et al. (1986). Cerebrospinal fluid lactate levels in term infants with perinatal hypoxia. *Pediatric Neurology*, **2**, 39–42.

18 Nylund L, Dahlin I and Lagercrantz H. (1987). Fetal catecholamines and the Apgar score. *Journal of Perinatal Medicine*, **15**, 340–354.

19 De Praeter C, Vanhaesebrouck P, Govaert P, et al. (1991). Creatine kinase isoenzyme BB concentrations in the cerebrospinal fluid of newborns: relationship to short-term outcome. *Pediatrics*, **88**, 1204–1210.

20 Hollander PI, Wright L, Nagey DA, et al. (1987). Indicators of perinatal asphyxia. *American Journal of Obstetrics and Gynecology*, **157**, 839–843.

21 Ezitis J, Finnstrom O, Hedman G, et al. (1987). CK_{BB}-enzyme activity in serum in neonates born after vaginal delivery and cesarean section. *Neuropediatrics*, **18**, 146–148.

22 Takeuchi T and Watanabe K. (1989). The EEG evolution and neurological prognosis of neonates with perinatal hypoxia. *Brain and Development*, **11**, 115–120.

23 Scher MS, Painter MJ, Bergman I, et al. (1989). EEG diagnosis of neonatal seizures: clinical correlations and outcome. *Pediatric Neurology*, **5**, 17–24.

24 Majnemer A, Rosenblatt B, Riley P, et al. (1987). Somatosensory evoked response abnormalities in high-risk newborns. *Pediatric Neurology*, **3**, 350–355.

25 Majnemer A, Rosenblatt B and Riley PS. (1990). Prognostic significance of multimodality evoked response testing in high-risk newborns. *Pediatric Neurology*, **6**, 367–374.

26 Stockard JE, Stockard JJ, Kleinberg F, et al. (1983). Prognostic value of brainstem auditory evoked responses in neonates. *Archives of Neurology*, **40**, 360–365.

27 Whyte HE, Taylor MJ, Menzies R, et al. (1986). Prognostic utility of visual evoked potentials in term asphyxiated neonates. *Pediatric Neurology*, **2**, 220–223.

28 Toet MC, Hellström-Westas L, Groenendaal F, et al. (1999). Amplitude integrated EEG 3 and 6 hours after birth in full term neonates with hypoxic–ischemic encephalopathy. *Archives of Diseases in Childhood Fetal and Neonatal Edition*, **81**, F19–F23.

29 Kuenzle C, Baenziger O, Martin E, et al. (1994). Prognostic value of early MR imaging in term infants with severe perinatal asphyxia. *Neuropediatrics*, **25**, 191–200.

30 Baenziger O, Martin E, Steinlin M, et al. (1993). Early pattern recognition in severe perinatal asphyxia: a prospective MRI study. *Neuroradiology*, **35**, 437–442.

31 Volpe JJ. (1995). Hypoxic–ischemic encephalopathy: clinical

aspects. In Volpe JJ, ed. *Neurology of the Newborn*, 3rd edn., pp. 314–369. Philadelphia: W. B. Saunders.

32 Hüppi PS, Murphy B, Maier SE, et al. (2001). Microstructural brain development after perinatal cerebral white matter injury assessed by diffusion tensor magnetic resonance imaging. *Pediatrics*, **107**, 455–460.

33 Robertson RL, Ben-Sira L, Barnes PD, et al. (1999). MR line-scan diffusion-weighted imaging of term neonates with perinatal brain ischemia. *American Journal of Neuroradiology*, **20**, 1658–1670.

34 Ahab-Barmada MA, Moossy J and Painter M. (1980). Pontosubicular necrosis and hyperoxemia. *Pediatrics*, **66**, 840–847.

35 Pryse-Davies J and Beard RW. (1973). A necropsy study of brain swelling in the newborn with special reference to cerebellar herniation. *Journal of Pathology*, **109**, 51–73.

36 Vannucci RC. (1990). Current and potentially new management strategies for perinatal hypoxic–ischemic encephalopathy. *Pediatrics*, **1990**, 961–968.

37 Mujsce DJ, Towfighi J, Stern D, et al. (1990). Mannitol therapy in perinatal hypoxic–ischemic brain damage in rats. *Stroke*, **21**, 1210–1214.

38 Eyre JA and Wilkinson AR. (1986). Thiopentone induced coma after severe birth asphyxia. *Archives of Disease in Childhood*, **61**, 1084–1089.

39 Goldberg RN, Moscoso P, Bauer CR, et al. (1986). Use of barbiturate therapy in severe perinatal asphyxia: a randomized controlled trial. *Journal of Pediatrics*, **109**, 851–856.

40 Ruth V, Virkola K, Paetau R, et al. (1988). Early high-dose phenobarbital treatment for prevention of hypoxic–ischemic brain damage in very low birthweight infants. *Journal of Pediatrics*, **112**, 81–86.

41 Hall RT, Hall FK and Daily DK. (1998). High-dose phenobarbital therapy in term newborns with severe perinatal asphyxia: a randomized, prospective study with three-year follow-up. *Journal of Pediatrics*, **132**, 345–348.

42 Gilman J, Gal P, Duchowny M, et al. (1989). Rapid sequential phenobarbital treatment of neonatal seizures. *Pediatrics*, **83**, 674–678.

43 Painter MJ, Scher MS, Stein ADA, et al. (1999). Phenobarbital compared with phenytoin for the treatment of neonatal seizures. *New England Journal of Medicine*, **341**, 485–489.

44 Vannucci RC and Perlman JM. (1997). Interventions for perinatal hypoxic–ischemic encephalopathy. *Pediatrics*, **100**, 1004–1014.

45 Battin RB, Dezoete A, Gunn TR, et al. (2001). Neurodevelopmental outcome of infants treated with head cooling and mild hypothermia after perinatal asphyxia. *Pediatrics*, **107**, 480–484.

46 Friede RL. (1989) *Developmental Neuropathology*, 2nd edn. New York: Springer-Verlag.

47 Rorke LB. (1992). Perinatal brain damage. In: Adams JH, Duchen LW, editors. *Greenfield's Neuropathology*, 5th edn. New York: Oxford University Press, pp. 639–709.

48 Norman MG. (1978). Perinatal Brain Damage. In Rosenberg HS, Bolande RP, eds. *Perspectives in Pediatric Neurology*, p. 41. Chicago: Year Book.

49 Myer JE. (1953). Uber die Lokalisation frühkindlicher Hirnshäden in arteriellen Grenzgebieten. *Archiv für Psychiatrie und Zeitschrift Neurologie*, **190**, 328–341.

50 Volpe JJ, Herscovitch P, Perlman JM, et al. (1985). Positron emission tomography in the asphyxiated term newborn: parasagittal impairment of cerebral blood flow. *Annals of Neurology*, **17**, 287–296.

51 Volpe JJ and Pasternak JF. (1979). Parasagittal cerebral injury in neonatal hypoxic–ischemic encephalopathy: clinical and neuroradiological features. *Journal of Pediatrics*, **91**, 472–476.

52 Voit T, Lemburg P, Neuen E, et al. (1987). Damage of thalamus and basal ganglia in asphyxiated full-term neonates. *Neuropediatrics*, **18**, 176–181.

53 Johnston MV and Hoon AH. (2000). Possible mechanisms in infants for selective basal ganglia damage from asphyxia, kernicterus, or mitochondrial encephalopathies. *Journal of Child Neurology*, **15**, 588–591.

54 Malamud N and Hirano A. (1974) *Atlas of Neuropathology*, 2nd edn. Berkeley: University of California Press.

55 Gilles FH. (1969). Hypotensive brain stem necrosis: selective symmetrical necrosis of tegmental neuronal aggregates following cardiac arrest. *Archives of Pathology*, **88**, 32–41.

56 Friede RL. (1972). Pontosubicular lesions in perinatal anoxia. *Archives of Pathology*, **94**, 343–354.

57 Rorke LB. (1982) *Pathology of Perinatal Brain Injury*. New York: Raven Press.

58 Roland EH, Hill A, Norman MG, et al. (1988). Selective brainstem injury in an asphyxiated newborn. *Annals of Neurology*, **23**, 89–92.

59 Pasternak JF and Gorey MT. (1998). The syndrome of acute near-total intrauterine asphyxia in the term infant. *Pediatric Neurology*, **18**, 391–398.

60 Natsume J, Watanabe K, Kuno K, et al. (1995). Clinical, neurophysiologic, and neuropathological features of an infant with brain damage of total asphyxia type (Myers). *Pediatric Neurology*, **13**, 61–64.

61 Barmada MA, Moossy J and Shuman RM. (1979). Cerebral infarcts with arterial occlusion in neonates. *Annals of Neurology*, **6**, 495–502.

62 Banker BQ. (1961). Cerebral vascular disease in infancy and

childhood. I. Occlusive vascular disease. *Journal of Neuropathology and Experimental Neurology*, **20**, 127–140.

63 Clancy R, Malin S, Laraque D, et al. (1985). Focal motor seizures heralding stroke in full-term neonates. *American Journal of Diseases of Childhood*, **139**, 601–606.

64 Koelfen W, Freund M and Varnholt V. (1995). Neonatal stroke involving the middle cerebral artery in term infants: clinical presentation, EEG and imaging studies, and outcome. *Developmental Medicine and Child Neurology*, **37**, 204–212.

65 Levine SC, Huttenlocher P, Banich MT, et al. (1987). Factors affecting cognitive function of hemiplegic children. *Developmental Medicine and Child Neurology*, **29**, 27–35.

66 Rivkin MJ, Anderson ML and Kaye EM. (1992). Neonatal idiopathic cerebral venous thrombosis: an unrecognized cause of transient seizures or lethargy. *Annals of Neurology*, **32**, 51–56.

67 Wong VK, LeMesurier J, Franceschini R, et al. (1987). Cerebral venous thrombosis as a cause of neonatal seizures. *Pediatric Neurology*, **3**, 235–237.

68 Leech RW and Alvord EC Jr. (1974). Glial fatty metamorphosis: an abnormal response of premyelin glia frequently accompanying periventricular leukomalacia. *American Journal of Pathology*, **74**, 603–612.

69 Gilles FH and Murphy SF. (1969). Perinatal telencephalic leucoencephalopathy. *Journal of Neurology, Neurosurgery and Psychiatry*, **32**, 404–413.

70 Banker BQ and Larroche JC. (1962). Periventricular leukomalacia of infancy. *Archives of Neurology*, **7**, 386–410.

71 Guzzetta F, Shackleford GD, Volpe S, et al. (1986). Periventricular intraparenchymal echodensities in the premature newborn: critical determination of neurologic outcome. *Pediatrics*, **78**, 995–1006.

72 Fawer CL, Calame A, Perentes E, et al. (1985). Periventricular leukomalacia: a correlation study between real-time ultrasound and autopsy findings. *Neuroradiology*, **27**, 292–300.

73 Trounce JQ, Rutter N and Levene MI. (1986). Periventricular leucomalacia and intraventricular haemorrhage in the preterm neonate. *Archives of Disease in Childhood*, **16**, 1196–1202.

74 Trounce JQ, Shaw DE, Leverne MI, et al. (1988). Clinical risk factors and periventricular leucomalacia. *Archives of Disease in Childhood*, **63**, 17–22.

75 Novotny EJ, Tharp BR, Coen RW, et al. (1987). Positive rolandic sharp waves in the EEG of the premature infant. *Neurology*, **37**, 1481–1486.

76 De Vries LS, Connell JA, Dubowitz LMS, et al. (1987). Neurological, electrophysiological and MRI abnormalities in infants with extensive cystic leukomalacia. *Neuropediatrics*, **18**, 61–66.

77 Dolfin T, Skidmore MB, Fong KW, et al. (1983). Incidence, severity, and timing of subependymal and intraventricular hemorrhages in preterm infants born in a perinatal unit as detected by serial real-time ultrasound. *Pediatrics*, **71**, 541–546.

78 Enzmann D, Murphy-Irwin K, Stevenson D, et al. (1985). The natural history of subependymal germinal matrix hemorrhage. *American Journal of Perinatology*, **2**, 123–133.

79 Scher MS, Wright FS, Lockman LA, et al. (1982). Intraventricular haemorrhage in the full-term neonate. *Archives of Neurology*, **39**, 769–772.

80 Volpe JJ. (1995). Intracranial hemorrhage: subdural, primary subarachnoid, intracerebellar, intraventricular (term infant), and miscellaneous. In Volpe JJ, ed. *Neurology of the Newborn*, 3rd edn, pp. 373–402. Philadelphia: W. B. Saunders.

81 Clancy RR, Tharp BR and Enzmann D. (1984). EEG in premature infants with intraventricular hemorrhage. *Neurology*, **34**, 583–590.

21

The use of the EEG in assessing acute and chronic brain damage in the newborn

Donald M. Olson and Jin S. Hahn

Stanford University Medical Center, Stanford, CA, USA

Introduction

The goal of this chapter is to help the reader understand the fundamentals of neonatal electroencephalogram (EEG), including the source of EEG signals and the technical aspects of a well-performed EEG. Particular attention will be paid to: (1) maturational features which correlate with the infant's conceptional age; (2) abnormal findings indicative of encephalopathies of various causes; and (3) value of the EEG in determining the prognosis for normal and abnormal neurological outcome. The role of EEG in neonatal seizures is covered more thoroughly in Chapter 37.

Value of the EEG

The EEG is a valuable tool for assessing neonatal brain function. It has unique properties compared to many other diagnostic tests of brain function. For example, it can resolve temporal aspects of brain function more effectively than computed tomography (CT), magnetic resonance imaging (MRI), or even the bedside neurological examination. There is no other test that can so precisely discriminate between epileptic seizures and nonepileptic events in the neonate. It provides information about the severity of brain dysfunction (encephalopathy). Serial EEGs provide information about the course and effectiveness of treatment. Sometimes the EEG helps distinguish between various etiologies of encephalopathy as well.

Indication for EEG

An EEG in the neonate should be considered when questions arise regarding the cause of the child's abnormal neurological responses. There are many scenarios in which the EEG provides much needed information that is otherwise difficult or impossible to obtain. For example, it is difficult to perform an adequate bedside neurological assessment of a neonate paralyzed due to neuromuscular blocking agents or an infant who is deeply sedated. The degree of neurological dysfunction may be addressed by means of the EEG. Some very ill infants would benefit from neuroimaging studies, but such studies might be difficult to obtain because of instability of the infant or due to the difficulty of moving an intubated and ventilated baby between the neonatal intensive care unit (NICU) and the radiology suite. Since the EEG is performed at the bedside, it can be helpful in these situations.

Another setting where the EEG is particularly valuable is when there is a question about seizures. In the case of the paralyzed or sedated infant, sudden and transient changes in vital signs may raise the suspicion of seizures though no obvious seizure-like movements are observed. The EEG is the only means of determining if frequent subtle (or "subclinical") seizures are present.[1,2] Even in non-paralyzed newborns, it is often difficult to distinguish neonatal seizures from other nonepileptic clinical behavior. Therefore, the EEG is helpful in most neonates who are having paroxysmal behavior changes that might represent seizures.

Timing of the EEG

An EEG should be obtained early in the course of an infant at risk for encephalopathy or seizures. First, it provides a starting point for later reference. If obtained when the baby is initially recognized as being neurologically "at risk," the EEG provides some prognostic information and can suggest the timing of the brain insult.[3–6] However, an EEG obtained within hours of an acute insult such as hypoxia or hypotension may only be transiently abnormal. Hence, serial EEGs are often of benefit.

Serial EEGs are valuable when prior EEGs show evidence of a severe encephalopathy, since persistence or improvement in the EEG findings has prognostic value and may provide evidence of the success (or failure) of various treatments.[7] Serial EEGs are also useful when previous recordings have identified frequent seizures and the treating physician needs to know whether the treatment has been adequate.

Technical considerations

General description

The EEG measures the "potential difference" (voltage) between areas on the baby's scalp. The electrical activity measured consists of the summed membrane potentials caused by many synapses on cortical neurons, not the individual, brief neuronal action potentials.[8] The activity recorded originates mainly from the cerebral cortex, particularly that close to the skull. However, some deeper centers act as pacemakers and cause changes in the EEG in various states of sleep and arousal. Scalp EEG abnormalities are sometimes strongly correlated with underlying pathology in deeper structures.[9–13] Other clinical neurophysiology tests directly measure neuronal activity from deeper structures such as the brainstem during brainstem auditory evoked responses or potentials (BAERs) or the spinal cord and brainstem during somatosensory evoked potentials (SEPs).[14,15]

Electrodes and application

Recording electrodes are usually applied with an electrolyte paste that holds the metal disk-shaped electrodes in place. The paste also has favorable electrical conduction properties. In order to keep the impedance low, the area to which the electrode will be attached needs to be cleaned. Sometimes, especially in very premature babies, particular care must be paid to the infant's thin, easily abraded skin during preparation for electrode application. A special glue (collodion) is occasionally used to secure the electrodes, particularly during more prolonged recordings, but in neonates gluing is seldom necessary.

The standard method of electrode placement is referred to as the "international 10–20 system".[16,17] This allows reliable electrode placements relative to the underlying brain structures, as well as consistent placements for serial EEG studies in a given infant. Standard electrode locations are designated by a combination of letters and numbers. *F, Fp, T, C, P,* and *O* correspond to frontal, frontopolar, temporal, central, parietal, and occipital locations, respectively. Odd numbers indicate the left side of the head, and even numbers the right. The letter "z" indicates the midline of the head. In neonates the number of electrodes is reduced because of the small head size and the relatively wide electrical fields of the activity measured in babies (Figure 21.1). For neonatal recordings the frontopolar electrodes are placed slightly posterior to their relative positions on the adult scalp and are sometimes designated *Fp3* and *Fp4*.[18,19] Placement often has to be modified slightly because of scalp intravenous lines, surgical dressings, or movement restricted by such procedures as carotid catheterization for extracorporeal membrane oxygenation (ECMO).

Neonatal EEG should almost always be accompanied by simultaneous polygraphic recording of physiologic variables, including eye movement, electromyogram (EMG: usually from the submental

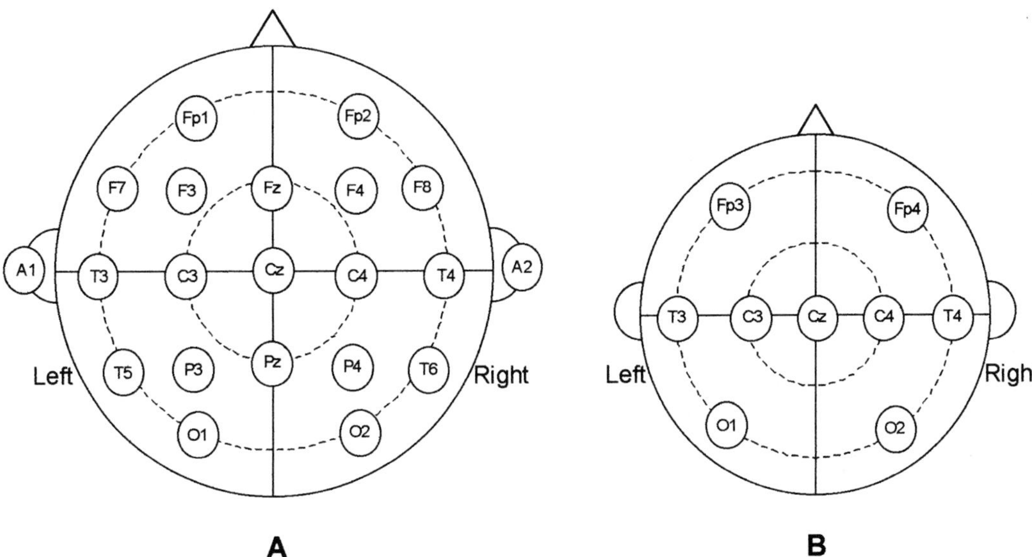

Figure 21.1 Electrode nomenclature using the International 10–20 system. (A) Most commonly used electrodes for recordings outside the neonatal period. (B) More limited set of electrodes used for neonates. Note the slightly more lateral placement of the frontopolar electrodes.

muscle on the chin, just below the lower lip), electrocardiogram (ECG), and respiration.[18] These tracings permit the interpreter to determine the baby's sleep state and, in the case of the respiration recording, correlate apnea with the presence or absence of seizures.[20,21]

Recordings in neonates can be performed using a single montage (arrangement of the EEG channels on the display) since there is a reduced number of electrodes compared with adult EEG recordings.[18,22] With modern digital EEG instruments, the EEG can be displayed in various other montages if the need arises. Other technical differences address the fact that the predominant frequencies of the EEG activity in neonates is much slower than older children and adults. Neonatal EEG recordings are often displayed using a compressed display with 20 s of EEG per page (slower paper speed). A display of at least 16 channels is recommended. Because slow-frequencies constitute the majority of neonatal EEG activity, slow-frequency filters should be minimal.[18]

Sedation

Sedation is seldom needed as a routine part of the neonatal EEG. While it is desirable to record awake, quiet, and active sleep states, careful preparation and communication with the NICU nursing team ahead of time, and a patient approach by the technologist, will usually suffice. If the neonate is taking oral feedings, timing the EEG shortly after a feeding can eliminate the need for sedation in the majority of cases. If sedation is required, chloral hydrate is most commonly used for EEG since it is relatively short-acting and has little effect on the EEG.[23] However some concerns about excessive sedation and possible toxicity of chloral hydrate metabolites have been raised.[24–26]

Duration to obtain sleep states

Most neonatal EEGs will last between 45 and 60 min.[19] To be considered adequate an EEG will ideally include all the stages of sleep that are likely to occur in a neonate of a given conceptional age. In the term infant these will include active rapid eye movement (REM) sleep onset, transitional sleep, quiet (non-REM) sleep, and postquiet sleep active sleep as well as wakefulness. By 32–34 weeks' conceptional age most normal infants have easily identifiable sleep states. The earliest stage of sleep, active sleep after wakefulness, may last up to 40 min; hence the duration of the recording may need to be as long as 60 min to try and record all sleep stages. Since this is longer than most recording done on adults and older children in the EEG laboratory, the EEG technologist and the NICU staff will have to plan accordingly.

Technologist

Working in challenging environment

The NICU is a far-from-ideal recording location. There are many pieces of electrical equipment that can cause electrical artifacts to appear on the EEG. Mechanical devices such as ventilator tubing may vibrate and cause rhythmic movement artifact that can be mistaken for seizures. Because of noise, bright lights, and the constant bustle of the NICU, getting a baby to sleep and keeping him or her asleep can be challenging. It is worthwhile for the technologist to contact the baby's nurse ahead of time and coordinate the EEG for just after a feeding or routine sedation – a time the infant is more likely to fall asleep.

Dealing with artifacts

Artifacts are a normal part of any EEG recording. A baby's movements are a common source of artifact and in fact constitute an important and necessary component of the recording in the neonate. The baby's sleep state is defined not by the EEG tracing from the scalp, but rather from physiologic channels that record respiration, ECG, eye movements, and muscle activity. Less desirable artifacts are caused by such things as movement near the child (e.g., a nurse working with the baby), fluid in ventilator tubing, and nearby electrical equipment introducing 60-Hz electrical noise. Many artifacts seen on EEG are rhythmic in appearance, such as those from high-frequency oscillating ventilators or ECMO pumps, and may be mistaken for seizures. An experienced technologist will carefully evaluate the tracing during the recording, and carefully document movements or things causing artifacts. He or she will work with the nursing staff in the NICU to decrease artifacts, e.g., by draining water from respirator tubing, moving nearby power cords, or turning off a high-frequency ventilator for a few seconds if medically safe.

Age of infant

Knowing the age of the infant is very important when interpreting the neonatal EEG. Because the EEG changes so dramatically between 24 weeks' gestational age and term, and because "dysmature" EEG findings are a frequently reported abnormality, correct assessment of the age of the neonate is critical. The "conceptional age" is the most important value to calculate: the baby's gestational age plus chronological (legal) age (in weeks) is noted at the beginning of the EEG. This permits the interpreting physician to look for characteristic patterns normally seen at a given conceptional age.[27]

Documenting behavior during recording

The neonatologist may be asking, "Are tongue thrusting or apneic spells seizures?" Correlating rhythmic or unusual body movements with paroxysmal EEG findings is frequently the most important aspect of EEG interpretation. Careful documentation of the baby's behavior and the staffs' movement near the bed is important when interpreting neonatal (and indeed all) EEGs. The corollary is the importance of documenting any movement (or lack of movement) while rhythmic, seizure-like patterns are present on the EEG. For example, a small amount of water condensed in ventilator tubing can induce a prominent rhythmic pattern (artifact) on the EEG that might be confused with a seizure.

Physiologic channels are sometimes not sufficient to pick up subtle movements that help the electroencephalographer score the sleep stage. Documentation of eye movements and body twitches during sleep help the electroencephalographer determine sleep state when the EEG's physiologic channels (respiration, eye movement, EMG) are not registering them. Notations such as "eye movement," "sucking," "mouth twitch," or "irregular respiration" can be valuable.

Seizures

The EEG is frequently ordered so the treating physicians can determine whether a particular observed behavior is epileptic or not. While simultaneous video recording is becoming a more common component of the "routine" bedside EEG, the technologist's observations of seizure-like behavior and physiologic changes are critical. In the sedated and paralyzed infant, sudden changes in transcutaneous oxygen saturation, blood pressure, and heart rate are not apparent on the EEG tracing, yet these sudden changes may be the very reason for obtaining the EEG.[2]

The technologist must be cognizant of the primary question leading to the EEG so appropriate observations can be made. Often some stereotyped movement is questioned as a "subtle seizure." It is incumbent on the technologist to note carefully such things as "tongue thrusting," "eye deviation," and rhythmic limb movements. At the same time, the technologist needs to watch the EEG carefully for electrographic seizure activity, and look carefully for coincident, subtle, and stereotyped behavior that is the clinical manifestation of the seizure. Apnea with or without bradycardia is often questioned as seizure.[21] Though apnea can sometimes be the sole manifestation of a seizure, "nonepileptic" apnea is more common in the NICU.[28] There is often some other subtle behavior which can be more specific, such as tonic eye deviation or rhythmic tongue thrusting. These important findings may only be detected because the technologist sees seizure activity on the EEG and looks for clinically subtle seizure behavior.

Interpretation by electroencephalographer

Experience

The accuracy of EEG interpretation is very dependent upon the skill and experience of the physicians reading the recording. They should be familiar with the normal maturational changes expected at various conceptional ages. Recognizing common artifacts will prevent interpreting these as abnormalities. Without experience in recognizing normal vs abnormal findings such as frequency of sharp waves or degree of "discontinuity" of the background, interpretation can be arduous despite the availability of good atlases of neonatal EEG. Electrographic seizures may be quite subtle on the EEG itself, and the interpreting physician should be experienced enough to differentiate normal rhythmic activity from brief, abnormal rhythmic activity and more sustained rhythmic evolving seizure activity.[29]

Report format

The EEG report should conform to a format well established by electroencephalographers.[30] The report should begin with identifying information such as name, medical record number, date of the recording, date of birth, conceptional age, and the conditions of recording (whether the recording is performed in the nursery or the EEG lab, whether EEG placement was altered because of scalp problems, what medications the child is receiving, and whether there are important features inhibiting full interpretation, such as paralysis preventing definition of sleep stages), and whether the baby has had previous EEGs. It should also contain a brief one- or two-sentence pertinent history and, if articulated by the ordering physicians, the question being asked of the EEG. The "Results" section of the report will describe in some detail the frequencies of the background EEG activity, the symmetry, the synchrony between hemispheres, and the presence of normal and abnormal patterns such as delta brushes and sporadic sharp waves. This will be highly technical and should communicate the appearance of the recording to other electroencephalographers more than other clinicians. The "Impression" section should state clearly whether the EEG is normal or abnormal. If abnormal, the reasons should be clearly stated and not merely refer to the descriptive "Results" section, since "Results" is not usually clear to most people not familiar with EEG jargon. A "Comments" or "Clinical Correlation" section should follow "Results" and should state in clear, jargon-free terms how the findings relate to the clinical question necessitating the EEG, how the EEG compares to prior EEGs, and whether the findings are specific or nonspecific with regard to etiology or prognosis. If additional EEGs are likely to be helpful, this should be stated under "Comments."

Maturational features

Introduction

Time of rapid anatomical maturation of the brain

Brain maturation occurs rapidly during the last trimester of fetal life and in the early weeks of postnatal life. The cortical surface is almost smooth with a simple sulcal pattern at 26–28 weeks' conceptional age. By contrast, the full-term newborn has a complex pattern of cortical gyri and sulci.[31] There are also rapid and dramatic changes in myelin formation.[32] The EEG features of normal newborns correlate well with the anatomic, MRI, and ultrasound-defined maturation of the brain.[33]

EEG changes correspond to brain maturation

It is not surprising, then, that the EEG undergoes similarly rapid and dramatic changes during the first weeks of life. Certain EEG patterns appear and others disappear during the last trimester and the first months of life. The most marked changes occur between 24 weeks' gestational age and 1 month after term.[34–36] These maturational changes are similar whether the infant is in utero or born prematurely.[27] In other words, the EEG of a 12-week-old infant born at 28 weeks' gestational age and that of a 2-day-old 40-week gestational age infant will be very similar. For this reason, it is important that the EEG technologist and interpreting physician have as accurate an idea as possible about the infant's gestational and legal age. The conceptional age should be clearly stated in the EEG report's introductory section. Specific EEG patterns are prominent features of normal neonates at particular ages. These include such features as "delta brushes," "frontal sharp transients," and "temporal theta bursts".[34–36] These patterns appear and disappear at various conceptional ages in a predictable fashion. Similarly, the overall background pattern of the EEG changes with conceptional age. In particular, the degree of "discontinuity" evolves in a predictable way[35,37] (Figure 21.2). Deviations in the evolution of these specific EEG patterns and the overall background pattern represent evidence of an encephalopathy.[38–41]

Ontogeny of sleep stage

Sleep states are important to identify in the newborn. Certain EEG patterns correlate with a given sleep state and a "discordance" between the EEG pattern and the sleep state is evidence of an encephalopathy. The two main sleep states in the neonate are active sleep and quiet sleep. Active sleep is the equivalent of REM sleep in older children and adults. Quiet sleep is the equivalent of non-REM sleep. It is important to understand that sleep states are identified by the physiologic changes observable in the infant, and not the EEG pattern.[36,42,43]

Active sleep can first be identified between 27 and 31 weeks' conceptional age.[34,35] It is characterized by rapid eye movements, irregular respirations, loss of muscle tone, and frequent small body and limb movements. The EEG background is continuous during active sleep.

Quiet sleep appears between 31 and 34 weeks' conceptional age. It is characterized by regular respiration, little motor activity, absence of eye movements, and subtle tonic muscle activity. The EEG background during quiet sleep is discontinuous, but becomes more continuous as the conceptional age increases (Figure 21.3).

Discontinuity of the background

The degree of discontinuity is one of the main features that distinguish among normal infants of varying conceptional ages.[40,42–44] Very premature infants between 24 and 28 weeks' conceptional age will normally have very discontinuous tracings.[35] The "interburst intervals," the low-amplitude portions of the tracing between bursts of brain activity, are virtually flat at 26 weeks' conceptional age. On the other hand, the discontinuity normally present in quiet sleep of a 42-week conceptional age infant will be fairly subtle, with the interburst intervals only slightly suppressed compared to the bursts (Figures 21.2 and 21.3). Discontinuity is limited to quiet sleep by 36 weeks' conceptional age.[36] Excessive discontinuity is a "dysmature feature" which indicates a degree of encephalopathy. It is not a very specific finding with regard to etiology or prognosis, however. It is important to realize that various neuroactive medications, such as barbiturates, may increase the interburst intervals and produce an excessively discontinuous pattern. If the infant is on such medications, the EEG must be interpreted with these caveats.

Another important feature of the discontinuity is the synchrony of the bursts. Even at a very early conceptional age, the bursts will almost entirely be simultaneous (synchronous) between the two hemispheres.[35] Poor interhemispheric synchrony also indicates an encephalopathy and may be useful in determining prognosis, but is not particularly specific for etiology, either.[5,44]

Specific patterns

Delta brushes

The delta brush is a pattern consisting of a short run of high-frequency EEG activity superimposed on a slower (delta frequency) wave (Figure 21.4). This rather distinct pattern is most frequent at about 32–34 weeks and is rarely present after 40–44 weeks. Furthermore, they will occur with more or less frequency in active or quiet sleep depending on the infant's conceptional age. The frequency with which delta brushes occur during active and quiet sleep at various conceptional ages has been carefully quantified.[36,45] Once again, an excessive number of delta brushes in a particular sleep state at a particular conceptional age is a nonspecific encephalopathic feature.

Frontal sharp transients and sporadic sharp waves

Sharp waves in the neonate do not have the same significance as they do in adults. In adults, sharp waves usually connote an increased risk of seizures. This is not the case with neonates. They normally have occasional sharp waves present during the EEG. Like other patterns already discussed, the frequency of their occurrence varies with sleep state and conceptional age. When they are repetitive or persistently focal, they can suggest an increased risk of seizures or a focal brain abnormality. More persistent repetitive bursts of sharp waves, especially if there is some evolution of the frequency and amplitude, have been characterized as "brief ictal rhythmic discharges," and suggest a higher risk of seizures.[46,47]

Another prominent sharp wave that is usually distinguished from the sporadic sharp waves described above is frontal sharp transients. These are high-amplitude monophasic or biphasic sharp waves which are, of course, maximum over the frontal regions (Figure 21.5). They are a prominent feature of active sleep and transitional sleep states in more mature neonates.[36,48]

Theta bursts

The temporal theta burst, or temporal "sawtooth" pattern, is a normal feature of the EEG of younger conceptional age infants. This sometimes dramatic pattern of rhythmic, sharply contoured theta waves is maximum between 27 and 32 weeks' conceptional age.[36] Other theta patterns described in EEGs of normal premature infants are maximum over the occipital and frontal regions.[49,50] The absence of these normally seen rhythms in the very premature infant suggests an encephalopathic process.[51]

(A)

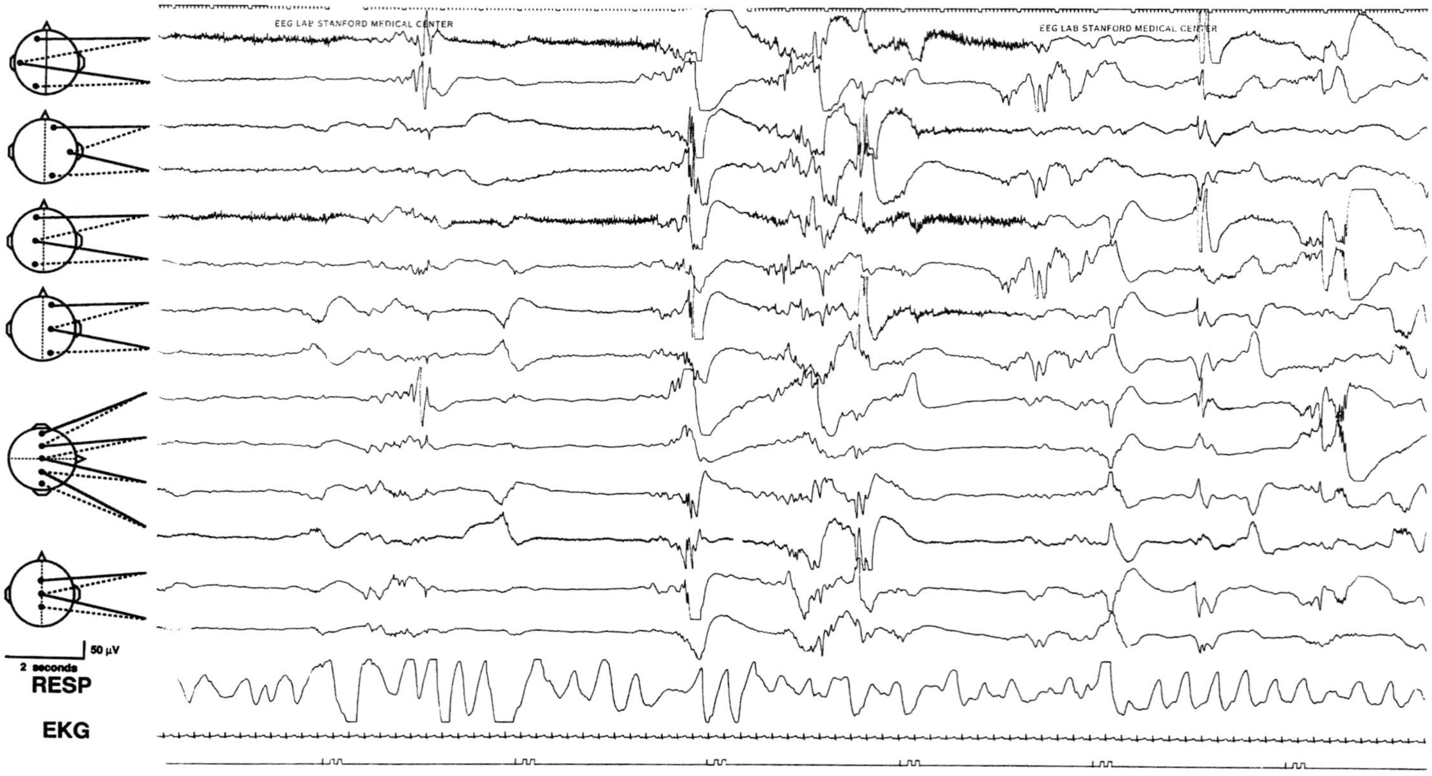

EEG LAB STANFORD MEDICAL CENTER

EEG LAB STANFORD MEDICAL CENTER

50 µV

2 seconds

RESP

EKG

(B)

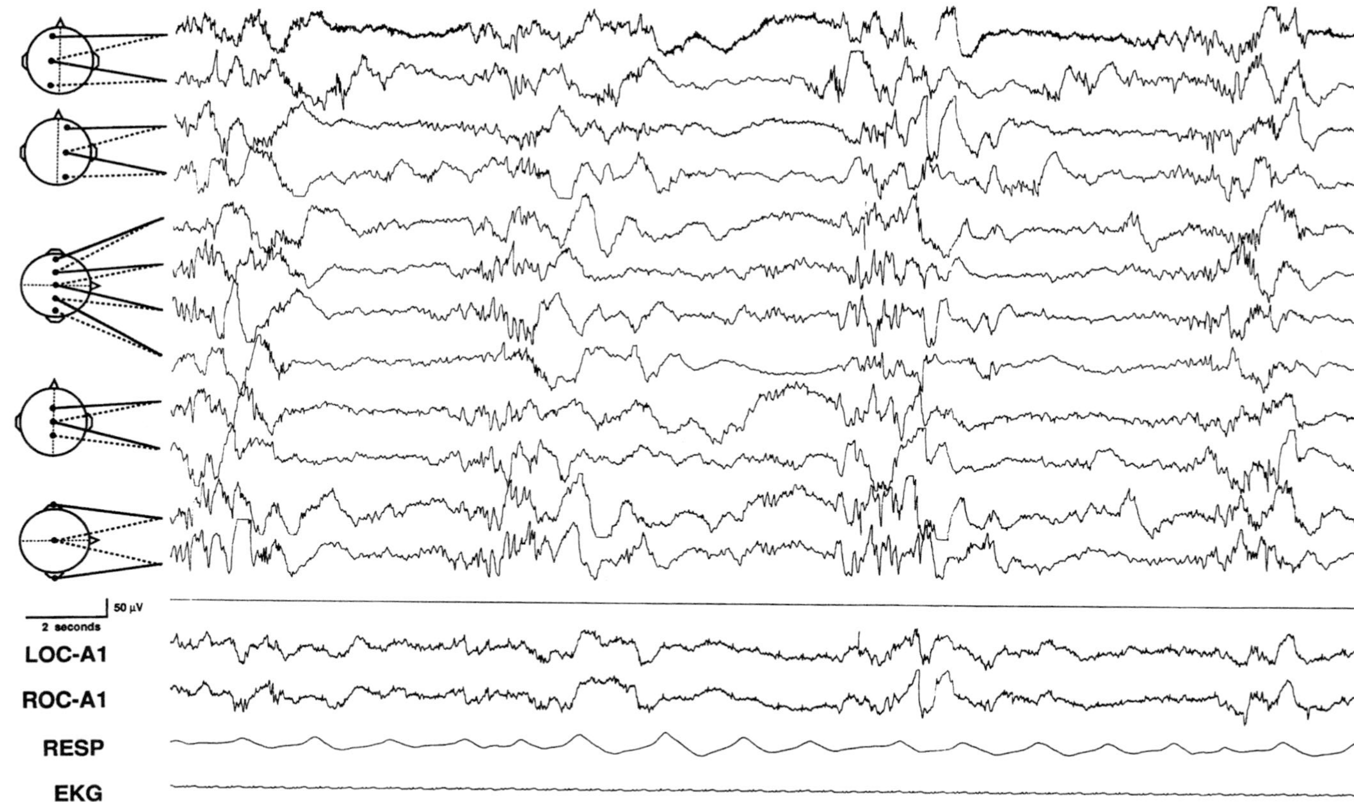

Figure 21.2 Normal discontinuous pattern in (A) a premature (24 weeks' conceptional age) infant and (B) a near-term (37 weeks' conceptional age) infant. In the very premature infant the interburst intervals are long and very flat (tracé discontinu). As premature infants approach term, the interburst intervals become shorter in duration and fill in with low-voltage activity (tracé alternant).

(A)

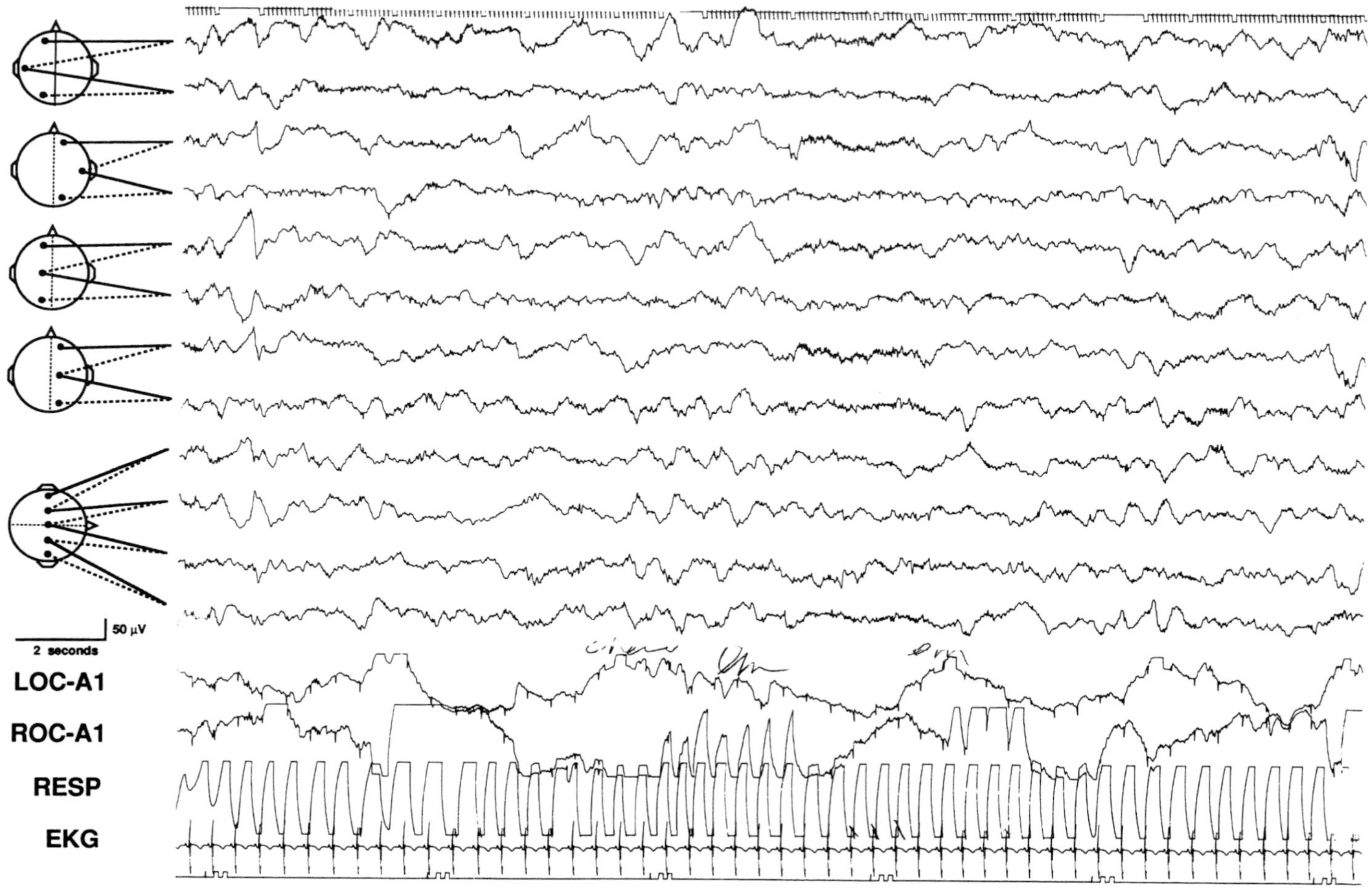

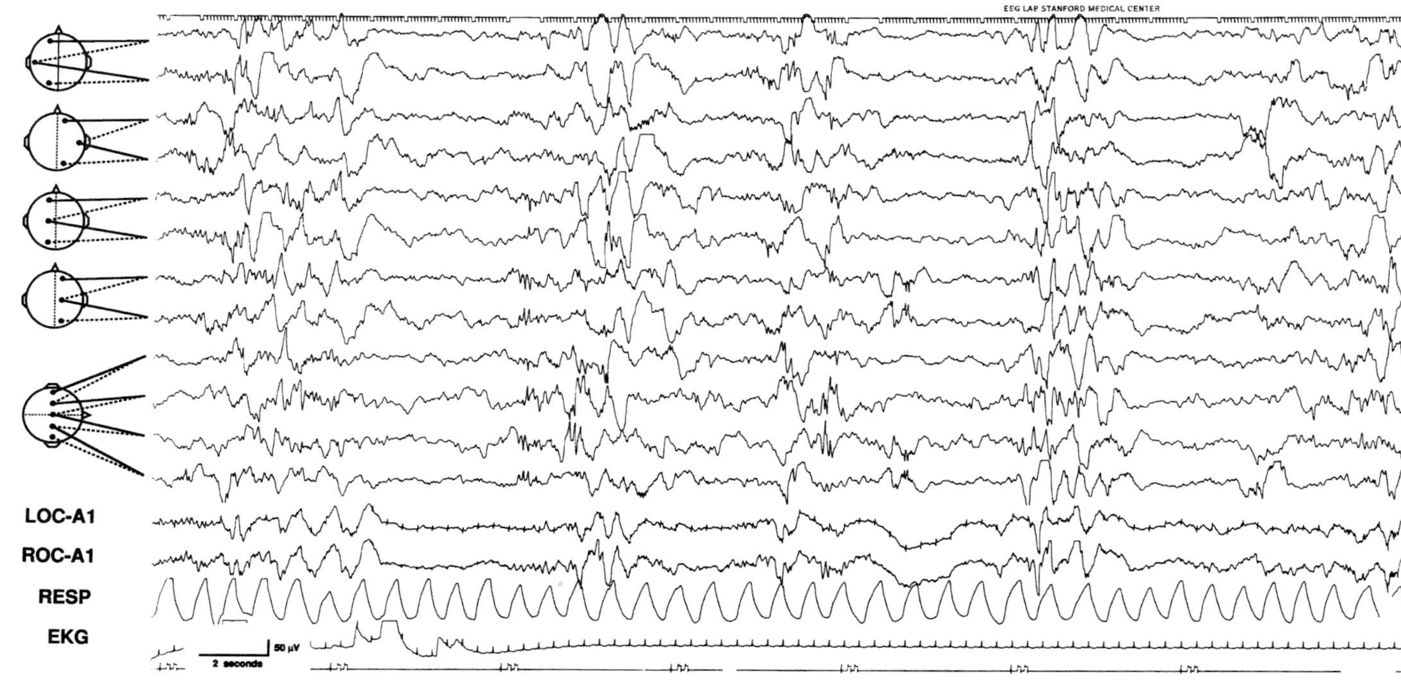

Figure 21.3 Normal electroencephalogram background activity in a term infant during (A) active sleep and (B) quiet sleep. Active sleep shows continuous mixed-frequency slow activity. Eye movements are noted by the technologist and can also be seen on the eye-lead channels. During quiet sleep there is a discontinous tracé alternant pattern with short interburst intervals.

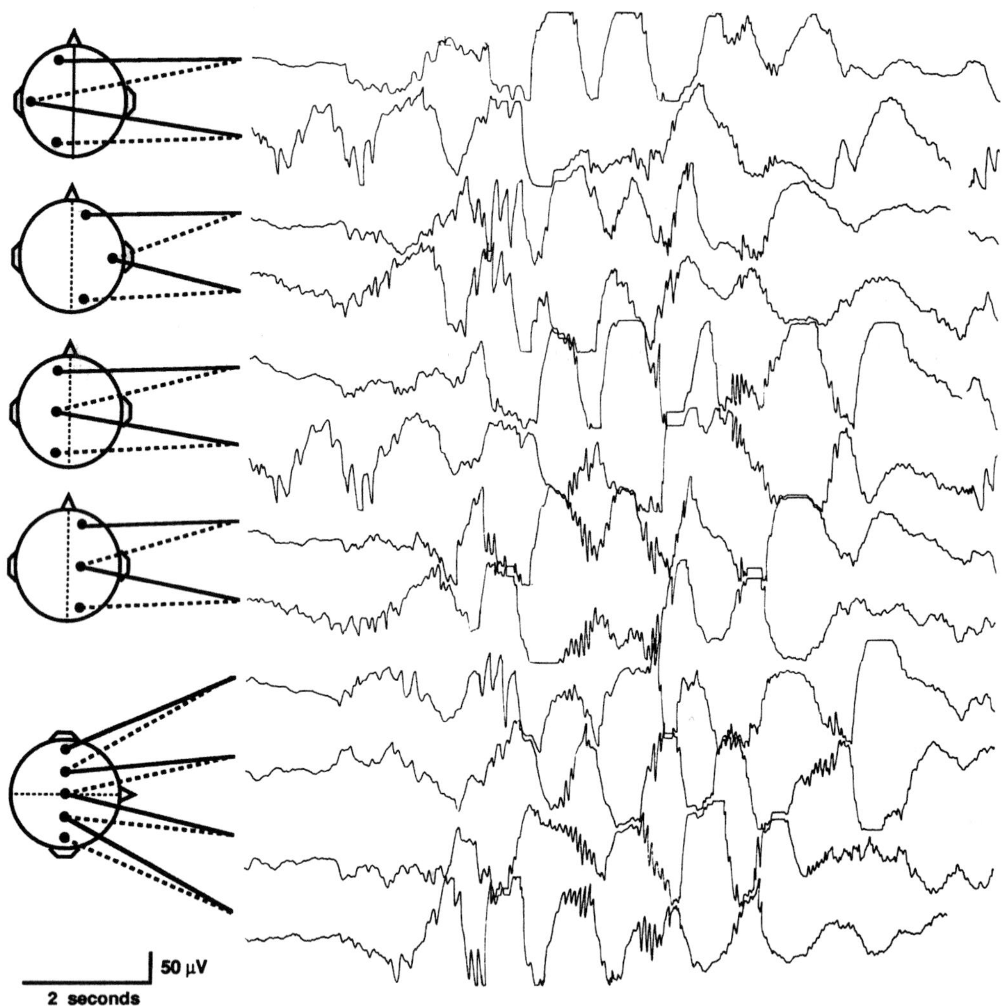

Figure 21.4 Example of delta brushes in a 28-week conceptional age infant. The brushes in this epoch are best seen in the central regions.

Midline rhythms

Various types of rhythmic or sharp EEG patterns occurring at the midline of the scalp can have a striking appearance but are still quite normal. Among these are single sharp waves, trains of 4–8 Hz sharp patterns, and runs of alpha-frequency waves lasting up to 3 s. They occur across a wide range of conceptional ages from 27 to 46 weeks. Though easily mistaken for abnormal rhythmic sharp EEG patterns, they are an occasionally seen feature of normal neonates and have been characterized as "Fz theta/alpha bursts".[52,53]

EEG in diffuse encephalopathy

EEG is often used to determine the severity and progression of encephalopathies in neonates. Most of the time, the EEG findings are not specific for a particular

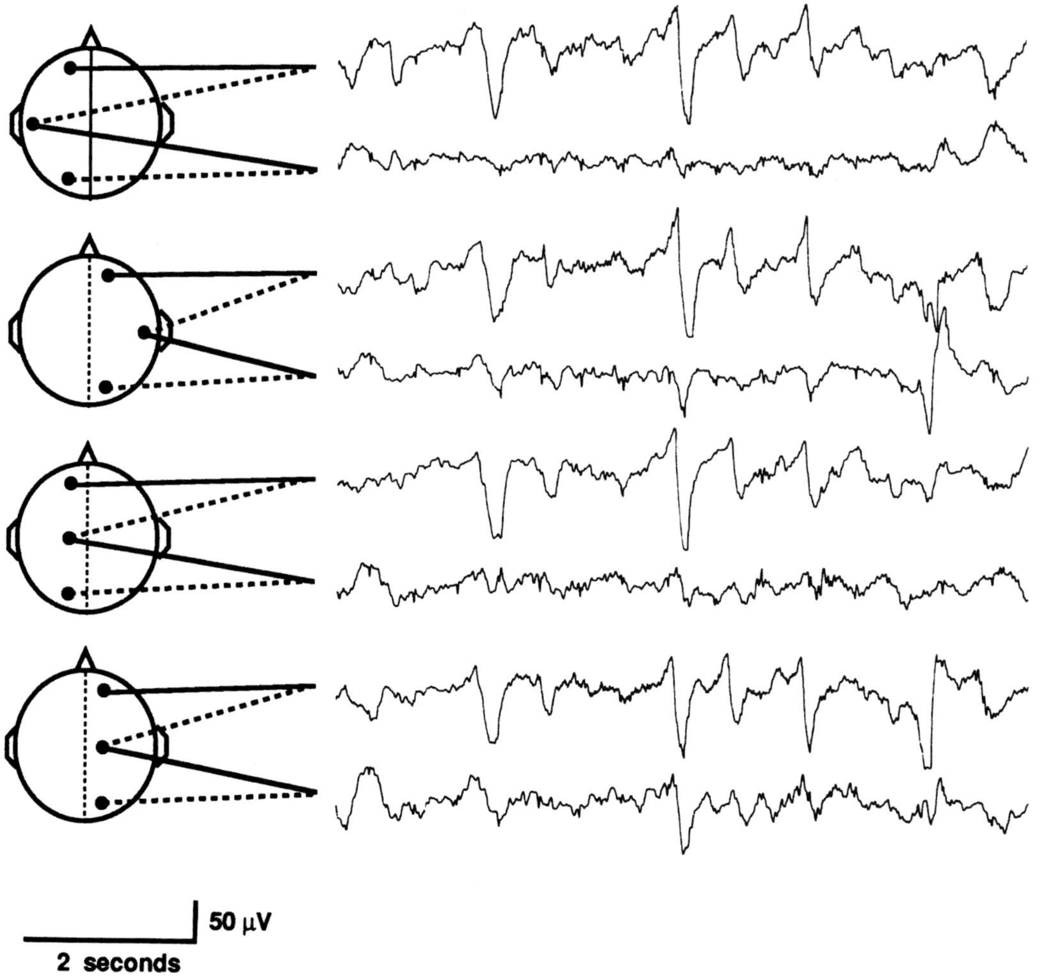

Figure 21.5 Example of frontal sharp waves in a term infant. They are bifrontal and fairly synchronous in this infant.

cause such as hypoxia or infection. Certain patterns, such as a dysmature background or burst-suppression, can occur in a variety of disorders. However, the degree of abnormality and the persistence or resolution of the abnormal finding are helpful in determining timing of an insult, the cause, and the prognosis.[54]

Grading encephalopathy using the EEG

The encephalopathy is most often referred to as "mild," "moderate," or "severe." The criteria for distinguishing between these categories may vary somewhat from one EEG laboratory to another, but it will generally be agreed that a severely abnormal EEG in a neonate comprises one of two patterns: burst-suppression or low-voltage undifferentiated (flat) pattern with no apparent EEG activity over 20 μV (Figures 21.6 and 21.7) These patterns are usually invariant, i.e., there is no spontaneous variability and very abnormal (or no) reactivity to vigorous stimulation.[40,55]

It is important to distinguish a burst-suppression

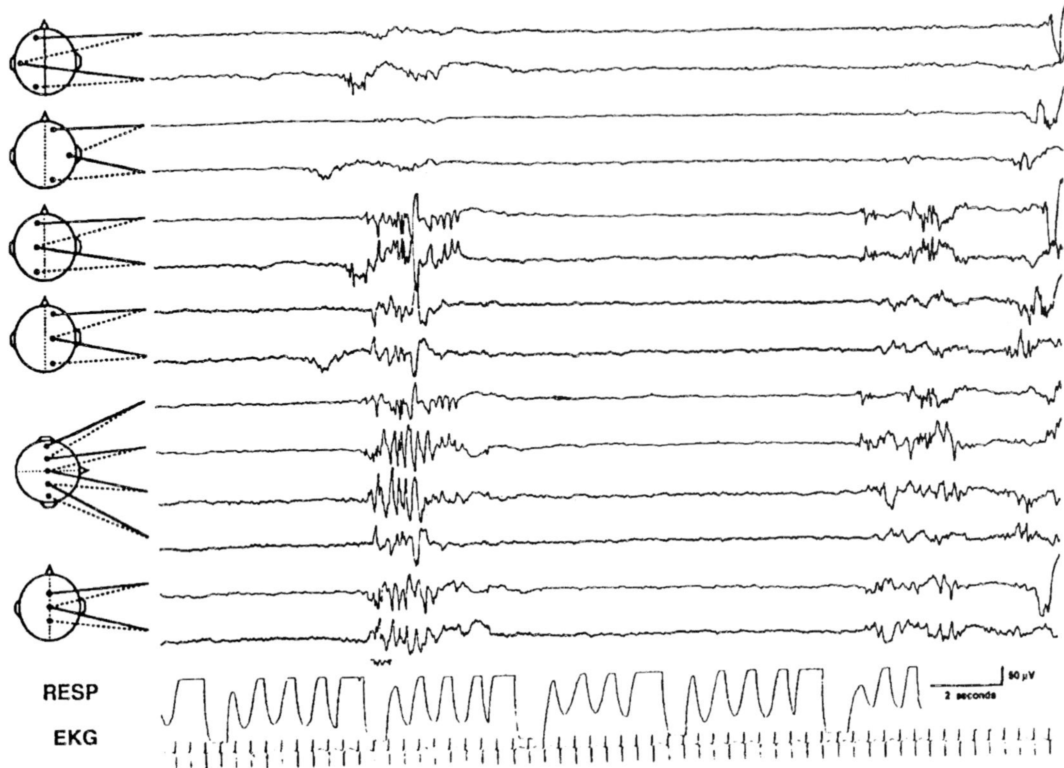

Figure 21.6 Burst-suppression pattern in a 1-day-old term infants with severe perinatal asphyxia, hypoxic–ischemic encephalopathy, and neonatal seizures.

pattern from normal discontinuity present in neonates at lower conceptional ages.[35,36] For instance, the interburst intervals of a 26-week conceptional age infant may appear very flat and suggest burst suppression (cf. Figures 21.2A and 21.6). However, there will generally be clear variability and reactivity if appropriate stimuli are administered during the recording. The bursts themselves will not look as abnormal in the normal premature infant as in a burst-suppression recording, since the latter will usually be very high in amplitude and contain bursts of abnormal repetitive sharp waves and will lack normal patterns.

An EEG may be considered severely abnormal because of other findings that have been shown to have prognostic significance: positive rolandic sharp waves, electrographic seizures, marked interhemispheric voltage asymmetry, or excessively slow background with absence of the patterns expected at the particular conceptional age.[54] The prognostic significance of these various EEG patterns as they relate to outcomes is provided in Table 21.1.

Specificity of the "encephalopathic" EEG

The cause of the encephalopathy will most often be apparent from the baby's history. The EEG itself seldom gives specific information about the underlying cause. A severely abnormal EEG may be seen in hypoxia,[44,56,57] various metabolic abnormalities,[58,59] infections,[60–63] and brain malformations.[64–66]

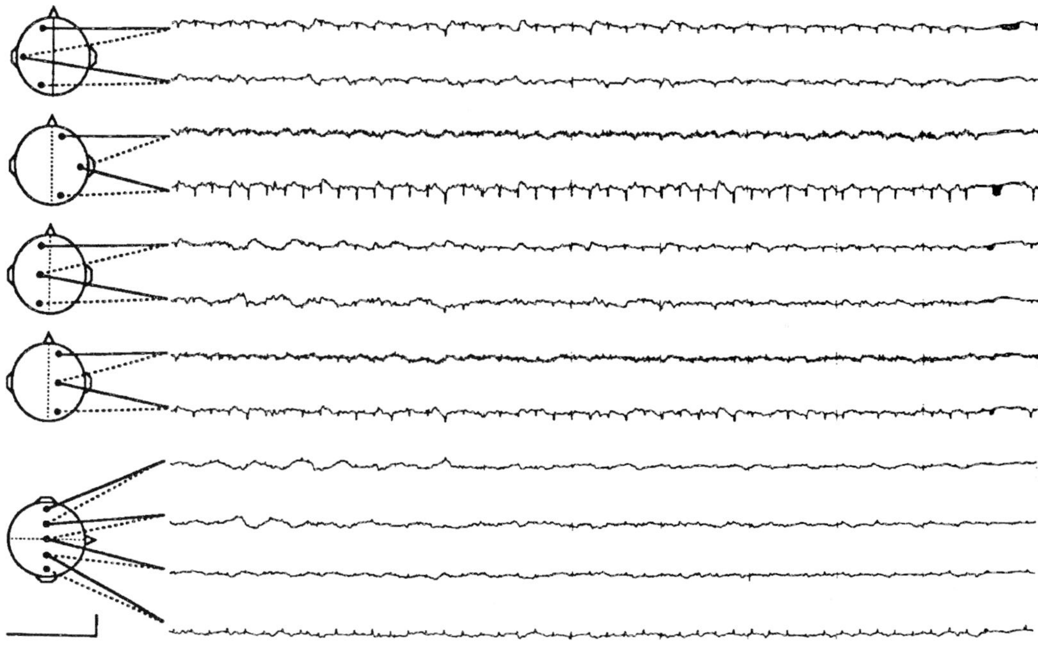

Figure 21.7 Low-voltage undifferentiated pattern seen in a 3-day-old term infant with perinatal asphyxia. Electrocardiographic artifacts are seen at this high sensitivity. Calibration: 20 μV, 2 s.

Table 21.1. Various encephalopathic electroencephalogram (EEG) patterns and their prognostic significance.

EEG background patterns	Percent with favorable outcome
Isoelectric	0–5
Suppression-burst	0–15
Low-voltage undifferentiated	15–30
Excessively discontinuous	40–50
Diffuse slow activity	15–20

Prognostic value of the encephalopathic EEG

A single severely abnormal EEG is usually indicative of an abnormal neurological outcome.[54] However, under certain circumstances, the prognostic value of a severely abnormal EEG is limited. For example, if an infant has received a large amount of neuroactive medication, the EEG may be flat or have a burst-suppression pattern. Immediately after an acute hypoxic event, hypotension, or other acute metabolic derangement (hypoglycemia, hypothermia), the EEG may appear severely abnormal although the cause is reversible and did not persist long enough to produce a significant degree of permanent brain injury.[57] Hence, it is important to know the clinical circumstances during and just prior to obtaining the EEG.

Serial EEGs, particularly in premature infants, may be a better way of determining the prognosis for neurological outcome.[54,58,67] Clancy and Chung[58] found that serial recordings provided more useful prognostic information than did any single recording. Aso and colleagues studied 32 infants who underwent autopsy and were found to have periventricular intraventricular hemorrhage.[68] Twenty-seven had parenchymal pathology including periventricular leukomalacia, ischemic neuronal sclerosis, pontosubicular necrosis, cerebral infarction, or cerebral hemorrhage. The severity of the pathological changes was highly correlated with the grading of the severity of the EEG background abnormalities. In a study of 119 near-term infants with severe respiratory failure, a burst-suppression pattern or electrographic seizures on two or more recordings was predictive of a poor prognosis (death, severely abnormal developmental score, or cerebral palsy), but a single such recording in this series was not predictive.[69]

Timing of a brain insult may be suggested by an abnormally dysmature EEG. Tharp described a case of an infant whose abnormal EEG at several hours of age showed many dysmature features.[27] The delivery was complicated by an abnormal fetal heart rate suggesting fetal distress, and the question was whether the intrapartum distress was the cause of the infant's severe encephalopathy. The infant died and the autopsy revealed changes that had occurred 7–10 days prior to death.

Timing of an insult may also be suggested by the changes (or lack of changes) that occur over time.[4,57] It takes several days for positive rolandic sharp waves (PRSW) to appear in cases of periventricular leukomalacia.[70] Hence, if such findings are present in the first days of life and persist with little change, it is suggested that the insult occurred prior to delivery. If the changes are more dynamic, i.e., appear then disappear on serial EEGs over several weeks, the likelihood is that the encephalopathy was more acute.

ECMO is a situation where EEG can be useful for helping follow the child's encephalopathic condition.[71] Infants undergoing ECMO are often quite encephalopathic from their original insult or are pharmacologically paralyzed, so clinical assessment can be difficult. In children undergoing ECMO, two or more severely abnormal EEG patterns (burst-suppression or electrographic seizure tracings) are strongly predictive of an abnormal neurological outcome.[72] The majority of the infants in this study by Graziani et al. had moderate-to-severe EEG abnormalities before ECMO. The authors concluded that fetal and neonatal complications related to the occurrence and treatment of severe cardiorespiratory failure are responsible in large part for the neurologic sequelae in ECMO survivors.

Another question specific to ECMO is whether cannulation of the right common carotid artery damages the right cerebral hemisphere. Studies looking at EEGs performed during ECMO have not shown a predilection for lateralized abnormalities over the right side, and therefore conclude that carotid artery cannulation is relatively safe.[69,71,73]

EEG can also be valuable in assessing the adequacy of therapy. Aside from the importance of EEG in assessing remission of subtle and subclinical seizures in neonates, it can also provide evidence that medical intervention has been helpful.[7,74]

Correlation with specific disorders

Brain malformation

Lissencephaly

Lissencephaly, a disturbance of neuronal migration associated with agyria or pachygyria, is associated with an abnormal EEG pattern in the neonatal period. Abnormal high-amplitude rhythmic fast frequencies have been described.[65,75] There may be poor reactivity to stimulation and absent sleep–wake changes.

Aicardi syndrome

Aicardi syndrome comprises agenesis of the corpus callosum, characteristic ocular lesions, and infantile spasms. EEG findings in the neonatal period include abnormal, poorly synchronized bursts, usually in the setting of burst-suppression.[64,66]

Holoprosencephaly

Holoprosencephaly, a malformation of the brain characterized by some degree of failure of separation of the forebrain, may show suggestive EEG changes in the neonatal period as well.[66] The EEG in the region of the dorsal cyst is low-voltage or isoelectric. The EEG in regions overlying the cortical tissue shows prolonged runs of rhythmic alpha and theta patterns, as well as fast beta (ictal) discharges. Multifocal spikes and polyspikes can also be seen, especially when cortical malformations accompany holoprosencephaly.

Metabolic encephalopathies

Maple syrup urine disease

A unique, mu-like rhythm has been described in association with maple syrup urine disease. This pattern, characterized by rhythmic 5–7-Hz activity, can be distinguished from similar patterns occurring in normal infants and those with other encephalopathies, so it may be relatively specific for maple syrup urine disease.[76]

Pyridoxine dependency

The EEG may be particularly suggestive of pyridoxine dependency in the setting of medically refractory neonatal seizures. In one study, burst-suppression and a pattern of high-amplitude bilateral slow waves were very suggestive of pyridoxine dependence.[77] Furthermore, the response to treatment (with pyridoxine) provides additional evidence for this disorder.[55]

Nonketotic hyperglycinemia

The EEG may be suggestive of nonketotic hyperglycinemia.[78] Burst-suppression pattern appears to be common, and may evolve over time to hypsarrhythmia.[67] A burst-suppression pattern with superimposed midline seizures and cortical myoclonus has been described in one study.[79]

Hyperammonemia

A burst-suppression pattern, excessive discontinuity (short of true burst-suppression), or a pattern of multifocal sharp waves may be present in the setting of citrullinemia or ornithine transcarbamylase deficiency. The improvement (or worsening) of the EEG during therapeutic interventions can provide evidence of the treatment efficacy.[58,80]

Intraventricular hemorrhage

The EEG has a limited role in the diagnosis of intraventricular hemorrhage, but has proven helpful in assessing the prognosis for neurological outcome.[68,81] The EEG can provide prognostic information beyond that apparent from brain-imaging studies.[82] In a series of 88 EEGs from 35 infants with autopsy-proven intraventricular hemorrhage, the EEG correlated better with the overall brain abnormalities than with the grade of intraventricular hemorrhage.[68] In another study, the continuity of background activity was not affected by intraventricular hemorrhage, but there was depression of the EEG background activity during the onset or extension of periventricular–intraventricular hemorrhage.[83]

Periventricular leukomalacia

PRSW are an EEG pattern associated with deep white-matter injury. A number of studies have shown the predictive value of PRSW.[84] PRSW have been associated with periventricular leukomalacia. In a study of 301 premature infants, the absence of PRSW was correlated with a favorable motor development in 98.2%.[11] When very frequent (2/min), they were strongly predictive of severe spastic diplegia. They were not specifically associated with social and language developmental abnormalities. PRSW also precede the appearance of the typical changes of cystic periventricular leukomalacia as detected by ultrasound, though ultrasound-detected echodensities may appear earlier.[70,85] Positive temporal sharp waves have also been associated with neurologically abnormal infants.[10] In another study, positive temporal sharp waves were less concerning if they were infrequent and not persistent.[86]

Stroke

Focal or hemispheric voltage attenuation may occur when infants have had large-vessel infarction.[63,87,88] In some cases EEG changes will precede those on ultrasound or CT.[88]

Infectious disease

Encephalitis

Herpes simplex meningoencephalitis is a potentially devastating infectious disease in infants. EEG changes are often nonspecific, but a pattern of temporal or multifocal periodic sharp waves has been described in infants (though this periodic pattern is more common in older children and adults).[61,89] EEG changes are likely to precede changes on neuroimaging studies,[90] and the imaging changes most characteristic of neonatal herpes may only be apparent late.[91–93]

The EEG in other forms of encephalitis often shows abnormalities, but most reports are case reports, and findings are usually nonspecific.[62,94–96] Presumably the background EEG changes again support a neurological prognostication.[55]

Meningitis

Meningitis can cause devastating brain injury in the neonate. The EEG has been a useful tool for helping predict long-term neurological outcome in neonates with meningitis.[97,98] In a study of 29 infants with culture-proven meningitis, the degree of background abnormality correlated with outcome. Infants with normal or mildly abnormal background EEGs were normal at follow-up, whereas those with markedly abnormal EEGs died or had severe neurological sequelae. EEG patterns were nonspecific, although some well-recognized patterns such as PRSW suggested more specific pathology.[63]

Maternal drug use

Scher and colleagues have reported the effects of cocaine and other illicit drugs on the EEG of neonates.[99] Cocaine produced abnormalities in the spectral correlations between homologous brain regions at birth, while alcohol, marijuana, and tobacco use were found to affect state regulation and cortical activities.

Conclusion

When obtained in a timely and considered way, the EEG will provide useful information about acute and chronic brain processes. This chapter has stressed the importance of looking at the EEG in the context of the clinical setting and in conjunction with other diagnostic studies. Not enough emphasis can be placed on the importance of clear communication between the clinicians caring for the infant, the EEG technologist, and the electroencephalographer.

REFERENCES

1 Mizrahi EM. (1999). Pediatric electroencephalographic video monitoring. *J Clin Neurophysiol*, **16**, 100–10.

2 Scher MS, Aso K, Beggarly ME, et al. (1993). Electrographic seizures in preterm and full-term neonates: clinical correlates, associated brain lesions, and risk for neurologic sequelae (see comments). *Pediatrics*, **91**, 128–34.

3 Itakura A, Kurauchi O, Hayakawa F, et al. (1996). Timing of periventricular leukomalacia using neonatal electroencephalography. *Int J Gynaecol Obstet*, **55**, 111–15.

4 Hayakawa F, Okumura A, Kato T, et al. (1999). Determination of timing of brain injury in preterm infants with periventricular leukomalacia with serial neonatal electroencephalography. *Pediatrics*, **104**, 1077–81.

5 Watanabe K, Hayakawa F and Okumura A. (1999). Neonatal EEG: a powerful tool in the assessment of brain damage in preterm infants. *Brain Dev*, **21**, 361–72.

6 Marret S, Jeannot E, Parain D, et al. (1989). Positive rolandic sharp waves, periventricular ischemia and neurologic outcome. Prospective study in 66 premature infants. *Arch Fr Pediatr*, **46**, 249–53.

7 Bellieni CV, Ferrari F, De Felice C, et al. (2000). EEG in assessing hydroxycobalamin therapy in neonatal methylmalonic aciduria with homocystinuria. *Biol Neonate*, **78**, 327–30.

8 Brazier MAB. (1977). *Electrical Activity of the Nervous System*, 4th edn. Baltimore: Williams and Wilkins.

9 Marret S, Parain D, Menard JF, et al. (1997). Prognostic value of neonatal electroencephalography in premature newborns less than 33 weeks of gestational age. *Electroencephalogr Clin Neurophysiol*, **102**, 178–85.

10 Chung HJ and Clancy RR. (1991). Significance of positive temporal sharp waves in the neonatal electroencephalogram. *Electroencephalogr Clin Neurophysiol*, **79**, 256–63.

11 Marret S, Parain D, Jeannot E, et al. (1992). Positive rolandic sharp waves in the EEG of the premature newborn: a five year prospective study. *Arch Dis Child*, **67**, 948–51.

12 Novotny EJ Jr, Tharp BR, Coen RW, et al. (1987). Positive rolandic sharp waves in the EEG of the premature infant. *Neurology*, **37**, 1481–6.

13 Cukier F, Andre M, Monod N, et al. (1972). Contribution of EEG to the diagnosis of intraventricular hemorrhages in the premature infant. *Rev Electroencephalogr Neurophysiol Clin*, **2**, 318–22.

14 Levy SR. (1997). Brainstem auditory potentials in pediatrics. In *Evoked Potentials in Clinical Medicine*, 3rd edn, Chiappa KH, (ed.), pp. 269–278. New York: Raven Press.

15 Levy SR. (1997). Somatosensory evoked potentials in pediatrics. In *Evoked Potentials in Clinical Medicine*, 3rd edn, Chiappa KH (ed.), pp. 453–470. Philadelphia: Lippincott-Raven.

16 Jasper HH. (1958). The ten twenty electrode system of the international federation. *Electroencephalogr Clin Neurophysiol*, **10**, 371–375.

17 Nuwer MR. (1987). Recording electrode site nomenclature. *J Clin Neurophysiol*, **4**, 121–33.

18 American Electroencephalographic Society. (1994). Guideline two: minimum technical standards for pediatric electroencephalography. *J Clin Neurophysiol*, **11**, 6–9.

19 Hrachovy RA, Mizrahi EM and Kellaway P. (1990). Electroencephalography of the newborn. In *Current Practice of Clinical Electroencephalography*, 2nd edn, Daly TA (ed.), pp. 201–242. New York: Raven Press.

20 Ramelli GP, Donati F, Bianchetti M, et al. (1998) Apnoeic attacks as an isolated manifestation of epileptic seizures in infants. *Eur J Paediatr Neurol*, **2**, 187–91.

21 Watanabe K, Hara K, Miyazaki S, et al. (1982). Apneic seizures in the newborn. *Am J Dis Child*, **136**, 980–4.

22 Hahn JS and Tharp B. (1999). Neonatal and pediatric electroencephalography. In *Electrodiagnosis in Clinical Neurology*, 3rd edn, Aminoff M (ed.), pp. 81–127. New York: Churchill Livingstone.

23 Thoresen M, Henriksen O, Wannag E, et al. (1997). Does a sedative dose of chloral hydrate modify the EEG of children with epilepsy? *Electroencephalogr Clin Neurophysiol*, **102**, 152–7.

24 Anyebuno MA and Rosenfeld CR. (1991). Chloral hydrate toxicity in a term infant. *Dev Pharmacol Ther*, **17**, 116–20.

25 Steinberg AD. (1993). Should chloral hydrate be banned? *Pediatrics*, **92**, 442–6.

26 Reimche LD, Sankaran K, Hindmarsh KW, et al. (1989). Chloral hydrate sedation in neonates and infants – clinical and pharmacologic considerations. *Dev Pharmacol Ther*, **12**, 57–64.

27 Tharp BR. (1990). Electrophysiological brain maturation in premature infants: an historical perspective. *J Clin Neurophysiol*, **7**, 302–14.

28 da Silva O, Collado Guzman GM and Young GB. (1998). The value of standard electroencephalograms in the evaluation of the newborn with recurrent apneas. *J Perinatol*, **18**, 377–80.

29 Wical BS. (1994). Neonatal seizures and electrographic analysis: evaluation and outcomes. *Pediatr Neurol*, **10**, 271–5.

30 American Electroencephalographic Society. (1994). Guideline eight: guidelines for writing EEG reports. *J Clin Neurophysiol*, **11**, 37–9.

31 Dooling EC, Chi JG and Gilles FH. (1983). Telencephalic development. In *The Developing Human Brain: Growth and Epidemiologic Neuropathology*, Dooling EC (ed.), pp. 117–182. Boston: Wright-PSG.

32 McArdle CB, Richardson CJ, Nicholas DA, et al. (1987). Developmental features of the neonatal brain: MR imaging. Part I. Gray-white matter differentiation and myelination. *Radiology*, **162**, 223–9.

33 Scher MS, Martin JG, Steppe DA, et al. (1994). Comparative estimates of neonatal gestational maturity by electrographic and fetal ultrasonographic criteria. *Pediatr Neurol*, **11**, 214–18.

34 Monod N and Tharp B. (1977). The normal EEG of the neonate (author's transl). *Rev Electroencephalogr Neurophysiol Clin*, **7**, 302–15.

35 Selton D, Andre M and Hascoet JM. (2000). Normal EEG in very premature infants: reference criteria. *Clin Neurophysiol*, **111**, 2116–24.

36 Torres F and Anderson C. (1985). The normal EEG of the human newborn. *J Clin Neurophysiol*, **2**, 89–103.

37 Van Sweden B, Koenderink M, Windau G, et al. (1991). Long-term EEG monitoring in the early premature: developmental and chronobiological aspects. *Electroencephalogr Clin Neurophysiol*, **79**, 94–100.

38 Biagioni E, Bartalena L, Biver P, et al. (1996). Electroencephalographic dysmaturity in preterm infants: a prognostic tool in the early postnatal period. *Neuropediatrics*, **27**, 311–16.

39 Hayakawa F, Okumura A, Kato T, et al. (1997). Disorganized patterns: chronic-stage EEG abnormality of the late neonatal period following severely depressed EEG activities in early preterm infants. *Neuropediatrics*, **28**, 272–5.

40 Biagioni E, Bartalena L, Boldrini A, et al. (1999). Constantly discontinuous EEG patterns in full-term neonates with hypoxic–ischaemic encephalopathy. *Clin Neurophysiol,* **110**, 1510–15.

41 Hahn JS and Tharp BR. (1990). Winner of the Brazier Award. The dysmature EEG pattern in infants with bronchopulmonary dysplasia and its prognostic implications. *Electroencephalogr Clin Neurophysiol,* **76**, 106–13.

42 Scher MS, Steppe DA, Banks DL, et al. (1995). Maturational trends of EEG-sleep measures in the healthy preterm neonate. *Pediatr Neurol,* **12**, 314–22.

43 Scher MS, Steppe DA, Dokianakis SG, et al. (1994). Maturation of phasic and continuity measures during sleep in preterm neonates. *Pediatr Res,* **36**, 732–7.

44 Wertheim D, Mercuri E, Faundez JC, et al. (1994). Prognostic value of continuous electroencephalographic recording in full term infants with hypoxic ischaemic encephalopathy. *Arch Dis Child,* **71**, F97–102.

45 Lombroso CT. (1979). Quantified electrographic scales on 10 pre-term healthy newborns followed up to 40–43 weeks of conceptional age by serial polygraphic recordings. *Electroencephalogr Clin Neurophysiol,* **46**, 460–74.

46 Oliveira AJ, Nunes ML, Haertel LM, et al. (2000). Duration of rhythmic EEG patterns in neonates: new evidence for clinical and prognostic significance of brief rhythmic discharges. *Clin Neurophysiol,* **111**, 1646–53.

47 Shewmon DA. (1990). What is a neonatal seizure? Problems in definition and quantification for investigative and clinical purposes. *J Clin Neurophysiol,* **7**, 315–68.

48 Nunes ML, Da Costa JC and Moura-Ribeiro MV. (1997). Polysomnographic quantification of bioelectrical maturation in preterm and fullterm newborns at matched conceptional ages. *Electroencephalogr Clin Neurophysiol,* **102**, 186–91.

49 Kuremoto K, Hayakawa F and Watanabe K. (1997). Rhythmic alpha/theta bursts in the electroencephalogram of early premature infants: (1). The features in normal early premature infants. *No To Hattatsu,* **29**, 239–43.

50 Hughes JR, Miller JK, Fino JJ, et al. (1990). The sharp theta rhythm on the occipital areas of prematures (STOP): a newly described waveform. *Clin Electroencephalogr,* **21**, 77–87.

51 Kuremoto K, Hayakawa F and Watanabe K. (1997). Rhythmic alpha/theta bursts in the electroencephalogram of early premature infants: (2). Correlation with background EEG activity. *No To Hattatsu,* **29**, 244–8.

52 Hayakawa F, Watanabe K, Hakamada S, et al. (1987). Fz theta/alpha bursts: a transient EEG pattern in healthy newborns. *Electroencephalogr Clin Neurophysiol,* **67**, 27–31.

53 Zaret BS, Guterman B and Weig S. (1991). Circumscribed midline EEG activity in neurologically normal neonates. *Clin Electroencephalogr,* **22**, 13–22.

54 Tharp BR, Cukier F and Monod N. (1981). The prognostic value of the electroencephalogram in premature infants. *Electroencephalogr Clin Neurophysiol,* **51**, 219–36.

55 Holmes GL and Lombroso CT. (1993). Prognostic value of background patterns in the neonatal EEG. *J Clin Neurophysiol,* **10**, 323–52.

56 Selton D and Andre M. (1997). Prognosis of hypoxic–ischaemic encephalopathy in full-term newborns – value of neonatal electroencephalography. *Neuropediatrics,* **28**, 276–80.

57 Pressler RM, Boylan GB, Morton M, et al. (2001). Early serial EEG in hypoxic ischaemic encephalopathy. *Clin Neurophysiol,* **112**, 31–7.

58 Clancy RR and Chung HJ. (1991). EEG changes during recovery from acute severe neonatal citrullinemia. *Electroencephalogr Clin Neurophysiol,* **78**, 222–7.

59 Taylor MJ and Robinson BH. (1992). Evoked potentials in children with oxidative metabolic defects leading to Leigh syndrome. *Pediatr Neurol,* **8**, 25–9.

60 Chang Y, Soffer D, Horoupian DS, et al. (1990). Evolution of post-natal herpes simplex virus encephalitis to multicystic encephalopathy. *Acta Neuropathol,* **80**, 666–70.

61 Sainio K, Granstrom ML, Pettay O, et al. (1983). EEG in neonatal herpes simplex encephalitis. *Electroencephalogr Clin Neurophysiol,* **56**, 556–61.

62 Schmitt B, Seeger J and Jacobi G. (1992). EEG and evoked potentials in HIV-infected children. *Clin Electroencephalogr,* **23**, 111–17.

63 Chequer RS, Tharp BR, Dreimane D, et al. (1992). Prognostic value of EEG in neonatal meningitis: retrospective study of 29 infants. *Pediatr Neurol,* **8**, 417–22.

64 Htsuka Y, Oka E, Terasaki T, et al. (1993). Aicardi syndrome: a longitudinal clinical and electroencephalographic study. *Epilepsia,* **34**, 627–34.

65 Bode H and Bubl R. (1994). EEG changes in type I and type II lissencephaly. *Klin Padiatr,* **206**, 12–17.

66 Shah KN, Rajadhyaksha S, Shah VS, et al. (1992). EEG recognition of holoprosencephaly and Aicardi syndrome. *Indian J Pediatr,* **59**, 103–8.

67 Markand ON, Garg BP and Brandt IK. (1982). Nonketotic hyperglycinemia: electroencephalographic and evoked potential abnormalities. *Neurology,* **32**, 151–6.

68 Aso K, Abdab-Barmada M and Scher MS. (1993). EEG and the neuropathology in premature neonates with intraventricular hemorrhage. *J Clin Neurophysiol,* **10**, 304–13.

69 Graziani LJ, Streletz LJ, Baumgart S, et al. (1994). Predictive value of neonatal electroencephalograms before and during extracorporeal membrane oxygenation. *J Pediatr,* **125**, 969–75.

70 Okumura A, Hayakawa F, Kato T, et al. (1999). Positive rolandic sharp waves in preterm infants with periventricular leukomalacia: their relation to background electroencephalographic abnormalities. *Neuropediatrics*, **30**, 278–82.

71 Streletz LJ, Bej MD, Graziani LJ, et al. (1992). Utility of serial EEGs in neonates during extracorporeal membrane oxygenation. *Pediatr Neurol*, **8**, 190–6.

72 Graziani LJ, Gringlas M and Baumgart S. (1997). Cerebrovascular complications and neurodevelopmental sequelae of neonatal ECMO. *Clin Perinatol*, **24**, 655–75.

73 Kumar P, Gupta R, Shankaran S, et al. (1999). EEG abnormalities in survivors of neonatal ECMO: its role as a predictor of neurodevelopmental outcome. *Am J Perinatol*, **16**, 245–50.

74 Mikati MA, Trevathan E, Krishnamoorthy KS, et al. (1991). Pyridoxine-dependent epilepsy: EEG investigations and long-term follow- up. *Electroencephalogr Clin Neurophysiol*, **78**, 215–21.

75 Worle H, Keimer R and Kohler B. (1990). [Miller-Dieker syndrome (type I lissencephaly) with specific EEG changes.] *Monatsschr Kinderheilkd*, **138**, 615–18.

76 Tharp BR. (1992). Unique EEG pattern (comb-like rhythm) in neonatal maple syrup urine disease. *Pediatr Neurol*, **8**, 65–8.

77 Nabbout R, Soufflet C, Plouin P, et al. (1999). Pyridoxine dependent epilepsy: a suggestive electroclinical pattern. *Arch Dis Child Fetal Neonatal Ed*, **81**, F125–9.

78 Seppalainen AM and Simila S. (1971). Electroencephalographic findings in three patients with nonketotic hyperglycinemia. *Epilepsia*, **12**, 101–7.

79 Scher MS, Bergman I, Ahdab-Barmada M, et al. (1986). Neurophysiological and anatomical correlations in neonatal nonketotic hyperglycinemia. *Neuropediatrics*, **17**, 137–43.

80 Brunquell P, Tezcan K and DiMario FJ Jr. (1999). Electroencephalographic findings in ornithine transcarbamylase deficiency. *J Child Neurol*, **14**, 533–6.

81 Clancy RR, Tharp BR and Enzman D. (1984). EEG in premature infants with intraventricular hemorrhage. *Neurology*, **34**, 583–90.

82 Watanabe K, Hakamada S, Kuroyanagi M, et al. (1983). Electroencephalographic study of intraventricular hemorrhage in the preterm newborn. *Neuropediatrics*, **14**, 225–30.

83 van de Bor M, van Dijk JG, van Bel F, et al. (1994). Electrical brain activity in preterm infants at risk for intracranial hemorrhage. *Acta Paediatr*, **83**, 588–95.

84 Hughes JR and Guerra R. (1994). The use of the EEG to predict outcome in premature infants with positive sharp waves. *Clin Electroencephalogr*, **25**, 127–35.

85 Baud O, d'Allest AM, Lacaze-Masmonteil T, et al. (1998). The early diagnosis of periventricular leukomalacia in premature infants with positive rolandic sharp waves on serial electroencephalography. *J Pediatr*, **132**, 813–17.

86 Vecchierini-Blineau MF, Nogues B, Louvet S, et al. (1996). Positive temporal sharp waves in electroencephalograms of the premature newborn. *Neurophysiol Clin*, **26**, 350–62.

87 Sreenan C, Bhargava R and Robertson CM. (2000). Cerebral infarction in the term newborn: clinical presentation and long-term outcome. *J Pediatr*, **137**, 351–5.

88 Koelfen W, Freund M and Varnholt V. (1995). Neonatal stroke involving the middle cerebral artery in term infants: clinical presentation, EEG and imaging studies, and outcome. *Dev Med Child Neurol*, **37**, 204–12.

89 Lai CW and Gragasin ME. (1988). Electroencephalography in herpes simplex encephalitis. *J Clin Neurophysiol*, **5**, 87–103.

90 Mikati MA, Feraru E, Krishnamoorthy K, et al. (1990). Neonatal herpes simplex meningoencephalitis: EEG investigations and clinical correlates. *Neurology*, **40**, 1433–7.

91 Enzmann D, Chang Y and Augustyn G. (1990). MR findings in neonatal herpes simplex encephalitis type II. *J Comput Assist Tomogr*, **14**, 453–7.

92 Shian WJ and Chi CS. (1996). Magnetic resonance imaging of herpes simplex encephalitis. *Zhonghua Min Guo Xiao Er Ke Yi Xue Hui Za Zhi*, **37**, 22–6.

93 Bale JF, Andersen RD and Grose C. (1987). Magnetic resonance imaging of the brain in childhood herpes virus infections. *Pediatr Infect Dis J*, **6**, 644–7.

94 Funk M, Joseph-Steiner J, Hernaiz-Driever P, et al. (1996). Nervous system manifestations in HIV infected children. *Klin Padiatr*, **208**, 299–303.

95 Haddad J, Messer J, Gut JP, et al. (1990). Neonatal echovirus encephalitis with white matter necrosis. *Neuropediatrics*, **21**, 215–17.

96 Kohyama J, Suzuki N, Kajiwara M, et al. (1993). A case of chronic epileptic encephalopathy of neonatal onset. A probable concern of human cytomegalovirus. *Brain Dev*, **15**, 448–52.

97 Berg U, Bohlin AB and Malmborg AS. (1981). Neonatal meningitis caused by *Haemophilus influenzae* type c. *Scand J Infect Dis*, **13**, 155–7.

98 Watanabe K, Hara K, Hakamada S, et al. (1983). The prognostic value of EEG in neonatal meningitis. *Clin Electroencephalogr*, **14**, 67–77.

99 Scher MS, Richardson GA and Day NL. (2000). Effects of prenatal cocaine/crack and other drug exposure on electroencephalographic sleep studies at birth and one year. *Pediatrics*, **105**, 39–48.

22

Structural and functional imaging of hypoxic–ischemic injury (HII) in the fetal and neonatal brain

Francis G. Blankenberg and Patrick D. Barnes

Lucile Packard Children's Hospital, Palo Alto, CA, USA

Introduction

In the twenty-first century neonatal neuroimaging will be classified as either "structural," that is, based on anatomic or morphologic data, or "functional," in which images will be generated based upon physiologic or metabolic data. Currently the major structural imaging modalities are ultrasound (US), computed tomography (CT), and magnetic resonance imaging (MRI). These are commonly used to screen for anatomic abnormalities associated with neonatal intracranial hemorrhage (ICH) and ischemia associated with hypoxic-ischemic injury (HII).[1–10] While US, CT, and MRI are technologically mature, few studies address the issue of which imaging protocols are most appropriate for the diagnosis of neonatal ICH and ischemia.[11–15] US, the most commonly employed imaging modality in neonates, is less sensitive and less specific for the detection of intracranial ischemia and hemorrhage compared with CT or MRI.[6,16–19] It is unclear, however, if the greater expense and logistical difficulties in obtaining CT and MRI examinations in critically ill neonates are justified.[20,21] Furthermore, the lack of white-matter myelinization and patterns of ischemic and hemorrhagic lesions are markedly different in premature infants as compared to term which complicates the interpretation of CT or MRI examinations.[16,19] The predictive value and clinical utility of US, CT, or MRI in neonates with HII have also been the subject of a number of longitudinal studies.[2–12,20–25] However, it is difficult from any of these investigations to distill out a uniform set of imaging protocols for the screening and management of neonates with HII and, more importantly, individual prognostication.

Newer functional imaging modalities such as MR proton spectroscopy,[26–30] diffusion-weighted imaging (DWI)[31–37] and radiolabeled markers of perfusion[38–41] and cell death[42] imaged by single-photon emission computed tomography (SPECT) and positron emission tomography (PET),[43–45] may offer potentially useful additional clinical information to that obtained from conventional US, CT, and MRI structurally based examinations. These and possibly other functional imaging techniques may dramatically impact short- and long-term management of neonates as well as prognostication as they can potentially provide diagnostic and prognostic information in the first hours after a cerebral insult.

In this chapter we will outline the diagnostic considerations and potential pitfalls of US, CT, and MRI for the neuroanatomic structural imaging of hypoxic–ischemic brain injury in both preterm and full-term infants. We will also discuss the latest advances in functional imaging with DWI and MR spectroscopy as well as SPECT and PET studies of cerebral perfusion and cell death that may profoundly impact upon the screening and follow-up of infants with suspected hypoxic–ischemic brain injury.

Neuroimaging of neonates

US and Doppler studies

The fundamentals of neurosonographic imaging

The fontanels in the newborn provide excellent acoustic windows through which sonographic anatomic (gray-scale) imaging of the brain can be obtained.[46] These gaps in the neonatal skull allow for the sound waves generated by the US probe to be transmitted and received while avoiding the severe losses of signal caused by the presence of air or bony structures in the path of the sound beam. US employs frequencies of sound between 5 and 13 MHz to yield images based on the degree of reflectance (backscatter) and attenuation of the primary sound wave by the soft tissues, fluids, and anatomic interfaces within the brain. Images are generated by placing a small (1–2-cm) solid-state transceiver probe over the fontanel of interest. In order to obtain an adequate impedance match with the scalp, a water-based gel is applied over a given fontanel. The resultant reflected sound signals from the original primary beam are computer-processed to yield a real-time wedged or fan-shaped image with a working focusing depth between 2 and 12 cm for a standard 8-MHz sector probe with a maximal resolution of approximately 1–2 mm. For higher resolution, increased sensitivity to flow, and better near-field focusing (several millimeters to 8 cm), linear phased-array probes designed with higher frequency ranges (8–15 MHz) and a larger number of detectors per unit area can be used. These probes, as opposed to sector probes, generate rectangular-shaped images of the underlying brain. The disadvantages of these probes, however, are their long length (5–6 cm), longer than the largest fontanel, permitting views of only the midline or slightly off-midline structures and the relative lack of tissue penetration at higher frequencies (i.e., the higher the frequency, the less penetration of the sound beam).

The relative reflectance of tissue (or fluid) in the region of sonographic interrogation provides the imaging contrast to resolve various intracerebral structures such as the cerebral and cerebellar sulci, midline structures such as the cavum septum pellucidum, the third and fourth ventricles, the posterior fossa and the detection of pathology such as hemorrhage, ischemia, or hydrocephalus.

Cerebrospinal fluid (CSF) is minimally echogenic (i.e., anechoic) and is usually the "darkest" component seen on US. The most echogenic normal structures in the neonatal brain are that of the choroid plexus and the germinal matrix (a fetal structure normally only found in preterm infants less than 33 weeks' gestational age). The choroid plexus located posteriorly in the lateral ventricles and in the roof of the third ventricle and the germinal matrix located in the caudothalamic groove of preterm neonates are both highly reflective due to the millions of tiny interfaces within these dense tangles of capillaries. These interfaces are approximately the same size of the wavelength of the sound beam, causing the beam to scatter in multiple directions, including back towards the transducer. Normal gray and white matter are of medium echogenicity, that is, a brightness somewhere in between that of CSF and the highly echogenic choroid plexus and germinal matrix.

Clotted blood within CSF or the brain parenchyma, containing millions of "miniature mirrors" in the form of clotted red blood cells, strongly reflects (backscatters) sound waves and therefore appears as brighter, sonographically speaking, than either CSF or normal gray or white matter. Hemorrhage in the CSF or brain parenchyma can also be isoechoic; that is, the same medium echogenicity as the surrounding soft tissue if unclotted (i.e., hyperacute bleed) or later on during the gradual involution of clot beginning several days after an acute bleed.

Curiously, regions of ischemia in either the gray or white matter are also strongly reflective and thus generate bright echoes. The reason for this apparent anomaly is that regions of ischemia also contain microscopic regions of red blood cells that have extravasated into the interstitium.

The most commonly described method for neurosonography is the so-called "anterior fontanel approach" in which the probe is placed against the anterior fontanel. Once placed, a sonographer slowly angles the probe from side to side and front to back so that a sweep of the entire brain is obtained in at least two different planes (i.e., coronal and sagittal). Care must be taken systematically to angle the sonographic beam of the sector probe as far lateral, anterior, and posterior as possible to insure that the lateral convexities of the cerebrum and the frontal and occipital-parietal regions are adequately visualized. Typically images are viewed real-time during neurosonography and prints are made of sagittal and coronal views.

Other approaches are now routinely employed to supplement the anterior fontanel view, including the typically small posterior fontanel[47] and the so-called "mastoid view[48]" obtained through the smaller posterior-lateral (mastoid) fontanels located immediately posterior to each ear. The posterior fontanel view provides excellent detail of the occipital horns to assess better for intraventricular hemorrhage (IVH) that may be layering posteriorly and difficult to distinguish from the echogenic choroid plexus in the anterior fontanel view. This view is also helpful in ruling out angle-dependent echogenic artifacts seen with the anterior fontanel approach caused by the orientation of tiny medullary vessels and nerve fibers within the deep periventricular white matter perpendicular to the path of the sound beam (e.g., the periventricular "halo"). The mastoid view gives an excellent view of the cerebellum, fourth ventricle, and the rest of the posterior fossa – structures that can sometimes be difficult to see from the more distant anterior fontanel.

Fundamentals of Doppler cerebral blood flow velocity studies

Doppler measurements during neurosonography can provide information about relative cerebral blood flow (CBF) of newborns.[46,49,50] Doppler signal is obtained by real-time rapid computer calculation of the frequency shift of the returning sound beam reflected by the red blood cells flowing in a vessel of interest as compared with that of the original pulse. Blood flowing away from the transducer will have a negative shift that is, less than the original frequency, whereas blood flowing towards the transducer will have a positive shift, that is, greater than the original sound beam. Doppler signals can be displayed as a continuous wave of the blood velocities obtained from a graphically determined volume of interest electronically superimposed on the corresponding neurosonographic anatomic gray-scale image (i.e., pulsed-wave Doppler). Doppler signals can also be displayed on a color scale, typically blue for blood flowing away from the transducer and red for blood flowing towards the transducer, and electronically superimposed on the sonographic images in a real-time fashion.[51] Another display of Doppler signal is the power Doppler mode, in which all flow, regardless of direction, is summed real-time to give a single color-encoded image of flow representing the magnitude or speed of blood flow within a sonographic image.

Although precise quantitation of CBF is not currently possible, other calculated Doppler flow indices have been correlated to neonatal brain pathology and neurodevelopmental outcome.[52] Relative changes in the measurements of flow velocities within the anterior or middle cerebral arteries correlate proportionately to changes in global and regional CBF.[53] Markers of CBF include measurements of area under the velocity curve and velocity amplitudes (systolic, diastolic, mean velocity).[54]

One calculated measure of cerebral vascular dynamics is the resistive index (RI or Pourcelot index), which is defined as: (peak systolic velocity − end-diastolic velocity)/peak systolic velocity.[49] RI measurements from the anterior cerebral artery are normally slightly higher in preterm infants as compared with term infants averaging 0.80 (range 0.5–1.0) and 0.71 (range 0.6–0.8), respectively. Increases in intracranial pressure caused by hypoxic–ischemic encephalopathy, brain edema, or hydrocephalus are accompanied by elevations in RI. When intracranial pressure exceeds that of the arterial perfusion pressure with brain death, a reversal of diastolic flow is noted with an eventual dampening of peak systolic flow. These Doppler flow findings have been used to support the difficult diagnosis of brain death in infants.

In order to improve the specificity for the diagnosis of hydrocephalus some institutions recommend serial measurements of RI with compression of the anterior fontanel with the ultrasound probe (less than 5 s of pressure).[55] The percent change in the RI with compression over time correlates with direct CSF pressure measurements within the ventricles.

The variation of blood flow velocities during the cardiac cycle can also be summarized by the calculation of the pulsatility index (PI) defined as: (peak systolic velocity − end-diastolic velocity)/mean velocity. Increased PI has been associated with the presence of a patent ductus arteriosius and may increase the risk for development of IVH.[56, 57]

Another pathophysiologic phenomenon that can be detected by serial Doppler measurements in the first few days of life is that of impaired cerebrovascular autoregulation following HII.[58–62] Preterm infants who otherwise would be able regionally to autoregulate vasomotor tone and vascular cross-sectional area transiently lose these autonomic functions, particularly in watershed regions such as found in the periventricular white matter.[63] The loss of autoregulation allows for pressure-passive flow in which the vascular bed is unable appropriately to constrict in response to increases in mean systemic arterial pressure or dilate in response to falls in mean arterial pressure. Pressure-passive flow in preterm infants with normal mean arterial pressures causes a significant rise in peak velocity within the thalamostriate vessels (the surrogate markers of the perfusion of the periventricular white matter in preterm infants) and the vascular bed cross-sectional area.[64] Both these findings are associated with an increased risk for the development of intracranial hemorrhage and periventricular leukomalacia (PVL).

Doppler studies have also been used to examine the effects of therapies on neonatal CBF.[65–68] One study suggested that sampling from high-lying umbilical arterial catheters had a more adverse effect on CBF velocity compared to sampling from low-lying ones[69] (although it should be pointed out that no significant differences in IVH rate were found in large prospective randomized trials examining umbilical arterial catheter positioning[70]).

Germinal matrix and intraventricular hemorrhage

The most common use of neurosonography in the neonatal intensive care unit is to detect the presence and evolution of ICH, especially in the premature newborn.[1,19,71,72] The incidence of ICH varies most significantly with gestational age and birth weight. Extremely low-birth-weight (ELBW) newborns (gestational age <27 weeks, birth weight <750 g) are estimated to have ICH at a rate of 10–30 per 100 surviving newborns.[1–3] The incidence of ICH decreases with gestational age, and is quite rare in newborns greater than 32 weeks' gestational age or 1500 g.

The precise mechanisms leading to neonatal ICH remain ill defined. It is generally felt however that the premature brain is at highest risk for ICH for a variety of factors associated with mild or subclinical partial perinatal asphyxia, that is, a transient decrease but not complete cessation of CBF.[73,74] Predisposing factors include: relatively late development of the end-arterial circulation during the last trimester; relatively decreased mesenchymal support for this vascular bed, particularly in the region of the germinal matrix (which normally does not completely involute until after the 33rd week of gestation); and decreased autoregulation of CBF, with the extremely premature infant having virtual "passive-pressure" CBF. The rare term newborn with ICH usually has some predisposing factor such as a history of profound asphyxia (complete or near-complete temporary cessation of CBF) or coagulation abnormalities. These coagulopathies may be intrinsic or secondary to anticoagulation therapy such as that used during ECMO.[6]

The most widely used classification system for ICH is that originally described by Papile et al.[71] consisting of four grades of hemorrhage of increasing clinical severity.

1. Grade 1 is sometimes referred to as a germinal matrix or subependymal hemorrhage. This subset of ICH is seen on neurosonography as an abnormally increased number of echoes in the caudothalamic groove (i.e., notch) in the expected location of the germinal matrix. Normally the germinal matrix echoes taper down smoothly as they

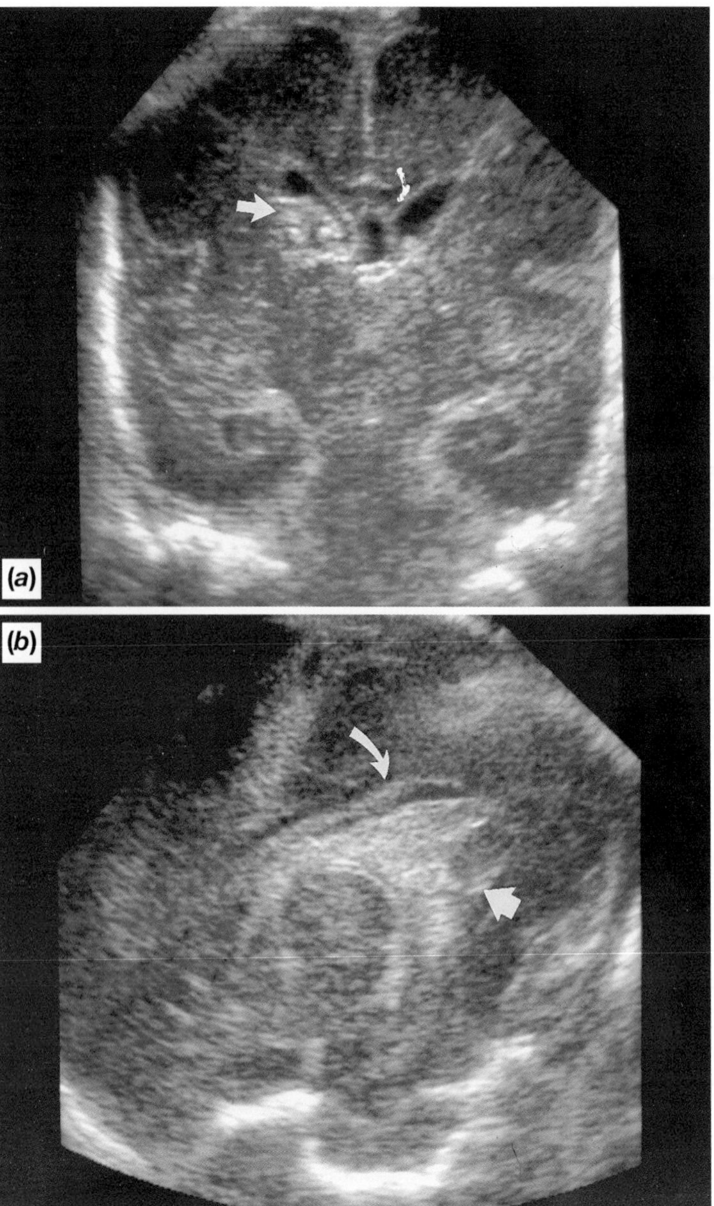

Figure 22.1 Right-sided grade 2 germinal matrix hemorrhage (GMH)/intraventricular hemorrhage (IVH) in a preterm infant on day 3 of life. (*a*) Coronal view obtained via the anterior fontanel shows a focal GMH seen as a focal globular (bulbous) increased echogenicity (arrow) in the region of the caudothalamic groove. (*b*) Sagittal posterior fontanel view demonstrating clot (short arrow) filling the occipital horn posterior to the calar avis (curved arrow), the normal limit to the posterior portion of the choroid plexus. This view also confirms the presence of GMH seen as an abnormal bulbous region of increased echogenicity in the expected location of the germinal matrix in the region of the caudothalamic groove. Note the lack of normal tapering of the germinal matrix as it courses anteriorly in the caudothalamic groove, suggesting the correct diagnosis of GMH.

course anteriorly in the caudothalamic groove. The germinal matrix is also never located anterior to the foramen of Monro. Echoes seen anterior to the foramen of Monro without tapering as they course anteriorly in the caudothalamic groove indicate a germinal matrix hemorrhage.

2. Grade 2 (Figure 22.1) describes an extension of a germinal matrix/subependymal hemorrhage into the ventricles, without any ventricular enlargement. The detection of IVH which is echogenic in the first several days after a bleed can be easily confused with normal choroid plexus (which normally can be amorphous with multiple echogenic lumps). The observation of echogenic material within the occipital horn (posterior to the calcar avis) is diagnostic of IVH, as the choroid plexus does not extend into the occipital lobe. The observation of an echogenic blood–CSF fluid level with the ventricular system is also diagnostic of IVH. The rare primary choroid plexus bleeds, 95% of which occur in full-term neonates, are considered as grade 2 bleeds (benign clinical significance) for purposes of prognostication. An ancillary sign of IVH is the presence of a hyperechoic thickened ependyma (so-called "ependymitis") which is a subacute reaction to intraventricular blood products occurring 3–5 days after a bleed and lasting several weeks.[75] This sign may be useful to diagnose posthemorrhagic hydrocephalus (PHH) in a patient with a long delay between birth and the first scan in which the original site of hemorrhage or the intraventricular blood component may have become isoechoic or completely reabsorbed.
3. Grade 3 (Figure 22.2) consists of a germinal matrix hemorrhage that extends into the ventricles with ventriculomegaly. It must be emphasized that IVH without accompanying hydrocephalus within the first 24 h after detection is classified as grade 2, even if the infant later develops PHH, as shown in Figures 22.2*c* and *d*.
4. Grade 4 (Figure 22.3) describes a germinal matrix hemorrhage that dissects and extends into the adjacent brain parenchyma, irrespective of the presence or absence of IVH. It is also referred to as an intraparenchymal hemorrhage (IPH) when found elsewhere in the parenchyma. Hemorrhage extending into the periventricular white matter in association with an ipsilateral GMH/IVH has been classified as periventricular hemorrhagic venous infarction (PHVI).

It is useful to note that 70% of all germinal matrix hemorrhages in premature infants happen by days 3 and 4 of life and that 90% of all germinal matrix hemorrhages occur within 1 week.[1,76] Once diagnosed, 90% of germinal matrix hemorrhages do not progress in severity after 24 h. Bleeds occurring 1 week after birth are invariably grade 1–2 and have minor-to-no clinical significance.

The final reading of a neurosonographic study for ICH should include narrative commentary beyond a specific grading, including description of both hemispheres as well as comparison to previous studies. For grade 2 ICH, it may be helpful to know how much volume of the ventricles is occupied by blood. Similarly, grade 3 ICH may have minimal-to-massive ventriculomegaly. Severe ventriculomegaly may require surgical intervention and placement of a ventricular shunt.

As stated previously, the severity of ICH, as reflected by the Papile or other grading systems, in general correlates with increasing risk of long-term neurodevelopmental abnormalities.[12,77–80] Premature infants with grade 1 and 2 germinal matrix hemorrhages are at a minimally increased risk of neurodevelopmental abnormalities compared to preterm neonates of the same size and gestation (a risk which is still higher than that of term newborns). Grade 3 ICH has a greater risk for central nervous system sequelae when the degree of hydrocephalus requires surgical drainage or shunting. Grade 4 ICH that is extensive or is found bilaterally has the most guarded prognosis for normal neurodevelopmental outcome.

Recommendations for timing for US in high-risk very-low-birth-weight (VLBW) newborns are quite varied and depend greatly upon the particular institution and clinical situation. If ICH is to occur, it will usually start within the first 24–72 h of life. Some clinicians suggest the first examination to be at 3–5

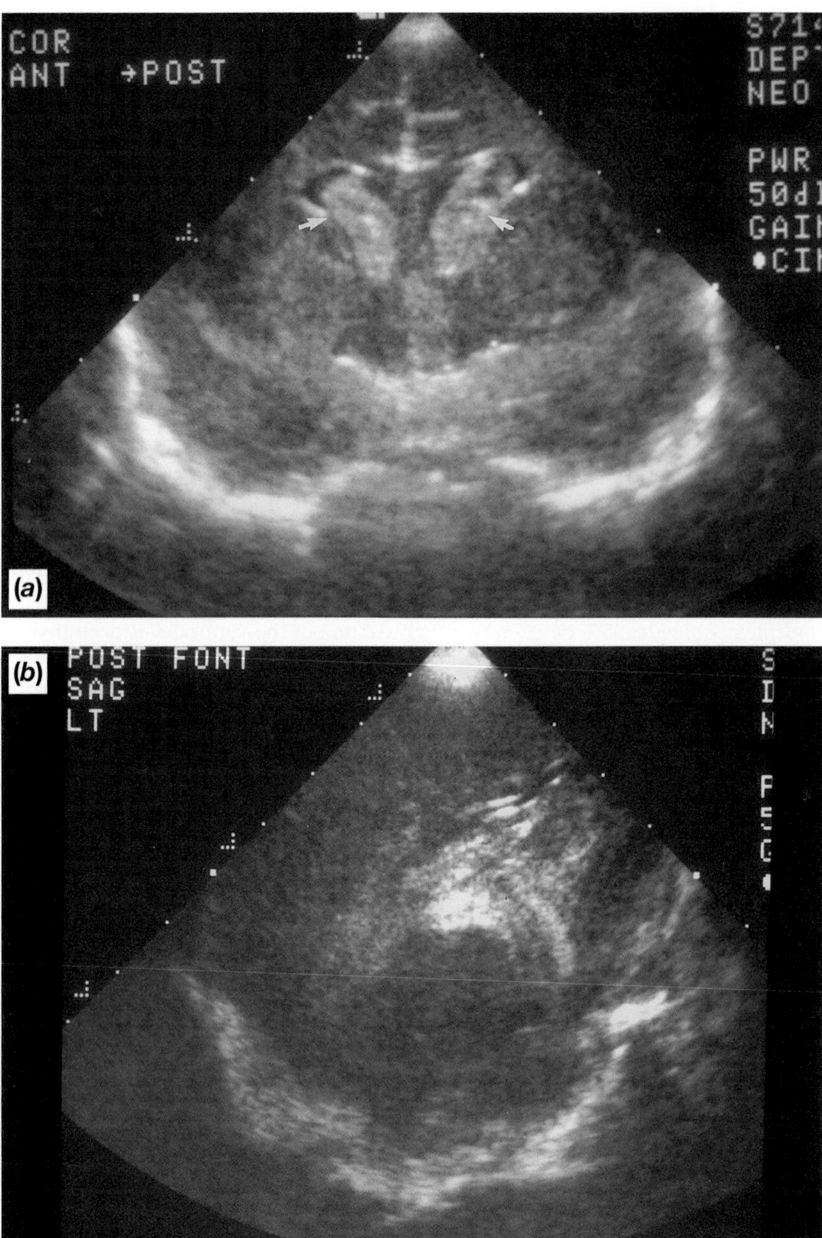

Figure 22.2 Bilateral grade 3 germinal matrix hemorrhage (GMH)/intraventricular hemorrhage (IVH) 3 and 10 days after birth. (*a*) coronal anterior fontanel and (*b*) posterior fontanel views on day 3 of life showing massive bilateral echogenic GMH and IVH completely filling the lateral and third ventricles with gross ventricular dilation. On day 10 of life (*c*) coronal anterior fontanel and

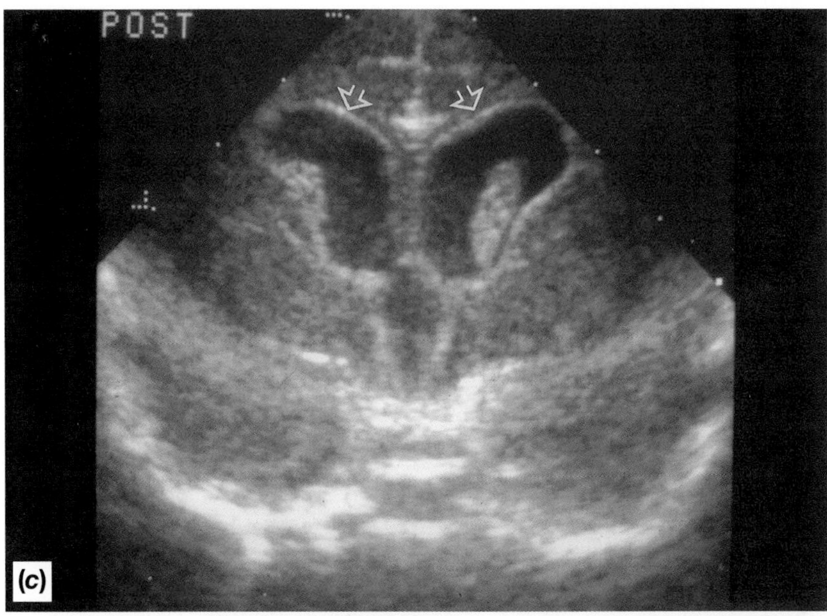

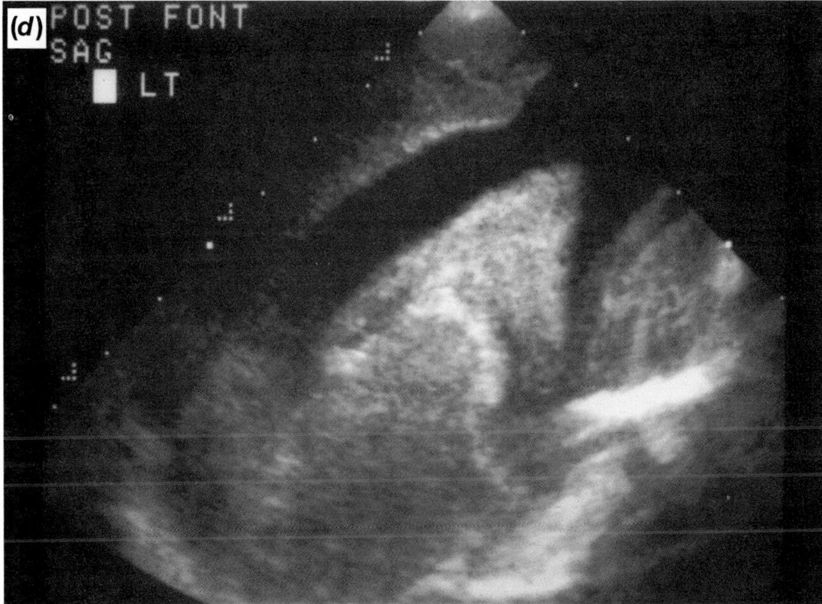

(*d*) sagittal posterior fontanel views show progressive posthemorrhagic hydrocephalus with partial involution of intraventricular clot. There has also been development of posthemorrhagic-induced ependymitis seen as increased echogenicity of the wall of the lateral ventricles.

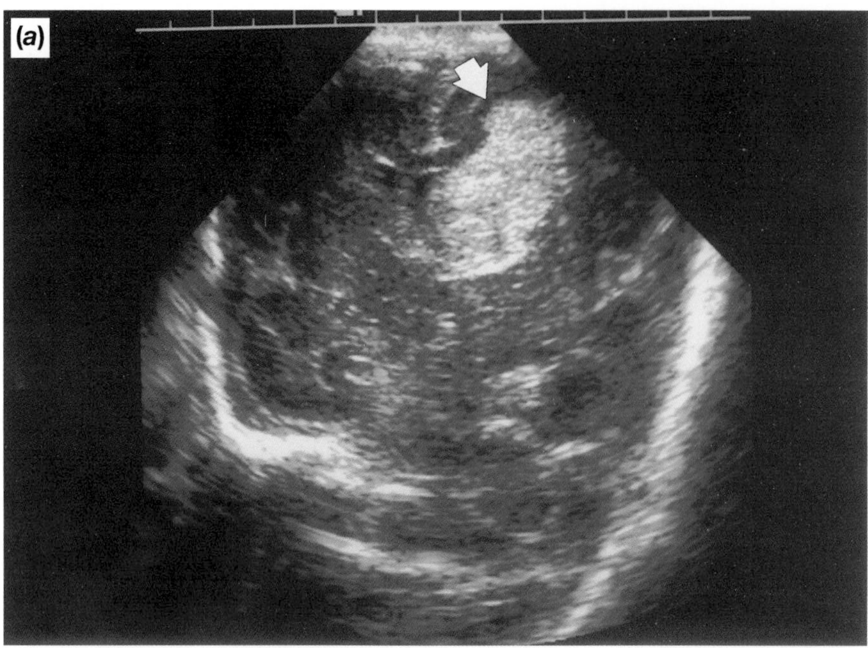

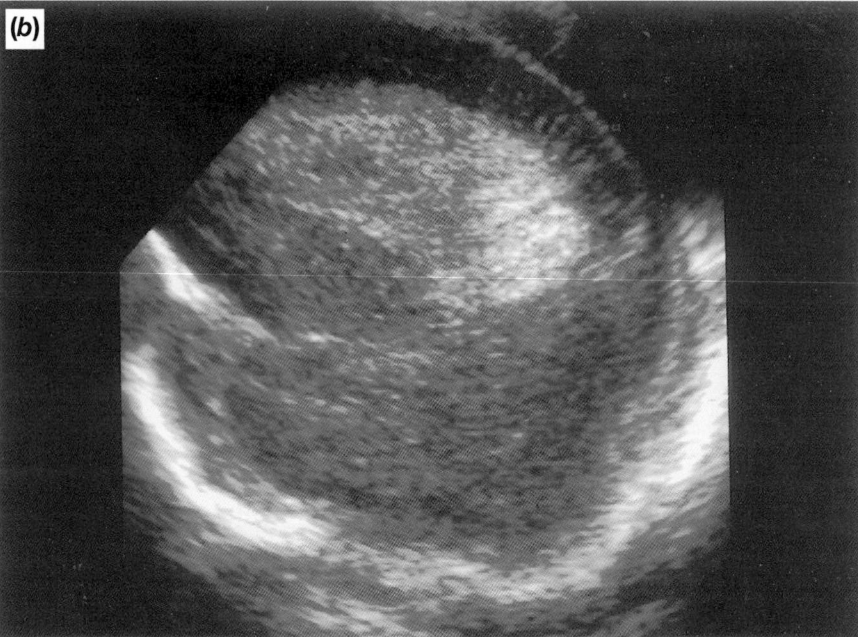

Figure 22.3 Grade 4 germinal matrix hemorrhage (GMH) on day 2 of life. (*a*) Coronal and (*b*) sagittal views through the anterior fontanel demonstrate a large echogenic region with mass effect in the region of the left caudothalamic groove with direct extension into the adjacent brain parenchyma (arrow).

days of life; others recommend deferring until 7–10 days. If such an exam were negative for ICH, it would be unlikely to find hemorrhage thereafter. Although there are no definitive data about the extension of ICH that theoretically could be caused by indometacin's effects on platelets, some medical centers use early neurosonography to aid in the decision between medical versus surgical intervention for patent ductus arteriosus (PDA). It has also been recommended to obtain a final neurosonogram closer to discharge, e.g., at 34–36 weeks' gestation, to look not only for ICH but also for PVL. However, recent studies suggest that MRI may be a more sensitive and specific measure of PVL and white-matter injury in premature infants, particularly just prior to discharge when there is substantially more myelinization than at birth.

Clinical circumstances may play an important role in the timing of neurosonography. In the very unstable premature infant, especially one with an unexplained drop in hematocrit, acidosis, or change in neurological status, an earlier study may be indicated. The presence of severe ICH may then be incorporated in decisions about the prolongation or escalation of intensive care support. If an initial neurosonogram has detected IVH, serial exams may be performed every 1–2 weeks until the IVH is felt to be stable.

Periventricular leukomalacia

PVL describes a characteristic pattern of white-matter ischemic injury (or infarction) found predominantly in premature newborns and is believed to be a response to partial perinatal asphyxia.[63,77–82] A temporary reduction of CBF first affects the watershed zone of end-artery distributions between the lenticulostriate arteries and the long deep penetrating arteries of the middle cerebral artery. Anatomically this watershed zone corresponds to the superolateral border of periventricular white matter. There is an association of PVL with ICH, which increases with more severe degrees of ICH. However, PVL can arise without ICH, and vice versa. On neurosonography PVL initially presents as numerous foci of increased periventricular echogenicity adjacent to the superolateral aspect of the ventricles which become evident within the first several days after the instigating insult (Figure 22.4). Classically these periventricular regions undergo cystic degeneration (or necrosis) over the next 2–3 weeks, resulting in a "Swiss cheese" pattern of white-matter loss that can be readily detected with neurosonography. PVL can also have a hemorrhagic component that is thought to represent more severe injury. The evolution of PVL can also be noncystic, manifested primarily by the irregular loss of the periventricular white matter with irregular ventricular dilation (Figure 22.5). This form of PVL is more difficult to detect with neurosonographic examination. After 2–3 months both cystic and noncystic PVL are characterized by variable degrees of ventricular dilation and the irregular scalloping of the ventricular walls (Figure 22.6). At 2–4 months MRI is the modality of choice for the detection of PVL. In affected infants MRI can detect not only the morphologic changes secondary to PVL but abnormal tissue signals within the periventricular white matter that will be discussed later on in this chapter.[83]

It is important to note however that even severe cystic PVL can have a normal sonographic appearance in the first week of life (Figure 22.7). Furthermore increased periventricular echogenicity seen in the first week of life can be due to artifact. Cystic PVL can also be seen in the first week of life presumably from in utero HII several weeks prior to birth (Figure 22.8).

PVL has been distinguished from PHVI by several investigators.[78,84] These studies note that PVL and PHVI can have a similar geographic distribution but subtle differences in the evolution of lesion echogenicity. PVL usually has echodensities that evolve into multiple smaller cysts that do not communicate with the lateral ventricle. Bass et al.[78] used these characteristics to classify 77% of white-matter lesions into either PVL or PVHI, with only 11% having overlapping features, with an equally small subgroup having echodensities without evolving cystic changes. Neurodevelopmental deficits were observed in all groups; however those patients with

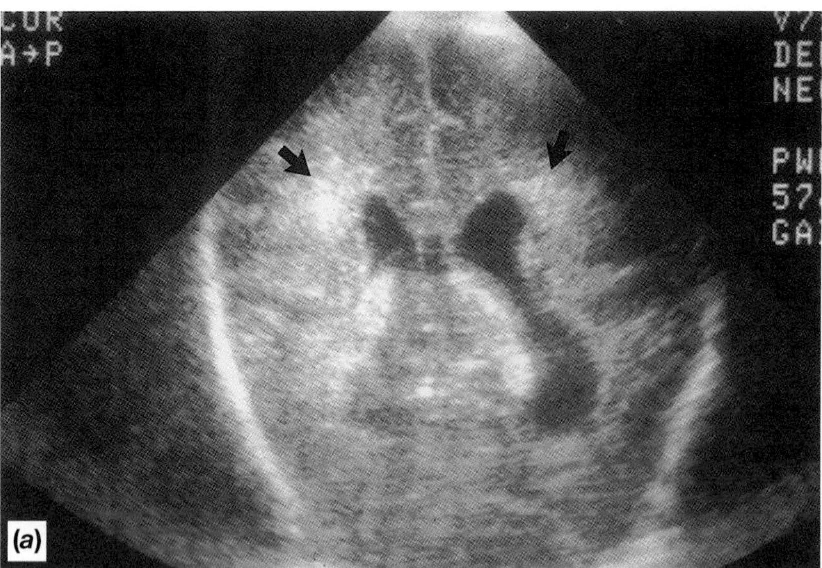

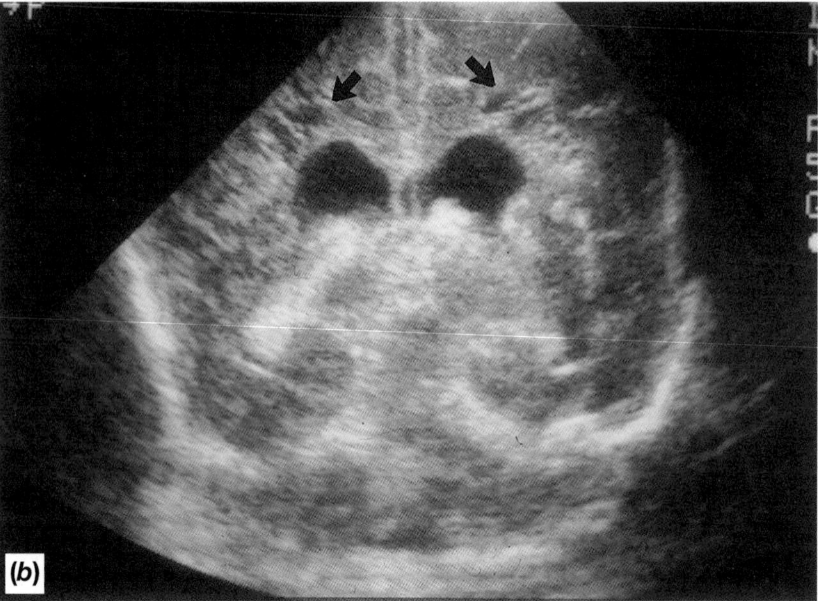

Figure 22.4 Periventricular leukomalacia seen in week 1 and 4 of life. Coronal views through the anterior fontanel of the choroid plexus posteriorly in (*a*) week 1 and (*b*) week 4 after birth. Note the abnormally increased echogenicity in the periventricular white matter (arrows) in week 1 evolving into areas of cystic degeneration at the same location in week 4 (arrows). There is also development of mild ventriculomegaly due to the diffuse loss of white matter. Axial T1-weighted magnetic resonance images through (*c*) the frontal and occipital horns and (*d*) the superior aspect of the lateral ventricles showing marked cystic periventricular leukomalacia (arrows) and ventriculomegaly 2 months after birth.

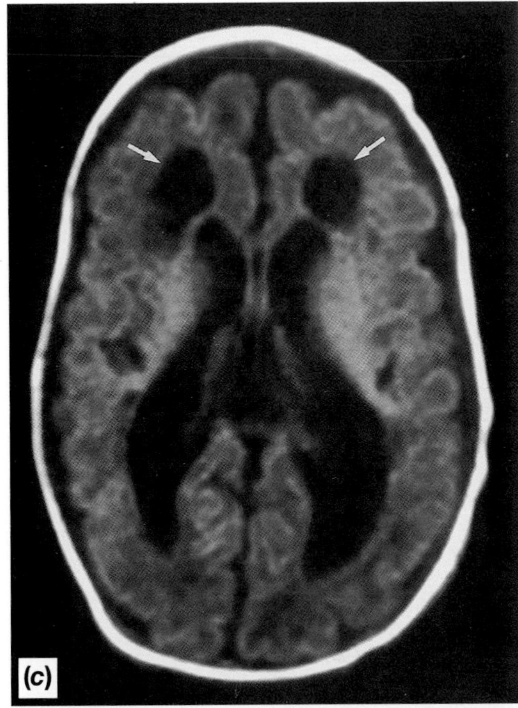

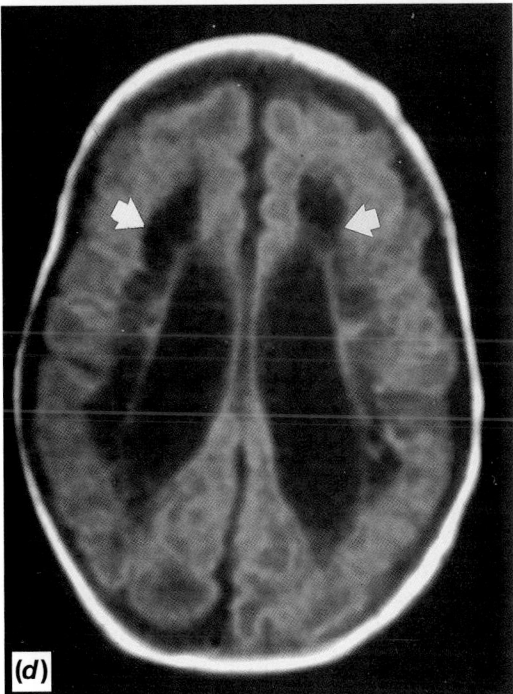

PVHI had a normal mean developmental quotient. One large series found PVL in 3.2% of infants with birth weights less than 1500 g, with most affected patients having benign clinical courses without identified risk factors for central nervous system insult.

Profound perinatal asphyxia/hypoxic–ischemic injury

HII in neonates may cause a wide range of central nervous system injury that can be seen by neurosonography. In both the preterm and term newborn profound perinatal asphyxia can initially lead to global ischemia with generalized cerebral edema seen sonographically as diffusely increased echogenicity throughout the brain with small, slit-like ventricles and poor gray–white-matter differentiation[46] (Figure 22.9). Care must be taken however not to diagnose generalized cerebral edema based solely on the observation of slit-like ventricles in the absence of increased brain echogenicity and poor gray–white-matter differentiation, as this finding can be seen in up to one-third of normal neonates.[85] Also of note, diffusely increased brain echogenicity can be quite subtle, particularly within the first 24 h after an ischemic insult, and difficult to differentiate from common artifacts due to high gain settings or poor probe-scalp contact. In this setting CT may be the modality of choice as it can be done rapidly and has a superior ability to distinguish normal and ischemic tissue[16,19] (Figure 22.10).

Profound perinatal asphyxia can also selectively affect the most metabolically active parts of the brain, including the basil ganglia, posterolateral thalami, and hippocampal regions, paradoxically sparing the less active cortical gray matter.[17] At neurosonography there is increased echogenicity of these deep structures, usually in a symmetric distribution[86] (Figure 22.11). Unfortunately, US can be quite insensitive to the presence of brainstem and basil ganglia ischemia and infarction despite the presence of severe neurologic disabilities. MRI, because of its superior tissue characterization, is more sensitive, though both modalities may detect

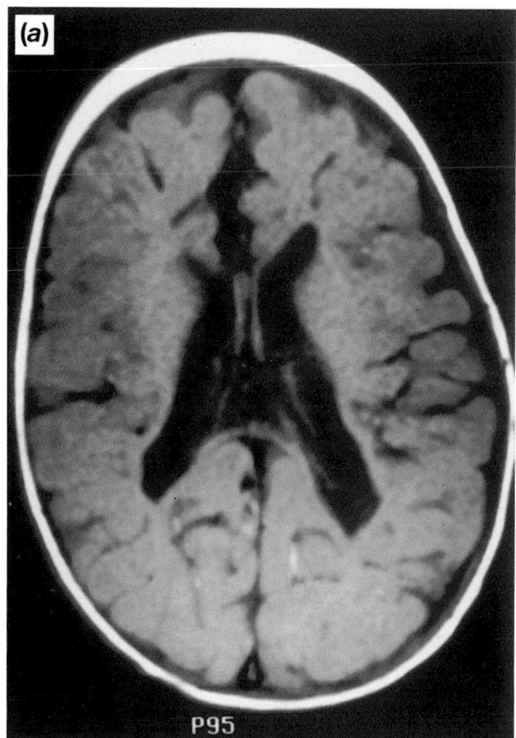

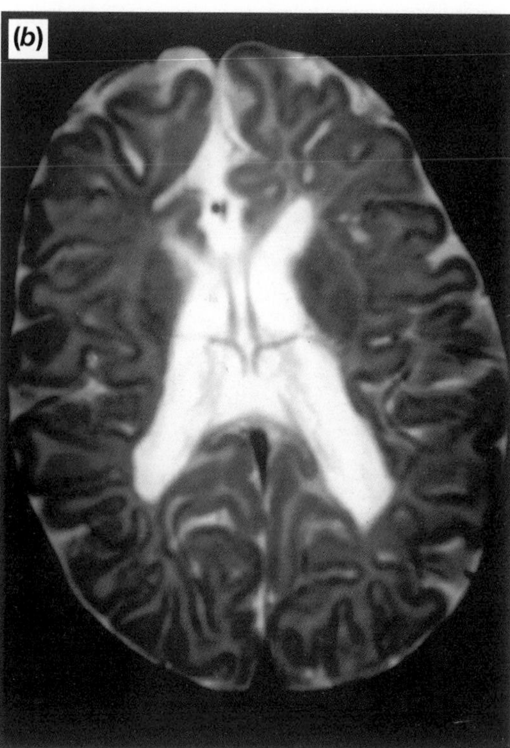

Figure 22.5 Noncystic periventricular leukomalacia 6 months after birth. (*a*) Axial T1-weighted and corresponding (*b*) T2-weighted magnetic resonance images through the lateral ventricles. Note the lack of cystic degeneration in the markedly irregularly thinned periventricular white matter. This marked irregular loss of white matter causes a scalloped appearance to the ventricle walls and moderate ventriculomegaly, and allows the cortical gray matter to come into abnormally close contact with the walls of the lateral ventricles.

less than 50% of these injuries in some series (Figure 22.12).

Severe HII has also been associated with focal IPH. At neurosonography IPH is seen as a highly echogenic lesion with local mass effect and shift of adjacent structures (Figure 22.13). IPH that infiltrates normal structures with poorly defined borders or without definite mass effect can be quite difficult to distinguish from sites of ischemic injury or infarction that also appear echogenic on US (Figure 22.14). In this situation CT or MR can readily differentiate IPH from ischemic injury and infarction.[16,19]

Term infants suffering from partial perinatal asphyxia with more mature deep centrifugal arterial circulation as compared with preterm infants tend to develop watershed ischemia/infarction in the subcortical white matter.[9] Again, CT and MRI are superior for the detection of ischemic lesions, particularly adjacent to the lateral convexities of the brain that are difficult to visualize with US (Figure 22.15).

Given the above it is important to emphasize that HII may lead to severe neurologic injury without any neurosonographic findings. At least one recent study of over 100 asphyxiated newborns was unable to correlate neonatal US findings with their outcome at 1 year of age.[77] A recent prospective study found both CT and MRI vastly superior to US for the detec-

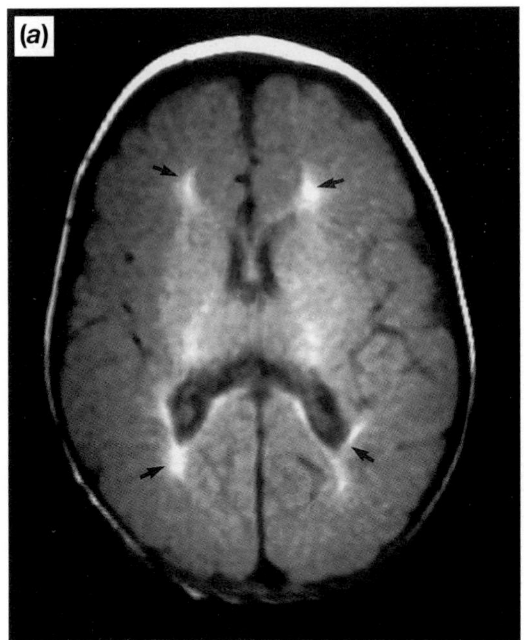

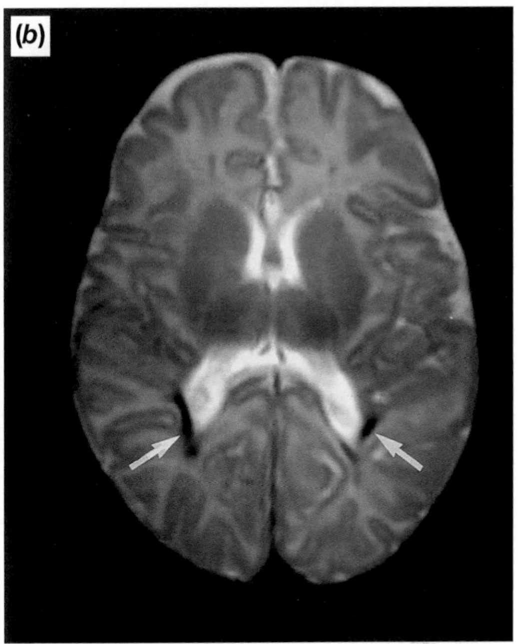

Figure 22.6 Subacute white-matter magnetic resonance (MR) signal changes with periventricular leukomalacia (PVL) 2 months after birth. (*a*) Axial T1-weighted and corresponding (*b*) T2-weighted MR images through the lateral ventricles. Note that the abnormally increased T1 signal in the periventricular white matter (arrows) in (*a*) and the abnormally low T2-weighted signal seen in the periventricular white matter of the occipital horns (arrows) is due to hemosiderin deposits that can sometimes be seen with the subacute stages of PVL.

tion of HII, particularly in the cortical and subcortical gray matter of the lateral cerebral convexities, the most difficult regions to examine adequately by ultrasound, especially via the anterior fontanel approach.[19] Whether infants should be screened with CT or MRI as opposed to US acutely following an episode of suspected HII is uncertain and is dependent on scan availability, the medical stability of the patient, and ultimately on cost–benefit analyses, which are beyond the scope of this chapter.

Limitations

As mentioned above, despite its advantages of being noninvasive and portable, neurosonography has technical considerations that limit clinical correlation and may require alternative neuroimaging modalities. More superficial structures beneath the skull, particularly adjacent to the lateral cerebral convexities, have limited resolution; for example, subarachnoid hemorrhage (SAH) is routinely missed on US. However, massive SAH may show up as prominent, thickened echogenicity within the normally anechoic subarachnoid space with intact bridging veins seen at color or power Doppler examination. Deeper structures of the brain, including the basal ganglia and brainstem, are generally less well seen by neurosonography as compared to more superficial structures due to losses of beam energy and scatter effects in the soft tissues. Supplemental views of these deep structures through the posterior and posterior-lateral fontanels may partially alleviate this difficulty, as there is less soft tissue that needs to be penetrated by the sound beam with

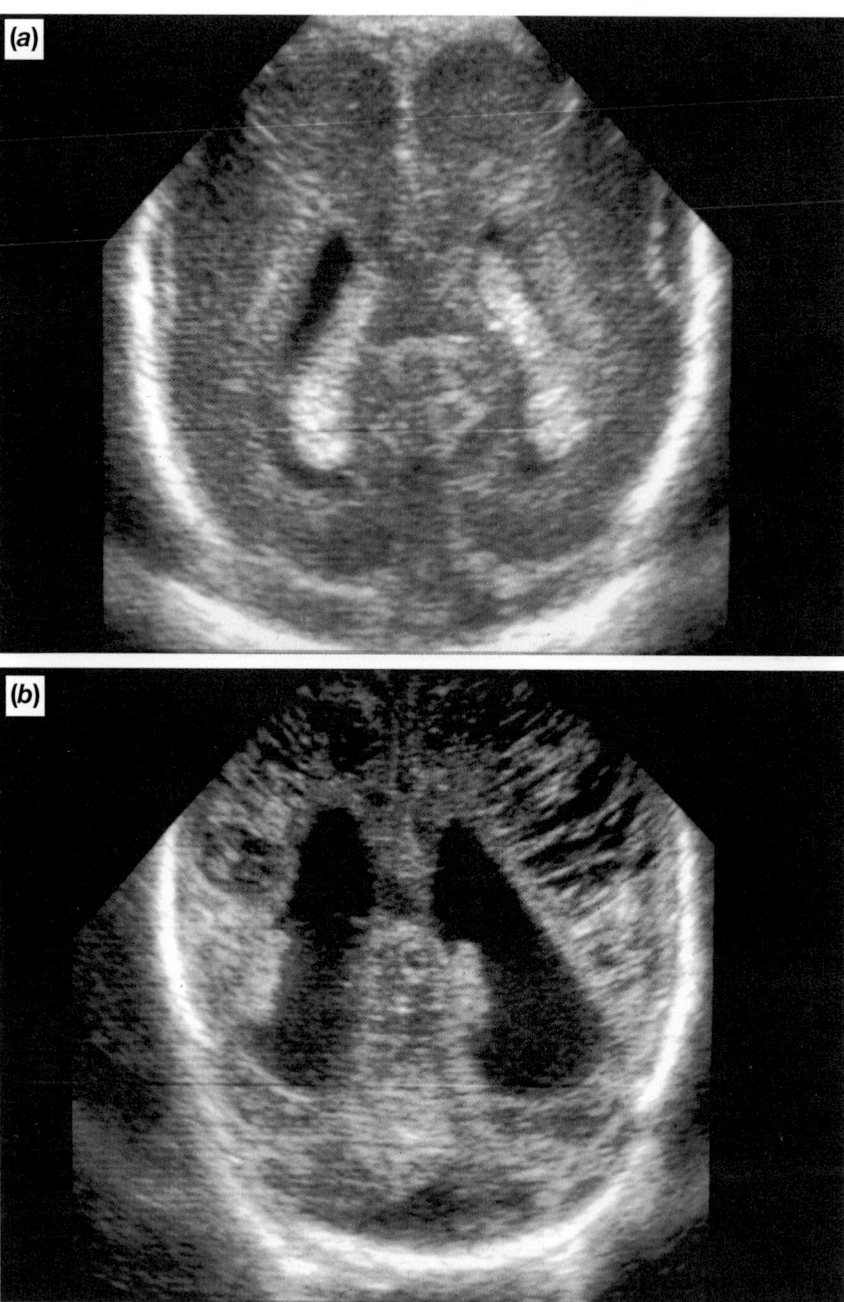

Figure 22.7 Massive cystic degeneration due to periventricular leukomalacia. Coronal views through the anterior fontanel at (*a*) week 1 and (*b*) 3 weeks after birth. All ultrasound exams in the first week of life were normal, without evidence of abnormally increased periventricular white-matter echogenicity. At week 3 there has been massive cystic degeneration, i.e., "Swiss cheese appearance," with marked ventriculomegaly due to white-matter loss.

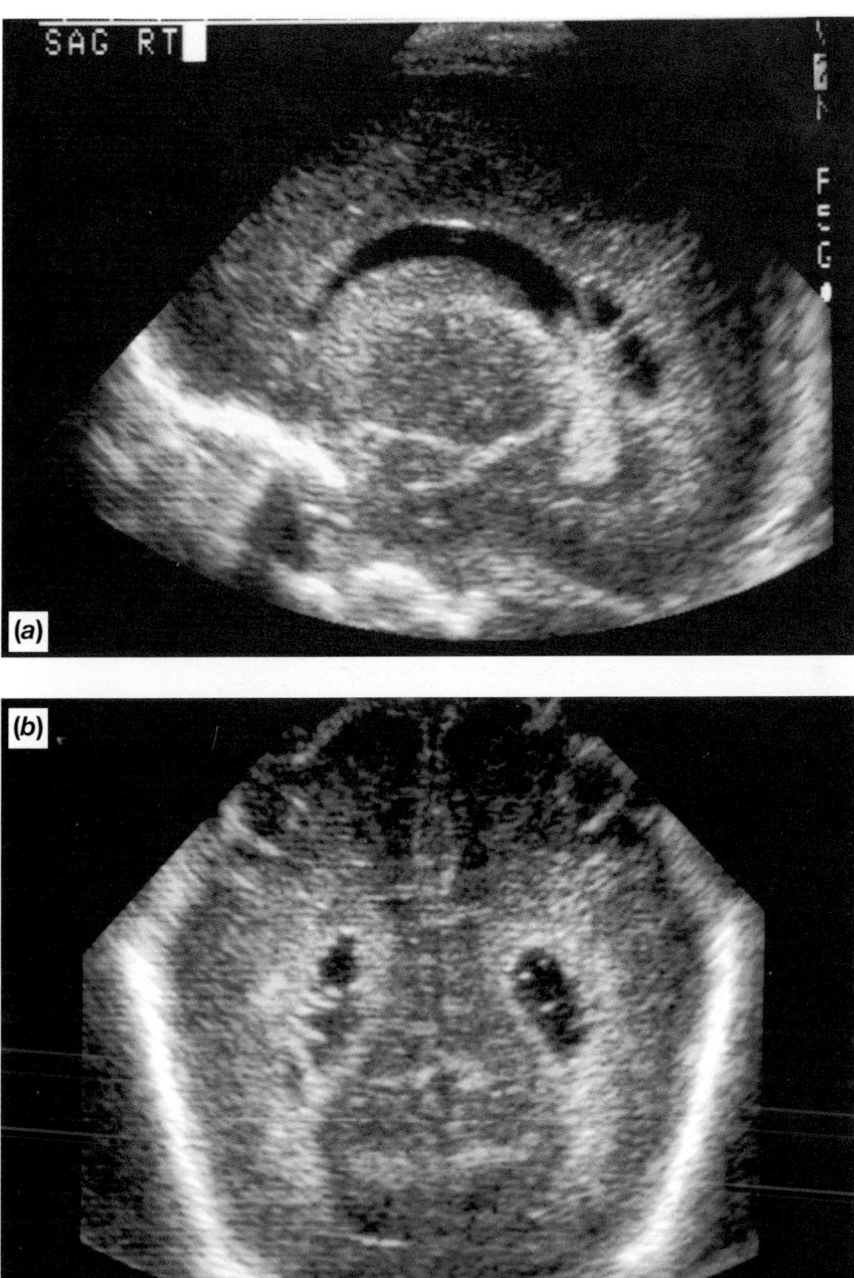

Figure 22.8 Cystic changes of periventricular leukomalacia (PVL) at birth. (*a*) Sagittal and (*b*) coronal views through the anterior fontanel at day 1 of life. There are bilateral cystic changes of the parietal-occipital periventricular white matter consistent with an uretero-PVL event occurring several weeks prior to birth.

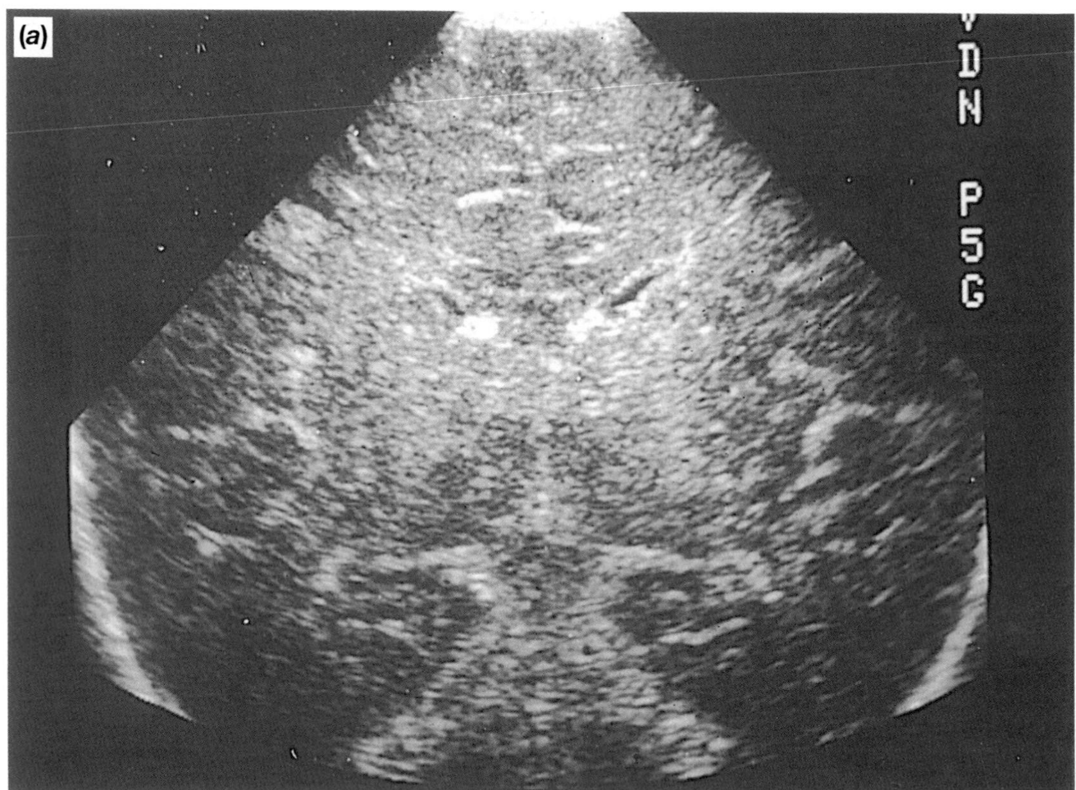

Figure 22.9 Global cerebral ischemia seen on ultrasound and computed tomography (CT). (*a*) Anterior fontanel coronal view though the midbrain showing diffusely increased echogenicity of the cerebral central gray and white matter on day 2 after birth. (*b*) Axial CT scan through the midbrain showing poor cortical and central gray–white-matter differentiation and diffusely low attenuation consistent with severe cerebral edema on day 3 of life.

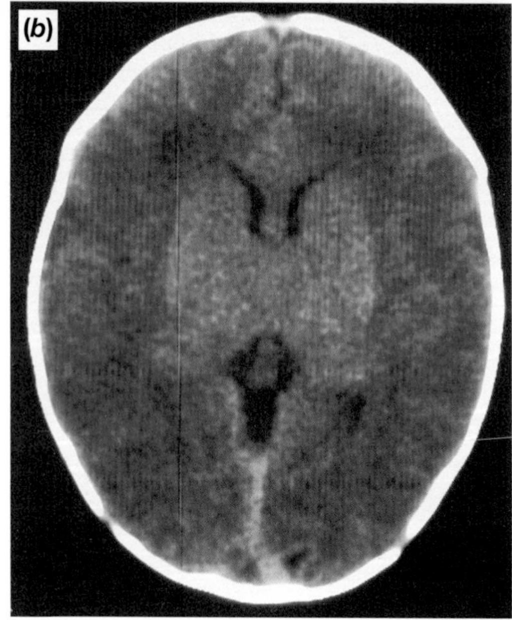

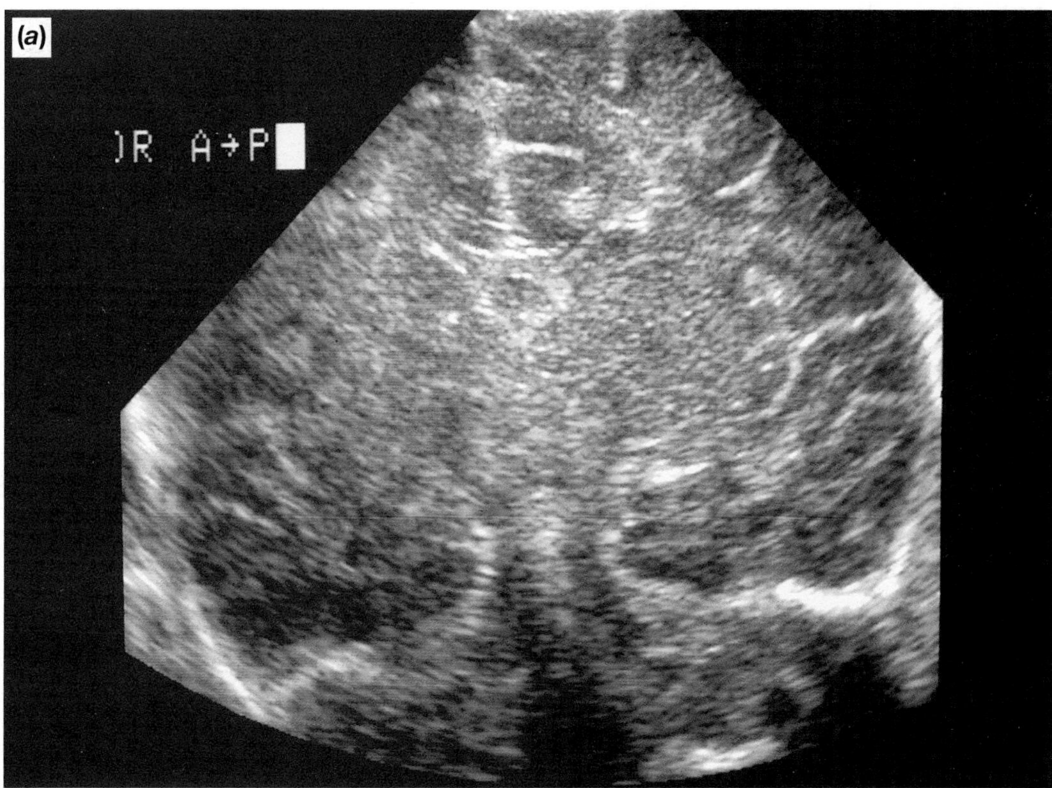

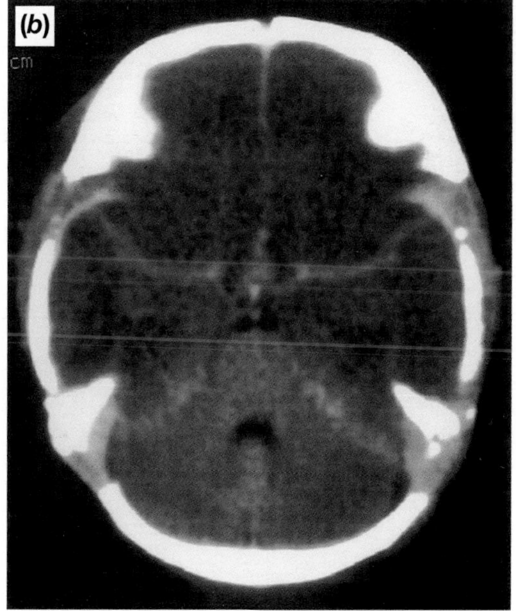

Figure 22.10 Ultrasound and computed tomography (CT) images of early diffuse cerebral edema 12 h after birth in a term infant with seizures. (*a*) Anterior fontanel coronal view though the midbrain showing subtle questionably increased diffuse echogenicity 12 h after birth. (*b*) Axial CT scan 1 h later showing no cortical and central gray–white-matter differentiation and starkly low cerebral attenuation consistent with severe cerebral edema. Note the normal attenuation of the cerebellum and brainstem consistent with relative sparing of these structures.

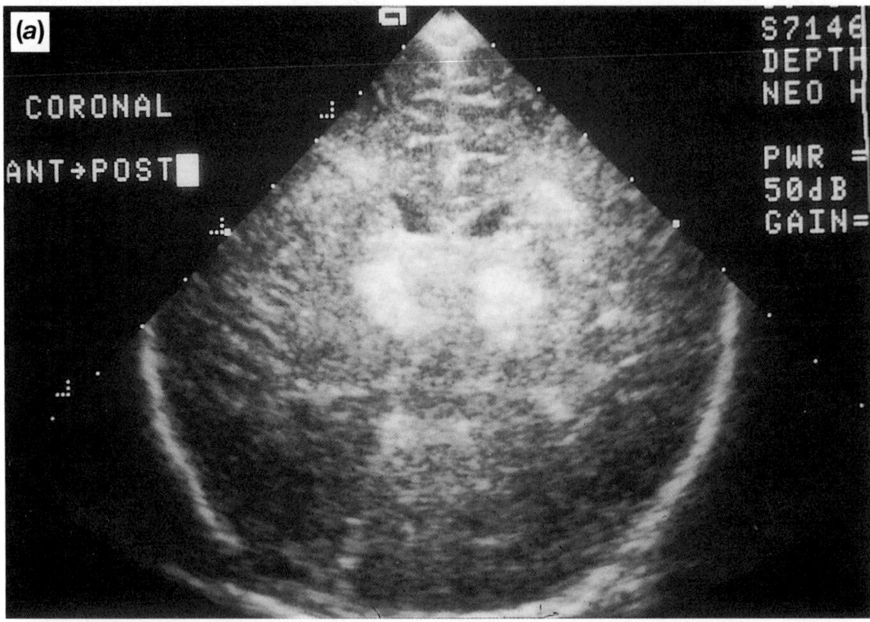

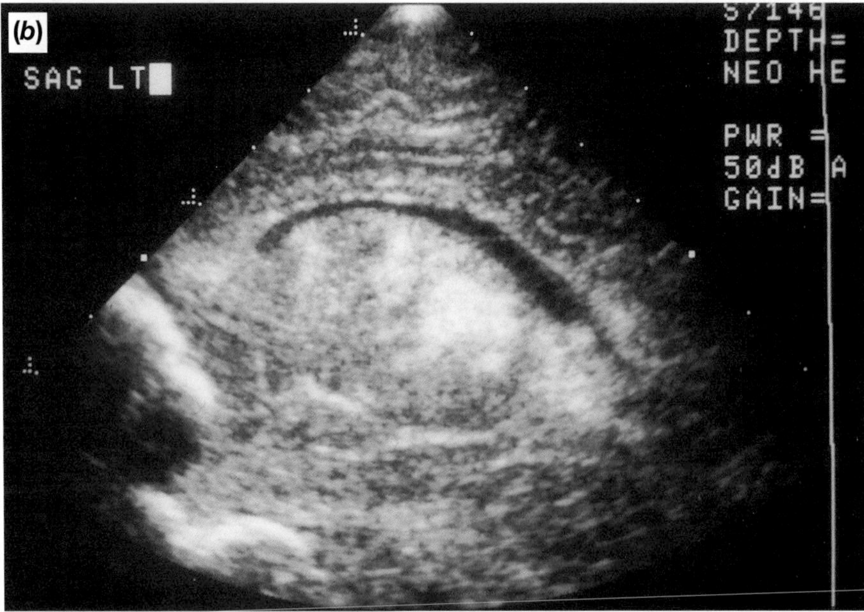

Figure 22.11 Ultrasound images of basal ganglia/thalamic ischemia–infarction. (*a*) Coronal and (*b*) sagittal views through the anterior fontanel demonstrating patchy markedly echogenic regions in the basal ganglia and thalami bilaterally, consistent with profound perinatal asphyxia.

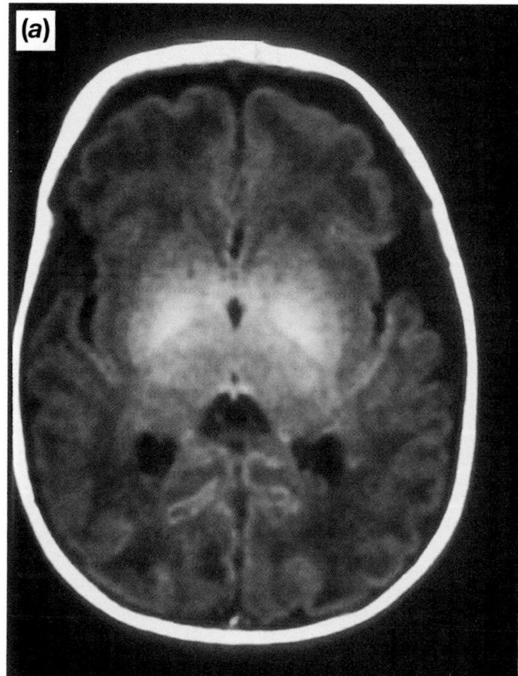

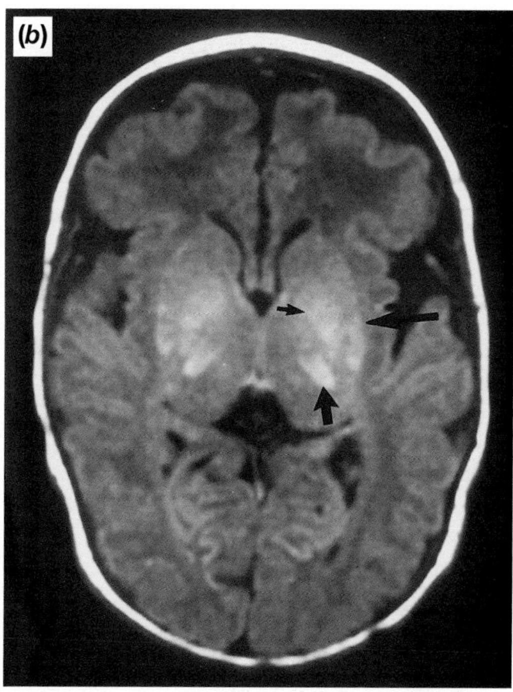

Figure 22.12 Profound perinatal asphyxia on magnetic resonance (MR). (*a*) Axial T1-weighted MR image in a normal month-old preterm infant showing normal symmetrically increased T1-weighted signal of myelinated white matter of the posterior limb of the internal capsule. Note that the rest of the white matter has not undergone myelinization at this stage of neurodevelopment. (*b*) Axial T1-weighted MR image of an infant suffering from profound perinatal asphyxia showing abnormally symmetrically increased T1-weighted signal of the putamen (arrow), globus pallidus, and posterior-lateral thalamus (small arrow) bilaterally. Note that the signal of these structures is greater than that of the normal myelinization of the posterior limb of the internal capsule.

these approaches (Figure 22.16). In addition, US in general has poorer tissue characterization capabilities as compared with CT or MRI as discussed earlier in this chapter (Figure 22.17). In the instance of IPH vs severe focal infarction, US will show an echogenic lesion with mass effect. CT or MRI however can easily distinguish IPH from the focal cerebral edema associated with ischemia or infarction. US is also surprisingly insensitive with respect to global and brainstem ischemia and focal cerebral infarction within the first 24–48 h after an HII. CT and MRI are vastly superior to US for the visualization of ischemia/infarction in this time period. CT and MRI are also superior in the follow-up of the complications of severe ischemia, such as transtentorial herniation (and other types of shifts due to massive edema), white- and gray-matter loss, etc. As mentioned earlier, several authors have tried to determine the relative accuracy of US findings compared to neurodevelopmental outcome or neuropathology. US findings that include significant bilateral periventricular changes have the greatest correlation with adverse neurologic outcome, i.e., cerebral palsy. In one study comparing US results to postmortem neuropathology, US correctly identified the primary central nervous system insult in only 59% of patients, sometimes due to imaging timing.[87] However, in nearly 25% of these study patients, US did not find the primary injury. Not every US abnormality represents significant neurological injury and

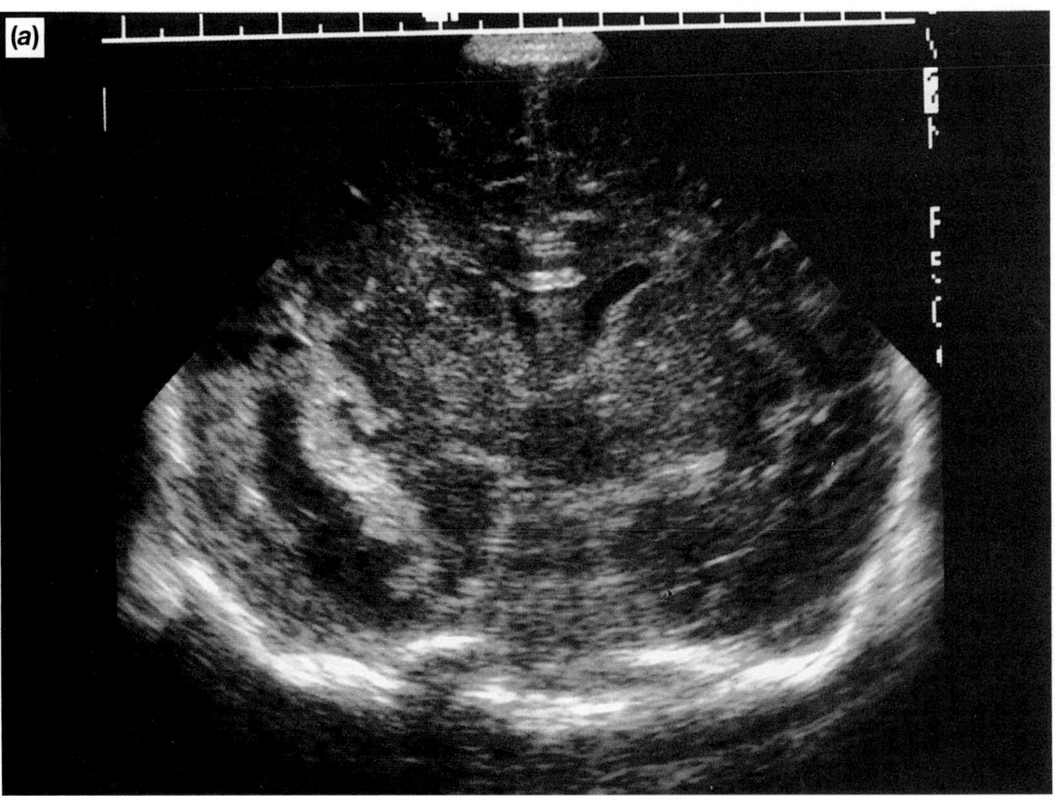

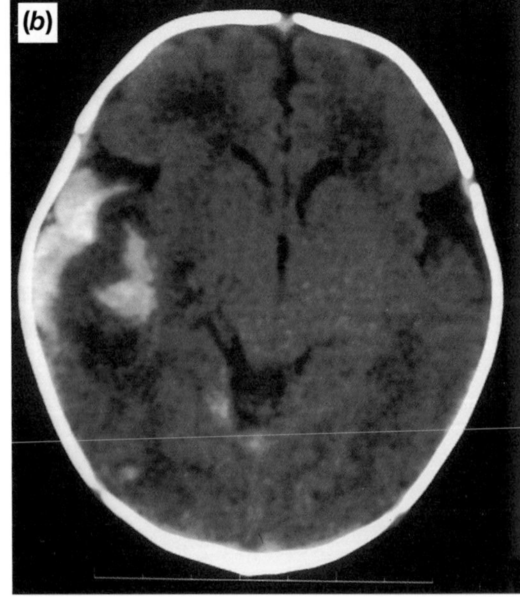

Figure 22.13 Right temporal lobe intraparenchymal hemorrhage ultrasound (IPH). (*a*) Coronal ultrasound view through the anterior fontanel showing a mixed echogenic intraparenchymal lesion of the right temporal lobe with mass effect and subarachnoid hemorrhage. (*b*) Axial computed tomography scan showing the same lesion with mixed attenuation consistent with IPH and surrounding edema. High-attenuation (clotted) blood is also seen in the subarachnoid space adjacent to the anterior portion of the right temporal lobe.

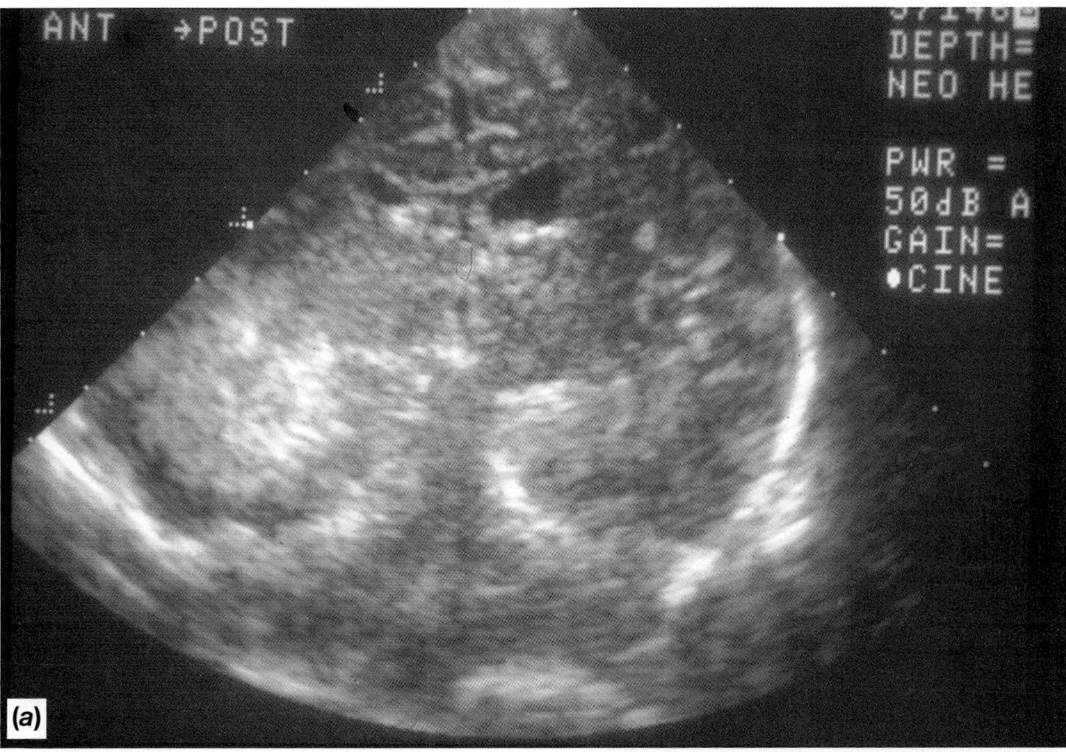

Figure 22.14 Massive bilateral temporal-occipital intraparenchymal hemorrhage (IPH). (*a*) Coronal ultrasound images obtained through the anterior fontanel showing right greater than left echogenic temporal lobe lesions. It is difficult to determine if these lesions are hemorrhagic or ischemic in nature as there is little mass effect. (*b*) Axial computed tomography scan of the same lesions, unequivocally demonstrating massive IPH with hyperattenuating clot bilaterally.

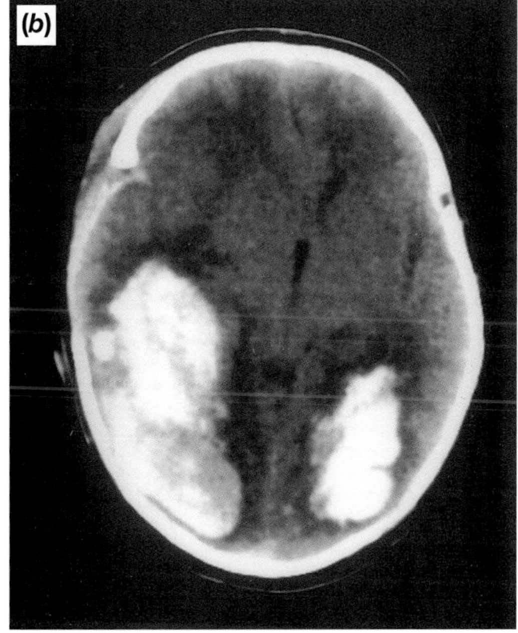

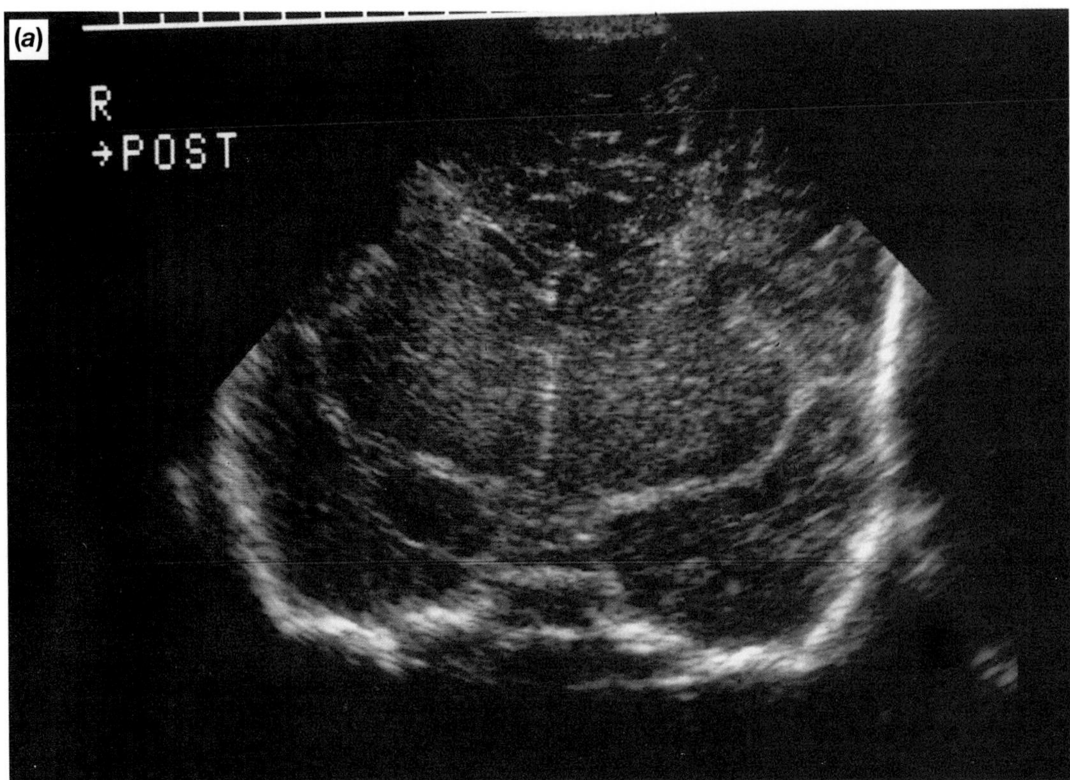

Figure 22.15 Left middle cerebral artery (MCA) infarction. (*a*) Coronal ultrasound view through the anterior fontanel showing subtly increased echogenicity in the left MCA distribution with partial effacement of the left frontal horn. (*b*) Axial computed tomography scan less than 24 h later showing a well-defined left MCA infarction characterized by markedly low attenuation, moderate mass effect, and virtually no gray-white differentiation within the lesion.

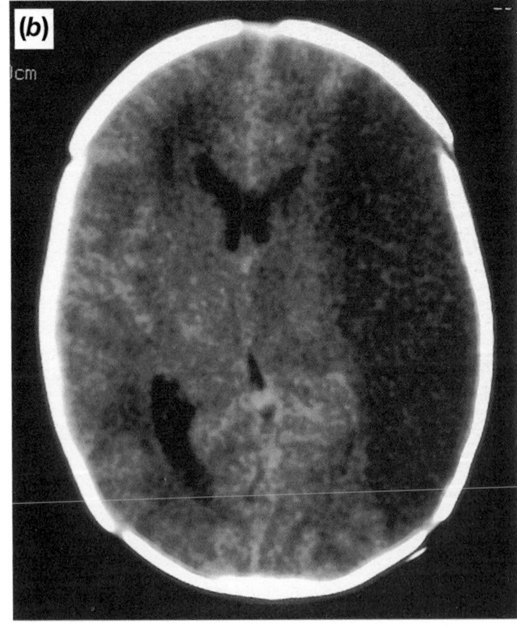

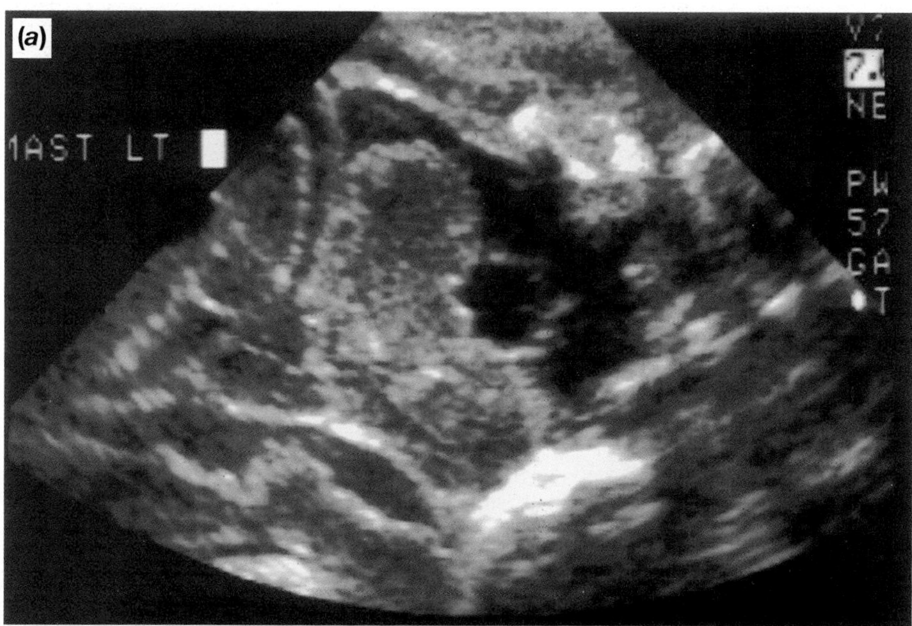

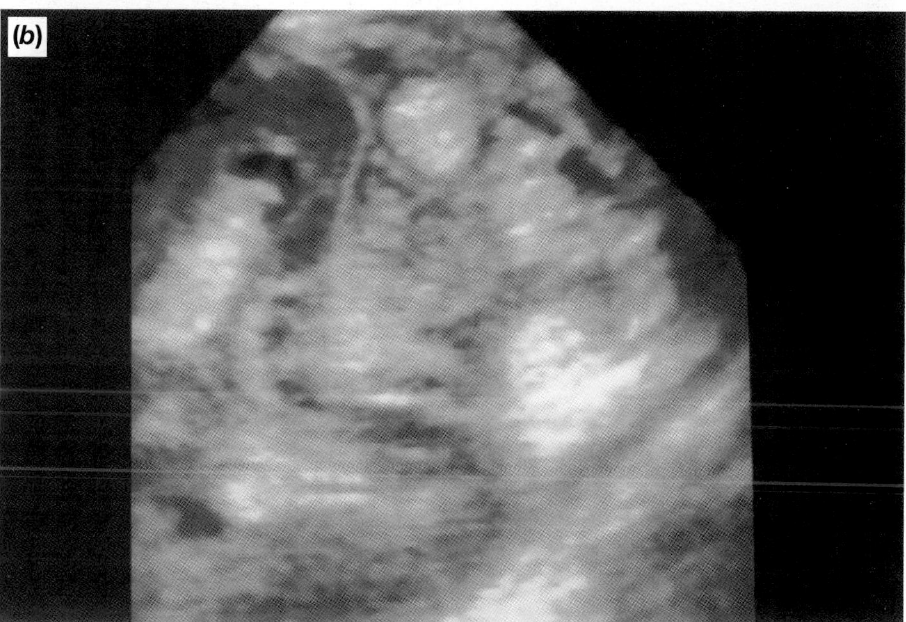

Figure 22.16 Posterior fossa hemorrhage. (*a*) Ultrasound image through the posterior-lateral ("mastoid") fontanel in a newborn term infant on day 1 of life showing an axial representation of the cerebellar hemispheres and the surrounding anechoic subarachnoid space of the posterior fossa. (*b*) Repeat mastoid view 2 days later demonstrating complete obliteration of the subarachnoid space by hemorrhage with regions of hemorrhage and/or ischemia in the cerebellar hemispheres.

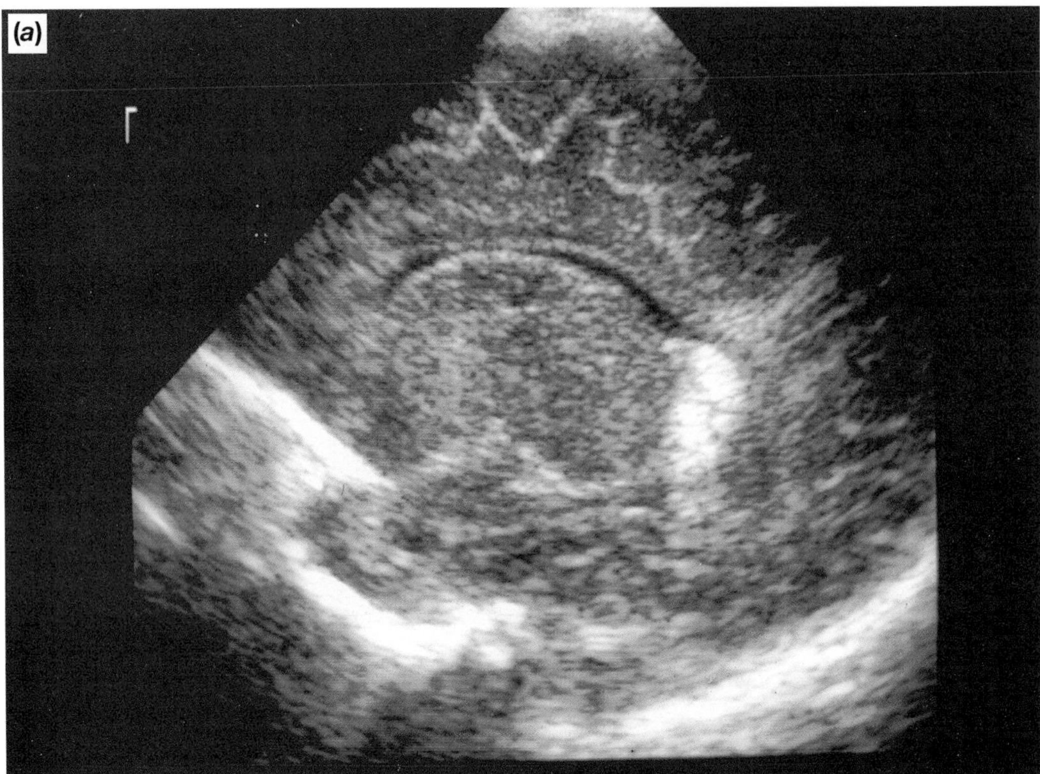

Figure 22.17 Choroid plexus hemorrhage on ultrasound (US) and magnetic resonance (MR). (*a*) Sagittal US image through the anterior fontanel showing a "lumpy" echogenic choroid plexus posteriorly vs a choroid plexus hemorrhage. (*b*) Axial T1-weighted MR 2 days prior to the US examination definitively demonstrating a focal hemorrhage with abnormally increased T1-weighted signal of the left choroid plexus.

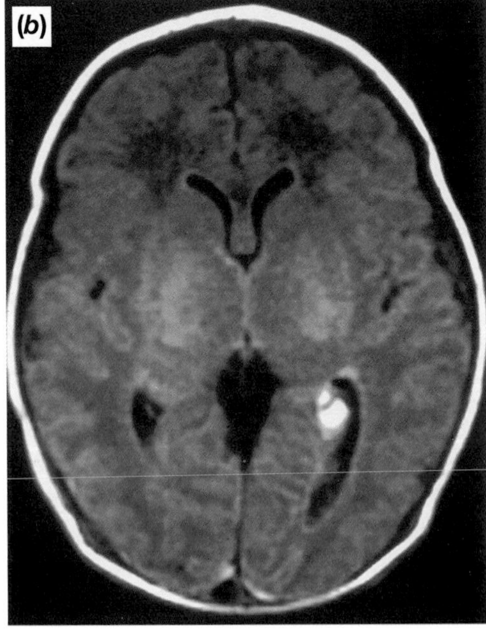

its technical limitations may lead to a significant false-negative predictive value for certain pathologies, e.g., SAH or subdural hemorrhage.

Computed tomography

As mentioned above, neuroimaging modalities may be classified as structural (macrostructural or microstructural) and functional.[49,81,82,88] US is primarily a macrostructural imaging modality with some functional capabilities (e.g., Doppler), as discussed in the previous section.[16,19,49,50,64,81,82,88–91] Probably the most important uses of US are: (1) fetal and neonatal screening; (2) screening of the infant who cannot be examined in the radiology department (e.g., premature neonate with intracranial hemorrhage, extracorporeal membrane oxygenation, intraoperative); (3) when important adjunctive information is quickly needed (e.g., cystic vs solid, vascularity, vascular flow, or increased intracranial pressure); and (3) for real-time guidance and monitoring of invasive diagnostic or therapeutic surgical and interventional procedures.

CT is also primarily a macrostructural imaging modality that has some functional capabilities (e.g., CT angiography).[16,19,49,81,82,88,89,92,93] Although using ionizing radiation, current-generation CT effectively collimates and restricts the X-ray exposure to the immediate volume of interest. Direct imaging is usually restricted to the axial or coronal plane (Figure 22.18). Reformatting from thin axial sections to other planes (e.g., coronal or sagittal) is the alternative. Projection scout images may provide information similar to plain films but with less spatial resolution. CT of the pediatric central nervous system is usually done using either the conventional or the helical/spiral technique. CT requires sedation in infants and young children more often than does US but less often than MRI. The neonate or very young infant, however, may be examined while asleep after a feed or during a nap. CT occasionally needs intravenous iodinated contrast enhancement, and sometimes cerebrospinal (CSF) contrast opacification. High-resolution bone and soft-tissue algorithms are important for demonstrating fine anatomy (e.g., skull base). Advances in computer display technology include image fusion, two-dimensional reformatting,

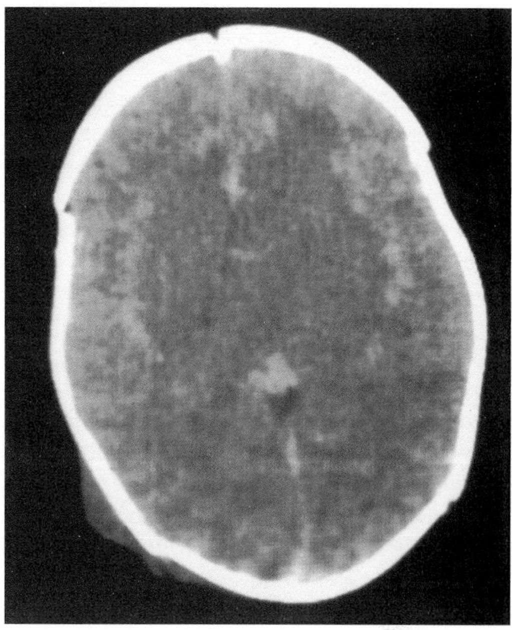

Figure 22.18 Nonenhanced axial computed tomography of acute term perinatal hypoxic–ischemic injury. There are extensive bilateral cerebral hemispheric and deep low densities with loss of gray–white-matter differentiation and small slit-like ventricles.

three-dimensional volumetric and reconstruction methods, segmentation, and surface-rendering techniques. These high-resolution display techniques are used for CT angiography and venography, craniofacial and spinal imaging for surgical planning, and for stereotactic image guidance of radiotherapy, interventional, and neurosurgical procedures. Newer multidetector CT technology provides ultrafast imaging and isotropic resolution for reformatting. This has dramatically reduced the need for sedation.

The role of CT has been redefined in the context of accessible and reliable US and MRI.[49,82,88] US is the procedure of choice for primary macrostructural imaging or screening of the brain and spinal neuroaxis in the neonate and young infant. When US does not satisfy the clinical inquiry, or an acoustic window is not available, then CT becomes the primary modality for brain imaging in children, especially in acute or emergent presentations. This is especially important for acute neurologic presentations. In these situations, CT is primarily used to screen for acute or subacute hemorrhage (Figure 22.14), edema, herniation, fractures, HII (Figure 22.18), focal infarction (Figure 22.15), hydrocephalus, tumor mass, or abnormal collection (e.g., abscess). Other primary indications for CT include the evaluation of bony or air-space abnormalities of the skull base, cranial vault, orbit, paranasal sinuses, facial bones, and the temporal bone. Additionally, CT is the definitive procedure for the detection and confirmation of calcification. It is also important in the bony evaluation of a localized spinal column abnormality (e.g., trauma). Contraindications to CT in childhood are unusual, particularly with the proper application of radiation protection, the appropriate use of nonionic contrast agents, the proper administration of sedation or anesthesia, and the use of vital monitoring.

When CT is used, intravenous enhancement for blood pool effect (e.g., CT angiography) or blood–brain barrier disruption is additionally recommended for the evaluation of suspected or known vascular malformation, infarction, neoplasm, abscess, or empyema.[49,82,88] Enhanced CT may help evaluate a mass or hemorrhage of unknown etiology and identify the membrane of a chronic subdural collection (e.g., child abuse). It may also help differentiate infarction from neoplasm or abscess, serve as an indicator of disease activity, for example, in degenerative or inflammatory disease and vasculitis, or provide a high-yield guide for stereotactic or open biopsy. Ventricular or subarachnoid CSF contrast opacification may further assist in evaluating or confirming CSF compartment lesions or communication (e.g., arachnoid cyst or ventricular encystment). As a rule, and except for suppurative infection, MRI is the preferred alternative to contrast-enhanced CT in the circumstances just enumerated.

Magnetic resonance imaging

Overview of MR techniques

MRI has macrostructural, microstructural, and functional imaging capabilities.[16,17–37,49,82,88,89,92,94–113] MRI uses magnetic fields and radio waves. It is one of the less invasive or relatively noninvasive imaging technologies. Furthermore, the MRI signal is exponentially derived from multiple parameters (e.g., T1, T2, proton density, T2*, proton flow, proton relaxation enhancement, chemical shift, magnetization transfer, and molecular diffusion). MRI also employs many more basic imaging techniques than other modalities (e.g., spin echo, inversion recovery, gradient echo, and chemical shift imaging methods). Advancing MRI capabilities have further improved its sensitivity, specificity, and efficiency.[49,82,88] These include the fluid attenuation inversion recovery technique (FLAIR), fat suppression short T1 inversion recovery imaging (STIR), and magnetization transfer imaging (MTI) for increased macrostructural resolution. Fast and ultrafast MRI techniques (fast spin echo, fast gradient echo, echo planar imaging) have also been developed to reduce imaging times and improve macrostructural resolution, as well as providing microstructural and functional resolution. Important applications include MR vascular imaging (MR angiography (MRA) and venography) and perfusion MRI (PMRI), diffusion imaging (DI), CSF flow and brain/cord motion imaging, brain activation techniques, and MR spectroscopy (MRS). Fast and ultrafast imaging techniques are also being used for fetal/obstetrical imaging (Figure 22.19), morphometrics, treatment planning, and "real-time" MRI-guided surgical and interventional procedures.[96–99]

Although, in general, MRI is more expensive than US or CT, it is less expensive than the more invasive modalities such as angiography which more often requires anesthesia. The role of MRI in imaging of the developing central nervous system is defined by its superior sensitivity and specificity in a number of areas as compared to US and CT.[49,81,82,88,89] MRI has also redefined the roles of invasive procedures like myelography, ventriculography, cisternography, and angiography. MRI provides multiplanar imaging with equivalent resolution in all planes without repositioning the patient. Bone does not interfere with soft-tissue resolution, although metallic objects often

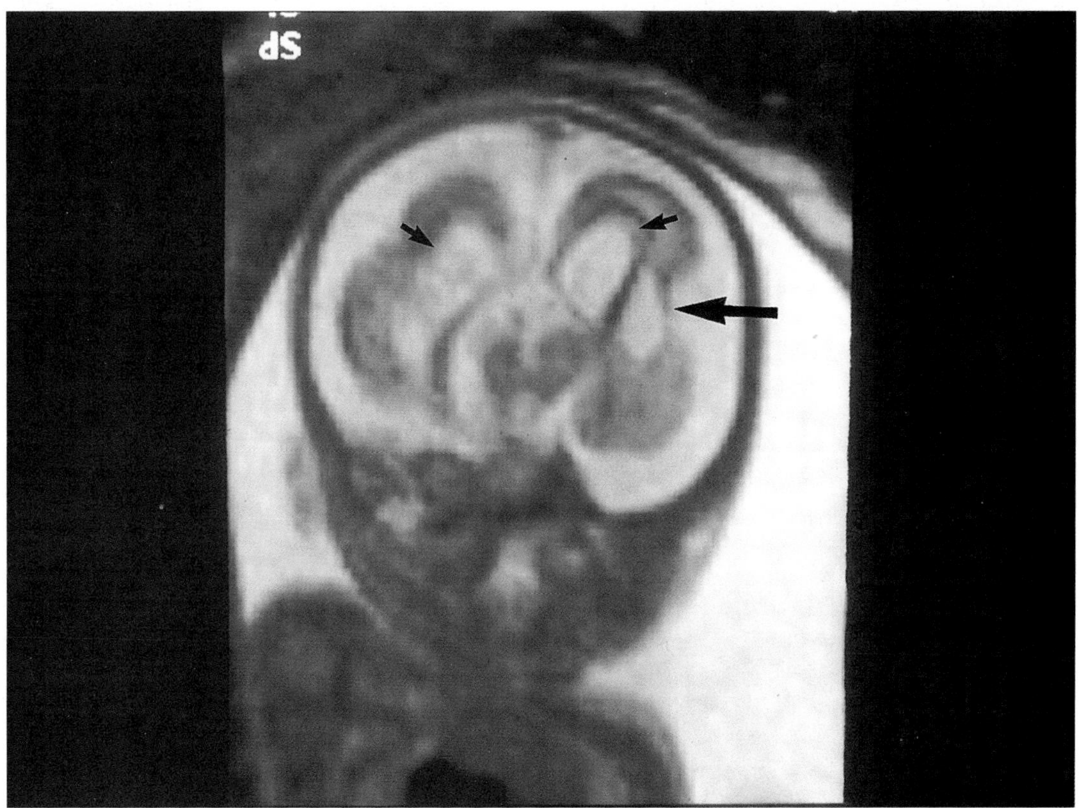

Figure 22.19 Coronal ultrafast magnetic resonance imaging (MRI) of early second-trimester fetal encephalomalacia. There is cerebral atrophy with high-intensity cavitations (large arrow), large ventricles (small arrows), and large extracerebral spaces.

produce signal void or field distortion artifacts. Some ferromagnetic or electronic devices (e.g., ferrous aneurysm clips and pacemakers) pose a hazard, and MRI is usually contraindicated in these cases. MRI is not as fast as US or CT, and patient sedation or anesthesia is often required in most infants and younger children, since image quality is easily compromised by motion. MRI may not be as readily accessible to the pediatric patient as is US or CT and may not be feasible in emergencies or for intensive care cases unless magnet-compatible vital monitoring and support are available. This is particularly important for the neonate.

MRI demonstrates superior sensitivity and specificity in a number of circumstances, particularly with the addition of new structural and functional techniques such as FLAIR, STIR, magnetization transfer contrast (MTC), DI, PMRI, and MRS.[49,82,88] The FLAIR sequence attenuates the signal from flowing water (i.e., CSF) and increases the conspicuity of nonfluid water-containing lesions (Figure 22.20). The STIR technique suppresses fat signal to provide improved conspicuity of water-containing lesions in regions where fat dominates (e.g., orbit, head and neck, spine). The MTI method suppresses background tissues and increases conspicuity for

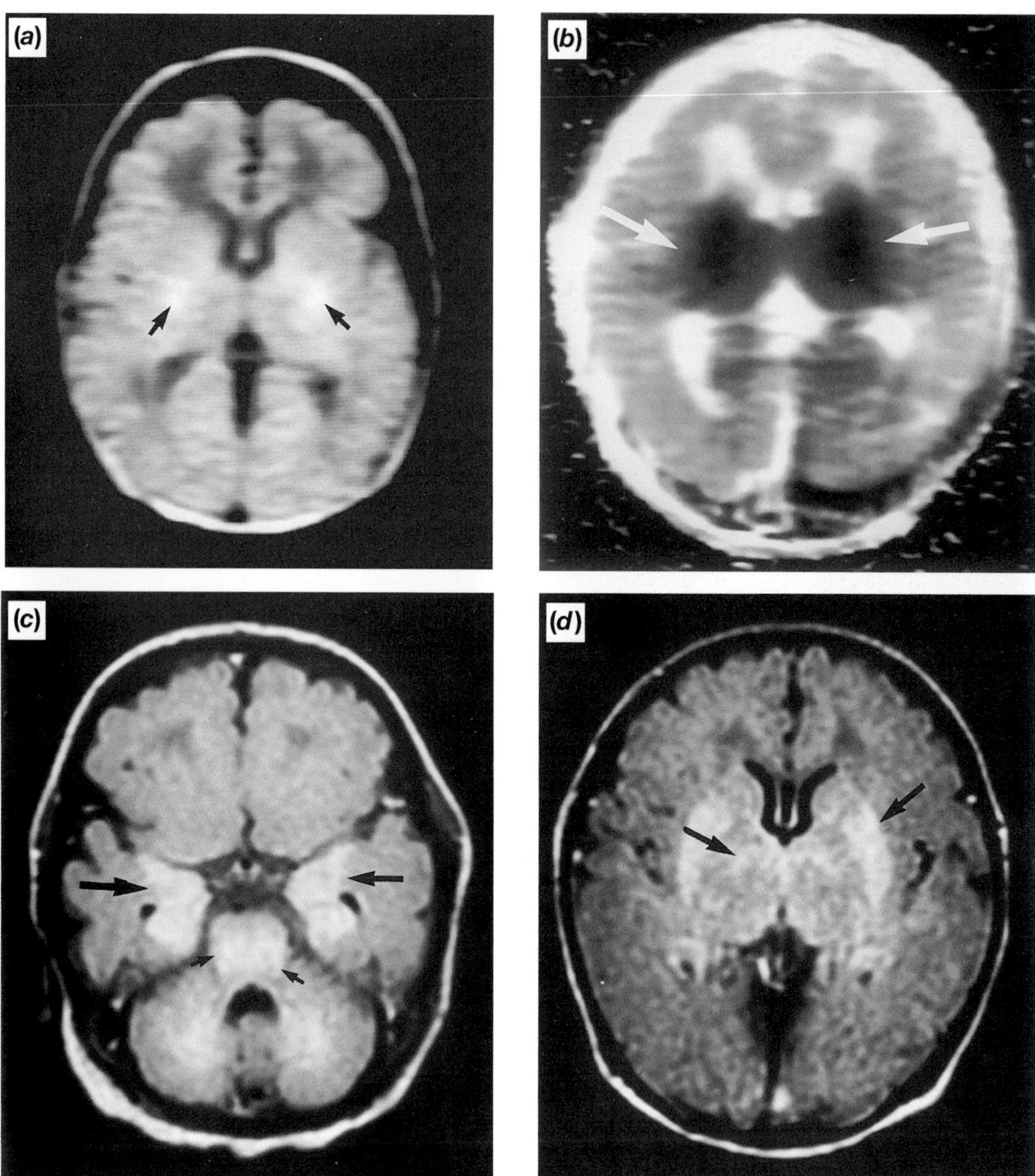

Figure 22.20 Magnetic resonance imaging of term perinatal profound hypoxic–ischemic injury. (*a*) Axial diffusion imaging in the acute phase shows increased intensity (restricted diffusion) of the basal ganglia (arrows). (*b*) Axial apparent diffusion coefficient map in another newborn in the acute phase shows decreased intensity (restricted diffusion) throughout the basal ganglia and thalami. (*c–e*). Axial fluid attenuation inversion recovery technique images in another neonate in the subacute phase show high intensities involving the pons (small arrows – *c*) and hippocampi (large arrows–*c*) , putamina and thalami (arrows – *d*), and paracentral cerebrum (arrows – *e*). (*f*) Axial T2 image in an older child in the chronic phase shows high intensities in the posterior putamina and ventrolateral thalami (arrows – *f*).

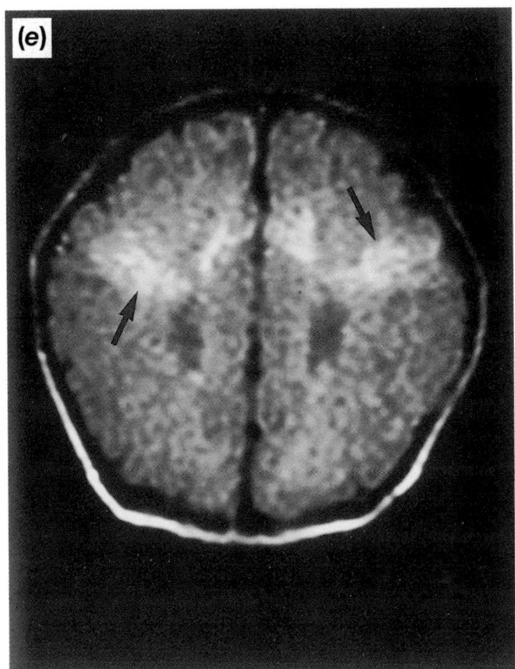

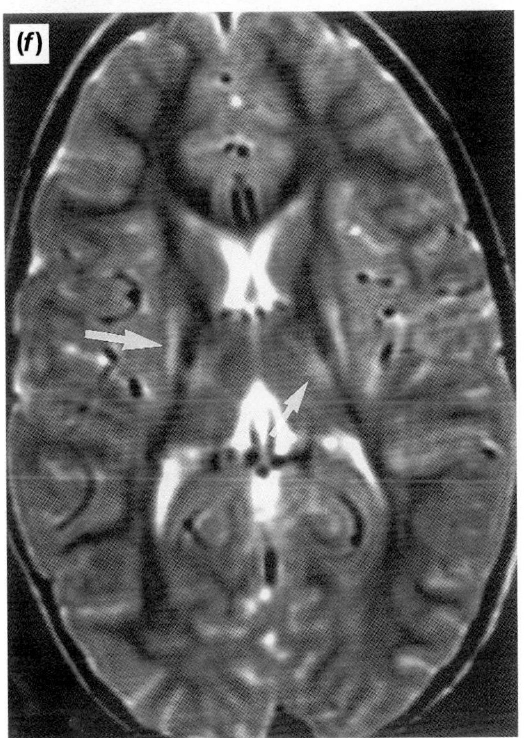

Table 22.1. Imaging patterns of diffuse or global hypoxic–ischemic encephalopathy (HIE)[a]

Hemorrhage
Germinal matrix – intraventricular hemorrhage
Choroid plexus – intraventricular hemorrhage
Subarachnoid hemorrhage
Partial HIE
Preterm: periventricular leukomalacia
Term/postterm: cortical/subcortical injury (border zone, watershed, parasagittal)
Intermediate: combined or transitional pattern
Ulegyria
Profound HIE
Thalamic and basal ganglia injury
Brainstem injury
Hippocampal injury
Cerebral white matter injury
Paracentral injury
Global injury (prolonged profound)
Combined profound and partial prolonged HIE

Note:
[a] Depends on gestational age, chronological age, duration, and severity of the insult.

vascular flow enhancement (e.g., MRA) and gadolinium enhancement.

MRI is the imaging modality of choice in a number of clinical situations.[49,82,88] MRI frequently offers greater diagnostic specificity than does CT or US for delineating vascular and hemorrhagic processes (Tables 22.1–22.3). This includes the clear depiction of vascular structures and abnormalities based on proton flow parameters and software enhancements not requiring the injection of contrast agents (e.g., MRA). MRA may further contribute to MRI in the differentiation of global HII from vascular occlusive infarction, and to distinguish HII from nonvascular disease.[49,81,82,88] Using gradient recalled echo (GRE, GE) magnetic susceptibility sequences, MRI also provides more specific identification and staging of hemorrhage and clot formation according to the evolution of hemoglobin breakdown. MRI is often

Table 22.2. Magnetic resonance imaging (MRI) of intracranial hemorrhage and thrombosis

Stage	Biochemical form	Site	T1-MRI	T2-MRI
Hyperacute* (+ edema) (<12 h)	Fe II oxy Hb	Intact RBCs	Iso-low I	High I
Acute (+ edema) (1–3 days)	Fe II deoxy Hb	Intact RBCs	Iso-low I	Low I
Early subacute (+ edema) (3–7 days)	Fe III metHb	Intact RBCs	High I	Low I
Late subacute (− edema) (1–2 weeks)	Fe III metHb	Lysed RBCs (extracellular)	High I	High I
Early chronic (− edema) (>2 weeks)	Fe III transferrin	Extracellular	High I	High I
Chronic (cavity)	Fe III ferritin and hemosiderin	Phagocytosis	Iso-low I	Low I

Notes:
[a] Computed tomography more sensitive and specific than MRI or ultrasound for hyperacute/acute hemorrhage in all compartments.
RBCs, red blood cells; I, signal intensity; + present; – absent; Hb, hemoglobin; Fe II, ferrous; Fe III, Ferric; Iso, isointense.
Sources: Modified from Barnes P and Wolpert SM (1992). MRI. In *Pediatric Neuroradiology*, Wolpert SM, ed. pp. 3–40. St Louis, MO: Mosby Year Book; and Kleinman P and Barnes P. (1992). Head trauma. In *Imaging of Child Abuse*, 2nd edn, Kleinman PK, ed. St Louis, MO: Mosby Year Book; chapter 15 does not include influence of fetal Hb.

reserved for more definitive evaluation of hemorrhage and as an indicator or guide for angiography.

Magnetic resonance spectroscopy

MRS offers a noninvasive in vivo approach to biochemical analysis.[26,27,29,30,49,82,88,94] Furthermore, MRS provides additional quantitative information regarding cellular metabolites since signal intensity is linearly related to steady-state metabolite concentration. MRS can detect cellular biochemical changes prior to the detection of morphological changes by MRI or other imaging modalities. MRS may therefore provide further insight into both follow-up assessment and prognosis. With recent advances in instrumentation and methodology, and utilizing the high inherent sensitivity of hydrogen-1, single-voxel and multivoxel proton MRS is now carried out with relatively short acquisitions to detect low concentration metabolites in healthy and

Table 22.3. Occlusive neurovascular disease in the fetus, neonate, and infant

Idiopathic	Thrombosis
Vascular maldevelopment	Meningitis
Atresia	HIE/DIC
Hypoplasia	Dehydration/hypernatremia
Vasculopathy	Sepsis/DIC
Familial proliferative	Polycythemia/hyperviscosity
Isoimmune thrombocytopenia	Protein S or C deficiency
Vasospasm	Antithrombin III deficiency
Maternal cocaine use	Antiphospholipid antibodies
Vascular distortion	Factor V deficiency
Extreme head and neck motion	*Thromboembolic*
ECMO	Placental vascular anastomoses
Emboli	Cotwin fetal death
Involuting fetal vessels	Fetofetal transfusion
Congenital heart disease	*HIE/thromboembolism*
Catheterized vessels	

Notes:
HIE, hypoxic–ischemic encephalopathy; DIC, disseminated intravascular coagulation; ECMO, extracorporeal membrane oxygenation.
Source: Modified from Volpe JJ. (1995). *Neurology of the Newborn*, 3rd edn, Philadelphia: WB Saunders, p. 302.

diseased tissues. Phosphorus-31 spectroscopy has also been developed for pediatric use. Currently, MRS has been primarily used in the assessment of brain development and maturation, perinatal brain injury (Figure 22.21), central nervous system neoplasia vs treatment effects, and metabolic and neurodegenerative disorders.

Alterations in metabolites are often displayed by MRS as a ratio relative to the reference metabolite, creatine (Cr), an energy marker. In disorders in which there is predominant neuronal degeneration (i.e., loss of cell bodies, axons) and atrophy, the major MRS finding is a decrease in *N*-acetyl-aspartate (NAA; Figure 22.21), a neuronal (neurons including axons) and immature oligodendroglial marker. In disorders in which there is predominant loss of myelin sheaths with secondary axonal degeneration and gliosis (e.g., demyelination), the characteristic spectral abnormalities are characterized by elevated lipids, a marker for myelin destruction; elevated choline (Cho), a marker of membrane turnover (e.g., myelin, glial); variable increases in lactate (L), a marker of anaerobic glycolysis; elevated glutamate/glutamine (G), neuroexcitatory amino acid markers; and, elevated myoinositols (M), also an osmolyte and glial marker.

Perfusion magnetic resonance imaging and functional MRI

PMRI is currently being used to evaluate cerebral perfusion dynamics through the application of a dynamic contrast-enhanced T2*-weighted MRI technique.[49,82,88,95] This new technique is undergoing further development to qualitate and quantitate normal and abnormal cerebrovascular dynamics of

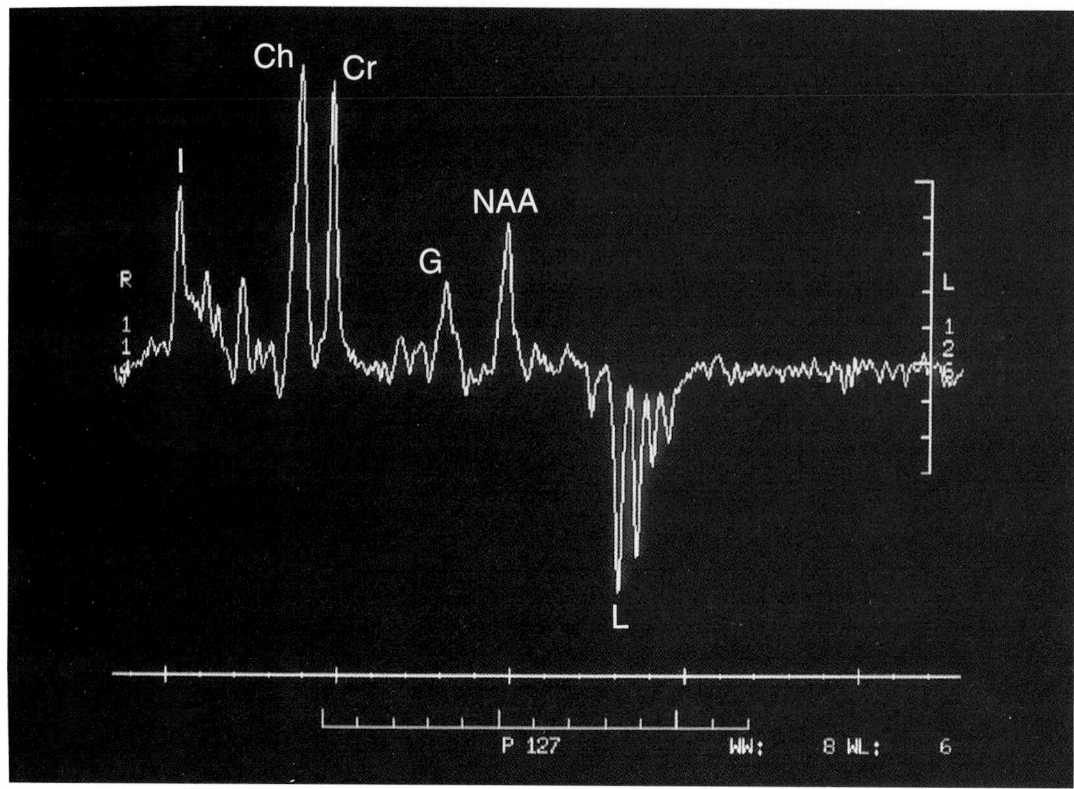

Figure 22.21 Magnetic resonance spectroscopy in acute term perinatal profound hypoxic–ischemic injury. The spectra obtained from the basal ganglia show decreased *N*-acetyl-aspartate (NAA) and a prominent inverted lactate (L) doublet. G, glutamate/glutamine; Cr, creatine; Ch, choline; I, myoinositol.

the developing brain by analyzing hemodynamic parameters, including relative cerebral blood volume, relative CBF, and mean transit time, all as complementary to conventional MRI. It is of limited use in the neonatal period because of venous access and safety issues. Current and advanced applications of this and other PMRI techniques not requiring contrast administration (e.g., flow-activated inversion recovery – FAIR; blood oxygen level determination – BOLD) include the evaluation of ischemic cerebrovascular disease (e.g., hypoxia–ischemia, moyamoya, sickle-cell disease), the differentiation of tumor progression from treatment effects, and brain activation imaging.[49,82,88] One of the most active areas of research is the localization of brain activity, an area previously dominated by nuclear medicine, including SPECT and PET.

Functional MRI (fMRI) is the terminology often applied to brain activation imaging in which local or regional changes in CBF are displayed that accompany stimulation or activation of sensory (e.g., visual, auditory, somatosensory), motor, or cognitive centers.[49,82,88] fMRI is providing important information regarding the spatial distribution of motor and cognitive function and functional impairment (Figure 22.22). Also, it may serve as a guide for safer and more effective interventions, including microneurosurgery or conformal radiotherapy, for example, the ablation of tumors, vascular malformations, and seizure foci.

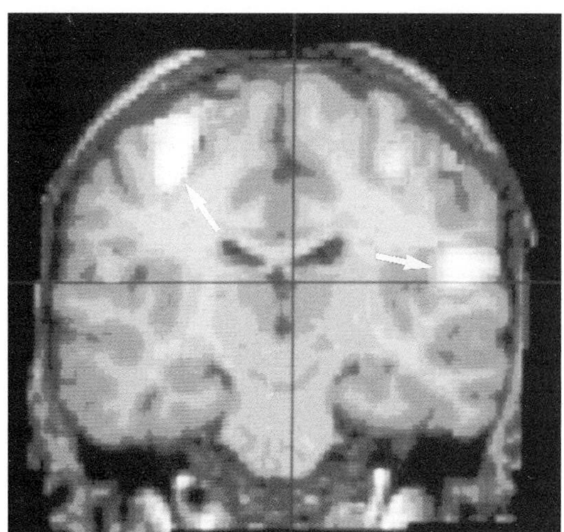

Figure 22.22 Coronal functional magnetic resonance imaging (blood oxygen level determination technique) in an older child. Bilateral cerebral cortical high intensities (arrows) associated with voluntary motor activation from auditory cues.

Diffusion-weighted MRI

Using echo planar or line-scan spin echo techniques, DI provides information based upon differences in the rate of diffusion of water molecules and is especially sensitive to intracellular changes.[31–37,49,82,88] The rate of diffusion, or apparent diffusion coefficient (ADC), is higher for free or pure water than for macromolecular bound water. The ADC varies according to the microstructural or physiologic state of a tissue. Current clinical applications include the assessment of brain maturation, the evaluation of acute ischemic injury (Figure 22.23), and the analysis of the sequelae of injury (Figure 22.24). A particularly important application of DI is in the early detection of diffuse and focal ischemic injury. The ADC of water is reduced within minutes of an ischemic insult and is progressive within the first hour. Bright signal is demonstrated on DI (dark signal on ADC maps) at a time when conventional imaging is negative and likely reflects cellular injury (e.g., necrosis). Further investigation is underway regarding the roles of DI, PMRI, and MRS in the early diagnosis and treatment of potentially reversible HII, as well as the roles of DI (e.g., relative or fractional anisotropy) and fMRI, respectively, in the microstructural and functional assessments of chronic injury (Figures 22.22 and 22.24).

CT and MR in neonates with perinatal hypoxic–ischemic injury

Neurovascular disease characteristically presents as an acute neurologic event (e.g., seizures, hypotonia). However, a recently discovered but fixed deficit (e.g., hemiplegia, spastic diplegia, congenital hypotonia) may be the first indication of a remote prenatal or perinatal neurovascular injury. Imaging assists in the clinical evaluation and differentiation of hypoxia–ischemia, hemorrhage, occlusive vascular disease, and nonvascular disease (Tables 22.1–22.3).[49,81,82,88,89] US and CT may provide important screening information, particularly with regard to gross macrostructural abnormalities (e.g., hemorrhage, encephalomalacia). However, current and advanced MRI techniques often provide more definitive macrostructural, microstructural, and functional imaging information in both the early and late assessment of fetal and neonatal central nervous system injuries.

In general, the pattern of HII associated with hypoxic–ischemic–reperfusion insults varies with severity and duration of the insult as well as with the gestational age (GA) of the fetus or infant at the time of the insult.[17,49,81,82,88,89,92,100–113] Different brain structures are more vulnerable than others to the different types of HII (e.g., partial prolonged, profound, combined) at different stages of brain development (e.g., formational vs postformational GA, preterm vs term vs full-term vs postterm GA). Brain tissues in the arterial border zones or watersheds, brain tissues with high metabolic demands, mature or actively maturing tissues, and tissues with higher concentrations of neuroexcitatory amino acids are particularly vulnerable to HII and to other insults (e.g., hypoglycemia, trauma, infection, seizures).[37,49,81,82,88,89,109] Prenatal or perinatal partial prolonged HII (e.g., one or more insults of

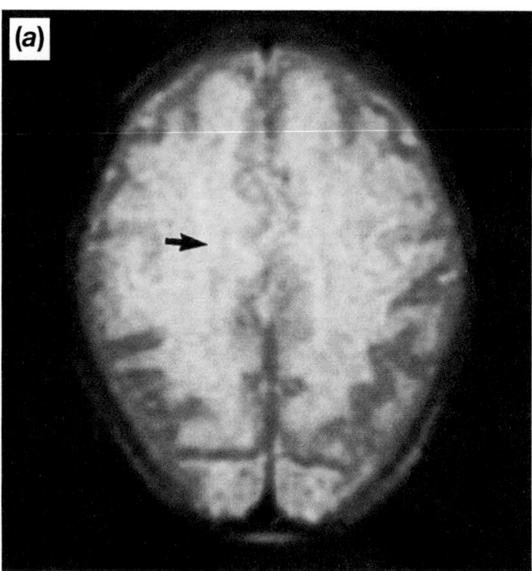

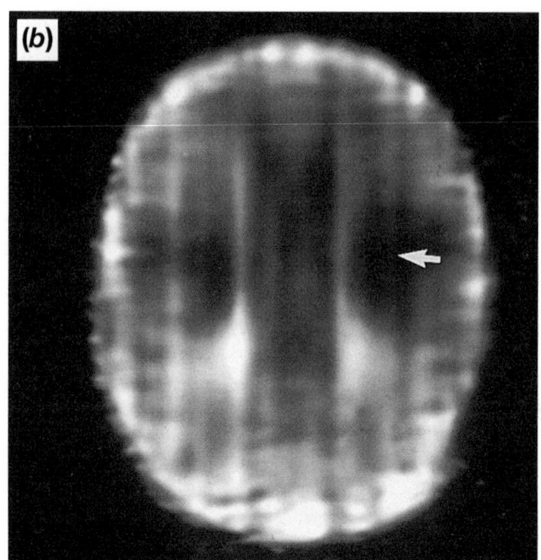

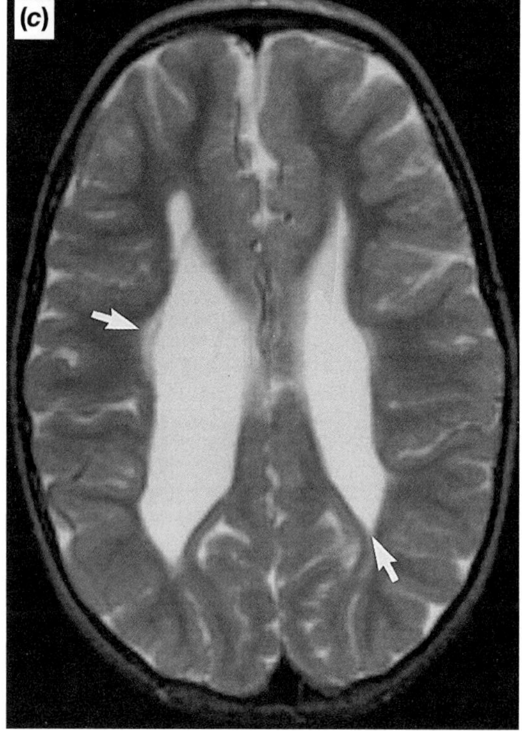

Figure 22.23 Magnetic resonance imaging of preterm perinatal hypoxic–ischemic injury and periventricular leukomalacia. (*a*) Axial T2 image in the acute phase shows nonspecific bilateral cerebral white-matter hyperintensities (arrow). (*b*) Axial apparent diffusion coefficient map in the same patient in the acute phase shows bilateral periventricular hypointensities (restricted diffusion – arrow). (*c*) Axial T2 image in an older child in the chronic phase shows irregular lateral ventricular enlargement, subependymal hyperintensities (arrows), and reduced volume of the periventricular white matter.

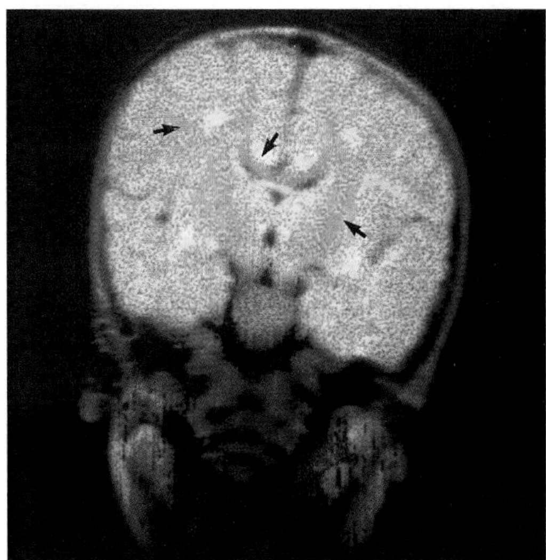

Figure 22.24 Diffusion tensor map. Coronal white-matter map derived from diffusion tensor magnetic resonance imaging techniques shows the fiber tracts (arrows) of the corpus callosum, the internal capsule, and the cerebral hemispheres derived from fractional anisotropic (FA) computations.[32,33]

hypoxia/hypoperfusion) may be associated with periventricular border-zone/watershed injury to the preterm fetus or neonate (e.g., 27–35 weeks' GA: Figure 22.23), or cortical and subcortical border-zone/watershed cerebral injury during term gestation (e.g., 37–42 weeks' GA: Figure 22.25). A combined partial prolonged HII pattern (cortical/subcortical/periventricular) may be seen in the late preterm to the early-midterm GA (e.g., 36–39 weeks). Fetal or neonatal brain injury may also occur with more profound HII insults (e.g., anoxia or circulatory arrest) and involve the thalami, basal ganglia (especially putamina), brainstem (especially midbrain), hippocampi, paraventricular white matter, and perirolandic cortex (Figure 22.20). This type of injury may also vary with GA (thalamic greater than putaminal involvement in the preterm GA; putaminal, hippocampal, and paracentral injury more common in the term GA). Combined patterns (i.e., partial prolonged plus profound HII) are also common (Figure 22.26).[17,49,81,82,88,89,92,100–113] CT or MRI (e.g., DI) may demonstrate evolving edema, necrosis, or hemorrhage in the hyperacute, acute, and subacute phases (Figure 22.18). There may be SAH, germinal matrix hemorrhage and IVH (e.g., premature fetus or neonate), choroid plexus/IVH (e.g., term fetus or neonate), or intracerebral hemorrhage (e.g., hemorrhagic infarction). The hemorrhage usually appears high-density on CT in the acute to subacute phases (range 3 h–7 days) unless there is associated coagulopathy (Figure 22.14). With evolution and resolution, the hemorrhage becomes isodense to low-density. MRI may offer more specific characterization of the hemorrhagic component with regard to timing (Table 22.2).

The edema (range 1–5 days) of nonhemorrhagic HII often peaks between 2 and 4 days after the insult. CT may show hypodensities with decreased gray–white-matter differentiation (Figure 22.18). In the early phases of the injury, the neuroimaging findings are often nonspecific as to specific causation (e.g., HII vs infection vs metabolic disorder).[49,81,82,88,89,109] MRI or US may provide greater sensitivity and specificity depending upon the techniques used and the timing of the imaging (Figures 22.20, 22.23, and 22.25). Conventional MRI may show characteristic T1 hypointensities/T2 hyperintensities (12–48 h), followed by T1 hyperintensities (about 3 days), and then T2 hypointensities (about 6 days).[17] DI may be abnormal before conventional MRI and show restricted diffusion with decreased ADC as increased intensity on diffusion images and decreased intensity on ADC maps[31–37,49,82,88] (Figures 22.20 and 22.23). Doppler with resistive indices (e.g., RI<60) or MRS (e.g., elevated lactate, elevated glutamate, elevated lipids, decreased NAA) may provide additional early indicators of timing and outcome[26,27,29,30,49,82,88,94,110] (Figure 22.21). The more subtle ischemic PVL lesions (e.g., cystic phase) are occasionally better delineated by US (2–6 weeks after insult) than by CT or MRI, in which the density and intensity character of immature white matter often obscures the injury. However, CT and MRI often show gray-matter injury better than US.[19,49,64,81,82,88,89] Further developments of PMRI, DI, and MRS may further improve diagnostic sensitivity

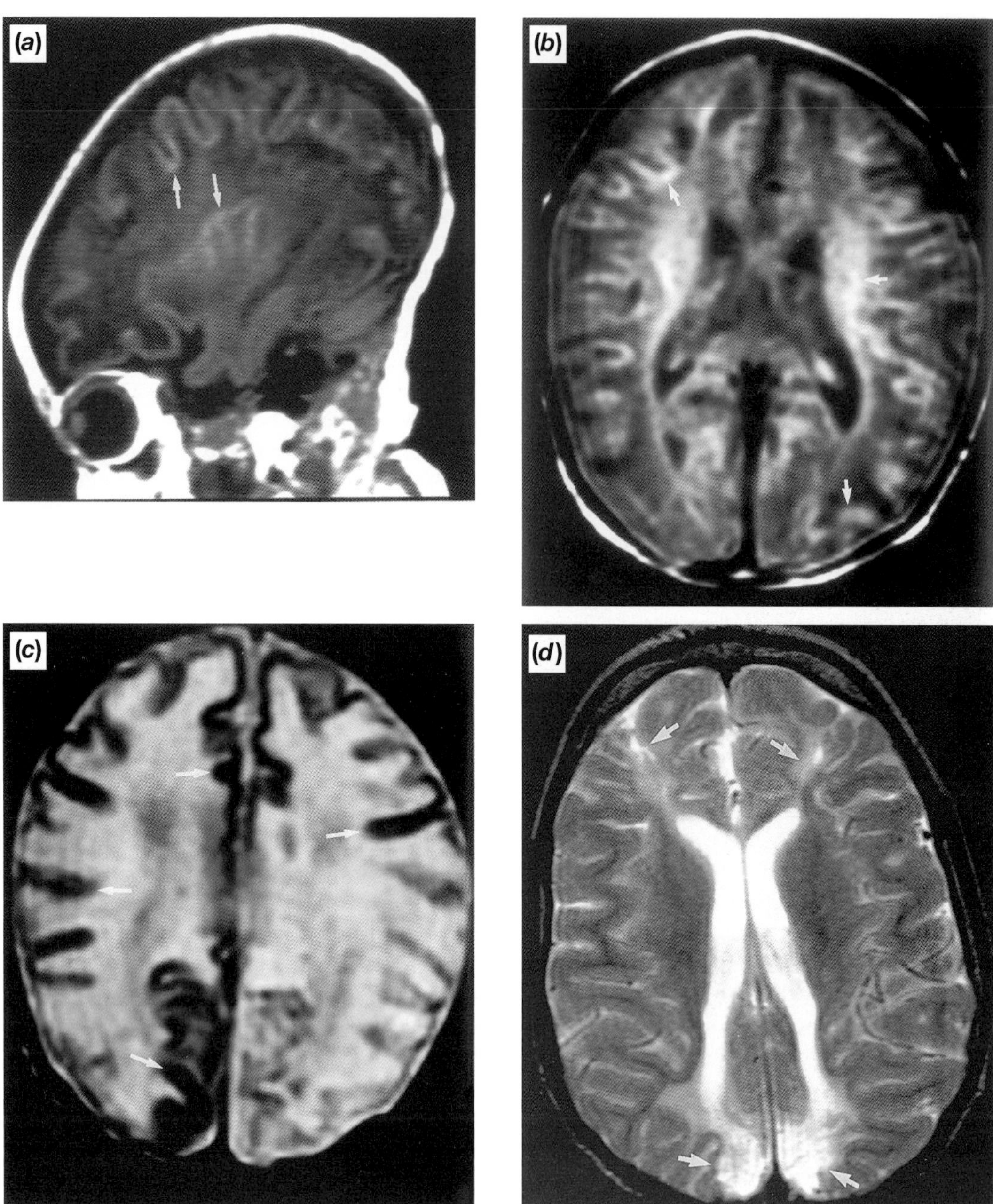

Figure 22.25 Magnetic resonance imaging of term perinatal watershed hypoxic–ischemic injury. (*a* and *b*). Sagittal and axial T1 images in the subacute phase show extensive cerebral white-matter hypointensities plus linear hyperintensities (arrows) at cortical, subcortical, and periventricular gray–white matter junctions. (*c*) Axial T2 image in the same newborn in the subacute phase shows extensive cerebral white-matter hyperintensities with cortical/subcortical band-like hypointensities (arrows). (*d*) Axial T2 image in an older child in the chronic phase shows bilateral hyperintense gliosis and atrophy in a parasagittal cerebral distribution.

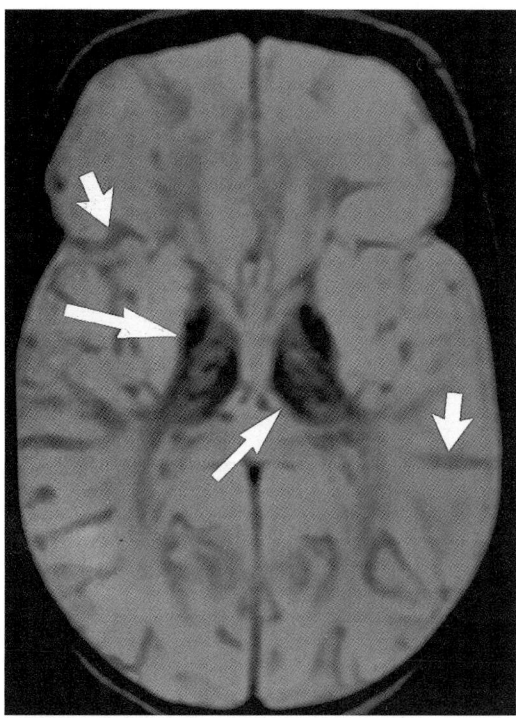

Figure 22.26 Magnetic resonance imaging of combined profound and partial prolonged hypoxic–ischemic injury in the chronic phase in an older child. Axial T2 image shows bilateral hyperintense cystic encephalomalacia with hypointense septations (short arrows) and hypointense basal ganglia and thalami (long arrows).

and specificity. In fact, DI has demonstrated restricted diffusion in the acute phase of PVL when US, CT, and conventional MRI were negative or nonspecific (Figure 22.23). Such advances may facilitate the early institution of neuroprotective measures to treat potentially reversible primary injury (necrosis, apoptosis) and secondary injury (transneural degeneration) in HII.[37] These advanced MRI techniques may also assist in distinguishing HII from other causes of encephalopathy, including other common metabolic disorders (e.g., hypoglycemia, hyperbilirubinemia), nonmetabolic conditions (e.g., infection), and other rarer disorders (e.g., inborn metabolic errors).

The long-term result of HII is a static encephalopathy (i.e., cerebral palsy) and imaging may demonstrate injury in the chronic phases (>14–21 days after the insult), including porencephaly, hydranencephaly, atrophy, chronic periventricular leukomalacia, cystic encephalomalacia, gliosis, or mineralization in a characteristic distribution as described above.[17,49,81,82,88,89,92,100–113] The chronic changes are best demonstrated by CT or MRI (Figures 22.20, 22.23, and 22.25).

SPECT/PET neuroimaging of neonatal brain injury

Uses of SPECT and PET have been limited to the study of cerebral vascular perfusion in both normal infants and in infants suffering from HII.[38–41,43–45] While SPECT and PET techniques in particular lend themselves to extremely sensitive and accurate measures of CBF and circulatory physiology they suffer from lack of portability, relatively long scanning times, and poor spatial resolution. Molecular imaging, a field that focuses on the unique properties of stressed and injured tissues, may fundamentally change the approach to the noninvasive assessment of the neonate with suspected HII. Animal model work has shown promising results in the detection of HII using a new clinically safe molecular probe, technetium^{99m}-annexin V. Annexin V is an endogenous human protein that localizes to neurons (and astrocytes) that are

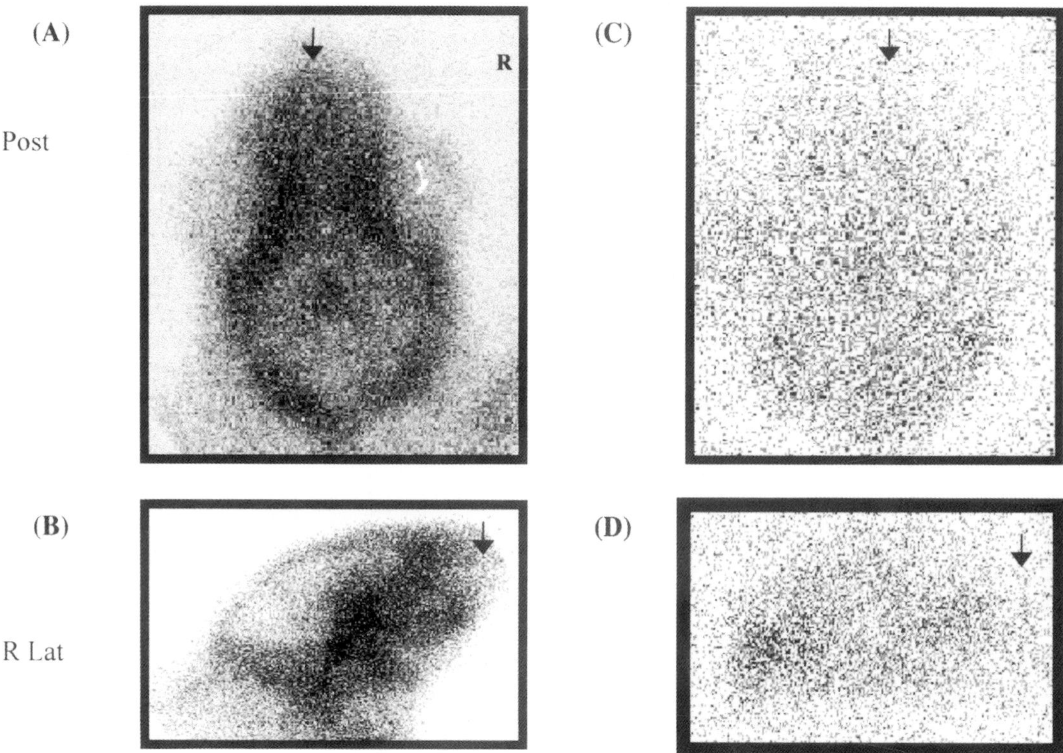

Figure 22.27 Annexin V imaging of a control (no hypoxia) neonatal rabbit after right carotid artery ligation. In vivo posterior (A), right lateral (B) in vivo and posterior (C), right lateral (D) ex vivo radionuclide pinhole images of a representative brain of a control animal demonstrating no abnormal increases in the cerebral uptake of annexin V 2 h after injection of 2 mCi of radiopharmaceutical. There is, however, slightly increased annexin V uptake of the cerebellum as compared to the rest of the brain, as seen in the posterior (C) and right lateral (D) ex vivo radionuclide images. Note the normal annexin V uptake of calvarial bone marrow and cranial soft tissues seen in the in vivo radionuclide images (A and B). The right side of the brain is indicated (R), while the arrow points to the position of the nose in A–C. Note that the arrow in D points to the cerebellum.

ischemically stressed, injured, or that are undergoing apoptotis (programmed cell death). Early studies suggested that annexin V radionuclide scans may be more sensitive than DWI MR at detecting regions at risk for ischemic injury; becoming positive within minutes of an insult (Figures 22.27 and 22.28). Annexin V scanning therefore could screen neonates immediately after birth, permitting the rapid institution of novel neuroprotective therapy. With advances in the understanding of the molecular markers of ischemic disease, other highly sensitive and biologically specific imaging tracers will undoubtedly follow.

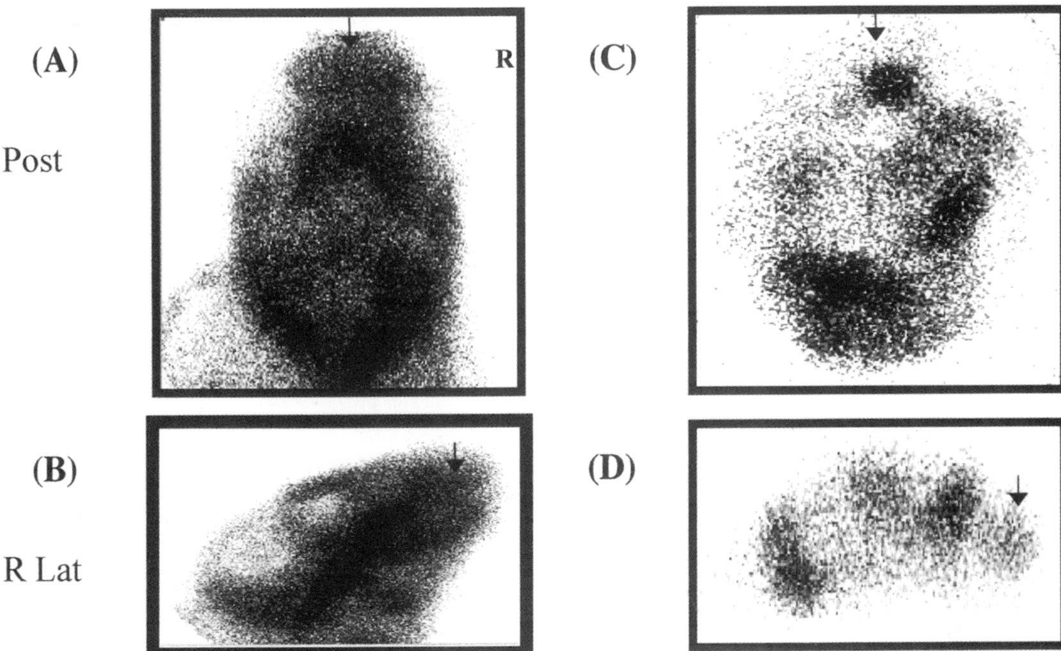

Figure 22.28 Annexin V imaging 10 hours after reversal of hypoxia (2 h at an Fio_2 of 10%) in a neonatal rabbit with right carotid artery ligation. In vivo posterior (A), right lateral (B) in vivo and posterior (C), right lateral (D) ex vivo radionuclide pinhole images of a representative animal 10 h after reversal of hypoxia. These images demonstrate marked multifocal uptake of annexin V in both hemispheres (right greater than left hemisphere) best seen on the ex vivo radionuclide images (C and D) 2 h after injection of 2 mCi of radiopharmaceutical. Corresponding diffusion-weighted imaging and gadolinium-DPTA bolus tracking magnetic resonance studies were entirely normal (images not shown) after reversal of hypoxia. Note again the normal overlying annexin V uptake in the normal calvarial bone marrow and soft tissues in the in vivo radionuclide images (A and B). Also note the increased cerebellar uptake of annexin V in the posterior (C) and right lateral (D) ex vivo radionuclide images. The right side of the brain is indicated (R), while the arrow points to the position of the nose in parts A, B, and C. Note that the arrow in part D points to the cerebellum.

REFERENCES

1 Enzmann D, Murphy-Irwin K, Stevenson D, et al. (1985). The natural history of subependymal germinal matrix hemorrhage. *Am J Perinatol*, **2**, 123–133.

2 Hay CT, Rumack CM and Horgan JG. (1989). Cranial sonography: intracranial hemorrhage, periventricular leukomalacia, and asphyxia. *Clin Diagn Ultrasound*, **24**, 25–42.

3 Cohen HL and Haller JO. (1994). Advances in perinatal neurosonography. *Am J Radiol*, **163**, 801–810.

4 Matamoros A, Anderson JC, McConnell J, et al. (1989). Neurosonographic findings in infants treated with extracorporeal membrane oxygenation (ECMO). *J Child Neurol*, **4**(suppl), 52–61.

5 Babcock DS and Matsumoto JS. (1991). Update on cranial sonography of the infant. In *Syllabus: A Special Course in Ultrasound 1991*, Rifkin MD, Charboneau JW and Laing FC, eds, pp. 337–345. Oak Brook, IL: Radiological Society of North America.

6 von Allmen D, Babcock D, Matsumoto J, et al. (1992). The

predictive value of head ultrasound in the ECMO candidate. *J Pediatr Surg*, **27**, 36–39.

7 Keeney SE, Adcock EW and McArdle CB. (1991). Prospective observation of 100 high-risk neonates by high-field (1.5 Tesla) magnetic resonance imaging of the central nervous system. I. Intraventricular and extracerebral lesions. *Pediatrics*, **87**, 421–430.

8 Keeney SE, Adcock EW and McArdle CB. (1991). Prospective observation of 100 high-risk neonates by high-field (1.5 Tesla) magnetic resonance imaging of the central nervous system. II. Lesions associated with hypoxic–ischemic encephalopathy. *Pediatrics*, **87**, 431–438.

9 Christophe C, Clercx A, Blum D, et al. (1994). Early MR detection of cortical and subcortical hypoxic–ischemic encephalopathy in full-term infants. *Pediatr Radiol*, **24**, 581–584.

10 Byrne P, Welch R, Johnson MA, et al. (1990). Serial magnetic resonance imaging in neonatal hypoxic–ischemic encephalopathy. *J Pediatr*, **117**, 694–700.

11 Pinto-Martin J, Paneth N, Witomski T, et al. (1992). The central New Jersey neonatal brain haemorrhage study: design of the study and reliability of ultrasound diagnosis. *Paediatr Perinatal Epidemiol*, **6**, 273–284.

12 Pinto-Martin JA, Riolo S, Cnaan A, et al. (1995). Cranial ultrasound prediction of disabling and nondisabling cerebral palsy at age two in a low birth weight population. *Pediatrics*, **95**, 249–254.

13 Bulas DL, Glass P, O'Donnell RM, et al. (1995). Neonates treated with ECMO: predictive value of CT and US neuroimaging findings on short-term neurodevelopmental outcome. *Radiology*, **195**, 407–412.

14 Aziz K, Vickar DB, Sauve RS, et al. (1995). Province-based study of neurologic disability of children weighing 500 through 1249 grams at birth in relation to neonatal cerebral ultrasound findings. *Pediatrics*, **95**, 837–844.

15 Boal DKB, Watterberg KL, Miles S, et al. (1995). Optimal cost-effective timing of cranial ultrasound screening in low-birth-weight infants. *Pediatric Radiol*, **25**, 425–428.

16 Blankenberg FG, Norbash AM, Barton L, et al. (1996). Neonatal intracranial ischemia and hemorrhage: diagnosis with US, CT and MR Imaging. *Radiology*, **199**, 253–259.

17 Barkovich JA, Westmark K, Partridge C, et al. (1996). Perinatal asphyxia: MR findings in the first 10 days. *Am J Neuroradiol*, **16**, 427–438.

18 Bulas DL, Taylor GA, O'Donnell RM, et al. (1996). Intracranial abnormalities in infants treated with extracorporeal membrane oxygenation: update on sonographic and CT findings. *Am J Neuroradiol*, **17**, 287–294.

19 Blankenberg FG, Loh N, Bracci P, et al. (2000). Sonography, CT, and MR imaging: a prospective comparison of neonates with suspected intracranial ischemia and hemorrhage. *Am J Neuroradiol*, **21**, 213–218.

20 van de Bor M, den Ouden L and Guit GL. (1992). Value of cranial ultrasound and magnetic resonance imaging in predicting neurodevelopmental outcome in preterm infants. *Pediatrics*, **90**, 196–199.

21 Skranes JS, Vik T, Nilsen G, et al. (1993). Cerebral magnetic resonance imaging (MRI) and mental and motor function of very low birth weight infants at one year of corrected age. *Neuropediatrics*, **24**, 256–262.

22 Scher MS, Belfar H, Martin J, et al. (1991). Destructive brain lesions of presumed fetal onset: Antepartum causes of cerebral palsy. *Pediatrics*, **88**, 898–906.

23 Allan WC and Riviello JJ. (1992). Perinatal cerebrovascular disease in the neonate. Parenchymal ischemic lesions in term and preterm infants. *Pediatr Clin North Am*, **39**, 621–650.

24 Menkes JH and Curran J. (1994). Clinical and MR correlates in children with extra pyramidal cerebral palsy. *Am J Neuroradiol*, **15**, 451–457.

25 Ford LM, Steichen J, Steichen Asch PA, et al. (1989). Neurologic status and intracranial hemorrhage in very-low-birth-weight preterm infants. *Am J Dis Child*, **143**, 1186–1190.

26 Tzika A, Vigneron D, Ball W, et al. (1993). Localized proton MR spectroscopy of the brain in children. *J MRI*, **3**, 719–729.

27 Wang Z, Zimmerman RA and Sauter R. (1996). Proton MR spectroscopy of the brain: clinically useful information obtained in assessing CNS diseases in children. *Am J Neuroradiol*, **167**, 191–199.

28 Chateil J-F, Quesson B, Brun M, et al. (1999). Localized proton magnetic resonance spectroscopy of the brain after perinatal hypoxia: a preliminary report. *Pediatr Radiol*, **29**, 199–205.

29 Holshouser BA, Ashwal S, Luh GY, et al. (1997). Proton MR spectroscopy after acute central nervous injury: outcome prediction in neonates, infants, and children. *Radiology*, **202**, 487–496.

30 Moore GJ. (1989). Proton magnetic resonance spectroscopy in pediatric neuroradiology. *Pediatr Radiol*, **28**, 805–814.

31 Forbes KPN, Pipe JG and Bird R. (2000). Neonatal hypoxic–ischemic encephalopathy: detection with diffusion-weighted MR imaging. *Am J Neuroradiol*, **21**, 1490–1496.

32 Huppi PS, Maier SE, Peled S, et al. (1998). Microstructural development of human newborn cerebral white matter

assessed in vivo by diffusion tensor magnetic resonance imaging. *Pediatr Res*, **44**, 584–590.
33 Huppi PS, Murphy B, Maier SE, et al. (2001). Microstructural brain development after perinatal cerebral white matter injury assessed by diffusion tensor magnetic resonance imaging. *Pediatrics*, **107**, 455–460.
34 Johnson AJ, Lee BCP and Lin W. (1999). Echoplanar diffusion-weighted imaging in neonates and infants with suspected hypoxic–ischemic injury. *Am J Roentgenol*, **172**, 219–226.
35 Neil JJ, Shiran SI and McKinstry RC. (1998). Normal brain in human newborns: apparent diffusion coefficient and diffusion anisotropy measured by using diffusion tensor MR imaging. *Radiology*, **209**, 57–66.
36 Phillips MD and Zimmerman RA. (1999). Diffusion imaging in pediatric hypoxic–ischemic injury. *Neuroimaging Clin North Am*, **9**, 41–52.
37 Robertson RL, Ben-Sira L, Barnes PD, et al. (1999). MR line scan diffusion imaging of term neonates with perinatal brain ischemia. *Am J Neuroradiol*, **20**, 1658–1670.
38 Park CH, Spitzer AR, Desai HJ, et al. (1992). Brain SPECT in neonates following extracorporeal membrane oxygenation: evaluation of technique and preliminary results. *J Nucl Med*, **33**, 1943–1948.
39 Konishi Y, Kuriyama M, Mori I, et al. (1994). Assessment of local cerebral blood flow in neonates with *N*-isopropyl-P-[^{123}I]iodoamphetamine and single photon emission computed tomography. *Brain Dev*, **16**, 450–453.
40 Haddad J, Constantinesco A, Brunot B, et al. (1994). A study of cerebral perfusion using single photon emission computed tomography in neonates with brain lesions. *Acta Paediatr*, **83**, 265–269.
41 Haddad J, Constantinesco A, Brunot B, et al. (1994). Cerebral perfusion studies during maturation using single photon emission computed tomography in the neonatal period. *Biol Neonate*, **65**, 281–286.
42 D'Arceuil H, Rhine W, de Crespigny A, et al. (2000). 99mTc annexin V imaging of neonatal hypoxic brain injury. *Stroke*, **31**, 2692–2700.
43 Volpe JS, Herscovitch P, Perlman JM, et al. (1983). Positron emission tomography in the newborn: extensive impairment of regional blood flow with intraventricular hemorrhage and hemorrhagic intracerebral involvement. *Pediatrics*, **72**, 589–601.
44 Azzarelli B, Caldemeyer KS, Phillips JP, et al. (1996). Hypoxic–ischemic encephalopathy in areas of primary myelinization: a neuroimaging and PET study. *Pediatr Neurol*, **14**, 108–116.
45 Chugani HT. (1992). Functional brain imaging in pediatrics. *Pediatr Clin North Am*, **39**, 777–799.
46 Barr LL. (1999). Neonatal cranial ultrasound. *Radiol Clin North Am*, **37**, 1127–1146.
47 Anderson N, Allan R, Darlow B, et al. (1994). Diagnosis of intraventricular hemorrhage in the newborn: value of sonography via the posterior fontanelle. *Am J Roentgenol*, **163**, 893–896.
48 Buckley KM, Taylor GA, Estroff JA, et al. (1997). Use of the mastoid fontanelle for improved sonographic visualization of the neonatal brain and posterior fossa. *Am J Roentgenol*, **168**, 1021–1025.
49 Barnes PD and Taylor GA. (1998). Imaging of the neonatal central nervous system. *Neurosurg Clin North Am*, **1**, 17–48.
50 Allison JW and Seibert JJ. (1999). Transcranial Doppler in the newborn with asphyxia. *Neuroimaging Clin North Am*, **9**, 11–16.
51 Rubin JM, Bude RO, Carson PL, et al. (1994). Power Doppler: a potentially useful alternative to mean-frequency based color Doppler sonography. *Radiology*, **190**, 853–856.
52 Morrison FK, Patel NB, Howie PW, et al. (1995). Neonatal cerebral arterial flow velocity waveforms in term infants with and without metabolic acidosis at delivery. *Early Hum Dev*, **42**, 155–168.
53 Horgan JG, Rumack CM, Hay T, et al. (1989). Absolute intracranial blood-flow velocities evaluated by duplex Doppler sonography in asymptomatic preterm and term infants. *Am J Roentgenol*, **152**, 1059–1064.
54 Taylor GA, Short LB, Walker LK, et al. (1990). Intracranial blood flow: quantification with duplex and color Doppler flow US. *Radiology*, **176**, 231–236.
55 Taylor GA and Madsen JR. (1996). Hemodynamic response to fontanelle compression in neonatal hydrocephalus: correlation with intracranial pressure and need for shunt placement. *Radiology*, **201**, 685–689.
56 Anderson JC and Mawk JR. (1988). Intracranial arterial duplex Doppler waveform analysis in infants. *Childs Nerv Syst*, **4**, 144–148.
57 Mullaart RA, Hopman JC, Rotteveel JJ, et al. (1997). Cerebral blood flow velocity and pulsation in neonatal respiratory distress syndrome and periventricular hemorrhage. *Pediatr Neurol*, **16**, 118–125.
58 Pryds O, Greisen G, Lou H, et al. (1990). Vasoparalysis associated with brain damage in asphyxiated term infants. *J Pediatr*, **117**, 119–125.
59 Frewen TC, Kissoon N, Kronick J, et al. (1991). Cerebral blood flow, cross-brain extraction, and fontanelle pressure after hypoxic–ischemic injury in newborn infants. *J Pediatr*, **118**, 265–271.

60 Pryds O. (1991). Control of cerebral circulation in the high risk neonate. *Ann Neurol*, **30**, 321–329.

61 Skov L, Pryds O, Greisen G, et al. (1993). Estimation of cerebral venous saturation in newborn infants by near infrared spectroscopy. *Pediatr Res*, **33**, 52–55.

62 Pryds O. (1994). Low neonatal cerebral oxygen delivery is associated with brain injury in preterm infants. *Acta Paediatr*, **83**, 1233–1236.

63 DeReuck J, Chattaha AS and Richardson EP. (1972). Pathogenesis and evolution of periventricular leukomalacia in infancy. *Arch Neurol*, **27**, 229–236.

64 Blankenberg FG, Loh N, Norbash AM, et al. (1997). Impaired cerebrovascular autoregulation after hypoxic–ischemic injury in extremely low birth weight neonates: detection with power and pulsed wave doppler US. *Radiology*, **205**, 563–568.

65 Cabanas F, Pellicer A, Garcia-Alix A, et al. (1997). Effect of dexamethasone therapy on cerebral and ocular blood flow velocity in premature infants studied by colour Doppler flow imaging. *Eur J Pediatr*, **156**, 41–46.

66 Rutter N and Evans N. (2000). Cardiovascular effects of an intravenous bolus of morphine in the ventilated preterm infant. *Arch Dis Child Fetal Neonatal Edn*, **83**, F101–F103.

67 Dani C, Bertini G, Reali MF, et al. (2000). Brain hemodynamic changes in preterm infants after maintenance dose caffeine and aminophylline treatment. *Biol Neonate*, **78**, 27–32.

68 Romagnoli C, De Carolis MP, Papacci P, et al. (2000). Effects of prophylactic ibuprofen on cerebral and renal hemodynamics in very preterm neonates. *Clin Pharmacol Ther*, **67**, 676–683.

69 Lott JW, Connor GK and Phillips JB. (1996). Umbilical artery catheter blood sampling alters cerebral blood flow velocity in preterm infants. *J Perinatol*, **16**, 341–345.

70 Barrington KJ. (2000). Umbilical artery catheters in the newborn: effects of position of the catheter tip. *Cochrane Database Syst Rev*, **2**, CD000505.

71 Papile LA, Burnstein J, Burstein R, et al. (1978). Incidence and evolution of subependymal and intraventricular hemorrhage: a study of infants less than 1500 gm. *J Pediatr*, **92**, 529–534.

72 Quisling RG, Reeder JD, Setzer ES, et al. (1983). Temporal comparative analysis of computed tomography with ultrasound for intracranial hemorrhage in premature infants. *Neuroradiology*, **24**, 205–211.

73 Volpe JJ. (1989). Intraventricular hemorrhage in the premature infant – current concepts. Part I. *Ann Neurol*, **25**, 3–11.

74 Volpe JJ. (1989). Intraventricular hemorrhage in the premature infant – current concepts. Part II. *Ann Neurol*, **25**, 109–116.

75 Rypens F, Avni EF, Dussaussois L, et al. (1994). Hyperechoic thickened ependyma: sonographic demonstration and significance in neonates. *Pediatr Radiol*, **24**, 550–553.

76 Perlman JM and Rollins N. (2000). Surveillance protocol for the detection of intracranial abnormalities in premature neonates. *Arch Pediatr Adolesc Med*, **154**, 822–826.

77 Boo NY, Chandran V, Zulfiquar MA, et al. (2000). Early cranial ultrasound changes as predictors of outcome during the first year of life in term infants with perinatal asphyxia. *J Pediatr Child Health*, **36**, 363–369.

78 Bass WT, Jones MA, White LE, et al. (1999). Ultrasonographic differential diagnosis and neurodevelopmental outcome of cerebral white matter lesions in premature infants. *J Perinatol*, **19**, 330–336.

79 Weiss HH, Goldtein RB and Piecuch RE. (1999). A critical review of cranial ultrasounds: is there a closer association between intraventricular blood, white matter abnormalities or cysts, and cerebral palsy? *Clin Pediatr*, **38**, 319–323.

80 Kuban K, Sanocka U, Leviton A, et al. (1999). White matter disorders of prematurity: association with intraventricular hemorrhage and ventriculomegaly. The Developmental Epidemiology Network. *J Pediatr*, **134**, 539–546.

81 Ball WS Jr and Franz DN. (1997). Neonatal brain injury. In *Pediatric Neuroradiology*, Ball WS, Jr ed., p. 239. Philadelphia: Lippincott-Raven.

82 Barnes PD and Robertson RL. (1998). Neuroradiologic evaluation of the cerebral palsies. In *The Cerebral Palsies: Causes, Consequences, and Management*, Miller G and Clark G, eds., pp. 109–150. Boston: Butterworth-Heinemann.

83 Schouman-Claeys E, Henry-Feugeas MC, Roset F, et al. (1993). Periventricular leukomalacia: correlation between MR imaging and autopsy findings during the first two months of life. *Radiology*, **189**, 59–64.

84 Guzzetta F, Shackelford GD, Volpe S, et al. (1986). Periventricular intraparenchymal echodensities in the premature newborn: critical determinant of neurologic outcome. *Pediatrics*, **78**, 995–1006.

85 Patel MD, Cheng AG and Callen PW. (1995). Lateral ventricular effacement as an isolated sonographic finding in premature infants: prevalence and significance. *Am J Roentgenol*, **165**, 155–159.

86 Connolly B, Kelehan P, O'Brien N, et al. (1994). The echogenic thalamus in hypoxic ischemic encephalopathy. *Pediatr Radiol*, **24**, 268–271.

87 Hope PL, Gould SJ, Howard S, et al. (1988). Precision of ultrasound diagnosis of pathologically verified lesions in the brains of very preterm infants. *Dev Med Child Neurol*, **30**, 457–471.

88 Huppi PS and Barnes PD. (1997). Magnetic resonance techniques in the evaluation of the newborn brain. *Clin Perinatol*, **24**, 693–723.

89 Barkovich A and Hallam D. (1977). Neuroimaging in perinatal hypoxic–ischemic injury. *Mental Retard Dev Disabilities Res Rev*, **3**, 28–41.

90 Chen CY, Chou TY, Zimmerman RA, et al. (1996). Pericerebral fluid collection: differentiation of enlarged subarachnoid spaces from subdural collections with color Doppler US. *Radiology*, **201**, 389–392.

91 Wilms G, Vanderschueren G, Demaerel PH, et al. (1993). CT and MR in infants with pericerebral collections and macrocephaly: benign enlargement of the subarachnoid spaces versus subdural collections. *Am J Neuroradiol*, **14**, 855–860.

92 Barkovich AJ. (1992). MR and CT evaluation of profound neonatal and infantile asphyxia. *Am J Neuroradiol*, **13**, 959–972.

93 Lupton BA, Hill A, Roland EH, et al. (1988). Brain swelling in the asphyxiated term newborn: pathogenesis and outcome. *Pediatrics*, **82**, 139–146.

94 Ashwal S, Holshouser BA, Tomasi LG, et al. (1997). Proton magnetic resonance spectroscopy determined cerebral lactate and poor neurological outcomes in children with central nervous system disease. *Ann Neurol*, **41**, 470–481.

95 Tzika A, Massoth R, Ball W Jr, et al. (1993). Cerebral perfusion in children: detection with dynamic contrast-enhanced T2-weighted images. *Radiology*, **87**, 449–458.

96 Levine D, Barnes PD, Madsen JR, et al. (1999). Fetal CNS anomalies revealed on ultrafast MR imaging. *Am J Roentgenol*, **172**, 813–818.

97 Levine D, Barnes PD, Madsen JR, et al. (1999). Central nervous system abnormalities assessed with prenatal magnetic resonance imaging. *Obstet Gynecol*, **94**, 1011–1019.

98 Levine D and Barnes PD. (1999). Cortical maturation in normal and abnormal fetuses as assessed with prenatal MR imaging. *Radiology*, **20**, 751–758.

99 Simon EM, Goldstein RB, Coakley FV, et al. (2000). Fast MR imaging of fetal CNS anomalies in utero. *Am J Neuroradiol*, **21**, 1688–1698.

100 Aida N, Nishimura G, Hachiya Y, et al. (1982). MR imaging of perinatal brain damage: comparison of clinical outcome with initial follow-up MR findings. *Am J Neuroradiol*, **19**, 1909–1922.

101 Barkovich AJ and Sargent SK. (1995). Profound asphyxia in the premature infant: imaging findings. *Am J Neuroradiol*, **16**, 1837–1846.

102 Barkovich AJ and Truwit CL. (1990). Brain damage from perinatal asphyxia: correlation of MR findings with gestational age. *Am J Neuroradiol*, **11**, 1087–1096.

103 Huppi PS, Warfield S, Kikinis R, et al. (1998). Quantitative magnetic resonance imaging of brain development in premature and mature newborns. *Ann Neurol*, **43**, 224–235.

104 Inder T, Huppi PS, Zientara GP, et al. (1999). Early detection of periventricular leukomalacia by diffusion-weighted magnetic resonance imaging techniques. *J Pediatr*, **134**, 631–634.

105 Inder TE, Huppi PS, Warfield S, et al. (1999). Periventricular white matter injury in the premature infant followed by reduced cerebral cortical gray matter volume at term. *Ann Neurol*, **46**, 755–760.

106 Rivkin MJ. (1997). Hypoxic–ischemic brain injury in the term newborn: neuropathology, clinical aspects, and neuroimaging. *Clin Perinatal*, **24**, 607–625.

107 Roland EH, Poskitt K, Rodriguez E, et al. (1998). Perinatal hypoxic–ischemic thalamic injury: clinical features and neuroimaging. *Ann Neurol*, **44**, 161–166.

108 Rorke LB and Zimmerman RA. (1992). Prematurity, postmaturity, and destructive lesions in utero. *Am J Neuroradiol*, **13**, 517–536.

109 Winkler P and Zimmerman RA. (2000). Perinatal brain injury. In *Neuroimaging: Clinical and Physical Principles*, Gibby WA and Carmody R, eds, pp. 531–583. New York: Springer.

110 Barkovich AJ, Baranski K, Vigneron D, et al. (1999). Proton MR spectroscopy in the evaluation of asphyxiated term neonates. *Am J Neuroradiol*, **20**, 1399–1405.

111 Ball WS Jr. (1997). Cerebrovascular disease. In *Pediatric Neuroradiology*, Ball WS Jr, ed., p. 505. Philadelphia: Lippincott-Raven.

112 Ball W Jr. (1994). Cerebrovascular occlusive disease in childhood. *Neuroimaging Clin North Am*, **4**, 393–421.

113 Boyer RS. (1994). Neuroimaging of premature infants. *Neuroimaging Clin North Am*, **4**, 241–261.

23

Near-infrared spectroscopy and imaging

Susan R. Hintz and Christopher H. Contag

Stanford University School of Medicine, Stanford, CA, USA

Theory of near-infrared spectroscopy and applications

Development of light-based diagnostic systems

Transillumination, or the passage of light through the body, is a concept that has been studied since the early 1800s. Initial attempts to image organs and tissues for the purpose of diagnosis and treatment have developed significantly over the years; light-based monitoring in the form of pulse oximetry is now relied upon daily in hospitals and clinics. Transillumination of the head, first described in 1831 by Richard Bright, would later be recognized as the first light-based diagnosis of hydrocephalus. The technique was modified and, although still crude, was used to diagnose intracranial hemorrhage in the neonate[1] at a time when head ultrasound was not yet in use, and computed tomography (CT) was extremely expensive and not widely available.

The early light-based devices for brain-imaging employed broad-spectrum visible light sources, whereas in more recent developments light over a narrower band of wavelengths has been used. However, in 1977, Jobsis showed that, if near-infrared (NIR) light, with a wavelength of 700–1000 nm, was used instead of visible light, absorption by tissue was low enough for spectral measurements to be made across the head of an animal with a diameter of 5–6 cm.[2] Using light in this wavelength band affords enormous potential diagnostic benefits far beyond those of very simple anatomic imaging possible with early devices. The absorption of this NIR light by particular pigments in the body changes as the oxygenation state of these pigments change. Thus, deoxyhemoglobin (Hb) absorbs light differently after it has bound oxygen and becomes oxyhemoglobin (HbO_2; Figure 23.1). This principle forms the basis for modern pulse oximetry, and for newer near-infrared spectroscopy (NIRS) devices which examine brain oxygenation and hemoglobin concentration. Cytochrome aa_3, the terminal enzyme in the mitochondrial electron transport chain, can also be detected using NIRS. Measurement of cytochrome aa_3 may allow assessment of oxygenation at the cellular level, with changes in oxidized and reduced cytochrome aa_3 concentrations (redox state) indicating changes in molecular oxygen availability; however, the validity of this signal is controversial.

In addition to measuring the inherent optical properties of tissues conferred by pigments that are naturally present in blood and tissues, exogenous dyes that absorb and emit light in the NIR can be used to sense changes in some biological processes that are not characterized by naturally occurring pigments. Although still experimental, dyes or contrast agents that can be activated by physiological processes or by expression of an endogenous or exogenous gene may enhance analyses of biological changes using optical measurements in the future.

NIRS devices

All NIR devices to study the brain have a few basic principles in common. Low-intensity light within

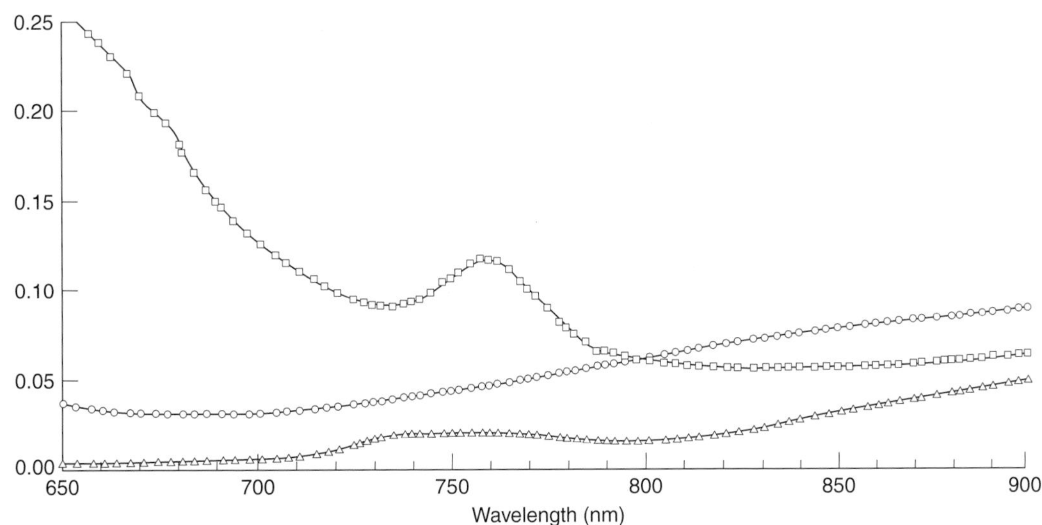

Figure 23.1 The absorption spectra of oxyhemoglobin (circles), deoxyhemoglobin (squares), and water (triangles), with absorption coefficients noted on the *y*-axis in 1/cm. Extinction coefficients taken from Wray et al.[64] Courtesy of ISS, Inc., Champaign, IL.

the NIR wavelengths is transferred from fiberoptic cables to optodes placed on the head (emitters). NIR light is a nonionizing form of radiation, and is known to penetrate several centimeters into tissue; thus the emitted light is transmitted through the neonatal scalp and skull and can reach the brain. As the photons of light interact with tissues they are scattered and absorbed to varying degrees based on the physical and chemical properties of the skin, bone, and brain. Other optodes (detectors) then collect the attenuated photons after they have traversed the tissue and the signals are transferred to an analyzer via fiberoptic cables. The depth of the tissue that is interrogated is a function of the emitter–detector separation distance on the tissue surface; the greater the distance between the two, the deeper the penetration. The photons are therefore transmitted through a portion of the brain between the emitter and detector, yielding information about the function, and in some cases structure, of the brain (Figure 23.2). An obvious corollary to the description of the device is that an adequate amount of light must reach the detector, a problem that can prevent the collection of satisfactory data in certain devices under particular circumstances. Photon absorption by superficial tissues or dark hair may also impact upon signal adequacy, although this is a more serious problem in studies of adults compared with those in neonates.[3]

There are several types of device currently in use in animal and human clinical studies. The most commonly used devices are "continuous-wave" devices in which two or more lasers generate NIR light at specific wavelengths. These light sources are connected to emitters from which the light is directed into the tissues. The transmitted nonabsorbed light is then detected and sent to a photomultiplier, and a computer calculates absorbance. Further calculations are made to obtain changes in chromophore concentrations (see Theory of Hemodynamic Evaluation by NIRS, below). These devices require that certain assumptions be made regarding scattering properties and homogeneity of the brain (see Assumptions and Potential Limitations, below).

Using this basic instrumentation format, additional

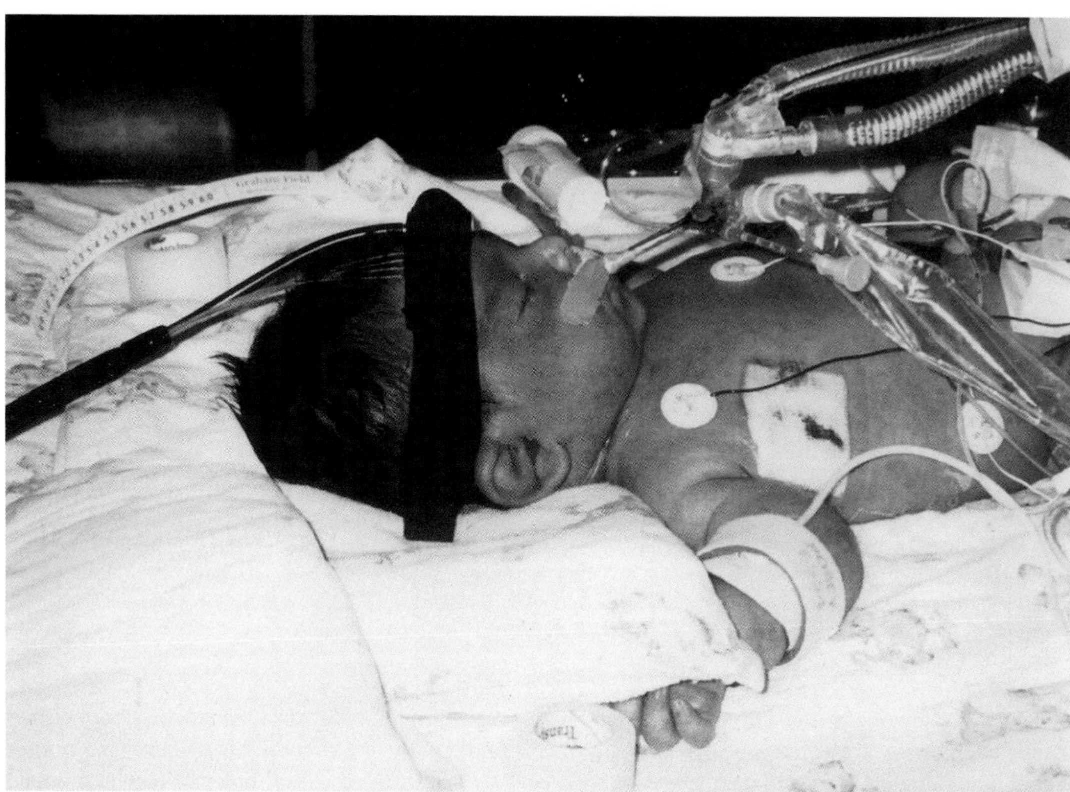

Figure 23.2 Near-infrared spectroscopy (NIRS) monitor probe in place on a critically ill term infant. Note that the headband has been constructed such that the emitter and detector fibers lie flat against the head. In this particular study, the optodes are positioned at the front of the infant's head. Fiber connections are made at the NIRS device, and information is displayed on a laptop computer. The infant shown is being monitored with an ISS Oximeter (Champaign, IL); numerous NIRS monitoring devices are currently available.

methods and devices have been developed. Phase-resolved spectroscopy devices utilize continuous-wave lasers, but light is intensity-modulated at a known frequency. Light which traverses the tissues is then detected, transmitted to a photomultiplier, and then to demodulators. A shift in the modulation phase of the detected signal, a phase shift, is determined by the device. Pathlength is computationally derived from phase shift, frequency of modulation, and the refractive index of the subject's tissue.[4] Studies using these types of devices have demonstrated the wide variability of tissue optical pathlength as a function of gestational and actual age, gender, and other factors.[5–7] This has reinforced the importance of either measuring factors that account for the subject-to-subject inconsistencies in scattering, or the actual optical pathlength at the initiation of each study. Time-of-flight spectroscopy uses pulsed laser light, and allows measurement of the time delay for each photon detected, rather than ensemble averages, within an early-arriving window over picoseconds.[8] This type of approach is independent of photon intensity, but relies on the peak time of photon detection and the time-vs-intensity curve to reveal information about the scattering and absorbance properties of the tissue (Figure 23.3).

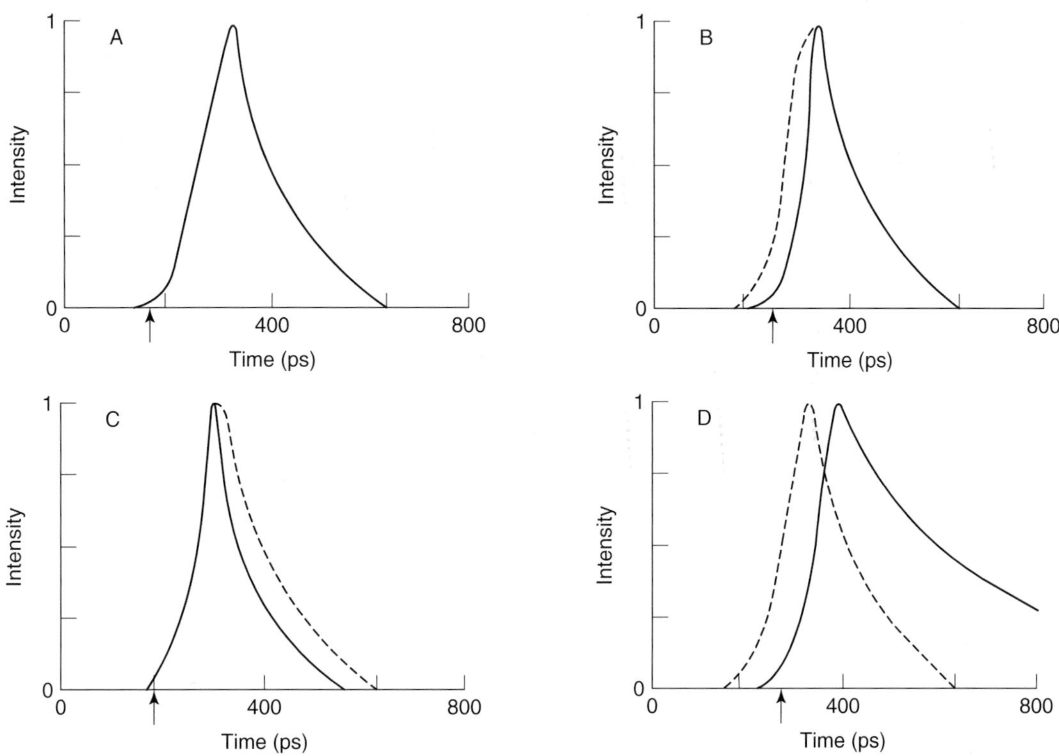

Figure 23.3 Normalized time-of-flight and absorbance (TOFA) curves through four tissue models. (A) Photon transmission through lipid alone yields a wide time-vs-intensity curve. Time of arrival of the first 1% of total transmitted light is indicated by the arrow. Blocking the direct optical path with rods (B) or a finger (D) results in loss of earliest-arriving photons as compared with curve through lipid, shown as dashed line. Blocking peripheral optical path (C) results in loss of later-arriving photons.

Time-resolved techniques are considered the most direct and accurate; however, they are also more expensive and potentially cumbersome than other NIRS approaches. Therefore, the development and clinical investigation of these types of devices have been limited.

Although seemingly complex, the benefits of light-based investigative and diagnostic technology are clear for the critically ill neonatal population. NIRS is a noninvasive bedside technology. It also has the potential to serve as a monitor, providing continuous real-time information rather than just a single static measurement. It also has the potential to act as a bedside functional imager. Current technologies which provide information regarding cerebral hemodynamics or oxygenation and attempt to identify evolving brain injury, such as functional magnetic resonance imaging (fMRI), magnetic resonance spectroscopy (MRS), and positron emission tomography (PET), are not available at every institution. If available, they are not amenable to frequent repeated scanning, and are thus not suited to unstable intensive care patients. In a rapidly changing critical care scenario, moving a patient to a distant radiology suite may be unwise or impossible. Furthermore, "snapshots" of brain function in an ill neonate, such as those provided by traditional imaging methods, may not be of optimal benefit in the approaching era of neuroprotective intervention.

Theory of hemodynamic evaluation by NIRS

There are known unique relative absorption coefficients for HbO_2 and Hb at each wavelength (Figure 23.1). By employing Beer–Lambert law, one may solve for the concentrations of HbO_2 and Hb, and thus for total hemoglobin (tHb) concentration by the relation:

$$A = \varepsilon CL \tag{23.1}$$

where A is absorbance, ε is the constant coefficient which represents the absorbance of the substance at a particular wavelength, C is the chromophore concentration, and L is distance traveled by light through the tissue (pathlength). As expressed in eqn 23.1, the Beer–Lambert law is highly simplified. This relation has been modified and described in numerous more complex ways, such as:

$$\mathrm{OD} = a[c]LB + \mathrm{G} \qquad (23.2)^{9-11}$$

where OD is optical density; a is the absorption coefficient of the chromophore (Hb or HbO_2) at a particular wavelength; c is the concentration of the chromophore; L is the interoptode distance (the measured distance between emitter and detector); and B is the differential pathlength factor (DPF). DPF is meant to be a measure of the variability in pathlength due to the scattering properties of the brain. G is a factor related to the optode geometry and scattering losses. Measuring total absorbance at more than one wavelength allows absorbance equations to be constructed and then solved simultaneously to allow determination of Hb and HbO_2. Changes in tHb may then be calculated by adding changes in Hb and HbO_2. Cerebral blood volume (CBV) has been calculated through modifications of equations based upon Fick's principle as follows:

$$\mathrm{CBV} = \frac{\mathrm{k}_1\,(\Delta \mathrm{HbO}_2 - \Delta \mathrm{Hb})}{2 \times H \times \Delta Sa\mathrm{o}_2} \tag{23.3}$$

where k_1 is a constant which includes factors describing the molecular weight of hemoglobin, the cerebral-to-large-vessel hematocrit ratio, and tissue density; ΔHbO_2 is the change in oxyhemoglobin; ΔHb is the change in deoxyhemoglobin; H is the arterial hemoglobin concentration; and ΔSao_2 is the change in arterial oxygen saturation.[12–14] Equations by which to extrapolate cerebral blood flow (CBF) by NIRS methods have also been published and reported in clinical investigations:

$$\mathrm{CBF} = \frac{\mathrm{k}_2\,(\Delta \mathrm{HbO}_2)}{H \times \int (\Delta Sa\mathrm{o}_2)\mathrm{dt}} \tag{23.4}$$

where k_2 is a constant incorporating the molecular weight of hemoglobin and tissue density. As the calculations include induced changes in Sao_2, these methods require use of the indicator dilution principle,[12–14] with HbO_2 acting as the intravascular indicator or tracer.

Assumptions and potential limitations

There are a number of potential pitfalls regarding the use of these equations with standard NIRS to assess cerebral hemodynamics. First, it may not be possible to induce changes in Sao_2 in every infant over a few seconds, which is a necessary component for these calculations. Also, the induced Sao_2 changes must not lead to changes in CBV or CBF; this assumption of stability is essential and inherent to the equations. Similarly, the hemoglobin concentration must be considered to be constant, and spatially unchanged, throughout the period of study. The brain is presumed to be optically homogeneous, and assumptions are also made regarding the scattering properties and therefore the optical pathlength.[11,13,15,16] Scattering is a major attenuator of photon intensity and an important factor in determining optical pathlength. It is assumed to be essentially the same between subjects of the same gestational age, but the assumption of constancy of transcranial optical pathlength across all clinical circumstances within a particular gestational age may not be valid.[17] The likelihood of a consistent optical pathlength is higher in a very quiet or paralyzed patient, with minor movements such as head tilting and leg positioning potentially leading to changes in pathlength due to changes in optical density.[18,19] Movement could also impact upon pathlength if the emitter–detector separation distance was altered.[5] The optical density characteristics of a traumatized, asphyxiated, or dead brain may also be substantially different from those of a healthy brain; these characteristics may also change with age, and therefore pathlength factors may differ significantly over time and from study to study.[5,6,20,21] Others, however, have reported relatively unchanged water content and optical density characteristics in animal models in the early phases of asphyxia[22,23] and after death in rodents.[11] It is nonetheless crucial that additional studies be undertaken to further the development of NIR techniques, such as time-of-flight and phase-shift modulation, capable of continuous pathlength measurements.[5,7,24,25] Combination systems that use both time-of-flight and phase-shift modulation may offer advantages over single-mode devices in the investigative stage of NIR technology. Moreover, instruments that combine optically based detectors with other modalities such as magnetic resonance imaging (MRI), CT, PET, or electroencephalogram (EEG) may reveal information that can be factored into the set of assumptions used in NIR spectroscopy and imaging.

Finally, it is also important to recognize that standard NIRS devices employing algorithms derived from the modified Beer–Lambert law have thus far been useful for the description of global, not focal, changes. Recent studies have shown that standard NIRS measurements of changes in HbO_2 and Hb during focal brain activation vary widely.[26] This may in part be due to positioning of the emitter–detector pairs resulting in a partial volume error due to the focal nature of the change. However, the variation observed is possibly the result of differential sensitivity of the wavelength measurement to the focal change, resulting in "cross-talk" between Hb and HbO_2 which could make a change in one appear to be a change in the other.[26–28] Therefore, standard NIRS may not be the best method by which to study suspected focal changes in HbO_2 and Hb caused by localized brain activation,[26,29] although other optical technologies exist which could offer exciting imaging alternatives (see Imaging section, below).

Neonatal clinical applications

Measurement and validity of cerebral hemodynamic parameters in the term and preterm infant

Although some controversy exists, numerous studies have concluded that NIRS-derived measurements of cerebral hemodynamic variables in the neonate are valid under optimal circumstances. CBF has been studied using ^{133}Xe clearance methods in neonates, and has been found to be comparable to NIRS results.[16,30–32] Further studies have recently compared NIRS estimations of CBF with microsphere quantitation in newborn piglets during steady state, ischemia, and reperfusion periods.[33] These studies demonstrated statistically similar results between the methods. Patel and colleagues compared CBF measurements in a small group of infants of varying gestational ages by two different NIRS-based, Fick principle-derived methods; the "standard" method using HbO_2 as a tracer, and another using indocyanine green (ICG) as a tracer.[34] The two methods were found to be in good agreement, and ICG allowed for rapid and repeated measurements without the need for Sao_2 alterations. In another recent report,[35] Kuebler and colleagues obtained estimates of CBF in pigs under a variety of clinical circumstances using NIRS with the tracer dye ICG, and compared findings with values assessed by radioactive microspheres. Although cortical blood flow measurements correlated significantly, the limits of agreement between the methods were wide. It has also been suggested by Newton et al. that CBF measurements, as obtained by NIRS in reflectance mode in dogs, are not valid at high CBF values.[36] However, others have countered that technical issues such as sample rate inadequacy, limitations of particular NIRS devices, and significant potential optical interference of the layers surrounding the brain in specific animal and adult models, may have led to inappropriate conclusions.[37] The importance of technical expertise and appropriate instrumentation is thus essential to proper study design and data collection in investigations of CBF using NIRS.

A detailed method for NIRS estimation of CBV was reported in 1990,[3] along with CBV values in normal and brain-injured infants. A close relationship between CBF and CBV has been demonstrated by some groups,[31] although results from others suggest that CBF and CBV may not have equivalent prognostic value.[5,12,38] Cyclical fluctuations in NIRS-derived estimates of CBV, which compared favorably to flow velocity fluctuations, as observed by Doppler ultrasound, have been reported.[39] In a small clinical study, Wickramasinghe et al. found CBF and CBV estimates by NIRS to be valid when compared against the method of jugular venous occlusion plethysmography.[40] Brun and colleagues later compared NIRS with radiolabel-based estimates of CBV in piglets, but they failed to demonstrate a correlation.[41] However, in a more recent study comparing NIRS-derived measurements of CBV with those obtained using radiolabeled red blood cells (^{51}Cr-RBC) and radioiodinated albumin ($^{1}2^{5}$I-RISA) in the immature lamb, the methodologies provided essentially identical results.[42]

The study of cerebral hemodynamic regulation in the potentially high-risk term and preterm infant by noninvasive NIRS may be of enormous value. Further assessment of the possible differences between technologic and methodological approaches in NIRS research would be helpful, but direct comparison of study results may be challenging because many clinical NIRS devices employing disparate analytical algorithms are now under investigation. In addition, the long-term implications of tHb, CBV, and estimated CBF changes monitored by NIRS are not yet clear. For instance, although changes in hemodynamic variables may be monitored using NIRS, the values below which death or severe disability may be expected are unknown.

NIRS-derived estimates of CBV in normal infants have been reported to range between 1.9 and 3.2 ml/100 g tissue[3,12] with a mean of 2.2 ml/100 g. This correlates well with observations in stable term and near-term infants by other investigators,[43] and with the recently reported mean CBV of 2.5 ml/100 g observed in NIRS studies of immature lambs.[42] A similar range of approximately 1–3 ml/100 g has been reported during the first 3 days of life in preterm infants.[44] Significantly higher CBV estimates (4.1–9.7 ml/100g) have been reported in severely asphyxiated newborns.[12] Neonatal CBF, as measured by NIRS, has generally been reported to be in range of 5–33 ml/100 g brain tissue/min.[13,30–32,34,44] Studies by Skov et al.[31] and Bucher et al.[32] found good correlation between NIRS CBF measurements and those of ^{133}xenon clearance in preterm and term infants. Much higher peak CBF in very-low-birth-weight preterm (66.1 ml/100 g tissue per min) and high-risk term infants (62.1 ml/100 g tissue per min) has been reported.[9,12,45] In the case of the perinatally asphyxiated term infants, a trend toward an association of higher CBF in the first 24 h of life with early death was noted, but the number of patients in this group was extremely small.[12] Similar CBF ranges in very-low-birth-weight preterm infants (approximately 7–25 ml/100 g tissue per min) have recently been reported using the ^{133}Xe clearance method.[46] In that study, however, an association of slightly lower CBF (15.2 ± 3.5 vs 13.0 ± 2.1 ml/100 g tissue per min) with nonsurvival was noted. Still others have reported that a CBF as low as 5 ml/100 g per min can be compatible with a normal neurodevelopmental outcome.[47,48]

Early clinical studies investigated CO_2 vasoreactivity in newborn preterm and term infants. A decrease in CBF with hyperventilation was first described in adults[49] and the phenomenon has now been studied by NIRS in term and preterm infants. Wyatt et al. found that cerebral blood volume reactivity to CO_2 (CBVR) increases with increasing gestational age from 0.07 ml/100 g tissue per kPa at 26 weeks' estimated gestational age (EGA) to 0.51 ml/100 g tissue per kPa at 40 weeks' EGA, indicating a maturational component to this process.[50] Further studies in healthy term infants by Dietz and colleagues suggested that CO_2 reactivity increases as postnatal age increases as well, although the change was not statistically significant.[51] Significantly lower CBVR values have been reported during the first 24 h in term and near-term infants who have sustained hypoxic–ischemic insult.[12] Median values of

0.10–0.17 ml/100 g tissue per kPa were observed in the first 24 h, but tended to return to normal, and did not appear to be associated with an increased likelihood of death or adverse neurodevelopmental outcome at 1 year in this small study.

Measurement and validity of cerebral oxygenation parameters in the term and preterm infant

Although an absolute "gold standard" does not exist for measurement of cerebral oxygenation, NIRS data have been compared to a number of methods. The method has been shown to compare well with jugular bulb oximetry data in children,[52] with an excellent correlation seen in infants undergoing cardiac surgery.[53] In that study of children with ages ranging from 2 weeks to 14 years, stratification revealed that regional cerebral oxygen saturation in patients less than 1 year of age as measured by NIRS compared extremely well with jugular bulb calculations ($r=0.85$, $P<0.0001$). Methodological correlation for individual patient data was even closer. This comparison assumes cerebral microcirculation is predominantly venous.[54,55] In addition, further studies have confirmed that cerebral oxygenation as measured by NIRS correlates with expected tissue oxygenation in piglets and infants, under both hypothermic and normothermic conditions.[56–58] Yoxall and Weindling reported cerebral oxygen consumption data, estimated through NIRS measures, in 20 term and preterm infants under a variety of clinical conditions.[59] The authors observed a range of values (0.52–1.76 ml/100 g per min) which increased with advancing gestational age. The data were also consistent with those obtained through more invasive methods such as ^{133}Xe clearance, PET imaging, and internal jugular vein sampling.[17,48,60] More recently, the capability of MRI and nuclear magnetic resonance (NMR) spectroscopy for mapping Hb concentration has allowed further combined study[61,62] and suggests future directions for comparative analyses.

However, intravascular oxygenation may not always accurately reflect intracellular oxygen availability, and this fact has led to the suggestion that cytochrome aa_3 or redox state could be assessed as more closely reflecting intracellular oxygenation status. Cytochrome aa_3 is the terminal enzyme in the mitochondrial electron transport chain; redox state is dependent on oxygen availability to the mitochondrion. However, caution has been recommended when interpreting data obtained with standard NIRS devices.[63] The signal of this chromophore is much weaker than that of hemoglobin and the algorithms used for calculation of cytochrome aa_3 by NIRS were derived from postmortem experiments of rat brains after exchange with fluorocarbon.[64] There is also overlap between the absorption spectra of hemoglobin and cytochrome aa_3.[65] None the less, there is evidence that NIRS-detected changes in oxidized cytochrome aa_3 reflect injury at the cellular level. In a piglet model of progressive hypoxia, Tsuji et al. studied changes in cerebral HbO_2, Hb, and oxidized cytochrome aa_3 by NIRS simultaneously with changes in phosphocreatine (PCr) and nucleoside triphosphate (NTP) concentrations by ^{31}P-labeled MRS.[66] Although HbO_2 decreased and Hb increased predictably during the study, intracellular injury as detected by loss of PCr and NTP was not observed until severe hypoxia was achieved. Decreases in oxidized cytochrome aa_3 and arterial blood pressure, but not changes in HbO_2 or Hb, correlated closely with these observed PCr and NTP decreases. A more recent study in a rat hypoxia model corroborated cytochrome aa_3 correlations with beta-adenosine triphosphate (ATP) and PCr to Fio_2 0.10.[67] A piglet cardiopulmonary bypass model has also been studied, revealing reductions in cytochrome aa_3 and HbO_2 correlated with decreases in ATP and PCr, with changes in cytochrome aa_3 and PCr showing the strongest correlation.[68] Further studies with animal models and humans have sought to improve spectral resolution and thus better separate the cytochrome aa_3 signal through use of charge-coupled device (CCD) camera-based full-spectrum NIRS systems.[69,70] Further studies will help to delineate challenges and validate the importance of measuring cytochrome aa_3 as a potentially crucial marker of impending cell death in clinical studies.

Neonatal cerebral hemodynamics and oxygenation during intensive care

The pressing need for noninvasive bedside diagnostic and monitoring instrumentation for the smallest and sickest patients, coupled with the unique applicability of light-based technology to the study of the brain in term and preterm infants, has driven numerous laboratories into the neonatal intensive care unit (NICU). Given that alterations in CBF and CBV, hypoxic–ischemic injury, and reperfusion events have all been implicated in the development of intraventricular hemorrhage, periventricular leukomalacia, and other brain injury leading to long-term neurodevelopmental delay,[71] the usefulness of such a strategy is clear. Unfortunately, clinical reports using NIRS have, to date, included only small numbers of patients. These studies have fallen into the categories of observation during "normal" periods, and during intensive care interventions or sensory stimulation. A recent study investigating changes in cerebral oxygenation and hemoglobin concentrations using full-spectrum NIRS immediately after delivery (commencing 70 s to 4 min after birth) suggested that significant dynamic changes occur in an infant's first quarter of an hour of life.[72] Although limited in size, with just seven term and near-term neonates as subjects, the report demonstrated that a rapid and dramatic increase in cerebral hemoglobin oxygen saturation, as well as an initial increase then decrease in cerebral hemoglobin concentration, may be included in neonatal adaptations to extrauterine life.

Several groups have also used NIRS to identify neonatal cyclical fluctuations in CBV.[39,73,74] Livera and colleagues[39] were the first to report on a single preterm infant with a cyclical CBV fluctuation of 3.5 cycles/min, which in that study compared well to strain-gauge plethysmography and to cyclical fluctuations of CBF velocity, as measured by Doppler ultrasound. Later studies with 58 full-term infants at 6–8 weeks of life during quiet daytime sleep further delineated cyclical CBV fluctuations with a frequency of 3–6 cycles/min.[73] In that report, no corresponding fluctuations in other parameters such as heart rate or Sao_2 were noted. Further studies by von Siebenthal et al.[74] showed that preterm infants (26–29 weeks' gestational age) in the first 36 h of life also demonstrated cyclical CBV fluctuations with a frequency of 2–4.7 cycles/min. They also observed slower cyclical fluctuations in heart rate and mean arterial blood pressure (MABP), and suggested that through the method of coherence analysis, a relationship between MABP and CBV fluctuations may exist. Importantly, although the authors used only 20 min of quiet, artifact-free measurements for data analysis, they demonstrated that up to 20 h of continuous NIRS monitoring was possible in even extremely-low-birth-weight premature infants in the first days of life. The etiology of these fluctuations is unknown; it has been suggested that it indicates an immaturity of autoregulation in the neonatal brain;[75] however the age at which this fluctuation is lost is undefined. The clinical importance of this fluctuation, and the quantification of normal amplitude and frequency parameters, remain for further study.

Breathing abnormalities and even crying have been shown to alter cerebral hemodynamics and oxygenation. In an early study of 20 healthy and 16 ill term and preterm infants ranging from 17 h to 24 days of age, Brazy[76] demonstrated that a majority of crying episodes resulted in an increase in CBV and Hb concentration, suggesting obstructed venous return. Apnea of prematurity and periodic breathing have also been shown to be associated with cerebral hemodynamic and oxygenation changes by NIRS. These findings were in agreement with previous studies using Doppler, which showed that CBF velocity decreases with apnea and bradycardia.[77] Jenni et al.[78] described differences in hemodynamic patterns using NIRS in 17 preterm infants with different types of apnea, indicating that obstructive apnea was associated with the most significant fall in cerebral tHb concentration. Later studies in 58 premature infants reinforced this finding, revealing decreases in CBV in a significant number of both short and long apneas, as well as consistent cerebral deoxygenation associated with apneas.[79]

CBF has also been studied by NIRS in critically ill

preterm infants in order to ascertain the validity of the "pressure-passive theory" of CBF in this patient population.[80] The authors found that no significant differences existed in CBF (12.3 ± 6.4 vs 13.9 ± 6.9 ml/100 g per min) between groups of preterm infants with significantly different MABP (27.2 vs 35.3 mm Hg, $P < 0.001$). Whether the difference in MABP, although statistically significant, is in fact clinically significant could be a matter of debate. Similarly, measurements of both CBF and MABP were made for a single relatively short period in the first 24 h, thus a dynamic and evolving process may have been overlooked. Interestingly, a significant correlation was noted with transcutaneous measurement of arterial carbon dioxide tension ($TcCO_2$) across the groups, suggesting that attentiveness to preventing hypocarbia in preterm infants may be of more importance to CBF than MABP. However, a recent report by Tsuji et al. investigated correlations between MABP and HbD, an NIRS-derived measure of cerebral oxygenation defined as $HbO_2 - Hb$, as well as later craniosonographic findings in ill preterm infants.[81] The study was unique in that multiple 30-min NIRS measurements over the first 3 days of life were examined through the method of coherence analysis, and further investigated in a frequency-specific manner. This group had previously demonstrated in a piglet model that induced systemic hypotension was correlated with decreases in CBF and HbD, and that HbD was a sensitive indicator of changes in CBF.[82] Concordant changes in MABP and HbD, as measured by ultralow-frequency coherence values of >0.5, were found in 17 of the 32 patients studied. This further suggested an impairment of cerebral autoregulation in these infants. Importantly, concordance values varied between measurements in these patients, perhaps indicating fluctuations in cerebrovascular stability. Ten of the 32 patients had severe intraventricular hemorrhage or periventricular leukomalacia; of those, eight had coherence scores of >0.5, indicating that infants with severe cranial ultrasound abnormalities were likely to have had evidence of impaired cerebral autoregulation. Although a small study, this report demonstrates both the importance of continuous and frequent NIRS monitoring in the assessment of dynamic processes, and the necessity for further large studies to identify confidently and prospectively high-risk patients and thus better to study potential neuroprotective agents and strategies. Changes in tHb and cerebral hemoglobin oxygenation have also been reported with removal of cerebrospinal fluid in neonates with hydrocephalus, and with increased intracranial pressure in a piglet model of hydrocephalus.[83,84] During the process of inducing acute hydrocephalus in seven neonatal piglets by intraventricular fluid infusion, significant decreases in HbD by NIRS and in CBF by microspheres were demonstrated.[84] A significant correlation between changes in HbD and CBF was also noted. Further investigations are required, but these findings suggest the potential utility of NIRS as an adjuvant monitoring tool for directing clinical interventions.

Events and interventions in the neonatal intensive care environment have also been shown to be associated with significant patient cerebral hemodynamic and oxygenation changes by NIRS. Unfortunately, the implications of these changes are unknown. In a small study of 10 preterm infants in which over 400 events were observed, Gagnon et al. showed that even common and presumably minor events such as rapidly opening an incubator door, inadvertent movement of a patient bed, or overhead announcements can cause dramatic changes in CBV and cytochrome aa_3 redox state.[85] Several groups have studied brain hemodynamic changes with NIRS in preterm infants after caffeine and aminophylline treatment. CBF and CBV have been reported by some to be decreased with aminophylline loading,[86,87] while a recent study indicates that CBV is increased after a maintenance dose of aminophylline but unaffected by caffeine.[88] However, the designs of these studies varied tremendously. The effects of indometacin, another commonly used medication in the NICU, have also been studied with respect to cerebral hemodynamics and oxygenation. In 1990, Edwards et al. reported the disturbing finding in 13 preterm infants that, regardless of rapidity of infusion, indometacin administration resulted in a sharp decrease in CBF, CBV, oxygen delivery, and CBV reactivity to carbon dioxide tension.[89] Later studies confirmed these findings, and further suggested that decreased intracellular oxygenation also resulted from indometacin administration through the measurement of oxidized cytochrome aa_3 and rat brain analyses.[90–92] A recent randomized controlled trial comparing indometacin with ibuprofen indicated that no significant change occurred in CBF, CBV, or oxygen delivery after ibuprofen, but that closure rate of the patent ductus arteriosus was slightly better in the indometacin group.[93] The long-term significance of these induced cerebral hemodynamic changes is unclear; further larger studies will be required to arrive at consensus regarding appropriate treatment regimen.

CBV changes during exchange transfusions were documented by NIRS in eight healthy term infants by van de Bor et al. in 1994.[43] Although the changes were moderate, the results were concerning, as they indicated that MABP-associated changes in CBV may occur in a clinically stable neonatal population. Liem and colleagues investigated the cerebral oxygenation changes associated with both blood transfusions for anemia in preterm infants and partial volume exchange transfusion for polycythemia in term and near-term infants.[94] The authors found that blood transfusions were associated with increases in cerebral HbO_2 while partial exchange was associated with decreases. However, this study was fairly small (13 preterm infants, 10 term or near-term infants), the patient groups were clinically quite different, and the technique used required that the DPF be considered constant throughout the procedures. In a case series of three patients examining the cerebral oxygenation changes during double volume exchange transfusions in ill septic newborns, increases in cerebral HbO_2 were observed upon initiation and continued throughout the procedure in all but one patient.[95] In that patient, who was later diagnosed with periventricular leukomalacia by autopsy, a marked increase in cerebral Hb and decrease in HbO_2 was noted during the exchange transfusion.

Another study by Liem et al. investigated cerebral oxygenation and hemodynamics by NIRS during induction of extracorporeal membrane oxygenation (ECMO) in 24 neonates.[96] The authors found that there was an increase in CBV in the majority of patients, and that changes in total cerebral hemoglobin were significantly positively correlated with changes in MABP. These findings suggest that a loss of cerebrovascular autoregulation could have occurred, which may have been associated with prolonged cerebral hypoxia or evolving ischemia prior to cannulation, rather than due to the initiation of ECMO itself. The study also reported unchanged cytochrome aa_3 concentrations with ECMO induction, leading to the speculation that intracellular oxygen availability was unchanged as a result of preserved cellular energy metabolism in the pre-ECMO period.

The effects of respiratory interventions, common in the NICU for both preterm and ill term infants, have been studied by NIRS and other methods for many years. Reports of significant increases in CBF velocity by Doppler associated with simple tracheal suctioning in preterm infants[97] led to further studies by NIRS in the 1990s. Significant decreases in cerebral HbO_2 and increases in cerebral Hb were observed with suctioning in most studies, but reported total cerebral hemoglobin concentration changes varied.[98–100] Bernert and colleagues suggested a possible reason for these differences, finding variations in cerebral hemodynamic and oxygenation fluctuations depending on the behavioral state of the patient at the time of suctioning.[101] In another small study of 15 preterm infants, a variable pattern of tHb concentration changes, but no differences in decreases in cerebral HbO_2 or increases in cerebral Hb were observed during suctioning between patients ventilated by conventional methods versus high-frequency oscillatory methods.[102] Surfactant administration has been associated with changes in CBF velocities, CBV, EEG changes, and systemic circulatory and oxygenation variability.[103–107] These findings sparked concerns that cerebral hemodynamic instability could result in treatment-associated brain injury. Studies undertaken using NIRS methodology have had mixed results. Some of these reports suggested a transient variable increase or decrease or relative stability in CBV and CBF,[108,109] while others suggested dramatic increases in CBV which were more evident with high-dose than with low-dose surfactant therapy.[110] It has been speculated that differences in surfactant administration methods leading to increased cerebral circulation resulting from elevation in $Paco_2$ may explain the apparently contradictory results.[105–110]

A recent study of 18 premature infants given low-dose surfactant with manual bag ventilation demonstrated no change in transcutaneous Pco_2 levels and a relatively stable tHb concentration.[111] The authors found that cerebral HbO_2 increased significantly and Hb decreased significantly in the first 2 min after surfactant administration, but that these values returned to baseline within the 30-min study period. Interestingly, both HbO_2 and tHb concentration were on the rise at the end of the study period, again suggesting longer-term monitoring of cerebral hemodynamic trends as a potentially fruitful area for further research.

Recent studies have focused on identifying regional cerebral hemodynamic and oxygenation changes in response to sensory stimuli. This area of research was first introduced through studies of adults, in which regional changes were observed with visual stimulation by both blood oxygen level-dependent (BOLD) MRI and NIRS.[29,112] When reviewing the available data, however, it is important to recall the recent concerns put forth regarding reliability of regional measurements from NIRS algorithms utilizing modifications of the Beer–Lambert law,[26–28] (see also Assumptions and Potential Limitations, above). Meek et al. were the first to report on functional hemodynamic changes to visual stimulation in the neonate using NIRS.[113] In that report, 10 infants were studied during visual stimulation with optical probes placed on the occipital region of the head, and 10 age-matched control infants were studied under the same conditions, but with optical probes over the frontoparietal region. The authors found that stimulation resulted in a marked but variable increase in tHb volume in the test group, but not the control group, indicating a region-specific response consistent with the sensory stimulus. This increase in regional CBV with visual stimulation was similar to that seen in previous adult studies. However, unlike adults where Hb decreased with stimulation, an increased Hb and HbO_2 was observed in neonates. These findings were in keeping with previous neonatal visual stimulation studies using MRI,[114,115] and suggested that regional oxygen consumption may exceed oxygen delivery capability during functional activation. A later visual stimulation report by Hoshi et al.[116] studied seven neonates, all term infant less than 1 week of age, whereas the previously described study enrolled term and preterm patients up to 14 weeks of age. The placement and number of optode pairs, the behavioral state of the infants, and the method of visual stimulation differed as well. The authors observed variable results. Increases in HbO_2 and tHb were observed in one of three optode pairs during stimulation, but the direction of the change in Hb differed between subjects and within the same subject between measurements. Decreases in HbO_2, Hb, and tHb were observed in surrounding optode pairs in five of seven cases; the authors suggested that this phenomenon, previously observed with functional stimulation,[117] might be explained by a deflection of blood flow to the area of activation. The differing findings between the two visual stimulation studies could be due to a number of factors, including level of alertness, age, and gestational age differences, technical variations, or normal human subject variability. Sakatani et al. were the first to measure changes induced by auditory stimulation in infants by NIRS.[118] Placing optodes over the frontal lobes, the authors found that over 90% of the subjects demonstrated increases in HbO_2 and tHb during stimulation; most, but not all of these showed concomitant increases in Hb. A later study, where probes were placed over the temporal area, again revealed increases in HbO_2 and tHb with stimulation, and accompanying increases in Hb in the majority of cases.[119] Hemodynamic responses to olfactory stimulation have also been recently studied by NIRS in 23 term infants.[120] The findings indicated a significant but slightly delayed increase in HbO_2 to vanilla, no change in HbO_2 to water (control) and an age-dependent increase in HbO_2 to colostrum. The authors further commented that changes in tHb were the same as for HbO_2, suggesting that there was no change in Hb during stimulation. Although the data were not presented, this would represent a potential difference in functional activation patterns in olfactory compared with other sensory stimuli studied to date.

Correlating cerebral NIRS measurements with outcome

Several important studies using non-NIRS methods attempted to identify prognostic cerebral hemodynamic and oxygenation factors associated with adverse short- and long-term outcome in preterm infants. Pryds[121] assessed cerebral oxygen delivery (COD) using CBF estimated by ^{133}Xe clearance in 93 preterm infants (25–34 weeks) within the first 2 days of life. He found that COD was related to gestational age, intrauterine growth restriction, $Pa\text{CO}_2$, and blood glucose concentration. He also found that lower CBF and COD were related to intraventricular hemorrhage or periventricular leukomalacia and subsequent neurological sequelae 1.7–4.6 years later. However, as discussed by the author, causation could not be assigned; the timing of the single CBF estimation and COD calculation in relation to the diagnosis of cerebral lesion was not specific, and the measurements were global. The infants studied were also broadly varied in terms of gestational age and severity of illness. Mueller et al., also using ^{133}Xe clearance, estimated cerebral CO_2 reactivity in 18 preterm infants within the first 36 h of age and related these findings to outcome.[122] Eight of the infants died, and 10 underwent Bayley Scales of Infant Development (BSID) assessment at 18 months' corrected age. The authors found that infants with higher BSID scores and those with normal brains on autopsy had higher CBF reactivity to CO_2 than did those with low BSID scores and cerebral pathology (median CO_2 reactivity 24.4%/kPa CO_2 vs 3.4%/kPa CO_2). This work suggested a possible role for using CO_2 reactivity to identify prospectively infants at risk for later neurodevelopmental abnormalities. However, these correlations were again based upon single measurements, and patient numbers were very small. The same group published a later much larger report[46] evaluating the potential role of CBF by ^{133}Xe clearance at three time periods within the first 10 days of life in predicting later neurodevelopmental abnormalities in preterm infants. Although the authors found a small but significant difference in CBF between survivors and nonsurvivors at all three time periods, there was no significant correlation between CBF and BSID at any time period, and no correlation between changes in CBF across the time periods and BSID scores. These and other important reports focused attention on the need and potential utility for further studies with a noninvasive and continuously monitoring technology such as NIRS.

Unfortunately, relatively few studies currently exist which correlate cerebral hemodynamic and oxygenation NIRS findings with outcome. Among these are two studies by Meek et al. The first of these reports[123] studied CBF as estimated by NIRS within the first 24 h of life in 24 preterm infants and correlated these results with cerebral ultrasound findings. The authors found that CBF was significantly lower in those infants later diagnosed with any intraventricular hemorrhage than in those with normal cerebral ultrasounds. Importantly, there were no differences in $Pa\text{CO}_2$ at the time of study. These findings were in agreement with the earlier work of Pryds.[121] Citing the concept of cerebral steal phenomenon, the authors further suggested that measurement of CBF by a noninvasive method such as NIRS, combined with assessment of ductal shunting, may be useful in identifying those infants most likely to benefit from early indometacin. NIRS measurements were performed in 21 of 27 term infants with clinical histories and signs consistent with perinatal asphyxia in a later study by the same group.[12] Increased CBV on the first day of life, considered to be greater than 2.6 ml/100 g based on previous findings in healthy neonates,[3] was found to be a sensitive (85%) but not specific (38%) predictor for death or severe disability at 1 year of age. The authors reported a wide range of CBV values in the infants who died, which may be explained by a failure of cerebral reperfusion in the most neurologically devastated. A trend toward higher CBF was also noted in infants with adverse outcomes. Finally, a reduction in CBVR was noted following asphyxia, but was not significantly associated with death or adverse outcome. In total, these findings appear to be in accordance with previous NIRS findings in, and proposed mechanisms of, severe perinatal injury, including reperfusion injury, vasodilatation, and vasoparalysis.[124,125] Unfortunately, as with most clinical NIRS studies to date, this report includes small numbers of subjects, especially for long-term follow-up analyses in which only 15 patients were included due to deaths. With larger patient numbers, these trends and correlations may become more significant and of even greater potential diagnostic impact.

Other NIRS studies indicate that cerebral oxygenation may be able to be used as a predictor of outcome. Tsuji and colleagues[81] studied a group of premature infants ranging from 23 to 31 weeks' gestational age to ascertain if a correlation existed between MABP and HbD ($HbD = HbO_2 - Hb$), an NIRS-obtained measure of cerebral oxygenation which has been noted to correlate with CBF in animal studies. Cerebral NIRS were performed and simultaneous MABP data were obtained for up to 6 h daily for the first 3 days of life. By the statistical method of coherence analysis, concordant changes in MABP and HbD were found in 17 infants. Eight members of this subset, but only two of the 15 "normal" premature infants, went on to be diagnosed with intraventricular hemorrhage or periventricular leukomalacia. This finding suggests that impaired cerebrovascular autoregulation could be identifiable by NIRS techniques, and that these data could be used to identify neonatal populations at risk for neurologic injury.

These reports are extremely important as they are the first to begin to use NIRS in critically ill infants to identify cerebral hemodynamic abnormalities, clinically silent using current monitoring techniques, in an attempt to correlate these findings with short- and long-term outcomes. Ultimately, of course, the evolution of neurodevelopmental disability in term and preterm infants and the development of intraventricular hemorrhage are likely to be extremely complex and multifactorial processes. However, in the future, use of cerebral NIRS monitoring systems coupled with measurements of cellular injury may help to direct neuroprotective therapies in the neonate.[125–127]

Applications in cardiovascular surgery

The technical successes of neonatal cardiovascular surgery have been increasingly impressive during the past several years. Unfortunately, neurodevelopmental sequelae remain a devastating complication encountered in 10–30% of these cases, particularly in complex repairs of cyanotic cardiac lesions.[128–130] Due to the portability and noninvasive nature of NIRS, as well as the potential to monitor continuously cerebral hemodynamic and oxygenation parameters in an environment where traditional monitoring techniques are often useless, NIRS has been the focus of intensive clinical research since the early 1990s. It has been hoped that intraoperative NIRS monitoring will help to provide much needed direction in the proper and timely application of neuroprotective strategies in this high-risk population.[131]

Greeley et al. were among the first to report cerebral oxygenation monitoring using NIRS during cardiopulmonary bypass in 15 pediatric patients ranging in age from 1 day to 6 years.[132] HbO_2, Hb, and oxidized cytochrome aa_3 (CytOx) were compared between nine patients who had undergone repairs during deep hypothermic (18 °C) with continuous cardiopulmonary bypass (CPB) and six patients who had undergone repairs during deep hypothermic circulatory arrest (DHCA). The authors found that, in the continuous bypass group, HbO_2 decreased during CPB and cooling, but returned to control levels during rewarming. However, in the DHCA group, both CytOx and HbO_2 decreased dramatically during circulatory arrest; CytOx did not return to baseline levels and Hb was elevated, even upon rewarming and initiation of CPB. These findings indicated that brain cellular metabolism may undergo sustained impairment after DHCA, even after presumably adequate flow and oxygenation had been established. Despite the controversies regarding CytOx measurement with NIRS, these findings concurred with previous work in children and neonates by the same group of investigators, which suggested disordered cerebral metabolism and oxygen utilization after DHCA but not after repairs under continuous CPB.[133]

In a later seminal study of 17 infants less than 1 month of age, Kurth et al. reported on changes in cerebral HbO_2 and tHb during cooling to 15 °C, undergoing DHCA, and upon rewarming.[134] Cytochrome aa_3 oxidation state could not be measured in this study due to device limitations. A significant decrease in tHb concentration was seen during the first minutes of CPB and cooling, likely due to hemodilution. Total cerebral hemoglobin remained constant throughout circulatory arrest until the time of recirculation. Kinetics of HbO_2 were variable in the first minute of CPB and cooling, with infants with profound preoperative cyanosis demonstrating a dramatic increase, and others relatively unchanged or minimally decreased. However, HbO_2 increased in all infants after 2 min of CPB, resulting in an overall increase in cerebral hemoglobin oxygen saturation (Sco_2). At the onset of circulatory arrest however, HbO_2 decreased in a curvilinear fashion for 40 min; no further desaturation was noted from that point. Upon recirculation, HbO_2 quickly returned to high precirculatory arrest levels, but then decreased to baseline. Of interest, two of the 17 infants experienced postoperative seizures 24–48 h after surgery; both of these had a circulatory arrest time of approximately 70 min. However, 12 other infants in the group had circulatory arrest times of 50–70 min and otherwise similar intraoperative courses, presenting no clear cause for seizures, as supported by NIRS or clinical data. Subsequent studies by the same group[135] revealed that the infants with early postoperative neurologic complications had a less pronounced increase in Sco_2 during CPB before DHCA. During DHCA, Sco_2 decreased dramatically in all patients, with no difference between patients with normal neurologic outcomes and those who later developed complications.

More recent studies have ignited controversy regarding the validity of reliance upon Sco_2 measurements alone. Du Plessis and colleagues elegantly studied the relationship between cerebral HbO_2 and CytOx in 63 infants and children aged 1 day to 9 months undergoing complex cardiac surgery.[136] Although HbO_2 increased during hypothermic CPB, as seen in previous studies,[134] oxidized CytOx paradoxically declined significantly, suggesting an uncoupling of intravascular and mitochondrial oxygenation. It was noted that infants older than 2 weeks of age had a greater decrease in CytOx than did those less than 2 weeks of age, consistent with the notion of increasing cerebral metabolic rate with age.[48] In addition, CytOx did not consistently or promptly return to baseline during reperfusion, despite rapid higher than baseline recovery of HbO_2. These findings have led to concern that the commonly held belief that the brain is protected during hypothermia may not be entirely accurate. The concept of "luxury perfusion" to the brain, as supported by increased intravascular Sco_2, may underestimate a metabolic impairment at the cellular level. In a later report utilizing a piglet bypass model,[137] data similar to these human cerebral oxygenation kinetics were demonstrated; cooling was associated with increased cerebral oxygenation but decreased CytOx, and DHCA was associated with significant decreases in HbO_2. Although differences in findings exist between this study and a previous study,[132] including timing of CytOx decline and direction of HbO_2 change during hypothermic CPB, disparities in patient population and intraoperative protocols may explain them. Finally, Skov and Greisen[63] described decreases in CytOx from the onset of CPB in spite of increased cerebral oxygenation during this time period in hypoxemic children only; similar findings were not noted in children with normal preoperative arterial saturations. Although others have suggested that observed total cerebral hemoglobin concentration differences between groups after initiation of CPB may have influenced this finding,[138] or that a more pronounced cellular disturbance was present in the hypoxemic group, the authors themselves questioned the validity of the CytOx signal.

More recent studies using NIRS have begun to examine particularly vulnerable periods in the cardiovascular surgery process, both before bypass and after the patient leaves the operating theatre. NIRS has also allowed for the opportunity to study cerebral hemodynamics and oxygenation parameters during relatively novel methods of surgical circulatory support, including low-flow perfusion. Cerebral fractional oxygen extraction (FOE) was measured using NIRS and jugular vein compression in 30 children undergoing hypothermic CPB with either circulatory arrest or low continuous flow.[139] FOE was reduced during cooling on bypass in all groups, but there was an increase in FOE on rewarming only in those patients who had been managed with continuous flow. Further NIRS studies suggested that temperature, specific flow variations, and hemodilution could alter cerebral oxygen extraction during CPB.[140] Daubeney et al.[141] suggested that surgical dissection and anesthetic complications prior to bypass may represent potential threats to cerebral oxygenation in pediatric patients, documenting decreases in cerebral hemoglobin oxygen saturation of greater than 15%. The immediate postbypass phase may also be a relatively unprotected period, as cerebral metabolic needs are increasing with possibly inadequate capability to meet them. This is of great interest, as recent animal studies have underscored ongoing concerns regarding disturbed cerebral vascular responses after DHCA and CPB. O'Rourke and colleagues found, in a piglet model, that cerebral vascular and oxgenation responses were altered after DHCA, but that only oxygenation response was altered after hypothermic CPB.[142] These data, coupled with previous reports of neuropathologic damage after DHCA,[143,144] suggest that ischemic episodes during cardiovascular surgery may not be well tolerated by the neonatal brain, even with benefit of deep hypothermia. Furthermore, resulting vascular instability may predispose postoperative cardiothoracic surgical patients to neurologic injury. A recent small report of neonates undergoing complex aortic arch reconstruction,[145] suggested that CBV and Sao_2 were significantly improved in those infants undergoing repair with deep hypothermic regional low-flow perfusion compared with DHCA. Although it has been speculated that maintenance of these NIRS-measured parameters during surgery may reduce adverse cognitive outcome, long-term studies comparing neurodevelopmental sequelae associated with each procedure will be required.

Finally, recent animal studies of NIRS parameters during cardiac surgery and correlations with MRS and histologic brain assessment may hold promise for future outcome studies in neonates.[68,146] Shin'oka and colleagues[68] studied 40 piglets during DHCA using NIRS and correlated these findings to MRS parameters of cellular metabolism (ATP, PCr and intracellular pH). Histologic scoring of brain injury was also made after the animals were sacrificed on postoperative day 4. Decreases in HbO_2 and CytOx were correlated with decreases in ATP, PCr, and intracellular pH, with the changes in CytOx and PCr demonstrating the strongest association. Furthermore, histologic brain injury was also correlated with reductions in CytOx and ATP. Although there are many potential pitfalls in the measurement of CytOx, and no animal model can adequately describe human neonatal clinical experience, these findings should stimulate considerable research into the utility of NIRS parameters as prognostic indicators and therapeutic directors in the cardiovascular surgical suite.

Antenatal applications

Hypoxic–ischemic insult to the fetus continues to be an important cause of long-term neurodevelopmental sequelae. Currently available technology and methods, such as fetal heart rate monitoring and surveillance of fetal scalp pH, have failed to identify reliably and prospectively fetuses at risk for poor outcome.[147–149] Electronic fetal monitoring (EFM), a commonly used technique, has poor specificity with a false-positive rate of 99.8% for the detection of subsequent development of cerebral palsy, and has been implicated in an increased relative risk for cesarean section.[149,150] Fetal arterial pulse oximetry has been investigated, but has generally focused on transvaginal monitoring.[151] Although recent reports have demonstrated the feasibility of transabdominal fetal pulse oximetry,[152] it would only provide information regarding fetal arterial saturation, not specific cerebral hemodynamic and oxygenation parameters. The potential for NIRS to provide more specific and possibly predictive information regarding fetal cerebral hemodynamics and oxygenation has led to a number of clinical studies.

In an early report of 50 term labors[153,154] by O'Brien and colleagues utilizing transvaginally placed NIRS probes on the fetal head with no direct attachment, two distinct patterns of change in cerebral hemodynamics and oxygenation with uterine contractions were observed. The C-pattern, present in approximately 45% of cases, showed covarying decreases in HbO_2, Hb, and tHb with uterine contractions. The D-pattern, marked by an increase in HbO_2, a rise in Hb, and a variable pattern in tHb, was seen in approximately 30% of the labors. The remainder of the cases demonstrated variable patterns, including rises in HbO_2, Hb, and tHb with contractions, as well as a relatively unresponsive pattern. These findings were in agreement with a previous smaller study by Peebles et al.[155] Subsequent studies of 10 term labors, however, demonstrated that if the contractions were associated with fetal heart rate decelerations,[156,157] an increase in Hb with a decrease in HbO_2 and tHb was witnessed, signifying a fall in fetal cerebral oxygenation. If there were late fetal heart rate decelerations, a more pronounced decrease in HbO_2 and increase in Hb was seen, indicating a significantly greater decrease in cerebral oxygenation. These findings were not associated with other clinical findings such as acidemia or poor outcome upon delivery. Changes in fetal cerebral hemoglobin changes have also been studied in relation to frequency of contractions.[158] In a report of 10 term labors, changes in cerebral HbO_2 were found to be correlated with the time interval between contractions, whereas changes in Hb were negatively correlated. It was concluded that shorter contraction intervals (<2.3 min) were associated with a decrease in fetal Sco_2. Aldrich et al. studied correlations of calculated Sco_2 by NIRS just prior to birth with acid–base status at delivery in 33 term and near-term infants.[159] The authors found that umbilical cord artery and vein pH showed significant positive correlation whereas base deficit and $P_a co_2$ showed significant negative correlation with mean cerebral oxygenation. However, as with previous studies, there was no correlation of NIRS parameters with short-term neonatal clinical outcomes such as encephalopathy. Due to a lack of randomized controlled trials comparing NIRS fetal monitoring with EFM or EFM with scalp pH assessment, a recent Cochrane Database review has concluded that there is insufficient evidence to comment upon the efficacy of antepartum surveillance by NIRS.[160]

Clearly, further research is required to evaluate properly the usefulness of NIRS in fetal monitoring, but many challenges exist. Among these is the fact that, due to the relatively small number of infants who suffer severe perinatal asphyxial incidents, a very large number of patients would need to be studied to assess accurately whether NIRS parameters correlate significantly with neonatal neurodevelopmental outcome. From the standpoint of NIRS methodology, transvaginal placement of fetal optodes may lead to poor contact with the fetal head, and movement may lead to artifact or optode displacement. Thus, the proportion of uninterpretable measurements reported in the studies above was as high as 30–40%. With these limitations in mind, other NIRS techniques, including intensity-modulated phase-resolved approaches, have been suggested for future fetal studies.[154,161] Ramanujam and colleagues have recently described preliminary studies of photon migration through the term and near-term fetal head using a continuous-wave NIRS device placed on the maternal abdomen.[162]

Imaging

Brain imaging

Although one of the earliest uses of medical light-based technology was transillumination of the skull, the further development of cerebral imaging devices has been relatively slow. Advances have been hampered primarily by the significant problem of photon scatter, resulting in poor image resolution. The source of this scattering in the brain is not entirely clear, although mitochondria and cell membranes may be major sources. It is also known that, although scattering effects are less in the neonatal brain than in the adult brain, temporal variations in scattering are likely to occur as a result of neural activation, temperature changes, cell injury, and water shifts.[163–166] However, NIR light-based imaging offers the prospect of noninvasive bedside imaging using a nonionizing form of radiation. Coupled with the functional detection and continuous monitoring capabilities of NIRS, the potential benefits afforded to the critically ill neonate have spurred research in the area of optical imaging.

Use of a time-resolved system, such as the time-of-flight and absorbance (TOFA) device[167] has been one approach to addressing the challenges of NIR light-based imaging. In general, time-resolved systems allow compensation for scattering effects due to the fact that these devices can measure the time delay, thus pathlength, for each photon detected. They are therefore considered to be the most quantitative systems, as assumptions regarding optical pathlength need not be made. However, reconstructed image resolution may be diminished if all late-arriving photons are included. Therefore, Benaron and colleagues used a variable-interval time window to collect a fixed percentage of transmitted photons for image reconstruction[8,18] in an attempt to ameliorate resolution difficulties due to scattering. Initial successful and accurate imaging studies with this technique included resin model systems (phantoms), small animals, and pathologic sheep and neonatal brain specimens using a tomographic stage-based scanner.[8,25,167,168] These were followed by the development of a clinically useful fiberoptic headband,[169] consisting of 34 custom-constructed optode pairs, each constructed from two very thin and flexible fibers terminating in a miniature mirrored prism. These were built into a comfortable, adjustable headband which could easily be secured on an infant's head (Figure 23.4). The headband was used in later diagnostic brain optical studies in premature and term infants in the NICU.[170] Eight optical scans were performed on six patients, aged 2–24 days, with gestational ages ranging from 23 to 39 weeks. These optical scans were compared with head ultrasound, CT, or MRI findings in a masked fashion. The optical scans compared favorably in terms of hemorrhage sensitivity, but the level of detail was much less than that of ultrasound, CT, or MRI, complicated by the effects of photon scattering. Imaging resolution is poorer as light penetrates further into a tissue, with the minimum detectable object increasing from 0.3 cm at a depth of 2 cm to 1.0 cm at a depth of 5 cm. Also, in order to obtain a complete circumferential TOFA scan, the system required hours of optical data collection prior to tomographic reconstruction. However, the study showed that, in term and premature infants, NIR light could penetrate to a depth of 3–5 cm, emerge bearing clues regarding the absorption and scattering properties of the brain, and the information could be used to reconstruct images of deep hemorrhage.

Other groups have continued to pursue accurate yet faster methods for detection of intracranial hematomas. Gopinath and others first reported on the identification of traumatic intracranial hemorrhages by NIRS, and discussed possible bedside applications for this technology in postoperative neurosurgical or postinjury scenarios.[171,172] Chance and colleagues have made significant contributions to the advancement of this technology. Although the group has shown that the most basic single-wavelength NIR spectrophotometer is capable of detecting hematomas, they have also pointed out the limitations of these simple devices.[173,174] These limitations include range of detection, validity in diagnosing deep intracranial hemorrhage, and interference or photon absorption by scalp hematoma or dark hair. A new pulsed-source, variable-intensity NIRS system was therefore recently developed by the group in order to overcome some of these problems.[175] Initial phantom and piglet hematoma model studies show that the system is

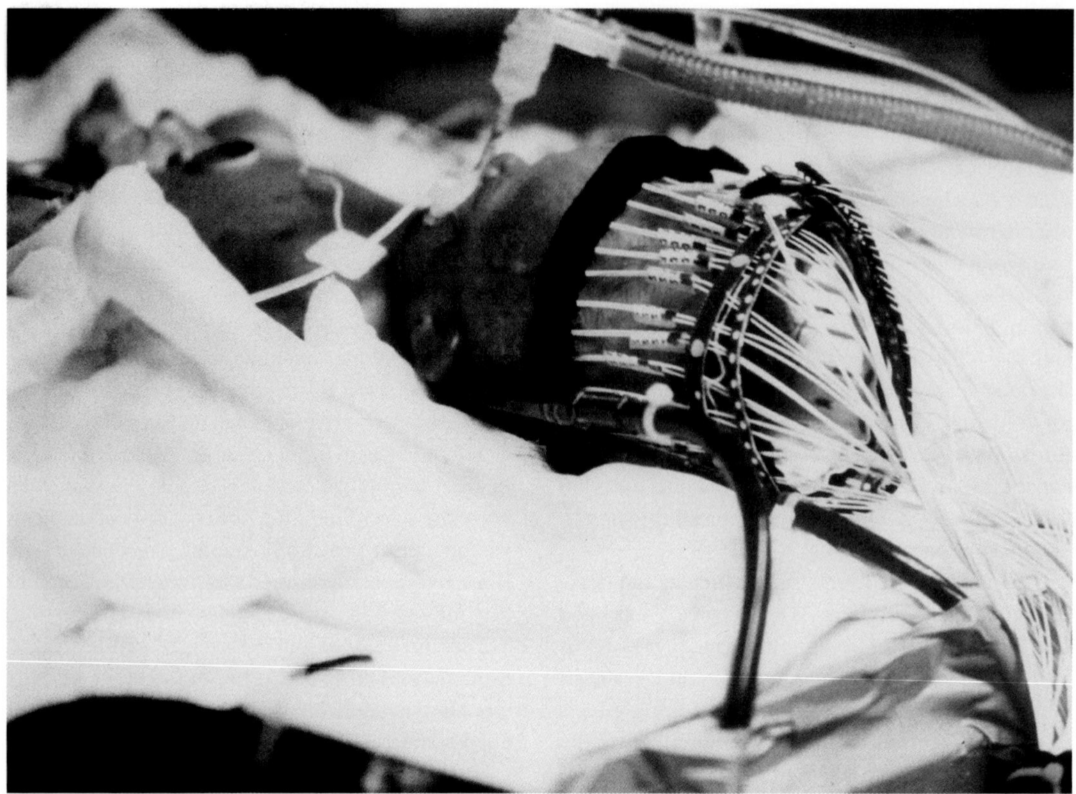

Figure 23.4 Time-of-flight and absorbance (TOFA) fiberoptic headband in place on critically ill neonate on extracorporeal membrane oxygenation.

effective, but that minor variances in the depth of an evolving hematoma may not be detectable.

Beyond proving that NIR light can simply penetrate deep within the brain, and emerge to be detected, information regarding cerebral function must be ascertained and combined with imaging to create an even more powerful diagnostic tool. Current nonlight-based methods of mapping brain function such as fMRI, MRS, and PET are not continuous or portable, not readily available in every hospital setting, and thus are not optimal diagnostic technologies for critically ill neonates; bedside, noninvasive and ideally real-time methods would be. To that end, "optical functional imaging studies" of the brain, essentially "mapping" cerebral oxygenation and hemodynamic parameters through reconstructed data, have been undertaken. Again using TOFA, NIRS brain functional images of adults during finger tapping have demonstrated excellent spatial agreement with fMRI, revealing localized contralateral hemoglobin oxygen saturation increases greater than 2 SD above the mean.[62] In an infant with a stroke, NIRS brain functional images revealed localized, quantifiable decreases in hemoglobin oxygen saturation.[62] When the optical image was reconstructed and highlighted for decreases in saturation greater than 2 SD below the mean, spatial correlation with a localized CT abnormality was found to be very good (Figure 23.5*a* and *b*, colour plates).

TOFA has the advantage of making precise and

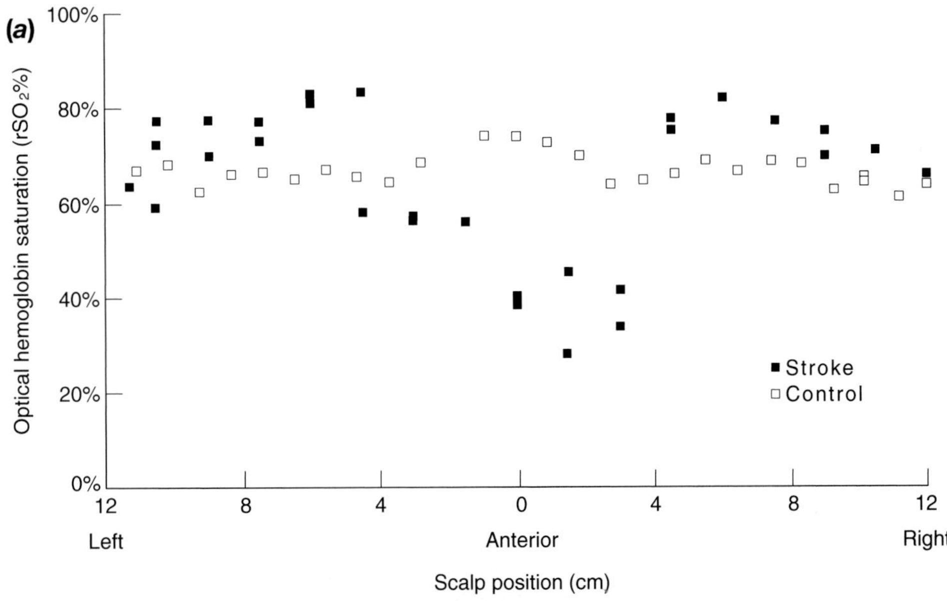

Figure 23.5 (*a*) Absolute saturations around the head of an infant with stroke (in filled squares) compared with those of control infant (in open squares),

quantitative measurements, but it is expensive and slower than the real-time target for clinical usefulness. Sacrificing quantitation, further methodology modifications have led to the emergence of much faster, less expensive continuous-wave systems. Chance and colleagues first reported cognitive brain functional images obtained in a large number of adult human subjects using a continuous-wave imager, establishing the validity of the technique;[176,177] however the resolution (2–4 cm^2) was relatively poor. The group has modified the device, employing amplitude and phase cancellation methodology and a phased-array imager with nine sources and four detectors, improving resolution to approximately 1 cm^2 with a data acquistion time of less than 30 s.[178] Preliminary observational neonatal brain functional studies with the imaging "pad" in place on the head during sensory stimulation and spontaneous movement revealed large-amplitude signal changes. A continuous-wave portable diffuse optical tomography (DOT) has also been developed by Siegel et al.[179] The system utilizes laser diodes at 780 and 830 nm wavelengths with a time-share sequence controlled by a portable laptop computer. Custom-built optical probes consist of nine source fibers arranged in a 3×3 grid and 16 dectector fibers arranged in a 4×4 grid embedded in silicone caps. The present system acquires data from all source-detector combinations in approximately 3 s per wavelength. Data reconstruction reveals images not unlike a topographic weather map. Images obtained using this system at 780 nm during right forefinger tapping in adults demonstrated activation-induced contralateral increase in absorption.[62] A preliminary functional optical study using the DOT system in premature infants has revealed interesting findings.[180,181] In a passive motor stimulation protocol, either the left or right arm of quiet and asleep infants was flexed and extended for 20–30 s followed by a 45–60 s rest period. In studies in which two wavelengths were used, contralateral increases in absorbance were noted at 830 nm, but even greater absorbance was observed at 780 nm, indicating an increase in blood volume to the area as well as an overall increase in Hb concentration (Figure 23.6, colour plate). This finding would correspond to studies which have shown inverse BOLD fMRI signal during visual stimulation in infants and young children,[115] as well as the finding of increased Hb observed by NIRS in response to visual stimulation in infants.[111] Further study is required to elucidate normal cerebral functional imaging changes in the neonate with age and gestational development, and to identify pathologic patterns which may correlate with outcome or signal a need for intervention. This portable combined technology is relatively inexpensive, simple to use, noninvasive, and produces essentially "real-time" results, making it a potentially excellent investigative tool for the neonatal population.

Use of exogenous dyes and contrast agents

There are several vital dyes that fluoresce in the NIR and these have been used as free dyes to mark the leaky vasculature of neoplasia, and as paired dyes that can be configured to be active only in the presence of a targeted enzyme or substrate. ICG is a clinically approved vital dye that excites and emits at wavelengths that penetrate mammalian tissues. Although not used in brain imaging or spectroscopy, this dye defines a principle that may have utility for sensing features of the central nervous system that are otherwise not detectable using NIR imaging and spectroscopy. Contrast agents have traditionally relied on differential uptake or selective retention in specific tissue or cellular compartments. Such strategies have been useful but are largely limited to structural analyses. Therefore, alternate strategies for sensing using NIR dyes are being investigated.

One alternate strategy that offers the potential of functional sensing and imaging is the use of complex molecules that contain paired dyes that are "dark" – do not have a detectable signal – until they come in contact with a molecular target. These agents employ modifications to traditional or novel compounds in which a dye is selected to absorb light emitted from an excited dye due to resonance energy transfer. Resonance energy transfer requires that the dyes be in close proximity, and the so-called "molecular beacons" must then be designed such that the activation event results in a spatial separation of the two dyes by either unfolding or cleavage. The absence of a detectable signature in tissue locations and circumstances that lack the specific molecular activation events reduces the background noise; this results in significantly improved signal-to-noise ratios as the contrast agents go from a relatively inactive state, or off-state, to an active state (on-state) in the presence of a specific molecular target. This strategy extends beyond the typical contrast agents that have been used to label individual pools of fluid, selectively bind to a given cell type or that concentrate in a given tissue. Labels or contrast agents that can be activated by a physiological process or by expression of an endogenous or exogenous gene allow the analyses of biological process that do not have an inherent optical signal. Molecular beacon strategies will allow analyses of gene activation, and permit the assessment of gene expression patterns in the context of intact organ systems.

To utilize resonance energy transfer, probes need to be designed with specific molecular targets in mind. The folding strategy has been utilized in DNA hybridization studies where the emitter and quencher are on each end of a DNA molecule that folds on to itself, placing the two dyes in close proximity. Unfolding occurs upon binding to the complementary strand of DNA and the fluorescent dye is separated from the quenching dye, resulting in a detectable signal.[182,183] This strategy has also been applied to enzyme assays that assess proteolysis. In this case two fluorochromes in their native state are in close proximity until they are cleaved from a specific peptide scaffold, or backbone, by the target protease. Sensor molecules have been generated that are specifically activated by caspase III activity, matrix metalloprotease II activity, cathepsin D activity, or cathepsin B and H activity.[184–186] One important feature of using paired dyes on peptide scaffolds is that any number of peptides can be inserted between

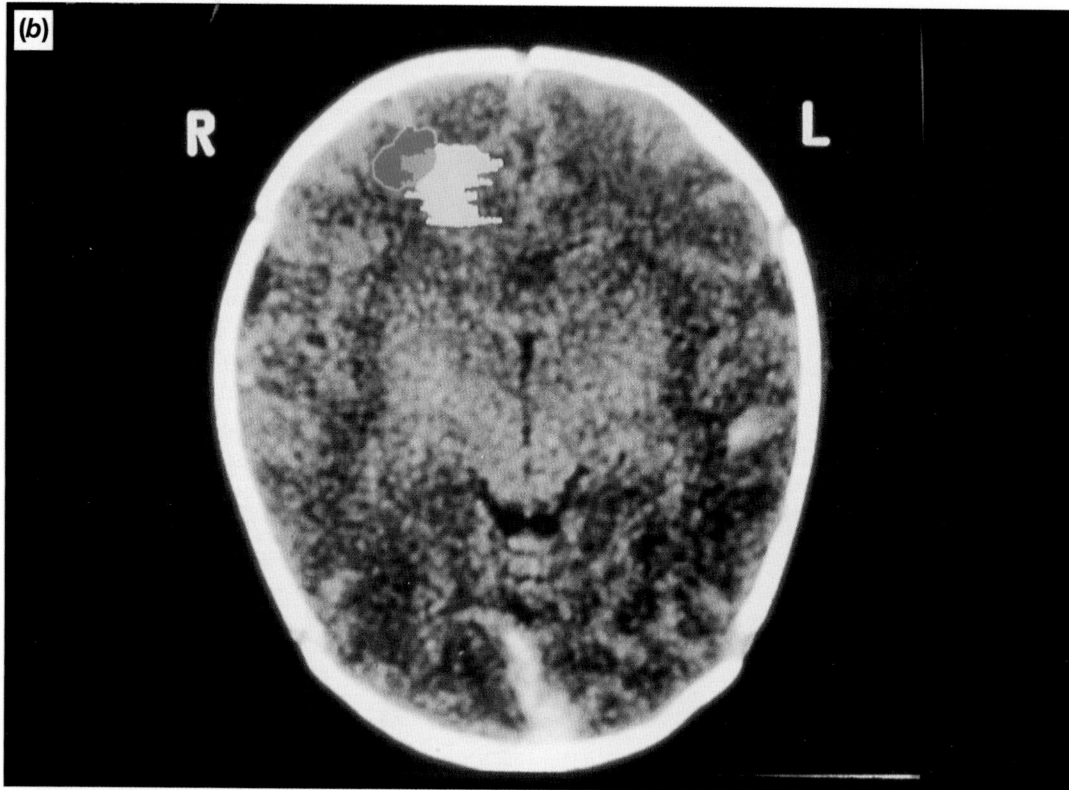

Figure 23.5 (*b*) Corresponding overlay of optical and computed tomographic (CT) images of infant with frontal stroke. The optical image was reconstructed from a tomographic optical scan ($n = 652$ measures) with the yellow area highlighting the focal area of mean hemoglobin saturation falling more than 2 SD below the nonstroke average. The CT image (gray) from the same plane shows a focal stroke, highlighted in red by a masked neuroradiologist. There is good spatial agreement of injury identification between the methods.

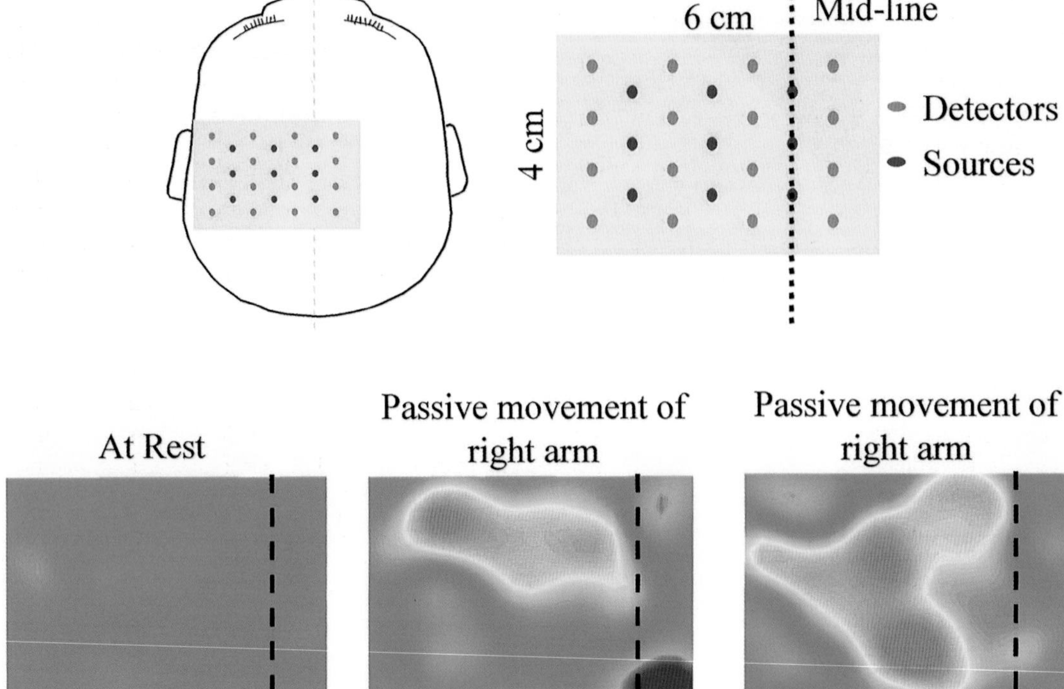

Figure 23.6 Functional images obtained at 830 nm using a diffuse optical tomography system described by Siegel et al.[179] during passive movement of the right arm in a 24-week gestational age infant. The prototype "patch probe" used for this study contained embedded emitter and detector fibers in a superimposed grid pattern. Note the increase in yellow to red color during passive motor stimulation, indicating increased absorbance in the region of the motor cortex contralateral to the side of movement.

the dyes, in a cassette manner, thus comprising a platform technology to interrogate any number of proteases, including those from viruses and bacteria. This approach lends itself to multiplexed assays using dyes of different colors to create reagents that are sensitive to different enzyme activities.

A variety of different imaging strategies can be envisioned that utilize modulation of resonance energy transfer. Many of these methods have been used in in vitro assays and only recently has an effort been made to move these into in vivo and then possibly to clinical scenarios. One difficulty of using fluorescent probes in vivo, is that light is absorbed in a wavelength-dependent manner, with blue and green light being largely absorbed and red being transmitted. Therefore, these probes must employ fluors that excite and emit in the range of 700–900 nm, the window where the light spectrum is not significantly affected.

Future challenges

NIRS is an exciting developing technology which has the potential to offer brain oxygenation and hemodynamic information noninvasively, continuously, and at the bedside of the most critically ill patients. As with any new medical technology, however, NIRS has a number of problems yet to be addressed before implementation can realistically be undertaken. Technological challenges remain, such as the accurate assessment of optical pathlength. Previous studies using time-resolved NIRS techniques have underscored the variability in this important parameter with clinical condition. Numerous investigators have already worked to modify and improve NIRS systems to obtain more accurate estimates of pathlength. However, if the goal of obtaining real-time cerebral oxygenation and hemodynamic measurements in a portable, easily used, and reasonably priced device is to be met, it would appear that the extremely expensive yet highly accurate time-resolved devices will not be implemented for wide-scale clinical use. Unfortunately, which system, or systems, should be used routinely for clinical studies is another important unanswered question. There are currently almost as many systems under development, under modification, or in use as there are laboratories studying clinical applications of NIRS. This fact makes study-to-study comparison extremely challenging as results are tempered by technical differences between systems and the experience and expertise of the operators. Those clinicians unfamiliar with the detailed variation in methodologies, but dedicated to finding ways to help their future patients, are left daunted by the apparent divergent results and skeptical as to the potential use of NIRS in their practice.

Advancements in contrast agent and probe design hold tremendous potential for revealing the nature of biological processes that do not possess, in and of themselves, optical properties. For example, it may be possible to image the juxtaposition of two proteins or two halves of a fusion protein offering the possibility of sensing protein–protein interactions and protein phosphorylation. It may one day be possible to assess the membrane potential of cells, or to follow functional activity in neurons by modulating the fluorescence of a molecular beacon by an endogenous protein. Expression of exogenous genes may be linked to reporter constructs such that their activity can be monitored in vivo and their effects on endogenous proteins assessed.

The published studies, which have attempted to evaluate the applicability of NIRS to clinical monitoring, have thus far contained very small numbers of patients. Given that the most exciting potential application for NIRS lies in early identification of the relatively small number of infants and fetuses at-risk for hypoxic–ischemic insult due to in utero, perinatal, and intrasurgical events, enrollment of many patients will be needed to power any study appropriately. Further, presently available reports have not included randomized trials of NIRS with any other mode of monitoring, making assessment of the comparative value of this technology difficult. In the future, this technology would ideally be used as a tool by which to identify those who could most benefit from neuroprotective agents. Therefore, evaluation of the advantages of NIRS should logically extend to its capabilities in predicting long-term outcome. It is clear that, as with ongoing trials of neuroprotective strategies in the neonatal population, a large multicenter approach should be taken in order efficiently and expeditiously to answer questions regarding the functionality and clinical benefit of NIRS monitoring.

REFERENCES

1 Donn, S.M., Sharpy, M.J., Kuhns, L.R., et al. (1979). Rapid detection of neonatal intracranial hemorrhage by transillumination. *Pediatrics*, **64**, 843–847.

2 Jobsis, F. (1977). Noninvasive, infrared monitoring of cerebral and myocardial oxygen sufficiency and circulatory parameters. *Science*, **198**, 1264–1267.

3 Wyatt, J.S., Cope, M., Delpy, D.T., et al. (1990). Quantitation of cerebral blood volume in newborn human infants by near infrared spectroscopy. *J Appl Physiol*, **68**, 1086–1091.

4 Sevick, E.M., Chance, B., Leigh, J., et al. (1991). Quantitation of time- and frequency-resolved optical spectra for the determination of tissue oxygenation. *Anal Biochem*, **195**, 330–351.

5 Benaron, D.A., Kurth, C.D., Steven, J.M., et al. (1995). Transcranial optical path length in infants by near-infrared phase-shift spectroscopy. *J Clin Monit*, **11**, 109–317.

6 Duncan, A., Meek, J.H., Clemence, M., et al. (1996). Measurement of cranial optical path length as a function of age using phase resolved near infrared spectroscopy. *Pediatr Res*, **39**, 889–894.

7 Duncan, A., Meek, J.H., Clemence, M., et al. (1995). Optical pathlength measurements on adult head, calf and forearm and the head of the newborn infant using phase resolved optical spectroscopy. *Phys Med Biol*, **40**, 295–304.

8 Benaron, D.A. and Stevenson, D.K. (1993). Optical time-of-flight and absorbance imaging of biologic media. *Science*, **259**, 1463–1466.

9 Adcock, L.M., Wafelman, L.S., Hegemier, S., et al. (1999). Neonatal intensive care applications of near-infrared spectroscopy. *Clin Perinatol*, **26**, 893–903.

10 Soul, J.S. and du Plessis, A.J. (1999). Near-infrared spectroscopy. *Semin Pediatr Neurol*, **6**, 101–110.

11 Delpy, D.T., Cope, M., van der Zee, P., et al. (1988). Estimation of optical pathlength through tissue from direct time of flight measurement. *Phys Med Biol*, **33**, 1433–1442.

12 Meek, J.H., Elwell, C.E., Mc Cormick, D.C., et al. (1999). Abnormal cerebral haemodynamics in perinatally asphyxiated neonates related to outcome. *Arch Dis Child Fetal Neonatal Edn*, **81**, F110–F115.

13 Edwards, A.D., Wyatt, J.S., Richardson, C., et al. (1988). Cotside measurements of cerebral blood flow in ill newborn infants by near infrared spectroscopy. *Lancet*, **2**, 770–771.

14 Reynolds, E.O., McCormick, D.C., Roth, S.C., et al. (1991) New non-invasive methods for the investigation of cerebral oxidative metabolism and haemodynamics in newborn infants. *Ann Med*, **23**, 681–686.

15 Wyatt, J.S., Cope, M., Delpy, D.T., et al. (1990). Measurement of optical path length for cerebral near-infrared spectroscopy in newborn infants. *Dev Neurosci*, **12**, 140–144.

16 Pryds, O. and Edwards, A.D. (1996). Cerebral blood flow in the newborn infants. *Arch Dis Child Fetal Neonatal Edn*, **74**, F63–F69.

17 Kurth, C.D., Steven, J.M., Benaron, D., et al. (1993). Near-infrared monitoring of the cerebral circulation. *J Clin Monit*, **9**, 163–170.

18 Skov, L., Pryds, O., Greisen, G., et al. (1993). Estimation of cerebral venous saturation and in newborn infants by near infrared spectroscopy. *Pediatr Res*, **33**, 52–55.

19 Benaron, D.A., Ho, D.C., Rubinsky, B., et al. (1988). Imaging (NIRI) and quantitation (NIRS) in tissue using time-resolved spectrophotometry: the impact of statically and dynamically variable optical path lengths. *SPIE*, **1888**, 10–20.

20 Lewis, S.B., Myburgh, J.A., Thornton, E.L., et al. (1996). Cerebral oxygenation monitoring by near-infrared spectroscopy is not clinically useful in patients with severe closed-head injury: a comparison with jugular bulb oximetry. *Crit Care Med*, **24**, 1334–1338.

21 Cruz, J. (1997). Relevant limitations of near-infrared spectroscopy. *Crit Care Med*, **25**, 555–556.

22 Yager, J.Y., Brucklacher, M. and Vanucci, R.C. (1992). Cerebral energy metabolism during hypoxia–ischemia and early recovery in immature rats. *Am J Physiol*, **262**, H672–H677.

23 Clemence, M., Springett, R., Thornton, J.S., et al. (1997). Near infra-red spectroscopy show path length changes which correlate with T2 in a piglet model of hypoxia–ischaemia. *Magn Reson Materials Phys, Biol Med*, **V**, 64A.

24 Benaron, D. and Stevenson, D. (1994). Resolution of near infrared time-of-flight brain oxygenation imaging. *Adv Exp Med Biol*, **345**, 609–617.

25 van Houten, J.P., Benaron, D.A., Spilman, S., et al. (1996). Imaging brain injury using time-resolved near infrared light scanning. *Pediatr Res*, **39**, 470–476.

26 Boas, D.A., Gaudette, T., Strangman, G., et al. (2001). The accuracy of near infrared spectroscopy and imaging during

focal changes in cerebral hemodynamics. *NeuroImage*, **13**, 76–90.

27 Mayhew, J., Zheng, Y., Hou, Y., et al. (1999). Spectroscopic analysis of changes in remitted illumination: the response to increased neural activity in brain. *NeuroImage*, **10**, 304–326.

28 Malonek, D. and Grinvald, A. (1996). Interactions between electrical activity and cortical microcirculation revealed by imaging spectroscopy: implications for functional brain mapping. *Science*, **272**, 551–554.

29 Kleinschmidt, A., Obrig, H., Requart, M., et al. (1996). Simultaneous recording of cerebral blood oxygenation changes during human brain activation by magnetic resonance imaging and near-infrared spectroscopy. *J Cereb Blood Flow Metab*, **16**, 817–826.

30 Pryds, O., Greisen, G., Skov, L.L., et al. (1990). Carbon dioxide-related changes in cerebral blood volume and cerebral blood flow in mechanically ventilated preterm neonates: comparison of near infrared spectrophotometry and ^{133}Xenon clearance. *Pediatr Res*, **27**, 445–449.

31 Skov, L., Pryds, O., Greisen, G. (1991). Estimating cerebral blood flow in newborn infants: comparison of near-infrared spectroscopy and ^{133}Xenon clearance. *Pediatr Res*, **20**, 570–573.

32 Bucher, H.U., Edwards, A.D., Lipp, A.E., et al. (1993). Comparison between near infrared spectroscopy and ^{133}Xenon clearance for estimation of cerebral blood flow in critically ill preterm infants. *Pediatr Res*, **33**, 56–60.

33 Goddard-Finegold, J., Louis, P.T., Rodriguez, D.L., et al. (1998). Correlation of near infrared spectroscopy cerebral blood flow estimations and microsphere quantitations in newborn piglets. *Biol Neonate*, **74**, 376–384.

34 Patel, J., Marks, K., Roberts, I., et al. (1998). Measurement of cerebral blood flow in newborn infants using near infrared spectroscopy with indocyanine green. *Pediatr Res*, **43**, 34–39.

35 Kuebler, W.M., Sckell, A., Habler, O., et al. (1998). Noninvasive measurement of regional cerebral blood flow by near-infrared spectroscopy and indocyanine green. *J Cereb Blood Flow Metab*, **18**, 445–456.

36 Newton, C.R., Wilson, D.A., Gunnoe, E., et al. (1997). Measurement of cerebral blood flow in dogs with near infrared spectroscopy in the reflectance mode is invalid. *J Cereb Blood Flow Metab*, **17**, 695–703.

37 Wolf, M., Baenziger, O., Keel, M., et al. (1998). Cerebral blood flow measurements by near infrared spectrophotometry in reflectance mode are valid in neonates. *J Cereb Blood Flow Metab*, **18**, 698–700.

38 Wyatt, J.S. (1993). Near-infrared spectroscopy in asphyxial brain injury. *Clin Perinatol*, **20**, 369–378.

39 Livera, L.N., Wickramasinghe, Y.A., Spencer, S.A., et al. (1992). Cyclical fluctuations in cerebral blood volume. *Arch Dis Child*, **67**, 62–63.

40 Wickramasinghe, Y.A., Livera, L.N., Spencer, S.A., et al. (1992). Plethysmographic validation of near infrared spectroscopic monitoring of cerebral blood volume. *Arch Dis Child*, **67**, 407–411.

41 Brun, N.C., Moen, A., Borch, K., et al. (1997). Near-infrared monitoring of cerebral tissue oxygen saturation and blood volume in newborn piglets. *Am J Physiol*, **273**, H682–H686.

42 Barfield, C.P., Yu, V.Y.H., Noma, O., et al. (1999). Cerebral blood volume measured using near-infrared spectroscopy and radiolabels in the immature lamb brain. *Pediatr Res*, **46**, 50–56.

43 van de Bor, M., Benders, M.J., Dorrepaal, C.A., et al. (1994). Cerebral blood volume changes during exchange transfusions in infants born at or near term. *J Pediatr*, **125**, 617–621.

44 Meek, J.H., Tyszczuk, L., Elwell, C.E., et al. (1998). Cerebral blood flow increases over the first three days of life in extremely preterm neonates. *Arch Dis Child Fetal Neonat Edn*, **78**, F33–F37.

45 Wafelman, L.S., Adcock, L.M., Moise, A.A., et al. (1996). Near infrared spectroscopic (NIRS) estimations of cerebral blood flow in very low birth weight (VLBW) infants. *Pediatr Res*, **39**, 382A.

46 Baenziger, O., Mueller, A.M., Morales, C.G., et al. (1999). Cerebral blood flow and neurological outcome in the preterm infant. *Eur J Pediatr*, **158**, 138–143.

47 Altman, D.I., Powers, W.J., Perlman, J.M., et al. (1988). Cerebral blood flow requirement for brain viability in newborn infants is lower than in adults. *Ann Neurol*, **24**, 218–226.

48 Altman, D.I., Perlman, J.M., Volpe, J.J., et al. (1993). Cerebral oxygen metabolism in newborns. *Pediatrics*, **92**, 99–104.

49 Kety, S.S. and Scmidt, C.F. (1946). The effects of active and passive hyperventilation on cerebral blood flow, cerebral oxygen consumption, cardiac output, and blood pressure of normal young men. *J Clin Invest*, **25**, 107–119.

50 Wyatt, J.S., Edwards, A. and Cope, M. (1991). Response of cerebral blood volume to changes in carbon dioxide tension in preterm and term infants. *Pediatr Res*, **29**, 553–557.

51 Dietz, V., Wolf, M., Keel, M., et al. (1999). CO_2 reactivity of the cerebral hemoglobin concentration in healthy term newborns measured by near infrared spectrophotometry. *Bio Neonate*, **75**, 85–90.

52 Yoxall, C.W., Dawani, N., Weindling, A.M., et al. (1995). Measurement of cerebral venous jugular venous oxyhaemoglobin saturation in children by near infrared

spectroscopy and partial jugular venous occlusion. *Pediatr Res*, **38**, 319–323.

53 Daubeney, P.E.F., Pilkington, S.N., Janke, E., et al. (1996). Cerebral oxygenation measured by near-infrared spectroscopy: comparison with jugular bulb oximetry. *Ann Thorac Surg*, **61**, 930–934.

54 Mchedlishvili, G.I. (1986). *Arterial Behavior and Blood Circulation in the Brain*, pp. 55–60. New York: Plenum Publishing.

55 Mukhtar, A.L., Frances, M.C. and Stothers J.K. (1982). Cranial blood flow and blood pressure changes during sleep in human neonates. *Early Hum Dev*, **6**, 59–64.

56 Nomura, F., Naruse, H., du Plessis, A., et al. (1996). Cerebral oxygenation measured by near infrared spectroscopy during cardiopulmonary bypass and deep hypothermic circulatory arrest in piglets. *Pediatr Res*, **40**, 790–796.

57 Hintz, S.R., Benaron, D.A., Robbins, R.C., et al. (1997). Brain functional imaging using time-of-flight optical spectroscopy. *SPIE Proc*, **3194**, 176–183.

58 Buchvald, F.F., Kesje, K. and Greisen, G. (1999). Measurement of cerebral oxyhaemoglobin saturation and jugular blood flow in term healthy newborn infants by NIRS and jugular venous occlusion. *Biol Neonate*, **75**, 97–103.

59 Yoxall, C.W. and Weindling, M. (1998). Cerebral oxygen consumption in the human neonate using near infrared spectroscopy: cerebral oxygen consumption increases with advancing gestational age. *Pediatr Res*, **44**, 283–290.

60 Garfunkel, J.M., Baird, H.W. and Zeigler, J. (1954). The relationship of oxygen consumption to cerebral functional activity. *J Pediatr*, **44**, 64–72.

61 Punwani, S., Ordidge, R.J., Cooper, C.E., et al. (1998). MRI measurements of cerebral deoxyhemoglobin concentration [dHb] – correlation with near infrared spectroscopy (NIRS). *NMR Biomed*, **11**, 281–289.

62 Benaron, D.A., Hintz, S.R., Villringer, A., et al. (2000). Noninvasive functional imaging of human brain using light. *J Cereb Blood Flow Metab*, **20**, 469–477.

63 Skov, L. and Greisen, G. (1994). Apparent cerebral cytochrome aa3 reduction during cardiopulmonary bypass in hypoxaemic children with congenital heart disease. A criticial analysis of in vivo near-infrared spectrophotometric data. *Physiol Meas*, **15**, 447–457.

64 Wray, S., Cope, M., Delpy, D., et al. (1988). Characterization of the near infrared absorption spectra of cytochrome aa3 and haemoglobin for the non-invasive monitoring of cerebral oxygenation. *Biochim Biophys Acta*, **933**, 184–192.

65 Cooper, C., Matcher, S., Wyatt, J., et al. (1994). Near-infrared spectroscopy of the brain: relevance to cytochrome oxidase bioenergetics. *Biochem Soc Trans*, **22**, 974–980.

66 Tsuji, M., Naruse, H., Volpe, J., et al. (1995). Reduction of cytochrome aa_3 measured by near-infrared spectroscopy predicts cerebral energy loss in hypoxic piglets. *Pediatr Res*, **37**, 253–259.

67 Matsumoto, H., Oda, T., Hossain, M.A., et al. (1996). Does the redox state of cytochrome aa3 reflect brain energy level during hypoxia? Simultaneous measurements by near infrared spectrophotometry and ^{31}P nuclear magnetic resonance spectroscopy. *Anesth Analg*, **83**, 513–518.

68 Shin'oka, T., Nollert, G., Shum-Tim, D., et al. (2000). Utility of near-infrared spectroscopic measurements during deep hypothermic circulatory arrest. *Ann Thorac Surg*, **69**, 578–583.

69 Springett, R., Newman, J., Cope, M., et al. (2000). Oxygen dependency and precision of cytochrome oxidase signal from full spectral NIRS of the piglet brain. *Am J Physiol Heart Circ Physiol*, **279**, H2202–H2209.

70 Heekeren, H.R., Kohl, M., Obrig, H., et al. (1999). Noninvasive assessment of changes in cytochrome-c oxidase oxidation in human subjects during visual stimulation. *J Cereb Blood Flow Metab*, **19**, 592–603.

71 Volpe, J.J. (1995). *Neurology of the Newborn*, 3rd edn, pp. 403–463. Philadelphia: WB Saunders.

72 Isobe, K., Kusaka, T., Fujikawa, Y., et al. (2000). Changes in cerebral hemoglobin concentration and oxygen saturation immediately after birth in the human neonate using full-spectrum near infrared spectroscopy. *J Biomed Optics*, **5**, 283–286.

73 Urlesberger, B., Trip, K., Ruchti, J.J.I., et al. (1998). Quantification of cyclical fluctuations in cerebral blood volume in healthy infants. *Neuropediatrics*, **29**, 208–211.

74 von Siebenthal, K., Beran, J., Wolf, M., et al. (1999). Cyclical fluctuations in blood pressure, heart rate and cerebral blood volume in preterm infants. *Brain Dev*, **21**, 529–534.

75 Anthony, M.Y., Evans, D.H. and Levene, M.I. (1991). Cyclical variations in cerebral blood flow velocity. *Arch Dis Child*, **66**, 12–16.

76 Brazy, J.E. (1988). Effects of crying on cerebral blood volume and cytochrome aa_3. *J Pediatr*, **112**, 457–461.

77 Perlman, J.M. and Volpe, J.J. (1985). Episodes of apnea and bradycardia in the preterm newborn: impact on cerebral circulation. *Pediatrics*, **76**, 333–338.

78 Jenni, O.G., Wolf, M., Hengartner, M., et al. (1996). Impact of central, obstructive and mixed apnea on cerebral hemodynamics in preterm infants. *Biol Neonate*, **70**, 91–100.

79 Urlesberger, B., Kaspirek, A., Pichler, G., et al. (1999). Apnea of prematurity and changes in cerebral oxygenation and cerebral blood volume. *Neuropediatrics*, **30**, 29–33.

80 Tyszczuk, L., Meek, J., Elwell, C., et al. (1998). Cerebral blood flow is independent of mean arterial blood pressure in preterm infants undergoing intensive care. *Pediatrics,* **102**, 337–341.

81 Tsuji, M., Saul, P., du Plessis, A., et al. (2000). Cerebral intravascular oxygenation correlates with mean arterial pressure in critically ill premature infants. *Pediatrics,* **106**, 625–632.

82 Tsuji, M., du Plessis, A., Taylor, G., et al. (1998). Near infrared spectroscopy detects cerebral ischemia during hypotension in piglets. *Pediatr Res,* **44**, 591–595.

83 du Plessis, A.J., Tsuji, M.K., Naruse, H., et al. (1995). Near infrared spectroscopy (NIRS) shows pronounced effects of CSF removal on cerebral hemodynamics in infantile hydrocephalus. *Pediatr Res,* **37**, 377A.

84 Soul, J.S., Taylor, G.A., Wypij, D., et al. (2000). Noninvasive detection of changes in cerebral blood flow by near-infrared spectroscopy in a piglet model of hydrocephalus. *Pediatr Res,* **48**, 445–449.

85 Gagnon, R.E., Leung, A. and Macnab, A.J. (1999). Variations in regional cerebral blood volume in neonates associated with nursery care events. *Am J Perinatol,* **16**, 7–11.

86 McDonnell, M., Ives, N.K. and Hope, P.L. (1992). Intravenous aminophylline and cerebral blood flow in preterm infants. *Arch Dis Child,* **67**, 416–418.

87 Bucher, H.U., Wolf, M., Keel, M., et al. (1994). Effect of aminophylline on cerebral hemodynamics and oxidative metabolism in premature infants. *Eur J Pediatr,* **153**, 123–128.

88 Dani, C., Bertini, G., Reali, M.F., et al. (2000). Brain hemodynamic changes in preterm infants after maintenance dose caffeine and aminophylline treatment. *Biol Neonate,* **78**, 27–32.

89 Edwards, A.D., Wyatt, J.S., Richardson, C., et al. (1990). Effects of indomethacin on cerebral haemodynamics in very preterm infants. *Lancet,* **35**, 1491–1495.

90 McCormick, D.C., Edwards, A.D., Brown, G.C., et al. (1993). Effect of indomethacin on cerebral oxidized cytochrome oxidase in preterm infants. *Pediatr Res,* **33**, 603–608.

91 Liem, K.D., Hopman, J.C., Kollee, L.A., et al. (1994). Effect of repeated indomethacin administration on cerebral oxygenation and haemodynamics in preterm infants: combined near infrared spectrophotometry and Doppler ultrasound study. *Eur J Pediatr,* **153**, 504–509.

92 Benders, M.J., Dorrepaal, C.A., van de Bor, M., et al. (1995). Acute effects of indomethacin on cerebral hemodynamics and oxygenation. *Biol Neonate,* **68**, 91–99.

93 Patel, J., Roberts, I., Azzopardi, D., et al. (2000). Randomized double-blind controlled trial comparing the effects of ibuprofen with indomethacin on cerebral hemodynamics in preterm infants with patent ductus arteriosus. *Pediatr Res,* **47**, 36–42.

94 Liem, K.D., Hopman, J.C.W., Oeseburg, B., et al. (1997). The effect of blood transfusion and haemodilution on cerebral oxygenation and haemodynamics in newborn infants investigated by near infrared spectrophotometry. *Eur J Pediatr,* **156**, 305–310.

95 Murakami, Y., Yamashita, Y., Nishimi, T., et al. (1998). Changes of cerebral hemodynamics and oxygenation in unstable septic newborns during exchange transfusion. *Kurame Med J,* **45**, 321–325.

96 Liem, K.D., Hopman, J.C.W., Oeseburg, B., et al. (1995). Cerebral oxygenation and hemodynamics during induction of extracorporeal membrane oxygenation as investigated by near infrared spectrophotometry. *Pediatrics,* **95**, 555–561.

97 Perlman, J.M. and Volpe, J.J. (1983). Suctioning in the preterm infant: effects on cerebral blood flow velocity, intracranial pressure and arterial blood pressure. *Pediatrics,* **72**, 329–334.

98 Shah, A.R., Kurth, C.D., Gwiazdowski, S.G., et al. (1992). Fluctuations in cerebral oxygenation and blood volume during endotracheal suctioning in premature infants. *J Pediatr,* **120**, 769–774.

99 Bucher, H.U., Blum-Gisler, M. and Duc, G. (1993). Changes in cerebral blood volume during endotracheal suctioning. *J Pediatr,* **122**, 324.

100 Skov, L., Ryding, J., Pryds, O., et al. (1992). Changes in cerebral oxygenation and cerebral blood volume during endotracheal suctioning in ventilated neonates. *Acta Paediatr,* **81**, 389–393.

101 Bernert, G., von Siebenthal, K., Seidl, R., et al. (1997). The effect of behavioural states on cerebral oxygenation during endotracheal suctioning of preterm babies. *Neuropediatrics,* **28**, 111–115.

102 Kohlhauser, C., Bernert, G., Hermon, M., et al. (2000). Effects of endotracheal suctioning in high-frequency oscillatory and conventionally ventilated low birth weight neonates on cerebral hemodynamics observed by near infrared spectroscopy (NIRS). *Pediatr Pulmonol,* **29**, 270–275.

103 Jorch, G., Rabe, H., Garbe, M., et al. (1989). Acute and protracted effects of intratracheal surfactant application on internal carotid blood flow velocity, blood pressure and carbon dioxide tension in very low birthweight infants. *Eur J Pediatr,* **148**, 770–773.

104 Cowan, F., Whitelaw, A., Wertheim, D., et al. (1991). Cerebral blood flow velocity changes after rapid administration of surfactant. *Arch Dis Child,* **66**, 1105–1109.

105 Skov, L., Hellstrom-Westas, L., Jacobsen, T., et al. (1992). Acute changes in cerebral oxygenation and cerebral blood volume in preterm infants during surfactant treatment. *Neuropediatrics*, **23**, 126–130.

106 Halliday, H. and Robertson, B. (1992). Cerebral blood flow velocity changes after rapid administration of surfactant. *Arch Dis Child*, **67**, 470.

107 Lundstrom, K. and Greisen, G. (1996). Changes in EEG, systemic circulation and blood gas parameters following two or six aliquots of porcine surfactant. *Acta Paediatr*, **85**, 708–712.

108 Skov, L., Bell, A. and Greisen, G. (1992). Surfactant administration and the cerebral circulation. *Biol Neonate*, **61**, 31–36.

109 Edwards, A.D., McCormick, D.C., Roth, S.C., et al. (1992). Cerebral hemodynamic effects of treatment with modified natural surfactant investigated by near infrared spectroscopy. *Pediatr Res*, **32**, 532–535.

110 Dorrepaal, C.A., Benders, M.J., Steendijk, P., et al. (1993). Cerebral hemodynamics and oxygenation in preterm infants after low- vs. high dose surfactant replacement therapy. *Biol Neonate*, **64**, 193–200.

111 Roll, C., Knief, J., Horsch, S., et al. (2000). Effect of surfactant administration on cerebral haemodynamics and oxygenation in premature infants – a near infrared spectroscopy study. *Neuropediatrics*, **31**, 16–23.

112 Belliveau, J.W., Kennedy, D.N., McKinstry, R.C., et al. (1991). Functional mapping of the human visual cortex by magnetic resonance imaging. *Science*, **254**, 716–719.

113 Meek, J.H., Firbank, M., Elwell, C.E., et al. (1998). Regional hemodynamic responses to visual stimulation in awake infants. *Pediatr Res*, **43**, 840–843.

114 Born, P., Rostrup, E., Leth, H., et al. (1996). Change of visually induced cortical activation patterns during development. *Lancet*, **347**, 543.

115 Born, P., Leth, H., Miranda, M.J., et al. (1998). Visual activation in infants and young children studied by functional magnetic resonance imaging. *Pediatr Res*, **44**, 578–585.

116 Hoshi, Y., Kohri, S., Matsumoto, Y., et al. (2000). Hemodynamic responses to photic stimulation in neonates. *Pediatr Neurol*, **23**, 323–327.

117 Hoshi, Y., Onoe, H., Watanabe, Y., et al. (1994). Non-synchronous behavior of neuronal activity, oxidative metabolism and blood supply during mental tasks in man. *Neurosci Lett*, **172**, 1229–1233.

118 Sakatani, K., Chen, S., Lichty, W., et al. (1999). Cerebral blood oxygenation changes induced by auditory stimulation in newborn infants measured by near infrared spectroscopy. *Early Hum Dev*, **55**, 229–236.

119 Zaramella, P., Freato, F., Amigoni, A., et al. (2001). Brain auditory activation measured by near-infrared spectroscopy (NIRS) in neonates. *Pediatr Res*, **49**, 213–219.

120 Bartocci, M., Winberg, J., Ruggiero, C., et al. (2000). Activation of olfactory cortex in newborn infants after odor stimulation: a functional near-infrared spectroscopy study. *Pediatr Res*, **48**, 18–23.

121 Pryds, O. (1994). Low neonatal cerebral oxygen delivery is associated with brain injury in preterm infants. *Acta Paediatr*, **83**, 1233–1236.

122 Mueller, A.M., Morales, C., Briner, J., et al. (1997). Loss of CO_2 reactivity of cerebral blood flow is associated with severe brain damage in mechanically ventilated very low birth weight infants. *Eur J Paediatr Neurol*, **1**, 157–163.

123 Meek, J.H., Tyszczuk, L., Elwell, C.E., et al. (1999). Low cerebral blood flow is a risk factor for severe intraventricular haemorrhage. *Arch Dis Child Fetal Neonatal Edn*, **181**, F15–F18.

124 Cope, M. and Delpy, D.T. (1988). A system for the long-term measurement of cerebral blood and tissue oxygenation in newborn infants by near infrared transillumination. *Med Biol Eng Comput*, **26**, 289–294.

125 Inder, T.E. and Volpe, J.J. (2000). Mechanisms of perinatal brain injury. *Semin Neonatol*, **5**, 2–16.

126 Berger, R. and Garnier, Y. (2000). Perinatal brain injury. *J Perinat Med*, **28**, 261–285.

127 Saliba, E. and Henrot, A. (2001). Inflammatory mediators and neonatal brain damage. *Biol Neonate*, **79**, 224–227.

128 Ferry, P.C. (1987). Neurologic sequelae of cardiac surgery in children. *Am J Dis Child*, **141**, 309–312.

129 Ferry, P.C. (1990). Neurologic sequelae of open-heart surgery in children: an irritating question. *Am J Dis Child*, **144**, 369–373.

130 Wernovsky, G., Jonas, R.A., Hickey, P.R., et al. (1993). Clinical neurologic and developmental studies after cardiac surgery utilizing hypothermic circulatory arrest and cardiopulmonary bypass. *Cardiol Young*, **3**, 308–316.

131 du Plessis, A.J. and Johnston, M.V. (1999). The pursuit of effective neuroprotection during infant cardiac surgery. *Semin Pediatr Neurol*, **6**, 55–63.

132 Greeley, W.J., Bracey, V.A., Ungerleider, R.M., et al. (1991). Recovery of cerebral metabolism and mitochondrial oxidation state is delayed after hypothermic circulatory arrest. *Circulation*, **84** (suppl. III), III400–III406.

133 Greeley, W.J., Kern, F.H., Ungerleider, R.M., et al. (1991). The effect of hypothermic cardiopulmonary bypass and total circulatory arrest on cerebral metabolism in neonates, infants and children. *J Thorac Cardiovasc Surg*, **101**, 783–794.

134 Kurth, C.D., Steven, J.M., Nicolson, S.C., et al. (1992). Kinetics of cerebral deoxygenation during deep hypothermic circulatory arrest in neonates. *Anesthesiology*, **77**, 656–661.

135 Kurth, C.D., Steven, J.M. and Nicolson, S.C. (1995). Cerebral oxygenation during pediatric cardiac surgery using deep hypothermic circulatory arrest. *Anesthesiology*, **82**, 74–82.

136 du Plessis, A.J., Newburger, J., Jonas, R.A., et al. (1995). Cerebral oxygen supply and utilization during infant cardiac surgery. *Ann Neurol*, **37**, 488–497.

137 Nomura, F., Naruse, H., duPlessis, A., et al. (1996). Cerebral oxygenation measured by near infrared spectroscopy during cardiopulmonary and deep hypothermic circulatory arrest in piglets. *Pediatr Res*, **40**, 790–796.

138 Nollert, G., Shin'oka, T. and Jonas, R.A. (1998). Near-infrared spectrophotometry of the brain in cardiovascular surgery. *Thorac Cardiovasc Surg*, **46**, 167–175.

139 Wardle, S.P., Yoxall, C.W. and Weindling, A.M. (1998). Cerebral oxygenation during cardiopulmonary bypass. *Arch Dis Child*, **78**, 26–32.

140 Kurth, C.D., Steven, J.M., Nicolson, S.C., et al. (1997). Cerebral oxygenation during cardiopulmonary bypass in children. *J Thorac Cardiovasc Surg*, **113**, 71–78.

141 Daubeney, P.E.F., Smith, D.C., Pilkington, S.N., et al. (1998). Cerebral oxygenation during paediatric cardiac surgery: identification of vulnerable periods using near infrared spectroscopy. *Eur J Cardio Surg*, **13**, 370–377.

142 O'Rourke, M.M., Nork, K.M. and Kurth, C.D. (2000). Neonatal cerebral oxygen regulation after hypothermic cardiopulmonary bypass and circulatory arrest. *Crit Care Med*, **28**, 157–162.

143 Fessatidis, I.T., Thomas, V.L., Shore, D.F., et al. (1993). Brain damage after profoundly hypothermic circulatory arrest: correlations between neurophysiologic and neuropathologic findings. An experimental study in vertebrates. *J Thorac Cardiovasc Surg*, **106**, 32–41.

144 Priestley, M.A., Golden, J.A., O'Hara, I.B., et al. (2001). Comparison of neurologic outcome after deep hypothermic circulatory arrest with alpha-stat and pH-stat cardiopulmonary bypass in newborn pigs. *J Thorac Cardiovasc Surg*, **121**, 336–343.

145 Pigula, F., Nemoto, E.M, Griffith, B.P., et al. (2000). Regional low-flow perfusion provides cerebral circulatory support during neonatal aortic arch reconstruction. *J Thorac Cardiovasc Surg*, **119**, 331–339.

146 Nollert, G., Jonas, R.A. and Reichart, B. (2000). Optimizing cerebral oxygenation during cardiac surgery: a review of experimental and clinical investigations with near infrared spectrophotometry. *Thorac Cardiovasc Surg*, **48**, 247–253.

147 MacDonald, D., Gran, A.M., Sheridan-Pereira, M., et al. (1985). The Dublin randomized controlled trial of intrapartum fetal heart rate monitoring. *Am J Obstet Gynecol*, **152**, 524–539.

148 Kruger, K., Hallberg, B., Blennow, M., et al. (1999). Predictive value of fetal scalp blood lactate concentration and pH as markers of neurologic disability. *Am J Obstet Gynecol*, **181**, 1072–1078.

149 Nelson, K.B., Dambrosia, J.M., Ting, J.Y., et al. (1996). Uncertain value of electronic fetal monitoring in predicting cerebral palsy. *N Engl J Med*, **334**, 613–618.

150 Thacker, S.B. (1987). The efficacy of intrapartum electronic fetal monitoring. *Am J Obstet Gynecol*, **156**, 24–30.

151 Dildy, G.A., Clark, S.L. and Loucks, C.A. (1993). Preliminary experience with intrapartum fetal pulse oximetry in humans. *Obstet Gynecol*, **81**, 630–635.

152 Zourabian, A., Siegel, A., Chance, B., et al. (2000). Trans-abdominal monitoring of fetal arterial blood oxygenation using pulse oximetry. *J Biomed Optics*, **5**, 391–405.

153 O'Brien, P.M.S., Koyle, P.M. and Rolfe, P. (1993). Near infrared spectroscopy in fetal monitoring. *Br J Hosp Med*, **49**, 483–487.

154 Hamilton, R., Hodgett, S.G. and O'Brien, P.M.S. (1996). Near infrared spectroscopy applied to intrapartum fetal monitoring. *Bailliere's Clin Obstet Gynaecol*, **10**, 307–324.

155 Peebles, D.M., Edwards, A.D., Wyatt, J.S., et al. (1992). Changes in human fetal cerebral hemoglobin concentration and oxygenation during labor measured by near-infrared spectroscopy. *Am J Obstet Gynecol*, **166**, 1369–1373.

156 Aldrich, C.J., D'Antona, D., Spencer, J.A., et al. (1995). Late fetal heart decelerations and changes in cerebral oxygenation during the first stage of labour. *Br J Obstet Gynaecol*, **102**, 9–13.

157 Aldrich, C.J., D'Antona, D., Spencer, J.A., et al. (1996). Fetal heart rate changes and cerebral oxygenation measured by near-infrared spectroscopy during the first stage of labour. *Eur J Obstet Gynecol Reprod Biol*, **64**, 189–195.

158 Peebles, D.M., Spencer, J.A., Edwards, A.D., et al. (1994). Relation bewteen frequency of uterine contractions and human fetal cerebral oxygen saturation studied during labour by near infrared spectroscopy. *Br J Obstet Gynaecol*, **101**, 44–48.

159 Aldrich, C.J., D'Antona, D., Wyatt, J.S., et al. (1994). Fetal cerebral oxygenation measured by near-infrared spectroscopy shortly before birth and acid-based status at birth. *Obstet Gynecol*, **84**, 861–866.

160 Mozurkewich, E. and Wolf, F.M. (2000). Near-infrared spectroscopy for fetal assessment during labour. *Cochrane Database Syst Rev*, **3**, CD002254.

161 Peebles, D.M. (1997). Cerebral hemodynamics and oxygenation in the fetus: the role of intrapartum near-infrared spectroscopy. *Clin Perinatol*, **24**, 547–565.

162 Ramanujam, N., Vishnoi, G., Hielscher, A., et al. (2000). Photon migration through fetal head in utero using continuous wave, near infrared spectroscopy: clinical and experimental model studies. *J Biomed Optics*, **5**, 173–184.

163 Cohen, L.B. (1973). Changes in neuron structure during action potential propagation and synaptic transmission. *Physiol Rev*, **53**, 373–418.

164 Grinvald, A., Lieke, E., Frostig, R.D., et al. (1986). Functional architecture of cortex revealed by optical imaging of intrinsic signal. *Nature*, **324**, 361–364.

165 Frostig, R.D., Lieke, E., Ts'o, D.Y., et al. (1990). Cortical functional architecture and local coupling between neuronal activity and the microcirculation revealed by in vivo high-resolution optical imaging of intrinsic signals. *Proc Natl Acad Sci*, **87**, 6082–6086.

166 Malonek, D. and Grinvald, A. (1996). Interactions between electrical and cortical microcirculation revealed by imaging spectroscopy: implications for functional brain mapping. *Science*, **272**, 551–554.

167 Benaron, D.A., Ho, D.C., Spilman, S., et al. (1994). Tomographic time-of-flight optical imaging device. *Adv Exp Med Biol*, **361**, 207–214.

168 Benaron, D.A., Ho, D.C., Spilman, S., et al. (1994). Non-recursive linear algorithms for optical imaging in diffusive media. *Adv Exp Med Biol*, **361**, 215–222.

169 Hintz, S.R., Benaron, D.A., van Houten, J.P., et al. (1998). Stationary headband for clinical time-of-flight optical imaging at the bedside. *Photochem Photobiol*, **68**, 361–369.

170 Hintz, S.R., Cheong, W.-F., van Houten, J.P., et al. (1999). Bedside imaging of infracranial hemorrhage in the neonate using light: comparison with ultrasound, computed tomography, and magnetic resonance imaging. *Pediatr Res*, **45**, 54–59.

171 Gopinath, S.P., Robertson, C.S., Grossman, R.G., et al. (1993). Near-infrared spectroscopic localization of intracranial hematomas. *J Neurosurg*, **79**, 43–47.

172 Robertson, C.S., Gopinath, S.P. and Chance, B. (1997). Use of near infrared spectroscopy to identify traumatic intracranial hematomas. *J Biomed Optics*, **2**, 31–41.

173 Villringer, A. and Chance, B. (1997). Non-invasive optical spectroscopy and imaging of human brain function. *Trends Neurosci*, **20**, 435–442.

174 Nioka, S., Luo, Q. and Chance, B. (1997). Human brain functional imaging with reflectance CWS. In *Oxygen Transport to Tissue*, vol. XIX, pp. 237–242, eds. D.K. Harrison and D.T. Delpy. New York: Plenum.

175 Zhang, Q., Ma, H., Nioda, S., et al. (2000). Study of near infrared technology for intracranial hematoma detection. *J Biomed Optics*, **5**, 206–213.

176 Luo, Q., Nioda, S. and Chance, B. (1997). Functional near-infrared image. In *Optical Tomography and Spectroscopy of Tissue: Theory, Instrumentation, Model, and Human Studies II*, pp. 84–93, eds. B. Chance and R. Alfano. Proceedings of SPIE 2979.

177 Chance, B., Luo, Q., Nioka, S., et al. (1997). Optical investigations of physiology: a study of biomedical intrinsic and extrinsic contrast. *Phil Trans R Soc Lond*, **B352**, 707–716.

178 Chance, B., Anday, E., Nioka, S., et al. (1998). A novel method for fast imaging of brain function, non-invasively, with light. *Optics Express*, **2**, 411–423.

179 Siegel, A.M., Marota, J.J.A. and Boas, D.A. (1999). Design and evaluation of a continuous-wave diffuse optical tomography system. *Optics Express*, **4**, 287–298.

180 Hintz, S.R., Benaron, D.A., Siegel, A.M., et al. (2001). Bedside functional imaging of the premature infant brain during passive motor stimulation. *J Perinat Med*, **29**, 335–343.

181 Hintz, S.R., Benaron, D.A., Siegel, A.M., et al. (1999). Bedside functional imaging of the premature infant brain. *SPIE Proc*, **3597**, paper #3597–31.

182 Sokol, D.L., Zhang, X., Lu, P., et al. (1998). Real time detection of DNA/RNA hybridization in living cells. *Proc Natl Acad Sci USA*, **95**, 11538–11543.

183 Tan, W., Fang, X., Li, J., et al. (2000). Molecular beacons: a novel DNA probe for nucleic acid and protein studies. *Chemistry*, **6**, 1107–1111.

184 Mahmood, U., Tung, C.H., Bogdanov, A. Jr, et al. (1999). Near-infrared optical imaging of protease activity for tumor detection. *Radiology*, **213**, 866–870.

185 Tung, C.H., Bredo, S., Mahmood, U., et al. (1999). Preparation of a cathepsin D sensitive near-infrared fluorescence probe for imaging. *Bioconjug Chem*, **10**, 892–896.

186 Weissleder, R., Tung, C.H., Mahmood, U., et al. (1999). *In vivo* imaging of tumors with protease-activated near-infrared fluorescent probes. *Nat Biotechnol*, **17**, 375–378.

Placental pathology and the etiology of fetal and neonatal brain injury

Geoffrey Altshuler

University of Oklahoma Health Sciences Center and the Children's Hospital of Oklahoma, Oklahoma City, OK, USA

Introduction

This article relates placental pathology to fetal and neonatal brain injury. In the author's experience, known causes of cerebral palsy have been substantially limited by deficient collaboration between clinicians, pathologists, epidemiologists, and basic scientists. Hence, in the following pages, there is advocacy for interdisciplinary investigations of neurologic and related disorders. The article is written by a pathologist who has practiced pediatric and placental pathology for more than 30 years and, including medicolegal consultations, has examined placentas from more than 450 cases of cerebral palsy. In reflection upon those experiences, there is no attempt to comment upon all relevant publications. Many more detailed aspects of the literature are provided in recent editions of Benirschke and Kaufmann,[1] and of Fox,[2] and there is convenient tabulated information in articles of Kaplan and colleagues[3] and Langston and colleagues.[4]

Clinical indications for placental examinations

Common sense should persuade one that any pregnancy which is sufficiently complicated to require "high-risk" management of the mother warrants sufficient concern to require gross and light microscopic placental examination. Similar consideration is applicable to the newborn. Indications for placental examination are provided in Table 24.1. This list, compiled by obstetricians, neonatologists, and pathologists,[3] is a reasonable guideline for colleagues to use or modify.

Pathology reports

In many hospitals, placentas from uncomplicated deliveries are stored at 4 °C for 1 week in seven bins. If clinical problems occur, procurement of placentas for examination is thus facilitated. Examples of gross placental findings are provided in Table 24.2. When clinical indications warrant placental examination by a pathologist, six or more microscopic slides insure meaningful clinicopathologic correlation. Tissues represented on light microscopic slides include umbilical cord, extraplacental membranes, and four or more placental locations with fetal and maternal surfaces therein.

Synopsis of placental pathology

The following paragraphs introduce considerations of relationships between placental pathology and fetal and neonatal brain damage.

Conditions associated with low uteroplacental blood flow

Terminology and histopathology

Ischemic change, infarction, fetal thrombi, avascular villi, and hemorrhagic endovasculopathy are histopathologic manifestations of low uteroplacental

Table 24.1. Indications which require a comprehensive gross and microscopic examination by a pathologist

Maternal conditions
Diabetes mellitus (or glucose intolerance)
Hypertension (pregnancy-induced)
Prematurity (less than 32 weeks)
Postmaturity (pregnancy longer than 42 weeks)
Maternal history of reproductive failure (defined as one or more previous stillbirths, spontaneous abortions, or premature births)
Oligohydramnios
Fever
Infection
Maternal history of substance abuse
Repetitive bleeding (other than minor spotting of the first trimester)
Abruptio placentae
Fetal and neonatal conditions
Stillbirth or perinatal death
Multiple birth
Congenital abnormalities
Fetal growth retardation
Prematurity (32 weeks' or less gestation)
Hydrops
Viscid/thick meconium
Admission to a neonatal intensive care unit
Severe central nervous system depression (Apgar score of 3 or less at 5 min)
Neurologic problems, including seizures
Suspected infection
Placental conditions
Any gross abnormality of the placenta, its membranes, or the umbilical cord

blood flow. Acute villous ischemic change is histopathologically characterized by agglutination of shrunken villi which have numerically increased syncytial knots; features of chronic villous ischemic change often include shrunken villi with villous knots and eosinophilic fibrinoid material (Figure 24.1, colour plate). Acute infarcts have ghost- like villi with obliteration of fetal blood vessels and villous connective tissue cells. Continuation of chronically reduced uterine blood flow leads to obliteration of fetal villous tissue by fibrin-like material and "X cells." Some of those last mentioned cells are seen in the pinkish fibrinoid material at the lower part of Figure 24.1. When these chronic features are focal, pathologists use the term "chronic infarct." Diffuse such change is called chronic ischemic change; it is often accompanied by fetal growth retardation. Although acute and chronic ischemic changes are morphologically different from one another, they have similar etiology. Maternal coagulopathy in maternal sinusoids is an important part of that pathogenesis. Additional to fetal growth retardation, morbidity, and mortality are major associated complications.

Fetal placental thrombi

Low uteroplacental blood flow may cause thrombosis in fetal stem vessels and in vessels of the superficial fetal plate (Figure 24.2, colour plate). These lesions range from the kind of thrombi which occur in any organ, to a characteristic "cushion" of

Table 24.2. Gross placental findings

GENERAL:

Trimmed weight: __________ g   **Complete** (Y/N): ____   **Fixed** (Y/N): ___   or   **Fresh** (Y/N): ___

Size: _ _._ × _ _._ × _ _._ cm   **Accessory lobe** (Y/N): __   (**Size** _ _._ × _ _._ × _ _._ cm)

MEMBRANES:

Placental sac rupture: ___ cm from margin   **Membranes edema:** (Y/N) ___

Membranes insertion site: ___ % marginal; ___ % circummarginate; ___ % circumvallate

Color: normal ❑ green (G) ❑ brown (B) ❑ yellow (Y) ❑ gray (G) ❑ combined colors __________

CORD:

Knots (number and type): true ___, variceal or false __; **Length:** ____ cm; **Vessels:** (3) __ or (2) __

Site of cord insertion: central ❑ marginal ❑ eccentric ❑ velamentous ❑

Color: normal ❑ green (G) ❑ brown (B) ❑ yellow (Y) ❑ gray (G) ❑ combined colors __________

PLACENTA:

Color: normal ❑ green (G) ❑ brown (B) ❑ yellow (Y) ❑ gray (G) ❑ combined colors __________

Superficial (e.g., tan-gray) fibrinoid material: none (Y/N) __, <25% ❑, 25–50% ❑, >50% ❑

Amnion nodosum or any other unusual superficial lesions (Y/N): __

Appearance of placental tissue: congested (Y/N) ___ very pale (Y/N) ___ unremarkable ___

Infarcts or infarction (including the distribution and the approximate amount of the placenta involved):
focal ❑ multifocal ❑ or diffuse ❑ <25% ❑, 25–50% ❑, >50% ❑

Abruption: (Y/N) _____ (approximate % of placental floor involved): ____ %
(approximate volume of blood clots: _______ ml)

Maternal floor calcification, degeneration, or infarction: (approximate % of floor involved) ____ %

OTHER INFORMATION:

COMMENTS:

fibrinous material across the endothelium of superficial placental vessels.

Avascular villi

Thrombosis in nutrient fetal arteries causes avascularity of villi. When that pathology is multifocal or diffuse, there is significant risk of associated fetal brain and other injury.

Nucleated red blood cells

Tissue storage and processing artifacts occasionally obscure the numerical extent of nucleated red blood cells (NRBCs). These cells are readily recognizable. In hematoxylin and eosin-stained sections, they have dark nuclei with distinctly regular or smooth nuclear membranes. Placental NRBCs signify fetal hypoxia. They are pathologic, even at 32 weeks' or less gestation, when I have often seen accompanying placental villous ischemic change and infarction.

Meconium staining

Gross and light microscopic meconium-induced morphologic changes are important means by which temporal aspects of fetal meconium exposure can be estimated. Three and more hours after exposure to meconium, the extraplacental membranes become edematous. They feel slippery, even with gloved fingers. Shortly after defecation, meconium has a green color. As time passes, the color progressively changes from green to tan-green, dark tan, and brown. The last two mentioned colors indicate 24 h or more exposure to meconium. Rarely, meconium causes digestion and absence of Wharton's jelly about umbilical vessels (Figure 24.3, colour plate). That is the most extreme placenta-related manifestation of meconium toxicity. Temporal light microscopic findings of fetal exposure to meconium include the following:

1. Numerous meconium-laden macrophages across the superficial placental chorionic plate indicate exposure to meconium for 3 h or more.
2. Abundant meconium-laden macrophages extensively beneath the amniotic epithelium of the extraplacental membranes are usually seen 6–12 h after fetal meconium discharge.
3. Meconium-induced umbilical vascular myocyte necrosis (Figures 24.4 and 24.5, colour plates) indicates 24–48 h or more of fetal meconium exposure (relative to the severity of the number of necrotic myocytes and to the number of the involved vessels).

Chorioamnionitis

This entity results from the ascent of microbes from the lower maternal genital tract to the decidual lining of the fetal sac and ultimately to the amniotic fluid. Because of chemoattractants in the amniotic fluid, leukocytes emigrate from chorionic tissue about the fetal sac, from superficial fetal placental vessels, and from vessels in the umbilical cord. Manifestations of this process include chorionitis, amnionitis, umbilical vasculitis, and inflammation in the Wharton's jelly of the umbilical cord (funisitis or funiculitis). Umbilical cord inflammation is almost never seen in umbilical cords of very immature fetuses. That remains true, even when there is severe superficial placental inflammation with fetuses of similar immaturity. Whereas infection singly with group B streptococcus produces little inflammation, *Escherichia coli* and diverse other microbes often cause severe inflammation. Because interleukin-8 is present in meconium, fetal meconium discharge often exacerbates microbially initiated chorioamnionitis.[5] This fact, and frequent polymicrobial cause of chorioamnionitis, confounds the interpretation of many pathologists who claim the ability to estimate chronicity of the process, according to the severity of its inflammation.

Villitis of unknown etiology

I encounter villitis of unknown etiology (VUE) 100 times more often than villitis caused by combined incidence of *E. coli, Listeria monocytogenes,* other bacteria, *Toxoplasma* cysts, rubella virus, cytomegalovirus, herpes simplex virus, and syphilis. Diverse light microscopic manifestations include lymphocytic, lymphohistiocytic, necrotizing, granulomatous, reparative, and evanescent villitis.[6] Diagnosis of VUE requires inflammation to be present within villi (Figure 24.6, colour plate). Pathologists often incorrectly diagnose this entity when maternal inflammatory cells are chemotactically attracted to ischemically induced necrosis of villi. Whereas VUE occurs in as many as 7% of placentas that I have examined, it has only rarely been accompanied by subsequent cerebral palsy. In my opinion, infection is the primary cause of villitis. I concede, however, that immunologically mediated influences may modify its morphological manifestations. Others have opined that it has an immunopathologic cause which manifests maternal antifetal immune response. These considerations have been recently discussed.[7]

Chorangiosis

Normal placental villi have only two to five villous capillaries. In chorangiosis, inspection with a 10× objective shows 10 or more villi, each with 10 or more capillaries, in 10 or more noninfarcted and nonischemic areas.[8] Often, during labor and delivery, obstruction of umbilical cord blood flow causes multifocal villous capillary hypervascularity, particularly in cotyledons near the insertion of the umbilical cord. Placental malperfusion is then most often associated with cesarean section, often as a result of the operative procedure itself or because of umbilical cord compressions which necessitated cesarean section. Placental malperfusion resultant from focal and even multifocal diverse ischemic and villous inflammatory damage frequently causes focal or multifocal villous capillary hypervascularity. Those features do not constitute chorangiosis (Figure 24.7, colour plate). To make that diagnosis, the capillary hypervascularity has to be present diffusely. With those criteria, I have seen chorangiosis in as many as 5% of newborns hospitalized in an intensive care unit. Mainly because of accompanying congenital anomalies, 35% of affected neonates expired.[8]

Hemorrhagic endovasculopathy (hemorrhagic endovasculitis)

When this lesion was initially named, an infectious etiology was considered to be likely.[9] Because there is no true (inflammatory) vasculitis in this lesion, the word "endovasculitis" is a misnomer. Obliterated vascular lumens herein include fragmented nucleated red blood cells and, often, fibrin. Silver and her colleagues observed similar findings in organ cultures of placentas from live-born infants, especially when organ explants were allowed to degenerate and sustain hypoxia.[10] As early as 1 day and for as long as 7 days, the lesions were particularly seen in fetal stem arteries.[10] That histopathology is frequently seen in placentas of macerated stillborns[11] and (in retrospect), I have occasionally seen it in placentas of patients who later developed cerebral palsy.

Use, abuse, and absence of the placenta in epidemiologic studies

The "Collaborative Study"

Between 1959 and 1966, the Collaborative Perinatal Study (CPS) of the United States National Institute of Neurological and Communicative Disorders and Stroke investigated more than 56 000 pregnancies in different regions of the USA.[12] In the introduction of his succinctly written book, Naeye summarized many organizational aspects of the investigation.[13] There and elsewhere, he did not clarify the total number of light microscopic placental examinations performed, nor the level of expertise and reliability of pathologists who reviewed slides from the 12 medical school-affiliated hospitals. This consideration and error in compilation of archived data may explain apparent major error in a recent publication: "Histologic chorioamnionitis is associated with fetal growth restriction in term and preterm infants."[14] In the opening sentence of the results section, the investigators stated that chorioamnionitis was found in 2579 (5.9%) of 43 940 evaluable deliveries of nonanomalous singleton infants.[14] This 5.9% figure is greatly less than the 21% incidence in our medical center[15] and in incidence figures of chorioamnionitis cited in earlier-mentioned textbooks.[1,2] I suspect that the wide discordance results from deficient interobserver reliability of the contributing pathologists.

Personal opinions

Some aspects of perinatal medicine have been disappointing:

1. There are very few experts in placental pathology.
2. Amongst those experts, there have been few intraobserver and interobserver reliability studies.
3. Placental pathology and associated patient outcome have never been examined relative to uniform clinical management. (Oncologists, for example, study patient outcome relative to precisely defined clinical management and histopathology.)
4. Other than for the now historic CPS, there has been deficient support for inclusion of pathologists in perinatal research.

Considerations of reliability studies

I am aware of only one study in which both intraobserver and interobserver reliability investigation was performed with numerous histopathologic considerations of numerous specimens. More than 15 features were examined for each of 74 intraobserver and 233 interobserver placental studies; each placenta was represented by six light microscopic slides.[16] Kappa statistics were used. A kappa value greater than 0.75 was considered to represent excellent agreement beyond chance; values between 0.40 and 0.75 were reported as fair to very good agreement. The intraobserver reliability of placental diagnoses was excellent for features other than chorangiosis (that kappa value being 0.58). Relative to the diagnoses of two investigators, interobserver reliability with inflammatory lesions was very good to excellent. When histopathologically evident low uteroplacental blood flow changes were subcategorized as acute, subacute, and chronic, there was poor agreement.[16]

Bendon and other experienced colleagues performed detailed examinations of histopathology in 628 placentas from preterm premature rupture of membranes cases and additional study of many diverse control specimens.[17] The cases and controls were scored for 40 histologic features by pathologists who were blinded to the identity of each sample (case or control). There were no histologic differences between preterm premature rupture of membranes cases treated with antibiotic and those receiving placebo, nor with respect to duration of membrane rupture greater or less than 48 h.[17] For features other than acute inflammation, however, concordance among pathologists was low.[17]

In a study of 70 microscopic slides, Khong and three pathologist colleagues investigated VUE. Intraobserver agreement was 84.7% (range 74–92%) and interobserver agreement was 81%.[18] The investigators concluded that experienced pathologists can show significant interobserver variation in assessing VUE.[18]

Five pathologists examined 24 light microscopic slides to assess placental immaturity by histology.[19] They concluded that experienced pathologists can have difficulty in assessing villous maturity of placentas by histology.[19]

In an interrater reliability study, five pathologists independently reviewed microscopic slides of 30 placentas.[20] There was moderate to substantial agreement among the raters for a variety of indicators of inflammation, presence of macrophages with pigment and indicators of villous maturity, increased syncytial knots, and maternal vasculopathy.[20] Substantial agreement was obtained for the presence of subchorionitis, chorionitis, and chorioamnionitis.[20]

Finally, in this brief review of placental reliability studies, I mention a most recent investigation which may have little relevance to diseases of the fetus and newborn. Six pathologists examined 30 slides to define and assess interobserver reliability in the diagnosis of chronic basal placental deciduitis.[21] The pathologists concluded that they were able to diagnose chronic deciduitis with sufficient concordance to be of value in clinical correlation studies.

Pathogenetic concepts in epidemiologic investigations

There is need of pathogenetic concepts in the construction of statistical analyses. When this is not done, important risk factors can be lost because of their frequent occurrence with other factors in the same data set.[22] Concepts of pathogenesis enable hypotheses which make epidemiologic findings reasonably predictable, e.g., the earlier-mentioned fact that chemoattractants in amniotic fluid cause leukocytes to emigrate from chorionic tissue about the fetal sac and from superficial fetal placental vessels and umbilical vessels. That phenomenon explains predictable associations between acute umbilical vasculitis, chorionic vasculitis, amnion epithelial necrosis, subchorionitis, chorionitis, and chorioamnionitis. This "clustering of morphologic characteristics" was recently demonstrated by Hansen and her colleagues in placentas of neonates with very low birth weight.[23] Not emphasized in that or in other epidemiologic investigations is the fact that it is remarkably rare for immature fetuses to have severe umbilical vasculitis and necrotizing funisitis. This fact remains true, even when there is severe chorioamnionitis in the accompanying placenta. My hypothetical explanation of that striking discordance is that an inflammatory suppressant is probably present in the Wharton's jelly of immature fetuses.

Differences of opinions

In a 1998 article of placental lesions associated with neurologic impairment and cerebral palsy in very-low-birth-weight infants, Redline and his colleagues reported that two types of "fetal placental vascular lesions" are associated with neurologic impairment: nonocclusive thrombi of chorionic plate vessels and severe villous edema.[24] By their comments, the authors seemingly supported Naeye's claim that, in neonates born before 28 weeks of gestation, villous edema is the most frequent cause of stillbirth, neonatal death, and neonatal morbidity.[25] Because the investigators did not include water-laden villous stromal macrophages in their diagnosis of edema,[24,25] I doubt their observations and conclusions. Not surprising, therefore, were the opinions published separately and later of Benirschke and Kaufmann,[1] and Fox.[2] Those authors indicated that alleged edema of villi in placentas of immature fetuses is actually attributable to normal intermediate villi – a consideration which was earlier suspected by Shen-Schwarz and her colleagues.[26]

In a study of cerebral palsy and neurologic impairment following term birth, Redline and O'Riordan found nine significantly associated lesions.[27] The authors stated that meconium-associated vascular necrosis, severe fetal chorioamnionitis, chorionic vessel thrombi, increased NRBCs, and findings consistent with abruptio placentae are generally considered to occur within days of delivery and that diffuse chronic villitis, extensive avascular villi, diffuse chorioamnionic hemosiderosis, and perivillous fibrin, have a much longer onset.[27] My findings, relative to term and more mature fetuses, have been slightly different. They are based upon epidemiologic analyses of placental diagnoses associated with clinically diagnosed perinatal asphyxia and separate experience of more than 450 cases of cerebral palsy. The latter mentioned cases involved medicolegal consultations made throughout the last 12 years. In those consultations I made light microscopic descriptions, morphologic diagnoses, and interpretations and was subsequently provided with related clinical information.

At and beyond term gestation, noninflammatory placental and umbilical cord pathology manifests the etiology of cerebral palsy. Typical features have been acute and chronic placental ischemic changes, infarction, associated oligohydramnios and cord compression, and resultant fetal defecation and exposure to meconium (Figure 24.8, colour plate). Accompanying manifestations of reduced uterine blood flow have often included fetal thrombotic lesions, fetal hemorrhagic endovasculopathy, avascular villi, and numerous fetal NRBCs. Even by univariate analysis, there has been no association between chorioamnionitis and clinically diagnosed perinatal asphyxia.[22] My experience has been that, when chorioamnionitis is histopathologically severe at and beyond term gestation, there is often the additional presence of meconium. Hence, I question if obscure meconium has complicated the alleged single association between severe fetal chorioamnionitis and neurologic impairment.[27] Relative to other findings of Redline and O'Riordan,[27] I have not found their observed "chorioamnionic hemosiderosis" to be significantly associated with cerebral palsy and neurologic impairment.[27] Two emphases need to be made about pathogenetic links between meconium and cerebral palsy. Recurrent and chronic fetal exposure to meconium staining is not at all rare. Because meconium-induced vascular necrosis has been reported to occur in umbilical cords of immature fetuses,[28] cerebral palsy may result from remote and recurrent fetal exposure to meconium.

Major differences in placental findings cause major differences of opinions. An example is readily forthcoming from two investigations of correlation between prenatal brain damage and placental pathology.[29,30] The study population in the first investigation included 61 spontaneous fetal demises, 24 terminations of pregnancy, and 13 liveborn neonates who survived for less than 1 h. The incidence of chorioamnionitis was therewith 22% (22 of 98 cases).[29] From 248 consecutive autopsies performed on fetuses dying after 20 weeks' gestation, 70 cases were light microscopically found to have ischemic brain injury.[30] Of those 70 cases, less than 3% had chorioamnionitis.[30] Even when one concedes that the populations differed in more than one respect, it is difficult to rationalize the major difference in the incidences of associated histopathologic chorioamnionitis.

The era of low uteroplacental blood flow

Prior to the early 1970s, histopathologic chorioamnionitis was often accompanied by clinically apparent chorioamnionitis, *Escherichia coli* infection, endotoxemia, and periventricular leukomalacia. Now, histopathologic signs of reduced uterine blood flow are more prevalent. In a study of 1252 placentas from selected singleton live births, the pathologic placental features were ischemic change (40%), meconium staining (27%), chorioamnionitis (21%), and placental abruption (21%); the incidence of villitis, chorangiosis, and other entities was no more than 4% for each.[15] The incidence of placental ischemic change was close enough to twice that of histopathologic chorioamnionitis and the combination of the two occurred in only 10%. The highest rates of placental ischemic change and infarction were observed in small term infants who weighed 1500–2499 g (65% and 23%, respectively).[15] In the afore-mentioned database of 1252 cases, whereas I saw diffuse ischemic features in 505 placentas, clinicians diagnosed preeclampsia in only 59 mothers. Expressed another way, histopathologic signs of reduced uterine blood flow have occurred 8½ times more often than clinically diagnosed preeclampsia.

Hansen and her colleagues found that 75% of placentas of very-low-birth-weight newborns, delivered because of severe pregnancy-induced hypertension or preeclampsia, had at least one sign of low uteroplacental blood flow.[31] Histopathology in an earlier report revealed that vascular lesions in maternal spiral arteries, multiple placental syncytial knots, placental infarcts, and placental weights of less than the 10th percentile represented a distinct subgroup among patients with preterm labor and preterm ruptured membranes.[32]

Citation of the afore-mentioned three investigations[15,31,32] requires acknowledgment of Naeye who earlier reported a relationship between pregnancy hypertension, placental evidence of low uteroplacental blood flow, and spontaneous premature delivery.[33]

The era of cytokines

During the writing of this manuscript, a literature search revealed references to 140 publications whose keywords include cytokine and chorioamnionitis. More than one-half of those articles originated from Dr. Roberto Romero and his colleagues. Recently, however, others have focused upon important pathogenetic links between low uteroplacental blood flow states, placental ischemic change, infarction, cytokines, and perinatal complications. As of now, there have been at least 210 articles whose keywords have included cytokine and preeclampsia.

Two articles directly relate cytokines to cerebral palsy.[34,35] They were enabled by preserved blood spot specimens which were obtained from the California Genetic Disease Program. The specimens were tested years after the birth of newborns who had later manifested cerebral palsy. The investigation was cleverly conceived, relative to knowledge that interferon-α, therapeutically administered to young children, had caused at least seven of those patients to develop spastic diplegia.[34,35] Cytokine production is influenced by a variety of factors, including infection, autoimmune states, trauma, ischemia, and neoplasia.[34] It is important to emphasize that cytokines are a consequence of disease, not a primary cause.

Conrad and Benyo evaluated the hypothesis that inflammatory cytokines may be overproduced by the placenta in response to local ischemia/hypoxia and that this could contribute to increased plasma levels, and subsequent maternal endothelial activation and dysfunction in preeclampsia.[36] They informed that, as early as 1924, Mayer was among the first investigators to provide direct evidence for endothelial involvement in preeclampsia. At least two items of pathogenetic import are noteworthy. Embolized placental syncytiotrophoblast has been implicated as causative of endothelial injury in preeclampsia and human placental trophoblast cells express erythropoietin. After providing much information, Conrad and Benyo offered a unifying hypothesis: "Briefly, inadequate trophoblast invasion and physiologic remodeling of spiral arteries initiate focal regions of placental ischemia/hypoxia, which in turn lead to overproduction of placental cytokines such as TNF-α . . . Elevated plasma levels of cytokines, such as TNF-α then contribute both directly and indirectly to endothelial cell dysfunction producing the disease manifestations."[36] An extension of this hypothesis is that primary maternal coagulopathy in uterine arteries and in placental sinusoids might account for the entire pathogenesis of eclampsia, including cytokines, embolized syncytiotrophoblast, and expression of erythropoietin by trophoblast cells.

Information in previous pages requires emphasis that histopathologically evident reduced uterine blood flow states are more common than chorioamnionitis and that they cause activity of cytokines.[15,31,36] It is thus very disappointing that, in the article "Fetal exposure to an intraamniotic inflammation and the development of cerebral palsy at the age of three years," there was no consideration of cytokines associated with placental ischemia or infarction.[37]

Epidemiology, epiphenomena, and need for placental examinations

Pathologic placental findings, later analyzed in conjunction with medical records, have often revealed that clinically observed abnormalities often have not been the primary cause of fetal damage. They have been secondary or incidental and, thus, epiphenomena. Nevertheless, many clinicians do not request placental examinations, even when there are obvious maternal and fetal indications to do so. Insightful Australian investigators appropriately asked: "Why is the placenta being ignored?"[38] Although 276 cases fulfilled multiple maternal, fetal, and placental indications for placental examination,[3] histopathologic findings were available for only 11.2%.[38] Attitudes which have caused a low percentage of placental examinations are not exclusive to Sydney. For example, Committee members of the American College of Obstetricians and Gynecologists issued the following statement: "When a skilled and systematic examination of the umbilical cord, membranes, and placenta is performed on properly prepared specimens, insight into antepartum pathophysiology may be gained under certain circumstances. In most of these instances, such as chorioamnionitis, the diagnosis already will have been made on clinical grounds, with the placental examination providing confirmation."[39] That statement is disturbingly incorrect. From investigation published 1 year before the Committee's opinion, Romero and his colleagues reported that only one of 11 mothers with positive amniotic microbial cultures had clinically recognizable chorioamnionitis.[40] Also, as mentioned earlier in the present placental article (in the paragraph titled "The era of low uteroplacental blood flow"): "histopathologic signs of reduced uterine blood flow occur 8½ times more frequently than clinically diagnosed preeclampsia." These facts exhort clinicians to include placental pathology in investigations of at-risk fetuses and newborns.

Meconium

Historical considerations

In 1945, Clifford studied 57 newborns with yellow staining of vernix caseosa, skin, nails and umbilical cord.[41] Although 93% had not manifested abnormal fetal recordings, 28% needed vigorous resuscitation at birth.[41] Clifford hypothesized that this "yellow vernix syndrome" resulted from asphyxial injury days or weeks before delivery and he concluded that the principal cause may well be revealed by microscopic examination of the placenta.[41]

In recent decades, literature concerning meconium aspiration syndrome has become "murky."[42] In a 1998 update of an earlier review by Cleary and Wiswell, meconium aspiration syndrome is stated to have occurred in 1.7–35.8% of infants born through meconium-stained amniotic fluid (median, 10.5%).[43] Two considerations probably account for this disturbingly wide range of clinical diagnosis: (1) few clinicians have exercised Clifford's enthusiasm for placental examinations; and thus, (2) few pathologists have developed expertise in interpretation of placentas.

In 1978, French investigators investigated the fact that newborns with clinical signs of meconium aspiration frequently pass dark urine.[44] By spectrophotometry, the investigators found that the causative water-soluble component is recognizable by an absorption band at about 405 nm.[44] Separate spectrophotometric determination of meconium concentration in amniotic fluid has also been well reported.[45]

In 1982, Abramovich and Gray reported the location of meconium in various parts of intestinal tract specimens from 31 midpregnancy fetuses.[46] They stated that anatomic studies of the anal canal suggested that "the fetus defecates routinely up to 16 weeks, after which time defecation becomes less common, finally ceasing after 20 weeks."[46] Several aspects of their methods and conclusion are questionable:

1. The investigators did not provide clinical or placental data to substantiate listed gestational ages.
2. There was no information as to the cause of the spontaneous abortions or reasons for the prostaglandin-induced abortions.
3. The gross studies did not include weights of meconium in various parts of the intestine.
4. The numbers of studied specimens were small.
5. Tabulated data and text were confusing. For example, whereas their Table 3 identifies a total of 21 spontaneous abortions and prostaglandin inductions, the materials and methods section of the article states that there was a total of 20 spontaneous abortions, nine prostaglandin terminations of pregnancy and two hysterotomy specimens.[46]

In 1985, Allen stated that "meconium-stained amniotic fluid during midtrimester genetic amniocentesis may not carry the ominous prognosis that originally might have been predicted."[47] In the discussion section of this article, Dr. Robert Resnik referred to a published claim that, in the course of fetal development, motilin does not appear until about 30 weeks' gestation. Ten years after Dr. Resnik's remark, Polish investigators published (in English) a statement that human fetuses at 19–21 weeks' gestation have blood levels of motilin that are 60% of those in their mothers.[48] Relative to the respective sizes of fetal and maternal intestinal tracts, fetal blood motilin levels seem to be more than sufficient to enable discharge of meconium.

Meconium and pulmonary pathology

In 1978, Manning and his colleagues reported neonatal death of a severely depressed, 38 weeks' gestation, 3450-g male whose Apgar scores had been 1 and 1.[49] Although the authors recognized that this was a case of massive intrauterine meconium aspiration, they considered that severity of the syndrome could be reduced by intrapartum and neonatal airway suctioning.[49] Later published literature helped to establish that this last-mentioned claim is incorrect. In 1987 Byrne and Gau reported a 40 weeks and 5 days' gestation fetus whose lungs featured "deep meconium aspiration with most alveoli lined with meconium." The title of their article was "In utero meconium aspiration: an unpreventable cause of neonatal death."[50] From a review of 14 527 deliveries between January 1985 and April 1987, Sunoo and colleagues documented 77 cases of meconium aspiration.[51] The authors included a report of four cases and suggested that meconium aspiration may occur before the onset of active labor and without evidence of fetal distress. They cited seven articles whose content supported their opinion.[51]

In an article of 1993, Falciglia et al. wrote: "To our knowledge, this is the first reported case of fatal intrauterine MAS [meconium aspiration syndrome] in an infant born at 27 weeks' gestation." [52] In 1996, from a review of 123 autopsies of humans, Burgess and Hutchins documented 19 cases with umbilical cord damage attributable to meconium.[53] The authors claimed that, in 37 cases (67%), there was inflammation secondary to meconium aspiration.[53] My experience of autopsies in humans has been that, whereas meconium augments inflammation caused by microbes, meconium is not a primary cause of inflammation. Perhaps the best evidence for this conclusion is that fetal autopsies not uncommonly reveal massive meconium aspiration unaccompanied by inflammation. Investigators who studied rabbits found that injections of sterile substances, including meconium, did not provoke granulocytic reaction.[54] Studies of meconium aspiration in guinea-pigs have also documented the absence of meconium-induced pneumonitis.[55] When investigators found "chemical pneumonitis" in an experimental adult rabbit model, my interpretation was that microbes were present in the lungs of the animals prior to the experiments.[56]

In 1999, Kearney reported three autopsies from which he interpreted that chronic intrauterine meconium aspiration had caused fetal lung infarcts, lung rupture, and meconium embolism.[57] He questioned the assertion that rarity of the cases might be explained by death occurring before the pathology had time to develop. His interpretation of the histopathology was that it resulted from meconium-induced vasoconstriction of peripheral preacinar arteries.[57]

Meconium and midtrimester fetuses

The first account of meconium-induced umbilical vascular necrosis in abortuses and immature fetuses was given in 1999. In that article three of four reported fetuses had gestational ages of 16, 19, and 29 weeks.[28] Necrotic cells in the umbilical vascular media manifested ovoid or globoid cells with dark nuclei and hypereosinophilic cytoplasm, accompanied by eosinophilic similarly shaped cells with ghost-like nuclei or no nuclei.[28] Autolytic umbilical vascular myocytes are distinctly different; they have elongated and narrow nuclei. With separate use of histochemical and immunocytochemical stains, macrophages near the necrotic myocytes stained positively for both bilirubin and the cytokine, interleukin-1ß. We suggested that cytokine may have contributed to the mechanism of fetal death.[28] Prior to this experience, meconium- induced vascular necrosis and superficial umbilical cord ulceration had only been reported in umbilical cords of term, postterm, and postmature fetuses.[58]

Affirmation of meconium-induced umbilical vascular necrosis in abortuses and immature fetuses was forthcoming at the 1999 annual meeting of the Paediatric Pathology Society. Kearney and Mortensen reported that, in a study of 68 midtrimester fetuses, they found eight unequivocal cases of intrauterine meconium aspiration.[59] The gestational ages ranged from 16 to 25 weeks (mean 20 weeks).[59]

Pharmacopathologic concepts of meconium

In 1988, during microscopic examination and report of routine pathology service, I encountered a remarkable specimen. A placenta and umbilical cord had necrosis in the muscle of superficial placental vessels, necrosis in umbilical vasculature, and meconium-laden macrophages in and near the blood vessels.[60] The observation led to the hypothesis that, before soluble components of meconium would have caused this damage, they probably would have produced vasoactivity and vasocontraction. To investigate whether meconium causes vasocontraction, Dr. Scott Hyde and I tested umbilical vein tissue with an isometric transducer connected to a polygraph.[60] Because meconium maximally produced 62.9% of serotonin-induced vasocontraction, we hypothesized that meconium may cause placental and umbilical vasocontraction, cerebral and other fetal hypoperfusion, and major poor outcome.[60]

A high incidence of stillbirth occurs with mothers who suffer cholestatic hepatopathy. On the assumption that chorionic vessels of the placental surface are particularly exposed to the increasing levels of bile acids accompanying maternal cholestatic hepatopathy, Sepúlveda and his colleagues investigated the effects of bile acids on isolated human placental chorionic veins.[61] Except for the fact that Hyde and I had investigated effects on umbilical venous tissue, the experimental procedures and results were similar to those that we had reported.[60] In addition, however, Sepúlveda and his colleagues found that bile acids cause dose-dependent vasoconstriction.[61] This was especially true for cholic acid.

After using significantly different methods from those of the above-mentioned reports,[60,61] Montgomery and his colleagues found that meconium inhibits the contraction of umbilical vessels induced by the thromboxane A_2 analog U46619.[62] Some reasons which may account for their contradictory finding include the following:

1. Whereas we eliminated prostaglandin effects by promptly using umbilical cords obtained from elective cesarean sections, Montgomery et al. used umbilical cords obtained after vaginal delivery or cesarean section done because of prolonged labor.
2. We promptly processed specimens into 37 °C Krebs solution transport media but Montgomery et al. "immediately" placed segments of cord into cold Krebs–bicarbonate solution. (In our opinion, immersion of vascular segments in cold Krebs solution would probably have altered the intrinsic properties of the vessels).
3. In our experiments, vascular segments were suspended in an organ bath under continuous aeration with 5% CO_2 and 95% O_2 at pH 7.4 and 37°C.[63] Montgomery et al. used an experimental tissue environment of unmentioned pH, temperature of 37°C, but 8.07% CO_2, 2.5% O_2 (and the balance of nitrogen). In the opinion of Montgomery and his colleagues, an environment of 5% CO_2 and 95% O_2 is not appropriate.[62]

In 1999, Holcberg et al. used a dual-perfusion technique to investigate the effect of meconium-stained amniotic fluid on the vasculature of isolated perfused human placental cotyledon.[64] A fetal artery and fetal vein from a single cotyledon were cannulated within 20 min of delivery. After establishing the fetal circulation, the placenta was mounted into a perfusion chamber, and the maternal circulation was simulated by placing four catheters into the intervillous space of the lobe corresponding to the perfused isolated cotyledon.[64] Maternal perfusate that returned from the intervillous space was continuously drained by a maternal venous catheter placed at the lowest level on the maternal decidual surface, to avoid significant pooling of perfusate. The experimental environment included pH 7.4, 95% O_2, 5% CO_2, and temperature 37 °C.[64] Bolus injections of 1.0 ml of meconium-stained amniotic fluid were made into the fetal circulation, at different concentrations. The investigators found that this caused a concentration-dependent increase in perfusion pressure. They thus concluded that meconium is a vasoconstrictive agent in the fetal–placental vasculature and that it has a concentration-dependent effect.[64]

Physiopathologic considerations of meconium

Earlier in this article, I mentioned that newborns with meconium aspiration syndrome have dark urine and that the causative water-soluble component is recognizable by an absorption band at 405 nm.[44] These observations indicate that newborns with meconium aspiration syndrome probably have soluble meconium components in their systemic circulation. All but one of the cited pharmacologic studies give evidence that meconium produces vasoconstrictive actions. Thus, I infer that this physiopathology contributes to the etiology of persistent fetal circulation in the meconium aspiration syndrome. It is noteworthy that, in newborn piglets, meconium aspiration induces a concentration-dependent pulmonary hypertensive response.[65] Relative to these considerations, important observations were made in an investigation of acute hemodynamic and respiratory effects of amniotic fluid embolism in a pregnant goat model: "The animals receiving amniotic fluid containing meconium had a marked acute elevation of the pulmonary capillary wedge pressure . . . the acute left ventricular failure may have been secondary to the markedly abnormal systemic vascular resistance . . . Oxygenation was profoundly adversely influenced by administration of amniotic fluid containing meconium."[66]

Enigmatic causes of meconium-induced effects

Severely elevated maternal serum bile acids are the major feature of intrahepatic cholestasis of pregnancy and Sepúlveda and his colleagues have found that cholic acid has a dose-dependent vasoconstrictive effect upon human placental chorionic veins.[61] Two facts, however, complicate this seemingly unchallengeable information. According to pharmacologists, bile acids have vasodilator properties, not vasoconstrictive properties.[67] Also, prolonged intravenous infusions of cholic acid into fetal lambs, even at high doses, has not been lethal or severely harmful to the fetuses.[68]

Earlier in this article, in a paragraph about chorioamnionitis, I mentioned chemotaxis and cited de Beaufort et al.[5] The results of that investigation indicate that interleukin-8, in sterile meconium, caused increased migration of neutrophils.[5] In the last 2 years, other publications related to cytokines and proinflammatory factors with meconium may become highly relevant to pharmacologic and physiopathologic actions of sterile meconium.[28,69–71] Certainly, because it is a major cause of perinatal morbidity and mortality, there is a great deal more that we need to learn about meconium.

Nucleated red blood cells

History

In a remarkably comprehensive article, Lippman cited publications which date back to 1876![72] He provided data on the blood of the newborn during the first 48 h after birth, in both absolute and percentage values.[72] Lippman cited Geissler and Japha, and Hayem and Loos, who had written that normoblasts in the blood of newborns are a pathologic finding.[72] In 1934, Ryerson and Sanes directed attention to a histologic method of determining the age of pregnancy early in its development.[73] They wrote that, if all the chorionic corpuscles are nucleated, the pregnancy is probably not older than 2 months.[73] If more than 1% are nucleated, the age is less than 3 months.[73] If fewer than 1% of the red cells are immature, pregnancy has passed beyond 3 months.[73] Ryerson and Sanes stated that the disappearance of erythroblasts takes place rapidly during 2 months and that NRBCs do not occur normally in the newborn or are very rare.[73] In 1939, Javert wrote an article which he titled "The occurrence and significance of nucleated erythrocytes in the fetal vessels of the placenta."[74] His major conclusion was that a diagnosis of prematurity should be considered when there are 10 or more nucleated erythrocytes per 100 white cells. Javert's conclusion implies that it is normal for premature newborns to have that number of NRBCs.[74] His data were entirely expressed as percentage values. (Expressed another way: he did not relate the number of NRBCs to absolute populations of white blood cells.) We now know that the commonest cause of prematurity is reduced uterine blood flow and that erythropoietin then causes an increase of NRBCs. Also, because of the same physiopathology, many newborns whose gestational ages exceed 37 weeks have increased NRBCs. Javert wrote that there is a gradual disappearance of NRBCs within 4 days of birth.[74] (Nowdays, presumably because of more effective therapy, NRBCs often disappear in less than 48 h). More than 60 years ago, Anderson stated that an increase of NRBCs points to pathologic states in the newborn, occurring during the course of delivery.[75] As will become readily apparent later in this review, we now know that an increase of NRBCs occurs prior to delivery. The absence of a placental histopathologic study may have contributed to Anderson's erroneous conclusion.[75] Prior to 1989, I, other pathologists, and probably most clinicians, had been unaware of this historic information.[22,76]

Nucleated red blood cells and placental histopathology

In 1967, Fox investigated the incidence and significance of fetal nucleated erythrocytes in mature placentas. He studied 574 placentas from a variety of cases, including uncomplicated full-term pregnancies, 64 premature deliveries, 50 prolonged but otherwise uncomplicated pregnancies, 159 cases of preeclampsia, 50 pregnancies with maternal essential hypertension, 50 cases of maternal diabetes, and 21 cases of nontoxemic antepartum hemorrhage.[77] Fox found increased nucleated erythrocytes in placentas from babies who had suffered from intrauterine distress, neonatal asphyxia, and fatal intrauterine anoxia.[77] In a study of neonatal asphyxia, placental histopathology was categorized according to whether it probably evolved throughout more than or less than 24 h.[22] After adjustment for influences from many placental histopathologic changes, NRBCs were found to be independently associated with clinical signs of neonatal asphyxia.[22] Maier and colleagues studied umbilical venous erythropoietin and umbilical arterial pH in relation to morphologic placental abnormalities.[78] Acute intervillous circulatory disturbance was diagnosed when premature placental separation or acute intervillous infarction was present; chronic intervillous circulatory disturbance was represented by intervillous and perivillous deposits of fibrin, villous fibrosis, and chronic intervillous infarction. Fetal vasculopathy consisted of fetal thrombi and villous obliterative angiopathy.[78] The investigators found increased erythropoietin with acute villous circulatory disturbance, fetal vasculopathy, and chorioamnionitis. Erythropoietin concentration in umbilical venous blood at birth correlated with the number of circulating NRBCs.[78]

Diagnosis, etiology, and timing of placental NRBCs

Nucleated erythrocytes which are more mature than erythroblasts typically have a smooth nuclear surface and a conspicuously smaller size than that of lymphocytes and mature red blood cells. In hematoxylin and eosin-stained microscopic slides, they have dark nuclei; the ratio of NRBCs to leukocytes is always pathological when it exceeds 2:3. Causes of NRBCs most often are reduced uterine blood flow states and maternal diabetes (which may both be clinically overt or clinically inapparent) and fetal blood loss (as with abruptio placentae, lacerated fetal vasculature, blood group incompatibility, and chronic fetal–maternal transfusion); and, rarely to very rarely, uterine hyper stimulation, severe umbilical cord compression, sepsis, chromosomal abnormality, and bleeding from stress-induced fetal esophagogastric ulceration.[79] Correlations between placental and clinical findings indicate that reduced uterine blood flow states and maternal diabetes are the commonest causes of clinically significant NRBCs.

With histopathologically evident reduced uterine blood flow states and maternal diabetes, high populations of fetal NRBCs do not occur in less than 48 h. Alternatively, with cases of obvious acute intrapartum fetal blood loss, I have seen more than twice the 90th percentile number of neonatal NRBCs (i.e., $>2 \times 10^9$ NRBCs per liter) in laboratory results of specimens collected less than 3 h after delivery. In those cases, the placenta and clinical findings did not include any other explanation for the increased NRBCs.

Mechanisms of increased NRBCs

In uncomplicated pregnancies, Widness and his colleagues found that the duration and intensity of labor are sufficient to cause an increase in the fetal erythropoietin level at delivery.[80] From correlation of placental microscopic findings with medical records (including laboratory results), uncomplicated labor and delivery rarely cause more than 1.5×10^9 NRBCs/l. That estimate is made from instances when known causes of increased NRBCs have occurred in newborns delivered after spontaneous vaginal deliveries. Acute severe asphyxia does not cause massive elevation of NRBCs. This conclusion is made from the personally observed file of a footling breech-delivered asphyxiated newborn, who had umbilical cord about the neck three times, and who also had a positive Coombs test and ABO blood group incompatibility. After the legs and trunk were delivered, the head had remained undelivered for approximately 20 min. Thirty minutes after delivery, the asphyxiated newborn had only 4×10^9 NRBCs/l. (Although that result is very high, it is much less than levels of 15×10^9 NRBCs/l, which I have seen with fetal growth retardation caused by reduced uterine blood flow.)

Clinicopathologic correlations establish that severe acute fetal stress and severe acute fetal blood loss may cause fetal nucleated erythrocytes to increase by 2×10^9 NRBCs/l within 2 h of delivery. This probably results from direct entrance of NRBCs into the circulation, from sites of extramedullary hematopoiesis. In cases of increased fetal NRBCs resultant from reduced uterine blood flow and/or maternal diabetes, erythropoietin-mediated increase of fetal erythrocytes occurs very slowly throughout days and weeks.[81–84] Green and Mimouni wrote an important article about nucleated erythrocytes in healthy infants and in infants of diabetic mothers.[83] They found that, when there is relative leukopenia, divergence from a control group can be inflated by laboratory result expressed per 100 leukocytes, rather than by the absolute population of NRBCs.[83] In their investigated population, the 90th percentile of the control group was 1×10^9 NRBCs/l.

The study of Nicolini and his colleagues included appraisal of fetal hypoxia and acidemia with sequential sonograms, in the prediction of fetal outcome.[82] They found that "the best prediction of perinatal outcome at one test was achieved by the combination of the degree of growth retardation and the nucleated-red-cell count."[82]

Although NRBCs correlate with the amount of hypoxia in the associated fetus, this does not mean that severely increased NRBCs necessarily cause anoxic–ischemic neuronal necrosis and resultant cerebral palsy. That statement is reinforced by Potter's findings in her historic account of Rh disease.[85]

Brief comments on recent articles on nucleated red blood cells

Thilaganathan et al. studied fetuses vaginally delivered at term, fetuses delivered by elective cesarean section, and fetuses delivered by emergency cesarean section.[86] Their findings indicated that, whereas leukocytosis is a nonspecific response of the fetus to labor, erythroblastosis reflects fetal tissue hypoxia.[86]

In 1995, Naeye and Localio reported an investigation of the time before birth when ischemia and hypoxemia initiate cerebral palsy.[87] The study examined NRBCs and lymphocytes in 16 newborns whose hypoxemia and ischemia were acute in 15 of the cases (abruptio placentae 11 cases; hemorrhage two cases; one case with a knot in the umbilical cord and another with cord prolapse[87]). The value of this investigation was limited by the fact that acute blood loss and acute severe stress cause rapid elevation of NRBCs.

Phelan and his colleagues performed at least three investigations in which they considered relationships between fetal NRBCs, fetal asphyxia, and brain injury.[88–90] Their studies increasingly contributed to knowledge of the significance of fetal immature erythrocytes, including the fact that the closer the time interval between asphyxia and birth, the lower the NRBCs.[88] From the vantage point of a pediatric and placental pathologist, three considerations are reasonable:

1. Their afore-mentioned finding was predictable.

2. Inclusion of placental histological findings would probably have revealed 15–20% of cases with more than one cause of elevated immature erythrocytes.
3. Absolute values of NRBCs may have increased the strength of their data.

Similar comments to the three statements in the immediately preceding paragraph are applicable to the articles of Leikin and her colleagues.[91,92] In their first article, they reported that NRBCs are not different in preterm infants with or without intraventricular hemorrhage and periventricular hemorrhage, even when there is control for gestational age and birth weight.[91] One year earlier, however, Green and his colleagues reported an investigation of average-for-gestational-age newborns at 32 weeks' gestational age or less, within the first 6 days of delivery. In prediction of grade III or IV intraventricular hemorrhage, they found that absolute count of NRBCs had a sensitivity of 63% and a specificity of 79%.[93] From a subsequent study, Leikin and her colleagues concluded that histologic chorioamnionitis produces an erythropoietic response in the fetus.[92] Perhaps the fetal erythropoietic response resulted from reduced uterine blood flow. In my experience, most general surgical pathologists are unlikely to recognize subtle light microscopic placental signs of subclinical reduced uterine blood flow.

In 1997, Hanlon-Lundberg and her colleagues attempted to correlate NRBCs in cord blood of singletons with various clinical conditions, including acidemia.[94] Two years later, the same journal published an investigation of NRBCs and acidemia from two of the same authors.[95] Related letters to the editor belatedly appeared in the June 2000 issue of the *American Journal of Obstetrics and Gynecology*. In that same year, a publication of the same authors reported an association of ABO incompatibility with elevation of NRBC counts in term neonates.[96] The investigators acknowledged that ABO blood group incompatibility rarely manifests hydrops fetalis. In Table II of their article,[96] throughout dyads relative to NRBC count, the largest "median" value was 9 (range 0–276). The matching "mean $\pm$ SD" was 22.82 ± 45.81. That data, absence of information of associated white blood cell counts, and absence of report about associated placental findings nullify the potential significance of the investigation.

From recent investigations, infants of smoking mothers were found to have median absolute NRBC counts of 0.5×10^9/l.[97] That result is not significant.[83]

The present review may facilitate the reader's decision as to whether additionally cited articles[98–102] and uncited articles offer anything truly new. My sense is that, if manuscripts continue to have absence of placental pathology, editors might be well advised to reject them.

NRBCs, lymphocytes, and platelets in the timing of fetal asphyxia

Because preterm infants have higher NRBCs than term neonates, authors have stated that elevated NRBCs in preterm infants are normal.[90] Information in the present review establishes that this opinion is erroneous. Prematurity results from pathologic causes. Placental histopathology reveals whether the pathogenesis is chronic or acute or resultant from both mechanisms. Investigators have studied lymphocytes and platelets in the temporal development of fetal brain damage.[87,90,103,104] Naeye and Lin recently acknowledged limitations of lymphocyte and platelet counts as reliable timers of antenatal hypoxic–ischemic fetal brain damage.[103] They itemized five considerations for study in a matrix analysis: (1) the etiology of the hypoxemia and ischemia; (2) the pattern of brain damage; (3) the presence or absence of hypoxic–ischemic damage in other organs; (4) the severity of metabolic-respiratory acidosis at birth; and (5) the time and difficulty in correcting the acidosis. In my opinion, lymphocytes and platelets may be helpful in maximally 15% cases whose affliction is acquired during labor and delivery. Unfortunately, however, clinicians have often not then submitted specimens for laboratory examination.

Closing considerations of the chronology of fetal and neonatal brain injury

Fetal and neonatal brain lesions result from clinicopathologic patterns of antenatal, intrapartum, and

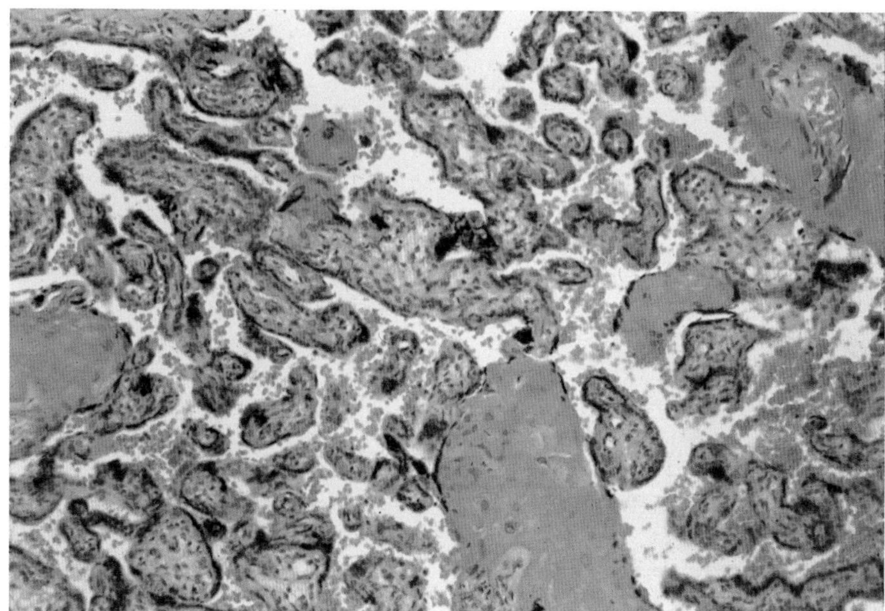

Figure 24.1 Placental ischemic change herein features small dark "syncytial knots" about superficial villous trophoblast and foci of eosinophilic fibrinoid material.

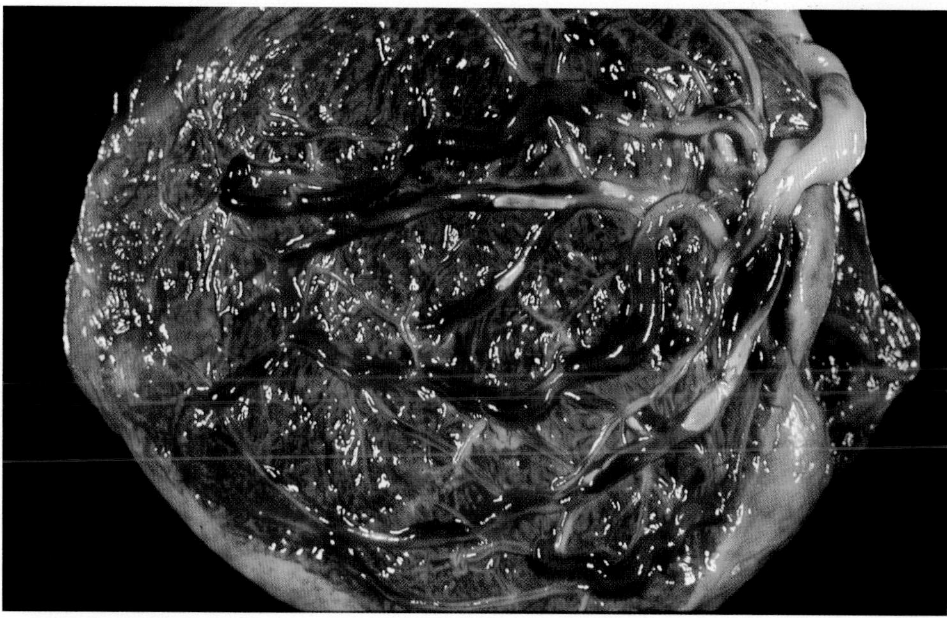

Figure 24.2 Above the central part of this picture, there is an apparent letter "7." That feature results from orange-tan thrombi in fetal plate blood vessels.

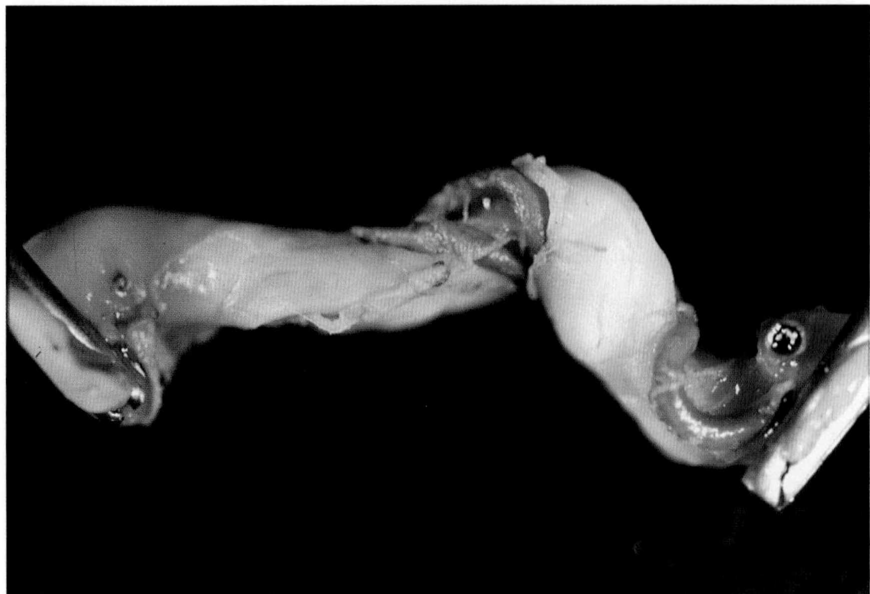

Figure 24.3 At the central part of the specimen and next to the clamp at the right, there are vessels devoid of surrounding Wharton's jelly.

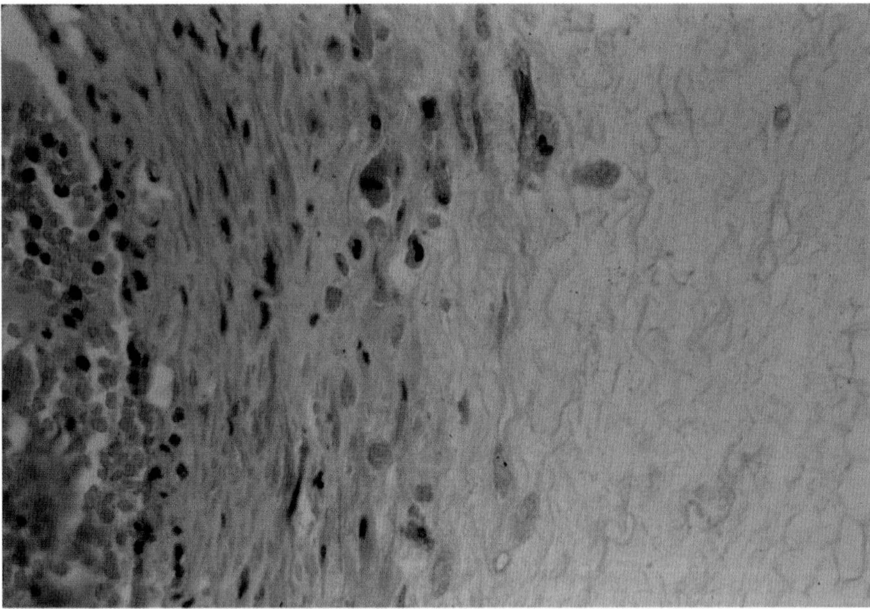

Figure 24.4 Umbilical vascular myocyte necrosis in the umbilical cord of an immature fetus. There are nucleated red blood cells at the far left, olive-brown meconium-laden macrophages at the right, and necrotic myocytes with black nuclei towards the middle and upper parts of the figure.

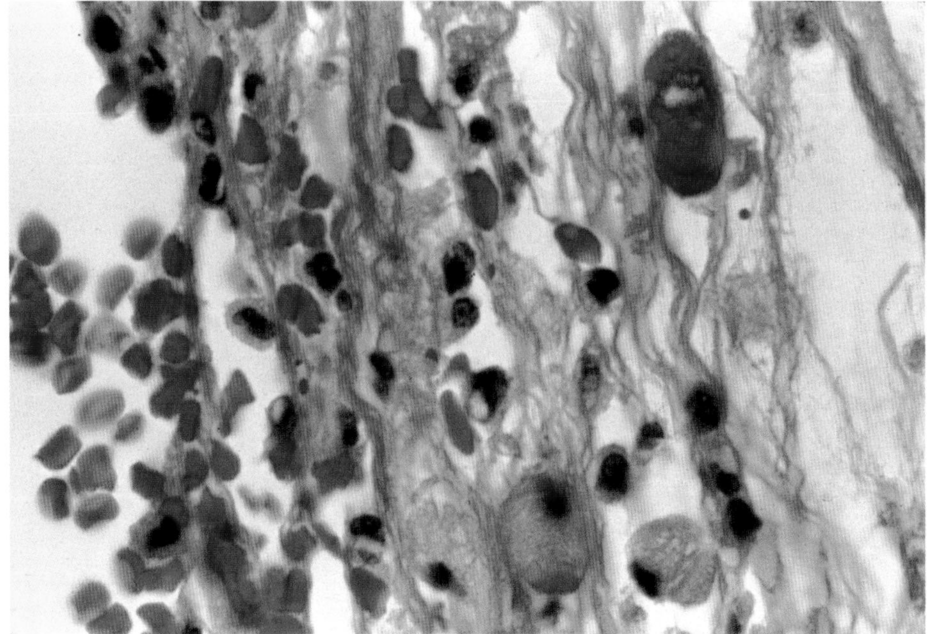

Figure 24.5 Umbilical vascular myocyte necrosis in the umbilical cord of a mature fetus. Meconium-laden macrophages herein have an olive-brown color, in comparison with the reddish-purple necrotic myocyte.

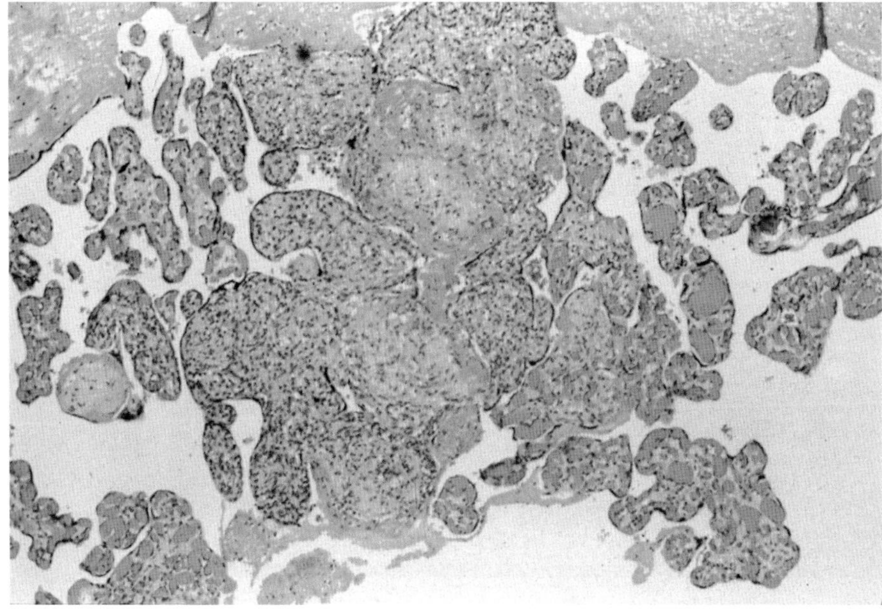

Figure 24.6 Abundant inflammatory cells in fetal villous tissue.

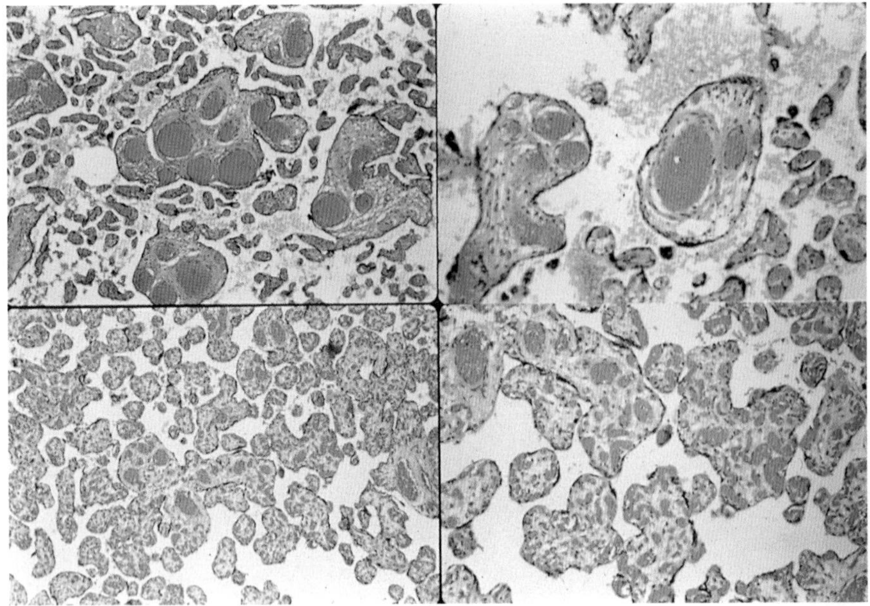

Figure 24.7 In this figure, lower and higher microscopic magnifications are seen, respectively, at the left and right aspects of the four panels. The top two pictures feature congestion and the lower two chorangiosis.

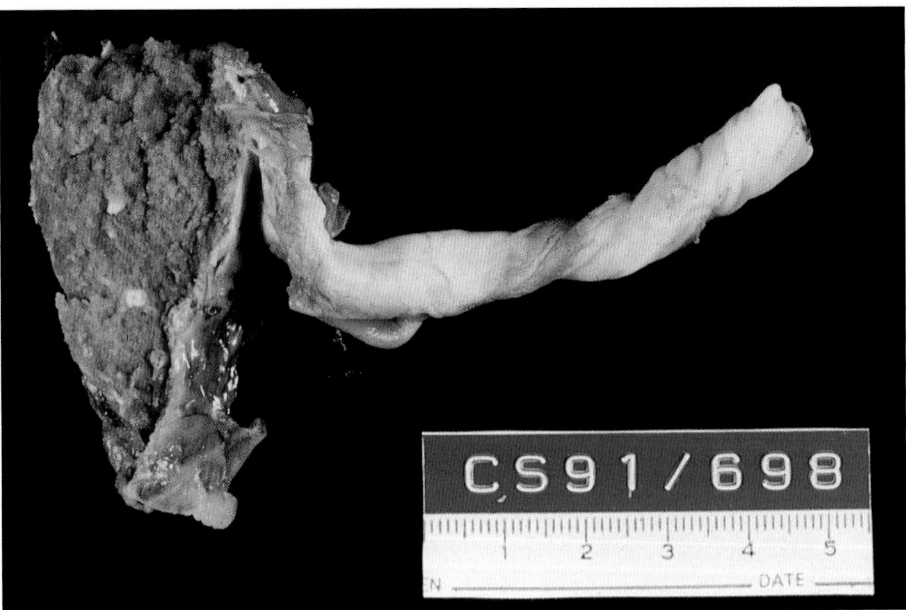

Figure 24.8 Towards the center of the umbilical cord segment seen here, there is olive-green ulceration of the umbilical cord. This resulted from oligohydramnios and cord compression.

postnatal causes. Myers wrote of "four patterns of perinatal brain damage and their conditions of occurrence in primates."[105] These patterns resulted from total asphyxia leading to severe brainstem injury, partial asphyxia leading to brain swelling and cortical injury, partial asphyxia leading to white-matter injury, and partial plus total asphyxia leading to basal ganglia injury.[105] In the context of humans, the placenta, and clinicopathologic correlations, cerebral palsy is classifiable into two pathogenetic patterns. My experience has been that more than 80% of cases involve two or more of: placental histopathologic signs of reduced uterine blood flow, increased fetal NRBCs, signs of acute, chronic, or recurrent fetal exposure to meconium, and chronic VUE. The major clinical profile of this group has been hypoxic–ischemic encephalopathy. Most cases have had abnormal ponderal index or other manifestations of nutritional deprivation. In less than 20% of cases, a normally grown fetus has sustained damage to its brain, kidneys, liver, heart (especially right ventricular papillary muscle), and hematopoietic system. Because of tissue necrosis in those multiple organs, protean laboratory abnormalities ensue. Severely elevated enzymes of the heart and liver are then accompanied by laboratory-evident coagulopathy, low blood glucose, and high creatinine. In my experience, those combined features, plus the need for cardiac pressor agents, are more reliable indicators of intrapartum asphyxia than are low umbilical cord pH and low Apgar scores.

Acknowledgment

Many thanks are expressed to Kurt Benirschke, M.D., for his review of the manuscript. His kindness in that gesture does not imply agreement with the entire content.

REFERENCES

1 Benirschke, K. & Kaufmann, P. (2000). *Pathology of the Human Placenta*, 4th edn, pp. 417–18. New York: Springer.

2 Fox, H. (1997). *Major Problems in Pathology*, vol. 7. *Pathology of the Placenta*, 2nd edn, pp. 168–70. Philadelphia: W.B. Saunders.

3 Kaplan, C., Lowell, D.M. & Salafia, C. (1991). College of American Pathologists Conference XIX on the examination of the placenta: report of the working group on the definition of structural changes associated with abnormal function in the maternal/fetal/placental unit in the second and third trimesters. *Arch. Pathol. Lab. Med.*, **115**, 709–16.

4 Langston, C., Kaplan, C., Macpherson, R. et al. (1997). Practice guideline for examination of the placenta. *Arch. Pathol. Lab. Med.*, **121**, 449–72.

5 de Beaufort, A.J., Pelikan, D.M.V., Elferink, J.G.R. & Berger, H.M. (1998). Effect of interleukin 8 in meconium on in-vitro neutrophil chemotaxis. *Lancet*, **352**, 102–5.

6 Altshuler, G. & Russell,P. (1975). The human placental villitides: a review of chronic intrauterine infection. *Curr. Top. Pathol.*, **60**, 64–112.

7 Altshuler, G. (1999). Placental pathology clues for interdisciplinary clarification of fetal disease. *Trophoblastic Res.*, **13**, 511–25.

8 Altshuler, G. (1984). Chorangiosis. An important placental sign of neonatal morbidity and mortality. *Arch. Pathol. Lab. Med.*, **108**, 71–4.

9 Sander, C.H. (1980). Hemorrhagic endovasculitis and hemorrhagic villitis of the placenta. *Arch. Pathol. Lab. Med.*, **104**, 371–3.

10 Silver, M.M., Yeger, H. & Lines, L.D. (1988). Hemorrhagic endovasculitis-like lesion induced in organ culture. *Hum. Pathol.*, **19**, 251–6.

11 Ornoy, A., Crone, K. & Altshuler, G. (1976). Pathological features of the placenta in fetal death. *Arch. Pathol. Lab. Med.*, **100**, 367–71.

12 The US Department of Health, Education and Welfare Public Health Service, National Institutes of Health. (1972). *The Women and Their Pregnancies. The Collaborative Perinatal Study of the National Institute of Neurological Diseases and Stroke*. Philadelphia: W.B. Saunders.

13 Naeye, R.L. (1992). *Disorders of the Placenta, Fetus, and Neonate: Diagnosis and Clinical Significance*. St. Louis: Mosby Year Book.

14 Williams, M.C., O'Brien, W.F., Nelson, R.N. & Spellacy, W.N. (2000). Histologic chorioamnionitis is associated with fetal growth restriction in term and preterm infants. *Am. J. Obstet. Gynecol.*, **183**, 1094–9.

15 Beebe, L.A., Cowan, L.D. & Altshuler, G. (1996). The epidemiology of placental features: associations with gestational age and neonatal outcome. *Obstet. Gynecol.*, **87**, 771–8.

16 Beebe, L.A., Cowan, L.D., Hyde, S.R. & Altshuler, G. (2000).

Methods to improve the reliability of histopathological diagnoses in the placenta. *Paediatr. Perinat. Epidemiol.*, **14**, 172–8.

17 Bendon, R.W., Faye-Petersen, O., Pavlova, Z. et al. (1999). Fetal membrane histology in preterm premature rupture of membranes: comparison to controls, and between antibiotic and placebo treatment. *Pediatr. Dev. Pathol.*, **2**, 552–8.

18 Khong, T.Y., Staples, A., Moore, L. & Byard, R.W. (1993). Observer reliability in assessing villitis of unknown aetiology. *J. Clin. Pathol.*, **46**, 208–10.

19 Khong, T.Y., Staples, A., Bendon, R.W. et al. (1995). Observer reliability in assessing placental maturity by histology. *J. Clin. Pathol.*, **48**, 420–3.

20 Grether, J.K., Eaton, A., Redline, R. et al. (1999). Reliability of placental histology using archived specimens. *Paediatr. Perinat. Epidemiol.*, **13**, 489–95.

21 Khong, T.Y., Bendon, R.W., Qureshi, F. et al. (2000). Chronic deciduitis in the placental basal plate: definition and interobserver reliability. *Hum. Pathol.*, **31**, 292–5.

22 Altshuler, G. & Herman, A. (1989). The medicolegal imperative: placental pathology and epidemiology. In *Fetal and Neonatal Brain Injury: Mechanisms, Management, and the Risks of Practice*, ed. D.K. Stevenson and P. Sunshine, 1st edn, pp. 250–63. Philadelphia, PA: B.C. Decker.

23 Hansen, A.R., Collins, M.H., Genest, D. et al. (2000). Very low birthweight placenta: clustering of morphologic characteristics. *Pediatr. Dev. Pathol.*, **3**, 431–8.

24 Redline, R.W., Wilson-Costello, D., Borawski, E., Fanaroff, A.A. & Hack, M. (1998). Placental lesions associated with neurologic impairment and cerebral palsy in very low-birth-weight infants. *Arch. Pathol. Lab. Med.*, **122**, 1091–8.

25 Naeye, R.L., Maisels, J., Lorenz, R.P. & Botti, J.J. (1983). The clinical significance of placental villous edema. *Pediatrics*, **71**, 588–94.

26 Shen-Schwarz, S., Ruchelli, E. & Brown, D. (1989). Villous oedema of the placenta: a clinicopathological study. *Placenta*, **10**, 297–307.

27 Redline, R.W. & O'Riordan, M.A. (2000). Placental lesions associated with cerebral palsy and neurologic impairment following term birth. *Arch. Pathol. Lab. Med.*, **124**, 1785–91.

28 Sienko, A. & Altshuler, G. (1999). Meconium-induced umbilical vascular necrosis in abortuses and fetuses: a histopathologic study for cytokines. *Obstet. Gynecol.*, **94**, 415–20.

29 Grafe, M.R. (1994). The correlation of prenatal brain damage with placental pathology. *J. Neuropathol. Exp. Neurol.*, **53**, 407–15.

30 Burke, C.J. & Tannenberg, A.E. (1995). Prenatal brain damage and placental infarction – an autopsy study. *Dev. Med. Child. Neurol.*, **37**, 555–62.

31 Hansen, A.R., Collins, M.H., Genest, D. et al. (2000). Very low birthweight infant's placenta and its relation to pregnancy and fetal characteristics. *Pediatr. Dev. Pathol.*, **3**, 419–30.

32 Arias, F., Rodriquez, L., Rayne, S.C. & Kraus, F.T. (1993). Maternal placental vasculopathy and infection: two distinct subgroups among patients with preterm labor and preterm ruptured membranes. *Am. J. Obstet. Gynecol.*, **168**, 585–91.

33 Naeye, R.L. (1989). Pregnancy hypertension, placental evidences of low uteroplacental blood flow, and spontaneous premature delivery. *Hum. Pathol.*, **20**, 441–4.

34 Nelson, K.B., Dambrosia, J.M., Grether, J.K. & Phillips, T.M. (1998). Neonatal cytokines and coagulation factors in children with cerebral palsy. *Ann. Neurol.*, **44**, 665–75.

35 Grether, J.K., Nelson, K.B., Dambrosia, J.M. & Phillips, T.M. (1999). Interferons and cerebral palsy. *J. Pediatr.*, **134**, 324–32.

36 Conrad, K.P. & Benyo, D.F. (1997). Placental cytokines and the pathogenesis of preeclampsia. *AJRI.* **37**, 240–9.

37 Yoon, B.H., Romero, R., Park, J.S. et al. (2000). Fetal exposure to an intra-amniotic inflammation and the development of cerebral palsy at the age of three years. *Am. J. Obstet. Gynecol.*, **182**, 675–81.

38 Badawi, N., Kurinczuk, J.J., Keogh, J.M., Chambers, H.M. & Stanley, F.J. (2000). Why is the placenta being ignored? *Aust. N.Z. J. Obstet. Gynaecol.*, **40**, 343–6.

39 ACOG Committee Opinion. (1993). *Placental Pathology.* Committee on Obstetrics: Maternal and Fetal Medicine. **125**, (Replaces #102, December 1991).

40 Romero, R., Mazor, M., Morrotti, R. et al. (1992). Infection and labor. VII. Microbial invasion of the amniotic cavity in spontaneous rupture of membranes at term. *Am. J. Obstet. Gynecol.*, **166**, 129–33.

41 Clifford, S.H. (1945). Clinical significance of yellow staining of the vernix caseosa, skin, nails and umbilical cord of the newborn. *Am. J. Dis. Child.*, **69**, 327–8.

42 Katz, V.L. and Bowes W.A. Jr. (1992). Meconium aspiration syndrome: reflections on a murky subject. *Am. J. Obstet. Gynecol.*, **166**, 171–83.

43 Cleary, G.M. & Wiswell, T.E. (1998). Meconium-stained amniotic fluid and the meconium aspiration syndrome. An update. *Pediatr. Clin. North Am.*, **45**, 511–29.

44 Dehan, M., Francoual, J. & Lindenbaum, A. (1978). Short reports. Diagnosis of meconium aspiration by spectrophotometric analysis of urine. *Arch. Dis. Child.*, **53**, 74–87.

45 Molcho, J., Leiberman, J.R., Hagay, Z. & Hagay, Y. (1986).

Spectrophotometric determination of meconium concentration in amniotic fluid. *J. Biomed. Eng.*, **8**, 162–5.

46 Abramovich, D.R. & Gray, E.S. (1982). Physiologic fetal defecation in midpregnancy. *Obstet. Gynecol.*, **60**, 294.

47 Allen, R. (1985). The significance of meconium in midtrimester genetic amniocentesis. *Am. J. Obstet. Gynecol.*, **152**, 413–17.

48 Kowalewska-Kantecka, B. (1995). Motilin in umbilical blood. *Roczniki Akademii Medycznej w Bialymstoku*, **40**, 662–6.

49 Manning, F.A., Schreiber, J. & Turkel, S.B. (1978). Fatal meconium aspiration "in utero": a case report. *Am. J. Obstet. Gynecol.*, **132**, 111–13.

50 Byrne, D.L. & Gau, G. (1987). In utero meconium aspiration: an unpreventable cause of neonatal death. *Br. J. Obstet. Gynaecol.*, **94**, 813–14.

51 Sunoo, C., Kosasa, T.S. & Hale, R.W. (1989). Meconium aspiration syndrome without evidence of fetal distress in early labor before elective cesarean delivery. *Obstet. Gynecol.*, **73**, 707–9.

52 Falciglia, H.S., Kosmetatos, N., Brady, K. & Wesseler, T.A. (1993). Intrauterine meconium aspiration in extremely premature infant. *Am. J. Dis. Child*, **147**, 1035–7.

53 Burgess, A.M. & Hutchins, G.M. (1996). Inflammation of the lungs, umbilical cord and placenta associated with meconium passage in utero. Review of 123 autopsied cases. *Pathol. Res. Pract.*, **192**, 1121–8.

54 Lauweryns, J., Bernat, R., Lerut, A. & Detournay, G. (1973). Intrauterine pneumonia. An experimental study. *Biol. Neonate*, **22**, 301–18.

55 Jovanovic, R. and Nguyen, V. (1989). Experimental meconium aspiration in guinea pigs. *Obstet. Gynecol.*, **73**, 652–6.

56 Tyler, D.C., Murphy, J. & Cheney, F.W. (1978). Mechanical and chemical damage to lung tissue caused by meconium aspiration. *Pediatrics*, **62**, 454–9.

57 Kearney, M.S. (1999). Chronic intrauterine meconium aspiration causes fetal lung infarcts, lung rupture, and meconium embolism. *Pediatr. Dev. Pathol.*, **2**, 544–51.

58 Altshuler, G., Arizawa, M. and Molnar-Nadasdy, G. (1992). Meconium-induced umbilical cord vascular necrosis and ulceration: a potential link between the placenta and poor pregnancy outcome. *Obstet. Gynecol.*, **79**, 760–6.

59 Kearney, M.S. & Mortensen, E. (2000). Intrauterine meconium aspiration in the second-trimester fetus. *Pediat. Dev. Pathol. Abstract from the 45th Annual Meeting of the Paediatric Pathology Society, Belfast, UK, September 9–11, 1999*, **3**, 395.

60 Altshuler, G. & Hyde, S. (1989). Meconium-induced vasocontraction: a potential cause of cerebral and other fetal hypoperfusion and of poor pregnancy outcome. *J. Child. Neurol.*, **4**, 137–42.

61 Sepúlveda, W.H., Gonzalez, C., Cruz, M.A. & Rudolph, M.I. (1991). Vasoconstrictive effect of bile acids on isolated human placental chorionic veins. *Eur. J. Obstet. Gynecol. Reprod. Biol.*, **42**, 211–15.

62 Montgomery, L.D., Belfort, M.A., Saade, G.R., Moise, K.J. Jr & Vedernikov, Y.P. (1995). Meconium inhibits the contraction of umbilical vessels induced by the thromboxane A_2 analog U46619. *Am. J. Obstet. Gynecol.*, **173**, 1075–8.

63 Hyde, S. & Altshuler, G. (1996). Need for placental and experimental pathologic examination to determine pathogenetic influences of chronically present intraamniotic meconium. *Am. J. Obstet. Gynecol.*, **174**, 1669–70.

64 Holcberg, G., Huleihel, M., Katz, M. et al. (1999). Vasoconstrictive activity of meconium stained amniotic fluid in the human placental vasculature. *Eur. J. Obstet. Gynecol. Reprod. Biol.*, **87**, 147–50.

65 Holopainen, R., Soukka, H., Halkola, L. & Kaapa, P. (1998). Meconium aspiration induces a concentration-dependent pulmonary hypertensive response in newborn piglets. *Pediatr. Pulmonol.*, **25**, 107–13.

66 Hankins, G.D.V., Snyder, R.R., Clark, S.L. et al. (1993). Acute hemodynamic and respiratory effects of amniotic fluid embolism in the pregnant goat model. *Am. J. Obstet. Gynecol.*, **168**, 1113–30.

67 Bomzon, A. & Ljubuncic, P. (1995). Commentary: bile acids as endogenous vasodilators? *Biochem. Pharmacol.*, **49**, 581–9.

68 Campos, G.A., Guerra, F.A. & Israel, E.J. (1986). Effects of cholic acid infusion in fetal lambs. *Acta. Obstet. Gynecol. Scand.*, **65**, 23–6.

69 Lally, K.P., Mehall, J.R., Xue, H. & Thompson, J. (1999). Meconium stimulates a pro-inflammatory response in peritoneal macrophages: implications for meconium peritonitis. *J. Pediatr. Surg.*, **34**, 214–17.

70 Yamada, T., Minakami, H., Matsubara, S. et al. (2000). Meconium-stained amniotic fluid exhibits chemotactic activity for polymorphonuclear leukocytes in vitro. *J. Reprod. Immunol.*, **46**, 21–30.

71 Yamada, T., Matsubara, S., Minakami, H. et al. (2000). Chemotactic activity for polymorphonuclear leukocytes: meconium versus meconium-stained amniotic fluid. *Am. J. Reprod. Immunol.*, **44**, 275–8.

72 Lippman, H.S. (1924). A morphologic and quantitative study of the blood corpuscles in the new-born period. *Am. J. Dis. Child.*, **27**, 473–526.

73 Ryerson, C.S. & Sanes, S. (1934). The age of pregnancy. Histologic diagnosis from percentage of erythroblasts in chorionic capillaries. *Arch. Pathol.* **17**, 648–51.

74 Javert, C.T. (1939). The occurrence and significance of nucleated erythrocytes in the fetal vessels of the placenta. *Am. J. Obstet. Gynecol.*, **37**, 184–94.

75 Anderson, G.W. (1941). Studies on the nucleated red cell count in the chorionic capillaries and the cord blood of various ages of pregnancy. *Am. J. Obstet. Gynecol.*, **42**, 1–14.

76 Salafia, C.M., Weigl, C.A. & Foye, G.J. (1988). Correlation of placental erythrocyte morphology and gestational age. *Pediatr. Pathol.*, **8**, 495–502.

77 Fox, H. (1967). The incidence and significance of nucleated erythrocytes in the foetal vessels of the mature human placenta. *J. Obstet. Gynaecol. Br. Commonwlth*, **74**, 40–3.

78 Maier, R.F., Gunther, A., Vogel, M., Dudenhausen, J.W. & Obladen, M. (1994). Umbilical venous erythropoietin and umbilical arterial pH in relation to morphologic placental abnormalities. *Obstet. Gynecol.*, **84**, 81–7.

79 Agarwal, A.K., Saili, A., Pandey, K.K. et al. (1990). Role of cimetidine in prevention and treatment of stress induced gastric bleeding in neonates. *Indian Pediatr.*, **27**, 465–9.

80 Widness, J.A., Clemons, G.K., Garcia, J.F., Oh, W. & Schwartz, R. (1984). Increased immunoreactive erythropoietin in cord serum after labor. *Am. J. Obstet. Gynecol.*, **148**, 194–7.

81 Philip, A.G.S. & Tito, A.M. (1989). Increased nucleated red blood cell counts in small for gestational age infants with very low birth weight. *Am. J. Dis. Child.*, **143**, 164–9.

82 Nicolini, U., Nicolaidis, P., Fisk, N.M. et al. (1990). Limited role of fetal blood sampling in prediction of outcome in intrauterine growth retardation. *Lancet*, **336**, 768–72.

83 Green, D.W. & Mimouni, F. (1990). Nucleated erythrocytes in healthy infants and in infants of diabetic mothers. *J. Pediatr.*, **116**, 129–31.

84 Salvesen, D.R., Brudenell, J.M., Snijders, R.J.M., Ireland, R.M. & Nicolaides, K.H. (1993). Fetal plasma erythropoietin in pregnancies complicated by maternal diabetes mellitus. *Am. J. Obstet. Gynecol.*, **168**, 88–94.

85 Potter, E.L. (1947). *Rh . . . Its Relation to Congenital Hemolytic Disease & to Intragroup Transfusion Reactions.* Chicago: Year Book.

86 Thilaganathan, B., Athanasiou, S., Ozmen, S. et al. (1994). Umbilical cord blood erythroblast count as an index of intrauterine hypoxia. *Arch. Dis. Child.*, **70**, F192–4.

87 Naeye, R.L. & Localio, A.R. (1995). Determining the time before birth when ischemia and hypoxemia initiated cerebral palsy. *Obstet. Gynecol.*, **86**, 713–19.

88 Phelan, J.P., Ahn, M.O., Korst, L.M. & Martin, G.I. (1995). Nucleated red blood cells: a marker for fetal asphyxia? *Am. J. Obstet. Gynecol.*, **173**, 1380–4.

89 Korst, L.M., Phelan, J.P., Ahn, M.O. & Martin, G.I. (1996). Nucleated red blood cells: an update on the marker for fetal asphyxia. *Am. J. Obstet. Gynecol.*, **175**, 843–6.

90 Phelan, J.P., Korst, L.M., Ahn, M.O. & Martin, G.I. (1998). Neonatal nucleated red blood cell and lymphocyte counts in fetal brain injury. *Obstet. Gynecol.*, **91**, 485–9.

91 Leikin, E., Verma, U., Klein, S. & Tejani, N. (1996). Relationship between neonatal nucleated red blood cell counts and hypoxic–ischemic injury. *Obstet. Gynecol.*, **87**, 439–43.

92 Leikin, E., Garry, D., Visintainer, P., Verma, U. & Tejani, N. (1997). Correlation of neonatal nucleated red blood cell counts in preterm infants with histologic chorioamnionitis. *Am. J. Obstet. Gynecol.*, **177**, 27–30.

93 Green, D.W., Hendon, B. & Mimouni, F.B. (1995). Nucleated erythrocytes and intraventricular hemorrhage in preterm neonates. *Pediatrics*, **96**, 475–8.

94 Hanlon-Lundberg, K.M., Kirby, R.S., Gandhi, S. & Broekhuizen, F.F. (1997). Nucleated red blood cells in cord blood of singleton term neonates. *Am. J. Obstet. Gynecol.*, **176**, 1149–56.

95 Hanlon-Lundberg, K.M. & Kirby, R.S. (1999). Nucleated red blood cells as a marker of acidemia in term neonates. *Am. J. Obstet. Gynecol.*, **181**, 196–201.

96 Hanlon-Lundberg, K.M. & Kirby, R.S. (2000). Association of ABO incompatibility with elevation of nucleated red blood cell counts in term neonates. *Am. J. Obstet. Gynecol.*, **183**, 1532–6.

97 Yeruchimovich, M., Dollberg, S., Green, D.W. & Mimouni, F. (1999). Nucleated red blood cells in infants of smoking mothers. *Obstet. Gynecol.*, **93**, 403–6.

98 Buonocore, G., Perrone, S., Gioia, D. et al. (1999). Nucleated red blood cell count at birth as an index of perinatal brain damage. *Am. J. Obstet. Gynecol.*, **181**, 1500–5.

99 Blackwell, S.C., Refuerzo, J.S., Wolfe, H.M. et al. (2000). The relationship between nucleated red blood cell counts and early-onset neonatal seizures. *Am. J. Obstet. Gynecol.*, **182**, 1452–7.

100 Minior, V.K., Bernstein, P.S. & Divon, M.Y. (2000). Nucleated red blood cells in growth-restricted fetuses: associations with short-term neonatal outcome. *Fetal Diagn. Ther.*, **15**, 165–9.

101 Minior, V.K., Shatzkin, E. & Divon, M.Y. (2000). Nucleated red blood cell count in the differentiation of fetuses with pathologic growth restriction from healthy small-for-gestational-age fetuses. *Am. J. Obstet. Gynecol.*, **182**, 1107–9.

102 Lim, F.T.H., Scherjon, S.A., van Beckhoven, J.M. et al. (2000). Association of stress during delivery with increased numbers

of nucleated cells and hematopoietic progenitor cells in umbilical cord blood. *Am. J. Obstet. Gynecol.*, **183**, 1144–51.

103 Naeye, R. & Lin, H-M. (2001). Determination of the timing of fetal brain damage from hypoxemia–ischemia. *Am. J. Obstet. Gynecol.*, **184**, 217–24.

104 Korst, L.M., Phelan, J.P., Wang, Y.M. & Ahn, M.O. (1999). Neonatal platelet counts in fetal brain injury. *Am. J. Perinatol.*, **16**, 79–83.

105 Myers, R.E. (1975). Four patterns of perinatal brain damage and their conditions of occurrence in primates. In *Advances in Neurology*, ed. B.S. Meldrum and C.D. Marsden. vol. 10, pp. 223–234. New York: Raven Press.

25

Correlations of clinical, laboratory, imaging and placental findings as to the timing of asphyxial events

Philip Sunshine, David K. Stevenson, and William E. Benitz

Stanford University Medical Center, Palo Alto, CA, USA

Following the birth of a depressed newborn, the infant's caretakers are involved in providing appropriate resuscitative techniques, stabilizing the infant's biochemical and physiological abnormalities, and evaluating the infant's response to these measures. The caretakers must also ascertain the cause of the infant's depression, attempt to determine when the event or events leading to the depression occurred, and develop a plan for follow-up evaluation and treatment that will be required. The determination of causation and timing not only has medical–legal implications, but is becoming extremely important in order to evaluate the types of therapy that may be utilized to mitigate the effects of a hypoxic–ischemic event. If the infant had suffered significant damage days or weeks prior to birth, then these rescue forms of therapy will have little, if any, beneficial effect on the infant's eventual outcome. In many situations, this determination is very difficult to make as there may be a myriad of events that could have occurred prior to the time of birth, and overlapping of significant problems makes this exercise an almost impossible task at times.

When an acute or sentinel event has taken place, such as a readily recognized prolapsed cord, an abruptio placentae, a ruptured uterus, or a disorder leading to acute and profound blood loss in the fetus, the timing of the event can be ascertained with a reasonable degree of accuracy. However, even in these circumstances, the time frame may not be known with certainty, especially if the process has been developing over a period of time. Often, the area of damage to the central nervous system can be found to correlate with this acute event, as it tends to involve the thalamus and the basal ganglia.[1,2] At times, when there is an occult prolapse of the cord, or if the infant is profoundly affected when the mother suffers from an amniotic fluid embolus that has an unusual form of presentation, the timing of an acute event cannot be made with precision.

There may also be overlapping of events leading to the infant's problems. Data from laboratory animals have demonstrated that even brief repeated episodes of cord occlusion can not only predispose the fetus to cerebral injury but can also lead to compromise of the cardiovascular system.[3–6] Thus, a fetus with intrauterine compromise may not be able to withstand the stresses of labor, and develop what would appear to be an acute catastrophic bradycardic episode and complicate an already preexisting neurological injury.

In addition, many infants who are depressed at birth or who are later found to have suffered neurological or intellectual impairment may have few, if any, indicators as to the cause, severity, or timing of the injury. Because we have limited capabilities of evaluating the neurological well-being of the fetus during the labor process, we use indirect indicators that may be of help in ascertaining the sequence of events leading to the birth of a depressed infant.

Table 25.1. Template for timing of neonatal brain injury

Maternal history of fetal activity
Use of biophysical profile
Fetal heart rate monitoring
Presence of meconium
Neonatal neurological examination
Electroencephalogram
Imaging studies
Ultrasound
CT scan
MRI
Laboratory studies
Cord blood gases and initial postnatal blood gases
Hematological studies
Biochemical evaluations
Examination of the placenta
Neuropathological evaluations
Follow-up evaluations of clinical and laboratory parameters

Notes:
CT, computed tomography; MRI, magnetic resonance imaging.

Many of these indicators are encountered in perfectly normal newborns, and the specificity and sensitivity of these findings are often inconclusive. Despite these shortcomings, neonatologists, perinatologists, pediatric neurologists, neuroradiologists, and pathologists are asked to perform retrospective analyses of data collected on the mother, the placenta, and the fetus in an attempt to create a reasonable theory as to the timing and severity of events leading to the infant's problems.[7]

The approach to such an exercise is outlined in Table 25.1, and can be used as a template for determining the timing. Realizing that many clinical signs may be subjective, one often has to evaluate numerous clues to determine the sequence of events that were involved. In most situations, timing of an injurious event can only be placed within broad periods such as during fetal development, the prelabor period, the intrapartum period, or the postpartum (neonatal) period.

Prepartum evaluation

Currently, most women with high-risk obstetrical problems are readily identified and have frequent and intensive monitoring of their pregnancies. With careful screening that is currently in place in obstetrical practices, many of these women are identified even prior to their pregnancies or in the early part of their gestation. The approach to antepartum evaluation is clearly delineated in Chapter 10. Also when a low-risk mother develops risk factors during her pregnancy, such as glucose intolerance, preeclampsia, decreased intrauterine growth, hydramnios, or postdatism, then, she too, will be evaluated more intensely and more frequently.[8] Women with a low-risk status will not have these evaluations and thus subjective signs to alert her caretakers to potential problems become important. The fetus who develops a marked increase in activity, such as writhing movements that do not stop, or as some women describe these, "as if the baby wanted to jump out of the uterus," may be an important sign of a fetus in distress.[9] This is especially true if the writhing movements are followed by a period of fetal inactivity. Similarly, the fetus that had been active and either gradually or suddenly stops moving is another important sign that may be helpful in the timing of an untoward event.[9,10] Since such findings are found in fetuses with perfectly normal outcomes, they may not be brought to the physician's attention or are regarded as variations of a normal pregnancy. Retrospective analyses of these findings may be helpful in determining the timing of the fetal injury. Similarly, the sudden onset of hydramnios may also be an important sign of fetal compromise.

Recognition of an acute event such as severe abdominal pain, sudden onset of cardiopulmonary insufficiency or arrest in the mother, or acute blood loss associated with vasa previa, abruptio placentae, or placenta previa can also be used to time the onset of an asphyxial event.

Fetal heart rate monitoring

The specifics of fetal heart rate monitoring are delineated in Chapter 11 and will not be covered here. However, Shields and Schifrin[11] and Phelan and Ahn[12] have identified an abnormal fetal heart rate pattern that is fixed and nonreactive that is highly suggestive of a neurological injury that occurred prior to the time that labor began. As early as 1985, Van der Moer et al. described a fixed fetal heart rate pattern with normal frequency and without decelerations and accelerations in a fetus who had suffered significant intrauterine brain damage 14 days prior to the time the mother went into labor.[13] Menticoglou and coworkers described two full-term infants with similar courses.[14] Schifrin et al. termed this as a "pattern of autonomic imbalance".[15] Phelan and Kim described this pattern in 45% of a population of 300 brain-damaged infants, and found it to be associated with a reduction in fetal activity, evidence of meconium-stained skin, and meconium aspiration syndrome.[16] When this heart rate pattern is found on the mother's admission to the labor unit and does not change, they suggest that this is consistent with a "static encephalopathy that antedated the patient's arrival to the hospital."

If a woman is admitted, is found to have a reactive fetal heart rate pattern, and then has a sudden and prolonged episode of fetal bradycardia, then an acute and catastrophic event is most likely occurring.

Other abnormalities that occur during labor, such as decelerations, tachycardias, and their relationship to fetal injury, are discussed in Chapter 11. Such abnormalities would suggest that, if the fetus is damaged, this damage occurred during the intrapartum period, especially if associated with significant fetal metabolic acidosis.[17] However, the sensitivities and specificities of the abnormalities to predict an adverse outcome are low.[18–22] The interpretations of these tracings vary from individual to individual and are greatly influenced by the interpreter's knowledge of the neonate's outcome.[23] It has always been a source of amazement to find "experts" point to a specific time on a fetal heart rate tracing and indicate that at that particular moment the fetus began to suffer intrauterine asphyxia, and had the infant been delivered within an appropriate time interval therein, the infant would have most likely been "perfectly normal." While there may be such occurrences, the use of the tracing to identify precise moments of injury to the fetus is speculative at best. While the use of electronic fetal heart rate monitoring has resulted in a decrease in intrauterine deaths, it has not resulted in a decrease in the incidence of cerebral palsy and/or mental retardation.

Meconium-stained amniotic fluid

This subject is discussed at length in Chapter 31 by Dr. Wiswell and to some extent in Chapter 24 by Dr. Altshuler. Infants who pass meconium in utero have a greater incidence of respiratory problems than those who do not, and also have a greater incidence of neurological sequelae.[24,25] Because meconium-stained amniotic fluid is encountered in a large number of deliveries and may be as frequent as 30–40% in postdates pregnancies, the association with neurological handicaps is enhanced when other factors, such as neonatal depression, acidemia, and low Apgar scores, are also present.

S.H. Clifford was one of the first to note an association of yellow staining of the vernix caseosa, skin, nails, and umbilical cord with an increased rate of neonatal morbidity and mortality.[26] He suggested that the "yellow vernix syndrome" was the result of an episode of fetal asphyxia occurring days to weeks prior to the onset of labor. Similar observations have been made by Phelan and Kim in patients who had persistently nonreactive fetal heart rate patterns, reduced fetal activity, and passage of "old meconium" at the time the membranes were ruptured.[16]

Sienko and Altshuler have demonstrated that meconium itself has vasoconstrictive properties when it is present in amniotic fluid for a period of time,[27] and those observations have been substantiated to some degree by Naeye.[28] The length of time that meconium has been present can be ascertained by evaluating the consistency of the meconium, which tends to be thick and tenacious when passed close to the time of delivery, and is thin with particulate matter when passed hours to days previously.[29] However, the infant may have had several episodes of meconium passage, and thus the timing of neurological injury to that of meconium passage is often difficult to make.

Seizures

Seizures associated with hypoxic–ischemic encephalopathy are associated with an adverse prognostic significance, and increase the risk of neurological sequelae two to five times as compared to those infants without seizures.[30] In most situations, the onset of these seizures is within the first 12 h of life, and they are often refractory to anticonvulsant therapy. The earlier the onset of seizures, usually the worse the outcome.[30] However, neither the time of the onset nor the severity of the seizures has been correlated with the timing of the event that led to the neurological insult affecting the fetus.[31] In some situations, the seizures may have occurred in utero and have not been fully recognized by either the mother or the physician. Such seizures have been reported in asphyxiated fetal lambs and have resulted in increased heart rate variability in the brain-damaged animal.[32]

Electroencephalogram

This aspect of evaluation is discussed in Chapter 21 by Dr. Olson. The electroencephalogram (EEG) is useful in identifying seizures in the neonatal period and is often helpful in determining the severity of the encephalopathy. Takeuchi and Watanabe have described a series of changes that occur in the EEG of asphyxiated term infants which initially demonstrate varying degrees of isoelectric or burst-suppression patterns, and which are often followed by increased degrees of discontinuity.[33] In the chronic stages, signs of dysmature and disorganized patterns evolve. There is also a sequence of evolution in the background of the EEG in infants with asphyxia that could also be used to time the injury. It would require that the EEG be evaluated very soon after birth and that frequent follow-up studies be performed to evaluate the progress of the patient, the response to antiepileptic medications, if required, and the evolution of the EEG pattern. Similar studies have also been reported in preterm infants by these authors.[34]

Using amplitude integrated EEGs, Toet and coworkers were able to evaluate infants with encephalopathy within 3 and 6 h after birth and to identify infants who had severe encephalopathic findings that could possibly benefit from interventional therapy as well as those who had mild changes and would not require such treatment.[35]

Laboratory findings

Lymphocytes and platelets

Hematological abnormalities have been used with increasing frequency to time the injury in affected newborns. Naeye and coworkers have utilized lymphocyte counts and nucleated red blood cell counts to determine the timing of neurological injury.[36,37] These authors have noted that lymphocyte counts increase to levels of greater than 10 000/mm^3 within 2 h of the initiation of the injurious event and return to normal within 14–18 h even if the hypoxic–ischemic event continues. In the more recent study, Naeye and Lin also showed that if cardiovascular or renal dysfunction was associated with the hypoxic event, the platelet count decreased by 30% at about 30 h and 50% by 60 h after the event causing hypoxic–ischemic encephalopathy occurred.[37] The use of this low value was especially helpful when an acute intrapartum event occurred. If the event was greater than 24 h prior to birth, the lymphocyte count was not elevated.

Nucleated red blood cell count (see Chapter 24)

We have found that elevation of normoblasts or nucleated red blood cells is of great help in identifying those infants who have evidence of intrauterine hypoxia that has been present for a period of time.[38–42] In most situations, if there has been sufficient in utero hypoxia, there is a stimulus to produce erythropoietin and increase the number of these cells. Based on data from laboratory animals and from human neonates, it has been suggested that it requires at least 48 h for erythropoietin to increase the number of nucleated red blood cells in the circulation. Thus, the finding of a markedly elevated nucleated red blood cell count would be indicative of problems that had been present for at least 48 h, although the exact duration of insult is often unknown.

Exceptions to this rule include the fetal or neonatal response to an acute hypovolemic event such as bleeding from the vasa previa or bleeding from an abruptio placentae, where the outpouring of nucleated red blood cells can occur in a matter of hours.[37,39] For a period of time it was thought that this type of response was due to the fetal response of "splenic contraction" and elaboration of immature cells. Studies by Calhoun et al. have shown that active hematopoiesis is not present in the spleen of the midgestation of the human fetus.[43] Thus, it is conceivable that the nucleated red blood cells in circulation, most likely from the liver or the bone marrow, are in response to a hypovolemic stimulus.

While it is usual to denote the elevation of nucleated red blood cells expressed per 100 white blood cells, we prefer to use the total number per cubic millimeter, as one might not appreciate an elevated count in those situations where there is also a leukocytic response as well. Thus, a number greater than 1500 nucleated red blood cells/mm^3 is abnormal, even in prematurely born infants.[44,45] Also, the more severe the hypoxic episode that is present, the longer the period of time that the nucleated red blood cell count remains elevated.[41] Table 25.2 lists the most frequent causes of elevated nucleated red blood cells in the circulatory blood volume of neonates.[39–46]

Table 25.2. Causes of elevated nucleated red blood cell counts[38–46]

Chronic intrauterine hypoxia
Prematurity – especially those with IVH
Hemolytic anemia
Rh incompatibility
ABO incompatibility
Homozygous α thalessemia
Chronic intrauterine anemia
Fetal–maternal bleeding
Twin-to-twin transfusion
Infants of poorly controlled diabetic mothers
Infants with intrauterine growth restriction
Infants of smoking mothers (mildly elevated)
Infants delivered associated with acute blood loss
Placenta abruptio
Vasa previa
Infants with diaphragmatic hernias
Severe placental insufficiency
Recurrent episodes of cord compression
Congenital infections (especially CMV)

Notes:
IVH, intraventricular hemorrhage; CMV, cytomegalovirus.

Biochemical markers of asphyxia

A list of laboratory studies that have been measured to assess the severity of hypoxemic–ischemic encephalopathy is found in Chapter 1 of this text and noted in Volpe's *Neurology of the Newborn* as well.[30] When these laboratory studies are markedly abnormal, there is good correlation with the severity of the asphyxic episode. Unfortunately, most of these assays are not readily available in many clinical laboratories, and samples have to be sent to specific centers in order to have them assayed. Most laboratories can measure ammonia in blood, and creatine phosphokinase (CPK) and lactate in serum. Even the measurement of brain-specific isozyme of CPK (CPK-BB) may not be available in many clinical laboratories. If CPK is to be utilized, it should be measured soon after birth and followed with frequent assays as it tends to rise and fall rapidly over a 1–2-day period.[47] In a recent study, Nagdyman and coworkers demonstrated that CPK-BB was found to be elevated at 2 h after birth in infants with moderate or severe hypoxic–ischemic encephalopathy and remained elevated for 12 h.[48]

Measurement of CPK-BB in cerebrospinal fluid may be an even better method of detecting asphyxial injury and abnormalities of this assay seems to correlate better with the severity of short-term outcome following an asphyxial event.[49] Again, this assay is not available in most clinical laboratories. Thus, an infant who is depressed at birth and is found to have a normal or minimally elevated CPK suggests that either the injury to the infant was mild or that it had occurred days prior to the intrapartum period.

The measurements of other parameters evaluating damage to other organs in an infant with asphyxia should also be elevated unless the asphyxic event was acute and there may not have been signs of multiorgan failure. If the infant has suffered from intrauterine damage, elevation of the liver enzymes aspartate aminotransferase (AST) and alanine aminotransferase (ALT) should be found.

These enzymes as well as lactic dehydrogenase (LDH) have been evaluated primarily in adults following myocardial infarction. There is a temporal pattern of enzyme release, with the ALT and AST rising and falling rapidly over a 2–3-day period. The LDH rises slowly during the first day after injury, peaking at 3–4 days and returning to normal levels in 14 days.[50] Such temporal data are not available for liver damage associated with acute hypoxic–ischemic injury in the newborn and thus often do not have the specificity to aid in the timing of the asphyxial event.

The serum creatinine will also increase over the first 1–2 days of life and remain elevated until renal function improves. The infant's initial serum creatinine measured soon after birth tends to parallel that of the mother's and then will increase if there has been significant renal involvement. If the infant's serum creatinine is found to be elevated soon after birth, is higher than the mother's level, and then begins to decrease, the injury to the infant most likely occurred days prior to the time the infant was born. Also the length of time that the creatinine remains elevated is often, but not always, correlative with the severity of the asphyxial episode.

Other markers of renal involvement include hematuria, proteinuria, and elevated urinary β_2-microglobulin.[51]

Although hypoglycemia can be encountered in infants following an asphyxial event and its finding should be anticipated as glycogen stores may be depleted, its onset and severity have not been useful in determining the timing of an adverse event.

Newborn neurological evaluations

This is discussed in Chapter 20 and the various stages of postasphyxial encephalopathy are described. It is also noted that some, but not all, infants may pass from one stage to another with overlapping findings. Infants who are found to have arthrogryposis have most likely developed this weeks to months prior to birth and this has nothing to do with intrapartum difficulties. Significantly increased tone encountered in the newborn period should suggest other diagnoses such as stiff-body syndrome, myotonia congenita, or infants born to mothers who abuse cocaine.

The infant who has marked hypotonia and without other findings of asphyxia should be evaluated for syndromes such as Prader–Willi syndrome, Zellweger's syndrome, Miller–Dieker syndrome, fragile X syndrome, myotonic dystrophy, and even congenital myasthenia gravis.

The infant with significant cerebral edema will have a full or bulging fontanel, spreading of the cranial sutures, and an enlarging head circumference (see Chapter 20). In most situations cerebral edema is not a prominent feature of hypoxic–ischemic encephalopathy in full-term infants.[52] If it is present, it usually requires 18–24 h to become recognizable clinically, and reaches a maximum pressure at 36–72 h after the cerebral insult.[52] Therefore, if an infant is born with cerebral edema already clinically evident, it would suggest that the damage had occurred at least 18 h previously.

It is also extremely important to evaluate intrauterine growth patterns of depressed newborns and identify those infants with asymmetric growth patterns. In most asymmetrically growth-restricted infants, the head growth is usually protected compared to the infant's weight and length. Thus, if an infant is born with decreased head growth compared to the infant's weight and especially the length, and has neonatal depression or is later found to have cerebral palsy, an adverse intrauterine event long before the onset of labor can be surmised.

Imaging studies

Blankenberg and Barnes describe neuroimaging techniques and studies in Chapter 22. The ultrasound examination can be used readily in the neonatal period without having to move the infant, and provides important screening information regarding gross structural anomalies, significant hemorrhage, hydrocephalus, and certain cystic changes. Its greatest value is in the preterm infant to detect interventricular hemorrhage, follow the infant for evidence of cystic periventricular leukomalacia, and follow the progression of hydrocephalus, should it develop. The ultrasound examination for demonstration of an acute hypoxemic event may not be helpful in evaluating the extent and the timing of the event. The brain may appear normal for the first 12–24 h, and then changes compatible with cerebral edema develop. There are often differences of opinion when evaluating "slit-like" ventricles in term infants and diffuse increased echogenicity throughout the brain tissue. In addition, studies using Doppler with resistive indices may also add some specificity to the physiological timing of the injuries. Low resistive indices are most marked 24–48 h after the injury. Ultrasound can also detect injury to the thalamus and basal ganglia, especially if accompanied by hemorrhage or hemorrhagic necrosis. Detection of subdural hemorrhage or hematoma is difficult with the ultrasound examination.

The computed tomography (CT) scan has also been useful in detecting various injuries to the central nervous system following asphyxial injury. It is superior to the ultrasound in many aspects, including the detection of focal and multifocal ischemic brain injury, as well as hemorrhagic lesions that accompany or complicate asphyxia.

Magnetic resonance imaging (MRI) is currently becoming the gold standard for fully evaluating the extent and severity of asphyxial injury to the brain.[53] In many, but not all, situations, it is of help in determining the timing of the asphyxial event, even if the study is carried out months to years after the birth of the infant.[53–60] It is the study of choice to detect developmental abnormalities, especially disorders of neuronal migration, disorders of myelination, abnormalities of the corpus callosum, and arteriovenous malformations. The MRI is also vastly superior to CT scanning in detecting cerebral infarcts, parasagittal cerebral injury, injury to the thalamus and basal ganglia, and hemorrhagic lesions.[53]

Periventricular white-matter injury associated with periventricular leukomalacia has been thought to occur only in preterm infants, and it has been suggested that if such findings were encountered in infants born at term, the injury most likely occurred prenatally during the 24th to 34th week of gestation. Such abnormalities have been found in as many as one-half of term infants with hypoxic–ischemic encephalopathy,[30] but whether the primary insult occurred during the intrapartum period or had been initiated previously is still debatable. Interestingly, Rutherford and coworkers described that the finding of an abnormal signal intensity in the posterior limb of the internal capsule on MRI in term infants with hypoxic–ischemic encephalopathy is associated with poor neurological outcome.[61] Whether this finding is associated with capsular white-matter injury only or is associated with thalamic or basal ganglia involvement is unclear at present.

Sie and coworkers studied 104 infants with evidence of bilateral posthypoxic–ischemic brain damage in the chronic phase of this illness.[62] They concluded that the severity of injury was the primary determinant of the location of the lesion rather than the postconceptual age at which the insult occurred. They describe three specific MR patterns in the infants: (1) periventricular leukomalacia; (2) predominant lesion of the basal ganglia and thalamus, in which 95% were preceded by acute profound asphyxia; and (3) multicystic encephalopathy. These lesions were found in both preterm and term infants. Interestingly, these authors found that the "common risk factors in the term infants with PVL [periventricular leukomalacia] patterns were dysmaturity or maternal pre-eclampsia and the majority had multiple risk factors for partial and/or relapsing hypoxia–ischemia."

There appears to be some disagreement in the literature regarding findings on MRI that can, in retrospect, define the timing of injury to the prenatal or the intrapartum period. Because clinically there is overlapping of the causes of hypoxic–ischemic encephalopathy, it is no wonder that the MRI may not determine with precision when the injury or injuries have taken place or whether they were confined to a single period of time. If one combines the use of continuous EEG monitoring with MRI findings, perhaps a more precise approach to timing will be forthcoming.[63]

Nevertheless, it is important to have an MRI study to detect developmental disorders, to ascertain the areas of involvement of damage associated with hypoxic–ischemic encephalopathy, and to document normal findings as well. It is important to document a normal MRI in a child who may have been depressed at birth and is later found to have severe mental retardation. The normal MRI would mitigate the diagnosis of an intrapartum event causing the retardation.

Placental pathology

In Chapter 24 Dr. Altshuler delineates the placental features of infants who have suffered from hypoxic–ischemic encephalopathy and notes the correlation of findings with the timing of these events. Unfortunately, much too often the placentas of depressed infants are not retained for examination or the examination is performed by pathologists who have little interest in this important organ. A great deal of information can be gathered by careful evaluation of the placenta, including the presence and location of meconium in various cells, the presence of thrombosis, edema, or degenerative changes, the presence and concentration of nucleated blood cells, evidence of infection, the presence of chorioamnionitis, and the location of acute and chronic inflammatory cells. If these data are available, timing of the event or events leading to the infant's difficulties can be made more readily, especially if they are correlated with clinical, laboratory, and imaging studies.

Neuropathological evaluations

As mentioned in Chapter 1, asphyxial insults that result in central nervous system damage are being recognized in preterm as well as term infants prior to the onset of labor. Sims et al. reported a 17% incidence of central nervous system injury in over 400 stillborn fetuses at the Los Angeles County/ University of Southern California Medical Center.[64] Ellis et al. reported that 25% of infants dying shortly after birth had pathological findings associated with prenatal damage,[65] and Low found evidence of antepartum injury in 17 of 30 infants who died in the neonatal period with the diagnosis of presumed asphyxia.[66] He also found five of 30 infants who had intrapartum problems who also died in the neonatal period. He devised a template to ascertain the timing of neuropathological features that appear following an asphyxial episode. If an infant or fetus dies within the first 18 h after the asphyxial event, the brain may appear normal, since it requires a minimum of 18 h before microscopic changes can be recognized. Low also documented a sequence of events leading from neuronal necrosis to microgleal response and astrocyte response or hypertrophy over a period of time. He also noted that macroscopic cavitation would appear after 4 days if the necrosis were severe. Table 25.3 outlines the sequence of events that occur and the interval between the onset of the insult and the neuropathology that ensued.

Conclusion

In many situations it is extremely difficult to ascertain the timing of an intrauterine event or events

Table 25.3. Sequence of observed neuropathic features and the interval between the asphyxial insult.

	Neuropathology			
Time	Neuronal necrosis	Microglial response	Astrocyte response	Cavitation
<18 h	0	0	0	0
18–36 h	+	0	0	0
36–72 h	+	+	0	0
72–96 h	+	+	+	0
>96 h	+	+	+	+

Source: Modified from Low[66] with permission.

that cause neurological damage to the developing fetus. Despite the improvement in monitoring of the progress of pregnancies, identifying and responding to abnormalities that develop, and in electronic monitoring of fetal heart rate prior to and during labor, the incidence of cerebral palsy and mental retardation has not been significantly altered. While the intrapartum death rate has declined, the complications secondary to these problems have not. When called upon to determine the causation and possible prevention of intrauterine problems, clinicians are often unable to identify the sequence of events that have occurred.

Using retrospective analyses and careful evaluation of subjective and objective parameters, one can often piece together a logical explanation of those adverse events. This is especially true if one carries out a careful analysis of the events of pregnancy, the results of electronic fetal heart rate monitoring, the condition of the infant at birth, and the biochemical and physiological abnormalities that may be present. Having access to the placenta for histological review is often of great help in identifying various lesions that affect the intrauterine milieu. Serial and, at times, continuous EEG evaluation can often help in the timing of events as well as offering appropriate approaches to therapy.[67] Lastly, using imaging studies, especially MRI, abnormalities of the central nervous system, their location, and severity can often determine the timing of adverse events to a reasonable degree.

Until we develop better indicators of intrauterine problems, are able to visualize changes in central nervous system function, and then apply these in a clinical situation that is easy to use and interpret, we are left with many indirect indicators that lack specificity and sensitivity in individual patients.

REFERENCES

1 Pasternak, J.F. and Gorey, M.T. (1998). The syndrome of acute near-total intrauterine asphyxia in the term infant. *Pediatr. Neurol.*, **18**, 391–398.

2 Roland, E.H. and Hill, A. (1992). MR and CT evaluation of profound neonatal and infantile asphyxia. *Am. J. Neuroradiol.*, **13**, 973–975.

3 Clapp, J.F. III, Peress, N.S., Welsley, M., et al. (1988). Brain damage after intermittent partial cord occlusion in the chronically instrumented fetal lamb. *Am. J. Obstet. Gynecol.*, **159**, 504–509.

4 Mallard, E.C., Williams, C.E., Johnston, B.M., et al. (1995). Repeated episodes of umbilical cord occlusion in fetal sheep lead to preferential damage to the striatum and sensitize the heart to further insults. *Pediatr. Res.*, **37**, 707–713.

5 De Haan, H.H., Gunn, A.J., Williams, C.E., et al. (1997). Brief repeated umbilical cord occlusions cause sustained cytotoxic cerebral edema and focal infarcts in near-term fetal lambs. *Pediatr. Res.*, **41**, 96–104.

6 Gunn, A.J., Maxwell, L., de Haan, H.H., et al. (2000). Delayed hypotension and subendocardial injury after repeated umbilical cord occlusion in near-term fetal lambs. *Am. J. Obstet. Gynecol.*, **183**, 1564–1572.

7 Hollier, L.M. (2000). Can neurological injury be timed? *Semin. Perinatol.*, **24**, 204–214.

8 Manning, F.A., Bondaji, W., Harman, C.R., et al. (1998). Fetal assessment based on fetal biophysical profile scoring. VIII The incidence of cerebral palsy in tested and untested perinates. *Am. J. Obstet. Gynecol.*, **178**, 696–706.

9 Rayburn, W.F. (1982). Clinical applications of monitoring fetal activity. *Am. J. Obstet. Gynecol.*, **144**, 967–980.

10 Goodlin, R.C. and Haesslein, H.C. (1977). When is it fetal distress? *Am. J. Obstet. Gynecol.*, **128**, 440–447.

11 Shields, J.R. and Schifrin, B.S. (1988). Perinatal anticedents of cerebral palsy. *Obstet. Gynecol.*, **71**, 899–905.

12 Phelan, J.P. and Ahn, M.O. (1994). Perinatal observations in

forty-eight neurologically impaired term infants. *Am. J. Obstet. Gynecol.*, **171**, 424–431.

13 Van der Moer, P., Gerresten, G. and Visser, G. (1985). Fixed heart rate pattern after intrauterine accidental decerebration. *Obstet. Gynecol.*, **65**, 125–127.

14 Menticoglou, S.M., Manning, F.A., Harman, C.R., et al. (1989). Severe fetal brain injury without evident intrapartum trauma. *Obstet. Gynecol.*, **74**, 457–461.

15 Schifrin, B.S., Hamilton-Rubenstein, T. and Shields, J.R. (1994). Fetal heart rate patterns and the timing of fetal injury. *J. Perinatol.*, **14**, 174–181.

16 Phelan, J.P. and Kim, J.O. (2000). Fetal heart rate observations in the brain-damaged infant. *Semin. Perinatol.*, **24**, 221–229.

17 Low, J.A., Victory, R. and Derrick, E.J. (1999). Predictive value of electronic fetal monitoring for intrapartum fetal asphyxia with metabolic acidosis. *Obstet. Gynecol.*, **93**, 285–291.

18 Nelson, K.B., Dambrosia, J.M., Ting, T.Y., et al. (1996). Uncertain value of electronic fetal monitoring in predicting cerebral palsy. *N. Engl. J. Med.*, **334**, 613–618.

19 Spencer, J.A.D., Badawi, W., Burton, P., et al. (1997). The intrapartum CTG prior to neonatal encephalopathy at term: a case-control study. *Br. J. Obstet. Gynaecol.*, **104**, 25–28.

20 Dellinger, E.H., Boehm, F.H. and Crane, M.M. (2000). Electronic fetal heart rate monitoring: early neonatal outcomes associated with normal rate, fetal stress and fetal distress. *Am. J. Obstet. Gynecol.*, **182**, 214–220.

21 Parer, J.T. and King, T. (2000). Fetal heart rate monitoring: is it salvageable? *Am. J. Obstet. Gynecol.*, **182**, 982–987.

22 Pschirrer, E.R. and Yeomans, E.R. (2000). Does asphyxia cause cerebral palsy? *Semin. Perinatol.*, **24**, 215–220.

23 Zain, H.A., Wright, J.W., Parrish, G.E., et al. (1998). Interpreting the fetal heart rate tracing. Effect of knowledge of neonatal outcome. *J. Reprod. Med.*, **43**, 367–70.

24 Dijxhoorn, M.J., Visser, G.H.A., Fidler, V.J., et al. (1986). Apgar score, meconium and acidaemia at birth in relation to neonatal neurological morbidity in term infants. *Br. J. Obstet. Gynaecol.*, **93**, 217–222.

25 Dijxhoorn, M.J., Visser, G.H.A., Touwen, B.C.L., et al. (1987). Apgar score, meconium and acidemia at birth in small for gestational age infants born at term, and their relationship to neonatal neurological morbidity. *Br. J. Obstet. Gynaecol.*, **94**, 873–879.

26 Clifford, S.H. (1945). Clinical significance of yellow staining of the vernix caseosa, skin, nails and umbilical cord of the newborn. *Am. J. Dis. Child.*, **69**, 327–328.

27 Sienko, A. and Altshuler, G. (1999). Meconium-induced umbilical vascular necrosis in abortuses and fetuses: a histopathologic study for cytokines. *Obstet. Gynecol.*, **94**, 415–420.

28 Naeye, R.L. (1995). Can meconium in the amniotic fluid injure the fetal brain? *Obstet. Gynecol.*, **86**, 720–724.

29 Meis, P.J., Hall, M. III, Marshall, J.R., et al. (1978). Meconium passage: a new classification for risk assessment during labor. *Am. J. Obstet. Gynecol.*, **131**, 509–513.

30 Volpe, J.J. (2001). Hypoxic-ischemic encephalopathy. In *Neurology of the Newborn* (ed J.J. Volpe), 4th edn, pp. 217–394. Philadelphia: W.B. Saunders.

31 Ahn, M.O., Korst, L.M., Phelan, J.P., et al. (1998). Does the onset of neonatal seizures correlate with the timing of fetal neurologic injury? *Clin. Pediatr.*, **37**, 673–676.

32 Westgate, J.A., Bennet, L. and Gunn, A.J. (1999). Fetal seizures causing increased heart rate variability during terminal fetal hypoxia. *Am. J. Obstet. Gynecol.*, **181**, 765–766.

33 Takeuchi, T. and Watanabe, K. (1989). The EEG evolution and neurological prognosis of perinatal hypoxic neonates. *Brain Dev.*, **11**, 115–120.

34 Watanabe, K., Hayakawa, F. and Okumura, H. (1999). Neonatal EEG: a powerful tool in the assessment of brain damage in preterm infants. *Brain Dev.*, **21**, 361–372.

35 Toet, M.C. Hellstrom-Westas, L., Groerendaal, F., et al. (1999). Amplitude integrated EEG 3 and 6 hours after birth in full term neonates with hypoxic–ischaemic encephalopathy. *Arch. Dis. Child. Fetal Neonatal Edn*, **81**, F19–F23.

36 Naeye, R.L. and Localio, A.R.L. (1995). Determining the time before birth when ischemia and hypoxemia initiated cerebral palsy. *Obstet. Gynecol.*, **86**, 713–719.

37 Naeye, R.L. and Lin, H-M. (2001). Determination of the timing of fetal brain damage from hypoxemia–ischemia. *Am. J. Obstet. Gynecol.*, **184**, 217–224.

38 Soothill, P.W., Nicolaides, K.H., and Campbell, S. (1987). Prenatal asphyxia, hyperlactic acidaemia, hypoglycaemia and erythroblastosis in growth retarded fetuses. *Br. Med. J.*, **294**, 1051–1053.

39 Benirschke, K. (1994). Placental pathology questions to the perinatologist. *J. Perinatal.*, **14**, 371–375.

40 Thilaganathan, B., Athanasiou, S., Ozmen, S., et al. (1994). Umbilical cord erythroblast count as an index of intrauterine hypoxia. *Arch. Dis. Child*, **70**, F192–F194.

41 Phelan, J.P., Korst, L.M., Ahn, M.O., et al. (1998). Neonatal nucleated red blood cell and lymphocyte counts in fetal brain injury. *Obstet. Gynecol.*, **91**, 485–489.

42 Buonocore, G., Perrone, S., Gioica, D., et al. (1999). Nucleated red blood cell count at birth as an index of perinatal brain damage. *Am. J. Obstet. Gynecol.*, **181**, 1500–1505.

43 Calhoun, D.A., Li, Y., Braylan, R.C., et al. (1996). Assessment of the contribution of the spleen to granulocytopoiesis and erythropoiesis of the mid-gestation human fetus. *Early Hum. Dev.*, **46**, 217–227.

44 Philip, A.G.S. and Tito, A.M. (1989). Increased nucleated red blood cell counts in small for gestational age infants with very low birth weight. *Am. J. Dis. Child.*, **143**, 164–169.

45 Green, D.W., Hendon, B. and Mimouni, F.B. (1995). Nucleated erythrocytes and intraventricular hemorrhage in preterm infants. *Pediatrics*, **96**, 475–478.

46 Yeruchimovich, M., Dollberg, S., Green, D.W., et al. (1999). Nucleated red blood cells in infants of smoking mothers. *Obstet. Gynecol.*, **93**, 403–406.

47 Lackmann, G.M. and Töllner, U. (1995). The predictive value of elevation in specific serum enzymes for subsequent development of hypoxic–ischemic encephalopathy or intraventricular hemorrhage in full term and premature asphyxiated newborns. *Neuropediatrics*, **26**, 192–198.

48 Nagdyman, N., Komen, W., Ko, H-K., et al. (2001). Early biochemical indicators of hypoxic–ischemic encephalopathy after birth asphyxia. *Pediatr. Res.*, **49**, 502–506.

49 De Praeter, C., Vanhaesebrouck, P., Govaert, P., et al. (1991). Creatine kinase isozyme BB concentrations in the cerebrospinal fluid of newborns: relationship to short-term outcomes. *Pediatrics*, **88**, 1204–1210.

50 Pincus, M.R., Zimmerman, H.J. and Henry, J.B. (1996). Clinical enzymology. In *Clinical Diagnosis and Management by Laboratory Methods* (ed J.B. Henry), pp. 268–295, Philadelphia: W.B. Saunders.

51 Tack, E.D., Perlman, J.M., and Robson, A.M. (1988). Renal injury in sick newborn infants: a prospective evaluation using urinary beta-2-microglobulin concentrations. *Pediatrics*, **81**, 432–440.

52 Lupton, B.A., Hill, A. and Roland, E.H. (1988). Brain swelling in the asphyxiated term newborn: pathogenesis and outcome. *Pediatrics*, **82**, 139–146.

53 Barnes, P.D. (2001). Neuroimaging and the timing of fetal and neonatal brain injury. *J. Perinatol.*, **21**, 44–60.

54 Barkovich, H.J. and Truwit, C.L. (1990). Brain damage from perinatal asphyxia: correlation of MR finding with gestational age. *Am. J. Neuroradiol.*, **11**, 1087–1096.

55 Truwit, C.L., Barkovich, A.J., Koch, T.K., et al. (1992). Cerebral palsy: MR findings in 40 patients. *Am. J. Neuroradiol.*, **13**, 67–78.

56 Kuenzle, B.C., Baenziger, O., Martin, E., et al. (1994). Prognostic value of early MR imaging in term infants with severe perinatal asphyxia. *Neuropediatrics*, **25**, 191–200.

57 Martin, E. and Barkovich, A.J. (1995). Magnetic resonance imaging in perinatal asphyxia. *Arch. Dis. Child.*, **72**, F62–F70.

58 Rademakers, R.P., Van der Knaap, M.S., Verbeeten, B. Jr, et al. (1995). Central cortico-subcortical involvement: a distinct pattern of brain damage caused by perinatal and postnatal asphyxia in term infants. *J. Comput. Assist. Tomogr.*, **19**, 256–263.

59 Okumura, A., Hayakawa, F., Kato, T., et al. (1997). MRI findings in patients with spastic cerebral palsy. I: Correlation with gestational age at birth. *Dev. Med. Child Neurol.*, **39**, 363–368.

60 Rutherford, M., Pennock, J., Schwieso, J., et al. (1996). Hypoxic–ischemic encephalopathy: early and late magnetic resonance imaging findings in relation to outcome. *Arch. Dis. Child*, **75**, F145–F151.

61 Rutherford, M.A., Pennock, J.M., Counsell, S.J., et al. (1998). Abnormal magnetic resonance signal in the internal capsule predicts poor neurodevelopmental outcome in infants with hypoxic–ischemic encephalopathy. *Pediatrics*, **102**, 323–328.

62 Sie, L.T.L., Van der Knaap, M.S., Oosting, J., et al. (2000). MR patterns of hypoxic–ischemic brain damage after prenatal, perinatal or postnatal asphyxia. *Neuropediatrics*, **21**, 128–136.

63 Biagioni, E., Mercuri, E., Rutherford, M., et al. (2001). Combined use of electroencephalogram and magnetic resonance imaging in full-term neonates with acute encephalopathy. *Pediatrics*, **107**, 461–468.

64 Sims, M.E., Turkell, S.B., Halterman, G., et al. (1985). Brain injury and intrauterine death. *Am. J. Obstet. Gynecol.*, **151**, 721–723.

65 Ellis, W.G., Goetzman, B.W. and Lindenberg, J.A. (1988). Neuropathologic documentation of prenatal brain damage. *Am. J. Dis. Child*, **142**, 858–866.

66 Low, J.A. (1993). Relationship of fetal asphyxia to neuropathology and deficits in children. *Invest. Med.*, **16**, 133–140.

67 Thornberg, E. and Ekström-Jodal, B. (1994). Cerebral function monitoring: a method of predicting outcome in term neonates after severe perinatal asphyxia. *Acta Paediatr.*, **83**, 596–601.

PART IV

Specific Conditions Associated with Fetal and Neonatal Brain Injury

Hypoglycemia in the neonate

Robert Schwartz,[1] Marvin Cornblath,[2] and Satish C. Kalhan[3]

[1]*Division of Pediatric Endocrinology and Metabolism, Brown University School of Medicine Rhode Island Hospital, Providence, RI, USA*

[2]*Division of Neonatology, Department of Pediatrics, The Johns Hopkins University School of Medicine, Baltimore, MD, USA*

[3]*Robert Schwartz Center for Metabolism and Nutrition, MetroHealth Medical Center and Department of Pediatrics, Case Western Reserve University School of Medicine, Cleveland, OH, USA*

Blood sugar measurements in neonates date back to the beginning of the twentieth century. By the 1920s it was known that concentrations of glucose were lower in premature (<2500 g birth weight) than in term infants, and both were less than those in older infants. In 1937, Hartmann and Jaudon first described a series of 286 neonates and infants with severe, recurrent, and/or persistent manifestations of hypoglycemia based on "true" blood sugar values.[1] Their definitions distinguished between degrees of hypoglycemia based on the concept that all deviations from biological norms represent a continuum of abnormality. Thus, "mild" hypoglycemia was arbitrarily defined between 40 and 50 mg/dl (2.2–2.8 mmol/l); "moderate" between 20 and 40 mg/dl (1.1–2.2 mmol/l); and "extreme" less than 20 mg/dl (<1.1 mmol/l). These "true" blood sugar values were marginally greater than the blood glucose values measured today.

These classical reports stimulated little interest. Furthermore, no clinical significance was attributed to these variations in blood sugar values, even if extremely low (<20 mg/dl: 1.1 mmol/l). In fact, only isolated cases of hypoglycemic neonates, usually from postmortem examination, appeared until 1954, when McQuarrie reported his experience with familial recurrent severe hypoglycemia.[2] In 1959, the report of transient symptomatic neonatal hypoglycemia in eight infants changed the concept and attitude to neonatal hypoglycemia.[3] Significant clinical manifestations occurred with laboratory blood or spinal fluid glucose values <20–25 mg/dl, and cleared after restoring the blood glucose concentration to normal (>40 mg/dl). These three components, i.e., clinical symptoms with low glucose concentrations and improvement with administration of glucose, were considered essential in establishing the diagnosis, and fulfilled the requirements of Whipple's triad.[4] The initial skepticism as to whether or not the entity existed was dispelled as verification was reported from nurseries around the world.

The definition of infants at risk was initially limited to small-for-gestational-age (SGA) males, often the smaller of twins, born to mothers with preeclamptic toxemia.[5] This was rapidly expanded to include the large-for-gestational age (LGA) infants of normal and diabetic mothers, infants with moderate to severe erythroblastosis, cold injury, adrenal hemorrhage, infection, or associated problems such as preexisting or coexisting central nervous system damage, and polycythemia.[6]

Concurrently, major advances in measuring glucose, insulin, alternate substrates and the metabolic, thermal and oxidative needs of the neonate were coupled with the development of the concepts of the SGA, LGA and appropriate-for-gestational age (AGA) infant. This further expanded the interest of pediatricians generally and neonatologists in particular in glucose and energy homeostasis and its regulation in the newborn infant. These studies compared the supply to the demand for glucose, the problems of accurately measuring blood glucose, the distinction between "primary" and "secondary" hypoglycemia, and the interrelationships among glucose, fat, oxygen, and temperature regulation,

The recognition of asymptomatic neonatal hypoglycemia prompted a definition based solely on statistical analysis of clinically observed blood glucose concentrations. Such definitions were arbitrarily based on blood glucose values 2 SD or more below the mean in apparently normal infants without any controlled outcome or evaluations. These "hypoglycemic" values also varied with gestation, birth weight, and age in hours and days. In the absence of any prospective clinically controlled trials to test the impact of hypoglycemia on ultimate neurologic and intellectual outcome, the definitions, concepts, and criteria for the diagnosis have undergone chaotic changes in the ensuing years. Statistical surveys of blood glucose values in "normal" term and preterm infants differed between the 1960s and 1980s; arbitrary decisions and definitions, inadequate screening techniques (and their interpretation), changing criteria for diagnosis, and increasing numbers of lawsuits have all contributed to this situation. In addition, these rough guidelines for "normoglycemia" were then converted to "cutoff" levels, below which brain damage was alleged to occur.

The revolutionary changes in care of preterm high-risk infants have made previously derived uncontrolled statistical standards no longer relevant to current premature populations. New functional definitions must determine plasma glucose concentrations that represent abnormal values for the very-low-birth-weight (VLBW) and sick low-birth-weight premature infant. The glucose requirements for these very immature and "sick" infants may be quite different from those of the term or near-term newborn making the normal metabolic adjustments to extrauterine life.[7]

As a result of these discrepancies, we propose to eliminate the term "hypoglycemia" in the neonate with transient low blood glucose values of uncertain etiology. In its place, we suggest the use of "operational thresholds" or levels of glucose at which clinical interventions may be considered.[7] As currently used and coded, "hypoglycemia" implies disease. "Operational thresholds" or "Glucose operational scales" imply action and represent conservative estimates of tolerable lower limits for normoglycemia. These ranges in glucose concentrations would differ for specific infants, at specific ages, and under a variety of established conditions. This proposal could serve as a basis for reconsidering the entire issue of blood glucose values and their significance in neonates.

This concept further supports the continuum of abnormality for low blood glucose values of varied duration and severity. The impact of the low plasma glucose concentration in any one infant depends on many other risk factors, such as hypoxia, asphyxia, sepsis, age, maturity, and ability to compensate by metabolic and endocrine adjustments.[8] Studies in both animals and humans confirm this complexity.

Definition

Several different approaches have been used to define clinically significant hypoglycemia in the newborn infant.[7] These have been based upon (1) clinical signs and symptoms; (2) glucose concentrations measured in large groups of infants with applied statistical methods, i.e., glucose levels more than 2 SD below the mean; (3) acute changes in metabolic and endocrine responses and neurological function; and (4) long-term neurological outcome.[9] None of these methods has been entirely satisfactory. The first method, i.e., based on clinical manifestations, is confounded by the fact that similar symptoms can occur with a number of clinical problems in the newborn infant and are not correlated with plasma glucose concentration. The second approach is an artificial statistical analysis without any relation to biology, and assumes that a plasma glucose level below a certain statistically defined value is likely to cause harm or requires intervention.[1,8,10,11] The approach relating endocrine and hormone responses is not easy to establish in a healthy newborn population because of ethical considerations, and the currently established definitions are based on very few data.[12] The data correlating long-term neurological sequelae are also confounded because of the lack of suitable normal controls, the small number of infants followed, and failure to consider the impact of other associated clinical problems.[13,14]

The diagnosis of hypoglycemia requires a reliable laboratory determination of a significantly low plasma or serum glucose value that may be present without (asymptomatic) or with (symptomatic) clinical signs and symptoms. All infants with clinical manifestations must respond to glucose therapy, as well, to fulfill a critical part of this definition.

During the first 24 h of age in both term and premature infants, a plasma glucose concentration less than 45 mg/dl (2.5 mmol/l) may be considered to be "hypoglycemia." This definition provides an indication to raise and sustain the plasma glucose levels to above 45–50 mg/dl (2.78 mmol/l). This represents a conservative definition of normoglycemia. Beyond 24 h of age, the threshold value plasma glucose concentration may be increased to 45–50 mg/dl (2.5–2.78 mmol/l). Values below this range are an indication to intervene; however, they do not necessarily imply pathological neuroglucopenia or potential risk for neurologic damage.

Whether or not plasma glucose concentrations between 25 and 45 mg/dl (1.39–2.50 mmol/l) are of any significance or consequence remains to be established. The evidence to date does not support the conclusion that these plasma values, alone, correlate with impaired neurologic or intellectual outcome. Yet, a number of pediatric neurologists, neonatologists, and other physician-scientists, believe that blood glucose values in the range of 36–45 mg/dl (2.00–2.50 mmol/l) can cause central nervous system damage within as short a time as 30 min. Experimental proof for these conclusions is lacking. The only report of such an association involved a retrospective analysis of several thousand glucose analyses in over 600 infants less than 1800 g birth weight who were the subjects in a well-designed prospective feeding trial.[14] Dubious correlations of isolated "low" (<46 mg/dl: 2.55 mmol/l) morning glucose values on 5 days or more (not necessarily consecutive) with handicaps in development were reported at 18-month follow-up in 1988.[15,16] The criterion for hypoglycemia was not defined and sampling bias was not avoided. Although a detailed follow-up of these data has not been published, the authors suggest, in response to a letter to the editor, that a "clinically significant" reduction in math and motor skills (approximately 0.5 SD reduction in scores adjusted for respiratory support, birth weight, and gestation) at 7.5–8 years of age was the only abnormality still associated with their definition of neonatal hypoglycemia.[15] This lack of persistence of the originally described developmental abnormalities in this group raises concern about the validity or interpretation of these results, or may be due to difficulties in neurological evaluation of the infants at an early age.

Based upon the currently available evidence in the literature, operational threshold values of plasma glucose concentration have been proposed at which the clinician should consider intervention.[7,17] These values are strictly meant to be "operational" rather than glucose concentrations at which clinical interventions aimed at raising the plasma glucose concentration should be instituted. These values do not represent the concentration of plasma glucose at which immediate or long-term sequelae will necessarily occur.

In clinically symptomatic infants, a plasma glucose concentration of 45 mg/dl (2.5 mmol/l) or less should be considered as the threshold for intervention. In asymptomatic babies and those at risk for hypoglycemia, irrespective of gestational or postnatal age, a plasma glucose concentration less than 36 mg/dl (2.0 mmol/l) should be considered as the threshold value. Since exclusively breast-fed babies maintain lower plasma glucose concentrations and higher concentrations of ketone bodies than formula-fed infants, the above threshold values may not be applicable to them.[7,17] These infants may well tolerate lower plasma glucose levels without any significant clinical manifestation or sequelae.

There are no recent data to support the adoption of different threshold values for preterm infants.

Infants on parenteral nutrition often have higher plasma insulin secretion due to the beta-cell stimulatory effect of administered glucose and amino acids. The higher insulin levels will also result in suppression of lipolysis and therefore lower concentration of alternate fuels, i.e., ketones and fatty acids. Therefore, these infants should be maintained at higher levels of plasma glucose (>45 mg/dl or 2.5 mmol/l) at all times.

Measurement of glucose

All of the glucose concentrations mentioned above are based on laboratory analysis of blood or plasma glucose obtained and kept in a manner to avoid the increased glycolysis by the blood cells. The blood should be handled expeditiously, similarly to samples obtained for measurements for blood gas analyses.

It should be emphasized that glucose oxidase reagent strip techniques should not be used as the basis for a diagnosis of hypoglycemia, and should be used only as a screening technique. Reasons for this include: (1) the result obtained depends upon the hematocrit; (2) the precision required for performance and timing is rarely achieved; (3) there is a wide variance of ±5–15 mg/dl (0.28–0.83 mmol/l) when compared to laboratory determinations; and (4) a striking lack of reproducibility.[16,18] This is especially true at blood glucose values less than 40–50 mg/dl (2.22–2.78 mg/dl), whether the strips are read by eye or by meters.

In contrast, screening at the bedside is possible by quantitative techniques (e.g., glucose oxidase analyzer or the newer optical bedside glucose sensors).[19]

At least two successive significantly low values should be obtained before making a definitive diagnosis of hypoglycemia in the neonate. A blood sample for laboratory analysis should be obtained before initiating parenteral therapy.

Frequency of neonatal hypoglycemia depends upon the criteria for diagnosis, the population surveyed as well as the method for blood collection and glucose analysis. Early intervention in high-risk and extremely-low-birth-weight (ELBW) infants will also modify occurrence figures.

Clinical manifestations

The clinical presentations of significant hypoglycemia are never specific, especially in the neonate, and include a wide range of local or generalized manifestations common in sick infants.

Episodes of changes in levels of consciousness, tremors, cyanosis, seizures, apnea, irregular respirations, irritability, apathy, limpness, hypothermia, difficulty in feeding, exaggerated Moro reflex, high-pitched cry, and coma have all been attributed to or have resulted from significant hypoglycemia. On occasion, vomiting, tachypnea, bradycardia and "eye-rolling" have also been associated with hypoglycemia.

The clinical manifestations should subside within minutes to hours in response to adequate treatment with intravenous glucose if hypoglycemia alone is responsible. If they do not, the signs and symptoms may well be secondary to a variety of neonatal problems, with or without hypoglycemia.

Some infants with hypoglycemia are rarely symptomatic for unexplained reasons. These include infants of diabetic mothers, those with transitional hypoglycemia in the first hours after birth and older infants with type I glycogen storage disease. Alternate substrates such as lactate, ketones, glycerol, and selected amino acids may support brain metabolism and prevent clinical manifestations in these neonates. Measurements of these substrates usually do not help in making clinical decisions about therapy.

Management of the neonate at risk

Clinical management of neonatal hypoglycemia is based on four basic principles:

1. monitoring infants at highest risk
2. confirming that the plasma glucose concentration is low and is responsible for the clinical manifestations and the metabolic and endocrine abnormalities present
3. demonstrating that all of the symptoms have responded following glucose therapy with restoration of the plasma glucose to normoglycemic levels and

4. observing and documenting all of these events

Routine monitoring for infants at the highest risk for developing significant hypoglycemia would include the following:

1. LGA as well as all infants of insulin-dependant and gestational diabetic mothers and massively obese mothers
2. SGA, especially the smaller of discordant twins
3. Apgar scores <5 at 5 min or later as well as those who require significant resuscitation
4. significant hypoxia and/or perinatal distress
5. ELBW infants (<1250 g)
6. severe erythroblastosis
7. infants of mothers on tocolytic therapies, oral hypoglycemic agents, β-adrenergic blockers, etc.

A rare but important group of neonates to screen because of the severity of their problems, if present, includes infants with:

1. isolated hepatomegaly
2. microphallus or anterior midline defect, especially with persistent hyperbilirubinemia
3. family history of neonate with hypoglycemia or unexplained death in infancy
4. exomphalos, macroglossia, and gigantism

In these high-risk infants, routine screening should be done on admission to the nursery or at 2–2.5 h of age and then before feedings for the next 24 h or until at least three normoglycemic values before the feed have been obtained.

Certainly, whenever any of the clinical manifestations noted above occur, the infant should be screened for hypoglycemia as a possible causative factor. Figure 26.1 provides a graphic flow sheet for screening, confirming, and treating the most common types of hypoglycemia currently encountered in neonates.

Some nurseries, especially in view of the national policy to discharge newborns within the first 24 h of life, now screen every newborn on admission. If the initial screen is low (<45 mg/dl or 2.5 mmol/l) or the infant fits into any of the risk categories noted above, screening should be continued until three preprandial values are "normal." Whether this approach will prove economical on cost–benefit analysis will depend on the number of litigations that will arise from poorly documented "false-positive" results vs those prevented by discovering otherwise undetected patients with hypoglycemic values.

Therapy

Preventive interventions that have been recommended include the early use of oral feedings,[20] parenteral fluids, and lipid supplementation.[21]

Once the diagnosis of hypoglycemia has been established by a reliable laboratory determination, therapy should be initiated promptly. In the asymptomatic infant during the first hours after birth, an oral feed of mixed nutrient (formula) may be given and another plasma glucose measurement obtained within 30–60 min after the feed. If still low, parenteral glucose therapy may be indicated. In the symptomatic infant, a blood sample can be obtained for a glucose determination when the parenteral glucose is started. If this initial plasma glucose value is significantly low and symptoms disappear following the restoration of normoglycemia, the diagnosis of symptomatic hypoglycemia has been established.

Parenteral glucose should be given as an initial minibolus of glucose 0.25 g/kg (1 ml/kg of 25% glucose in water or 2.5 ml/kg of 10% glucose in water) intravenously,[22] followed immediately by a continuous infusion of glucose at the rate of 6–8 mg/kg per min. The concentration of glucose to be used is determined by the total daily fluid requirements, which depend upon the age, weight, and maturity of the infant. For a term infant weighing 3000 g body weight, it corresponds to 80–110 ml/kg per day of 10–12.5% dextrose solution.

Plasma glucose concentrations should be measured at 1–3-h intervals initially to determine the effectiveness of the therapy. Once stable, plasma glucose may be monitored at 4–8-h intervals. If levels of plasma glucose cannot be maintained over 45–50 mg/dl (2.5–2.78 mmol/l) after 3–6 h of parenteral glucose, increase the rate to 8, then 10, 12 to 15 mg/kg per min over the next 24 h, as necessary to achieve normoglycemia. The rate can be increased by 1–2 mg/kg per min at 1–2-h intervals safely. After 12 h of fluid therapy, the addition of 1–2 mmol/kg per day as a hypotonic NaCl (40 mmol/l or "quarter-strength

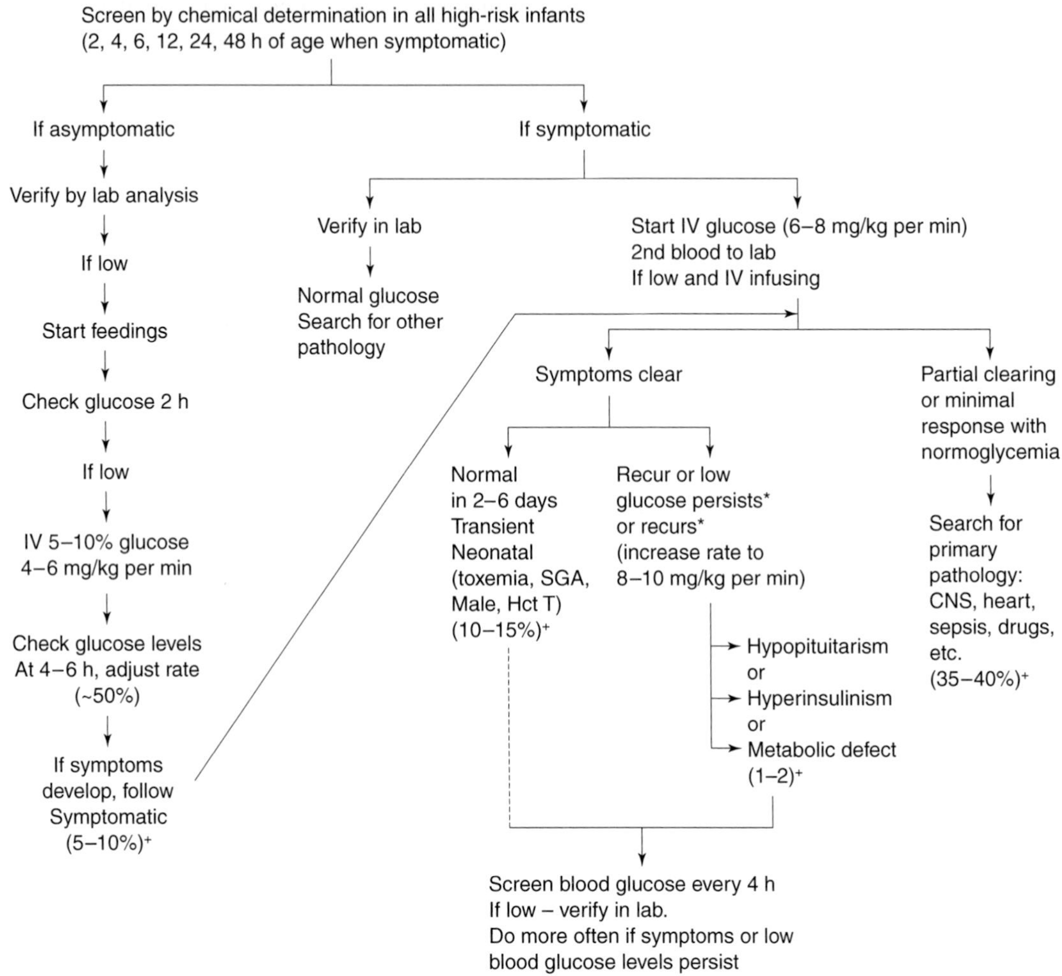

Figure 26.1 Flow diagram for detection and management of suspected hypoglycemia. SGA, small-for-gestational-age; Hct, hematocrit; CNS, central nervous system. Modified from Cornblath and Schwartz.[27]

saline") is indicated to prevent edema[23] or iatrogenic hyponatremia.[24,25] After 24 h, 1–2 mmol/kg per day of potassium (KCl or buffered potassium phosphate) should be added to the parenteral fluids.

Oral feedings can be introduced as soon as possible after clinical manifestations subside. If the rate of glucose infusion exceeds 10–12 mg/kg per min for a prolonged period, the infant may have a persistent type of hypoglycemia.

When normoglycemia has been established, the concentration of parenteral glucose can be decreased gradually to 5% so the rate of infusion is reduced to 6 mg/kg per min, then to 4 mg/kg per min and slowly discontinued over 4–6 h, while oral feedings, adequate in calories, are taken. If the intravenous glucose infiltrates or is stopped abruptly, a reactive hypoglycemia may occur and symptoms recur.

Failure to respond fully to therapy

Persistence of the clinical manifestations after normalization of the plasma glucose concentration indicates that the hypoglycemia may have been associated with or secondary to other primary abnormalities. A systematic clinical and laboratory diagnostic evaluation to determine the primary disease is important since hypoglycemia may be secondary to a variety of neonatal conditions that in themselves may be life-threatening or debilitating.

Monitoring is indicated in infants with:

1. central nervous system pathology, including intrauterine or perinatal infections, congenital defects, and hemorrhage
2. sepsis – especially bacterial, Gram-negative
3. congenital heart disease, especially left-sided abnormalities
4. hypoxia and/or asphyxia, especially with ischemia
5. adrenal hemorrhage
6. hypothyroidism
7. multiple congenital anomalies
8. neonatal tetany
9. postexchange transfusion
10. drugs taken by or given to mother
11. abrupt cessation of parenteral glucose
12. misplaced umbilical catheter (resulting in infusion in celiac axis)

Although support of the plasma glucose level is indicated, the primary disease is often the cause of morbidity or mortality in these infants. There is little evidence at present to attribute adverse outcomes to the associated or resulting hypoglycemia.

Transient hyperinsulinemia

Transient hyperinsulinemia occurs in newborn infants of diabetic mothers,[26] or as a consequence of intrapartum maternal hyperglycemia caused by administration of glucose or some pharmacologic agents or tocolytic drugs. Hypoglycemia is rarely seen in infants of diabetic mothers when maternal glucose control is normalized in the third trimester and/or during labor. Since hypoglycemia may be asymptomatic, it is prudent to measure blood (plasma) glucose concentration in the newborn. Therapeutic principles utilizing operational thresholds should be applied.

Recurrent or persistent neonatal hypoglycemia (Table 26.1)

Recurrent or persistent (>7 days) neonatal hypoglycemia, although rare, is associated with high mortality and morbidity. A definite pathophysiologic classification can often be determined even though specific molecular defects for every type are still not known. Only a brief discussion of those syndromes resulting from either hormone deficiencies or hormone excess, such as hyperinsulinemia, is presented here. A more detailed discussion of these syndromes as well as the hereditary defects in carbohydrate, amino acid, and/or fatty acid metabolism have been reviewed elsewhere.[8,27,28]

This category of neonatal hypoglycemia may be suspected as either requiring infusions of large amounts of glucose (>12–16 mg/kg per min) to maintain normoglycemia or low blood glucose levels persisting or recurring beyond the first 7–14 days of life. These infants require specific diagnostic determinations as well as a rapid trial of therapeutic intervention to determine etiology and effective therapy.

If persistent or recurrent hypoglycemia is anticipated or suspected, a diagnostic blood sample should be taken for the determination of plasma glucose, insulin, and beta-hydroxybutyrate concentrations prior to initiating parenteral therapy. Analyses for growth hormone, adrenocorticotropic hormone (ACTH), cortisol, thyroxine (T_4), glucagon, somatomedins (insulin-like growth factor (IGF)-I and II and their binding proteins), as well as for other substrates, such as lactate, pyruvate, uric acid, quantitative amino acids (especially glutamine and alanine) are also indicated. These blood samples, if obtained before and after glucagon administration at the time when the patient is hypoglycemic, are often diagnostic.[28]

In addition, urine collections for the determination of catecholamines, amino acids, organic acids and

Table 26.1. Recurrent or persistent hypoglycemia

Hormone deficiencies	
Multiple endocrine deficiencies or congenital hypopituitarism	
"Aplasia" anterior pituitary	Hypothalamic hormone deficiencies
Hypoplastic pituitary	
Congenital optic nerve hypoplasia	Midline CNS malformations
Primary endocrine deficiency	
Growth hormone: isolated	Thyroid
ACTH: ACTH unresponsiveness	Epinephrine
Cortisol: (a) hemorrhage, (b) adrenogenital syndrome	Glucagon
Hormone excess hyperinsulinism	
EMG syndrome of Beckwith–Wiedemann	
Islet cell adenoma	
Beta-cell hyperplasia or dysplasia	
Adenomatosis	
Hereditary defects in carbohydrate metabolism	
Glycogen storage disease, type I	
Fructose intolerance	
Galactosemia	
Glycogen synthase deficiency	
Fructose, 1–6 diphosphatase deficiency	
Hereditary defects in amino acid metabolism	
Maple syrup urine disease	
Propionic acidemia	
Methylmalonic acidemia	
Tyrosinosis	
3-hydroxy, 3-methyl glutaryl coenzyme A lyase deficiency	
Hereditary defects in fatty acid metabolism	
Dehydrogenase – medium- and long-chain deficiency	

Notes:
CNS, central nervous system; ACTH, adrenocorticotropic hormone; EMG, electromyogram.

specific reducing sugars should be done promptly. Specific intolerances to galactose, fructose, or leucine can be documented by eliminating these substances from the diet for 2–3 days while definitive diagnostic tests are done. Glycogen storage disease, type I, the exomphalos–macroglossia–gigantism syndrome of Beckwith–Wiedemann,[29] and leprechaunism have diagnostic physical stigma, as do many neonates with congenital hypopituitarism.

The diagnostic-therapeutic trial can be initiated and maintained until laboratory results are available. In addition to infusions of glucose, it consists of the sequential use of specific hormone or other therapies, e.g., diazoxide, glucocorticoids, etc. As additional therapeutic courses are added, it is not necessary to discontinue the previous unsuccessful agent, e.g., the patient with hyperinsulinemic hypoglycemia may be given hydrocortisone and diazoxide concurrently. During therapeutic trials, all blood samples to monitor glucose concentrations should also be assayed for insulin. With this approach, infants with severe hypoglycemia due to hyperinsulinemia can have definitive surgery, if medical therapy fails, as early as 2–3 weeks after birth. When an endocrine deficiency or metabolic error is identified, specific therapy should be initiated at once.

Hormone deficiencies

Multiple hormone deficiencies or congenital hypopituitarism syndromes may be associated with severe, even fatal, hypoglycemia during the first days of life. The concepts of their origin and pathogenesis have expanded significantly within this past decade. Congenital hypopituitarism, once attributed to hypothalamic hormone deficiencies or "aplasia" or hypoplasia, is now well established to be associated with congenital optic nerve hypoplasia (CONH), both unilateral and bilateral, with or without agenesis of the septum pellucidum and/or other structural abnormalities of the brain.[30] Congenital hypopituitarism has also been reported in a number of other syndromes, e.g., Russell–Silver, midline craniofacial defect with congential heart disease, choanal atresia, and cleft palate (CHARGE association) and Johanson-Blizzard syndrome of aplasia of the alae nasi, deafness, dwarfism, and hypothyroidism. The advanced imaging techniques of the central nervous system,[31] pituitary, and optic nerves and the specificity and ready availability of sensitive endocrine hormone assays have resulted in the recognition of a variety of pituitary malfunctions in a number of syndromes.

The frequency of congenital hypopituitarism has ranged from 1:29 000 in Oregon[32] to 1:100 000 reported at the Second International Conference on Neonatal Screening.[33]

In 1975, Patel et al.[34] were one of the first to emphasize the association of CONH, hypopituitarism, hypoglycemia, and hyperbilirubinemia. In addition, they provided a useful guide to the clinical picture of these syndromes at different ages: "In the newborn period there may be apnea, hypotonia, hypoglycemia, with or without seizures, and hyperbilirubinemia. At the age of 3 months, patients have hypotonia, psychomotor retardation, defective visual fixation, and seizures. A firm, nontender liver may be palpable and, in one case, there was mild jaundice. A receding lower jaw and, occasionally, a high-arched palate may be present. The general appearance is otherwise normal. The fasting blood glucose level may be mildly depressed, and results of the liver function tests may be abnormal. The older child in this series had psychomotor retardation, growth failure, defective vision, and seizures." With CONH and other forms of congenital hypopituitarism, the frequency of hypoglycemia appears to be associated with the severity of the hormone deficiencies. The high incidence of neurologic and developmental disabilities is related to the underlying cerebral developmental anomalies. The contribution of hypoglycemia to outcome appears to be minimal.

A number of additional problems have been identified with reasonable frequency in these babies to alert the physician to the possibility of hypopituitarism. Infants with symptomatic hypoglycemia, hyperbilirubinemia (often conjugated), microphallus in males and midline defects, especially in girls, often LGA (25% >95th percentile) should suggest investigation. They also may have thrombocytopenia, alone or associated with other hematologic abnormalities, and an abnormal T_4 on the neonatal screen. Recently, free water intolerance and a lack of thymic involution were noted as well.

A critical blood sample during hypoglycemic episodes, the results of substrate and hormones levels, followed by a prompt response to the Diagnostic Therapeutic Trial after the addition of cortisol and biosynthetic human growth hormone should establish the diagnosis.

The central nervous system, midline (medial cleft palate syndrome), genital (microphallus in the male), optic, and growth abnormalities usually do not require immediate attention. Nevertheless, the severe recurrent hypoglycemia, often unresponsive to intravenous glucose alone, the persistent jaundice[35] and the frequently associated hypothyroidism emphasize the importance of early recognition and therapy.

Hyperinsulinemic (organic) hypoglycemia

The concept of hyperinsulinemic hypoglycemia is not new. Subtotal pancreatectomy introduced by Graham and Hartmann[36] had been utilized in infants who could not be managed by the contemporary therapies. The major advance in diagnosis occurred in 1960 when Yalow and Berson[37] described the radioimmunoassay of insulin, allowing for micro- and then rapid analysis (within hours to days) of plasma insulin concentrations in infants. The simultaneous analysis of plasma glucose and insulin has permitted rapid diagnosis and early definitive therapy. Recent studies also indicate that hyperinsulinemia, especially with diffuse islet cell abnormalities, is inherited as an autosomal recessive.[38,39] The gene locus for this rare autosomal recessive "disease" of persistent hyperinsulinemic hypoglycemia of infancy has been identified at the region of chromosome 11p between markers D11S1334 and D11S899.[38,40,41] The beta-cell sulfonylurea receptor (SUR) has been cloned.[42] Furthermore, studies of individuals with hyperinsulinemic hypoglycemia were found to have two separate SUR gene site mutations.[38,41] In addition, functional candidate genes are being investigated in an autosomal dominant form of this disorder. Glaser[40] has recently reported on the etiology as well as the molecular biology of this disorder. The diagnosis of hyperinsulinemia can even be made in utero, as well, by analyzing insulin concentrations in amniotic fluid in subsequent pregnancies and this permits treatment to begin soon after birth.[43]

Medical therapy has been the most effective with diazoxide, which inhibits insulin secretion.[44] Pharmacologic agents such as somatostatin and/or glucagon have permitted preoperative stabilization but have not usually provided long-term effective therapy. Octreotide (a long-acting somatostatin preparation) has been used with mixed success in conjunction with frequent feedings and raw corn starch at night for long-term therapy to avoid pancreatectomy and the potential of subsequent diabetes mellitus.[40,45]

Surgical outcome improved with preservation of the spleen to avoid delayed major infections but was not consistently successful with subtotal pancreatectomy. As a result, Harken et al. strongly recommended near-total (95–99%) or total pancreatectomy.[46] Over time, this form of aggressive therapy has become accepted at early stages (weeks) after diagnosis and failed medical therapy.

A detailed report of the clinical features of 52 neonates with hyperinsulinism was presented by deLonlay-Debeney et al.[47] Their studies were unique because of preoperative pancreatic vein catheterization with insulin measurements and intraoperative histologic studies. Surgical resection was partial pancreatectomy for focal lesions but near-total resection for diffuse lesions. To date, the outcome for patients with focal lesions was satisfactory, i.e., normal parameters of glucose metabolism. In contrast, patients with diffuse pancreatic lesions had a variety of defects in glucose metabolism (hypoglycemic or hyperglycemia) in the year after surgery. The neurologic outcome of these plus 48 patients was reported recently.[48] These data show that, in spite of early and aggressive treatment, psychomotor retardation and epilepsy were often seen in patients with neonatal onset of hyperinsulinemic hypoglycemia.

The frequency of hyperinsulinemic hypoglycemia is unknown. Birth weights have been normal, but are usually increased. Both sexes are affected and familial occurrence has been reported on a number of occasions.[49] Aggressive, early medical or surgical intervention does not assure a successful outcome.[50] In the past decade, of 12 infants who have been operated on between 5 and 18 days after birth, 10 were reported with normal mental status. However, five had seizures, one was retarded, and another died.[51] This limited outcome may relate to the severity and duration of the hypoglycemia or to other congenital metabolic factors. However, the data, at present, do not show a clear relationship between the duration or severity of hypoglycemia, type of underlying pathology, type of therapy and the outcome.

Diagnostic studies are necessary to document the hypoglycemia and the hyperinsulinemia. This is best achieved by analyzing plasma samples obtained simultaneously for insulin and glucose concentrations at the time of clinical manifestations of hypoglycemia and pre- and postfeeding on multiple occasions. Hypoglycemia rarely poses problems in interpretation. In those reported, the blood glucose levels were all less than 35 mg/dl (1.94 mmol/l) and usually were 20 mg/dl (1.11 mmol/l) or less. In contrast, hyperinsulinemia may be relative rather than absolute. This relationship has been quantified by the insulin (μU/ml)-to-glucose (mg/dl) ratio which does not exceed 0.30 in the normal infant, child, or adult under basal conditions. This simple ratio, if positive, has proven to be especially useful in establishing the diagnosis. In addition, low concentrations of plasma ketones are associated with the hypoglycemia.

If the plasma insulin levels are elevated excessively (>200 μU/ml), it is critical to obtain a C-peptide level to establish its endogenous origin and to rule out the administration of exogenous insulin.[52] Recently, we have been consulted on four infants with "abnormal" hyperinsulinemia. Three were ELBW infants being given total parenteral nutrition (TPN) in the neonatal intensive care unit and one was a 6-month-old with a recent onset of profound hypoglycemia (plasma glucose concentrations between 10 and 20 mg/dl: 0.6–1.1 mmol/l) at the time of symptoms. The ELBW infants, two of whom were being given small quantities of insulin for symptomatic hyperglycemia and one was given TPN without insulin, had all apparently been given excessive quantities of insulin in their TPN solutions by error. The 6-month-old infant had extremely high plasma insulin concentrations (>400–>500 μU/ml). An exogenous source of the insulin was subsequently detected. Insulin was surreptitiously being injected into the central venous line. C-peptide determinations would have established the exogenous source of the insulin in all four instances. In three, analysis of the parenteral fluid confirmed the source of the insulin.

Medical therapy must be reviewed regularly and obvious failure is an indication for surgery. The treatment of choice currently is near-total pancreatectomy, retaining the spleen and duodenum. Immediately postoperatively, glucose control commonly becomes erratic because of secondary diabetes. The principles used in managing new type I diabetes mellitus apply here. However, because the source of glucagon has also been removed, there may be insulin sensitivity. It is unusual to see ketoacidosis in this situation. The degree and persistence of the hyperglycemia are highly variable and usually transient. C-peptide analyses (plasma and urine) may give the first indication that the islets are regenerating.[53]

Prognosis and follow-up

The prognosis in newborns with hypoglycemia represents a complex and a multifaceted problem. Of primary concern is the effect on survival. Mortality has been associated with severe unrecognized hypoglycemia ("nesidioblastosis," islet cell adenoma, congenital hypopituitarism). In addition, neuropathologic changes have been noted in the brain in the SGA infant with inadequately or untreated "classical" hypoglycemia.[54,55] A profoundly low plasma glucose level recurring or persisting over prolonged periods of time unrecognized and/or untreated can be lethal.

On the other hand, the effects of hypoglycemia on long-term mental or neurodevelopmental outcome are far from clear. The long-term consequences of significant neonatal hypoglycemia are poorly understood because it is often associated with, or secondary to, such devastating problems as hypoxic–ischemic encephalopathy,[56] congenital anomalies, cerebral pathology, or sepsis. While a number of dire consequences have been attributed to even brief periods of asymptomatic hypoglycemia, the available data do not support such conclusions. In an attempt to clarify this dilemma, it is necessary to review pertinent animal data as well as the clinical studies reported to date.

Animal data

Siesjo and associates have studied the effects of hypoglycemia alone on the electroencephalogram (EEG), brain energy metabolism, neurophysiology, and neuropathology in adult rats. Their elegant model was controlled for hypotension, anoxia, ischemia, and acidosis.[57,58]

Their studies clearly indicated that both profound (EEG isoelectric, glucose <18 mg/dl: 1.0 mmol/l) and prolonged (>30 min) hypoglycemia were necessary to demonstrate cell necrosis in the brain. Hypoglycemic neuronal damage required that cellular energy states be perturbed, suggesting that cell necrosis was the consequence of energy failure and membrane depolarization. The energy failure was characterized by decreases in concentrations of phosphocreatine and adenosine phosphates; and membrane depolarization, by an influx of calcium, an efflux of potassium, with an ensuing acceleration of proteolytic and lipolytic reactions.

The distribution of the hypoglycemic neuronal necrosis was unique, differed from that in ischemia or seizures, and suggested the involvement of a fluid-borne extracellular toxin as well. This could be an excitatory amino acid, such as glutamate or aspartate. These accelerated cell death by causing a dendrosomatic lesion attributed to calcium influx. Hypoglycemia in the newborn rat is also associated with increased activation of the cerebral *N*-methyl-D-aspartate (NMDA) receptor ion channel by glutamate.[59] In the neonatal pig, a prolonged period of profound hypoglycemia (<10 mg/dl) and the presence of an isoelectric EEG (as in the adult rat) was necessary before there is glutamate release (an early marker of activation of the NMDA receptor ion channel).[60]

Vannucci and his collaborators[61] have investigated the effects of hypoglycemia alone or in association with either hypoxemia (8% oxygen) or anoxia (100% nitrogen) in neonatal rats[61,62] and puppies.[63] In contrast to the adult rat, newborn animals tolerated as long as 60–120 min of blood glucose concentrations under 18 mg/dl (<1.0 mmol/l) without changes in behavior or untoward pathologic or pathophysiologic consequences. If then exposed to anoxia (100 % nitrogen), hypoglycemic rats died sooner than normoglycemic rats (5 vs 25 min). However, if given glucose prior to exposure to anoxia, no significant differences in survival times were noted.[62]

In contrast, 3–7-day-old-dogs, after similar periods of hypoglycemia (<18 mg/dl: 1 mmol/l), showed identical rates of demise and changes in acid–base parameters, $P\text{CO}_2$, heart rate, and blood pressure as normoglycemic controls following asphyxiation. Again, this indicates the resistance of the neonatal animal to low levels of plasma glucose.

Increase in cerebral blood flow and utilization of alternate substrates as well as a more permeable blood–brain barrier have been implicated as the explanation for these differences or resistance to hypoglycemia. However, the data on whole brain versus regional cerebral blood flow and measurements of energy sources and utilization in these young animals still require further study. Recent studies in newborn piglets indicate that hypoglycemia (10–18 mg/dl: 0.55–1.0 mmol/l) promotes increases in cerebral adenosine concentrations which contribute to pial dilatation and parenchymal hyperemia with local cerebral blood flow increase of 36±12%.[64]

The long-term consequences of prolonged hyperinsulinemic hypoglycemia have been studied in newborn rhesus monkeys by Schrier et al. They utilized an in utero model of hyperinsulinemia[65] to produce neonatal hypoglycemia by the continuous subcutaneous delivery of insulin for up to 4 h after birth. This resulted in plasma glucose concentrations of 14±4 mg/dl (0.78 mmol/l) for 6.5±1 h in one group of experimental animals and 16±4 mg/dl (0.89 mmol/l) for 10±1 h in another. The control placebo group maintained plasma glucose concentrations of 45±10 mg/dl (2.5 mmol/l). The animals were randomized at birth and then transferred to an experimental psychologist with experience in primate behavioral assessment. A cognitive and behavioral testing program was begun under blind conditions when each animal was 8 months of age. There were no neurologic abnormalities. Testing continued for 22 months, or the equivalent of late childhood in the human. None of the measures of cognitive abilities or behavior distinguished experimental animals with 6.5 h of hypoglycemia from controls. Ten hours of hypoglycemia resulted in motivational and adaptability problems that made it impossible for some animals to learn even the simplest tasks. However, when provided with additional attention and adequate motivation, these same experimental animals performed as well as controls in all tests designed to measure cognitive abilities. These investigators concluded that neonatal hypoglycemia of 10 h duration results in adaptive difficulties in rhesus monkeys, but if special attention is devoted to these animals, there are no enduring cognitive effects or behavioral deficits.

Follow-up studies

There have been at least 13 series of cases correlating subsequent neurodevelopmental outcome of neonates with neonatal hypoglycemia, but without controls.[14,66] The definition of hypoglycemia varied among studies, being <20 mg/dl (1.11 mmol/l) in seven, ≤20 mg/dl (1.11 mmol/l) in three, <25 mg/dl (1.39 mmol/l) in two and unknown in one. In summarizing the case series, of the total of 158 symptomatic infants with significantly low blood glucose values, in 70%, no criterion of response of symptoms to glucose therapy was noted (the only clinical criteria that permit a diagnosis); in only 13% of infants did the criteria for inclusion describe clearing of symptoms; and in 17%, symptoms did not respond to therapy. In this latter group, it was quite likely that the clinical manifestations and outcomes were due to associated or underlying pathology. In addition to the lack of nonhypoglycemic controls, failure to consider other pathology, and the small numbers of asymptomatic infants followed up raise serious questions about the validity and precision of any inference based on these reports. The prognosis and relative risk for neurodevelopmental abnormality in neonatal hypoglycemia cannot be determined by case studies alone.

A long-term prospective controlled study is necessary to resolve these objections and to allow a correlation between neonatal hypoglycemia and outcome.

Such a prospective study would require, at a minimum, the following:

1. A sound epidemiologic and statistical design to assure adequate numbers in cohorts, to avoid sampling bias, to provide complete follow-up assessed blindly, and to adjust for extraneous prognostic factors.
2. Reliable accurate plasma glucose determinations and clinical criteria for defining hypoglycemia, both with and without symptoms.
3. A prospective study to include normoglycemic controls with a follow-up of 7–9 years.
4. Either a controlled intervention at predetermined plasma glucose concentrations or a controlled prevention of hypoglycemia.
5. A specific definition of outcome to include, in addition to precise developmental and mental achievements and neurologic status, metabolic, endocrine, and physical growth criteria.

Only in this way will it ever be possible to establish the prognosis and relative risk of neonatal hypoglycemia as a primary causative factor in abnormal outcome. No such study exists and only fragments of this total objective have been reported. Therefore, only general conclusions, but no precise estimates of adverse outcome, in infants with neonatal hypoglycemia are possible at this time.

While seven controlled studies have evaluated neurodevelopmental outcomes of both hypoglycemic and nonhypoglycemic controls, none included a randomized trial of intervention for either the treatment or prevention of neonatal hypoglycemia. Three were follow-ups of infants of diabetic mothers who usually had transient asymptomatic hypoglycemia. None showed an association between neonatal hypoglycemia and outcome in this group.

The other four studies were concerned exclusively or primarily with low-birth-weight infants in whom hypoglycemia is usually associated with symptoms. Three of these controlled studies[67,68] were reported in the 1970s and were based on infants diagnosed in the 1960s. The latest study and the largest was included in a multicenter feeding study.[14] While a protocol for obtaining plasma glucose samples was included, there was none for assessing therapy or any precautions in handling the blood specimens to prevent glycolysis.

Two of the three early controlled studies reported a risk for subsequent neurodevelopmental abnormalities associated with neonatal hypoglycemia (blood glucose values <20 mg/dl: 1.11 mmol/l) in low-birth-weight infants.[68,69] The risk was substantial with symptomatic but not asymptomatic hypoglycemia.[68] The third study found no significant association of neonatal hypoglycemia with later cerebral abnormalities.[67] All three studies, while designed to address specifically the problem of neonatal hypoglycemia, contain serious deficiencies, e.g., sampling bias, small sample size, and incomplete follow-up. These raise serious questions about the validity of their findings concerning the prognosis of neonatal hypoglycemia.

The study by Lucas et al.[14] has enlarged the area of uncertainty from neonates with blood sugar values <20 mg/dl (1.11 mmol/l) or, at most, <30 mg/dl (1.67 mmol/l) and usually symptomatic to a plasma level <47 mg/dl (2.61 mmol/l) regardless of symptoms. In addition, duration of low glucose concentrations in days over the first 9 weeks of life have now been introduced as an independent variable. However, the fact that hypoglycemia was *not* a primary concern of this prospective controlled feeding study is apparent from the data, which indicate that some infants were permitted to have plasma glucose values less than 20 mg/dl (1.11 mmol/l) for as long as 3–7 days. In addition, the glucose values reported and used in their analysis for prognosis were the first one obtained each day and the number of days with any specific glucose value were usually not consecutive days. The adjustment for confounding factors and the large sample size were positive aspects of this study. In these high-risk infants under 1850 g birth weight, a first glucose value <47 mg/dl (2.61 mmol/l) on 5 days or more correlated positively with abnormal neurologic and developmental outcome at 18 months of age. The significance of this relationship is obscure and requires a prospective controlled intervention study for clarification. It is noteworthy that, 7 years after the initial report and with preliminary follow-up data presented at a conference in 1989,[16] no subsequent report has been forthcoming.

Pathogenesis and pathophysiology

Hypoglycemia essentially represents an imbalance between glucose production or input and glucose utilization or uptake. The regulation and complexity of glucose metabolism throughout fetal development have been detailed elsewhere.[27]

Hypoglycemia is the end result of multiple altered regulatory mechanisms. Some may have occurred or begun before birth, such as falling or low estriols or intrauterine hypoxia, resulting in reduced glucose transport across the placenta and in lower fetal hepatic glycogen. Fetal hypoglycemia early in labor has been associated with growth retardation, pre-eclampsia, accidental hemorrhage, and maternal hypoglycemia, but not with reduced fetal oxygen concentration or acidosis. Ketones and amino acids, which readily traverse the normal placenta, may be abnormal with maternal toxemia or diabetes. The placental transfer of free fatty acids, ketones, and glycerol and their metabolism and utilization in sparing glucose can influence extrauterine adaptation.

With all of these variables, plus the dynamic changes in energy requirements for air breathing and temperature maintenance, as well as circulatory changes and increased activities of both digestive and excretory functions, the concepts of excess utilization or uptake of glucose or inadequate intake or production of glucose are, indeed, complex.

Excess utilization or uptake of glucose may result from:

1. an absolute or relative hyperinsulinism – infants of diabetic mothers, erythroblastosis, LGA, SGA, or islet cell or other endocrine pathology, e.g., increased hormone receptor activity or failure of downregulation of insulin receptors
2. neonatal adaptation, stress, and/or incomplete aerobic oxidation with hypoxia, asphyxia, or infection
3. relatively excessive amounts of glucose-dependent tissues – brain-to-liver ratio in SGA
4. inadequate glucose-sparing substrates – free fatty acids, ketones, glycerol, amino acids, lactate

Inadequate production or input may result from:

1. inadequate or delays in feedings or providing parenteral calories and glucose
2. aberrant control mechanisms that regulate effective glucose transport across the blood–brain barrier,[70] gluconeogenesis, glycolysis, lipolysis; also hypothalamic, pituitary, and peripheral endocrine function
3. transient developmental immaturity of critical metabolic pathways reducing endogenous production of glucose and/or other substrates
4. deficient metabolic reserves of precursors or glucose-sparing substrates

Kalhan and Parimi[71] have recently provided a detailed analysis of gluconeogenesis (GNG) in the fetus and neonate. GNG, a key metabolic process, involves the formation of glucose and glycogen from nonglucose precursors via pyruvate. In the strict sense, it also includes the contribution of glycerol as well as recycled glucose carbon (Cori's cycle). The developmental expression of GNG in the fetus and newborn and the quantitative contribution of GNG to glucose has been extensively investigated in humans and other mammalian species. Data from studies in rodents, rabbits, and sheep fetuses show that the development of GNG is a well-orchestrated process that is regulated by enzymes, which catalyze GNG. These transcription factors and the genes for gluconeogenic enzymes are expressed at specific time periods during development. Although the fetus has the potential for GNG in vivo, the rate-limiting enzyme, phosphoenolpyruvate carboxykinase, appears only after birth in the immediate newborn period. Several tracer isotope methods have been employed to quantify the contribution of

GNG to glucose. Of these, the recently developed stable isotope techniques with deuterium-labeled water and the mass isotopomer distribution analysis appear to be the most precise and easily applicable in human studies. The available data show that, in the human newborn, GNG appears soon after birth and contributes 30–70% to glucose produced. Application of new molecular biology techniques, in combination with sensitive tracer isotopic methods, will allow us to identify and examine metabolic disorders that impact GNG and help develop intervention strategies.

An exciting development in the past decade has been the discovery of specific membrane proteins known as Glut-1, -2, etc., which are responsible for the entrance and exit of glucose from specific cells.[72] In fetal rats, Glut-2, which predominantly transports glucose out of the hepatocyte, may be decreased in both SGA and LGA pups, thus contributing to hypoglycemia.[73] Glucose transporter proteins 1 and 4 have been studied in fetal sheep in whom fetal hypoglycemia and hypoinsulinemia result in tissue-specific and time-dependent increases in Glut-1 and Glut-4 levels. When the availability of glucose is limited, "normalization" of fetal Glut expression might reflect a fetal cellular adaptation to limit glucose utilization.[74] Ten-day-old rats with septic shock have an increase in Glut-1 mRNA in liver, muscle, and fat, but not brain. This may be an important cause of increased tissue glucose uptake.[75]

In preliminary studies of hypoglycemia in infants and children, Koh et al.[12] observed abnormalities in auditory and somatic evoked potentials in 10 of 17 patients at glucose levels ranging from 25 to 47 mg/dl (1.4–2.6 mmol/l). These changes were transient. Similar findings have been reported in adults utilizing insulin-glucose clamp techniques with plasma glucose values between 60 and 72 mg/dl (3.3–4 mmol/l). The neurologic aberrations were transient and readily reversible.[76,77] The relationship between these changes and subsequent development in the infants has not been determined.

With the recent availability of noninvasive techniques to measure changes in cerebral function,[78] cerebral blood flow,[79,80] catecholamine responses,[80] and glucose utilization directly in the neonate, data should become available to define better those concentrations of plasma glucose that are correlated with abnormal responses and outcomes. Kinnala et al. have summarized newer neuroradiologic techniques to study neonatal hypoglycemia.[81]

Pryds et al.[80] compared cerebral blood flow and plasma epinephrine and norepinephrine responses in 13 hypoglycemic infants (mean birth weight 1500 g; mean gestational age 31.2 weeks) and 12 normoglycemic controls (mean birth weight 1310 g, mean gestational age 29.5 weeks). Hypoglycemia was defined as a blood glucose concentration <30 mg/dl (<1.7 mmol/l). There was a statistically significant increase in cerebral blood flow in the hypoglycemic group, but not in plasma epinephrine concentrations; norepinephrine levels remained constant throughout the range of blood glucose values. In a comparable study, Pryds et al.[79] reported cerebral function estimated by EEG and visual evoked potentials was normal during short periods of low glucose values. They concluded that blood glucose concentrations should be maintained above 30–45 mg/dl (1.7–2.5 mmol/l) to avoid cerebral hyperperfusion and epinephrine secretion. They suggested that previously unperfused capillaries are recruited to maintain the glucose transport into neurons.[82]

Correlating these acute changes in cerebral blood flow, cerebral blood volume, hormone responses, and EEG findings with long term neurodevelopmental outcomes will be the challenge for the future. More precise direct measurements of cerebral function, metabolic perturbations, blood flow, glucose uptake and utilization, and correlations with both immediate and long-term outcomes should ultimately resolve some of the current uncertainties.

Summary

Low blood glucose values in the neonate are not uncommon and require careful evaluation to determine their significance, persistence, or relevance to the clinical condition of the infant. Thus, plasma glucose concentrations represent an estimate of the metabolic milieu of a particular infant at a specific point in time. While restoration of the plasma glucose concentration to normoglycemic values is desirable, the urgency to do so and the methods to be employed depend upon the entire clinical evaluation of the infant, including the age in hours, the presence of clinical manifestations, and multiple other risk factors.

In contrast, severe and persistent hypoglycemia may be associated with high risk for both short- and long-term morbidity and mortality. Diagnostic studies at onset for hormones and substrates may provide the basis for the etiology. Aggressive medical therapy is indicated with parenteral dextrose, hormones, and pharmacologic agents. In organic hyperinsulinemic hypoglycemia, the failure of medical therapy mandates prompt surgical intervention, usually with near-total pancreatectomy.

The outcome for survival of severe or recurrent hypoglycemia has improved significantly. However, while prognosis for neurologic and mental outcome in these infants has improved, a significant risk still remains.

REFERENCES

1 Hartmann AF and Jaudon JC. (1937). Hypoglycemia. *J Pediatr*, **11**, 1–36.

2 McQuarrie I. (1954). Idiopathic spontaneously occurring hypoglycaemia in infants. *Am J Dis Child*, **4**, 399–428.

3 Cornblath M, Odell GB and Levin EY. (1959). Symptomatic neonatal hypoglycemia associated with toxemia of pregnancy. *J Pediatr*, **55**, 545–562.

4 Whipple AO and Fratz DK. (1935). Adenoma of islet cells with hyperinsulinism: a review. *Ann Surg*, **101**, 1299–1310.

5 Pildes RS, Forbes AD and Cornblath M. (1967). Blood glucose levels and hypoglycemia in twins. *Pediatrics*, **40**, 69–77.

6 Heck LJ and Erenberg A. (1987). Serum glucose levels in term neonates during the first 48 hours of life. *J Pediatr*, **110**, 119–122.

7 Cornblath M, Hawdon JM, Williams AF, et al. (2000). Controversies regarding definition of neonatal hypoglycemia: suggested operational thresholds. *Pediatrics*, **105**, 1141–1145.

8 Cornblath M and Ichord R. (2000). Hypoglycemia in the neonate. *Semin Perinatol*, **24**, 136–149.

9 World Health Organization. (1997). *Hypoglycaemia of the Newborn: Review of the Literature*. Geneva, Switzerland: World Health Organization. http://www.who.int.chd.pub.imci/bf/hyogly/hypoglyc.htm.

10 Cornblath M. (1996). Neonatal hypoglycemia 30 years later: does it injure the brain? Historical summary and present challenges. *Acta Paediatr Jpn*, **1**, S7–S11.

11 Stanley CA, Anday EK, Baker L, et al. (1979). Metabolic fuel and hormone responses to fasting in newborn infants. *Pediatrics*, **64**, 613–619.

12 Koh THHG, Aynsley-Green A, Tarbit M, et al. (1988). Neural dysfunction during hypoglycaemia. *Arch Dis Child*, **63**, 1353–1358.

13 Sinclair JC. (1997). Approaches to the definition of neonatal hypoglycemia. *Acta Paediatr Jpn*, **39**, S17–S20.

14 Lucas A, Morley R and Cole JJ. (1988). Adverse neuro developmental outcome of moderate neonatal hypoglycemia. *Br Med J*, **297**, 1304–1308.

15 Cornblath M and Schwartz R. (1999). Outcome of neonatal hypoglycaemia. Complete data are needed. *Br Med J*, **318**, 194–195.

16 Cornblath M, Schwartz R, Aynsley-Green A, et al. (1990). Hypoglycemia in infancy: the need for a rational definition. A Ciba Foundation discussion meeting. *Pediatrics*, **95**, 834–837.

17 Kalhan S and Peter-Wohl S. (2000). Hypoglycemia: what is it for the neonate? *Am J Perinatol*, **17**, 11–18.

18 Lin HC, Maguire C, Oh W, et al. (1989). Accuracy and reliability of glucose reflectance meters in the high-risk neonate. *J Pediatr*, **115**, 998–1000.

19 Conrad PD, Sparks JW, Osberg I, et al. (1989). Clinical application of a new glucose analyzer in the neonatal intensive care unit: comparison with other methods. *J Pediatr*, **114**, 281–287.

20 Smallpeice V and Davies PA. (1964). Immediate feeding of premature infants with undiluted breast milk. *Lancet*, **2**, 1349–1352.

21 Sann L, Mousson B, Rousson M, et al. (1988). Prevention of neonatal hypoglycaemia by oral lipid supplementation in low birth weight infants. *Eur J Pediatr*, **147**, 158–161.

22 Lilien LD, Pildes RS, Srinivasan G, et al. (1980). Treatment of neonatal hypoglycemia with minibolus and intravenous glucose infusion. *J Pediatr*, **97**, 295–298.

23 Raivio KO and Hallman N. (1968). Neonatal hypoglycemia. 1. Occurrence of hypoglycemia in patients with various neonatal disorders. *Acta Paediatr Scand*, **57**, 517–521.

24 Brown RJ and Wallis PG. (1963). Hypoglycemia in the newborn infant. *Lancet*, **1**, 1278–1282.

25 Gutberlet RL and Cornblath M. (1976). Neonatal hypoglycemia revisited – 1975. *Pediatrics*, **58**, 10–17.

26 Schwartz R and Teramo KA. (2000). Effects of diabetic pregnancy on the fetus and newborn. *Semin Perinatol*, **24**, 120–135.

27 Cornblath M and Schwartz R. (1991). *Disorders of Carbohydrate Metabolism in Infancy*, 3rd edn. Cambridge, MA: Blackwell Scientific Publications.

28 Cornblath M and Poth M. (1982). Hypoglycemia. In *Clinical Pediatric and Adolescent Endocrinology*, ed. Kaplan S, pp. 157–170. Philadelphia: W.B. Saunders.

29 DeBaun MR, King AA and White N. (2000). Hypoglycemia in Beckwith–Wiedemann syndrome. *Semin Perinatol*, **24**, 164–171.

30 Cornblath M and Schwartz R. (1993). Hypoglycemia in the neonate. *J Pediatr Endocrinol*, **6**, 113–129.

31 Van Hauthem H, Toppem V and Van Viiet G. (1992). Congenital hypopituitarism: results of pituitary stimulation tests and of magnetic resonance imaging in a newborn girl. *Eur J Pediatr*, **151**, 174–176.

32 Hanna CE, Krainz PL, Skeels MR, et al. (1986). Detection of congenital hypopituitary hypothyroidism: ten-year experience in the Northwest Regional Screening Program. *J Pediatr*, **109**, 959–964.

33 Fisher DA. (1983). Second international conference on neonatal screening: progress report. *J Pediatr*, **102**, 653–654.

34 Patel H, Tze WJ, Crichton JU, et al. (1975). Optic nerve hypoplasia with hypopituitarism. *Am J Dis Child*, **129**, 175–180.

35 Krahe J, Hauffa BP, Wolimann HA, et al. (1992). Transient elevation of urinary catecholamine excretion and cholestatic liver disease in a neonate with hypopituitarism. *J Pediatr Gastroent Nutr*, **14**, 153–159.

36 Graham EA and Hartmann AF. (1934). Subtotal resection of the pancreas for hypoglycemia. *Surg Gynecol Obstet*, **59**, 474–479.

37 Yalow RS and Berson SA. (1960). Immunoassay of endogenous plasma insulin in man. *J Clin Invest*, **39**, 1157–1175.

38 Glaser B, Chin KC, Anker R, et al. (1994). Familial hyperinsulinism maps to chromosome 11p14–15.1. *Nat Gen*, **7**, 185–188.

39 Thomas PM, Cote GJ, Hallman DM, et al. (1995). Homozygosity mapping to chromosome 11p, of the gene for familial persistent hyperinsulinemic hypoglycemia of infancy. *Am J Hum Genet*, **56**, 416–421.

40 Glaser B. (2000). Hyperinsulinism of the newborn. *Semin Perinatol*, **24**, 150–163.

41 Thomas PM, Cote GJ, Wahlick N, et al. (1995). Mutations in the sulfonylurea receptor gene in familial persistent hyperinsulinemic hypoglycemia in infancy. *Science*, **268**, 426–429.

42 Aguilar-Bryan L, Nichols CG, Wechsler SW, et al. (1995). Cloning of the ß cell high affinity sulfonylurea receptor: a regulator of insulin secretion. *Science*, **268**, 423–426.

43 Aparicio L, Carpenter MW, Schwartz R, et al. (1993). Prenatal diagnosis of familial neonatal hyperinsulinemia. *Acta Paediatr Scand*, **82**, 683–686.

44 Wolff FW and Parmeley WW. (1963). Aetiological factors in benzothiadiazine hyperglycemia. *Lancet*, **2**, 69.

45 Glaser B, Hirsch HJ and Landau H. (1993). Persistent hyperinsulinemic hypoglycemia of infancy: long term octreotide treatment without pancreatectomy. *J Pediatr*, **12**, 644–650.

46 Harken AH, Filler RM, AvRuskin TW, et al. (1971). The role of "total" pancreatectomy in the treatment of unremitting hypoglycemia of infancy. *J Pediatr Surg*, **6**, 284–289.

47 deLonlay-Debeney P, Poggi-Travert F, Fournet J-C, et al. (1999). Clinical features of 52 neonates with hyperinsulinism. *N Engl J Med*, **340**, 1169–1175.

48 Menni F, de Lonlay P, Sevin C, et al. (2001). Neurologic outcomes of 90 neonates and infants with persistent hyperinsulinemic hypoglycemia. *Pediatrics*, **108**, 476–479.

49 Thornton PS, Sumner AE, Ruchalli ED, et al. (1991). Familial and sporadic hyperinsulinism histopathologic findings and segregation analysis support a single autosomal recessive disorder. *J Pediatr*, **119**, 721–724.

50 Horev Z, Ipp M, Levey P, et al. (1991). Familial hyperinsulinism: successful conservative management. *J Pediatr*, **119**, 717–720.

51 Thomas CF Jr, Cuenca RE, Azizkhan RC, et al. (1988). Changing concepts of islet cell dysplasia in neonatal and infantile hyperinsulinism. *World J Surg*, **12**, 598–609.

52 Dershewitz R, Vestal B, MacLaren NK, et al. (1976). Transient hepatomegaly and hypoglycemia – a consequence of malicious insulin administration. *Am. J Dis Child*, **130**, 998–999.

53 Schonau E, Deeg KH, Huemmer HP, et al. (1991). Pancreatic growth and function following surgical treatment of nesidioblastosis in infancy. *Eur J Pediatr*, **150**, 550–553.

54 Anderson JM, Milner RDG and Strich SJ. (1967). Effects of neonatal hypoglycaemia on the nervous system: a pathological study. *J Neurol Neurosurg Psychiatry*, **30**, 295–310.

55 Banker BQ. (1967). The neuropathological effects of anoxia and hypoglycaemia in the newborn. *Devel Med Child Neurol*, **9**, 544–550.

56 Volpe JJ. (1987). *Neurology of the Newborn*, 2nd edn. Philadelphia: WB Saunders.

57 Auer RN and Siesjo BK. (1988). Biological differences between ischemia, hypoglycemia and epilepsy. *Ann Neurol*, **24**, 699–708.

58 Siesjo BK. (1988). Hypoglycemia, brain metabolism and brain damage. *Diab Metab Rev*, **4**, 113–144.

59 McGowan JE, Mishra OP, Kubin J, et al. (1995). Alteration of the cerebral kainate receptor during hypoglycemia in newborn piglets. *Pediatr Res*, **37**, abstract 2280.

60 Ichord RN, Northington FJ, Van Wylen DG, et al. (1999). Brain O_2 consumption and glutamate release during hypoglycemic coma in piglets are temperature sensitive. *Am J Physiol*, **276**, H2053–H2062.

61 Vannucci RC and Vannucci SJ. (2000). Glucose metabolism in the developing brain. *Semin Perinatol*, **24**, 107–115.

62 Vannucci RC and Vannucci SJ (1978). Cerebral carbohydrate metabolism during hypoglycemia and anoxia in newborn rats. *Ann Neurol*, **4**, 73–79.

63 Vannucci RC, Nardis EE, Vannucci SJ, et al. (1981). Cerebral carbohydrate and energy metabolism during hypoglycemia in newborn dogs. *Am J Physiol*, **240**, R192–R199.

64 Ruth VJ, Park TS, Gonzales ER, et al. (1993). Adenosine and cerebrovascular hyperemia during insulin-induced hypoglycemia in newborn piglet. *Am J Physiol*, **265**, H1762–H1768.

65 Schrier AM, Wilhelm PB, Church RM, et al. (1990). Neonatal hypoglycemia in the rhesus monkey: effect on development and behavior. *Infant Behav Dev*, **13**, 189–207.

66 Sinclair JC and Bracken MB. (1992). *Effective Care of the Newborn Infant. Part 111. Diseases, Abnormal Glucose Homeostasis.* Oxford: Oxford University Press.

67 Griffiths AD. (1968). Association of hypoglycaemia with symptoms in the newborn. *Arch Dis Child*, **43**, 688–694.

68 Koivisto M, Blanco-Sequerios M and Krause U. (1972). Neonatal symptomatic and asymptomatic hypoglycaemia: a follow-up study of 151 children. *Dev Med Child Neurol*, **14**, 603–614.

69 Pildes RS, Cornblath M, Warren L, et al. (1974). A prospective controlled study of neonatal hypoglycemia. *Pediatrics*, **54**, 5–14.

70 DeVivo DC, Trifiletti RR, Jacobson RI, et al. (1991). Defective glucose transport across the blood–brain barrier as a cause of persistent hypoglycorrhachia, seizures and developmental delay. *N Engl J Med*, **325**, 703–709.

71 Kalhan S and Parimi P. (2000). Gluconeogenesis in the fetus and neonate. *Semin Perinatol*, **24**, 94–106.

72 Gould GW and Bell GI. (1990). Facilitative glucose transporters: an expanding family. *Trends Biomed Sci*, **15**, 18–23.

73 Lane RH, Florzak HS, Ogata ES, et al. (1955). Hepatic glucose transporter gene expression in altered fetal growth. *Pediatr Res*, **37**, abstract 1855.

74 Das UG, Schroeder RE, Hay WW Jr, et al. (1995). Chronic hypoglycemia causes time-dependent and tissue-specific changes in ovine fetal Glut1 and Glut4 proteins. *Pediatr Res*, **37**, abstract 347.

75 Battelino T, Goto M, Topaloglu AK, et al. (1995). Tissue glucose uptake during septic shock in 10 day old rats. *Pediatr Res*, **37**, abstract 238.

76 DeFeo P, Gallai V, Mazzotta G, et al. (1988). Modest decrements in plasma glucose concentration cause early impairment in cognitive function and later activation of glucose counterregulation in the absence of hypoglycemic symptoms in normal man. *J Clin Invest*, **82**, 436–444.

77 Jones TW, McCarthy G, Tamborlane WV, et al. (1990). Mild hypoglycemia and impairment of brain stem and cortical evoked potentials in healthy subjects. *Diabetes*, **39**, 1550–1555.

78 Chugani HT and Phelps ME. (1986). Maturational changes in cerebral function in infants determined by ^{18}FDG positron emission tomography. *Science*, **231**, 840–843.

79 Pryds O, Greisen G and Friis-Hansen B. (1988). Compensatory increase of CBF supports cerebral metabolism in preterm infants during hypoglycemia. *Acta Paediatr Scand*, **77**, 632–637.

80 Pryds O, Christensen NJ and Friis-Hansen B. (1990). Increased cerebral blood flow and plasma epinephrine in hypoglycemic, preterm neonates. *Pediatrics*, **85**,172–176.

81 Kinnala A, Korvenranta H and Parkkola R. (2000). Newer techniques to study neonatal hypoglycemia. *Semin Perinatol*, **24**, 116–119.

82 Skov L and Pryds O. (1992). Capillary recruitment for preservation of cerebral glucose influx in hypoglycemic, preterm newborns: evidence for a glucose sensor? *Pediatrics*, **90**, 193–195.

Hyperbilirubinemia and kernicterus

David K. Stevenson and Phyllis A. Dennery

Stanford University Medical Center, Palo Alto, CA, USA

Introduction

The term "kernicterus" was originally used to describe the deposition of bilirubin in the basal ganglia. It was first described in 1903 by Schmorl.[1] More recently, the term has also been used in reference to the neurological manifestations of hyperbilirubinemia. Another acronym, BIND, has been adopted to describe any bilirubin-induced neurologic dysfunction.[2] Although technically the diagnosis of kernicterus can only be confirmed at autopsy, brain magnetic resonance imaging (MRI) studies may now aid in the confirmation of the diagnosis in a living child with severe jaundice. The MRI signature for kernicterus includes high signal intensity on T1-weighted (T1W) images in the globus pallidus (GP), internal capsule, thalamus, and hippocampi. The associated T2W images have abnormal increased signal in the GP and thalamus in the same regions as the high signal on the T1W images. Loss of demarcation between GP, internal capsule, and the anterior thalamus was the major finding[3] (Figures 27.1 and 27.2). The source of these abnormal signals has not been definitively identified and therefore, the MRI findings should not be considered diagnostic in themselves, but only consistent with the diagnosis of kernicterus in the context of severe neonatal jaundice and the acute clinical features of kernicterus (Table 27.1).

Neonatal jaundice and neurotoxicity

Most often a benign condition, a majority of term neonates develop neonatal jaundice which is a consequence of relatively increased bilirubin production (two- to threefold higher in a neonate compared to an adult) and limited ability to conjugate bilirubin in the transitional time after birth. Compared to healthy term infants, polycythemic infants or babies with hemolysis can produce significantly increased amounts of bilirubin.[4] By convention, a serum bilirubin concentration higher than 17 mg/dl at its peak is considered pathologic. Moreover, there is not any "safe" level of bilirubin that can be universally agreed upon because the level at which neurotoxicity develops and the conditions under which toxicity develops remain incompletely understood. Importantly, BIND, including kernicterus, does not occur in the absence of hyperbilirubinemia. Among the survivors with BIND, the long-term features of kernicterus are listed in Table 27.1. Importantly, each infant may not have all of the features of the syndrome, and the permanent injuries may vary in severity and include subtle neurologic deficits, suggesting that there may be a spectrum of injuries caused specifically by bilirubin.

The topic of bilirubin neurotoxicity has also been reviewed recently by Volpe.[5] That bilirubin is toxic is undisputed, and a variety of cellular toxic effects of bilirubin have been described.[6–9] From a clinical perspective, there are a variety of factors that influence empirically the neurotoxic effects of bilirubin. However, the exact mechanism(s) by which bilirubin injures the brain, and in particular what contributes to injury in an individual infant, is poorly understood.

Most of the experimental work on bilirubin toxicity has been done in vitro. In such systems the

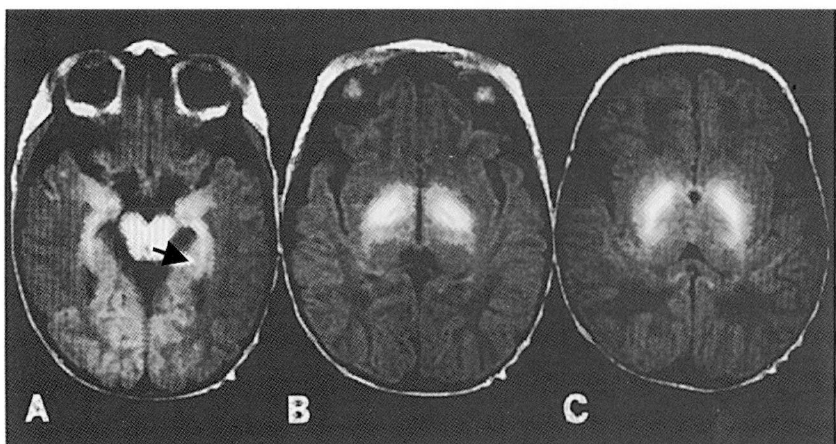

Figure 27.1 Series of three axial T1-weighted (T1W) images showing the following anatomy: (A) the hippocampus and temporal lobe; (B) the basal ganglia and subthalamus; and (C) the lenticular nuclei and thalamus. The major abnormality on these T1W images was the abnormal high signal intensity seen in the hippocampus in the medial temporal lobe (arrow, A). This was confirmed on sagittal images. This abnormal high signal intensity was also noted in the globus pallidus but not the putamen (B, C). The thalamus was less involved, but some increased signal intensity was present in the ventroposterolateral nucleus. The findings were bilateral and symmetrical in these structures and typical of regions of the brain damaged in kernicterus. Source: Reproduced with permission from Penn et al.[3]

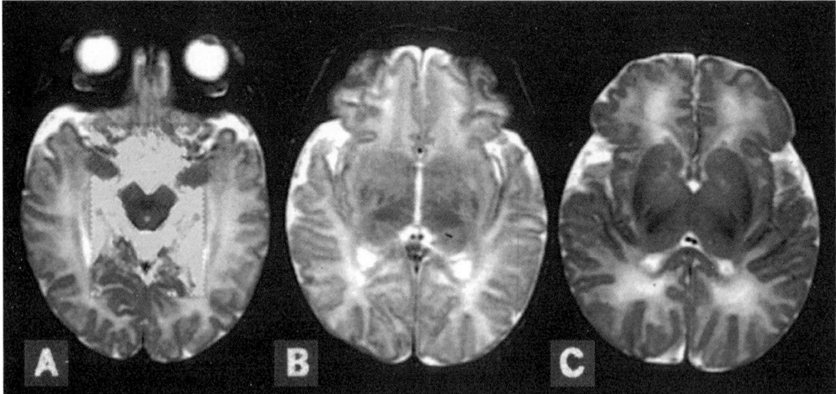

Figure 27.2 T2-weighted images at the same anatomic levels as the T1-weighted (T1W) images shown in Figure 27.1. Findings on these images are more subtle than the T1W abnormalities and are characterized by increased signal intensity in the same regions: the globus pallidus and anterior thalamus are best seen in image C. The basal ganglia abnormality is seen primarily as a loss of demarcation between the globus pallidus, internal capsule, and thalamus. The increased signal in the hippocampi is also subtle and best seen in image A as an area of increased signal intensity paralleling the temporal horn medially. Source: Reproduced with permission from Penn et al.[3]

Table 27.1. Clinical features of bilirubin encephalopathy

Acute	
Phase 1 First 1–2 days	Poor sucking, stupor, hypotania, seizures
Phase 2 Mid first week	Hypertonia of extensor muscles, opisthotonus, retrocollis, fever
Chronic	
First year of life	Hypotonia, active deep tendon reflexes, obligatory tonic neck reflexes, delayed motor skills
After first year	Extrapharyngeal movement abnormalities (choreoathetosis, ballismus, tremors), gaze abnormalities (upward gaze), auditory impairment (sensorineural hearing loss)

Source: Reproduced with permission from Dennery et al.[25]

binding of bilirubin to albumin is a critical phenomenon for understanding bilirubin toxicity.[10,11] However, its relevance to toxicity in intact animals or humans remains uncertain or is not known in most cases.[12] Nothing is known with certainty with respect to where bilirubin acts and how it acts. Overall, the in vitro studies of bilirubin toxicity are inconclusive, and extrapolation to in vivo conditions is uncertain because of confounding uncontrolled factors. Additionally, recent data suggest a beneficial antioxidant role of bilirubin,[13,14] although it is not clear whether this is of physiologic relevance in neonates. Conjugating capacity (hence the ability to excrete bilirubin) probably varies significantly in the general population and is further influenced by genetic conditions like Gilbert syndrome which is associated with a mildly decreased uridine diphosphate glucuronosyl transferase activity, attributed to an expansion of thymine-adenine (TA) repeats in the promoter region of the UG1TA gene, the principal gene in coding this enzyme.[15] There may also be racial variation in the number of TA repeats, thus suggesting a reason for differences in bilirubin metabolism between certain ethnic groups.[16] Recently, a DNA sequence variant (Gly71Arg) has also been associated with decreased uridine diphosphate glucuronosyl transferase activity and neonatal hyperbilirubinemia in Asians.[17] Even more interesting is the potential for gene interaction suggested in a report on glucose-6-phosphate dehydrogenase (G6PD) deficiency and Gilbert's syndrome.[15]

One of the major risk factors for severe neonatal hyperbilirubinemia and kernicterus is severe hemolysis.[18] Under such conditions (Rh disease), a serum bilirubin level of 20 mg/dl or greater has been empirically associated with a risk for neonatal brain injury or death. Thus, "vigintiphobia" has a historical and not a scientific basis, but extrapolation to other hyperbilirubinemic conditions besides Rh disease is not clear.[19] One historical exception to the role of hemolysis in severe hyperbilirubinemia is the clinical experience reported by Silverman et al. in 1956[20] with premature infants treated with sulfisoxazole. This tragedy suggested that great caution should be exercised in using any new drug in a neonate. In fact, all drugs considered for use in neonates should be tested for their capacities to displace bilirubin from albumin in order to avoid history repeating itself. Practically, the prediction of severe jaundice is now possible by combining an hour-specific bilirubin level with an estimate of the degree of bilirubin production with breath carbon monoxide analysis.

Prediction of hyperbilirubinemia

With early discharge, it is often difficult to observe infants long enough to detect pathologic hyperbilirubinemia. Although not perfect, hour-specific bilirubin levels can assist in the prediction of which infants might develop severe neonatal jaundice according to predetermined thresholds.[2] An hour-specific bilirubin level represents the interaction of increased bilirubin load and the ability to excrete the load. Hemolysis can be diagnosed sensitively by estimating bilirubin production noninvasively. Breath carbon monoxide detection (end-tidal measurement of carbon monoxide (CO) corrected for ambient CO

($ETCO_c$)) is a useful technique that has been used experimentally to estimate hemolysis and the risk for hyperbilirubinemia.[21] This early detection tool may help in deciding which infant should be observed more frequently and treated because jaundice associated with hemolysis has represented one of the most common serious threats. The importance of identifying increased bilirubin production as a contributing cause of neonatal jaundice cannot be overemphasized. Empirically, the rate of rise of the bilirubin level serves as a surrogate for this bilirubin load phenomenon. The risk of injury associated with hyperbilirubinemia is dependent upon how much bilirubin gets into tissues. This varies with the capacity to keep bilirubin in circulation (mainly determined by the albumin concentration),[10,22] the amount of bilirubin produced over time relative to what can be eliminated, and the metabolic state of the infant.[8,23] Thus, the bilirubin level by itself may not always reflect the magnitude of risk, but the higher the bilirubin level associated with increased production of the pigment, the higher the risk. An estimate of the magnitude of the bilirubin load using an index of bilirubin production, like exhaled CO, combined with an hour-specific bilirubin level provides even more information about the nature of the infant's transitional hyperbilirubinemia. Such a diagnostic approach could allow clinicians to make better judgments about which infants could be discharged early, which should be followed more closely over the first week of life, and which might require therapy, including home phototherapy. With the burden still on physicians to exclude hemolytic disease for compliance with the practice guideline for management of hyperbilirubinemia in the healthy term newborn, infants who are discharged before 48 h should probably have more than a direct Coombs test in order to determine if they have hemolysis. A positive direct Coombs test does not make this diagnosis. Only 50% of infants with a positive Coombs test actually hemolyze, and up to 25% of those with an ABO blood type incompatibility with their mother and lacking a positive Coombs test will have evidence of hemolysis based on a more sensitive test, the $ETCO_c$.[24]

Management of neonatal hyperbilirubinemia

Neonatal hyperbilirubinemia has been reviewed recently.[25] Moreover, the American Academy of Pediatrics has attempted to address the management of hyperbilirubinemia in the healthy term newborn.[26] However, the latter practice parameter does not apply to term infants with a variety of complicating conditions, and does not apply to near-term (35–37-week gestation) infants or preterm infants. These guidelines have been critiqued, pointing out their important limitations. None the less, until these guidelines are changed, they should be followed with the appropriate exclusions and recommendations for the healthy term newborn. When newborn infants are discharged before the serum bilirubin level is likely to have peaked, the medical responsibility for follow-up of the infant cannot be shifted to the parents without clear recommendations for follow-up by a physician or an appropriately trained individual 2–3 days after discharge.

The practice in many communities suggests that most infants with serum total bilirubin levels between 20 and 25 mg/dl are managed without exchange transfusion, but according to guidelines all should be treated with intense phototherapy. The many nomograms for guiding the decision-making of practitioners with respect to the treatment of hyperbilirubinemia should not be considered irrefutable standards, but rather recommendations for practice that need to be adapted and modified on an individual basis. Furthermore, there is no absolute standard level at which phototherapy should be applied, although the American Academy of Pediatrics recommendations are reasonable in this regard. In premature infants, some investigators have recommended the use of phototherapy at very low bilirubin levels because kernicterus has been diagnosed in such infants at bilirubin levels between 5 and 8 mg/dl.[27] Common sense usually weighs heavily in the decision to start phototherapy in an effort to avoid exchange transfusion – a procedure that carries a small but definite risk. Another factor that needs to be considered is duration of exposure to high serum bilirubin levels and this may also influence the decision to intervene earlier or more aggressively in a context where a level remains high despite intensive phototherapy.

In the presence of hemolysis, a total serum bilirubin level of 20 mg/dl or greater has been associated with an increased risk of neonatal brain injury or death. Therefore, exchange transfusion should be seriously considered in the infant under such circumstances. Exchange transfusion should be considered in any infant with bilirubin levels greater than 25 mg/dl if the bilirubin level does not decrease rapidly under intense phototherapy. An infant with jaundice associated with breast-feeding is a typical example. Such infants should not have markedly increased bilirubin production. However, despite the assumed benign nature of jaundice associated with breast-feeding, some practitioners would recommend exchange transfusion for any infant with a serum total bilirubin level greater than 25 mg/dl that does not respond to intense phototherapy. Moreover, exchange transfusion might be considered at a lower level if the infant were preterm or sick in any way, in particular, if the infant were asphyxiated or infected or had cardiorespiratory or metabolic instability. Infants with bilirubin levels greater than 30 mg/dl should definitely be exchanged if technically possible. Occasionally, an exchange might reasonably be avoided if the bilirubin level dropped dramatically below 25 mg/dl under intense phototherapy while preparing for the exchange. Exchange transfusion can be considered with lower bilirubin in any infant who is sick, in particular if the infant is asphyxiated or infected or has cardiorespiratory or metabolic instability. The use of drugs capable of displacing bilirubin from albumin in general should be avoided in the newborn. The use of intralipid as a continuous infusion at a rate to prevent central fatty acid deficiency is not dangerous, because free fatty acid albumin ratios are not elevated into the range at which displacement of bilirubin from albumin would be expected. Breast-feeding of any infant with a propensity for increased bilirubin production (e.g., bruising, hematoma, prematurity) represents an increased risk for hyperbilirubinemia and warrants close follow-up of the infant throughout the first week and into the second week of life. Early discharge of an infant from the hospital requires that a practitioner follow the American Academy of Pediatrics practice guideline.[26]

Reemergence of kernicterus

In the 1980s and 1990s, kernicterus had become a rare occurrence. However, with discharge from the hospital occurring sooner after birth, the peak of neonatal hyperbilirubinemia more often occurs outside the hospital observed by parents and not by physicians or other trained personnel. Thus, there has been a reemergence of reported kernicterus in the USA and possibly elsewhere.[3,28–31]

There are some particular clinical problems that get practitioners into trouble more often than others. Most of them can be related to the early discharge of infants from the hospital. One example is the breast-feeding infant with increased bilirubin production. The source of the increased bilirubin production may be unrecognized hemolytic disease or simply bruising or hematoma formation. The increased bilirubin production, combined with a lack of a decrease in the enterohepatic circulation, may contribute to a very rapid early rise in the total serum bilirubin level over the first several days of life, which can be missed if the infant is discharged before the time of peak hyperbilirubinemia at approximately 3–4 days. The peak may also be later, as is often the case when increased bilirubin production is a major factor contributing to jaundice or a conjugating defect is present, such as in a certain proportion of Asians.[32,33] Even a large premature or near-term infant who is breast-feeding, and does not have an obvious complication predisposing to increased bilirubin production, may have more difficulty in lowering the bilirubin level and should be followed closely throughout the first 2 weeks of life. Currently, term newborns are rarely seen by a practitioner in this period once discharged from the hospital. This is not a good practice. In hemolytic disease, late anemia is a complication that should also be overlooked once hyperbilirubinemia has been successfully managed. Such anemia may be so severe as to require transfusion by the second to fourth week of life. An estimate of bilirubin production will help in the recognition of this problem in the absence of hyperbilirubinemia.

In summary, kernicterus and BIND are real entities that have been more frequently reported in the last decade due to relaxed vigilance in the treatment of neonatal hyperbilirubinemia. These conditions are easily preventable by the use of predictive tools and aggressive intervention when appropriate.

REFERENCES

1 Schmorl G. (1903). Zur Kenntis des Icterus Neonatorum. *Verh Dtsch Ges Pathol*, **6**, 109.

2 Bhutani VK, Johnson L and Sivieri EM. (1999). Predictive ability of a predischarge hour-specific serum bilirubin for subsequent significant hyperbilirubinemia in healthy term and near-term newborns. *Pediatrics*, **103**, 6–14.

3 Penn AA, Enzmann DR, Hahn JS, et al. (1994). Kernicterus in a full term infant. *Pediatrics*, **93**, 1003–6.

4 Bartoletti AL and Johnson JD. (1977). Carbon monoxide excretion as an index of bilirubin production in newborn infants. *Pediatr Res*, **11**, 531.

5 Volpe JJ. (2000). Bilirubin and brain injury. In *Neurology of the Newborn*, ed. Volpe JJ, 2nd edn, pp. 490–514. Philadelphia, PA: W.B. Saunders.

6 Amato M. (1995). Mechanisms of bilirubin toxicity. *Eur J Pediatr*, **154**, S54–9.

7 Amit Y, Chan G, Fedunec S, et al. (1989). Bilirubin toxicity in a neuroblastoma cell line N-115: I. Effects on Na^+K^+ ATPase, $[^3H]$-thymidine uptake, L-$[^{35}S]$-methionine incorporation, and mitochondrial function. *Pediatr Res*, **25**, 364–8.

8 Wennberg RP, Gospe S Jr, Rhine WD, et al. (1993). Brainstem bilirubin toxicity in the newborn primate may be promoted and reversed by modulating $P\text{CO}_2$. *Pediatr Res*, **34**, 6–9.

9 Wennberg RP. (1991). Cellular basis of bilirubin toxicity (see comments). *N Y State J Med*, **91**, 493–6.

10 Ahlfors CE. (2000). Measurement of plasma unbound unconjugated bilirubin. *Anal Biochem*, **279**, 130–5.

11 Ahlfors CE. (2000). Unbound bilirubin associated with kernicterus: a historical approach. *J Pediatr*, **137**, 540–4.

12 Levine RL, Fredericks WR and Rapoport SI. (1985). Clearance of bilirubin from rat brain after reversible osmotic opening of the blood brain barrier. *Pediatr Res*, **19**, 1040–3.

13 Stocker R, Yamamoto Y, McDonagh AF, et al. (1987). Bilirubin is an antioxidant of possible physiological importance. *Science*, **235**, 1043–6.

14 Dennery PA, McDonagh AF, Spitz DR, et al. (1995). Hyperbilirubinemia results in reduced oxidative injury in neonatal Gunn rats exposed to hyperoxia. *Free Rad Biol Med*, **19**, 395–404.

15 Kaplan M, Renbaum P, Levy-Lahad E, et al. (1997). Gilbert syndrome and glucose-6-phosphate dehydrogenase deficiency: a dose-dependent genetic interaction crucial to neonatal hyperbilirubinemia. *Proc Natl Acad Sci USA*, **94**, 12128–32.

16 Beutler E, Gelbart T and Demina A. (1998). Racial variability in the UDP-glucuronosyltransferase 1 (UGT1A1) promoter: a balanced polymorphism for regulation of bilirubin metabolism? *Proc Natl Acad Sci USA*, **95**, 8170–4.

17 Akaba K, Kimura T, Sasaki A, et al. (1998). Neonatal hyperbilirubinemia and mutation of the bilirubin uridine diphosphate-glucuronosyltransferase gene: a common missense mutation among Japanese, Koreans and Chinese. *Biochem Mol Biol Int*, **46**, 21–6.

18 Mollison PL and Cutbush M. (1954). Haemolytic disease of the newborn. In *Recent Advances in Pediatrics*, ed. Gairdner D, p. 110. New York: Blakinston.

19 Watchko JF and Oksi FA. (1983). Bilirubin 20 mg/dl = vigintiphobia. *Pediatrics*, **71**, 660–3.

20 Silverman WA, Anderson DH, Blanc WA, et al. (1956). A difference in mortality rate and incidence of kernicterus among premature infants alloted to two prophylactic antibiotic regimens. *Pediatrics*, **18**, 614–26.

21 Vreman HJ, Stevenson DK, Oh W, et al. (1994). Semiportable electrochemical instrument for determining carbon monoxide in breath. *Clin Chem*, **40**, 1927–33.

22 Brodersen R and Stern L. (1990). Deposition of bilirubin acid in the central nervous system – a hypothesis for the development of kernicterus. *Acta Paediatr Scand*, **79**, 12–19.

23 Bratlid D, Cashore WJ and Oh W. (1984). Effects of acidosis on bilirubin deposition in rat brain. *Pediatrics*, **73**, 431–4.

24 Stevenson DK, Vreman HJ, Oh W, et al. (1994). Bilirubin production in healthy term infants as measured by carbon monoxide in breath. *Clin Chem*, **40**, 1934–9.

25 Dennery PA, Seidman DS and Stevenson DK. (2001). Neonatal hyperbilirubinemia. *N Engl J Med*, **344**, 581–90.

26 American Academy of Pediatrics. Provisional Committee for Quality Improvement and Subcommittee on Hyperbilirubinemia. (1994). Practice parameter: management of hyperbilirubinemia in the healthy term newborn. *Pediatrics*, **94**, 558–65.

27 Gartner LM, Snyder RN, Chabon RS, et al. (1970).

Kernicterus: high incidence in premature infants with low serum bilirubin concentrations. *Pediatrics*, **45**, 906–17.

28 Perlman JM, Rogers BB and Burns D. (1997). Kernicteric findings at autopsy in two sick near term infants. *Pediatrics*, **99**, 612–15.

29 Newman TB and Maisels MJ. (2000). Less aggressive treatment of neonatal jaundice and reports of kernicterus: lessons about practice guidelines. *Pediatrics*, **105**, 242–5.

30 Johnson L and Brown A. (1999). A pilot registry for acute and chronic kernicterus in term and near-term infants. *Pediatrics*, **104**, 736.

31 Maisels MJ and Newman TB. (1995). Kernicterus in otherwise healthy, breast-fed term newborns. *Pediatrics*, **96**, 730–3.

32 Fischer AF, Nakamura H, Uetani Y, et al. (1988). Comparison of bilirubin production in Japanese and Caucasian infants. *J Pediatr Gastroenterol Nutr*, **7**, 27–9.

33 Stevenson DK, Vreman HJ, Oh W, et al. (1994). Bilirubin production in healthy term infants as measured by carbon monoxide in breath. *Clin Chem*, **40**, 1934–9.

28

Polycythemia

Ted S. Rosenkrantz[1] and William Oh[2]

[1]*University of Connecticut Health Center, Farmington, CT, USA*
[2]*Department of Pediatrics, Brown University, Providence, RI, USA*

Introduction

Polycythemia and hyperviscosity were first associated with adverse neurologic events and sequelae in a series of case reports. The first case often referenced was published by Wood in 1952[1] and was followed by a small series of infants with polycythemia and hyperviscosity who displayed multiple problems, including cerebral dysfunction.[2–5] Since those early reports it has become clear that polycythemia has multiple etiologies which influence whether and which problems may be associated with it in the newborn period. In addition more recent animal and human studies have clarified the relationship between polycythemia and alterations in function of various organs.[6–33]

Definition

Polycythemia is usually defined in the literature as a hematocrit value ≥ 65% when the blood sample is obtained from a free-flowing, large venous blood vessel such as the inferior vena cava (umbilical vein sample) spun in a centrifuge.[34] Sampling from small vessels with low flow or capillary samples will have higher values. In addition, hematocrits calculated by a Coulter counter will yield comparatively lower values.[35–37] Independent of sample site or measurement technique, the hematocrit increases over the first 2–4 h of life, gradually returning to the birth value by 12–24 h of age.[34,38,39]

Incidence

The incidence of polycythemia varies by definition, altitude of the population, pregnancy risk factors, and techniques involved in the delivery of the fetus, and timing and sampling sites of blood samples. Studies by Wirth et al. have demonstrated that higher altitude is associated with a higher incidence of polycythemia in the general newborn population. At sea level the incidence is 1–2% while at 1600 ft (430 m), it has been documented to be 5%.[40,41]

Causes of polycythemia

A number of fetal and birth complications are known to increase the hematocrit. These problems can usually be attributed to acute or chronic fetal hypoxia, or placental transfusion due to delayed clamping of the umbilical cord (Table 28.1).[2,6,41–54]

Effects of increased hematocrit on organ blood flow and function

Using in vitro techniques, increases in hematocrit are associated with increases in whole-blood viscosity.[55,56] This observation led many to believe that very high hematocrit levels would be associated with decreased organ blood flow, particularly in the brain. It has been hypothesized that this reduction in blood flow would lead to organ hypoxia and damage. A detailed examination of the data from

Table 28.1. Etiologies and high-risk groups

Delayed cord clamping
Acute hypoxia
Meconium-stained infants
Postterm infants
Chronic hypoxia
Placental insufficiency
Infants of diabetic mothers
Large-for-gestational age infants
Twin-to-twin transfusion
Other
Trisomy 21
Beckwith–Wiedemann syndrome
Fetal/neonatal hyperthyroidism

several sources will clarify the relationship between hematocrit, blood viscosity, organ blood flow, and oxygenation.

Viscosity

Fluids can be categorized as newtonian and non-newtonian.[57,58] Blood is a nonhomogeneous, non-newtonian fluid. This means that there is not a reciprocal relationship between shear stress and shear rate as with newtonian fluids such as water.[57–59] There are numerous factors that affect whole-blood viscosity, including pH, plasma protein concentration, red cell deformity, white blood cell, fibrinogen, and platelet concentration, blood vessel diameter, and blood velocity.[14,56,60–66] However, in the newborn, the single most important factor is red cell concentration or hematocrit. When measured in vitro by a Wells viscometer, blood viscosity will increase as hematocrit increases.[60] In the newborn the increase becomes exponential at hematocrit values ≥ 65%. However, in small tubes and the capillaries, blood viscosity becomes similar to the viscosity of the plasma, independent of the hematocrit.[58,59,67,68] This suggests that changes in organ blood flow are not likely to be affected by hematocrit alone or blood viscosity as determined by in vitro techniques.

Relationship between polycythemia, blood viscosity, and organ oxygenation

Based on the stipulation that polycythemia is associated with an increase in blood viscosity that results in decreased blood flow, many individuals have assumed that polycythemia and hyperviscosity result in organ – particularly brain – ischemia and hypoxia. However, a series of experiments performed between 1980 and 1995 have now clarified the changes in blood flow, oxygen delivery, and utilization of the brain of the newborn with polycythemia.

Since Wood's first report, it has been assumed that infants with polycythemia had a reduction of brain blood flow due to sludging of red blood cells within the small blood vessels and capillaries of the brain. Utilizing Doppler techniques, we demonstrated that infants with polycythemia did have a reduction in brain blood flow that returned to normal baseline values following a partial exchange transfusion to reduce the hematocrit.[9] In order to understand the factors that were responsible for the reduction of brain blood flow, our group studied a series of newborn lambs in which hematocrit, whole blood viscosity, and arterial oxygen content were independently varied.[19] The data demonstrated that the changes in brain blood flow were due to changes in oxygen content which change in parallel with the changes in the hematocrit in the newborn. This is a normal physiologic response. Viscosity did not influence brain blood flow in this study. This finding has been confirmed by others.[69] Additional studies found that the usual reciprocal relationship between arterial oxygen content and brain blood flow which results in a consistent delivery of oxygen to the brain existed in conditions of increased hematocrit.[18,20,70,71] Further, brain uptake of oxygen was unaffected by polycythemia. These data strongly suggest that the elevated hematocrit alone cannot account for the neurologic abnormalities observed in infants with polycythemia and hyperviscosity.

Blood flow and functional changes in other organs related to increases in hematocrit

As noted, there are numerous signs and symptoms attributed to polycythemia. These are listed in Table 28.2. Cardiac output, as reflected clinically by heart rate, is decreased.[7,9,72,73] Systemic oxygen delivery is normal due to the reciprocal relationship between increased arterial oxygen content and cardiac output. Systemic blood pressure is not affected by polycythemia. Respiratory distress and cyanosis are likely due to decreased pulmonary blood flow.[10,21,74] Decreased pulmonary blood flow and increased pulmonary vascular resistance associated with shunting have been documented in human and animal investigations. Feeding intolerance, as evidenced by poor suck and oral feeding, is probably due to neurologic dysfunction.[75] On the other hand there is an increased risk of lower gastrointestinal dysfunction, including ileus and necrotizing enterocolitis.[7,10,23,24,76–79] Nowicki et al. have documented changes in gastrointestinal blood flow and oxygen delivery and utilization in the unfed and fed state.[7] A study by Black et al. has suggested that partial exchange transfusion may contribute significantly to the development of necrotizing enterocolitis.[24] Renal function is compromised, as evidenced by a decreased renal plasma flow and glomerular filtration rate, and decreased urine output in those infants with normovolemic polycythemia.[13] Newborn infants with polycythemia are at increased risk for hypoglycemia.[26,27] It is not clear whether this is due to decreased gluconeogenesis or increased glucose utilization. Of concern is the finding that cerebral glucose delivery and uptake at whole blood or plasma glucose concentrations are somewhat greater than concentrations that are generally accepted as normal.[71] This is due to the fact that glucose only exists in the plasma fraction of the blood. This fraction is reduced in polycythemia. Therefore the glucose-carrying capacity of the blood is reduced. When taken in combination with the decreased cerebral blood and plasma flow, cerebral glucose delivery, the limiting determinant of cerebral glucose uptake, reaches its lower limit for normal cerebral glucose uptake at higher concentrations of glucose compared to normal infants. This may have some implication for impaired cerebral function in infants with polycythemia.

Table 28.2. Signs and symptoms associated with polycythemia

Cyanosis
Plethora
Tremulousness/jitteriness
Seizures
Respiratory distress
Cardiomegaly
Lethargy
Poor suck and feeding
Hyperbilirubinemia
Thrombocytopenia
Hypoglycemia
Hypocalcemia

Effects of polycythemia on neurologic function

Information about neurologic function is limited by study design and selection process for subjects. A number of studies have examined neurologic function in the newborn period while others have concentrated on long-term development outcome. Of those examining symptomatic newborns, only two studies have been prospective and randomized. To date, there are no controlled randomized studies of asymptomatic polycythemic infants to determine their long-term neurologic outcome with reference to treatment. However, as cited in the discussion below, some of the studies, such as those by Bada et al.[75] and Høst and Ulrich,[79] included asymptomatic infants as well as those exhibiting sign and symptoms that are associated with polycythemia.

Symptomatic infants

Problems in the newborn period

Symptoms associated with polycythemia are listed in Table 28.2.[5,76,77,80] The first controlled study of symptomatic infants and the effects of a partial exchange transfusion to reduce the hematocrit were reported by Goldberg et al.[77] Prechtl and Brazelton examinations were initially abnormal in the polycythemic population compared to control infants. Normalization of these examinations in the polycythemic infants who received therapy to reduce the hematocrit was not accelerated. Van der Elst et al. performed a study of similar design in which the Brazelton score alone was used to evaluate the infants.[78] While the polycythemic infants were different from control infants, again, therapy to reduce the hematocrit did not alter outcome in the newborn period.

There have been some studies that have specifically examined the outcome of small-for-gestational-age infants. As a group, the small-for-gestational-age infants have an increased incidence of polycythemia and an outcome that is inferior to those infants who have normal intrauterine growth.[52,81] Polycythemia, likely a compensatory mechanism for chronic hypoxia, does not appear to be an independent factor in the outcome of this group of infants.[53,75]

Long-term sequalae

Goldberg et al. were able to reexamine a subset of the original study population at 8 months of age.[77] Abnormalities were found in 67% of the infants treated with partial exchange transfusion, 50% of the untreated infants, and 17% of the control infants. These findings are in contrast to those of van der Elst et al., who found that all of the infants had normal neurologic examinations.[78] There were no differences in the developmental scores of the three groups.

Black et al. have performed two studies to determine the long-term outcome of infants with polycythemia. In the first study 111 infants with polycythemia and 110 control infants were studied.[80] The infants with polycythemia were not randomized as to observation or treatment. Follow-up examinations were performed between 1 and 3 years of age. Control infants had fewer abnormalities compared to the polycythemia group. The polycythemic infants were characterized by a 25% incidence of motor abnormalities, especially spastic diplegia. Forty percent had some type of handicap. However, there were no differences in outcome when the two subsets of polycythemic infants (observed vs treated) were compared.

In 1985 Black and colleagues published data on a group of 93 infants with polycythemia who were randomized to treatment or observation.[82] The total population included infants who were symptomatic and asymptomatic in the newborn period. At 1 year 59% of the infants were available for follow-up and no differences between the groups were found. At 2 years 61% of the original group was examined and the treated group had fewer abnormalities. This same group was called back again at school age (7 years of age).[83] At that time only 49 of the original 93 infants were available for evaluation. Significant differences between the control and polycythemic infants persisted. However, the observed and treated polycythemic groups were virtually identical.

Høst and Ulrich revealed the outcome of 635 infants as part of a public health project.[79] Screening in the newborn period revealed that 117 (18%) had venous hematocrit >60%, 30 (4.7%) had hematocrit >65%, and seven had hematocrit greater than 70%. Only 13 had any symptomatology that could be ascribed to polycythemia. None received an exchange transfusion to reduce the hematocrit. Over 80% of the infants were available for follow-up at age 6 years. Of those restudied, 104 of 113 polycythemic infants were normal. The remainder had minor problems, such as febrile convulsions, that could not be attributed to polycythemia in the newborn period.

Lastly, Bada et al. examined a group of infants with asymptomatic and symptomatic polycythemia and a control group of infants.[75] Follow-up at 30 months of age revealed no differences between the three groups of infants. However, when multivariant analysis was performed using multiple perinatal factors, it became clear that these other perinatal risk factors were highly related to outcome in all groups of infants and polycythemia fell out as a nonsignificant factor.

When the results of these studies are taken together with our current knowledge of adaptive fetal physiology, several conclusions can be made. First, polycythemia appears to be an adaptive mechanism for chronic and acute fetal hypoxia. Hypoxia alone is known to be responsible for irreversible brain injury. Second, exchange transfusion does not appear to have an appreciable influence on the long-term neurologic function of infants with elevated hematocrits at birth, although the polycythemia is clearly a marker for increased risk of cerebral dysfunction. The demographic data from the studies of Black et al. and Bada et al. clearly indicate that these infants, particularly those who are symptomatic in the newborn period and in later life, are those infants that experience an adverse fetal environment.[75,82,83] Therefore it would appear that the events, particularly hypoxia–ischemic events, that result in an increase in hematocrit, are likely to be responsible for the observed cerebral dysfunction. This would explain the failure of postnatal reduction of the hematocrit to alter the long-term prognosis.

Asymptomatic infants

There are still institutions that screen either all or high-risk infants for polycythemia. There are no large population studies of the long-term outcome of this type of population. Based on the findings in the studies cited in the preceding section, these infants may be at some nonquantifiable increased risk for long-term sequelae; however, current data strongly suggest that there is no evidence that an exchange transfusion to reduce the hematocrit will change the outcome, as these sequelae appear to be due to other adverse perinatal events.

Recommendations for therapy

Partial exchange transfusion may be of benefit for those infants who exhibit signs and symptoms or complications that have been demonstrated to be related to physiologic abnormalities caused by polycythemia. Such manifestations or clinical conditions include respiratory distress with cyanosis, renal failure, and hypoglycemia. Before considering therapy, the infant should be evaluated for other temporal and clinical events which may, in fact, be responsible for the problems observed. A partial exchange transfusion should not be done in the hope of correcting neurologic abnormalities in the immediate newborn period or preventing future neurologic dysfunction.

As there are no adequate scientific data to demonstrate any benefit for polycythemic infants who are asymptomatic in the newborn period, simple observation alone would seem prudent. In situations when there are subtle signs and symptoms or in the presence of an extremely high hematocrit (e.g. >70%), the decision to perform a partial exchange transfusion may be initiated on individual clinical judgment based on the level of hematocrit, certainty of interpreting clinical symptoms, and the potential risk of the treatment (partial exchange transfusion). For those who develop neurologic abnormalities at a later time, the events during the prenatal and perinatal period should be examined carefully to verify an etiology, other than polycythemia, that might explain the cerebral dysfunction.

Summary

This chapter was originally written 6 years ago. Since that time there have been no new studies or follow-up data available on patients from the studies that have been cited in the body of this chapter. As such, our previous thoughts on the effects of polycythemia and the newborn have not changed. The data do not support a direct relationship between polycythemia and neurologic dysfunction. Polycythemia appears to be a marker for adverse prenatal and perinatal events that are known to cause mild to catastrophic neurologic injury. Postnatal exchange transfusion has not been shown to be of long-term benefit to infants who are symptomatic in the newborn period. There are no data to support the efficacy of this therapy in the infant with an elevated hematocrit and who is otherwise normal.

REFERENCES

1 Wood JL. (1952). Plethora in the newborn infant associated with cyanosis and convulsions. *J Pediatr*, **54**, 143–151.

2 Michael A and Mauer AM. (1961). Maternal–fetal transfusion as a cause of plethora in the neonatal period. *Pediatrics*, **28**, 458–461.

3 Minkowski A. (1962). Acute cardiac failure in connection with neonatal polycythemia in monovular twins and single newborn infants. *Biol Neonate*, **4**, 61–74.

4 Danks DM and Stevens LH. (1964). Neonatal respiratory distress with a high hematocrit. *Lancet*, **2**, 499–500.

5 Gross CP, Hathaway WE and McCaughey HR. (1973). Hyperviscosity in the neonate. *J Pediatr*, **82**, 1004–1012.

6 Oh W, Oh MA and Lind J. (1966). Renal function and blood volume in newborn infants related to placental transfusion. *Acta Paediatr Scand*, **56**, 197–210.

7 Nowicki P, Oh W, Yao A, et al. (1984). Effect of polycythemia on gastrointestinal blood flow and oxygenation in piglets. *Am J Physiol*, **247** (*Gastrointest. Liver Physiol.* **10**), G220–G225.

8 Surjadhana A, Rouleau J, Boerboom L, et al. (1978). Myocardial blood flow and its distribution in anesthetized polycythemic dogs. *Circ Res*, **43**, 619–631.

9 Rosenkrantz TS and Oh W. (1982). Cerebral blood flow velocity in infants with polycythemia and hyperviscosity: effects of partial exchange transfusion with plasmanate. *J Pediatr*, **101**, 94–98.

10 Fouron JC and Hebert F. (1973). The circulatory effects of hematocrit variations in normovolemic newborn lambs. *J Pediatr*, **82**, 995–1003.

11 Gatti RA, Muster AJ, Cole RB, et al. (1966). Neonatal polycythemia with transient cyanosis and cardiorespiratory abnormalities. *J Pediatr*, **69**, 1063–1072.

12 Kotagal VR, Keenan WJ, Reuter JH, et al. (1977). Regional blood flow in polycythemia and hypervolemia. *Pediatr Res*, **11**, 394.

13 Kotagal VR and Kleinman LI. (1982). Effect of acute polycythemia on newborn renal hemodynamics and function. *Pediatr Res*, **16**, 148–151.

14 Bergqvist G and Zetterman R. (1974). Blood viscosity and peripheral circulation in newborn infants. *Acta Paediatr Scand*, **63**, 865–868.

15 Linderkamp O, Strohhacker I, Versmold HT, et al. (1978). Peripheral circulation in the newborn: interaction of peripheral blood flow, blood pressure, blood volume and blood viscosity. *J Pediatr*, **129**, 73–81.

16 Gustafsson L, Applegren L and Myrvold HE. (1980). The effect of polycythemia on blood flow in working and non-working skeletal muscle. *Acta Physiol Scand*, **109**, 143–148.

17 Waffarn F, Cole CD and Huxtable RF. (1984). Effects of polycythemia on cutaneous blood flow and transcutaneous po_2 and pco_2 in the hyperviscosity neonate. *Pediatrics*, **74**, 389–394.

18 Jones MD, Traystman RJ, Simmons MA, et al. (1981). Effects of changes in arterial O_2 content on cerebral blood flow in the lamb. *Am J Physiol*, **240** (*Heart Circ. Physiol.* **9**), H209–H215.

19 Rosenkrantz TS, Stonestreet BS, Hansen NB, et al. (1984). Cerebral blood flow in the newborn lamb with polycythemia and hyperviscosity. *J Pediatr*, **104**, 276–280.

20 Rosenkrantz TS, Philipps AF, Skrzypczak PS, et al. (1988). Cerebral metabolism in the newborn lamb with polycythemia. *Pediatr Res*, **23**, 329–333.

21 Oh W, Wallgren G, Hanson JS, et al. (1967). The effects of placental transfusion on respiratory mechanics of normal term newborn infants. *Pediatrics*, **40**, 6–12.

22 Hakanson DO and Oh W. (1977). Necrotizing enterocolitis and hyperviscosity in the newborn infant. *J Pediatr*, **90**, 458–461.

23 LeBlanc MH, D'Cruz C and Pate K. (1984). Necrotizing enterocolitis can be caused by polycythemic hyperviscosity in the newborn dog. *J Pediatr*, **105**, 804–809.

24 Black VD, Rumack CM, Lubchenco LO, et al. (1985). Gastrointestinal injury in polycythemic term infants. *Pediatrics*, **76**, 225–231.

25 Herson VC, Raye JR, Rowe JC, et al. (1982). Acute renal failure associated with polycythemia in a neonate. *J Pediatr*, **100**, 137–139.

26 Leake RD, Chan GM, Zakauddin S, et al. (1980). Glucose perturbation in experimental hyperviscosity. *Pediatr Res*, **14**, 1320–1323.

27 Creswell JS, Warburton D, Susa JB, et al. (1981). Hyperviscosity in the newborn lamb produces perturbation in glucose homeostasis. *Pediatrics*, **15**, 1348–1350.

28 Rivers RPA. (1975). Coagulation changes associated with a high haematocrit in the newborn infant. *Acta Paediatr Scand*, **64**, 449–456.

29 Katz J, Rodriquez E, Mandani G, et al. (1982). Normal coagulation findings, thrombocytopenia, and peripheral hemoconcentration in neonatal polycythemia. *J Pediatr*, **101**, 99–102.

30 Henriksson P. (1979). Hyperviscosity of the blood and haemostasis in the newborn infant. *Acta Paediatr Scand*, **68**, 701–704.

31 Shaikh BS and Erslev AJ. (1978). Thrombocytopenia in polycythemic mice. *J Lab Clin Med*, **92**, 765–771.

32 Jackson CW, Smith PJ, Edwards CC, et al. (1979). Relationship between packed cell volume platelets and

platelet survival in red blood cell-hypertransfused mice. *J Lab Clin Med*, **94**, 500–509.

33 Meberg A. (1980). Transitory thrombocytopenia in newborn mice after intrauterine hypoxia. *Pediatr Res*, **14**, 1071–1073.

34 Rosenkrantz TS and Oh W. (1986). Neonatal polycythemia and hyperviscosity. In *Advances in Perinatal Medicine*, vol. 5, eds. A Milunsky, EA Friedman and L Gluck, pp. 93–123. New York: Plenum Medical Book.

35 Cornbleet J. (1983). Spurious results from automated hematology cell counters. *Lab Med*, **14**, 509–514.

36 Penn D, Williams PR, Dutcher TF, et al. (1979). Comparison of hematocrit determination by microhematocrit electronic particle counter. *Am J Clin Pathol*, **72**, 71–74.

37 Pearson TC and Guthrie L. (1982). Trapped plasma in the microhematocrit. *Am J Clin Pathol*, **78**, 770–772.

38 Oh W and Lind J. (1966). Venous and capillary hematocrit in newborn infants and placental transfusion. *Acta Paediatr Scand*, **55**, 38–40.

39 Shohat M, Reisner SH, Mimouni F, et al. (1984). Neonatal polycythemia. II. Definition related to time of sampling. *Pediatrics*, **73**, 11–13.

40 Wirth FH, Goldberg KE and Lubchenco LO. (1979). Neonatal hyperviscosity I. Incidence. *Pediatrics*, **63**, 833–836.

41 Stevens K and Wirth FH. (1980). Incidence of neonatal hyperviscosity at sea level. *J Pediatr*, **97**, 118–119.

42 Oh W, Blankenship W and Lind J. (1966). Further study of neonatal blood volume in relation to placental transfusion. *Ann Paediatr*, **207**, 147–159.

43 Yao AC, Moinian M and Lind J. (1969). Distribution of blood between infants and placenta after birth. *Lancet*, **2**, 871–873.

44 Linderkamp O. (1981). Placental transfusion: determinants and effects. *Clin Perinatol*, 9, 559–592.

45 Saigal S and Usher RH. (1977). Symptomatic neonatal plethora. *Biol Neonate*, **32**, 62–72.

46 Philip AGS, Yee AB, Rosy M, et al. (1969). Placental transfusion as an intrauterine phenomenon in deliveries complicated by fetal distress. *Br Med J*, **2**, 11–13.

47 Flod NE and Ackerman BD. (1971). Perinatal asphyxia and residual placenta blood volume. *Acta Paediatr Scand*, **60**, 433–436.

48 Yao AC and Lind J. (1969). Effect of gravity on placental transfusion. *Lancet*, **2**, 505–508.

49 Oh W, Omori K, Emmanouilides GC, et al. (1975). Placenta to lamb fetus transfusion in utero during acute hypoxia. *Am J Obstet Gynecol*, **122**, 316–321.

50 Sacks MO. (1959). Occurrence of anemia and polycythemia in phenotypically dissimilar single ovum human twins. *Pediatrics*, **24**, 604–608.

51 Schwartz JL, Maniscalco WM, Lane AT, et al. (1984). Twin transfusion syndrome causing cutaneous erythropoiesis. *Pediatrics*, **74**, 527–529.

52 Humbert JR, Abelson H, Hathaway WE, et al. (1969). Polycythemia in small for gestational age infants. *J Pediatr*, **75**, 812–819.

53 Widness JA, Garcia JA, Oh W, et al. (1982). Cord serum erythropoietin values and disappearance rates after birth in polycythemic newborns. *Pediatr Res*, **16**, 218A.

54 Philipps AF, Dubin JW, Matty PJ, et al. (1982). Arterial hypoxemia and hyperinsulinemia in the chronically hyperglycemic fetal lamb. *Pediatr Res*, **16**, 653–658.

55 Wells RE, Penton R and Merrill EW. (1961). Measurements of viscosity of biologic fluids by core plate viscometer. *J Lab Clin Med*, **57**, 646–656.

56 Linderkamp O, Versmold HT, Riegel KP, et al. (1984). Contributions of red cells and plasma to blood viscosity in preterm and full-term infants and adults. *Pediatrics*, **74**, 45–51.

57 Poiseuille JLM. (1840). Recherches expérimentales sur le mouvement des liquides dans les tubes de très petits diameters. *C R Acad Sci*, **11**, 961–1041.

58 van der Elst CW, Malan AF and de v. Heese H. (1977). Blood viscosity in modern medicine. *S Afr Med J*, **52**, 526–528.

59 Dintenfass L. (1968). Blood viscosity, internal fluidity of the red cell, dynamic coagulation and the critical capillary radius as factors in the physiology and pathology of circulation and microcirculation. *Med J Aust*, **1**, 688–696.

60 Wells RE and Merrill EW. (1962). Influence of flow properties of blood upon viscosity–hematocrit relationships. *J Clin Invest*, **41**, 1591–1598.

61 Bergqvist G. (1974). Viscosity of the blood in the newborn infants. *Acta Paediatr Scand*, **63**, 858–864.

62 Wells R. (1970). Syndromes of hyperviscosity. *N Engl J Med*, **283**, 183–186.

63 Smith CM, Prasler WJ, Tukey DP, et al. (1981). Fetal red cells are more deformable than adult red cells. *Blood*, **58**, 35a.

64 Lichtman MA. (1970). Cellular deformability during maturation of the myeloblast. Possible role in marrow egress. *N Engl J Med*, **283**, 943–948.

65 Lichtman MA. (1973). Rheology of leukocytes, leukocyte suspensions, and blood in leukemia. *J Clin Invest*, **52**, 350.

66 Miller ME. (1975). Developmental maturation of human neutrophil motility and its relationship to membrane deformability. In *The Phagocytic Cell in Host Resistance*, eds. UA Bellanti and DH Dayton, p. 295. New York: Raven Press.

67 Burton AC. (1966). Role of geometry, of size and shape, in the microcirculation. *Fed Proc*, **25**, 1753–1760.

68 Fahraeus R and Lindqvist T. (1931). The viscosity of the blood in narrow capillary tubes. *Am J Physiol*, **96**, 561–568.

69 Goldstein M, Stonestreet BS, Brann BS 4th, et al. (1988). Cerebral cortical blood flow and oxygen metabolism in normocythemic hyperviscous newborn piglets. *Pediatr Res*, **24**, 486–489.

70 Massik J, Tang YL, Hudak ML, et al. (1987). Effect of hematocrit on cerebral blood flow with induced polycythemia. *J Appl Physiol*, **62**, 1090–1096.

71 Rosenkrantz TS, Philipps AF, Knox I, et al. (1992). Regulation of cerebral glucose metabolism in normal and polycythemic newborns. *J Cereb Blood Flow Metab*, **12**, 856–865.

72 LeBlanc MH, Kotagal UR and Kleinman LI. (1982). Physiological effects of hypervolemic polycythemia in newborn dogs. *J Appl Physiol: Respir Environ Exercise Physiol*, **53**, 865–872.

73 Murphy DJ Jr, Reller MD, Meyer RA, et al. (1985). Effects of neonatal polycythemia and partial exchange transfusion on cardiac function: an echocardiographic study. *Pediatrics*, **76**, 909–913.

74 Brashear RE. (1980). Effects of acute plasma for blood exchange in experimental polycythemia. *Respiration*, **40**, 297–306.

75 Bada HS, Korones SB, Pourcyrous M, et al. (1992). Asymptomatic syndrome of polycythemic hyperviscosity: effect of partial plasma exchange transfusion. *J Pediatr*, **120**, 579–585.

76 Ramamurthy RS and Brans YW. (1981). Neonatal polycythemia. I. Criteria for diagnosis and treatment. *Pediatrics*, **68**, 168–174.

77 Goldberg K, Wirth FH, Hathaway WE, et al. (1982). Neonatal hyperviscosity. II. Effect of partial plasma exchange transfusion. *Pediatrics*, **69**, 419–425.

78 van der Elst, CW, Molteno CD, Malan AF, et al. (1980). The management of polycythemia in the newborn infant. *Early Hum Dev*, **4**, 393–403.

79 Høst A and Ulrich M. (1982). Late prognosis in untreated neonatal polycythemia with minor or no symptoms. *Acta Paediatr Scand*, **71**, 629–633.

80 Black VD, Lubchenco LD, Luckey DW, et al. (1982). Developmental and neurologic sequelae of neonatal hyperviscosity syndrome. *Pediatrics*, **69**, 426–431.

81 Hakanson DO and Oh W. (1980). Hyperviscosity in the small-for-gestational age infant. *Biol Neonate*, **37**, 109–112.

82 Black VD, Lubchenco LO, Koops BL, et al. (1985). Neonatal hyperviscosity: randomized study of effect of partial plasma exchange on long-term outcome. *Pediatrics*, **75**, 1048–1053.

83 Black VD, Camp BW, Lubchenco LO, et al. (1988). Neonatal hyperviscosity is associated with lower achievement and IQ scores at school age. *Pediatr Res*, **23**, 442A.

29

Hydrops fetalis

David P. Carlton

University of Wisconsin and Meriter Hospital, Madison, WI, USA

Hydrops fetalis is the term applied to the presence of excess body water in the fetus resulting in skin edema or effusions in the pleural, peritoneal, or pericardial space. Because surveillance during most pregnancies in the USA includes fetal ultrasound, most cases of hydrops will be recognized before birth. An associated abnormality can be diagnosed either antenatally or postnatally in the majority of patients who have hydrops. The prognosis for survival is generally poor. Over 50% of fetuses diagnosed with hydrops die in utero, and of those that survive to delivery, over half will die postnatally despite aggressive support.[1,2]

Immune hydrops

Immune hydrops is a late manifestation of the destruction of fetal erythrocytes and resultant anemia caused by transplacentally acquired maternal antibodies to fetal red cell antigens. The degree of anemia that causes hydrops is unpredictable, but hydrops most commonly occurs when the hematocrit is less than 20%.[3] Immune hydrops not treated with intrauterine red cell transfusion is associated with a significant risk of fetal death.

Historically, the most common antigen causing an antibody-mediated hemolytic anemia was the Rh D. Anemia as a function of sensitization to the D antigen is infrequent today because of the routine use of passive immunization with Rh immunoglobulin in the management of women who are Rh D-negative.[4,5] Sensitization to other red cell antigens, including Kell, e and c, also cause fetal hemolytic anemia and immune hydrops.[6]

Nonimmune hydrops

Nonimmune hydrops occurs in approximately 1 per 2000–4000 deliveries, and it occurs more frequently than immune hydrops.[7] Observational studies suggest that postnatal mortality averages ~50%, but the risk of death is significantly influenced by the accompanying disorder.[1,8]

Well over 100 different conditions are referred to as "causing" nonimmune hydrops, but only in a limited number of these disorders is there an understandable pathophysiologic link between the condition and the development of hydrops.[9] Approximately 60–80% of the cases of nonimmune hydrops in the USA occur in association with an identifiable disorder. In 20–40% of patients, an associated condition will not be found despite a thorough investigation.[1,10] These patients are considered to have "idiopathic" nonimmune hydrops (Table 29.1).

Proposed mechanisms of edema formation in patients with hydrops

The relative rates of fluid entry into and clearance from the interstitial space govern whether edema formation occurs. Excess fluid will leave the circulation if vascular surface area is increased, endothelial barrier integrity is compromised, hydrostatic pressure difference from the vascular to interstitial space is increased, or protein oncotic pressure difference between the vascular and interstitial spaces is decreased.[11] Fluid clearance from the interstitial

Table 29.1. Conditions associated with nonimmune hydrops

Idiopathic	*Urinary tract abnormalities*
Nonimmune anemias	Kidney dysplasia
Homozygous α-thalassemia (Hb Bart's hydrops)	Urinary tract malformations and obstructions
Erythrocyte enzyme abnormalities	*Intracranial abnormalities*
Fetal hemorrhage	Developmental brain malformations
Fetal–maternal hemorrhage	Intracranial hemorrhage
Twin-to-twin transfusion sequence (donor or recipient)	Arterial or venous intracranial malformations
Parvovirus infection	Encephalocele
Red cell aplasia	*Lymphatic and vascular abnormalities*
Chromosomal/syndromic/genetic abnormalities	Intravascular thrombosis
Trisomy 21, 18, 13	Chylothorax
Turner syndrome	Cystic hygroma
Chromosomal deletions/rearrangements	*Placental or umbilical cord abnormalities*
Noonan syndrome	Chorioangioma
Myotonic dystrophy	*Fetal tumors*
Tuberous sclerosis	Rhabdomyosarcoma
Cardiovascular abnormalities	Sacrococcygeal teratoma
Arrhythmias (congenital heart block and supraventricular tachycardias)	Neuroblastoma
Structural heart disease	Hemangioendothelioma
Chest masses	Hepatoblastoma
Congenital cystic adenomatoid malformation	*Infections*
Congenital lymphangiectasis	Parvovirus B19
Sequestration	TORCH infections
Bronchogenic cyst	Enteroviruses
Gastrointestinal abnormalities	*Metabolic abnormalities*
Diaphragmatic hernia	Storage diseases
Meconium peritonitis	Skeletal dysplasias
Intestinal atresias	*Maternal-specific associations*
	Antepartum indometacin
	Diabetes mellitus

Note:
TORCH, *Toxoplasma*, syphilis, rubella, cytomegalovirus, and herpes simplex.

space is impaired when lymphatic drainage is impeded.

A variety of hypotheses have been suggested to explain the pathophysiology of hydrops, one of which is an elevation of central venous pressure. Processes that increase right atrial and central venous pressures are common in hydropic infants and provide the basis for an increase in upstream microvascular hydrostatic pressure which will increase transvascular fluid filtration into the interstitium. An elevation in central venous pressure will also impede lymphatic drainage of interstitial fluid back into the central circulation. In experiments in fetal sheep, even minimal increases in lymphatic outflow pressure impair lymphatic drainage.[12,13] Because central venous pressure is the relevant outflow pressure for lymphatic drainage in the fetus, even small increases in central venous pressure may reduce the effectiveness of interstitial fluid clearance. Thus, in conditions that increase central venous pressure, hydrops may be caused, or at least aggravated, by two distinct mechanisms: increased transvascular fluid entry and impaired fluid clearance.

Tachyarrhythmias or myocardial dysfunction may be associated with an elevated central venous pressure. Myocardial dysfunction is the presumed basis for hydrops in fetuses who have an elevation in umbilical venous pressure.[14,15] Packed red blood cell transfusion not only reduces umbilical venous pressure, it also prevents hydrops formation, perhaps by improving cardiac function, and thus lowering right-sided venous pressures. Even in fetuses who are not anemic, there is evidence of myocardial dysfunction and elevated umbilical venous pressure, although in many of these fetuses the etiology of myocardial dysfunction is obscure.[14,15]

Another mechanism that has been proposed to account for hydrops is an increase in endothelial permeability. However, albumin flux studies in infants with Rh hemolytic anemia are similar in hydropic and nonhydropic infants, suggesting no difference in vascular integrity between these two groups of patients.[16] Similarly, tachyarrhythmias increase central venous pressure and total body water, but vascular permeability is unaffected.[17] Thus, there is insufficient evidence to confirm or refute the notion that increased vascular permeability is one of the pathophysiologic mechanisms underlying the formation of hydrops.

Another possible explanation for hydrops is hypoalbuminemia. Indeed, information from infants with Rh hemolytic disease and hydrops demonstrates that serum albumin concentration correlates with the degree of body water.[16] Likewise, pericardial fluid accumulation has been shown to be related to the presence of hypoalbuminemia, not myocardial dysfunction.[18] On the other hand, observations from infants who are born with inherited abnormalities of serum proteins suggest that hypoproteinemia alone need not result in hydrops. Patients who have congenital nephrotic syndrome or analbuminemia do not consistently have hydrops in utero or at the time of birth, although they may become edematous postnatally.[19,20] Similarly, in fetal lambs made hypoproteinemic, total body water is relatively unaffected.[21] Taken together, the role of hypoproteinemia in the pathophysiology of hydrops remains uncertain.

Neurologic injury associated with hydrops

Neurologic compromise in patients who have hydrops may occur under several different scenarios. First, abnormalities of the central nervous system such as porencephaly, absence of the corpus callosum, and encephalocele may be primary lesions associated with hydrops.[22] Second, occult neurological injury may also be present in patients who have no obvious cause of their hydrops. The neuropathologic changes of antenatal anoxia have been observed in patients who died with idiopathic nonimmune hydrops, suggesting that some types of neurologic injury may be present, but undiagnosed, in otherwise "idiopathic" cases of nonimmune hydrops.[23] Most commonly, however, brain injury occurs in nonimmune hydrops in conjunction with the underlying disorder that accompanies the hydrops. Genetic and chromosomal syndromes, congenital infections, and metabolic diseases are examples of disorders that are seen in association with hydrops and that often have abnormal neurologic sequelae as a feature of their symptom complex. Other brain injury syndromes are more directly linked to hydrops. For instance, the presence of severe platelet alloimmunization has been linked to intracranial hemorrhage in utero and resultant fetal anemia which then causes hydrops; intracranial hemorrhage in the absence of thrombocytopenia has also been associated with hydrops.[24,25] An anecdotal report has linked maternal parvovirus infection to fetal stroke and seizures.[26] Parvovirus is a common infectious agent linked to nonimmune hydrops.

Antenatal management

Antenatal management of the hydropic fetus is focused initially on establishing the diagnosis of an associated condition. Therapeutic options are limited in most cases. Intravascular infusion of packed red blood cells is the most consistently successful strategy available to treat hydrops, but its usefulness is limited to fetuses who have anemia.[27,28] Intrauterine therapy is unavailable for most patients with nonimmune hydrops. Only in limited circumstances does it appear that intrauterine treatment may be of benefit in patients with nonimmune hydrops. Successful treatment of fetal supraventricular tachycardia, evacuation of pleural fluid collections, and fetal surgical repair of lesions such as congenital cystic adenomatoid malformation or sacrococcygeal teratoma have resulted in the resolution of hydrops.[29–31]

Management of the hydropic fetus around the time of birth

Although the most appropriate time for delivery of a hydropic fetus cannot be discerned from the available observational studies, early delivery does not appear to convey a survival advantage.[1,8,32] Timing of delivery for the hydropic fetus should be based on several factors, including the degree of fetal lung development and maturation, general fetal health, and whether the hydrops is progressing. Antenatal steroids should be administered to accelerate fetal lung maturation if they are otherwise indicated. Although there is no information available to allow for firm recommendations as to mode of delivery, most hydropic fetuses are delivered by cesarean section. Regardless of mode of delivery, fetuses who have nonimmune hydrops often have some degree of birth depression, and for this reason delivery should occur at a tertiary neonatal center.[33] Tracheal intubation is almost always needed in patients who have significant hydrops, and edema of the face and oropharynx can make this procedure difficult for even experienced clinicians.[1] Diminished thoracic compliance often requires drainage of the pleural and peritoneal spaces in the delivery room to improve gas exchange. Pleural effusions are more common in patients who die soon after birth than in patients who survive, presumably as a result of associated pulmonary hypoplasia.[1,8]

Postnatal diagnostic studies

The postnatal investigation of patients with hydrops centers on studies that will establish the presence of an associated condition and on studies that will help in the therapeutic management of the patient.[9,34,35] The choice of diagnostic studies should be guided by history and neonatal examination, but in a significant proportion of patients who have had a thorough fetal evaluation no associated disorder will be discovered postnatally. Diagnostic studies should include karyotype and high-resolution chromosomal banding, as well as other studies to exclude genetic syndromes. Echocardiography should be performed to evaluate the presence of structural heart disease and assess myocardial function. Electrocardiography will be necessary if a rhythm disturbance is suspected. Imaging studies are often necessary and may include plain film radiography of the chest and abdomen or ultrasonography of the head and abdomen. These investigations will sometimes reveal occult abnormalities that will help clarify whether a genetic syndrome is present. Subspecialty consultation with an expert in clinical genetics may be helpful if further evaluation of the patient is necessary .

Pathological examination of the placenta is important. Some conditions associated with hydrops are readily diagnosed by placental examination but are difficult to diagnose in the newborn in the absence of invasive procedures. For example, some inborn errors of metabolism are associated with hydrops and have characteristic pathological features on placental examination.[36]

Postnatal management

If the patient survives the initial resuscitative period, numerous complications may occur that can be life-threatening, including infections, airleak syndromes, and hypotension. All of these complications can result in direct or indirect neurological injury, predominantly because they cause or aggravate cardiorespiratory instability. Cardiorespiratory instability may result in ischemia and hypoxemia and thus increase the risk for neurological injury in a manner similar to other conditions in high-risk patients in the newborn intensive care unit who suffer from physiological instability.

Respiratory failure is common, not infrequently requiring aggressive conventional mechanical ventilation or high-frequency ventilation.[37] Extracorporeal membrane oxygenation (ECMO) has been used successfully in hydropic infants, but selection of patients who are likely to have good outcome from treatment with ECMO remains problematic because lung growth sufficient to provide for adequate gas exchange may not occur during the period of ECMO treatment.[38] Although there is no information regarding surfactant content or function in newborn infants who have hydrops, if exogenous surfactant replacement is otherwise indicated in a nonhydropic infant of similar gestational age, surfactant should be administered.

Cardiovascular instability is frequent and will be exacerbated if high mean airway pressure is necessary to provide adequate gas exchange. Fluid infusions are often needed to help maintain circulating volume and catecholamines may be required to treat hypotension and myocardial depression. In patients with structural heart disease, therapy is directed towards correcting the abnormal physiology as it would be in a nonhydropic infant who has a similar lesion. Prostaglandin E_1 infusion should be used to maintain ductal patency if otherwise indicated.

Intravenous fluids should be administered with the goal of promoting sodium and water loss during the first week after birth. Serum electrolytes and body weight measurements should be used to help guide fluid therapy. After the initial period of fluid stabilization, parenteral nutrition will be necessary. The goal of intravenous nutrition should be to provide targeted calorie and nutrient requirements while limiting fluid administration to the greatest extent possible, at least until body edema has resolved. Patients who have hydrops will often lose 20–30% of birth weight during the first 2 weeks after birth before the nadir of postnatal weight is reached, but clinical examination should guide this assessment.[1]

If significant asphyxia complicates the hospital course, coagulopathy is common and prothrombin and partial thromboplastin times should be measured. Treatment for clinically important coagulopathy consists of the administration of fresh frozen plasma or, if indicated, cryoprecipitate.

Most patients who have nonimmune hydrops will be hypoproteinemic and hypoalbuminemic. Diminished serum protein concentration at the time of birth increases the risk of early death.[1] Although there is no evidence to suggest that outcome is improved by the infusion of colloid solutions, infusion of 5% or 25% albumin is a common therapeutic maneuver. Whether maintaining serum albumin in the range usually found in nonhydropic infants improves outcome is unclear.

Many of the comments above regarding postnatal management of patients with hydrops apply to those who have either immune or nonimmune hydrops. However, additional management issues are relevant for the infant who has immune hydrops, specifically if hemolysis continues to complicate the postnatal course. Intravenous immune globulin decreases the rate of erythrocyte destruction and reduces the likelihood that exchange transfusion will be necessary. Intravenous immune globulin can be administered at 0.5 g/kg body weight and may have to be repeated within 24–48 h after the initial infusion.[39,40] Other complications encountered in patients with immune hydrops include thrombocytopenia and hypoglycemia, either of which may lead to neurologic injury.

Outcome of hydropic infants

In selected patients who have nonimmune hydrops, the electroencephalogram (EEG) shows marked abnormalities, including burst-suppression, abnormal background patterns, multifocal sharp waves, and seizure activity.[41] Patients who have significant abnormalities on EEG also show severe abnormalities neuropathologically, at least some of which appear to be antenatal in origin. Of interest, cranial ultrasound examination fails to demonstrate anatomic abnormalities in the majority of these patients. In a series of patients with hydrops who died in utero or shortly after birth, neuropathological findings of antenatal hypoxic–ischemic injury were found in over 50% of patients.[42]

Only limited information is available documenting the long-term neurological outcome of hydropic infants. In patients who receive intrauterine transfusions for severe hemolytic disease, neurologic outcome appears to be independent of the presence of hydrops at initial fetal presentation.[27,28] Of course, in this population, survival of hydropic infants is reduced compared to nonhydropic infants, so selection bias may contribute to the apparent equivalence in outcome. If patients survive to delivery, 90–95% will have normal neurological exam and 80–85% will have a normal developmental outcome at follow-up between 6 months and 6 years.[27,28] These outcomes compare favorably with other high-risk infants managed in the neonatal intensive care unit. As might be expected, perinatal asphyxia is significantly related to abnormal neurologic outcome.[28] Because hydropic infants who are anemic do not tolerate the hypoxemia that accompanies vaginal delivery, cesarean section is frequently the most prudent route of delivery.[43] The long-term neurologic outcome for patients with nonimmune hydrops is limited, but observational data would suggest normal neurologic outcome in 65–85%.[8,32]

Summary

Many patients who have hydrops will die soon after delivery because of pulmonary hypoplasia and the inability to establish adequate gas exchange. Of those patients that survive the immediate postnatal period, many will succumb to the underlying condition associated with their hydrops. In patients who have nonimmune hydrops and who survive to discharge, neurologic outcome appears to be favorable, with most patients having a normal neurologic exam on follow-up. The risk of neurologic impairment appears to increase in association with birth at earlier gestational ages and with underlying disorders in which neurologic dysfunction is an expected feature.

REFERENCES

1 Carlton DP, McGillivray BC and Schreiber MD. (1989). Nonimmune hydrops fetalis: a multidisciplinary approach. *Clin Perinatol,* **16**, 839–851.

2 Ismail KM, Martin WL, Ghosh S, et al. (2001). Etiology and outcome of hydrops fetalis. *J Matern Fetal Med,* **10**, 175–181.

3 Nicolaides KH, Soothill PW, Clewell WH, et al. (1988). Fetal haemoglobin measurement in the assessment of red cell isoimmunisation. *Lancet,* **1**, 1073–1075.

4 Adams MM, Marks JS, Gustafson J, et al. (1981). Rh hemolytic disease of the newborn: using incidence observations to evaluate the use of RH immune globulin. *Am J Public Health,* **71**, 1031–1035.

5 Clarke CA, Mollison PL and Whitfield AG (1985). Deaths from rhesus haemolytic disease in England and Wales in 1982 and 1983. *Br Med J (Clin Res Ed),* **291**, 17–19.

6 Wenk RE, Goldstein P and Felix JK. (1985). Kell alloimmunization, hemolytic disease of the newborn, and perinatal management. *Obstet Gynecol,* **66**, 473–476.

7 Maidman JE, Yeager C, Anderson V, et al. (1980). Prenatal diagnosis and management of nonimmunologic hydrops fetalis. *Obstet Gynecol,* **56**, 571–576.

8 Nakayama H, Kukita J, Hikino S, et al. (1999). Long-term outcome of 51 liveborn neonates with non-immune hydrops fetalis. *Acta Paediatr,* **88**, 24–28.

9 Jones DC. (1995). Nonimmune fetal hydrops: diagnosis and obstetrical management. *Semin Perinatol,* **19**, 447–461.

10 Holzgreve W, Holzgreve B and Curry CJ. (1985). Nonimmune hydrops fetalis: diagnosis and management. *Semin Perinatol,* **9**, 52–67.

11 Apkon M. (1995). Pathophysiology of hydrops fetalis. *Semin Perinatol,* **19**, 437–446.

12 Brace RA. (1989). Effects of outflow pressure on fetal lymph flow. *Am J Obstet Gynecol,* **160**, 494–497.

13 Gest AL, Bair DK and Vander Straten MC. (1992). The effect of outflow pressure upon thoracic duct lymph flow rate in fetal sheep. *Pediatr Res,* **32**, 585–588.

14 Johnson P, Sharland G, Allan LD, et al. (1992). Umbilical

venous pressure in nonimmune hydrops fetalis: correlation with cardiac size. *Am J Obstet Gynecol*, **167**, 1309–1313.

15 Weiner CP. (1993). Umbilical pressure measurement in the evaluation of nonimmune hydrops fetalis. *Am J Obstet Gynecol*, **168**, 817–823.

16 Phibbs RH, Johnson P and Tooley WH. (1974). Cardiorespiratory status of erythroblastotic newborn infants. II. Blood volume, hematocrit, and serum albumin concentration in relation to hydrops fetalis. *Pediatrics*, **53**, 13–23.

17 Gest AL, Hansen TN, Moise AA, et al. (1990). Atrial tachycardia causes hydrops in fetal lambs. *Am J Physiol*, **258**, H1159–H1163.

18 DeVore GR, Acherman RJ, Cabal LA, et al. (1982). Hypoalbuminemia: the etiology of antenatally diagnosed pericardial effusion in rhesus-hemolytic anemia. *Am J Obstet Gynecol*, **142**, 1056–1057.

19 Cormode EJ, Lyster DM and Israels S. (1975). Analbuminemia in a neonate. *J Pediatr*, **86**, 862–867.

20 Hallman N, Norio R and Rapola J. (1973). Congenital nephrotic syndrome. *Nephron*, **11**, 101–110.

21 Moise AA, Gest AL, Weickmann PH, et al. (1991). Reduction in plasma protein does not affect body water content in fetal sheep. *Pediatr Res*, **29**, 623–626.

22 Hutchison AA, Drew JH, Yu VY, et al. (1982). Nonimmunologic hydrops fetalis: a review of 61 cases. *Obstet Gynecol*, **59**, 347–352.

23 Kobori JA and Urich H. (1986). Intrauterine anoxic brain damage in nonimmune hydrops fetalis. *Biol Neonate*, **49**, 311–317.

24 Bose C. (1978). Hydrops fetalis and in utero intracranial hemorrhage. *J Pediatr*, **93**, 1023–1024.

25 Stanworth SJ, Hackett GA and Williamson LM. (2001). Fetomaternal alloimmune thrombocytopenia presenting antenatally as hydrops fetalis. *Prenat Diagn*, **21**, 423–424.

26 Craze JL, Salisbury AJ and Pike MG. (1996). Prenatal stroke associated with maternal parvovirus infection. *Dev Med Child Neurol*, **38**, 84–85.

27 Doyle LW, Kelly EA, Rickards AL, et al. (1993). Sensorineural outcome at 2 years for survivors of erythroblastosis treated with fetal intravascular transfusions. *Obstet Gynecol*, **81**, 931–935.

28 Janssens HM, de Haan MJ, van Kamp IL, et al. (1997). Outcome for children treated with fetal intravascular transfusions because of severe blood group antagonism. *J Pediatr*, **131**, 373–380.

29 Ahmad FK, Sherman SJ, Hagglund KH, et al. (1996). Isolated unilateral fetal pleural effusion: the role of sonographic surveillance and in utero therapy. *Fetal Diagn Ther*, **11**, 383–389.

30 Bullard KM and Harrison MR. (1995). Before the horse is out of the barn: fetal surgery for hydrops. *Semin Perinatol*, **19**, 462–473.

31 Simpson LL. (2000). Fetal supraventricular tachycardias: diagnosis and management. *Semin Perinatol*, **24**, 360–372.

32 Haverkamp F, Noeker M, Gerresheim G, et al. (2000). Good prognosis for psychomotor development in survivors with nonimmune hydrops fetalis. *Bjog*, **107**, 282–284.

33 McMahan MJ and Donovan EF. (1995). The delivery room resuscitation of the hydropic neonate. *Semin Perinatol*, **19**, 474–482.

34 Poeschmann RP, Verheijen RH and Van Dongen PW. (1991). Differential diagnosis and causes of nonimmunological hydrops fetalis: a review. *Obstet Gynecol Surv*, **46**, 223–231.

35 Steiner RD. (1995). Hydrops fetalis: role of the geneticist. *Semin Perinatol*, **19**, 516–524.

36 Beck M, Bender SW, Reiter HL, et al. (1984). Neuraminidase deficiency presenting as non-immune hydrops fetalis. *Eur J Pediatr*, **143**, 135–139.

37 Wy CA, Sajous CH, Loberiza F, et al. (1999). Outcome of infants with a diagnosis of hydrops fetalis in the 1990s. *Am J Perinatol*, **16**, 561–567.

38 Bealer JF, Mantor PC, Wehling L, et al. (1997). Extracorporeal life support for nonimmune hydrops fetalis. *J Pediatr Surg*, **32**, 1645–1647.

39 Alpay F, Sarici SU, Okutan V, et al. (1999). High-dose intravenous immunoglobulin therapy in neonatal immune haemolytic jaundice. *Acta Paediatr*, **88**, 216–219.

40 Rubo J, Albrecht K, Lasch P, et al. (1992). High-dose intravenous immune globulin therapy for hyperbilirubinemia caused by Rh hemolytic disease. *J Pediatr*, **121**, 93–97.

41 Laneri GG, Claassen DL and Scher MS. (1994). Brain lesions of fetal onset in encephalopathic infants with nonimmune hydrops fetalis. *Pediatr Neurol*, **11**, 18–22.

42 Larroche JC, Aubry MC and Narcy F. (1992). Intrauterine brain damage in nonimmune hydrops fetalis. *Biol Neonate*, **61**, 273–280.

43 Phibbs RH, Johnson P, Kitterman JA, et al. (1972). Cardiorespiratory status of erythroblastotic infants. 1. Relationship of gestational age, severity of hemolytic diseases, and birth asphyxia to idiopathic respiratory distress syndrome and survival. *Pediatrics*, **49**, 5–14.

30

Acidosis/alkalosis

Robert C. Vannucci

Pennsylvania State University College of Medicine, Hershey, PA, USA

Introduction

The pH regulation of the blood is a critical physiologic process necessary to maintain optimum metabolism of body tissues, including the brain. Accordingly, the maintenance of a normal blood pH is of paramount importance for physicians to prevent the untoward effects of acidosis or alkalosis. Respiratory acidosis and alkalosis, as well as metabolic acidosis, are frequently encountered in sick premature and full-term newborn infants. Respiratory acidosis occurs as a consequence of respiratory distress syndrome and other pulmonary disease, while respiratory alkalosis typically occurs as an iatrogenic component of the hyperventilation necessary to oxygenate adequately a critically ill newborn infant. Metabolic acidosis with or without respiratory acidosis typically arises from systemic hypoxia or asphyxia in the fetus or newborn infant. The present chapter will review available information regarding pH regulation of cerebral blood flow (CBF) and metabolism under physiologic conditions and the contribution of acidosis/alkalosis to brain damage, especially that arising from cerebral hypoxia–ischemia.

Effect of respiratory acidosis/alkalosis on cerebral blood flow

Cerebral blood vessels are known to be sensitive to changes in $Paco_2$, such that CBF is increased during respiratory acidosis and decreased during respiratory alkalosis. These CBF responses to changes in $Paco_2$ exist in the fetus and newborn animal, including the newborn infant, although the sensitivity of immature cerebral blood vessels is not as well developed as in the adult. Investigations have been conducted in a variety of animal species, including dogs, pigs, sheep, and monkeys. In our own laboratory, anesthetized, paralyzed, and artificially ventilated newborn dogs were subjected to either hyperventilation or to a gas mixture rich in carbon dioxide. CBF during steady-state hypocapnia or hypercapnia was determined by the classic Kety–Schmidt technique[1] (Figure 30.1). Linear regression analysis revealed a close relationship between CBF and $Paco_2$; blood flow corresponded to changes in $Paco_2$ tensions by an average of 0.6 ml/100 g per min per mmHg CO_2. This value was only one-fifth that reported for adult dogs.[2] The cerebral vascular responses to changes in $Paco_2$ have also been reported to be lower in newborn sheep and monkeys compared to adults.[3,4] These studies indicate that, in the early stages of postnatal development, CBF responses to hypocapnia and hypercapnia are less well developed than in adults.

Hypercapnia is also associated with an increased CBF in fetal animals.[4–7] Maximal responses of CBF to $Paco_2$ elevations in fetal sheep occur at values minimally greater than 55 mmHg,[5,7] tensions which are lower than those reported for newborn and adult animals.[1–3] When $Paco_2$ is 40–45 mmHg (the normal range for fetuses), cerebral vascular resistance ranges from 0.5 to 0.7 resistance units (ml/100 g per min per mmHg $Paco_2$). These low resistance values suggest that, at physiologic gas tensions, the fetal

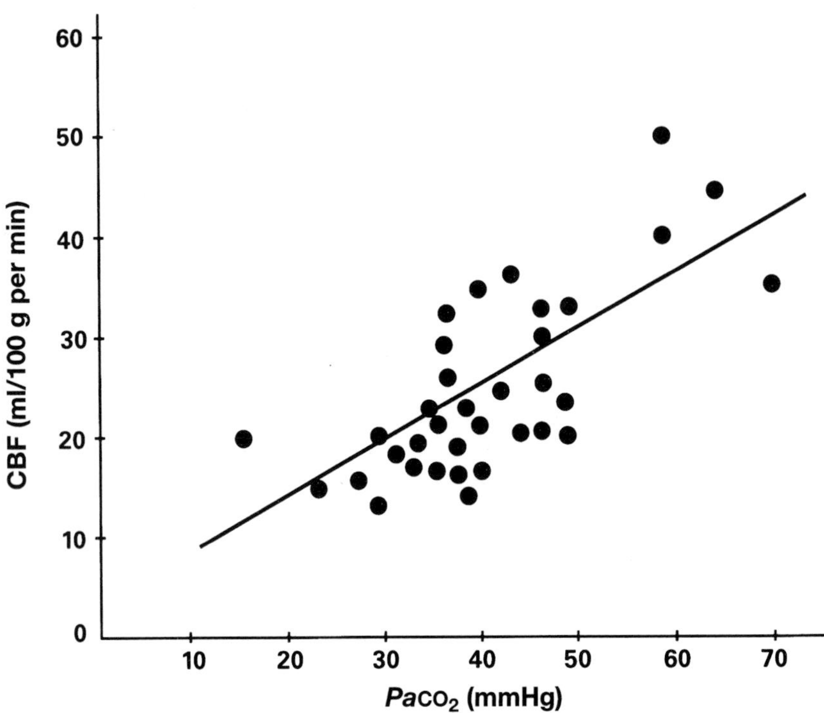

Figure 30.1 Cerebral blood flow (CBF)–carbon dioxide sensitivity in newborn dogs. CBF was determined using the Kety–Schmidt technique with ^{133} xenon as the radioactive indicator. Individual CBF values are plotted as a function of $Pa\text{CO}_2$. The line was drawn from a linear regression equation, with a slope which equated to CBF = 1.3 ± 0.6 $Pa\text{CO}_2$; $r = 0.61$; $P < 0.01$. Derived from data of Hernandez et al.[1]

cerebral vasculature is relatively widely dilated with little vasodilatory reserve remaining, although regional differences exist.[6] Thus, hypercapnia when combined with hypoxia produces only a minimal augmentation of CBF over that found during hypoxia alone (see below).

Regional responses of CBF to changes in $Pa\text{CO}_2$ have been investigated in perinatal animals.[6–10] In general, CBF–CO_2 sensitivity is greater in gray-matter structures compared to white matter and is also greater in brainstem structures than in diencephalic regions (basal ganglia; thalamus) or cerebral cortex. The latter finding is in keeping with the general observation that more mature structures (e.g., brainstem) prior to or at birth exhibit greater CBF–CO_2 sensitivities than less developed structures (e.g., cerebral cortex) at the same period of development. The finding is also in keeping with the general rule that phylogenetically older structures develop earlier than phylogenetically more recent ones.[11]

The observations described above are exemplified by the investigation of Cavazzuti and Duffy[9] in newborn dogs. Using iodo-[^{14}C]-antipyrine as the CBF marker, these investigators measured regional CBF at $Pa\text{CO}_2$ ranging from 27 to 77 mmHg. Regional CBF was then plotted as a function of $Pa\text{CO}_2$ for a total of 32 gray-matter ($n = 28$) and white-matter ($n = 4$) structures (Figure 30.2). A positive linear correlation was obtained in each of the 32 regions analyzed. The responses to CO_2 varied widely among the individual brain structures, ranging from 0.15 ml/100 g per

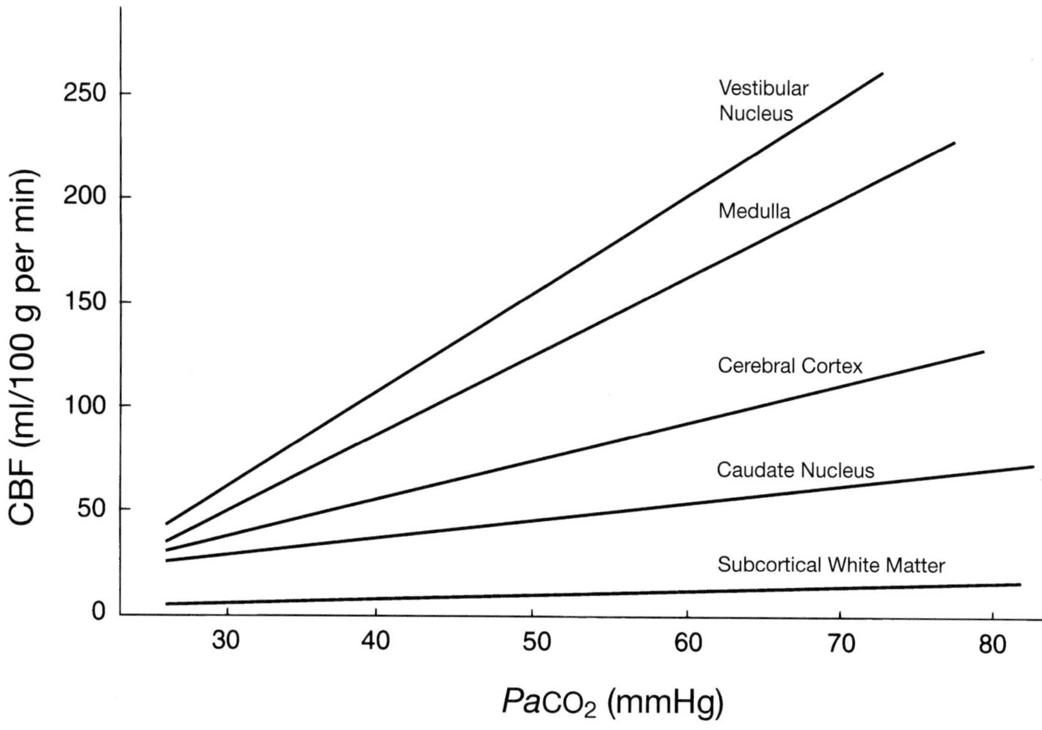

Figure 30.2 Regional cerebral blood flow (CBF)–carbon dioxide sensitivity in newborn dogs. Regional CBF was determined using the indicator fractionation technique with ^{14}C-iodoantipyrine as the radioactive indicator. The lines were drawn from linear regression analyses, the slopes of which all differed significantly ($P<0.05$) from one another by analysis of covariance. Derived from data of Cavazzuti and Duffy.[9]

min per mmHg in subcortical white matter to 4.8 in the vestibular and superior olivary nuclei of the brainstem. Thus, white-matter blood flow in the newborn dog brain was only marginally responsive to changes in $Pa\text{CO}_2$, whereas the sensitivity to CO_2 of specific brainstem nuclei was more than twice that reported for the adult dog cerebral cortex. Another interesting finding of the study was the fact that, when the mean normocapnic blood flow of each brain region was plotted as a function of CO_2 sensitivity, a positive correlation was observed for all structures, indicating that the higher the physiologic blood flow to a particular structure, the greater will be its vasodilatory response to increasing $Pa\text{CO}_2$. In other words, the lower the intrinsic CBF, the less responsive the structure to changes in $Pa\text{CO}_2$. A parallel observation in newborn dogs by Shapiro et al.[8] indicated that the maximal CBF–CO_2 sensitivity in white matter occurs at a lower $Pa\text{CO}_2$ than those of gray-matter structures (Figure 30.3). The difference in CBF–CO_2 sensitivity of gray and white matter during the perinatal period might account for the selective vulnerability of these structures to hypoxic–ischemic brain damage in the human fetus and newborn infant.

Studies have also been conducted in newborn animals to ascertain the CBF responses to profound or prolonged hypocapnia. Species differences in CBF–CO_2 sensitivity have been reported, depending upon the functional maturity of the animal shortly following birth. In newborn dogs, hypocapnia to $Pa\text{CO}_2$ tensions as low as 10 mmHg is associated with

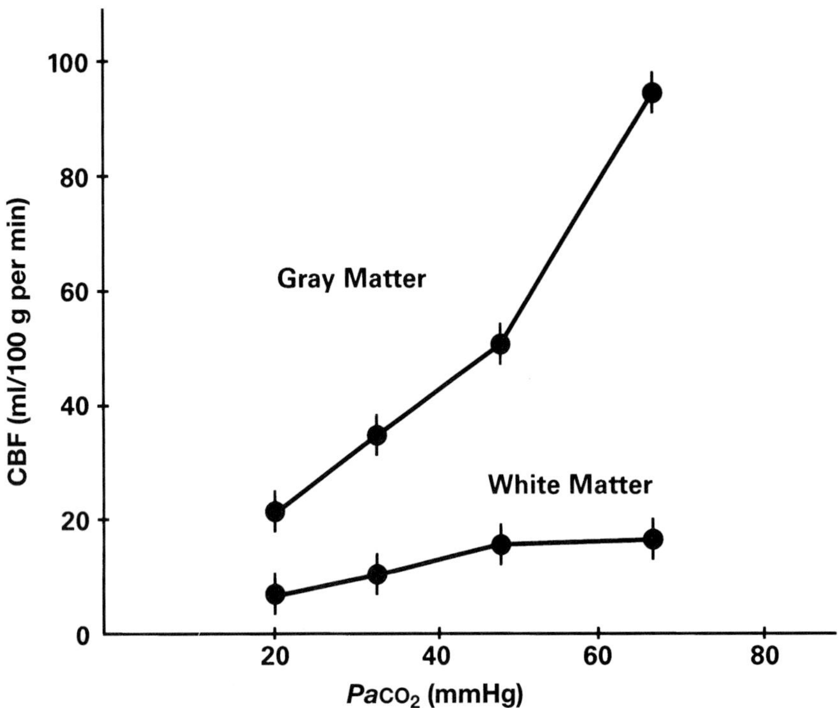

Figure 30.3 Regional cerebral blood flow (CBF)–carbon dioxide sensitivity in newborn dogs. Regional CBF was determined using the indicator fractionation technique with ^{14}C-iodoantipyrine as the radioactive tracer. Symbols represent mean CBF values for 3–7 animals. Vertical lines denote ±1 SE. Derived from data of Shapiro et al.[8]

decreases in both global and regional CBF, with the greatest reduction observed in the brainstem and diencephalic structures[12,13] (Figure 30.4). Less dramatic reductions occur in cerebral cortex and subcortical white matter. In newborn lambs, a more mature species at birth than dogs, hypocapnia to $Paco_2$ tensions as low as 12 mmHg is associated with decreases in CBF which are similar in all of seven gray-matter structures analyzed, including cerebral cortex, diencephalon, and brainstem.[14] By contrast, CBF to brainstem, cerebellum, and thalamus of newborn pigs is not altered by $Paco_2$ tensions as low as 15 mmHg, with a minimal decrease in CBF of cerebral cortex.[10] The latter finding is surprising in light of data in newborn animals of other species. Taken together, the published reports would suggest that, like hypercapnia, hypocapnia is associated with substantial changes in CBF in perinatal animals and that the associated reductions are most dramatic in gray-matter structures, especially the brainstem.

An interesting, clinically relevant investigation has been conducted by Gleason et al.[15] which simulates the situation in newborn human infants who initially are hyperventilated for persistent fetal circulation (PFC) but who then are rapidly rendered normocapnic when subjected to extracorporeal membrane oxygenation (ECMO). To simulate the human situation, the investigators subjected six newborn lambs to hyperventilation for 6 h with a resultant $Paco_2$ of 15 mmHg, following which the hyperventilation was abruptly terminated. Thirty minutes of hypocapnia was associated with 34–36% decreases in CBF of the cerebral hemispheres, brain-

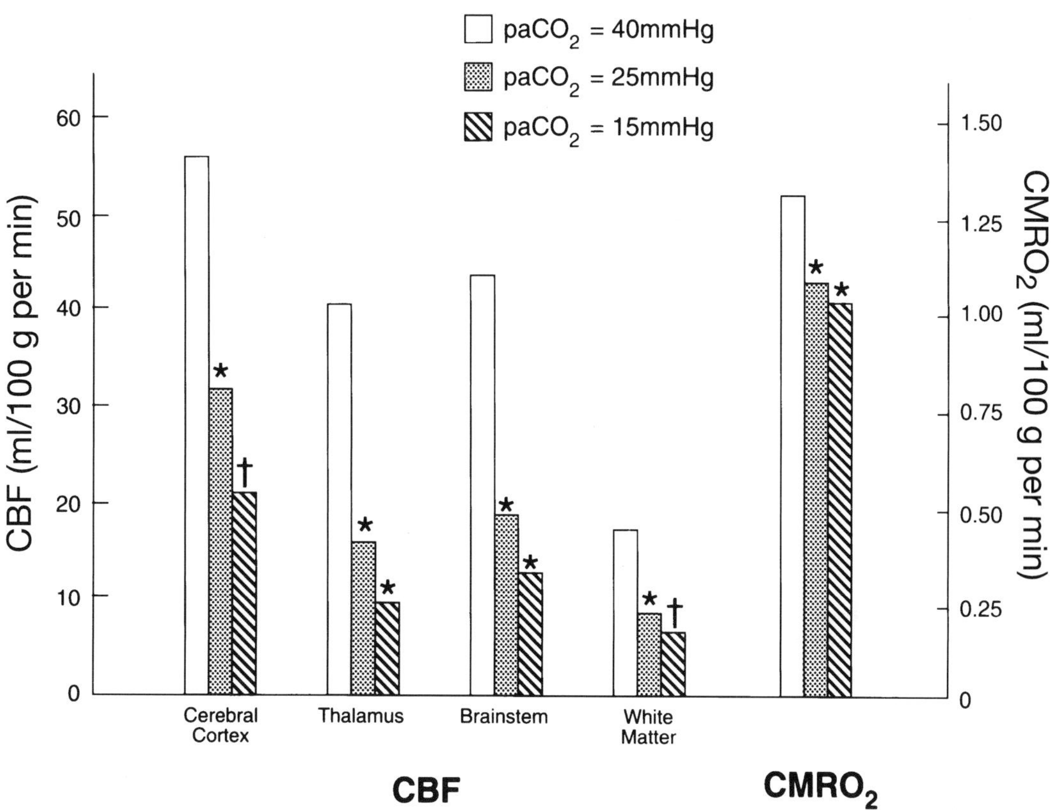

Figure 30.4 Regional cerebral blood flow (CBF) and the cerebral metabolic rate for oxygen ($CMRO_2$) during hypocapnia in newborn dogs. Regional CBF was determined using radioactive microspheres. $CMRO_2$ was calculated from total CBF × arteriovenous O_2. Columns represent means of six animals. * $P<0.05$ compared to 40 mmHg; † $P<0.05$ compared to 25 mmHg. Derived from data of Reuter and Disney.[13]

stem, and cerebellum, and these flows essentially reverted to baseline by 6 h. Upon abrupt restitution of normocapnia ($Paco_2$ = 36 mmHg), blood flows to all analyzed structures dramatically increased by 110–141% and this persisted for 90 min or more. The investigators speculated (probably rightly) that the posthypocapnic brain hyperemia results from compensatory changes in cerebrospinal fluid (CSF) and perivascular pH, which tends to normalize during prolonged hypocapnia because of an accumulation of organic acids, especially lactate, and a concurrent decrease in CSF bicarbonate. When the hyperventilation is abruptly discontinued, the low CSF/perivascular bicarbonate produces an acidotic pH with resultant cerebrovascular vasodilation and hyperemia. The investigators further emphasize that such a hyperemia in sick newborn human infants might contribute to the occurrence of intracranial hemorrhage which is frequently observed during ECMO therapy.

The response of the cerebral circulation to changes in $Paco_2$ has also been investigated in newborn human infants, especially those born prematurely. Using the Kety–Schmidt technique to measure CBF, Greisen and his coworkers have determined CBF–CO_2 sensitivity in a large number of premature infants with gestational ages of 32 weeks or less.[16–20] Despite low CBF values at normocapnia (approx. 20 ml/100 g per min) relative to more mature newborn infants,[16] CBF responds appropriately to either spontaneous or ventilator-induced changes in $Pa\text{CO}_2$.[17–20] On the first day of postnatal life, mechanically ventilated but stable premature infants exhibit a CBF–CO_2 sensitivity of 0.66 ml/100 g per min per mmHg CO_2, a value near identical to that reported for newborn dogs.[1] In spontaneously breathing newborn infants, CBF–CO_2 sensitivity actually approaches that of adult humans, i.e., approximately 1.5 ml/100 g per min per mmHg CO_2. Indometacin, a cyclooxygenase inhibitor, attenuates the responsivness of CBF to changes in $Pa\text{CO}_2$.[21] Accordingly, the cerebral circulation of even premature newborn infants reacts appropriately to either hyper- or hypocapnia despite the immaturity of their brains and an intrinsic vulnerability to hypoxic–ischemic and hemorrhagic damage (see below).

The mechanism by which CO_2 influences CBF is not entirely understood but presumably involves specific receptor activation, either directly or indirectly, of the smooth muscles of the resistance vessels of the brain. As a gas, CO_2 readily diffuses across the endothelium of cerebral blood vessels and, therefore, could conceivably act directly on vascular smooth muscle, possibly by lowering extra- or intracellular pH. In this regard, the vascular smooth muscle of isolated pial vessels responds appropriately to CO_2 even in the absence of endothelial cells.[22,23] An alternative mechanism is an activation of specific receptors on the luminal or abluminal side of the vascular endothelium; in turn, this signals an activation of specific receptors on the vascular smooth muscle. Whatever the precise mechanism, other CBF modulators might act synergistically with CO_2 to regulate the cerebral circulation during respiratory acidosis or alkalosis.

Recent investigations, especially in newborn piglets, suggest that CO_2 modulates CBF, at least in part, via prostanoid production. Both in vitro and cranial window techniques indicate that CO_2 enhances the production of vasodilator prostanoids, presumably derived from the endothelium, and that the cyclooxygenase inhibitor indometacin completely abolishes the vasodilatory response to hypercapnia.[24,25] The prostanoids then act on smooth muscle receptors, possibly mediating specific intracellular signals, including cyclic adenosine monophosphate (cAMP), cyclic guanosine monophosphate (cGMP), or Ca^{2+}. Increases in CBF during hypercapnia also appear to be dependent on the production of endothelium-derived relaxing factor, now known to be nitric oxide (NO).[26] In adult rats, inhibitors of the NO-synthesizing enzyme, NO synthase, attenuate the hyperemic response to hypercapnia, and the effect is reversed by the NO substrate donor, L-arginine.[27] Since NO synthase is located not only in endothelial cells but also in perivascular nerves supplying major brain arteries and arterioles,[28] the endothelial or perivascular production of NO might contribute substantially to the cerebral circulation's response to changes in $Pa\text{CO}_2$ as well as to basal CBF.

Effect of metabolic acidosis/alkalosis on cerebral blood flow

Unlike CO_2, which either acts directly on the endothelium of cerebral resistance vessels or readily crosses the blood–brain barrier to influence CBF, organic acids appear to influence CBF little or not at all. It has been generally assumed that nonvolatile, organic acids have little or no effect on CBF, at least in adult animals and humans.[29] That metabolic acidosis (acidemia) or alkalosis (alkalemia) does not perturb physiologic CBF also appears to be the case in perinatal animals, although discrepancies in the experimental data exist. Investigations on alterations in blood metabolic acid–base homeostasis have been conducted largely in newborn dogs, goats, and piglets. In newborn dogs, neither an infusion of unbuffered lactic acid (blood pH = 7.1–7.2) nor buffered lactic acid (blood pH = 7.3–7.4) adversely influences CBF or attenuates CBF autoregulation.[30,31] Likewise, blood metabolic alkalosis, produced by the infusion of sodium bicarbonate, does not affect CBF.[7,32] By contrast, in both newborn goats and piglets, unbuffered lactic acid infusions to

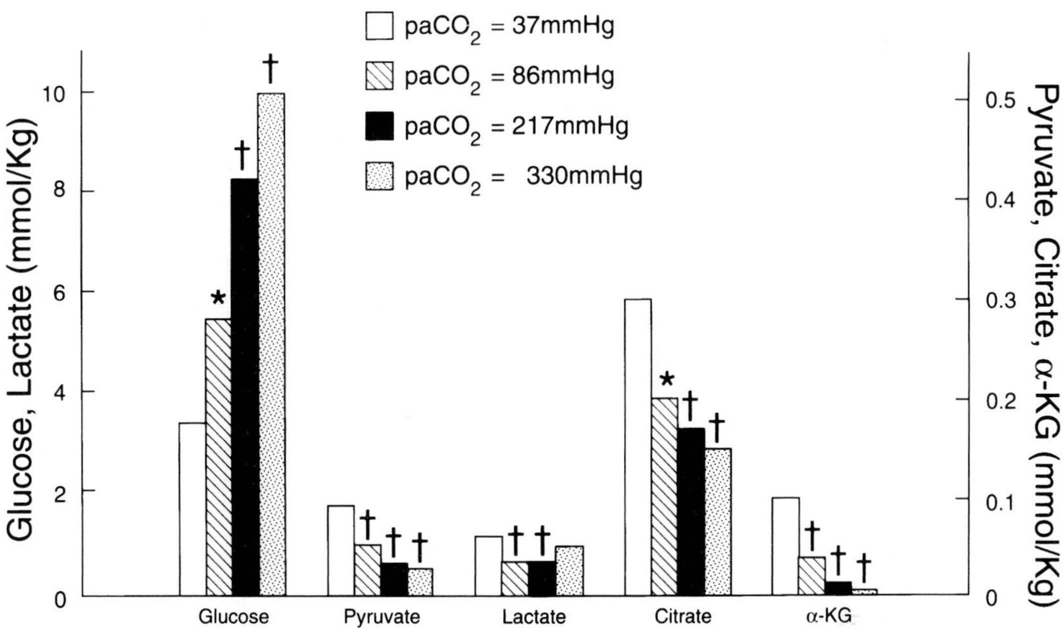

Figure 30.5 Cerebral glycolytic and tricarboxylic acid intermediates during hypercapnia in adult rats. Columns represent mean tissue concentrations of five to six animals. α-KG, α-ketoglutarate. * $P<0.05$; † $P<0.001$ compared to normocapnia ($Paco_2=37$ mmHg). Derived from data of Folbergrová et al.[39–41]

reduce arterial pH (pHa) by 0.2–0.4 units are associated with approximately 50% increases in CBF, despite the maintenance of normocapnia.[33,34] However, buffered lactic acid infusion to maintain pHa constant leads to a similar elevation in CBF in the piglets,[34] suggesting that the CBF increase is not the result of a lower pHa but rather the consequence of plasma hyperosmolality. Given the available evidence, the experimental data suggest that, like adults, metabolic alterations in pHa minimally influence perinatal CBF.

Effect of respiratory acidosis/alkalosis on cerebral metabolism

CO_2 has been shown, largely in adult animals, to have substantial effects on cerebral metabolism *per se*. Hypercapnia leads to a generalized suppression of oxidative metabolism, as indicated by an inhibition of cerebral energy utilization and a curtailment of glycolytic and tricarboxylic acid flux.[35–38] In adult dogs, the $CMRO_2$ is decreased by 7 and 11% at $Paco_2$ tensions of 80 and 100 mmHg, respectively.[38] Increasing $Paco_2$ to 80 mmHg results in a 25% decrease in $CMRO_2$ in adult monkeys.[36] The suppression in oxidative metabolism is associated with major changes in the concentrations of key glycolytic and tricarboxylic acid intermediates in brain, as determined by direct tissue analysis (Figure 30.5). Increasing hypercapnia with $Paco_2$ ranging from 50 to 350 mmHg is associated with progressive increases in the tissue concentrations of glucose and glucose-6-phosphate, with concurrent decreases in pyruvate and lactate.[39–41] Essentially all of the tricarboxylic acid metabolites, including citrate, α-ketoglutarate, fumarate, and malate, are decreased during hypercapnia.[39–41] Several critical amino acids are also decreased by hypercapnia, including the excitatory amino acids, glutamate, and aspartate, and the inhibitory amino acid, γ-aminobutyric acid (GABA). The changes in the oxidative intermediates during hypercapnia presumably result from H^+ inhibition of the glycolytic regulatory enzyme, phosphofructokinase; this activity is pH-dependent. Inhibition of this enzyme, in turn, would cause a downstream partial depletion in tissue metabolites.[42] That the overall rate of oxidative metabolism is suppressed by hypercapnia is also demonstrated by a reduction in the cerebral metabolic rate for glucose (CMRglucose) by as much as 50% of the rate at normocapnia.[42] A 50% reduction in CMRglucose has also been shown in developing rats during hypercapnia.[43] It is noteworthy that, despite the suppression of oxidative metabolism, no perturbations in cerebral energy reserves (concentrations of adenosine triphosphate and phosphocreatine) occur,[40,41] indicating that, even with extreme hypercapnia, the energy status of brain tissue is maintained. In this regard, the observed changes in cerebral metabolism which occur with hypercapnia are similar to those seen with anesthesia, especially barbiturates, and probably account for the anesthetic effect of high concentrations of CO_2 (CO_2 narcosis).

Recent in vitro investigations from several laboratories have shown that hypercapnic acidosis of the brain extracellular compartment blunts the action of excitatory amino acid neurotransmitters, especially glutamate, via an inhibition of the *N*-methyl-D-aspartate (NMDA) cell surface receptor.[44–46] Furthermore, hypercapnia actually reduces brain tissue concentrations of glutamate (see above) and possibly inhibits the secretion of the excitatory amino acid into the synaptic cleft, especially during neuronal stimulation, as occurs during seizures or hypoxia–ischemia (see below). The manner in which extracellular acidosis inhibits NMDA receptor activation is not entirely clear, but in vitro studies suggest a downregulation of NMDA-gated ion channel currents with a secondary reduction in intracellular calcium accumulation.[47]

The changes in cerebral metabolism which result from respiratory alkalosis are complex and not simply the reverse of those seen in respiratory acidosis. The alterations in metabolism which occur appear in large part to reflect the occurrence of tissue hypoxia induced by extreme hypocapnia and its vasoconstriction of cerebral resistance vessels leading to reduced CBF. In adult experimental animals and humans, acute hypocapnia causes mental confusion and occasional seizures with an associated slowing of the electroencephalogram; these clinical and electrical disturbances can be reversed by the concurrent administration of 100% oxygen.[48,49] Additional support for the concept that extreme hyperventilation produces brain tissue hypoxia includes the following: (1) brain and cerebral venous blood $P\text{O}_2$ is decreased; (2) brain and CSF lactate and lactate/pyruvate ratios are increased; (3) brain tissue $NADH/NAD^+$ ratios are increased; and (4) CMRglucose is increased, the latter suggesting a stimulation of anaerobic glycolysis.[50–52] At the brain cellular level, graded hypocapnia to $Pa\text{CO}_2$ as low as 10 mmHg is associated with increased concentrations of glucose, pyruvate, and lactate and associated elevations in the lactate/pyruvate and $NADH/NAD^+$ ratios, findings which suggest not only a stimulation of anaerobic glycolysis but the accumulation of cellular metabolic acids as well[51,52] (Figure 30.6). Thus, the alkaline intracellular pH which is observed at moderate levels of hypocapnia ($Pa\text{CO}_2 = 26$ mmHg) reverts to normal or even mildly subnormal (acidosis) when $Pa\text{CO}_2$ falls below 20 mmHg.[51] Despite these alterations, high-energy phosphate reserves are relatively well preserved even during extreme hypocapnia, owing in part to a suppression of cerebral energy utilization.[52]

Findings similar to those of adult animals have been observed in newborn dogs and lambs exposed to hyperventilation.[12–14] In newborn dogs, hypocapnia to $Pa\text{CO}_2$ of 15–17 mmHg leads to a 20% reduction in $CMRO_2$, which occurs in association with an increase in brain tissue lactate and a negative cerebral arteriovenous difference for lactate.[12,13] Taken together, the findings suggest a partial shift from aerobic to anaerobic glycolysis to maintain tissue energy stores normal; the shift in metabolism pre-

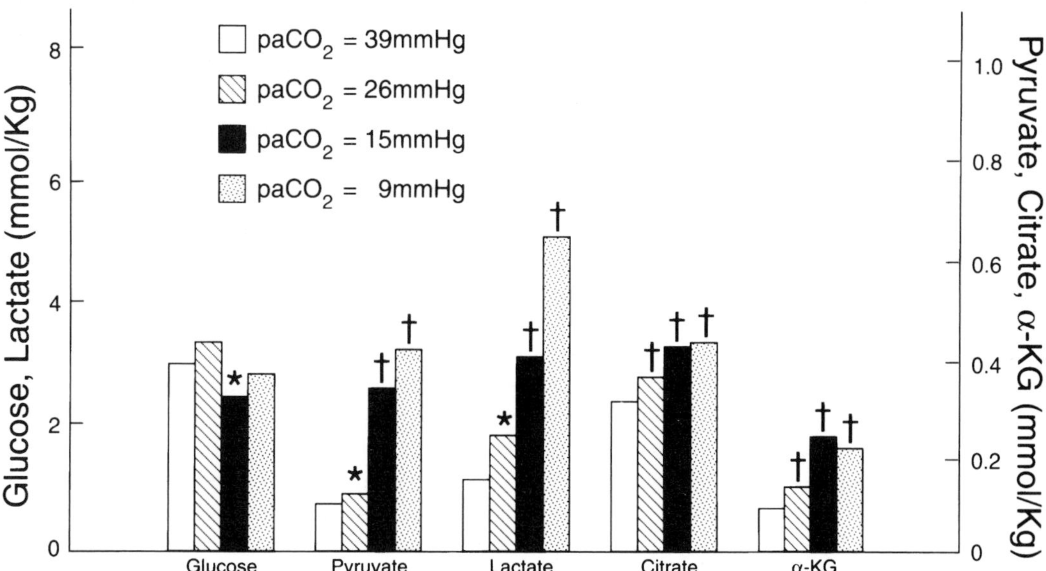

Figure 30.6 Cerebral glycolytic and tricarboxylic acid intermediates during hypocapnia in adult rats. Columns represent mean tissue concentrations of five to six animals. α-KG, α-ketoglutarate. * $P<0.05$; † $P<0.001$ compared to normocapnia ($Paco_2=39$ mmHg). Derived from data of MacMillan and Siesjö.[51]

sumably occurs as a consequence of tissue hypoxia produced by severe cerebral vasoconstriction. Interestingly, the canine electroencephalogram is not adversely influenced by hypocapnia, unlike that of adult animals and humans.

Although tissue hypoxia appears to occur during extreme hypocapnia, there is no experimental or clinical evidence to suggest that hypocapnia *per se* and any associated hypoxia would be severe enough to produce brain damage. It is difficult to imagine that the mammalian brain would be stupid enough to allow itself to be injured by a physiologic process, namely vasoconstriction produced by hypocapnia. Rather, the evidence indicates that, when hypocapnia is extreme and CBF falls below a critical level, a compensatory change in the form of a stimulation of anaerobic glycolysis occurs with the production of cellular metabolic acids, especially lactic acid, and this presence would tend to relax cerebral resistance vessels. Accordingly, a balance would be achieved between the vasoconstriction effect of low $Paco_2$ and the vasodilation effect of brain tissue acidosis (see above). This conclusion is supported by the fact that during even prolonged hypocapnia (hours) the metabolic alterations which occur in the brain are not progressive and that cellular energy reserves are always preserved in uncomplicated hypocapnia (but see below).

Effect of metabolic acidosis/alkalosis on cerebral metabolism

Unlike the wealth of information which is available regarding the brain-modulating effect of respiratory acidosis/alkalosis, little is known regarding the effect of metabolic acidosis/alkalosis on brain metabolism. The paucity of information relates in part to the ability of even the immature blood–brain barrier to impede the influx of H^+ ions into the brain and to the brain's own buffering capacity. Thus, while H^+ ions are either restricted to the vascular compartment or rapidly buffered within brain tissue, the organic component of the acid might be readily transported across the blood–brain barrier to be utilized by oxidative processes. That buffered organic compounds can be oxidized is especially apparent in the immature brain, in which blood–brain transport mechanisms for monocarboxylic acids are well developed.[53] Thus, both lactic acid and the ketone bodies, acetoacetate and β-hydroxybutyrate, are readily transported into the immature brain and undergo oxidation for energy production; as such, they become substitute fuels for glucose. My research colleagues and I have determined that, in the suckling immature rat, up to 30% of cerebral energy production is provided by ketone bodies and the percentage contribution is probably even higher during fasting when blood ketone body concentrations increase two- to threefold.[54,55] In hypoglycemic newborn dogs, lactic acid becomes the preferred cerebral energy fuel, accounting for over 50% of oxidative metabolism.[56,57] Thus, under conditions of both lactacidemia and ketonemia, brain oxidative and energy metabolism are well preserved so long as the tissue is well oxygenated and in osmolar balance.

As mentioned previously, the influence of metabolic acidosis/alkalosis on cerebral metabolism has received little attention in the experimental setting, owing primarily to the existence of the blood–brain barrier and specific acid–base-regulating mechanisms in even the immature brain. Accordingly, brain pH remains relatively normal, even when blood pH fluctuates widely as a result of the disappearance or accumulation of organic acids. To bypass the blood–brain barrier, investigators have used ventriculocisternal perfusion to cause local changes in brain pH without adversely influencing blood pH. By the perfusion of mock CSF of varying pH, Van Nimmen et al.[58] have demonstrated that CMRglucose is depressed in acidotic tissue while it is strongly increased in alkalotic tissue. The changes in CMRglucose parallel those seen in respiratory acidosis and alkalosis (see above) and are probably mediated through the pH-sensitive glycolytic enzyme, phosphofructokines, the modulation of which serves to regulate brain pH through the formation or consumption of organic acids.[29,59]

Hypoxic–ischemic brain damage and metabolic acidosis

Hypoxia–ischemia of a degree sufficient to produce brain damage is always associated with a tissue acidosis owing to the accumulation of lactic acid.[60–62] The cellular lactacidosis results from a shift in glucose utilization from oxidative metabolism to either partial or total anaerobic glycolysis. The question remained as to whether or not the tissue lactacidosis causes or contributes to neuronal injury, when Myers and Yamaguchi[63] demonstrated in juvenile monkeys that the brain damage that arises from cardiopulmonary arrest is influenced by the nutritional status of the animal. Specifically, monkeys fasted before cerebral ischemia exhibited far less brain damage than animals that were fed or received an intravenous infusion of glucose before arrest. Myers[64] attributed the difference in neuropathologic outcome to a varying degree of cerebral lactacidosis in the two groups; the fasted animals had substantially lower tissue lactate levels than either the fed or glucose-infused animals. Controlled studies from several other research laboratories have confirmed and extended the original observation that glucose pretreatment of mature animals accentuates hypoxic–ischemic brain damage.[65–67] Indeed, Pulsinelli et al.[66] have demonstrated that glucose supplementation of rats subjected to severe forebrain ischemia actually converts selective neuronal necrosis into infarction. Clinical studies in adult stroke patients also support the notion that hyperglycemia accentuates ischemic neuronal injury.[68–70] The pathophysiologic mechanism by which glucose accentuates brain damage has been attributed to an excessive production of tissue lactic acid or to an associated derangement in pH homeostasis.[64,71–73] Some investigators have suggested that brain lactacidosis enhances hypoxic–ischemic injury in vulnerable regions and that a minimum concentration of 15–20 mmol lactate/kg brain is required for irreversible damage to occur. Furthermore, it has been demonstrated that the injection of lactic acid into the cerebral cortex of adult rats leads to histologic alterations resembling ischemic infarction – an injury that does not occur following injection of other organic acids of comparable pH.[74–76] Presumably, excessive lactate production during hyperglycemic cerebral hypoxia–ischemia relates to a greater acceleration of anaerobic glycolytic flux than that which occurs when the circulating glucose concentration is not increased. Hyperglycemia *per se* does not substantially increase cerebral glucose utilization (CGU) via the glycolytic pathway;[77] however, determinations of CGU during hyperglycemic cerebral hypoxia–ischemia have not been practical because of difficulties in measuring accurately glucose consumption under such a pathologic condition.[78,79]

Whereas lactic acid appears to contribute to the brain damage resulting from hypoxia–ischemia in adult animals and humans, the question remained as to the contribution of lactic acid to perinatal hypoxic–ischemic brain damage. To answer this question, my research colleagues and I have conducted a series of experiments to ascertain the effect of glucose supplementation and lactacidosis on hypoxic–ischemic brain damage in the immature rat. Our findings indicate that mild hyperglycemia (blood glucose = 350–400 mg/dl) does not influence neuropathologic outcome in immature rats subjected to cerebral hypoxia–ischemia and that moderate hyperglycemia (blood glucose >450 mg/dl) is highly protective.[80,81] Metabolic experiments have been conducted in parallel with the neuropathologic investigations. In mildly hyperglycemic immature rats undergoing cerebral hypoxia–ischemia, cerebral glucose concentrations are persistently higher than those of normoglycemic controls, reflecting enhanced transport of the substrate from blood into brain in association with an unchanging rate of glucose consumption.[82] Brain lactate increases to a similar degree in both the hyperglycemic and normoglycemic rat pups and is actually slightly higher in the normoglycemic animals at the terminus of hypoxia–ischemia. Thus, mild hyperglycemia combined with hypoxia–ischemia is associated with increased glucose transport into brain but not with enhanced glucose utilization or lactate accumulation over that of hypoxia–ischemia alone.

A more severe degree of hyperglycemia with blood glucose concentrations ranging from 450 to 650 mg/dl in immature rats subjected to cerebral hypoxia–ischemia is associated with persistently high tissue and intracellular glucose concentrations throughout the course of hypoxia–ischemia compared to negligible concentrations in normoglycemic controls.[83] Concurrent with the increased brain glucose concentrations in the hyperglycemic rat pups, brain tissue and intracellular concentrations of lactate increase progressively to very high values during hypoxia–ischemia, and these values ultimately exceed the level in the normoglycemic animals by over 200% (Figure 30.7). The finding of an extremely high brain lactate concentration in immature rats in which hypoxic–ischemic brain damage is minimized by glucose supplementation provides evidence that lactic acid *per se* does not cause or contribute to perinatal hypoxic–ischemic brain damage.

However, it must be emphasized that cerebral hypoxia–ischemia leads to cellular acidosis via sources of H^+ ions in addition to lactic acid. Major sources of reducing equivalents include products of the acid hydrolysis of adenosine triphosphate and the formation of NADH ($+H^+$) which accumulates during cellular oxygen debt.[84] In this regard, Welsh et al.[85] examined the oxidation–reduction (redox) state of immature rat brain undergoing hypoxia–ischemia by the technique of reflectance fluorometry. Alterations in regional fluorescence, representing the intracellular accumulation of NADH, were prominent in the cerebral cortex and the CA1 sector of the hippocampus during the first hour of hypoxia–ischemia. The pattern of NADH fluorescence mimicked closely the distribution of selective neuronal necrosis observed in this model of perinatal brain injury. The close correspondence between altered NADH fluorescence and neuropathologic outcome suggests an important role for intracellular acidosis in the pathogenesis of hypoxic–ischemic brain damage, albeit not necessarily lactacidosis. There is no question that a cellular acidosis occurs during the course of cerebral hypoxia–ischemia in the immature rat, as is also indicated by a calculation

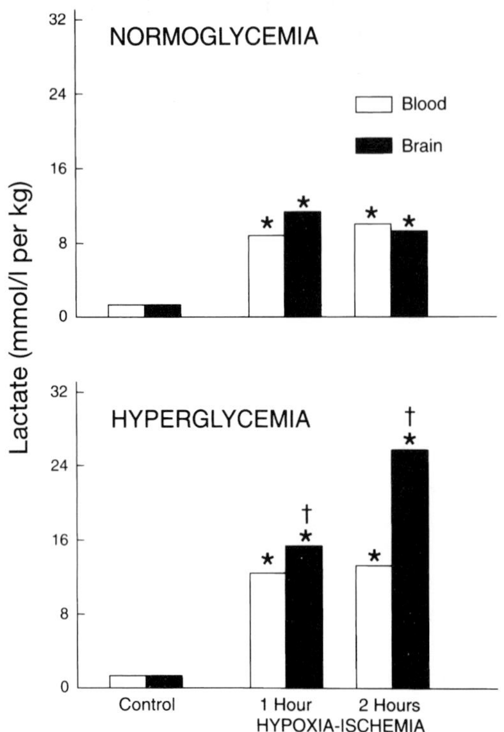

Figure 30.7 Brain glucose and lactate concentrations during hypoxia–ischemia in hyperglycemic and normoglycemic immature rats. Seven-day postnatal rats were rendered hyperglycemic with subcutaneous glucose, immediately following which they were subjected to cerebral hypoxia–ischemia; normoglycemic controls received normal (N) saline prior to hypoxia–ischemia. Columns represent mean tissue concentrations of five to six animals. * $P<0.01$ compared to controls; † $P<0.001$ compared to normoglycemia at same interval. Derived from data of Vannucci et al.[83]

of intracellular pH from the tissue concentrations of high-energy phosphate reserves.[81,86]

Cellular acidosis can be responsible for or contribute to neuronal necrosis in the setting of hypoxia–ischemia by a variety of mechanisms, including inhibition of mitochondrial function, derangement of ionic homeostasis, intracellular calcium accumulation, or enhanced edema formation.[87,88] Combs et al.[89] reported a dissociation between intracellular acidosis and lactate concentration during cerebral ischemia in adult gerbils, such that increasing lactic acid does not affect intracellular pH until a threshold is reached, beyond which intracellular pH falls precipitously. Paschen et al.[84] also emphasized the importance of distinguishing between tissue lactosis and acidosis in a variety of pathologic states, including hypoxia–ischemia.

Hypoxic–ischemic brain damage and respiratory acidosis/alkalosis

As is well known, there are two forms of acidosis which occur in both perinatal experimental animals and human fetuses and newborn infants suffering hypoxia–acidosis (asphyxia) – metabolic and respiratory acidosis. In this regard, recent clinical investigations suggest that premature infants who require mechanical ventilation to prevent or minimize hypoxemia arising from respiratory distress syndrome are at increased risk for the development of brain damage in the form of periventricular leukomalacia if hypocapnia occurs during the course of respiratory management.[90–92] The clinical setting is reminiscent of the alterations in systemic acid–base homeostasis which occur in immature rats undergoing hypoxic–ischemic brain damage.[85] When 7-day postnatal rats are exposed to 8% oxygen, the hypoxemia leads to lactacidemia. The animals hyperventilate to an extent that produces hypocapnia; in turn, this completely compensates for the metabolic acidemia; and blood pH remains normal. The question remained as to the contribution of the hypocapnia to the severity of the hypoxic–ischemic brain damage. To answer this important question, my research colleagues and I conducted experiments whereby immature rats were subjected to cerebral hypoxia–ischemia with or without CO_2 added to the hypoxic gas mixture to which the animals were exposed.[93]

As in our previous experiments,[94] 7-day postnatal rats underwent unilateral common carotid artery occlusion following which they were subjected to hypoxia at 37°C for 2.5 h. The combination of the unilateral carotid artery occlusion and systemic hypoxia causes brain damage in the cerebral hemisphere ipsilateral to the arterial occlusion. The hypoxic gas mixture contained 8% oxygen combined with 0, 3, 6, or 9% CO_2-balance nitrogen. There was a minimum mortality in any of the groups during the hypoxic exposure. Thereafter, the rat pups were returned to their dams until 30 days of postnatal age, at which time their brains underwent neuropathologic analysis. Individual brains were grouped into one of five categories, specifically, grade 0 = normal; grade 1 = mild brain atrophy; grade 2 = moderate brain atrophy; grade 3 = atrophy with cystic cavitation <3 mm; and grade 4 = atrophy with cystic cavitation >3 mm.

Blood gas analysis during the course of hypoxemia indicated that those immature rats breathing 8% oxygen without supplemental CO_2 were hypocapnic, as previously demonstrated[84] (Table 30.1). Rat pups exposed to 3% CO_2 were normocapnic during hypoxemia, while those animals exposed to 6 and 9% CO_2 were progressively hypercapnic. Blood oxygen tensions were essentially identical in all hypoxic groups.

A composite of the neuropathologic findings is shown in Table 30.2. The data show a protective influence of CO_2 inhalation during hypoxemia on the severity of hypoxic–ischemic brain damage. Specifically, rat pups exposed to 3% CO_2 exhibited less brain damage than those not exposed to CO_2 ($P < 0.01$), while rat pups exposed to 6% CO_2 were less brain-damaged than those exposed to 3% CO_2 ($P < 0.001$). Indeed, the greatest reduction in hypoxic–ischemic brain damage occurred in those immature rats exposed to 6% CO_2, with no further protection at a higher concentration. In fact, the rat pups exposed to 9% CO_2 exhibited severities of brain damage comparable to those of rat pups exposed to 3% CO_2, i.e., normocapnia. The results indicate that, in an immature rat model, normocapnic cerebral hypoxia–ischemia is associated with less severe brain damage than is hypocapnic hypoxia–ischemia and that mild hypercapnia is more protective than normocapnia.

In a more recent experiment, we subjected 7-day postnatal rats to hypoxia–ischemia during which they inhaled either 12 or 15% CO_2.[95] In this experiment, control animals were subjected to the same

Table 30.1. Blood carbon dioxide and oxygen tensions in immature rats subjected to hypoxia–ischemia

Variable	P_{CO_2} (mmHg)	P_{O_2} (mmHg)
Control	44	60
Hypoxia–ischemia		
0% CO_2	26	38
3% CO_2	39	28
6% CO_2	59	37
9% CO_2	71	35
12% CO_2	85	43
15% CO_2	102	39

Note:
Values represent means for five to six animals in each hypoxia–ischemia group and 11 controls.
Source: Derived from data of Vannucci et al.[93,95]

Table 30.2. Severity of brain damage in rats previously subjected to cerebral hypoxia–ischemia with or without supplemental carbon dioxide inhalation

Variable	Normal	Atrophy	Infarct
0% CO_2	11	40	49
3% CO_2	29	61	10
6% CO_2	70	30	0
9% CO_2	65	18	17
12% CO_2	72	14	14
15% CO_2	36	7	57

Note:
Animals were categorized as no damage, atrophy without infarct, or infarct. Columns represent the percent of the total number of brains analyzed in each category and according to the concentration of inhaled carbon dioxide.
Source: Data derived from Vannucci et al.[93,95]

interval of hypoxia–ischemia breathing 3% CO_2 (normocapnia). No neuropathologic difference was noted in those animals breathing 12% CO_2 compared to controls exposed to 2 h of hypoxia–ischemia. However, animals breathing 15% CO_2 showed greater brain damage than controls breathing 3% CO_2. Indeed, the severity of brain damage seen in the 15% CO_2 animals was comparable to that previously seen in hypocapnic immature rats (Table 30.2).

Numerous mechanisms potentially exist whereby CO_2 protects the perinatal brain from hypoxic–ischemic brain damage. As discussed previously, such mechanisms would entail hematologic, cardiovascular, cerebrovascular, and metabolic factors. To resolve the issue of the CO_2 effect on perinatal cerebral hypoxia–ischemia, we performed metabolic studies in addition to our neuropathologic experiments.[96] Seven-day postnatal rats were subjected to hypoxia–ischemia (see above), during which they were rendered hypocapnic, normocapnic, or mildly hypercapnic by the inhalation of 0, 3, or 6% CO_2. Cerebral blood flow during hypoxia–ischemia was better preserved in the normo- and hypercapnic rat pups compared to hypocapnic littermates; these animals also exhibited a stimulation of cerebral glucose utilization (Table 30.3). Brain glucose concentrations were higher and lactate lower in the normo- and hypercapnic animals, indicating that glucose was consumed oxidatively in these groups rather than by anaerobic glycolysis, as apparently occurred in the hypocapnic animals. The high-energy phosphate reserves, adenosine triphosphate, and phosphocreatine, were better preserved in the normo- and hypercapnic rats compared with the hypocapnic animals. CSF glutamate, as a reflection of the brain extracellular fluid concentration, was lowest in the hypercapnic rats at 2 h of hypoxia–ischemia. From the findings, we concluded that during hypoxia–ischemia in the immature rat, CBF is better preserved during normo- and mild hypercapnia, and the greater oxygen delivery promotes cerebral glucose utilization and oxidative metabolism for optimum maintenance of tissue high-energy phosphate reserves. An inhibition of glutamate secretion into the synaptic cleft, thereby attenuating postsynaptic receptor activation, would further protect the mildly hypercapnic animal from hypoxic–ischemic brain damage.

Table 30.3. Cerebral blood flow (CBF) and glucose utilization (CGU) during hypoxia–ischemia in immature rats at varying carbon dioxide tensions

Variable	CBF	CGU
0% CO_2	59%	114%
3% CO_2	71%	166%
6% CO_2	75%	155%
12% CO_2	75%	
15% CO_2	62%	

Note:
Values represent percentages of control values in each CO_2 group.
Source: Derived from data of Vannucci et al.[93,95]

Although metabolic studies have not been conducted in immature rats exposed to higher blood CO_2 tensions, cerebral blood flow measurements have been ascertained during hypoxia–ischemia in immature rats exposed to 12 or 15% CO_2. Rat pups breathing 12% CO_2 have CBF values comparable to littermates breathing 3% CO_2, while CBF in animals breathing 15% CO_2 is the lowest of the three groups (Table 30.3). Presumably, the low CBF accentuated the cerebral ischemia, producing greater brain damage than seen in the 3 or 12% CO_2-exposed animals.[95]

Acidosis and perinatal hypoxic–ischemic brain damage

Our past and present experiments in the immature rat pertaining to cerebral hypoxia–ischemia at variable CO_2 tensions are relevant to the situation in human fetuses and newborn infants. As mentioned previously, clinical investigations suggest that premature infants who require mechanical ventilation to prevent or minimize hypoxemia arising from respiratory distress syndrome are at increased risk for the development of periventricular leukomalacia if hypocapnia occurs during the course of respiratory management.[90–92] In this regard, mild hypercapnia (permissive hypercapnia) during the course of management of respiratory distress syndrome has recently been advocated,[97] but any beneficial effect of mild hypercapnia on the immature human brain has yet to be determined.

Obstetricians have long used blood acid–base status to ascertain the presence or absence of systemic hypoxia–acidosis (asphyxia) in the fetus during the intrapartum period. Early studies found only a poor-to-fair correlation between the presence of acidosis, determined by measurement of either fetal scalp or umbilical cord blood pH, with either neonatal depression (low Apgar scores) or encephalopathy,[98–101] but little or no correlation with long-term neurologic outcome.[102,103] The lack of a strong correlation between these variables related, at least in part, to the use of pH values (pH<7.15–7.20) not indicative of severe acidosis or to the failure to discern whether the acidosis was respiratory, metabolic, or mixed in origin. More recently, investigators have concentrated on more severe degrees of acidosis than previously reported and on the extent to which the altered pH reflects an underlying respiratory or metabolic (lactic) acidosis. In the study of Goldaber et al.,[104] 2.5% of 3506 full-term newborn infants exhibited an umbilical artery pH of <7.00, of whom 66.7% had a metabolic component to their acidosis. Significantly more of the severely acidotic newborn infants exhibited low (<3) 1- and 5-min Apgar scores compared to infants with higher umbilical artery pH values. In addition, neonatal death was significantly more frequent in the severely acidotic group. Low et al.[105] compared 59 full-term fetuses exhibiting metabolic acidosis to 59 fetuses with normal umbilical blood acid–base status and 51 fetuses exhibiting only a respiratory acidosis at birth. A variety of newborn complications, including encephalopathy, was apparent in 54% of the newborn infants experiencing a metabolic acidosis compared to very low complication rates in those infants with either respiratory acidosis or no acidosis at all.[106–108] Furthermore, Low et al.[109] have previously demonstrated a positive correlation between the severity and duration of intrapartum metabolic acidosis and neurodevelopmental outcome at 1 year. However, Van den Berg et al.[110] have demonstrated that fetuses undergoing acute asphyxiation and exhibiting an umbilical artery pH <7.0 with a prominent respiratory component ($P\text{CO}_2 = 92$ mmHg) are more likely to exhibit neurologic, respiratory, cardiovascular, and gastrointestinal complications than newborn infants with an umbilical artery pH >7.24. With increasing hypercapnia, the proportion of neonates with neurologic complications increases.[111] Further clinical investigations are required to resolve the issue of the effect of severe hypercapnia on perinatal hypoxic–ischemic brain damage.

Conclusions

In summary, the present review has focused on current knowledge regarding the effects of respiratory and metabolic acidosis/alkalosis on CBF and metabolism with or without associated systemic and cerebral hypoxia–ischemia. Past and recent animal experiments suggest that glucose supplementation is protective to the perinatal brain subjected to cerebral hypoxia–ischemia and that excessive tissue lactic acid formation does not aggravate hypoxic–ischemic brain damage. Furthermore, mild respiratory acidosis is neuroprotective, while severe respiratory acidosis is deleterious. These findings in the immature rat are corroborated to some extent by clinical data in the human fetus or newborn human infant undergoing perinatal hypoxia or asphyxia.

Acknowledgments

Dr. Vannucci's past research endeavors have been supported by grants from the National Institute of Child Health and Human Development, the American Heart Association, the Diabetes Association, and the United Cerebral Palsy Foundation. Dr. Vannucci's present research endeavors are supported by Program Project

#HD30704 from the National Institute of Child Health and Human Development.

REFERENCES

1 Hernandez MJ, Brennan RW, Vannucci RC, et al. (1978). Cerebral blood flow and oxygen consumption in the newborn dog. *Am J Physiol*, **234**, R209–R215.

2 Häggendal E and Johansson B. (1965). Effects of arterial carbon dioxide tension and oxygen saturation on cerebral blood flow autoregulation in dogs. *Acta Physiol Scand*, **66** (suppl. 258), 27–53.

3 Reivich M, Brann AW and Shapiro H. (1971). Reactivity of cerebral vessels to CO_2 in the newborn rhesus monkey. *Eur Neurol*, **6**, 132–136.

4 Rosenberg AA, Jones MD, Traystman RJ, et al. (1982). Response of cerebral blood flow to changes in $P\text{CO}_2$ in fetal, newborn and adult sheep. *Am J Physiol*, **242**, H862–H866.

5 Purves MJ and James IM. (1969). Observations on the control of cerebral blood flow in the sheep fetus and newborn lamb. *Circ Res*, **25**, 651–667.

6 Ashwal S, Dale PS and Longo LD. (1984). Regional cerebral blood flow: studies in the fetal lamb during hypoxia, hypercapnia, acidosis, and hypotension. *Pediatr Res*, **18**, 1309–1316.

7 Reddy GD, Gootman N, Buckley NM, et al. (1974). Regional blood flow changes in neonatal pigs in response to hypercapnia, hemorrhage and sciatic nerve stimulation. *Biol Neonate*, **25**, 249–262.

8 Shapiro HM, Greenberg JH, Naughton KVH, et al. (1980). Heterogeneity of local cerebral blood flow – $P\text{aCO}_2$ sensitivity in neonatal dogs. *J Appl Physiol*, **49**, 113–118.

9 Cavazzuti M and Duffy TE. (1982). Regulation of local cerebral blood flow in normal and hypoxic newborn dogs. *Ann Neurol*, **11**, 247–257.

10 Hansen NB, Nowicki PT, Miller RR, et al. (1986). Alterations in cerebral blood flow and oxygen consumption during prolonged hypocarbia. *Pediatr Res*, **20**, 147–150.

11 Himwich HE. (1951). *Brain Metabolism and Cerebral Disorders*. Baltimore: Williams and Wilkins.

12 Young RSK and Yagel SK. (1984). Cerebral physiological and metabolic effects of hyperventilation in the neonatal dog. *Ann Neurol*, **16**, 337–342.

13 Reuter JH and Disney TA. (1986). Regional cerebral blood flow and cerebral metabolic rate of oxygen during hyperventilation in the newborn dog. *Pediatr Res*, **20**, 1102–1106.

14 Rosenberg AA. (1988). Response of the cerebral circulation to profound hypocarbia in neonatal lambs. *Stroke*, **19**, 1365–1370.

15 Gleason CA, Short BL and Jones MD. (1989). Cerebral blood flow and metabolism during and after prolonged hypocapnia in newborn lambs. *J Pediatr*, **115**, 309–314.

16 Greisen G. (1986). Cerebral blood flow in preterm infants during the first week of life. *Acta Pediatr Scand*, **75**, 43–51.

17 Greisen G and Trojaborg W. (1987). Cerebral blood flow, $P\text{aCO}_2$ changes, and visual evoked potentials in mechanically ventilated, preterm infants. *Acta Pediatr Scand*, **76**, 394–400.

18 Pryds O and Greisen G. (1989). Effect of $P\text{aCO}_2$ and haemoglobin concentration on day to day variation of CBF in preterm neonates. *Acta Pediatr Scand Suppl*, **360**, 33–36.

19 Pryds O, Greisen G, Lou H, et al. (1989). Heterogeneity of cerebral vasoreactivity in preterm infants supported by mechanical ventilation. *J Pediatr*, **115**, 638–645.

20 Pryds O, Greisen G, Skov LL, et al. (1990). Carbon dioxide-related changes in cerebral blood volume and cerebral blood flow in mechanically ventilated preterm neonates: comparison of near infrared spectrophotometry and ^{133}Xenon clearance. *Pediatr Res*, **27**, 445–449.

21 Levene MI, Shortland D, Gibson N, et al. (1988). Carbon dioxide reactivity of the cerebral circulation in extremely premature infants: effects of postnatal age and indomethacin. *Pediatr Res*, **24**, 175–179.

22 Toda N, Hatano Y and Mori K. (1989). Mechanisms underlying response to hypercapnia of isolated dog cerebral arteries. *Am J Physiol*, **257**, H141–H146.

23 Wang Q, Pellegrino DA and Koenig HM. (1993). The role of endothelium in rat pial arteriolar dilatory responses. *Soc Neurosci Abstr*, **500**, 13.

24 Parfenova H, Shibata M, Zuckerman S, et al. (1994). CO_2 and cerebral circulation in newborn pigs: cyclic nucleotides and prostanoids in vascular regulation. *Am J Physiol*, **266**, H1494–H1501.

25 Wagerle LC and Degiulio PA. (1994). Indomethacin-sensitive CO_2 reactivity of cerebral arterioles is restored by vasodilator prostaglandin. *Am J Physiol*, **266**, H1332–H1338.

26 Faraci FM and Brian JE. (1994). Nitric oxide and the cerebral circulation. *Stroke*, **25**, 692–703.

27 Pellegrino DA, Koenig HM and Albrecht RF. (1993). Nitric oxide synthesis and regional cerebral blood flow responses to hypercapnia and hypoxia in the rat. *J Cereb Blood Flow Metabol*, **13**, 80–87.

28 Nozaki K, Moskowitz MA, Maynard KI, et al. (1993). Possible origins and distribution of immunoreactive nitric oxide synthase-containing nerve fibers in cerebral arteries. *J Cereb Blood Flow Metabol*, **13**, 70–79.

29 Siesjö BK. (1978). *Brain Energy Metabolism*. Chichester, England: Wiley.

30 Hermansen MC, Kotagal UR and Kleinman LI. (1984). The effect of metabolic acidosis upon autoregulation of cerebral blood flow in newborn dogs. *Brain Res*, **324**, 101–105.
31 Powell CL, Hernandez MJ and Vannucci RC. (1985). The effect of lactacidemia on regional cerebral blood flow in the newborn dog. *Dev Brain Res*, **17**, 314–316.
32 Young RSK, Yagel SK and Woods CL. (1984). The effects of sodium bicarbonate on brain blood flow, brain water content, and blood–brain barrier in the neonatal dog. *Acta Neuropathol*, **65**, 124–127.
33 Bucciarelli RL and Eitzman DV. (1979). Cerebral blood flow during acute acidosis in perinatal goats. *Pediatr Res*, **13**, 178–180.
34 Laptook AR, Peterson J and Porter AM. (1988). Effects of lactic acid infusions and pH on cerebral blood flow and metabolism. *J Cereb Blood Flow Metabol*, **8**, 193–200.
35 Kogure K, Busto R, Scheinberg P, et al. (1975). Dynamics of cerebral metabolism during moderate hypercapnia. *J Neurochem*, **24**, 171–178.
36 Fliefoth AB, Grubb RL and Raichle ME. (1979). Depression of cerebral oxygen utilization by hypercapnia in the rhesus monkey. *J Neurochem*, **32**, 661–663.
37 Berntman L, Dahlgeren N and Siesjö BK. (1979). Cerebral blood flow and oxygen consumption in the rat brain during extreme hypercarbia. *Anesthesiology*, **50**, 299–305.
38 Artru AA and Michenfelder JD. (1980). Effects of hypercarbia on canine cerebral metabolism and blood flow with simultaneous direct and indirect measurement of blood flow. *Anesthesiology*, **52**, 466–469.
39 Folbergrová J, MacMillan V and Siesjö BK. (1972). The effect of hypercapnic acidosis upon some glycolytic and Krebs cycle-associated intermediates in the cat brain. *J Neurochem*, **19**, 2507–2517.
40 Folbergrová J, Ponté U and Siesjö BK. (1974). Patterns of changes in brain carbohydrate metabolites, amino acids, and organic phosphates at increased carbon dioxide tensions. *J Neurochem*, **22**, 1115–1125.
41 Folbergrová J, Norberg K, Quistorff B, et al. (1975). Carbohydrate and amino acid metabolism in rat cerebral cortex in moderate and extreme hypercapnia. *J Neurochem*, **25**, 457–462.
42 Miller AL, Hawkins RA and Veech RL. (1975). Decreased rate of glucose utilization by rat brain in vivo after exposure to atmospheres containing high concentrations of CO_2. *J Neurochem*, **25**, 553–558.
43 Miller AL and Corddry DH. (1981). Brain carbohydrate metabolism in developing rats during hypercapnia. *J Neurochem*, **36**, 1202–1210.
44 Tombaugh GC and Sapolsky RM. (1990). Mild acidosis protects hippocampal neurons from injury induced by oxygen and glucose deprivation. *Brain Res*, **506**, 343–345.
45 Takadera T, Shimada Y and Mohri T. (1992). Extracellular pH modulates *N*-methyl-D-aspartate receptor-mediated neurotoxicity and calcium accumulation in rat cortical cultures. *Brain Res*, **572**, 126–131.
46 Kaku DA, Giffard RG and Choi DW. (1993). Neuroprotective effects of glutamate antagonists and extracellular acidity. *Science*, **260**, 1516–1518.
47 Tombaugh GC and Sapolsky RM. (1993). Evolving concepts about the role of acidosis in ischemic neuropathology. *J Neurochem*, **61**, 793–803.
48 Reivich M, Kohen PJ and Greenbaum L. (1966). Alterations in the electroencephalogram of awake man produced by hyperventilation: Effects of 100% oxygen at 3 atmospheres (absolute) pressure. *Neurology*, **16**, 304.
49 Plum F, Posner JB and Smith WW. (1968). Effect of hypocarbic-hyperoxic hyperventilation on blood, brain and CSF lactate. *Am J Physiol*, **215**, 1240–1244.
50 Plum F and Posner JB. (1967). Blood and cerebrospinal fluid lactate during hyperventilation. *Am J Physiol*, **212**, 864–870.
51 MacMillan V and Siesjö BK. (1973). The influence of hypocapnia upon intracellular pH and upon some carbohydrate substrates, amino acids and organic phosphates in the brain. *J Neurochem*, **21**, 1283–1299.
52 Kogure K, Busto R, Matsumoto A, et al. (1975). Effect of hyperventilation on dynamics of cerebral energy metabolism. *Am J Physiol*, **228**, 1862–1867.
53 Cremer JE. (1982). Substrate utilization and brain development. *J Cereb Blood Flow Metab*, **2**, 394–407.
54 Vannucci RC, Christensen MA and Stein DT. (1989). Regional cerebral glucose utilization in the immature rat: effect on hypoxia–ischemia. *Pediatr Res*, **26**, 208–214.
55 Yager JY, Heitjan DF, Towfighi J, et al. (1992). Effect of insulin-induced and fasting hypoglycemia on perinatal hypoxic–ischemic brain damage. *Pediatr Res*, **31**, 138–142.
56 Hernandez MJ, Vannucci RC, Salcedo A, et al. (1980). Cerebral blood flow and metabolism during hypoglycemia in newborn dogs. *J Neurochem*, **35**, 622–628.
57 Hellmann J, Vannucci RC and Nardis EE. (1982). Blood–brain barrier permeability to lactic acid in the newborn dog: lactate as a cerebral metabolic fuel. *Pediatr Res*, **16**, 40–44.
58 Van Nimmen D, Weyne J, Demeester G, et al. (1986). Local cerebral glucose utilization during intracerebral pH changes. *J Cereb Blood Flow Metab*, **6**, 584–589.
59 Weyne J, Demeester G and Leusen I. (1970). Effects of carbon dioxide, bicarbonate, and pH on lactate and pyruvate in the brain of rats. *Pflugers Arch*, **314**, 292–311.

60 Siesjö BK. (1981). Cell damage in the brain: a speculative synthesis. *J Cereb Blood Flow Metab*, **1**, 155–185.
61 Hossmann K-A. (1982). Treatment of experimental cerebral ischemia. *J Cereb Blood Flow Metab*, **2**, 275–297.
62 Raichle ME. (1983). The pathophysiology of the brain ischemia. *Ann Neurol*, **13**, 2–10.
63 Myers RE and Yamaguchi S. (1977). Nervous system effects of cardiac arrest in monkeys. Preservation of vision. *Arch Neurol*, **34**, 65–74.
64 Myers RE. (1979). A unitary theory of causation of anoxic and hypoxic brain pathology. In *Cerebral Hypoxia and Its Consequences*, eds. Fahn S, Davis JN, Rowland LP, pp. 195–213. New York: Raven Press.
65 Kalimo H, Rehncroná S, Söderfeldt B, et al. (1981). Brain lactic acidosis and ischemic cell damage: 2. Histopathology. *J Cereb Blood Flow Metab*, **1**, 313–327.
66 Pulsinelli WA, Waldman S, Rawlinson D, et al. (1982). Hyperglycemia converts neuronal damage into brain infarction. *Neurology*, **32**, 1239–1246.
67 Duverger D and MacKenzie ET. (1988). The quantification of cerebral infarction following focal ischemia in the rat: influence of strain, arterial pressure, blood glucose concentration and age. *J Cereb Blood Flow Metab*, **8**, 449–461.
68 Pulsinelli WA, Levy DE, Sigsbee B, et al. (1983). Increased damage after ischemic stroke in patients with hyperglycemia with or without diabetes mellitus. *Am J Med*, **74**, 540–544.
69 Berger L and Hakim AM. (1986). The association of hyperglycemia with cerebral edema in stroke. *Stroke*, **17**, 865–871.
70 Levine SR, Welsh KMA, Helpern JA, et al. (1988). Prolonged deterioration of ischemic brain energy metabolism and acidosis associated with hyperglycemia: human cerebral infarction studies by serial ^{31}P NMR spectroscopy. *Ann Neurol*, **23**, 416–418.
71 Rehncroná S, Rosén I and Siesjö BK. (1981). Brain lactic acidosis and ischemic cell damage: 1. Biochemistry and neurophysiology. *J Cereb Blood Flow Metab*, **1**, 297–311.
72 Welsh FA, Ginsberg MD, Rieder W, et al. (1980). Deleterious effect of glucose pretreatment on recovery from diffuse cerebral ischemia in the cat. II. Regional metabolite levels. *Stroke*, **11**, 355–363.
73 Pulsinelli WA, French J, Rawlinson D, et al. (1982). Cerebral ischemia damages neurons despite lowered brain lactate levels. *Ann Neurol*, **12**, 86.
74 Kraig RP, Petito CK, Plum F, et al. (1987). Hydrogen ions kill brain at concentrations reached in ischemia. *J Cereb Blood Flow Metab*, **7**, 379–386.
75 Petito CK, Kraig RP and Pulsinelli WA. (1987). Light and electron microscopic evaluation of hydrogen ion-induced brain necrosis. *J Cereb Blood Flow Metab*, **7**, 625–632.
76 Goldman SA, Pulsinelli WA, Clarke WY, et al. (1989). The effects of extracellular acidosis on neurons and glia in vitro. *J Cereb Blood Flow Metab*, **9**, 471–477.
77 Orzi F, Lucignani G, Dow-Edwards D, et al. (1988). Local cerebral glucose utilization in controlled graded levels of hyperglycemia in the conscious rat. *J Cereb Blood Flow Metab*, **8**, 346–356.
78 Tanaka K, Welsh FA, Greenberg JH, et al. (1985). Regional alterations in glucose consumption and metabolite levels during postischemic recovery in cat brain. *J Cereb Blood Flow Metab*, **5**, 502–511.
79 Lockwood AH, Peek KE, Izumiyama M, et al. (1989). Effects of moderate hypoxemia and unilateral carotid artery ligation on cerebral glucose metabolism and acid–base balance in the rat. *J Cereb Blood Flow Metab*, **9**, 342–349.
80 Voorhies TM, Rawlinson D and Vannucci RC. (1986). Glucose and perinatal hypoxic–ischemic brain damage in the rat. *Neurology*, **36**, 1115–1118.
81 Vannucci RC and Mujsce DJ. (1992). Effect of glucose on perinatal hypoxic–ischemic brain damage. *Biol Neonate*, **62**, 215–224.
82 Vannucci RC, Vasta F and Vannucci SJ. (1987). Cerebral metabolic responses of hyperglycemic immature rats to hypoxia–ischemia. *Pediatr Res*, **21**, 524–529.
83 Vannucci RC, Brucklacher RM and Vannucci SJ. (1996). The effect of hyperglycemia on cerebral metabolism during hypoxia–ischemia in the immature rat. *J Cereb Blood Flow Metab*, **16**, 1026–1033.
84 Paschen W, Djuricic B, Mies G, et al. (1987). Lactate and pH in the brain: association and dissociation in different pathophysiological states. *J Neurochem*, **48**, 154–159.
85 Welsh FA, Vannucci RC and Brierley JB. (1982). Columnar alterations of NADH fluorescence during hypoxia–ischemia in immature rat brain. *J Cereb Blood Flow Metab*, **2**, 221–228.
86 Vannucci RC and Yager JY. (1992). Glucose, lactic acid, and perinatal hypoxic–ischemic brain damage. *Pediatr Neurol*, **8**, 3–12.
87 Hakim AM and Stoubridge EA. (1989). Cerebral acidosis in focal ischemia. *Cerebrovasc Brain Metab Rev*, **1**, 115–132.
88 Hillered L, Smith ML and Siesjö BK. (1985). Lactic acidosis and recovery of mitochondrial function following forebrain ischemia in the rat. *J Cereb Blood Flow Metab*, **5**, 259–266.
89 Combs DJ, Dempsey RJ, Maley M, et al. (1990). Relationship between plasma glucose, brain lactate and intracellular pH during cerebral ischemia in gerbils. *Stroke*, **21**, 936–942.

90 Greisen G, Munck H and Lou H. (1987). Severe hypocarbia in preterm infants and neurodevelopmental deficit. *Acta Pediatr Scand*, **86**, 401–404.

91 Graziani L, Spitzer AR, Mitchell DG, et al. (1992). Mechanical ventilation in preterm infants: neurosonographic and developmental studies. *Pediatrics*, **90**, 515–522.

92 Ikonen RS, Janas MO, Koidikko MJ, et al. (1992). Hyperbilirubinemia, hypocarbia and periventricular leukomalacia in preterm infants: relationship to cerebral palsy. *Acta Pediatr Scand*, **81**, 802–807.

93 Vannucci RC, Towfighi J, Heitjan DF, et al. (1995). Carbon dioxide protects the perinatal brain from hypoxic–ischemic damage: an experimental study in the immature rat. *Pediatrics*, **95**, 868–874.

94 Rice JE, Vannucci RC and Brierley JB. (1981). The influence of immaturity on hypoxic–ischemic brain damage in the rat. *Ann Neurol*, **9**, 131–141.

95 Vannucci RC, Towfighi J, Brucklacher RM, et al. (2001) Effect of extreme hypercapnia on hypoxic–ischemic brain damage in the immature rat. *Pediatr Res*, **49**, 799–803.

96 Vannucci RC, Brucklacher RM and Vannucci SJ. (1997). Effect of carbon dioxide on cerebral metabolism during hypoxia–ischemia in the immature rat. *Pediatr Res*, **42**, 24–29.

97 Mariani G, Cifuentes J and Carlo WA. (1999). Randomized trial of permissive hypercapnia in preterm infants. *Pediatrics*, **104**, 1082–1088.

98 Bowen LW, Kochenour NK, Rehm NE, et al. (1986). Maternal–fetal pH difference and fetal scalp pH as predictors of neonatal outcome. *Obstet Gynecol*, **67**, 487–495.

99 Page FO, Martin JN, Palmer SM, et al. (1986). Correlation of neonatal acid–base status with Apgar scores and fetal heart rate tracings. *Am J Obstet Gynecol*, **154**, 1306–1311.

100 Vintzileos AM, Gaffney SE, Salinger LM, et al. (1987). The relationships among the fetal biophysical profile, umbilical cord pH, and Apgar scores. *Am J Obstet Gynecol*, **157**, 627–631.

101 Winkler CL, Hauth JC, Tucker JM, et al. (1991). Neonatal complications at term as related to the degree of umbilical artery acidemia. *Am J Obstet Gynecol*, **164**, 637–641.

102 Dennis J, Johnson A, Mutch L, et al. (1989). Acid–base status at birth and neurodevelopmental outcome at four and one-half years. *Am J Obstet Gynecol*, **161**, 213–220.

103 Fee SC, Malee K, Deddish R, et al. (1990). Severe acidosis and subsequent neurologic status. *Am J Obstet Gynecol*, **162**, 802–806.

104 Goldaber KG, Gilsterap LC, Leveno KJ, et al. (1991). Pathologic fetal acidemia. *Obstet Gynecol*, **78**, 1103–1107.

105 Low JA, Panagiotopoulos C and Derrick EJ. (1994). Newborn complications after intrapartum asphyxia with metabolic acidosis in the term fetus. *Am J Obstet Gynecol*, **170**, 1081–1087.

106 Perlman JM and Risser R. (1993). Severe fetal acidemia: neonatal neurologic features and short-term outcome. *Pediatr Neurol*, **9**, 277–282.

107 Socol ML, Garcia PM and Riter S. (1994). Depressed Apgar scores, acid–base status, and neurologic outcome. *Am J Obstet Gynecol*, **170**, 991–999.

108 Low JA, Panagiotopoulos C and Derrick EJ. (1995). Newborn complications after intrapartum asphyxia with metabolic acidosis in the preterm fetus. *Am J Obstet Gynecol*, **172**, 805–810.

109 Low JA, Galbraith RS, Muir DW, et al. (1984). Factors associated with motor and cognitive deficits in children after intrapartum fetal hypoxia. *Am J Obstet Gynecol*, **148**, 533–539.

110 Van den Berg PP, Nelen WLDM, Jongsma HW, et al. (1996). Neonatal complications in newborns with an umbilical artery pH <7.00. *Am J Obstet Gynecol*, **175**, 1152–1157.

111 Goodwin TM, Belai I, Hernandez P, et al. (1992). Asphyxial complications in the term newborn with severe umbilical acidemia. *Am J Obstet Gynecol*, **162**, 1506–1512.

31

Meconium staining and the meconium aspiration syndrome

Thomas E. Wiswell

SUNY Stony Brook, Stony Brook, NY, USA

Introduction

Meconium-stained amniotic fluid (MSAF) occurs in approximately 10–15% of all pregnancies.[1] The presence of MSAF has been recognized as being associated with adverse fetal and neonatal outcomes for centuries.[2] In fact, Aristotle gave the substance the name *meconium-arion,* meaning "opium-like," as he believed it induced fetal sleep. The philosopher likely recognized fetal deaths and neonatal depression as being associated with meconium, hence the appellation. Obstetricians and pediatricians recognize the relationship of MSAF with stillborn infants, abnormal fetal heart rate tracings, neonatal encephalopathy, respiratory distress, and an abnormal neurologic outcome in some survivors. Nevertheless, the vast majority of infants born through MSAF do not have apparent antenatal, intrapartum, or postnatal problems. Thus, we have somewhat limited ability to be able to predict and prognosticate from the presence of MSAF. Health-care providers should be appropriately concerned about both MSAF and meconium-stained neonates who subsequently develop respiratory distress, the meconium aspiration syndrome (MAS). However, despite the frequent occurrence of MSAF and MAS, there remains a distinct paucity of literature describing the neurological development of either children born through MSAF or those with MAS. In this chapter, I will present what is currently known about the substance and its association with adverse outcomes.

Historical aspects

More than 75 years ago, Schulze[3] reviewed several controversies concerning MSAF, including whether its presence reflected fetal asphyxia vs a physiologic process, as well as whether MSAF represented a grave prognostic omen. She referred to publications from the 1600s in which MSAF was considered a sign of death or impending death of the fetus. In addition, Schulze quoted several publications from the 1800s in which MSAF portended an endangered condition of the fetus. She refered to Jesse's 1888 report in which MSAF was found in 9.5% of pregnancies. In this latter report, of 314 pregnancies in which MSAF was found, 74 of the infants were stillborn, while 74 were described as "asphyxiated." Grant[4] refered to the work of Kennedy in 1833 in which MSAF was described as a harbinger of stillbirth or fetal distress. In 1918 Reed[5] proposed that in utero anoxia would relax the anal sphincter and result in meconium passage. Reed was the first individual to describe in utero aspiration of meconium. Clifford[6] reported a 6% mortality rate and a 60% morbidity rate among infants born through MSAF. He specifically commented on the frequent need for resuscitation of such infants. Brews[7] subsequently hypothesized that meconium passage was a result of increased intestinal peristalsis as a response to asphyxia. The degree of hypoxia needed for meconium passage was first described by Walker.[8] He found that meconium passage was associated with umbilical venous oxygen saturations $<30\%$.

Some data concerning MSAF and MAS were reported from the National Institute of Neurological and Communicative Disorders and Stroke Collaborative Perinatal Project (CPP) of the late 1950s and 1960s. In this study, more than 42 000 children were followed from birth for the development of cerebral palsy (CP), mental retardation, and other neurologic disorders.[9,10] Fujikura and Klionsky reported that 10.3% of all live-born infants in the CPP had meconium staining.[9] They found the stained group to have a neonatal mortality death rate of 3.3% compared to 1.7% among nonmeconium-stained babies. Fully 18.1% of the babies that died in the CPP were born through MSAF. In a little-known aspect of the study, Naeye reported that 64% of the cases of meconium in the amniotic fluid were associated with the presence of acute chorioamnionitis.[10] Naeye found that MAS occurred in 8.7% of the infants in the CPP who were born through MSAF. Of those babies with such respiratory distress, 63% died.

In the 1950s, Desmond and colleagues addressed several important issues concerning MSAF and MAS.[11,12] They initially described the amount of time it took for color changes to occur in the finger- and toenails of babies, as well as in vernix, during exposure to meconium-stained fluid. The following year, these authors reported an overall 22.8% incidence of MAS following exposure to MSAF. Babies with MAS had a 16% mortality rate. They also noted a less frequent occurrence of MSAF among women with preterm compared to term-gestation deliveries. The overall mortality rate among meconium-stained infants was 3.4% compared to a 1.5% rate among children born through clear amniotic fluid. Furthermore, these authors found meconium-stained babies to be more likely to have abnormal neurologic findings.

During the 1970s several articles appeared supporting the benefits of aggressive airway management in meconium-stained neonates.[13–15] Although they represented anecdotal experience and not randomized controlled trials, these three works led to virtually universal practices of obstetrical naso- and oropharyngeal suctioning, as well as postpartum intratracheal suctioning, of meconium-stained infants in the delivery room. However, in the year 2000 the results of a large randomized, controlled trial were published in which it was established that intratracheal intubation and suctioning did not improve the respiratory outcomes of apparently vigorous meconium-stained neonates.[16] The current recommendation of the Neonatal Resuscitation Program of the American Academy of Pediatrics (AAP) and the American Heart Association[17] is to provide expectant care to the apparently vigorous meconium-stained infant (i.e., no intratracheal suctioning). At the time of writing of this chapter, I was aware of several other large trials assessing the validity of several interventions commonly applied in the presence of MSAF (amnioinfusion, obstetrical naso- and oropharyngeal suctioning).

Meconium-stained amniotic fluid and fetal distress

Despite the many publications concerning adverse outcomes associated with MSAF, several authors have questioned whether MSAF is an independent marker of fetal distress.[18,19] They largely argue that in the absence of abnormal fetal heart rate (FHR) patterns, neonatal outcome of infants born through MSAF is similar to that of babies born through clear fluid. What is the evidence supporting the association of MSAF with fetal distress? Unquestionably, babies born through MSAF and those who subsequently develop MAS have a higher frequency of abnormal FHR tracings.[20–27] The classic work of Walker[8] revealed the markedly low fetal oxygen saturations related to meconium passage. White[28] found one-third of meconium-stained infants required delivery room resuscitation. Others have found meconium-stained infants to be more likely to have lower scalp pHs or low umbilical cord artery pHs.[19,29–35] Additionally, meconium-stained infants have lower 1-min and 5-min Apgar scores.[21,36,37] When we previously reviewed the literature,[1] we found approximately one-third of all reported babies (10 studies) were "depressed" at birth. Additionally, it is likely than in some cases the lower Apgar scores in meconium-stained babies are due to the intubation procedure itself.[16]

Can there be abnormal outcomes in babies born through MSAF who have normal antenatal testing or normal FHR tracings? Various authors have found from 29% to 60% of infants with meconium-associated respiratory distress had normal FHR tracings.[16,20,22,24,38] Smith and colleagues[39] reviewed a series of fetal deaths which followed antepartum heart rate testing. They found 16 of 53 stillborn infants had passed meconium. Thirteen of these 16 had had normal, reactive nonstress tests (NSTs). Finally, Fleischer's group[40] reported that, even with the presence of normal intrapartum FHR tracings and normal 5-min Apgar scores, infants with MSAF had an incidence of respiratory complications many times greater than those born through clear amniotic fluid. I conclude that the finding of MSAF is associated with many markers of fetal distress. The evidence definitely supports that one should not be at ease in cases of MSAF with normal FHR tracings – adverse outcomes may still occur.

Nonneurologic adverse outcome

Fleischer and colleagues[40] found meconium-stained, term-gestation infants to be 100 times more likely to develop respiratory distress than their counterparts born through clear amniotic fluid. MAS is the most frequently noted adverse outcome found among infants subsequent to being born through MSAF. I use the term "meconium aspiration syndrome" to refer to infants born through MSAF who have respiratory distress and whose symptoms cannot be otherwise explained. In two large reviews of the disorder,[2,41] we have found approximately 5% of infants born through MSAF will subsequently develop MAS, one-third to one-half of those with MAS will require mechanical ventilation, one-quarter will develop pneumothoraxes, and one in 20 will die. The death rate has varied over time, from as many as 63% of those in the CPP to as low as 0% in more recent, smaller populations. The death rate has declined over time,[1] a finding which likely has been influenced by aggressive airway management in the delivery room, better ventilatory techniques, and improvements in supportive care (thermoregulation, parenteral nutrition, etc.). Two-thirds of neonates with persistent pulmonary hypertension have MAS as an associated disorder.[42] The proportion of babies admitted to neonatal intensive care units (NICUs) is increased among those born through MSAF compared to those born through clear amniotic fluid. Nathan et al.[23] found 24% of meconium-stained babies were admitted to their NICU compared to 7% of those born through clear fluid. Anyaegbunam et al.[31] found a similar increase in NICU admissions (31% vs 3%), as did Mahomed and colleagues (18.2% vs 2.2%).[23] Among premature infants born through MSAF, Wagner and associates[43] found lower 1- and 5-min Apgar scores, as well as a fourfold higher mortality rate. Thus, among babies born through MSAF there is considerable morbidity not related to neurologic outcome.

Adverse neurologic outcomes

There are no prospective investigations that have specifically followed a group of meconium-stained infants, nor even the sicker group of children with MAS, for a minimum of at least 2–6 years to assess adequately how such children develop. None the less, there exists abundant literature which links some adverse neurologic findings with meconium. In a light note, if one views freshly passed meconium under light microscopy (Figure 31.1), one finds an eerie resemblance to the human brain.

Desmond and colleagues found infants born through MSAF to be more likely to have hypotonia, lethargy, and seizures.[12] Several investigators have examined data from the CPP. Naeye[10] reported that, if infants were born through MSAF, they had a significantly increased risk for neurologic abnormalities at 7 years of age, including quadriplegic CP, chronic seizures, and severe mental retardation. These children were also more likely to have hyperactivity at this age. Nelson and Broman[44] assessed a group of 50 children from the CPP who had marked neurological abnormalities, characterized by moderate or severe motor disability and severe mental retardation, and compared them to a large control population. Those with severe handicaps were more than twice as likely

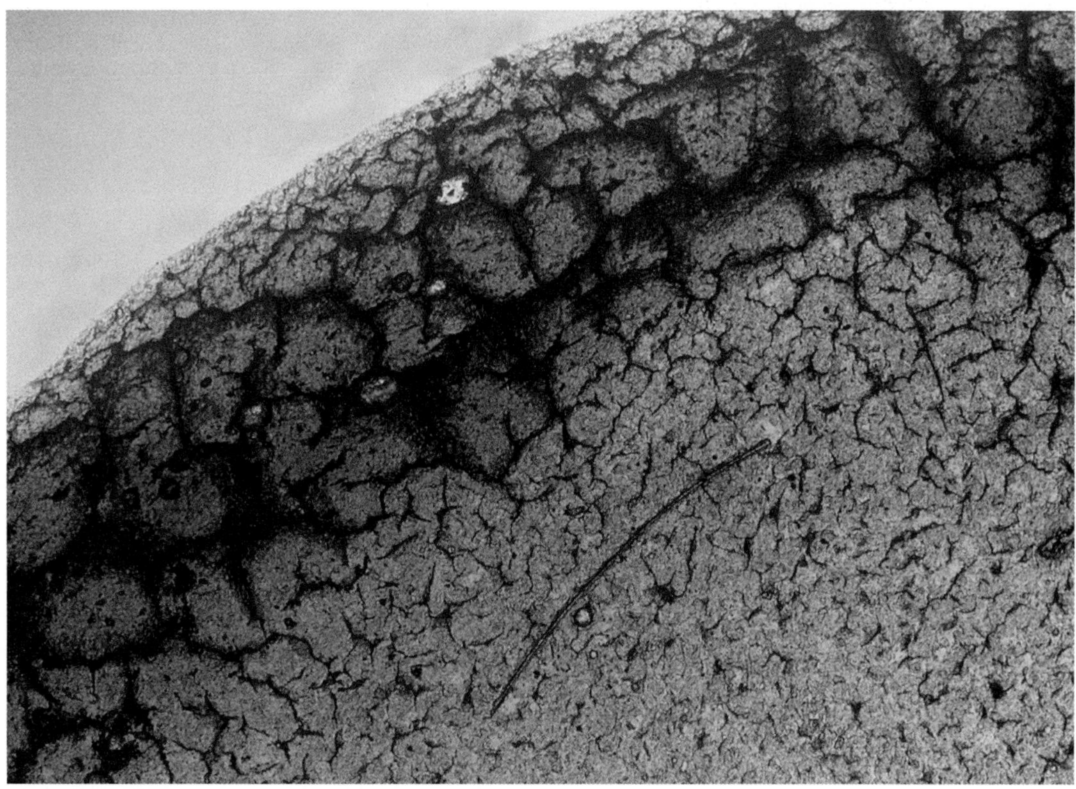

Figure 31.1 An unstained smear of freshly passed meconium from a term-gestation neonate. A piece of hair is noted in the specimen. There is a distinct resemblance of this smear to cerebral cortex.

to have been born through MSAF (40.8% vs. 19.1 %). Nelson[45] found the rate of CP among the children with birth weight >2500 g in the project to be approximately 3/1000 if there was no history of obstetrical complications. When there was a history of MSAF and no other complications, 4/1000 survivors developed CP. However, when there was a history of MSAF and a 5-min Apgar score <3, the rate of CP increased to 94/1000. Finally, among CPP infants of birth weight <2500 g born through MSAF, Nelson and Ellenberg[46] reported the frequency of CP to be 15/1000. Additionally, 12/1000 of the low-birth-weight babies had no CP but developed seizures.

Shields and Schifrin[47] examined a group of 75 babies with CP who had been born between 1976 and 1983. They found that 41% had been born through MSAF. Moreover, 21% of the 75 babies had been affected with MAS. Gaffney and colleagues[48] in England similarly examined a group of infants with CP ($n=141$). They found MSAF to be significantly more common in those with CP versus control (non-CP) infants (24.2% vs 9.9%). Erkkola et al.[22] reported that 7% of babies with MAS had permanent neurological sequelae (including CP). We[49] reported an increased incidence of adverse outcomes (cystic periventricular leukomalacia (PVL) and CP) among premature infants <30 weeks' gestation born through MSAF. Spinillo et al.[50] subsequently confirmed the increased risk for CP among meconium-stained premature infants. This group also demonstrated that meconium-stained premature infants were more likely to develop PVL.[51]

Table 31.1. Neurodevelopmental test scores over time in babies with meconium aspiration syndrome (MAS) who were treated with extracorporeal membrane oxygenation.

Test (age)	Normal range	Mean score in MAS children
Bayley (age 1 year)		
Mental Developmental Index	100 ± 15	104.6
Psychomotor Developmental Index	100 ± 15	96.7
Bayley (age 2 years)		
Mental Developmental Index	100 ± 15	98.4
Psychomotor Developmental Index	100 ± 15	98.3
Mullen (age 3–5 years)		
VRO	50 ± 10	51.5
VEO	50 ± 10	48.4
LRO	50 ± 10	46.7
LEO	50 ± 10	46.0
McCarthy (age 4–6 years)	50 ± 10	51.2
WPPSI-FIQ (age 5–6 years)	100 ± 15	88.6

Notes:
Testing consisted of: (1) Bayley Scales of Infant Development (Mental Developmental Index and Psychomotor Developmental Index) at 1 and 2 years of age; (2) Mullen Scales of Early Learning at 3–5 years; and (3) the motor portion of the McCarthy, as well as the Wechsler Preschool and Primary Scale of Intelligence – Revised (WPPSI-FIQ) at 5–6 years. VRO, visual receptor organization; VEO, visual expressive organization; LRO, language receptor organization; LEO, language expressive organization.
Source: Data from Desai, S., Stanley, C., Wiswell, T. E., Graziani, L. J. (1995). Long-term neurodevelopmental outcome following ECMO in congenital diaphragmatic hernia (CDH) survivors: improvement over time. *Pediatric Research*, **37**, 253A(#1505).

Seizures during the neonatal period are an important predictor of subsequent neurological handicap. Neonatal seizures occur in approximately 0.4–0.8% of all liveborn infants. Berkus et al.[20] found a sevenfold increased risk for neonatal seizures, as well as a fivefold increased risk for hypotonia, among infants born through moderately thick or thick MSAF. Similarly, Nathan et al.[23] found a fivefold increased risk for seizures during the first 24 h of life if infants had been born through MSAF (2.0% vs 0.4%). Mahomed et al.[24] found the increased risk for seizures to be 16-fold (1.6% if MSAF vs 0.1% if clear amniotic fluid). Usta and colleagues[52] reported 1.3% of 937 infants born through MSAF developed neonatal seizures. Lien et al.[53] reviewed a group of term-gestation infants that had neonatal seizures. Of 40 such infants, 40% had been born through MSAF, while 12.5% had a history of MAS. As many as 50% of newborns who have severe hypoxic–ischemic encephalopathy (HIE) develop neonatal seizures.[54] Finer's group[55] reviewed 95 infants of >37 weeks' gestation that had evidence of HIE. Almost half of these children (48.4%) had a history of MAS, while 28% of those with MAS subsequently developed moderate-to-severe neurologic handicaps.

Matsuishi et al.[56] prospectively evaluated the inci-

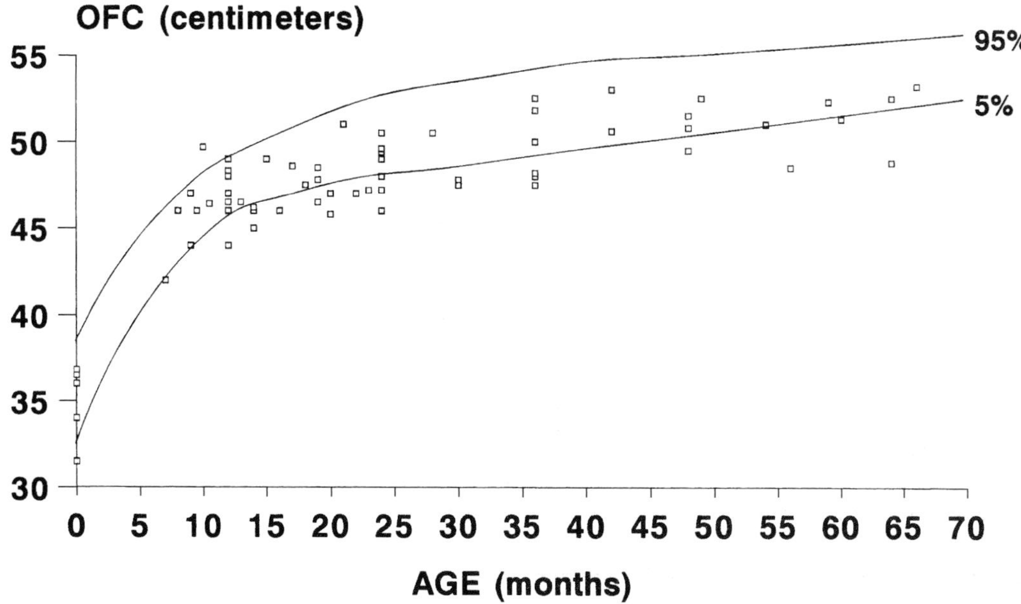

Figure 31.2 The head circumferences of a series of infants who had meconium aspiration syndrome and required extracorporeal membrane oxygenation. There is an apparent drop-off over time in the occipital–frontal circumference (OFC) in the older children.

dence of autistic disorder among 5271 survivors of an NICU. The children were assessed sequentially for neurodevelopmental disorders for a 5-year period following discharge. Autistic disorder was identified in 18 of the infants, while 57 had CP. The authors found that a history of MAS was significantly higher in children with autistic disorder (22%) or CP (8.8%) compared to the control population of NICU graduates without MAS.

At Thomas Jefferson University in Philadelphia, more than 300 infants were treated with extracorporeal membrane oxygenation (ECMO) between 1985 and 1994. Complete neurodevelopmental information is available for 209 survivors >2 years of age. Ninety-two of these infants had MAS as their primary disorder of respiratory failure. Eight (9%) of these infants have CP. Furthermore, of 25 non-CP infants with MAS managed with ECMO who survived at least 5 years, neurodevelopmental test scores have seemingly dropped over time (Table 31.1).[57] Moreover, the head circumferences of these infants appear to be decreasing over time from the average range to lower levels (Figure 31.2, unpublished data).

The data I have discussed in this section indicate a relationship between certain adverse neurodevelopmental outcomes and MSAF/MAS. Presumably, most infants born through MSAF will ultimately be neurologically intact. Unfortunately, because there are no prospective epidemiologic studies of various adverse neurodevelopmental outcomes and MSAF, one cannot generally prognosticate about infants either born through MSAF or those who develop MAS.

Pathophysiology of meconium passage

Meconium is a viscous green liquid consisting of gastrointestinal secretions, bile, bile acids, mucus, pancreatic juice, cellular debris, amniotic fluid, and swallowed vernix caseosa, lanugo, and blood.[2] Between the 10th and 16th weeks of gestation, the substance may first be noted in the fetal gastrointestinal tract. Typically, 60–200 g of the substance is found in a term-gestation infant's intestine. Because of the lack of strong peristalsis, as well as the presence of good anal sphincter tone and a terminal cap of particularly viscous meconium, in utero passage of the substance is uncommon.

In utero passage of meconium has generally been thought to reflect ante- or intrapartum asphyxia. Reed[5] suggested that hypoxia would relax anal sphincter tone, while Brews[7] hypothesized that hypoxia would increase intestinal peristalsis. In addition, it has been speculated that compression of the fetal head or umbilical cord (often seen in the postterm infant with oligohydramnios) could cause a vagal response and result in meconium passage.[58] Both Hobel[33] and Walker[8] documented hypoxia causing meconium passage. The finding of fetal acidosis among infants with MSAF is consistent with a hypoxic environment.[29,31,32] Nevertheless, for most infants passage of meconium is likely a physiologic maturational event. Meconium passage is rare before 37 weeks' gestation, but may occur in 35% or more of pregnancies lasting longer than 42 weeks.[23,59–61] In addition, motilin is a hormone responsible for bowel peristalsis and defecation. Motilin levels are higher in term and postdates infants than in premature infants,[62] additionally supporting the maturity concept of the physiologic passage of meconium.

A seldom recognized mechanism causing fetal defecation is that of intrauterine infection. Naeye[10] reported that 64% of cases of MSAF were associated with acute chorioamnionitis. Wen and colleagues[63] found a significantly higher rate of clinical intra-amniotic infection in women with MSAF compared to those with clear amniotic fluid, while Markovitch et al.[64] found MSAF to be associated with maternal infectious morbidity in women with preterm delivery. Romero and associates[65] presented evidence that bacterial endotoxin is a cause of meconium passage. In addition, Romero's group[66] found the prevalence of positive amniotic fluid cultures to be significantly higher among women with MSAF than those with clear fluid. Others[38,67] have found a high proportion of infants with MAS to have a history of maternal chorioamnionitis. Most recently, Piper and colleagues[68] reported MSAF to be associated with higher rates of clinical maternal infection both pre- (chorioamnionitis) and post- (endometritis) delivery. As inflammation plays an important role in the course of neonates with meconium-associated respiratory distress, the infectious mechanism of meconium passage needs to be further explored.

Unfortunately, for any given fetus, neither obstetricians nor pediatricians may be able to ascertain prenatally the specific mechanism of passage, nor is the rationale readily apparent postnatally. Indeed, conceivably a combination of mechanisms could affect any given fetus. Whatever the reason for fetal defecation, it will occur in 10–15% of all deliveries. In the USA alone, this would result in a half-million meconium-stained infants annually. Health-care providers should not make the glib assumption that the presence of MSAF is generally a benign finding – the consequences could be a severely ill neonate and a delay in appropriate therapy.

Potential mechanisms of neurologic injury

I have previously discussed the association of MSAF and adverse neurologic outcomes, such as neonatal seizures and CP. What are the potential mechanisms of injury in these children? Because of the dearth of prospective data on a large group of infants born through MSAF or who develop MAS, I can only speculate. The infants at highest risk appear to be those who have prolonged postpartum depression. Data from the CPP indicate that the combination of MSAF and a 5-min Apgar score <3 resulted in a 9.4% incidence of CP among surviving infants >2500 g birth weight.[69] Very real culprits which one must consider include the events potentiating meconium passage. Meconium staining among infants in the CPP was strongly associated with disorders which could affect the fetus: chorioamnionitis, premature rupture of membranes, abruptio placentae, and large placental infarcts.[10] Acute asphyxiating events, such as abruption of the placenta, can be associated with severe in utero hypoxia and acidosis. More subtle disorders, such as chorioamnionitis or chronic asphyxia, may not result in a neonate who is severely depressed at birth. Additionally, one must recognize the concept of in utero recovery. Some fetuses suffer acute or chronic episodes which are severe enough to cause neurological injury but not severe enough to result in death. The stress may disappear and the fetus resumes its normal status. Such an infant may not demonstrate postpartum depression with low umbilical cord pHs or low Apgar scores, and may appear neurologically intact for months after birth, only to end up with major neurodevelopmental disabilities.

The postdates fetus is at high risk for oligohydramnios, uteroplacental insufficiency, and meconium passage.[70] These fetuses may suffer from chronic insults insufficient to cause death or even signs of fetal distress, but sufficient to cause neurologic damage. The pathophysiologic mechanisms that cause CP remain elusive and usually cannot be ascribed to birth injury or hypoxic–ischemic insults during delivery.[71] Recurrent neonatal seizures predict CP better than other perinatal characteristics.[44,54,71,72] However, although such seizures are significantly more likely in infants born through MSAF, they are likely the consequence, rather than the cause, of the processes leading to CP. Similarly, an abnormal FHR tracing or persistently low Apgar scores may be reflective of an insult that occurred long before birth (hours to days to even weeks or months), rather than of more immediate intrapartum difficulties.

Are there substances in the meconium itself which make it harmful? I have previously addressed the relationship between intraamniotic infection and MSAF. Hyde et al.[73] has described a mechanism of vasoconstriction of the umbilical vessels by intraamniotic bacterial products. Could such a mechanism directly cause fetal ischemia because of vasoconstriction of placental or umbilical vessels? Moreover, could these vasoactive substances cross into the circulation of the fetuses and cause ischemia of cerebral vessels or make pulmonary vessels more reactive, hence persistent pulmonary hypertension of the newborn (PPHN)? Two compelling articles are those of Altshuler and Hyde.[74,75] These investigators initially performed an in vitro experiment in which they exposed excised umbilical venous tissue to solutions of meconium and found substantial vasoconstriction. Although no specific constituent in the substance was identified as the vasoactive substance, they found the agent to be heat-labile. They hypothesized that MSAF could cause in vivo placental and umbilical cord vasoconstriction. Additionally, the vasoconstricting agents could cross into the fetal circulation and lead to cerebral or other organ hypoperfusion. Additionally, this group has described meconium-induced necrosis of placental and umbilical cord vessels. Holcberg and colleagues[76] have recently confirmed the vasoconstrictive effects of meconium on the fetal–placental vasculature. Altshuler[75] has commented that meconium discharge and aspiration may occur many hours or days before delivery and that the mechanism of fetal death in many of these cases is completely unknown. He has stated that, with the presence of meconium in the fetal sac, it takes a minimum of 4–12 h for the meconium to diffuse to and into the lumens of placental and umbilical cord vessels and become a pathogenetic means of inducing placental and umbilical vasoconstriction. Additionally, this author has cogently commented about the incomplete investigation of meconium's role in adverse fetal outcomes.[74,75,77,78]

Burgess and Hutchins[79] have presented further evidence implicating meconium's role in producing direct injury to the umbilical cord. In a series of 123 autopsied cases in which there was meconium passage, these investigators described substantial placental and fetal lung inflammation due to the meconium, as well as abundant umbilical cord pathology. Kaspar and colleagues[80] recently assessed the relationship between the immediate neonatal outcome and the presence of placental lesions in 96 pregnancies complicated by MSAF. They found an increased prevalence of severe placental lesions (vascular thromboses, placental infarcts, etc.) and adverse immediate neonatal outcomes (lower 5-min Apgar scores, lower umbilical artery pHs, and more NICU admissions) associated with the duration of exposure to meconium. We[81] have examined the effect of intraamniotic meconium over time in an in vivo model. We injected various concentrations of meconium into fetal gestational sacs of rabbits and followed changes over intervals from 15 min to 96 h. No concurrent hypoxia was induced. Seventeen of 107 rabbit fetuses aspirated meconium, as early as 15 min after injection. Of the 32 fetal rabbits exposed to meconium for >24 h, 28 (88% died). Ischemic changes were found in both the placenta and the umbilical cords of virtually all of these latter fetuses. Our findings further support the concept that meconium itself is not an innocuous substance.

Kojima et al.[82] have described meconium-induced oxidant injury to the lungs caused by activation of alveolar macrophages, while Jones et al.[83] found increased production of proinflammatory cytokines in MAS (including tumor necrosis factor and interleukin-8). Moreover, both human infants and piglets with MAS may have increased levels of eicosanoids such as leukotriene B_4 and thromboxane B_2, substances that may cause pulmonary vasoconstriction.[84,85] Both oxidant- and cytokine-induced injury could also damage the brain, while eicosanoids could result in ischemia of the brain. We know little about the potentially deleterious effects on neural tissue by the increased levels of oxidants, cytokines, and eicosanoids found with MAS.

Naeye[10] suggested that meconium-induced brain damage may be a subacute rather than an acute process. He reported that only three of 31 non-CPP children with meconium-associated spastic quadriplegia whose cases he had reviewed had more than brief occurrences of neonatal renal or myocardial failure. The latter entities are often seen concurrently with acute hypoxic damage and neonatal encephalopathy.[86] Naeye and Localio[87] studied 43 infants with quadriplegic CP who were born through MSAF. These authors concluded that meconium-induced vasoconstriction sometimes leads to ischemic, hypoxemic injury.

Benirschke[88] has commented about the important toxic vasoconstrictive properties of meconium, suggesting this as an etiology of fetal hypoperfusion and PPHN, as well as brain injury. He commented that meconium's damage to the umbilical cord vessels occurs after the "noxious agent" seeps through Wharton's jelly. He has also suggested[89] that umbilical venous and placental vessel vasoconstriction may reduce the venous return of oxygenated blood from the placenta to the child. Benirschke[88] has commented that we know virtually nothing about the long-term function of meconium-injured vessels, nor of meconium's diffusion or transportation through the umbilical cord and placental membranes. He also reminds us about the effect of cytokines and other infection-related factors which may additionally affect vascular injury in the presence of MSAF. Benirschke and Kaufmann[89] commented on the overrepresentation of infants with CP who have a history of chorioamnionitis and funisitis, again reminding us that bacterial products may produce umbilical cord vessel constriction. Benirschke[90] has recently written a comprehensive review concerning the fetal consequences of amniotic fluid meconium.

During the past 5 years, much data has been accumulated indicating the role of in utero infection in the propagation of brain injury in children.[91] The increased incidence of chorioamnionitis in the presence of MSAF, as well as the frequent finding of inflammatory changes in the placenta, umbilical cord, and fetal membranes, and lungs suggest that inflammation may play an important role in brain injury in this population. The precise mechanisms, however, remain unclear. Theoretically, vasoconstriction or cytokine-mediated injury likely play a role. Sienko and Altshuler[92] assessed four cases of meconium-induced umbilical vascular necrosis. These were in three fetal demises and one live-born, growth-retarded infant. Bilirubin was found in macrophages between umbilical vascular myocytes and in the Wharton's jelly. Additionally, immunocytochemical staining revealed the presence of interleukin-1β in these same macrophages. These authors speculated that cytokines and other meconium-associated factors may contribute to the pathogenesis of fetal death or neonatal morbidity (such as PVL).

Neonates with severe MAS, particulary those with concomitant PPHN, may be severely hypoxic and acidotic due to the lung disorder itself, factors which of themselves may contribute to neurologic injury.[93,94] Some authors have reported a high incidence of seizures, cerebral infarction, and intracranial hemorrhage among infants with PPHN.[93,95,96] Additionally, therapies used for the management of MAS could potentially injure a child's brain. Hyperventilation is often used to treat MAS, particularly if PPHN is evident.[93] The aim of this therapy is to achieve respiratory alkalosis, often with arterial pHs above 7.55 and/or hypocapnia to $Pa\text{CO}_2$ levels of 25 mmHg or less. Hyperventilation to these extremes has been shown to decrease cerebral blood flow and oxygen consumption in animal models and adult humans.[97–99] The so-called "gentle ventilation" management of PPHN consists of accepting modest levels of acidosis, hypoxemia, and hypercapnia.[100] Follow-up data from children managed with hyperventilation have shown impairment in neurological outcomes (e.g., CP) and sensorineural hearing loss.[95,101–104] However, it is unclear whether or not the changes can be attributed to the hyperventilation or to preexisting damage due to the effects of the child's illness or the degree of acidosis, hypoxemia, and hypercapnia often present. Moreover, it is similarly unclear whether or not accepting a greater degree of acidosis, hypoxemia, and hypercarbia during gentle ventilation may contribute to neurological injury. Infants with MAS tend to do relatively less well when treated conventionally compared to other term-gestation infants with respiratory failure due to other disorders.[105] Adjunctive therapies have the potential of being deleterious to infants with MAS. Administration of exogenous surfactant could potentially cause hypoxemia and bradycardia.

High-frequency ventilation is often used to manage infants with MAS. There are several reports of severe brain injury being associated with this therapy when it is applied in premature infants.[106–108] However, to date there are no trials that have assessed neurological outcomes among infants with MAS who are treated with high-frequency vs conventional ventilation. In addition, inhaled nitric oxide (iNO) is used for the management of infants with MAS who have severe respiratory failure, typically with PPHN. The substance is a potent pulmonary vasodilator. The toxicity of iNO and its metabolites in the newborn bears careful study, particularly with regard to long-term exposure. In the gaseous phase nitric oxide (NO) combines with oxygen to form nitrogen dioxide (NO_2), a volatile and highly toxic miasma (or vapor). Careful monitoring of both NO and NO_2 levels during administration are required. Delivery systems that allow for careful titration of doses are also necessary. NO itself is toxic at higher concentrations and potential side-effects include methemoglobinemia, pulmonary edema, and platelet dysfunction.[109] Methemoglobin levels in excess of 5–7% have been noted in 10% of patients treated with 80 parts per million (p.p.m.), but not at levels of 40 or 20 p.p.m. NO reacts with superoxide anion to form peroxynitrite which potentially can cause lipid peroxidation and other oxidative injury to membranes.

The therapy of last resort for PPHN is ECMO,[93] a form of long-term cardiopulmonary bypass used when children failing conventional therapy have a projected high rate of mortality. Many children requiring this therapy have been profoundly acidotic, hypoxemic, and hypotensive. The most common way of performing ECMO over the past two decades involves permanent ligation of the right carotid artery and jugular vein. There are relatively scant data concerning survivors of ECMO, particularly concerning neurodevelopmental outcome beyond 1–2 years of age. At least 60% of survivors are intact, approximately 25% have substantial neurodevelopmental impairment, and 15% have findings which are potentially indicative of neurologic damage.[110,111] ECMO has been used in children with MAS for approximately 25 years. Children with MAS make up the largest proportion of newborn infants who are treated with this therapy (approximately 35%). This proportion has not changed over the years, although the absolute number of babies treated annually with ECMO has declined markedly since 1995.[112] Additionally, of neonates treated with ECMO, those with MAS have the shortest ECMO courses and the highest survival rates compared to those with other disorders (Table 31.2). Moreover,

Table 31.2. Diagnosis-related duration of extracorporeal membrane oxygenation (ECMO) course and survival rate (335 patients treated pre-1986, the remainder between 1986 and the first quarter of 2001)

Principal diagnosis	Total number	Mean duration of ECMO course (h)	Number survived (%)
Meconium aspiration syndrome	5831	128	5476 (94%)
Congenital diaphragmatic hernia	3699	223	2012 (54%)
Idiopathic persistent pulmonary hypertension	2382	141	1878 (79%)
Sepsis	2223	138	1678 (75%)
Respiratory distress syndrome	1318	133	1109 (84%)
Pneumonia	215	209	127 (59%)
Air leak syndrome	83	154	58 (70%)
Other	930	169	617 (66%)

Sources: Data courtesy of Robert E. Schumacher, M.D. and the ECMO Registry of the Extracorporeal Life Support Organization (ELSO), Ann Arbor, Michigan, July 2001.

the occurrence of adverse neurological findings among infants treated with ECMO is significantly lower in babies with MAS compared to those with other disorders (Table 31.3).[113] Unfortunately, there are no long-term data comparing neurological outcomes (such as the occurrence of CP) or developmental testing in a large population of infants who were managed with ECMO.

We reviewed our findings concerning more than 300 babies we have managed with ECMO at Thomas Jefferson University Hospital in Philadelphia between 1985 and 1995 (unpublished data). Of these, 209 surviving infants were followed for more than 2 years. Seventeen (8%) of these infants had CP, 14 had cognitive and language development in the mentally retarded range (including 10 of the 17 with CP). Eleven infants had sensorineural hearing loss. We compared these 11 with a control group of 26 ECMO-treated infants without such findings, as well as with the 17 with CP. We found those with hearing loss to be significantly more likely to have had profoundly lower $Pa\text{CO}_2$ levels prior to initiation of ECMO (a mean of 13 mmHg compared to 23 and 27 mmHG, in the nonhearing loss and CP groups, respectively). Three hundred and four neonates managed with ECMO had serial head ultrasounds during and after ECMO; 200 additionally had computed tomography or magnetic resonance imaging of their brains within 3 weeks of ECMO termination. A total of 68/304 (22%) had major intracranial lesions. Of grade 3 intraventricular bleeds, one was left-sided, nine were bilateral. Of parenchymal bleeds, 11 were right-sided, eight were left-sided, while seven were bilateral. Six hemorrhagic infarcts were right-sided, while six were left-sided. Two ischemic infarcts were right-sided, three were left-sided, and four were bilateral. Cystic periventricular leukomalacia was found on the right side in two instances, on the left in three, and bilaterally in one. Finally, five infants had marked diffuse cerebral atrophy. These findings are not consistent with lateralization of injury to side of carotid ligation. Moreover, we evaluated 65 survivors who were at least 5 years of age using the Wechsler Preschool and Primary Scale of Intelligence (WPPSI). Thirty of these infants had MAS. The entire group had a mean WPPSI full-scale IQ of 90.5. The mean score of MAS infants was similar (89.7). Of note, however, were the

Table 31.3. Adverse neurological findings in neonates requiring extracorporeal membrane oxygenation (ECMO). Those with meconium aspiration syndrome (MAS) are compared to those with all other disorders (included are all infants in the Extracorporeal Life Support Organization registry through early 2001)

	MAS	Other disorders	Significance
Total number of infants	5754	10649	
Seizures (%)	642 (11.2%)	1308 (12.3%)	P=0.034
Cerebral infarct (%)	374 (6.5%)	1262 (11.9%)	P<0.0001
Cerebral hemorrhage (%)	125 (2.2%)	666 (6.3%)	P<0.0001
Brain death (%)	48 (0.8%)	126 (1.2%)	P=0.015

Sources: Data courtesy of Robert E. Schumacher, M.D. and the ECMO Registry of the Extracorporeal Life Support Organization (ELSO), Ann Arbor, Michigan, April 2001.

findings of the subset testing: performance IQs compared to verbal IQs. The results of subset testing from a group of 25 MAS ECMO-survivors are presented in Figure 31.3. These findings are similar to those in the remaining 40 infants. We found the verbal scores to be substantially higher than the performance scores, with a difference of at least 10 points in nine of 25 babies. We are intrigued, as the performance IQ generally reflects right-sided brain activity, while the verbal IQ reflects left-sided brain activity. These findings could indicate subtle right-sided brain injury which has not been previously noted. All of these children had been managed with venoarterial ECMO and had their right carotid arteries and jugular veins ligated.

Timing of meconium passage

Can one make estimates of the amount of time that has passed from fetal defecation to delivery? There are some elements which may, perhaps, assist estimation of this interval: the color of the MSAF, the consistency of the MSAF, staining of the neonate, and placental/membrane alterations due to the meconium. Freshly passed meconium in a healthy newborn is a thick, viscous shimmering black-green colored substance. When passed by a fetus, the early color of MSAF is also black-green. However, the dilutional effect of the amount of amniotic fluid plays a role in the visually appreciated color of the MSAF.[114] As time progresses, the color of MSAF will progress to a brown and then to tan or yellow. Classically, yellow-brown MSAF has been considered to reflect "old" meconium.[6,9,12,115,116] Some believe the tan/yellow color change is due to the concomitant presence of vernix caseosa, the white cheesy substance whose presence may "lighten up" the darker meconium (K. Bernischke, personal communication). Altshuler[117] comments that the color of placental staining reflects duration since fetal defecation: "acute" staining is slimy and has a dark-green appearance, "chronic" staining is muddy-brown in appearance, while "very remotely passed" meconium is light tan. Recently, Sienko and Altshuler[92] have correlated the degree of meconium-associated placental and umbilical cord damage, as well as the color of the meconium staining, with the duration of time the fetus was exposed to the meconium. The "fresh" meconium staining was green-brown in color and was not associated with substantial changes. Long-term placental staining (greater than 6 h of exposure) progressively manifested in color as greeenish-tan, muddy-brown, and then light-tan. The latter colored membranes and fetal surfaces

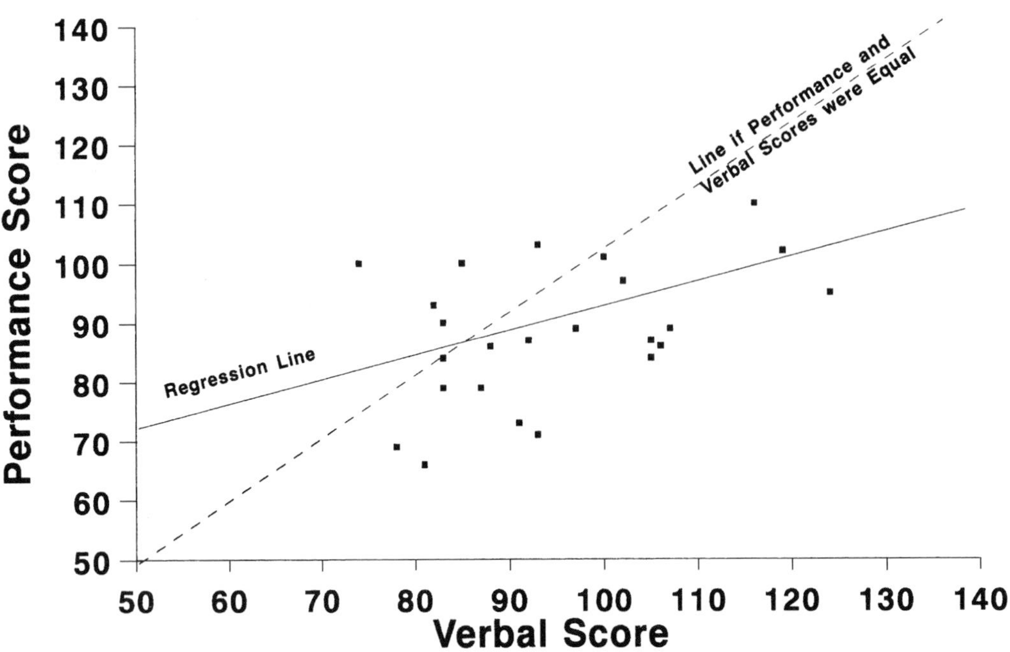

Figure 31.3 A plotting of scores from the Weschler Preschool and Primary Scale of Intelligence (WPPSI) from a series of 25 infants with meconium aspiration syndrome who were managed with extracorporeal membrane oxygenation. The children were tested at 5–6 years of age. There is a discrepancy in the verbal scores and the performance scores. The latter scores generally reflect right brain function.

were more likely to be associated with adverse placental, membrane, and umbilical cord findings.

We performed a prospective in vitro study to assess the effect of time and other factors on the color changes of meconium.[114] We sought to evaluate factors which might influence the color changes of MSAF. We obtained uncontaminated amniotic fluid from women at the time of elective cesarean sections and mixed it with human meconium to produce concentrations of 10% and 40% by volume. To 5-ml aliquots of these solutions we added (1) nothing (control); (2) 2 g of human vernix; (3) antibiotics (ampicillin and gentamicin); (4) 1 mmol $NaHCO_3$; or (5) 1 ml of 12–Normal hydrochloric acid. Specimens were placed in an incubator at 37 °C and serially examined for color changes at 0, 6, 12, 24, 48, 72, 96, 168, and 336 h. Photographs were taken at each time point. We used a nine-point color gradation scale (from black-green to yellow-tan) to score the specimens. Seven individuals blinded to solution content and time of photograph assigned color scores for the specimens. The 10% specimens were lighter in color than the 40% solutions at all periods. Regardless of meconium concentration, the specimens containing vernix were lighter throughout the study. All specimens became progressively lighter over time, most notably between 24 and 72 h. Neither the presence of antibiotics nor pH changes independently affected the color changes of the solutions. A factor we could not assess was the influence of natural, in vivo uptake and degradation of meconium by living tissue. Nonetheless, the color changes of MSAF are independently affected by meconium concentration, the presence of vernix, and the duration of time since initial passage.

When meconium is passed and diluted by a normal

volume of amniotic fluid, it will be of thin consistency. If there is oligohydramnios, often seen with postmaturity[70] or chronic uteroplacental insufficiency, the MSAF will be thicker in consistency. This will often result in the tenacious, "pea-soup" consistency seen in these children. In addition, in the presence of a normal or near-normal amount of amniotic fluid, when greater quantities of meconium are passed the fluid becomes thicker in consistency. A term-gestation infant may have as much as 60–200 g of meconium in its intestinal tract – a considerable amount, indeed. Furthermore, meconium will be absorbed after several days;[75,118] this may be reflected in decreased fluid consistency and a thinner, more watery appearance. There may be repeated defecations by a fetus under stress. This could progressively increase the thickness of the MSAF. A clinician may not be able to appreciate that there were repeated defecations. Thus, the thickness of the MSAF is a relatively unreliable marker of the interval since passage.

Staining of the external fetus is a better indicator of the amount of time since the child passed the substance. Desmond et al.[11] immersed the feet of normal babies into rubber gloves containing meconium-stained solutions. They found that it took at least 4–6 h for the toenails to mainfest yellow staining. They further assessed the amount of time it took for vernix placed into MSAF to become stained. Desmond and colleagues found that it took at least 12–14 h for vernix to achieve definite yellow staining. In an in vitro experiment, Miller et al.[119] obtained umbilical cords from normal term newborn infants. They also obtained meconium samples from normal term infants less than 18 h of age and froze these specimens at 4 °C for later evaluation. The authors subsequently exposed transverse sections of the umbilical cords to various concentrations of meconium (5%, 10%, and 20%). They found minimal staining after 1 h and maximal staining of all specimens at 3 h. We do not know if cold storage of the meconium or exposure of the fluid to diverse antibiotics could have affected the uptake of the pigment, causing the cords to become colored.

Examination of the placenta and membranes may assist in timing meconium's passage. One should recognize, however, that if a placenta sits unrefrigerated with meconium covering the membranes, postpartum transport in macrophages may proceed for some time.[89] Benirschke and Kaufmann remark that repeated meconium discharge may occur in utero, causing a spectrum of changes which would make it difficult to assess the time of passage accurately. Altshuler[78] refers to this scenario's clinical appearance when nurses sequentially observe MSAF with differing color over time. The in vitro study of Miller et al.[119] is a frequently cited work delineating changes due to meconium over time in the placenta and membranes. They exposed placentas and membranes to various meconium solutions. Within 1 h, meconium pigment-laden macrophages could be found in the amnion. After 3 h, pigmented macrophages could be found in all of the chorions. In addition, Miller and colleagues found a time correlation with amniotic epithelial degeneration: pseudostratification was exhibited in the epithelium after 1–3 h. Epithelial disorganization was present after 3 h of exposure. These investigators found the depth of penetration and uptake by macrophages to be related to length of exposure and to be independent of meconium concentration. Finally, these authors stated that meconium may be cleared from the amniotic fluid by both fetal swallowing and macrophage uptake. In such an instance, although the amniotic fluid would be seemingly clear, they felt that one could detect meconium in placental macrophages for at least a week after initial meconium passage. Altshuler[75] has expressed his concern about the Miller investigation, commenting that the temporal development of meconium-induced tissue changes may be influenced by coexisting conditions such as chorioamnionitis. Almost 25 years before the Miller report, Bourne[120] performed a similar experiment. He exposed amniotic membranes to varying concentrations of meconium. Bourne found gross staining of the amnion to occur in 2–6 h. Furthermore, although 10% formalin apparently removed or dissolved the gross pigment, the pigment could still be found within the vacuoles of the macrophages of the amnion. Bourne conjectured that meconium from different fetuses may be phagocytized at different rates in such an artificial situation, and cautioned readers concerning any conclusions from an in vitro experiment.

We examined the issue in our in vivo fetal rabbit model.[81] Initial meconium staining could be seen at 3 h in the amnion. However, it took 6–12 h for macrophages in both the chorion and amnion to exhibit meconium staining, with no differences in rate of uptake between the two concentrations (10% and 40%) of meconium-stained fluid. The amnion initially became reactive and edematous and would disappear, probably due to the toxicity of the meconium. We first found epithelial degeneration at 3 h, with some vacuolization within 3 h. We found squamous regeneration of the epithelium at 24 h. The chorion responded to the meconium by becoming edematous at 1–3 h and accumulating macrophages with vacuoles.

Altshuler opines[75] that, in the presence of MSAF, acute amniotic epithelial necrosis is the light microscopic counterpart of grossly observed acute (<4 h since passage) meconium staining. He states chronic meconium staining is manifested by amniotic epithelial vaculozation and balloon degeneration, as well as by the presence of balls of squamous epithelium across the placental surface and meconium-laden macrophages within the extraplacental membranes, placenta, and umbilical cord. He states that, in the absence of chorioamnionitis, meconium-laden macrophages deep within the umbilical cord indicate meconium has been in the fetal sac for at least 2 days. Benirschke[88] is not as definite, stating that there is less certainty as to the chronology of umbilical cord staining and the temporal evolution of meconium-induced vascular injury.

The timing of meconium passage is complex. We must keep in mind that the majority of babies who subsequently are noted to have CP, as well as those who are stillborn, are not born through MSAF. Clearly, severe enough stress to result in brain injury, or even death, may not always result in meconium passage. Furthermore, the vast majority of babies born through MSAF apparently do not suffer any neurologic morbidity. Again, there are no specific longitudinal follow-up studies concerning the neurodevelopmental outcome of this latter group of infants. I wonder if there could be more subtle neurologic changes which would only manifest later in life, such as learning disorders, behavior problems, or attention deficit disorders. Conceivably, with in utero recovery, a fetus could suffer a substantial insult, pass meconium, suffer brain injury, recover over a period of days, have some or all of the meconium resorbed, be born through either MSAF or apparently clear amniotic fluid, appear completely normal neurologically in the neonatal period, and subsequently manifest long-term neurodevelopmental abnormalities.

Other elements used to assess timing of injury

Meconium passage is not the sole marker of fetal distress. The AAP and the American College of Obstetricians and Gynecologists (ACOG) have published joint *Guidelines for Perinatal Care.* They comment on markers of damaging acidemia, hypoxia, and metabolic acidosis in the intrapartum period. In the 1997 edition of the guidelines,[121] they state that a neonate who had hypoxia proximate to delivery severe enough to result in hypoxic encephalopathy will show other evidence of hypoxic damage, including all of the following:

1. profound metabolic or mixed acidemia (pH< 7.00) on an umbilical cord arterial blood sample, if obtained
2. persistence of an Apgar score of 0–3 for longer than 5 min
3. neonatal neurologic sequelae such as seizures, coma, or hypotonia
4. multiorgan system dysfunction, i.e., cardiovascular, gastrointestinal, hematologic, pulmonary, or renal system

These guidelines are largely based on the opinions of Nelson.[45] In a fashion similar to the AAP/ACOG guidelines, an international task force[122] recently published a consensus statement addressing the relationship between acute intrapartum events and CP. The task force consisted of 49 individuals from seven countries. The consensus was that three essential criteria must all be present to consider

Table 31.4. Criteria to define an acute intrapartum hypoxic event (established by the International Cerebral Palsy Task Force)

Essential criteria	Criteria that together suggest an intrapartum timing but by themselves are nonspecific
Evidence of a metabolic acidosis in intrapartum fetal, umbilical arterial cord, or very early neonatal blood samples (pH<7.00 and base deficit >12 mmol/l)	A sentinel (signal) hypoxic event occurring immediately before or during labor
Early onset of severe or moderate neonatal encephalopathy in infants of 34 weeks' gestation	A sudden, rapid, and sustained deterioration of the fetal heart rate pattern usually after the hypoxic sentinel event where the pattern was previously normal
Cerebral palsy of the spastic quadriplegic or dyskinetic type	Apgar scores of 0–6 for longer than 5 min
	Early evidence of multisystem involvement
	Early imaging evidence of acute cerebral abnormality

Source: MacLennan, A. for the International Cerebral Palsy Task Force (1999). A template for defining a causal relation between acute intrapartum events and cerebral palsy: international consensus statement. *British Medical Journal*, **319**, 1054–1059, with permission from the BMJ Publishing Group.

intrapartum hypoxia as a cause of the CP (Table 31.4). Five additional criteria were agreed upon as being helpful in timing a hypoxic event to the intrapartum period.

A diminution or complete stoppage of maternal perception of gross fetal movements may be indicative of in utero compromise.[123] A fetus reduces its oxygen requirements by reducing activity. However, there are many false-positive perceptions of decreased movements. There are no investigations which have clearly delineated the time period from the perception of decreased fetal movements to when substantial neurologic injury may occur. Additionally, although many abnormal or nonreassuring fetal heart rate patterns have been touted as markers of acute or ongoing fetal distress, there are no data confirming that such patterns can be used to time precisely a specific in utero event. In a series of 44 children with CP, frequent fetal heart rate findings included absent variability and small variable decelerations, with overshoot, all occurring from the onset of monitoring during labor.[124] The pattern was frequently found in association with meconium staining. Nelson and colleagues noted characteristic fetal heart rate findings in 21 of 78 infants with CP who had undergone electronic monitoring of the fetal heart rate. The findings included multiple late decelerations and decreased variability.[125] However, these 21 infants only represented 0.2% of all infants with such fetal heart rate patterns (i.e., 99.8% of fetuses with these patterns did not develop CP). To date there is no evidence that obstetricians acting upon any type of abnormal fetal heart rate pattern will prevent neurologic injury. Many authors are of the opinion that by the time decreased fetal movements or an abnormal fetal heart rate are noted, damage to the fetal brain has already occurred.[69] Low and colleagues[30] reviewed 20 antepartum and intrapartum risk factors to assess their predictive value. They found that a significant proportion of intrapartum fetal asphyxia occurred in pregnancies with no risk factors, while the positive predictive value of clinical risk factors was only 3% (a 97% false-positive rate). Thus, although clinicians seek to recognize asphyxia before damage to the fetus occurs in order to intervene, there are no clearcut markers with good sensitivity and specificity, as well as high positive predictive values. Children born by cesarean section have no documented reduced risk of cerebral palsy.[126]

Richie and colleagues[127] explored the relationship of markers of acute and chronic asphyxia in infants with MSAF. There was no correlation between several of the markers (umbilical artery cord blood pH, lactate, or hypoxanthine) and meconium. However, erythropoietin levels were significantly elevated in newborns with MSAF. Multiple other groups have corroborated the presence of elevated fetal erythropoietin levels among meconium-stained infants.[128–130] Adult and fetal animal data indicate that 3–4 h of hypoxemia are needed before blood erythropoietin levels increase.[131] A response to increased erythropoietin would be the presence of increased nucleated red blood cells (NRBC) in the fetal or neonatal circulation. Meconium-stained babies are more likely to have elevated NRBC levels compared to those born through clear amniotic fluid.[132] We[133] found elevated NRBC counts in infants with MAS who required ECMO compared to healthy infants. Phelan and colleagues[134] have addressed the issue by examining cord blood NRBC levels of neonates who were neurologically impaired compared to normal newborns. They found elevated levels of cord blood NRBC counts compared to the healthy controls. In addition, this group[135] subsequently confirmed their finding and assessed possible relationships with the timing of fetal neurological injury. Essentially, they found the longer the NRBCs persisted, the greater the period of time prior to delivery the injury occurred. The closer the asphyxia event was to birth, the smaller the rise in NRBCs. These authors suggest that the clearance time of NRBCs may help characterize the timing of the hypoxic insult.

Other groups have confirmed the association between elevated NRBC counts and perinatal brain injury.[136,137] Blackwell's group[138] recently explored the relationship between NRBC counts and early-onset neonatal seizures. Forty percent of infants with neonatal seizures had been meconium-stained, compared to 11% of control infants without seizures. Moreover, the majority of meconium-stained infants with early-onset seizures had elevated NRBC counts. Similarly, nonmeconium-stained neonates with seizures also had elevated NRBC counts compared to controls without seizures. Studies in animals suggest that, from the initial onset of hypoxic exposure, it takes at least 48 h to be able to detect increased NRBC production in the bone marrow.[138] Similarly, Altshuler and Hermann[77] have estimated that in human fetuses the elevation of NRBCs takes at least 12–48 h in response to provocative levels of hypoxia.

I am intrigued by the work by Naeye and Localio.[87] They have examined information concerning the courses of infants in which there was a reasonably accurate timing of injury (acute placental abruption). These authors found an elevated lymphocyte count in the infants' peripheral blood (to levels above 10000 per μl) to occur within an hour of the insult. This elevation in lymphocytes does not persist beyond 24 h. Naeye and Lin[139] have explored this issue further. They examined a series of 55 children ultimately diagnosed with CP. These authors noted lymphocytosis to appear approximately 25 min after unexpected unremitting fetal bradycardia first began. In all cases, the bradycardia persisted through the time of delivery. The lymphocytosis disappeared approximately 14–18 h after it first appeared. All infants were considered to have hypoxic–ischemic encephalopathy. In addition, thrombocytopenia initially appeared between 20 and 28 h after the beginning of fetal bradycardia. It took a mean of 61 h for the platelet count to decrease by 50%. Of considerable interest is that Naeye and Lin reported that meconium was the cause of the hypoxemia–ischemia in fully 60% of the 55 neonates. These authors postulated that meconium-induced vasoconstriction led to the hypoxemia–ischemia.

In this section I have delineated several factors which may be useful in assessing the time of fetal compromise. Confounding the issue is the possibility that there could be a single catastrophic insult, multiple catastrophic insults, or chronic insults, all of which can damage a developing fetus's brain. Altshuler[75,77] has listed placental signs of fetal hypoxia and outlined whether these processes reflect acute damage (fewer than 24 h preceding delivery) or chronic damage (greater than 24 h preceding delivery). From my perspective, the pathologist is a key individual in searching for explanations of neurodevelopmental disorders. Currently, in most centers placentas are only examined under specific circumstances (low Apgar scores, premature delivery, etc.). However, the majority of children who develop CP are apparently normal in the neonatal period and do not have any of the risk factors for which their placentas would be routinely examined. Because the information may be important, my opinion is that the placentas of all neonates should be examined and that representative sections of these specimens should be saved for a minimum of 5–10 years. Medicolegal cases often address whether or not a cesarean section should have been performed earlier, typically 1–12 h prior to the actual delivery. The presumption is that such an action could have prevented some or all of a child's neurologic injury. Again, however, there is no evidence that performing a cesarean section will prevent CP.[126] As precise an assessment of the actual time an insult or insults occurred is critically important to assist in the accuracy of the final medicolegal decision.

Thick- versus thin-consistency meconium

What does the thickness of meconium represent? There are several factors which come into play, most importantly the total quantity of defecated material and the amount of amniotic fluid present. However, one should consider that the meconium at the most distal end of the intestinal tract is more viscous and likely to result in a thicker-consistency MSAF. Additionally, if meconium is present for a period of time, it will gradually be resorbed by surrounding tissue, or swallowed by the fetus. Is "thick" meconium clinically worse than "thin" or watery meconium? Clearly, infants born through "thick" MSAF are more likely to develop MAS.[24,38,140] Presumably, the thicker substance is more likely to cause obstructive airway problems. However, as many as 44% of those who develop MAS were born through "thin-consistency" MSAF.[1] Those born through thin-consistency meconium may still develop substantial respiratory distress, need ECMO, or die.[141,142] We do not know if the severity of respiratory disease associated with the thinner substance is less or more severe than that of infants born through thicker MSAF. Benirschke[88] conjectures that the thinner-consistency MSAF may be even more injurious than the thicker form – the toxic elements of meconium may be more accessible to the host tissue. Furthermore, if we accept that chronic hypoxemia (over at least several days) may result in pulmonary vascular remodeling, a fetus with such changes would likely have defecated at least several days before birth. Presumably, most of the meconium which was passed early in the course of hypoxemia will have been resorbed and the MSAF will be of watery consistency.

Estimating the consistency of MSAF is a very subjective matter. I have seen many different clinicians apply the appellations "thin, moderate, and thick" in an almost capricious manner, with no two individuals giving the same fluid the same name. Reasonable definitions are: (1) thin (synonymous with "watery" or "light"): only discoloration of the fluid. One could read through this liquid; (2) moderate (synonymous with "moderately thick"): particulate suspension present. The solution would be opaque and you could not read through it; and (3) thick (synonymous with "heavy"): tenacious fluid of pea-soup viscosity and appearance. There have been attempts to quantitate objectively the consistency of MSAF. Weitzner and colleagues[143] developed a method of centrifuging MSAF in a manner similar to centrifuging blood to determine a percentage of red cells (hematocrit). They claimed the "meconium-crit" was directly proportional to meconium concentration by weight. However, as this was an in vitro experiment using vortexed stock solutions, I cannot envision that thick particulate meconium was easily drawn up by capillary into the slender hematocrit tubes. Quite simply, with the thickest MSAF some meconium will be present in chunks or in particles too large to enter collecting tubes. Trimmer and Gilstrap[144] tried to correlate the meconium-crit to clinical markers of birth asphyxia (umbilical artery pH$<$7.20, low Apgar scores, and newborn seizures). In a small group of 106 women with MSAF, these authors found no correlation of meconium-crit with neonatal asphyxia. Although babies born through thicker-consistency meconium are more likely to have lower Apgar scores and umbilical cord artery pHs,[20,140] there are no data comparing the long-term neurodevelopmental outcome on the basis of MSAF consistency. Until such investigations are performed, I believe clinicians have to be wary with infants born through any consistency of MSAF.

Summary

Meconium-staining of the amniotic fluid is an everyday occurrence for health-care providers. The last several decades have resulted in an increased understanding of meconium passage, the pathophysiology of MAS, and mechanisms of brain injury associated with MSAF and MAS. We are learning more about how the substance itself may be both directly and indirectly toxic to tissue. Unfortunately, our knowledge is still scant. I remain of the opinion that we need a new project on the scale of the CPP in order to assess factors involved in the development of CP, mental retardation, and other abnormal neurodevelopmental outcomes. This is not just because of meconium-related issues. The current rate of CP is virtually the same among term-gestation neonates in the four decades since babies were enrolled in the study. I wonder if the same types of babies in the year 2002 develop CP as did those in the early 1960s? Perhaps babies who would have died during the time of the CCP will now survive and manifest CP, while those who were found to have CP in the late 1950s and early 1960s will have had improved prenatal care, nutrition, and intra- and postpartum care and not develop CP. Thus, while the overall percentage of babies who have CP would remain the same, the characteristics of the children would be different.

We continue to make incredible technological advances in how we support and manage critically ill infants. Our resuscitative skills have improved since the early 1960s, while our methods of managing neonatal pulmonary disease have also considerably improved. With one single disorder, MAS, we have decreased the death rate 10-fold (from >60% to <5%). Smaller and smaller premature infants are surviving. We have made huge advances in our ability to image the brain of term and preterm-gestation neonates, as well as in interpreting other techniques of assessing brain injury (near-infrared spectroscopy, electroencephalography, etc.) I believe our understanding of brain injury and development of methods to prevent such injury could only be enhanced by a future study enrolling at least as many infants as the CPP.

Despite our best efforts, a finite number of infants will be harmed by the effects of meconium. We may not be able to predict or prevent the stresses which lead to meconium passage. Moreover, babies who suffer in utero aspiration or those who develop remodeling of the pulmonary vasculature may not be responsive to current therapies. There is no evidence that current obstetrical management of women who exhibit MSAF has resulted in improved neurodevelopmental outcomes of their progeny. Moreover, although we have decreased the death rate due to MAS, there is no evidence that improved delivery room or NICU management has led to improved neurologic outcomes in infants born through MSAF. As MSAF and MAS are such common entities, further research efforts need to be made to increase our knowledge and, hopefully, to develop therapies to prevent or mitigate the consequences of meconium. I continue to reflect on how much we do not understand about MSAF and MAS. One fact remains a certainty – the greatest importance of MSAF is to alert us to the potential for problems.

REFERENCES

1 Wiswell, T.E., Tuggle, J.M., Turner, B.S. (1990). Meconium aspiration syndrome: have we made a difference? *Pediatrics*, **85**, 715–721.

2 Wiswell, T.E., Bent, R.C. (1993). Meconium staining and the meconium aspiration syndrome: unresolved issues. *Pediatric Clinics of North America*, **50**, 955–981.

3 Schulze, M. (1925). The significance of the passage of meconium during labor. *American Journal of Obstetrics and Gynecology*, **10**, 83–88.

4 Grant, A. (1989). Monitoring the fetus during labor. In *Effective Care in Pregnancy and Childbirth*, eds. I.

Chalmers, M. Enking, and M.J.N.C. Keirse, pp. 846–882. Oxford: Oxford University Press.

5 Reed, C.B. (1918). Fetal death during labor. *Surgery, Gynecology and Obstetrics*, **26**, 545–551.

6 Clifford, S.H. (1945). Clinical significance of yellow staining of the vernix caseosa, skin, nails, and umbilical cord of the newborn. *American Journal of Diseases of Children*, **69**, 327–328.

7 Brews, A. (1948). Fetal asphyxia. In *Eden and Holland's Manual of Obstetrics*, 9th edn, ed. A. Brews, pp. 609–612. London: J & A Churchill.

8 Walker, J. (1954). Foetal anoxia. *Journal of Obstetrics and Gynecology of the British Empire*, **61**, 162–180.

9 Fujikura, T., Klionsky, B. (1975). The significance of meconium staining. *American Journal of Obstetrics and Gynecology*, **121**, 45–50.

10 Naeye, R.L. (1992). *Disorders of the Placenta, Fetus, and Neonate: Diagnosis and Clinical Significance*, pp. 257–268, 330–352. St. Louis: Mosby Year Book.

11 Desmond, M.M., Lindley, J.E., Moore, J., et al. (1956). Meconium staining of newborn infants. *Journal of Pediatrics*, **49**, 540–549.

12 Desmond, M.M., Moore, J., Lindley, J.E., et al. (1957). Meconium staining of the amniotic fluid: a marker of fetal hypoxia. *Obstetrics and Gynecology*, **9**, 91–103.

13 Gregory, G.A., Gooding, C.A., Phibbs, R.H., et al. (1974). Meconium aspiration in infants: a prospective study. *Journal of Pediatrics*, **85**, 848–852.

14 Ting, P., Brady, J.P. (1975). Tracheal suction in meconium aspiration. *American Journal of Obstetrics and Gynecology*, **122**, 767–771.

15 Carson, B.S., Losey, R.W., Bowes W.A., et al. (1976). Combined obstetric and pediatric approach to prevent meconium aspiration syndrome. *American Journal of Obstetrics and Gynecology*, **126**, 712–715.

16 Wiswell, T.E., Gannon C.M., Jacob, J.J., et al. (2000). Delivery room management of the apparently vigorous meconium-stained neonate: results of the multicenter, international collaborative trial. *Pediatrics*, **105**, 1–7.

17 Kattwinkel, J., Short, J., Niermeyer, S. et al. (2000). *Neonatal Resuscitation Textbook*, 4th edn, pp. 2–9. Elk Village, IL: American Academy of Pediatrics.

18 Katz, V.L., Bowes,W.A. (1992). Meconium aspiration syndrome: reflections on a murky subject. *American Journal of Obstetrics and Gynecology*, **166**, 171–183.

19 Woods, J.R., Glantz, J.C. (1994). Significance of amniotic fluid meconium. In *Maternal–Fetal Medicine: Principles and Practice*, 3rd edn, eds. R.K. Creasy, R. Resnik, pp. 413–422. Philadelphia: W.B. Saunders.

20 Berkus, M.D., Langer, O., Samueloff, A., et al. (1994). Meconium-stained amniotic fluid: increased risk for adverse neonatal outcome. *Obstetrics and Gynecology*, **84**, 115–120.

21 Baker, P.N., Kilby, M.D., Murray, H. (1992). An assessment of the use of meconium alone as an indication for fetal blood sampling. *Obstetrics and Gynecology*, **80**, 792–796.

22 Erkkola, R., Kero, P., Suhonen-Polvi, H., et al. (1994). Meconium aspiration syndrome. *Annales Chirugiae et Gynaecologiae*, **83**, 106–109.

23 Nathan, L., Leveno, K.J., Carmody, T.J., et al. (1994). Meconium: a 1990s perspective on an old obstetric hazard. *Obstetrics and Gynecology*, **83**, 329–332.

24 Mahomed, K., Nyoni, R., Masona, D. (1994). Meconium staining of the liquor in a low-risk population. *Paediatric and Perinatal Epidemiology*, **8**, 292–300.

25 Krebs, H.B., Petres, R.E., Dunn, L.J., et al. (1980). Intrapartum fetal heart rate monitoring. III. Association of meconium with abnormal fetal heart rate patterns. *American Journal of Obstetrics and Gynecology*, **137**, 936–941.

26 Meis, P.J., Hall, M., Marshall, J.R., et al. (1978). Meconium passage: a new classification for risk assessment during labor. *American Journal of Obstetrics and Gynecology*, **131**, 509–513.

27 Kariniemi, V., Harrela, M. (1990). Significance of meconium staining of the amniotic fluid. *Journal of Perinatal Medicine*, **18**, 345–349.

28 White, V.T. (1955). The significance and management of meconium in the liquor amnii during labour. *Medical Journal of Australia*, **1**, 641–644.

29 Mitchell, J., Schulman, H., Fleischer, A., et al. (1985). Meconium aspiration and fetal acidosis. *Obstetrics and Gynecology*, **65**, 352–355.

30 Low, J.A., Simpson, L.L., Tonni, G., et al. (1995). Limitations in the clinical prediction of intrapartum fetal asphyxia. *American Journal of Obstetrics and Gynecology*, **172**, 801–804.

31 Anyaegbunam, A., Fleischer, A., Whitty, J., et al. (1991). Association between umbilical artery cord pH, five-minute Apgar scores and neonatal outcome. *Gynecologic and Obstetric Investigation*, **32**, 220–223.

32 Ramin, K., Leveno, K., Kelly, M., et al. (1994). Observations concerning the pathophysiology of meconium aspiration syndrome. *American Journal of Obstetrics and Gynecology*, **170**, 312.

33 Hobel, C.J. (1971). Intrapartum clinical assessment of fetal distress. *American Journal of Obstetrics and Gynecology*, **110**, 336–342.

34 Miller, F.C., Sack, D.A., Yeh, S-Y., et al. (1975). Significance of meconium during labor. *American Journal of Obstetrics and Gynecology*, **122**, 573–580.

35 Starks, G.D. (1980). Correlation of meconium-stained amniotic fluid, early intrapartum fetal pH, and Apgar scores as predictors of perinatal outcome. *Obstetrics and Gynecology*, **56**, 604–609.

36 Bouchner, C.J., Medearis, A.L., Ross, M.G., et al. (1987). The role of antepartum testing in the management of postterm pregnancies with heavy meconium in early labor. *Obstetrics and Gynecology*, **69**, 903–907.

37 Steer, P.J., Eigbe, F., Lissauer, T.J., et al. (1989). Interrelationships among abnormal cardiotocograms in labor, meconium staining of the amniotic fluid, arterial cord blood pH, and Apgar scores. *Obstetrics and Gynecology*, **74**, 715–721.

38 Coughtrey, H., Jeffery, H.E., Henderson-Smart, D.J., et al. (1991). Possible causes linking asphyxia, thick meconium, and respiratory distress. *Australian and New Zealand Journal of Obstetrics and Gynaecology*, **31**, 92–102.

39 Smith, C.V., Nguyen, H.N., Kovacs, B., et al. (1987). Fetal death following antepartum fetal heart rate testing: a review of 65 cases. *Obstetrics and Gynecology*, **70**, 18–20.

40 Fleischer, A., Anyaegbunam, A., Guidetti, E., et al. (1992). A persistent clinical problem: profile of the term infant with significant respiratory complications. *Obstetrics and Gynecology*, **79**, 185–190.

41 Cleary G.M., Wiswell, T.E. (1998). Meconium-stained amniotic fluid and the meconium aspiration syndrome: an update. *Pediatric Clinics of North America*, **45**, 511–529.

42 Abu-Osa, Y.K. (1991). Treatment of persistent pulmonary hypertension of the newborn: update. *Archives of Diseases in Childhood*, **66**, 74–77.

43 Wagner, W., Druzin, M., Rond, A., et al. (1991). Meconium stained amniotic fluid (MSAF) ≤32 weeks predicts poor perinatal outcome. *American Journal of Obstetrics and Gynecology*, **164**, 357.

44 Nelson, K.B., Broman, S.H. (1977). Perinatal risk factors in children with serious motor and mental handicaps. *Annals of Neurology*, **2**, 371–377.

45 Nelson, K.B. (1989). Perspective on the role of perinatal asphyxia in neurologic outcome: its role in developmental deficits in children. *Canadian Medical Association Journal*, **141** (suppl.), 3–10.

46 Nelson K.B., Ellenberg, J.H. (1984). Obstetric complications as risk factors for cerebral palsy or seizure disorders. *Journal of the American Medical Association*, **251**, 1843–1848.

47 Shields, J.R., Schifrin, B.S. (1988). Perinatal antecedents of cerebral palsy. *Obstetrics and Gynecology*, **71**, 899–905.

48 Gaffney, G., Sellers, S., Flavell, V., et al. (1994). Case-control study of intrapartum care, cerebral palsy, and perinatal death. *British Medical Journal*, **308**, 743–750.

49 Wiswell, T.E., Graziani, L.J., Gannon, C.M., et al. (1996). Premature infants <30 weeks gestation born through meconium-stained amniotic fluid (MSAF) have an increased risk for cerebral palsy (CP): a prospective study. *Pediatric Research*, **39**, 253A.

50 Spinillo, A., Fazzi E., Capuzzo, E., et al. (1997). Meconium-stained amniotic fluid and risk for cerebral palsy in preterm infants. *Obstetrics and Gynecology*, **90**, 519–523.

51 Spinillo, A., Capuzzo, E., Stronati, M., et al. (1998). Obstetric risk factors for periventricular leukomalacia among preterm infants. *British Journal of Obstetrics and Gynaecology*, **105**, 865–871.

52 Usta, I.M., Mercer, B.M., Aswad, N.K., et al. (1995). The impact of a policy of amnioinfusion for meconium-stained amniotic fluid. *Obstetrics and Gynecology*, **85**, 237–241.

53 Lien, J.M., Towers, C.V., Quilligan, E.J., et al. (1995). Term early-onset neonatal seizures: obstetric characteristics, etiologic classifications, and perinatal care. *Obstetrics and Gynecology*, **85**, 163–169.

54 Strafstrom, E.E. (1995). Neonatal seizures. *Pediatrics in Review*, **16**, 248–255.

55 Finer, N.N., Robertson, C.M., Richards, R.T., et al. (1981). Hypoxic ischemic encephalopathy in term neonates: perinatal factors and outcome. *Journal of Pediatrics* **98**, 112–117.

56 Matsuishi, T., Yamashita, Y., Ohtani, Y., et al. (1999). Brief report: incidence of and risk factors for autistic disorder in neonatal intensive care unit survivors. *Journal of Autism and Developmental Disorders*, **29**, 161–166.

57 Desai, S., Stanley, C., Wiswell, T.E., et al. (1995). Long-term neurodevelopmental outcome following ECMO in congenital diaphragmatic hernia (CDH) survivors: improvement over time. *Pediatric Research*, **37**, 253A.

58 Miller, F.C., Read, J.A. (1981). Intrapartum assessment of the postdate fetus. *American Journal of Obstetrics and Gynecology*, **141**, 516–520.

59 Eden, R.D., Seifert, L.S., Winegar, A., et al. (1987). Perinatal characteristics of uncomplicated postdate pregnancies. *Obstetrics and Gynecology*, **69**, 296–299.

60 Ostrea, E.M., Naqvi, M. (1982). The influence of gestational age on the ability of the fetus to pass meconium in utero. *Acta Obstetricia et Gynecologica Scandinavica*, **61**, 275–277.

61 Usher, R.H., Boyd, M.E., McLean, F.H., et al. (1988). Assessment of fetal risk in postdate pregnancies. *American Journal of Obstetrics and Gynecology*, **158**, 259–264.

62 Lucas, A., Adrian, T.E., Christofides, N., et al. (1980). Plasma

motilin, gastrin, and enteroglucagon and feeding in the human newborn. *Archives of Diseases in Childhood*, **55**, 673–677.

63 Wen, T.W., Eriksen, N.L., Blanco, J.D., et al. (1993). Association of clinical intra-amniotic infection and meconium. *American Journal of Perinatology*, **10**, 438–440.

64 Markovitch, O., Mazor, M., Shoham-Vardi, I., et al. (1993). Meconium stained amniotic fluid is associated with maternal infectious morbidity in preterm delivery. *Acta Obstetrica et Gynecologica Scandinavica*, **72**, 538–542.

65 Romero, R., Mazor, M., Sepulveda,W., et al. (1992). Is bacterial endotoxin a cause of meconium passage in utero? *American Journal of Obstetrics and Gynecology*, **166**, 290.

66 Romero, R., Hanaoka, S., Mazo, M., et al. (1991). Meconium-stained amniotic fluid: a risk factor for microbial invasion of the amniotic cavity. *American Journal of Obstetrics and Gynecology*, **164**, 859–862.

67 Hernandez, C., Little, B.B., Dax, J.S., et al. (1993). Prediction of the severity of meconium aspiration syndrome. *American Journal of Obstetrics and Gynecology*, **169**, 61–70.

68 Piper, J.M., Newton, E.R., Berkus, M.D., et al. (1998). Meconium: a marker for peripartum infection. *Obstetrics and Gynecology*, **91**, 741–745.

69 Nelson, K.B. (1989). Relationship of intrapartum and delivery room events to long-term neurologic outcome. *Clinics in Perinatology*, **16**, 995–1007.

70 Crowley, P. (1989). Post-term pregnancy: induction or surveillance? In *Effective Care in Pregnancy and Childbirth*, eds. I. Chalmers, M. Enking, and M.J.N.C. Keirse, pp. 776–791. Oxford: Oxford University Press.

71 Kuban, K.C.K., Leviton, A. (1994). Cerebral palsy. *New England Journal of Medicine*, **330**, 188–195.

72 Finer, N.N., Robertson, C.M., Peters, K.R.N., et al. (1983). Factors affecting outcome in hypoxic–ischemic encephalopathy in term infants. *American Journal of Diseases of Children*, **137**, 21–25.

73 Hyde, S., Smotherman, J., Moore, J.l., et al. (1989). A model of bacterially induced umbilical vein spasm, relevant to fetal hypoperfusion. *Obstetrics and Gynecology*, **73**, 966–970.

74 Altshuler, G., Hyde, S. (1989). Meconium-induced vasocontraction: a potential cause of cerebral and other fetal hypoperfusion and of poor pregnancy outcome. *Journal of Child Neurology*, **4**, 137–142.

75 Altshuler, G. (1995). Placental insights into neurodevelopmental and other childhood diseases. *Seminars in Pediatric Neurology*, **2**, 90–99.

76 Holcberg, G., Huleihel, M., Katz, M., et al. (1999). Vasoconstrictive activity of meconium stained amniotic fluid in the human placental vasculature. *European Journal of Obstetrics and Gynecology and Reproductive Biology*, **87**, 147–150.

77 Altshuler, G., Hermann, A.A. (1989). The medicolegal imperative: placental pathology and epidemiology. In *Fetal and Neonatal Brain Injury*, eds. D.K. Stevenson and P. Sunshine, pp. 250–263. Toronto: B.C. Decker.

78 Altshuler, G. (1993). A conceptual approach to placental pathology and pregnancy outcome. *Seminars in Diagnostic Pathology*, **10**, 204–221.

79 Burgess, A.M., Hutchins, G.M. (1996). Inflammation of the lungs, umbilical cord, and placenta associated with meconium passage in utero: review of 123 autopsied cases. *Pathology, Research and Practice*, **192**, 1121–1128.

80 Kaspar, H.G., Abu-Musa, A., Hannoun, A., et al. (2000). The placenta in meconium staining: lesions and early neonatal outcome. *Clinical and Experimental Obstetrics and Gynecology*, **27**, 63–66.

81 Wiswell, T.E., Popek, E., Barfield, W.D., et al. (1994). The effect of intra-amniotic meconium on histologic findings over time in a fetal rabbit model. *Pediatric Research*, **35**, 261A.

82 Kojima, T., Hattori, K., Fujiwara, T., et al. (1994). Meconium-induced lung injury mediated by activation of alveolar macrophages. *Life Sciences*, **54**, 1559–1562.

83 Jones, C.A., Cayabyab, R.G., Hamdan, H., et al. (1994). Early production of proinflammatory cytokines in the pathogenesis of neonatal adult respiratory distress syndrome (ARDS) associated with meconium aspiration. *Pediatric Research*, **35**, 339A.

84 Bui, K.C., Martin, G., Kammerman, L.A., et al. (1992). Plasma thromboxane and pulmonary artery pressure in neonates treated with extracorporeal membrane oxygenation. *Journal of Thoracic and Cardiovascular Surgery*, **104**, 124–129.

85 Wu, J-M., Yeh, T-F., Lin, Y.-J., et al. (1995). Increases of leukotriene B_4 (LTB_4) and D_4 (LTD_4) and cardio-hemodynamic changes in newborn piglets with meconium aspiration (MAS). *Pediatric Research*, **37**, 357A.

86 Perlman, J.M. (1989). Systemic abnormalities in term infants following perinatal asphyxia: relevance to long-term neurologic outcome. *Clinics in Perinatology*, **16**, 475–484.

87 Naeye, R.L., Localio, A.R. (1995). Determining the time before birth when ischemia and hypoxemia initiated cerebral palsy. *Obstetrics and Gynecology*, **86**, 713–719.

88 Benirschke, K. (1994). Placenta pathology questions to the perinatologist. *Journal of Perinatology*, **14**, 371–375.

89 Benirschke, K., Kaufmann, P. (2000). Legal considerations.

In *Pathology of the Human Placenta*, 4th edn, eds. K. Benirschke and P. Kauffmann, pp. 903–916.

90 Benirschke, K. (2001). Fetal consequences of amniotic fluid meconium. *Contemp Ob/gyn*, **46**, 76–83.

91 Grether, J.K., Nelson, K.B. (1997). Maternal infection and cerebral palsy in infants of normal birth weight. *Journal of the American Medical Association*, **278**, 207–211.

92 Sienko, A., Altshuler, G. (1999). Meconium-induced umbilical vascular necrosis in abortuses and fetuses: a histopathologic study for cytokines. *Obstetrics and Gynecology*, **94**, 415–420.

93 Walsh-Sukys, M.C. (1993). Persistent pulmonary hypertension of the newborn: the black box revisited. *Clinics in Perinatology*, **20**, 127–143.

94 Walsh-Sukys, M.C., Cornell, D.J., Houston, L.N., et al. (1994). Treatment of persistent pulmonary hypertension of the newborn without hyperventilation: an assessment of diffusion of innovation. *Pediatrics*, **94**, 303–306.

95 Klesh, K.W., Murphy, T.F., Scher, M.S., et al. (1987). Cerebral infarction in persistent pulmonary hypertension of the newborn. *American Journal of Diseases in Children*, **141**, 852–857.

96 Oelberg, D.G., Temple, D.M., Haskins, K.S., et al. (1988). Intracranial hemorrhage in term or near-term newborns with persistent pulmonary hypertension. *Clinical Pediatrics*, **27**, 14–17.

97 Hansen, N.B., Nowicki, P.T., Miller, R.R., et al. (1986). Alterations in cerebral blood flow and oxygen consumption during prolonged hypocarbia. *Pediatric Research*, **20**, 147–150.

98 Reuter, J.H., Disney, T.A. (1986). Regional blood flow and cerebral metabolic rate of oxygen during hyperventilation in the newborn dog. *Pediatric Research* **20**, 1102–1106.

99 Hauge, A., Thoresen, M., Walloe, L. (1980). Changes in cerebral blood flow during hyperventilation and CO_2-breathing measured by a bidirectional, pulsed, ultrasound Doppler blood velocitymeter. *Acta Paediatrica Scandinavica*, **110**, 167–173.

100 Wung, J.T., James, L.S., Kilchevsky, E., et al. (1985). Management of infants with severe respiratory failure and persistence of the fetal circulation. *Pediatrics*, **76**, 488–494.

101 Hendricks-Muñoz, K.D., Walton, J.P. (1988). Hearing loss in infants with persistent fetal circulation. *Pediatrics*, **81**, 650–656.

102 Bifano, E.M., Pfannenstiel, A. (1988). Duration of hyperventilation and outcome in infants with persistent pulmonary hypertension. *Pediatrics*, **81**, 657–661.

103 Sell E.J., Gaines J.A., Gluckman C., et al. (1985). Persistent fetal circulation: neurodevelopmental outcome. *American Journal of Diseases in Children*, **139**, 25–28.

104 Graziani, L.J., Baumgart, S., Desai, S., et al. (1997). Clinical antecedents of neurologic and audiologic abnormalities in survivors of neonatal extracorporeal membrane oxygenation. *Journal of Child Neurology* **12**, 415–419.

105 Davis, P.J., Shekerdemian, L.S. (2001). Meconium aspiration syndrome and extracorporeal membrane oxygenation. *Archives of Disease in Childhood Fetal and Neonatal Edition*, **84**, F1–F3.

106 HiFi Study Group (1989). High-frequency oscillatory ventilation compared with conventional mechanical ventilation in the treatment of respiratory failure in preterm infants. *New England Journal of Medicine*, **320**, 88–93.

107 HiFO Study Group (1993). Randomized study of high-frequency oscillatory ventilation in infants with severe respiratory distress syndrome. *Journal of Pediatrics*, **122**, 609–619.

108 Wiswell, T.E., Graziani, L.J., Kornhauser, M.S., et al. (1996). High-frequency jet ventilation in the early management of respiratory distress syndrome is associated with a greater risk for adverse outcomes. *Pediatrics*, **98**, 1035–1043.

109 Zapol, W.M., Rimar S., Gilles, N., et al. (1994). Nitric oxide and the lung. *American Journal of Respiratory and Critical Care Medicine*, **149**, 1375–1380.

110 Page J., Frisk V., Whyte H. (1994). Developmental outcome of infants treated with extracorporeal membrane oxygenation (ECMO) in the neonatal period: is the evidence all in? *Paediatric and Perinatal Epidemiology*, **8**, 123–139.

111 Walsh-Sukys, M.C., Bauer, R.E., Cornell, D.J., et al. (1994). Severe respiratory failure in neonates: mortality and morbidity rates and neurodevelopmental outcomes. *Journal of Pediatrics*, **125**, 104–110.

112 ECMO Registry of the Extracorporeal Life Support Organization (ELSO). (2001). Ann Arbor, Michigan: Extracorporeal Life Support Organization.

113 ECMO Registry of the Extracorporeal Life Support Organization (ELSO). (2001). Ann Arbor, Michigan: Extracorporeal Life Support Organization.

114 Wiswell, T.E., Tencer, H.L. (1994). What causes the color changes of meconium-stained amniotic fluid? *Pediatric Research*, **35**, 261A.

115 Vidyasagar, D., Yeh, T.F., Harris, V., et al. (1995). Assisted ventilation in infants with meconium aspiration syndrome. *Pediatrics*, **56**, 208–213.

116 Abramovici, H., Brandes, J.M., Fuchs, K., et al. (1974). Meconium during delivery: a sign of compensated fetal distress. *American Journal of Obstetrics and Gynecology*, **118**, 251–255.

117 Altshuler, G. (1991). Placenta within the medicolegal imperative. *Archives of Pathology and Laboratory Medicine*, **115**, 688–695.

118 Naeye, R.L. (1987). Functionally important disorders of the placenta, umbilical cord, and fetal membranes. *Human Pathology*, **18**, 680–691.

119 Miller, P.W., Coen, R.W., Benirschke, K. (1985). Dating the time interval from meconium passage to birth. *Obstetrics and Gynecology*, **66**, 459–462.

120 Bourne, G. (1962). Meconium transport. In *The Human Amnion and Chorion*, ed. G. Bourne, pp. 143–154, Chicago: Year Book.

121 American Academy of Pediatrics, American College of Obstetricians and Gynecologists. (1997). Assessment of infants in the delivery room. In *Guidelines for Perinatal Care*, 4th edn, pp. 122–125. Elk Grove Village, Ill: American Academy of Pediatrics.

122 MacLennan, A. for the International Cerebral Palsy Task Force. (1999). A template for defining a causal relation between acute intrapartum events and cerebral palsy: international consensus statement. *British Medical Journal*, **319**, 1054–1059.

123 Baskett, T.F., Liston, R.M. (1989). Fetal movement monitoring: clinical application. *Clinics in Perinatology*, **16**, 613–625.

124 Schifrin B.S., Hamilton-Rubinstein, T., Shields, J.R. (1994). Fetal heart rate patterns and the timing of fetal injury. *Journal of Perinatology*, **14**, 174–181.

125 Nelson, K.B., Dambrosia, J.M., Ting, T.Y., et al. (1996). Uncertain value of electronic fetal monitoring in predicting cerebral palsy. *New England Journal of Medicine*, **334**, 613–618.

126 Scheller, J.M., Nelson, K.B. (1994). Does cesarean delivery prevent cerebral palsy or other neurologic problems of childhood? *Obstetrics and Gynecology*, **83**, 624–630.

127 Richey, S.D., Ramin, S.M., Bawdon, R.E., et al. (1995). Markers of acute and chronic asphyxia in infants with meconium-stained amniotic fluid. *American Journal of Obstetrics and Gynecology*, **172**, 1212–1215.

128 Jazayeri, A., Politz, L., Tsibris, J.C.M., et al. (2000). Fetal erythropoietin levels in pregnancies complicated by meconium passage: does meconium suggest fetal hypoxia? *American Journal of Obstetrics and Gynecology*, **183**, 188–190.

129 Maier, R.F., Böhme, K., Dudenhausen, J.W., et al. (1993). Cord blood erythropoietin in relation to different markers of fetal hypoxia. *Obstetrics and Gynecology*, **81**, 575–580.

130 Manchanda, R., Vora, M., Gruslin, A. (1999). Influence of postdatism and meconium on fetal erythropoietin. *Journal of Perinatology*, **19**, 479–482.

131 Widness, J.A., Teramo, K.A., Clemons, G.K., et al. (1986). Temporal responses of immunoreactive erythropoietin to acute hypoxemia in fetal sheep. *Pediatric Research*, **20**, 15–19.

132 Hanlon-Lundberg, K.M., Kirby, R.S. (1999). Nucleated red blood cells as a marker of acidemia in term neonates. *American Journal of Obstetrics and Gynecology*, **181**, 196–201.

133 Wiswell, T.E., Rohatsch, R.R., Mathur, G.V., et al. (1995). Absolute nucleated red blood cell count (ANRBC) reflects *in-utero* hypoxia and correlates with survival in neonates with congenital diaphragmatic hernia (CDH). *Pediatric Research* **37**, 246A.

134 Phelan, J.P, Ahn, M.O., Korst, L.M., et al. (1995). Nucleated red blood cells: a marker for fetal asphyxia? *American Journal of Obstetrics and Gynecology*, **173**, 1380–1384.

135 Korst, L.M., Phelan, J.P., Ahn, M.O., et al. (1996). Nucleated red blood cells: an update on the marker for fetal asphyxia. *American Journal of Obstetrics and Gynecology*, **175**, 843–846.

136 Buonocore, G., Perrone, S., Gioia, D., et al. (1999). Nucleated red blood cell count at birth as an index of perinatal brain damage. *American Journal of Obstetrics and Gynecology*, **181**, 1500–1505.

137 Minior, V.K., Bernstein, P.S., Divon, M.Y. (2000). Nucleated red blood cells in growth-restricted fetuses: associations with short-term neonatal outcome. *Fetal Diagnosis and Therapy*, **15**, 165–169.

138 Blackwell, S.C., Refuerzo, J.S., Wolfe, H.M., et al. (2000). The relationship between nucleated red blood cell counts and early-onset neonatal seizures. *American Journal of Obstetrics and Gynecology*, **182**, 1452–1457.

139 Naeye, R.L., Lin, H-L. (2001). Determining the time before birth when ischemia and hypoxemia initiated cerebral palsy. *American Journal of Obstetrics and Gynecology*, **184**, 217–224.

140 Rossi, E.M., Philipson, E.H., Williams, T.G., et al. (1989). Meconium aspiration syndrome: intrapartum and neonatal attributes. *American Journal of Obstetrics and Gynecology*, **161**, 1106–1110.

141 Wiswell, T.E., Henley, M.A. (1992). Intratracheal suctioning, systemic infection, and the meconium aspiration syndrome. *Pediatrics*, **89**, 203–206.

142 Valencia, P., Sosa, R., Wyble, C., et al. (1993). Accuracy of admission chest x ray (CXR) in the prediction of sickness severity in infants with meconium aspiration syndrome (MAS). *Clinical Research*, **41**, 736A.

143 Weitzner, J.S., Strassner, H.T., Rawlins, R.G., et al. (1990). Objective assessment of meconium content of amniotic fluid. *Obstetrics and Gynecology*, **76**, 1143–1144.

144 Trimmer, K.J., Gilstrap, L.C. (1991). "Meconium-crit" and birth asphyxia. *American Journal of Obstetrics and Gynecology*, **165**, 1010–1013.

32

Persistent pulmonary hypertension of the newborn

Krisa P. Van Meurs, William D. Rhine, and William E. Benitz

Stanford University Medical Center, Palo Alto, CA, USA

Persistent pulmonary hypertension of the newborn (PPHN) is characterized by markedly elevated pulmonary vascular resistance and pulmonary arterial pressure, along with striking pulmonary vasoreactivity, which produces right-to-left shunting through the ductus arteriosus and foramen ovale.[1,2] With severe PPHN, this extrapulmonary shunting results in severe hypoxemia, which typically is poorly responsive to treatment with high concentrations of inspired oxygen, assisted ventilation, and pharmacologic manipulation of the circulation. Elevated pulmonary vascular resistance with right-to-left extrapulmonary shunting also often occurs in association with severe pulmonary parenchymal disease, including meconium aspiration syndrome, bacterial pneumonia, lung hypoplasia, or hyaline membrane disease, and may be compounded by coexistent impairment of systemic cardiac output and/or systemic arterial pressures due to impaired myocardial function, hypovolemia, or systemic vasodilation.[3] In addition, pulmonary hypertension is often very difficult to distinguish from total anomalous pulmonary venous return, and may complicate a variety of other congenital cardiac malformations. These associated conditions may occur with or without intrinsic structural and functional abnormalities of the pulmonary vascular bed, and treatment needs not only to be specific for the underlying or associated conditions, but also must account for the expected normal or abnormal behavior of the pulmonary blood vessels. As a consequence, infants with pulmonary hypertension present one of the most difficult diagnostic and therapeutic challenges in neonatal intensive care. The complexity of these relationships has also led to a complicated and inconsistent nosology in the medical literature;[4] while some clinicians apply the label of PPHN to nearly all neonates with hypoxemia unresponsive to administration of 100% oxygen, excluding only those with cyanotic congenital heart disease, some use this term for all infants with elevated pulmonary artery pressures and right-to-left shunting, and others reserve this terminology for only those with excessive pulmonary arterial reactivity associated with pathognomonic excessive muscularization of the pulmonary arteries, with or without associated parenchymal disease (e.g., meconium aspiration) or other congenital malformations (e.g., pulmonary hypoplasia, congenital diaphragmatic hernia, or cardiac disease). The following discussion addresses the latter, more narrowly defined, syndrome of PPHN, for which some authors have reserved the label of "persistent fetal circulation." Because the fetal circulation includes the placenta, however, this is somewhat of a misnomer for a description of abnormal physiology in the infant after birth.

Infants with PPHN are among the most critically ill patients cared for in a neonatal intensive care unit, and until recently, the mortality rate was as high as 50%.[5] They often have a wide variety of preexisting perinatal conditions, such as low Apgar scores or fetal distress, which may place them at high risk for abnormal neurodevelopmental outcomes. Severe hypoxemia, often complicated by impaired cardiac function, is a hallmark of this disease, placing these neonates at high risk for acquisition of cerebral injuries in the postnatal period. Furthermore, treatment of PPHN may include use of aggressive therapies such as hyperventilation, extracorporeal membrane oxygenation (ECMO), or inhaled nitric oxide, which also have the potential to affect outcome adversely, either directly or because of iatrogenic complications, such as pneumothorax or hemorrhagic diatheses, for example. Therefore, there may be multiple reasons for neurodevelopmental abnormalities in infants diagnosed with PPHN, and they may be extremely difficult to disentangle when it becomes apparent that the long-term outcome is less than optimal. Because severe PPHN occurs in as many as 1 of every 1000 live births,[5] infants with this condition have the potential to contribute substantially to prevalence of neurodevelopmental disorders. Further, recent improvements in treatment have resulted in significant reduction in mortality rates, but there is concern that this may have been achieved at the expense of increasing the number of survivors with neurodevelopmental impairments. The pathogenesis, pathophysiology, and management of PPHN have been the subject of detailed, excellent reviews,[6,7] and will be reiterated only briefly in the following discussion.

Differential diagnosis of persistent pulmonary hypertension of the newborn

The diagnosis of PPHN must be considered in any infant who remains hypoxemic, with a Pao_2 less than 100 mmHg, while breathing 100% oxygen.[3] This clinical observation provides strong evidence for right-to-left shunting, but provides no information regarding the location or cause of such shunting. The prerequisites for right-to-left shunting include pressures on the right (pulmonary) side of the circulation exceeding those on the left (systemic) side, along with a communication between the right and left sides through which shunting can occur. In addition to the fetal channels (ductus arteriosus and foramen ovale), which are present and patent in almost every infant, shunting may occur at atrial or ventricular septal defects, aortopulmonary windows, or at other sites where cardiac malformations permit admixture of venous and arterial blood (e.g., atrioventricular canal, truncus arteriosus). Since right-to-left shunting may result from reduced systemic pressures even if pulmonary arterial pressures are normal, pulmonary hypertension should not be considered until it has been established that systemic cardiac output is adequate. Because the right ventricle can sustain systemic pressures, it is essential that normal systemic arterial pressures should not be taken as proof of adequacy of left ventricular output.

Presently, color Doppler echocardiography provides the most direct approach to assessment of systemic blood flow, allowing diagnosis of structural obstructions (covering the entire spectrum of hypoplastic left heart syndromes) as well as intrinsic (hypoglycemia, hypocalcemia, asphyxial or toxic cardiomyopathy) and extrinsic (tamponade, hypovolemia) left ventricular dysfunction. If these conditions have been excluded, and there is echocardiographic evidence of elevated pulmonary arterial pressures, such as color Doppler confirmation of right-to-left shunting at the foramen or ductus, high-velocity regurgitant flow through an incompetent tricuspid valve, hypertensive flow–velocity profiles in the pulmonary arteries, or increased preejection period to ejection time ratios, the cause of the elevation in pulmonary artery pressures must be ascertained. Since high pressures may result from increased flow as well as from increased resistance, conditions which may produce an obligatory increase in pulmonary blood flow, such as intracardiac left-to-right shunts or large arteriovenous malformations, must be identified or excluded. Hyperviscosity, most commonly due to a hematocrit greater than 65%, has a larger effect on pulmonary than on systemic vascular resistance and pressures, and may produce intractable right-to-left shunting until corrected by partial exchange transfusion. Constriction of otherwise normal pulmonary arteries may occur with any significant pulmonary parenchymal process, mediated by reflex vasoconstriction of blood vessels in poorly ventilated and hypoxic regions of the lungs. The management of impaired systemic cardiac output or refractory hypoxemia secondary to pulmonary parenchymal disease is discussed in Chapter 34; however, specific diagnosis is important, since adequate treatment of the primary process will ameliorate secondary pulmonary vasoconstriction, increase systemic cardiac output, and reduce or eliminate right-to-left shunting and these conditions do not require interventions primarily intended to alter pulmonary vascular tone.

Intrinsic disease of the pulmonary arteries may be recognized by its association with other congenital malformations, especially pulmonary hypoplasia (e.g., congenital diaphragmatic hernia, thoracic dystrophies, chronic intrauterine pleural effusions),[8,9] or by the infant's characteristic response to induction of systemic alkalosis, typically by acute hyperventilation.[10] Infants with mild-to-moderately-severe pulmonary arterial disease respond to this stimulus with at least a transient pulmonary vasodilation, reflecting the dynamic component of their pulmonary vascular obstruction, which is clinically evident as a reduction in pulmonary pressures to below systemic levels, reversal of right-to-left shunting, and a marked increase in Pao_2 to well above 100 mmHg. Typically, these infants exhibit a pH threshold below which they have right-to-left shunting and are hypoxemic and above which they have a well-saturated arterial blood; this threshold may be as low as 7.48–7.50 early in the course of mild disease, but may be much higher (7.65–7.70) later in the course or in infants with severe disease. Infants with severe pulmonary vascular disease, however, may fail to respond perceptibly to alkalosis, either because structural remodeling of the pulmonary vessels is so advanced that vasodilation is impossible or insufficient, or because early intrauterine growth failure has produced not only pulmonary hypoplasia but also a deficient number of arteries and arterioles beyond the third or fourth branching generation,[9] so that the maximal cross-sectional area of the pulmonary arterial tree is severely compromised, even with maximal dilation of these vessels. In summary, clinical diagnosis of PPHN requires exclusion of other causes of right-to-left shunting, confirmation of elevated pulmonary artery pressures (usually by echocardiography), and demonstration of a threshold response to elevation of the systemic pH.

Pathogenesis of persistent pulmonary hypertension of the newborn

PPHN, defined narrowly as above, is characterized by striking intrinsic structural and functional abnormalities of the pulmonary arteries.[6] During normal pulmonary development, the muscular investment of the pulmonary arteries extends from proximal to distal vessels, and the thickness of the medial smooth-muscle layer increases in the already muscular proximal vessels. In normal infants at term, the arteries and arterioles found within the respiratory acinus (distal to terminal bronchioles) are all nonmuscular, and a muscular arterial media is present only in the more proximal, extraacinar arteries. Infants with PPHN exhibit precocious development of the muscular investment of the pulmonary arteries, with extension of the smooth muscular investment into smaller and more peripheral intraacinar arteries, as far peripherally as the pleura, and the thickness of the muscular media in more proximal vessels is markedly increased.[11] In addition, there is marked thickening of the adventitial connective tissue surrounding the pulmonary arteries, with increased deposition of adventitial collagen and elastin. These changes are associated with abnormal pulmonary vascular sensitivity to a variety of stimuli, ranging from hypercarbia, acidosis, and hypoxia to stimulation from tracheal suctioning, handling, or a noisy environment. Excessive vasoconstrictive responses appear to be mediated by excessive production of endothelin and possibly other vasoconstrictive substances, and by deficient local production of nitric oxide (NO), presumably due to loss of NO synthase activity in these pulmonary vessels.[7] Normal activity of these vasoregulatory mechanisms appears to recover a few days after birth, accounting for the clinical observation that pulmonary vasoconstriction becomes much less problematic at about 4 days of age in infants with PPHN who can be supported through that period.[12] On the other hand, the structural abnormalities in the pulmonary arteries of these infants probably resolve much more slowly, and normal pulmonary arterial structure may be achieved only after months or years, when lung development catches up with the precocious arteries.

The antecedents of accelerated arterial development and abnormal vasoregulatory function remain uncertain.[6] Clinical observations suggest that antenatal hypoxia or increased intrauterine pulmonary blood flow may be important predisposing factors. The archetypal infant with PPHN is a meconium-stained postterm baby with wasted subcutaneous fat and epidermal peeling, suggesting chronic placental insufficiency. Infants with intrauterine closure or constriction of the ductus arteriosus (resulting from exposure to nonsteroidal antiinflammatory agents) or with cardiac malformations that impose increased pulmonary blood flow and elevated pulmonary arterial pressures in utero have been associated with both pulmonary arterial remodeling and clinical pulmonary hypertension in the immediate postnatal period. Increased sensitivity of the ductus to the constrictor effects of prostaglandin synthetase inhibitors and the more advanced development of the pulmonary arteries with increasing gestation, particularly near term, may both contribute to the lower risk of PPHN in preterm infants and the predilection for this disorder to occur in postterm infants, especially those of greater than 42 weeks' gestation. In many cases, however, no predisposing intrauterine condition can be identified.

In sheep, fetal hypoxia resulting from maternal hypotension,[13] placental embolization,[14] or umbilical cord compression[15] produces pulmonary arterial remodeling, elevated pulmonary vascular resistance and pressures, and accentuated and more prolonged vasoconstrictor responses to asphyxial stimuli, but pulmonary arterial pressures remain substantially below systemic levels during normoxic ventilation in these models. Ligation of the ductus arteriosus several days before delivery in fetal lambs,[16–18] or partial occlusion of the ductus using an inflatable occluder for 9–14 days in fetal calves,[19] with consequent diversion of right ventricular output into the lungs, causes an acute increase in pulmonary artery flow and pressure. Although the elevated pressure is sustained, the increment in flow is reversed as the pulmonary vascular resistance increases, and these animals exhibit elevation of pulmonary artery pressures to equal or exceed those in the aorta, along with the right-to-left extrapulmonary shunting and refractory hypoxemia that is characteristic of infants with PPHN. These animals also have increased muscularity of the pulmonary arteries, analogous to that observed in infants who die with PPHN. Notably, these structural and functional changes in the pulmonary arteries occur only 5–8 days (or more) after induction of the hypoxic or pulmonary hypertensive condition, and there is no evidence that even repeated or severe acute asphyxial episodes can rapidly elicit the intractable pulmonary vasoconstriction that epitomizes this condition. These observations have several implications for infants with PPHN who subsequently manifest neurodevelopmental impairments. It is clear that these infants have been subject to a significantly disturbed intrauterine environment for a period of at least several days. Reduced arterial oxygen content, due to impaired placental function or increased arteriovenous admixture at the atrial level with premature constriction of the ductus, may impair cerebral oxygen delivery, placing these infants at increased risk for intrauterine hypoxic–ischemic cerebral insults. Redistribution of cardiac output in a fetus who is hypoxic or has reduced flow from the ductus into the descending aorta may impair renal perfusion, causing oligohydramnios, increasing the risk of cord compression events prior to and during labor and delivery. The primary events may also reduce the capacity for the fetus to tolerate the stress of labor and delivery, either directly or by blunting the metabolic and endocrine responses to this stress, enhancing the potential for intrapartum insults. Abnormal developmental outcomes in these infants therefore often have several antecedents, most of which are not amenable to diagnosis or treatment, and attribution of a poor outcome exclusively to intrapartum or obstetrical events is not easily justified.

Treatment of persistent pulmonary hypertension of the newborn

Recent review articles demonstrate the wide variety of practice patterns in the treatment of PPHN.[7,20–23] As there is no singular cause of PPHN, nor a singular pathophysiologic effect on the body, there is clearly no defined strategy to treat it. Whenever PPHN is secondary, such as in severe respiratory distress syndrome or sepsis, therapeutic intervention must include addressing the underlying disease. Similarly, when there are secondary effects from PPHN, e.g., pulmonary hemorrhage, treatment must also correct those perturbations.

Nonrespiratory interventions

The initial approach to treat PPHN includes normalization of physiologic perturbations that can exacerbate PPHN, including normalization of serum glucose, calcium, and reduction exchange transfusion for polycythemia. Optimization of cardiac function may require colloid volume infusion or inotropic pressor support, e.g., dopamine or dobutamine infusions. Intravenous vasodilators, e.g., tolazoline or nitroprusside, are usually nonselective and affect both systemic and pulmonary vascular resistance, so are often not successful in reversing right-to-left shunting associated with PPHN. Oxygen-carrying capacity may be improved by red blood cell transfusion. Sedation may be useful to decrease agitation and resistance to mechanical ventilation. Intravenous administration of magnesium sulfate has been suggested to be helpful in treating neonates with PPHN,[24–26] although in a newborn pig model magnesium did not show vasodilatory effects selective to the pulmonary vascular bed.[27]

Ventilator management

Ventilator management is the most controversial arena for the treatment of PPHN. Alkalosis by hyperventilation and hypocapnia has been shown to reduce the pulmonary vascular resistance in PPHN,[10,28] and for many physicians this represents the cornerstone of the treatment of severe PPHN.[20] However, the excessive barotrauma and/or volutrauma that may be necessary to achieve hyperventilation may delay lung repair or even cause further injury such as pneumothorax and pulmonary edema. Furthermore, extremely low $Paco_2$ has been shown to reduce cerebral blood flow (CBF) in human adults and animal models.[29] In neonatal humans, this response might not be fully present or it may be transient, with subsequent adjustment of CBF at a reduced $Paco_2$. If there is a reduction in CBF, any improvement in oxygen content in the blood by hyperventilation may be more than counterbalanced by a reduction in CBF, leading to a net overall reduction in cerebral oxygen delivery and consumption. Regional CBF reduction and accompanying oxygen deficits might account for specific neurologic injury in PPHN, e.g., sensorineural hearing loss. Measurement of the relative effects of hyperventilation and other strategies upon cerebral metabolism and integrity will require development of portable bedside monitoring techniques such as near-infrared optical spectroscopy. An alternative to extreme hyperventilation is more modest hypocapnia ($Paco_2$ = 25–35 mmHg or 3.3–4.7 kPa) combined with more aggressive alkali (bicarbonate or tromethamine) administration. It should be noted that, according to the review by Walsh-Sukys et al.[23] achieving alkalosis by alkali administration was associated with a fivefold increase in the use of ECMO, while hyperventilation seemed to reduce the risk of ECMO without increasing the use of oxygen at 28 days of age. Peak inspiratory pressures to achieve hyperventilation may be reduced with the implementation of high-frequency ventilation or synchronous ventilator techniques.

An alternative approach to ventilator management advocated by Wung and others is that of "gentle ventilation," with more modest blood gas goals such as Pao_2 = 50–70 mmHg (6.7–9.3 kPa) and $Paco_2$ = 40–60 mmHg (5.3–8.0 kPa), along with avoidance of paralysis.[30,31] This strategy, which seeks to minimize ventilator-induced injury, has been shown in several uncontrolled reports to help neonates with severe PPHN avoid ECMO, and to recover with favorable neurologic outcomes, including intact sensorineural hearing.[32]

The absence of any controlled trials comparing hyperventilation to "gentle ventilation" or any other specific ventilator strategy makes it impossible to state definitely which approach is superior. Furthermore, an individual's experience with one such strategy might predispose to a less favorable outcome if there is a radical change in therapeutic style.

Recent advances in the treatment of pulmonary hypertension

Exogenous surfactant

Patients with severe PPHN may have several reasons to have inadequate surfactant activity. Meconium, infection-related inflammation, and pulmonary hemorrhage may decrease surfactant effectiveness. In patients with congenital diaphragmatic hernia or severe respiratory distress syndrome, there may be insufficient surfactant present.[33,34] Improving alveolar expansion via surfactant administration may be important in optimizing the effect of inhaled NO.[35] Lotze et al. have shown that surfactant replacement reduces duration of ECMO bypass in noncongenital diaphragmatic hernia (CDH) patients with PPHN.[36] Given the relatively rare, limited, and transient adverse side-effects seen with surfactant administration, some advocate at least a test dose in patients with severe PPHN approaching ECMO. A large multicenter randomized trial has shown that administration of surfactant led to a 30% reduction in the need for ECMO in a high-risk population of neonates, most of whom had PPHN.

High-frequency ventilation

The use of high-frequency ventilation (HFV), be it by flow-interruption, oscillation, or jet ventilation, has been advocated for neonatal respiratory disease.[37–40] HFV maintains lung expansion and achieves ventilation with rapid (5–15 Hz) delivery of breaths at tidal volumes that may be smaller than the nominal physiological dead space. The maximal distension during HFV is less than in conventional tidal volume ventilation, thereby decreasing barotrauma. In patients nearing or meeting ECMO criteria, HFV strategies seem to reduce the need for bypass in 10–50% of patients, depending in large part upon the underlying lung disease.[41–43] HFV may also improve alveolar expansion and thereby improve response to inhaled NO (iNO).[44]

Inhaled nitric oxide

The intracellular mediator of vascular smooth-muscle dilation released by the neighboring endothelial cell appears to be NO.[45] Within the smooth muscle, NO activates guanylate cyclase to form cyclic guanosine monophosphate, which causes muscle relaxation. Administration of exogenous NO by inhalation reduces pulmonary vascular resistance (PVR).[46,47] In neonates with severe PPHN, reduced PVR should decrease right-to-left shunting at the foramen ovale or patent ductus arteriosus and thereby improve oxygenation. Besides reducing extrapulmonary right-to-left shunting, iNO may also improve intrapulmonary ventilation perfusion matching. iNO is rapidly metabolized by conversion of hemoglobin to methemoglobin, and has little or no effect on systemic vascular resistance and cardiac output.

Initial clinical trials of iNO in neonates with respiratory failure and PPHN have shown dramatic improvements in oxygenation, and often an apparent decrease in the subsequent need for ECMO.[22,48,49] Two recent multicenter randomized controlled trials demonstrated that iNO decreased the incidence of ECMO or death in newborns with PPHN,[50,51] which led to its Food and Drug Administration (FDA) approval in December 1999.

iNO is not without potential risks that could possibly affect prognosis and neurologic outcome. Methemoglobinemia and hypoxia can result from excess NO administration or in the rare patient with decreased methemoglobin reductase. NO and its metabolites, including nitrogen dioxide and peroxynitrites, may cause lung injury. iNO increases bleeding time in normal adult humans[52] presumably through platelet-mediated effects. However, in patients with acute respiratory distress syndrome, NO affected platelet aggregation tests without changing the bleeding time.[53] Effects of NO on coagulation could theoretically put neonatal iNO recipients at higher hemorrhagic risk, although this has not been seen to be a significant side-effect in the clinical trials to date. Given these potential risks, it is understandable that the clinical trials of iNO in neonates with severe PPHN are also examining secondary outcomes, including neurodevelopment. In a follow-up to one of the pivotal studies used for FDA approval, nitric oxide was not associated with an increase in neurodevelopmental, behavioral, or medical abnormalities at 2 years of age.[54] In two smaller studies in prematures, presumably a population at greater risk of intracranial hemorrhage, iNO use did not adversely affect intracranial hemorrhage rate[55] or neurodevelopment at 30 months.[56]

Other pharmacologic approaches to treat pulmonary hypertension

Tolazoline administration via the endotracheal tube has been used to target this vasodilator therapy more selectively to the pulmonary vascular bed.[57–59] However, no prospective randomized studies have investigated its effects on major outcomes, such as the need for ECMO. Adenosine infusion has been shown to dilate the pulmonary vessels of fetal and newborn lambs,[60] and has also been associated with improved oxygenation in a small series of newborns with PPHN.[61] Because adenosine presumably acts upon adenylate cyclase, its action may be additive to that of iNO, as suggested by the data of Aranda et al. in an experimental model of PPHN.[62]

Other pharmacologic manipulations have been aimed at the NO pathway without the use of iNO. As L-arginine is the precursor for the formation of NO, it has been given as an infusion to stimulate NO production. L-arginine infusion has been shown to dilate the pulmonary vasculature in a lamb model of PPHN[63] and in a small series of five human infants with PPHN, a single dose of L-arginine led to improved oxygenation in four patients. iNO leads to the formation of cyclic guanosine monophosphate, which is vasodilatory until it is degraded by phosphodiesterase (PDE). There are several types of PDE, of which type V dominates in the pulmonary vascular bed. Inhibitors of PDE, e.g., dypyramidole, have been used to potentiate the effects of iNO,[64] although their use has been associated with deleterious side-effects, including severe hypotension. Recently, more type V selective PDE inhibitors such as Zaprinast and E4021, have been used to affect pulmonary vasodilation, often to potentiate the effects of iNO.[65–67]

Extracorporeal membrane oxygenation

ECMO is a form of heart–lung bypass providing cardiorespiratory support for days to weeks, which is available at approximately 100 US centers and another 20 outside the US.[68] Venoarterial (VA) ECMO bypass, using right jugular venous drainage and right carotid arterial return, can provide respiratory and cardiac support; the latter is often needed in patients with PPHN associated with sepsis or cardiac disease. Venovenous (VV) ECMO, usually performed via a double-lumen catheter placed in the right jugular vein with the tip in the right atrium, returns oxygenated blood preferentially towards the right ventricle, thereafter relying on the patient's cardiac function to achieve adequate systemic oxygen delivery. Once on bypass, ventilator settings are weaned dramatically, thereby avoiding or minimizing further oxygen toxicity and barotrauma, and permitting pulmonary healing and reversal of PPHN.

Both VA and VV ECMO require systemic heparinization titrated based on bedside coagulation studies to prevent circuit clotting. This puts ECMO patients at increased risk for hemorrhagic complications, including risk for intracranial hemorrhage, which occurs in approximately 10–20% of patients, but varies depending on gestational age, diagnosis, and coagulation status.[69,70] Strategies to decrease the incidence of intracranial hemorrhage of ECMO include administration of aminocaproic acid, a fibrinolysis inhibitor,[71] as well as the use of cephalad venous drainage catheters.[72] Besides pre-ECMO and hemorrhagic risks for neurologic sequelae, ECMO patients have additional risks, including nosocomial and transfusion-related infection, thromboembolism, and potential effects of neck vessel ligation. Jugular venous ligation may impair cerebral venous drainage and lead to superior vena cava syndrome. Carotid artery ligation leads to collateral flow to the right side of the brain. VV ECMO obviates the need for carotid artery ligation as in VA bypass. Some centers advocate post-ECMO carotid artery repair, but there may be subsequent stenosis, and there are no data to date demonstrating improved neurobehavioral outcomes with such repair.

Given the relatively invasive nature of ECMO therapy and its attendant risks, ECMO is used for neonates with severe PPHN or other forms of cardiorespiratory disease only after failure of presumably less risky medical management. Criteria predicting high mortality rates (60–80%) have been developed based on arterial blood gases and ventilator settings. It is also important that there must be adequate time to transport such critically ill patients to an ECMO center and to place them on bypass before cardiac arrest or hypoxic brain injury occurs. Despite the critical nature and high predicted mortality rates for ECMO patients, survival rates are quite high, averaging over 80%.[73]

Liquid ventilation

The newest frontier for neonatal respiratory failure, possibly including PPHN, is the use of perfluorocarbon (PFC) liquid ventilation. When placed into the lungs, PFC allows diffusion-mediated oxygenation and ventilation. The perfluorocarbon most extensively tested to date is perflubron (LiquiVent). In total liquid ventilation, there is slow tidal volume filling and emptying of the lungs with preoxygenated, hypocarbic PFC. Alternatively, partial liquid ventilation entails filling the alveoli with PFC and then using either conventional or high-frequency mechanical ventilation to oxygenate and ventilate through the PFC. These PFCs maintain alveolar expansion with decreased transmitted pressure and volume, thereby decreasing injury. PFCs also improve pulmonary toilet, which can be helpful in the recovery from meconium aspiration, pneumonia, and other inflammatory insults.

In several animal models of lung injury, including meconium aspiration and oleic acid-induced ARDS, liquid ventilation provided good oxygenation and ventilation.[23,74–80] Survival was better, and histopathology was remarkably improved compared to conventional mechanical ventilation. PFCs are also permeable to iNO, allowing for a combination of therapies that might be particularly helpful when PPHN accompanies other lung disease. Initial studies have shown additive benefits when both liquid ventilation and iNO were used in experimental models of meconium aspiration syndrome.[81] Although the vast bulk of perflubron and other PFCs dissipates within hours to days after discontinuation of use, the long-term effects of the albeit small local and systemic absorption of these products remain uncertain. Ultimately, liquid ventilation strategies will need to be subjected to controlled randomized trials comparing them to other possible interventions for severe neonatal respiratory failure and PPHN.

Outcome of persistent pulmonary hypertension of the newborn

Outcome of PPHN survivors treated with conventional medical therapy

Conventional medical therapy for PPHN often includes lengthy periods of mechanical ventilation with high pressure and high concentrations of oxygen, which increase the risk for chronic lung disease (CLD). CLD has been shown to be associated with poorer cognitive outcome.[82,83] Hyperventilation with production of a respiratory alkalosis is also frequently used in treating PPHN. Hyperventilation has been shown to decrease pulmonary artery pressures and increase arterial Pao_2.[10] Although hyperventilation has been shown to attenuate pulmonary vasoconstriction, the resulting hypocarbia can produce cerebrovascular vasoconstriction with a subsequent reduction in CBF.[84,85] Concern exists that decreased CBF can result in cerebral hypoxia and cerebral atrophy with subsequent neurodevelopmental sequelae.[29,85] Whether hyperventilation is specifically responsible for the neurodevelopmental sequelae seen in PPHN survivors is difficult to determine due to the multitude of potential causes of injury present in this population. The following studies have documented the outcome for survivors of PPHN and the results are summarized in Table 32.1.

PPHN follow-up studies

Cohen et al.[86] examined 29 survivors of PPHN treated with tolazoline between 1974 and 1978. Fifty percent had abnormal electroencephalograms or seizures in the neonatal period. Neurologic examination performed between the ages of 1 and 3 years found 3.5% with bilateral hearing impairment, 17% with cerebral palsy, 3.5% with a seizure disorder, and 35% with microcephaly. Stanford–Binet IQ testing of 12 children at age 3 yielded a mean score of 98. Five children had mean IQ scores of 101 when compared to their sibling's scores of 108. Only one child had CLD. In summary, the authors concluded that 28% of the children at age 3 had evidence of significant neurologic impairment. Examination of children with perinatal hypoxia and an Apgar score less than 6 revealed a similar incidence of significant handicapping conditions. Cohen et al. attributed the morbidity from PPHN to the degree of perinatal hypoxia.

Brett et al.[87] reported on the neurologic and developmental assessment of nine infants with PPHN treated with hyperventilation. The infants were exposed to a $Paco_2$ less than 20 mmHg for 51 h, to a $Paco_2$ less than 15 mmHg for 11.8 h, to a pH greater than 7.5 for 64.4 h, and to a pH greater than 7.6 for 6.1 h. All had normal neurologic examinations and seven of the eight had normal development quotient (DQ) on testing performed between the ages of 1 and 3 years. The one infant with a DQ of 89 was a small-for-gestational-age twin with Apgar scores of 1 and 4 and a history of fetal distress. The authors felt that the neurologic and developmental outcome following hyperventilation in this study was reassuring.

Bernbaum et al.[88] evaluated 11 surviving children treated for PPHN with hyperventilation. The authors attempted to correlate neurologic and neurodevelopmental outcome with physiologic parameters such as pH, $Paco_2$, Pao_2 and blood pressure. Testing was performed between the ages of 6 months and 4 years. Eight of the children had normal neurologic examinations. Two had mildly increased tone or reflexes and one had a mild hemiparesis. Nine children had normal developmental scores while two were mildly delayed with mean Bayley Mental Developmental Index (MDI) and Psychomotor Developmental Index (PDI) scores of 72. Comparison of the three patients with abnormal neurologic outcome to the remainder of the group showed significant differences in the duration of blood pressure less than 50 mmHg and $Paco_2$ less than 25 mmHg. The authors speculated that hypocarbia may potentiate hypoxic–ischemic encephalopathy by further compromising CBF.

In a review of the developmental follow-up of PPHN in their institution, Ballard and Leonard[89] reported on the outcome of 11 infants with PPHN treated with hyperventilation. The neurologic outcome was found to be normal in all children. Cognitive development was assessed using the McCarthy scales performed between the ages of 4 and 6 years; the mean General Cognitive Index (GCI) was 95, with scores ranging from 79 to 120. They concluded that there was no evidence for a specific negative effect of hyperventilation. The presence of a specific motor or mental deficit was felt to be more attributable to perinatal asphyxia.

Ferrara et al.[90] studied the efficacy and outcome of 23 infants treated with hypocapneic alkalosis for PPHN. Eighty-seven percent responded with an

Table 32.1. Outcome following conventional medical therapy

Study	Description	Age	*n*	Neurologic outcome	*n*	Cognitive outcome	
Cohen et al. 1980[86]	PPHN Tolazoline	1–3 years	29	Deaf: 3.5% Seizures: 3.5% CP: 10% Microcephaly: 34%	12	Stanford–Binet IQ 97.7 (range 66–132)	
Brett et al. 1981[87]	PPHN Hyperventilation	1–3 years	9	Normal: 100%	8	Developmental quotient 107.6 (range 89–130)	
Bernbaum et al. 1984[88]	PPHN Hyperventilation	6 months to 4 years	11	Normal: 73% Abnormal: 27% (1 hemiparesis, 2 increased tone/ reflexes)	11	Developmental quotient 92 (range 70–110)	
Ferrara and Leonard 1984[90]	PPHN Hyperventilation	1 year	16	Normal: 88% Abnormal: 12% (1 hemiparesis, 1 gross motor delay)	11	Bayley MDI 106	Bayley PDI 93
Ballard et al. 1984[89]	PPHN Hyperventilation	4–6 years	11	Normal: 100%	9	McCarthy GCI 95 (range 76–120)	
Sell et al. 1985[91]	PPHN Hyperventilation	1–4 years	40	Normal: 40% Hearing loss: 20% CP: 15% Severely impaired: 7.5%	12	Bayley MDI 116 (1 year) 102 (2 years) McCarthy GCI 110 (3 years) 103 (4 years)	Bayley PDI 102 (1 year) 91 (2 years)
Leavitt et al. 1987[94]	PPHN Hyperventilation	1–2 years	12	Normal: 50% Suspect: 8% Abnormal: 42% (3 hearing loss, 1 mild abnormality)	12	Bayley MDI 95	Bayley PDI 102
Bifano and Pfannenstiel 1988[82]	PPHN Hyperventilation	1 year	21	Normal: 52% Suspect: 29% Abnormal: 19% (4 CP)	21	Bayley MDI 106	Bayley PDI 91
Hageman et al. 1988[98]	PPHN Hyperventilation	1 year	10	Not reported	10	Bayley MDI 98 for $AaDO_2$ >600 93 for $AaDO_2$ <599	
Marron et al. 1992[32]	PPHN Gentle ventilation	2–6 years	27	Normal: 63% Mild abnormality: 22% Severe abnormality: 15%	13	Stanford–Binet IQ 96 (for children with normal or mildly abnormal neurologic examination)	

Notes:
Unless otherwise noted, all scores are mean values. PPHN, persistent pulmonary hypertension of the newborn; CP, cerebral palsy; MDI, Mental Developmental Index; PDI, Psychomotor Developmental Index; GCI, General Cognitive Index.

increase in $Pa\text{O}_2$. Electroencephalograms done during hyperventilation were abnormal in all 11 patients studied. Fourteen of 16 infants seen for neurologic follow-up had a normal examination by 1 year of age, despite transient hypotonia in nine infants. One infant had mild hemiparesis and one had a moderate gross motor delay. Eleven infants received a Bayley examination at 1 year with mean MDI of 106 and PDI of 93. Due to the transient hypotonia, high incidence of electroencephalographic abnormalities during hyperventilation and the wide discrepancy in Bayley MDI and PDI scores, Ferrara et al. urged further long-term studies to determine the effects of hyperventilation.

Sell et al.[91] examined the neurodevelopmental and hearing status of 40 patients between the ages of 1 and 4 years hyperventilated for PPHN. Forty percent were found to be normal with hearing loss in 20%, cerebral palsy in 15%, profound impairment in 7.5%, and mild motor delay in 2%. Mean Bayley and McCarthy scores for the 37 functional children were within the normal range. Thirty percent had CLD. This study was the first to note an increased incidence of hearing abnormalities in the PPHN population. Sell et al. concluded that the incidence of sensorineural hearing loss was dramatically increased over that seen in high-risk infants without PPHN. They were unable to identify any other associated factors to explain this phenomenon.

Several studies have specifically addressed the hearing outcome of PPHN survivors. Naulty et al.[92] found three of 11 infants (27%) with progressive sensorineural hearing loss (SNHL). A subsequent study by Hendricks-Munoz and Walton[93] reported a 52.5% incidence of hearing impairment in a study of 40 infants treated for PPHN. In this study, a longer duration of hyperventilation and ventilation was highly associated with hearing loss. Leavitt et al.[94] corroborated the high incidence of SNHL in children with PPHN treated with hyperventilation. Twenty-five percent were found to have sensorineural hearing impairment. Cheung et al.[95] reported that 62% of their CDH population had SNHL on long-term follow-up. The incidence of SNHL was 65% in the ECMO-treated group and 59% in the conventionally treated group. Survivors with SNHL had a higher cumulative exposure to pancuronium bromide. This finding was unexpected and requires further study. An important aspect of the hearing loss seen in PPHN survivors is the delayed onset and progressive nature of the problem, which make diagnosis difficult. As described by Hutchin et al.[96] and Desai et al.,[97] the hearing loss seen in PPHN survivors occurs in children who have had normal hearing documented in the newborn period. For this reason, PPHN survivors should have regular audiologic monitoring until age 3 years. The most recent position statement from the Joint Committee on Infant Hearing does not recognize PPHN as a risk factor for delayed-onset SNHL, but revision is anticipated.

Bifano and Pfannenstiel[82] examined 21 PPHN survivors treated with hyperventilation at 1 year of age. Using stepwise regression analysis a correlation was found between the duration of hyperventilation and abnormal neurodevelopmental outcome. Although the mean Bayley MDI and PDI scores were within the normal range, the infants with abnormal neurologic examinations or below-average Bayley scores were found to have spent a significantly greater period of time with their $Pa\text{CO}_2$ less than 25 mmHg than did the other infants. The authors concluded that prolonged hypocarbia was associated with poor outcome.

Hageman et al.[98] studied the highest AaDO_2 in relationship to outcome. They found that alveolar arterial oxygen difference (AaDO_2) values were significantly higher in nonsurvivors when compared to survivors. Analysis of Bayley scores failed to show any relationship between neurodevelopmental outcome at age 1 and AaDO_2 values.

A study by Marron et al.[32] of infants with PPHN treated without hyperventilation or paralysis reported on the neurologic, intelligence, and hearing status of 27 infants managed with this conservative regimen. Testing was performed between the ages of 4 and 6 years. They found 63% to have a normal neurologic examination, while 22% and 15% had mild and severe abnormalities, respectively. A significant relationship was found between low Apgar scores at 1 and 5 min and poor neurologic outcome. Three of the four children with severe neurologic impairment had biochemical evidence of asphyxia at birth with low pH and high base excess measurements. No SNHL was found in the 25 children examined. Neurodevelopmental evaluation was attempted in 17 children. Four were untestable; one was profoundly impaired, one was Spanish-speaking, and two had significant behavior problems with hyperactivity and inattention. The mean value of Stanford–Binet scores for the 13 children tested was 96. Chronic lung disease was diagnosed in two of the 27 infants (7%). Marron et al. concluded that conservative management without hyperventilation resulted in no SNHL and a good neurologic outcome. They speculated that hyperventilation or alkalosis may be the causative factor for the high incidence of SNHL seen in other studies of PPHN survivors. Animal studies have shown that one of the highest areas of blood flow is the auditory nucleus.[99] Decreased blood flow with hyperventilation may cause injury to the auditory nucleus. Alkalosis also could potentially induce hearing abnormalities by affecting the sodium-potassium pump in the cochlea or the chemical composition of the endolymph.[100]

Outcome of PPHN survivors treated with ECMO

In 1975 Dr. Robert Bartlett successfully supported the first ECMO survivor at University of California, Irvine. During the 1980s a rapidly increasing number of medical centers began to use ECMO for infants with PPHN failing conventional medical management. Although life-saving, ECMO is an invasive therapy with many potential complications.

Risks associated with ECMO

Systemic heparinization accounts for the majority of the complications related to ECMO. There are many hemorrhagic complications reported, but the most common and potentially devastating is intracranial hemorrhage.[101–107] The incidences of intracranial hemorrhage and cerebral infarction are 4.9 and 9.9% respectively,[108] but selected patients are at higher risk due to risk factors such as prematurity, pre-ECMO acidosis, and asphyxia or coagulopathy.

Numerous studies have attempted to correlate head ultrasound, head computed tomography (CT), and cranial magnetic resonance imaging (MRI) findings with later neurodevelopmental outcome.[109–112] Some authors have suggested that a strong correlation exists between the severity of abnormality on neuroimaging and neurodevelopmental outcome. Although individual outcomes cannot be predicted, neuroimaging can be useful in assigning ECMO survivors to different risk categories. The presence of abnormalities is associated with an increased risk of developmental delay, but the sensitivity and specificity values for normal neuroimaging in predicting normal developmental outcome are relatively low.[109] Cerebrovascular injury in the ECMO population is likely to be multifactorial. Prematurity, hypoxemia, asphyxia, and mechanical ventilation have all been associated with intracranial hemorrhage and infarction in critically ill newborns. Thus, even before ECMO, these infants are at high risk for cerebrovascular injury.

Ligation of both the right carotid artery and jugular vein was required for all patients receiving ECMO prior to the development of the double-lumen venovenous catheter in 1990. Ligation of the right carotid artery has been shown to result in decreased right and increased left hemispheric flow. After right carotid artery ligation, the vertebrobasilar and the contralateral internal carotid systems are the main sources of flow for the right hemisphere via the circle of Willis. The circle of Willis provides a unique anatomic arrangement; it is able to redistribute and balance flow and thereby theoretically can avoid any deficit in cerebral perfusion due to unilateral carotid ligation. Numerous studies have attempted to determine if hemispheric brain injury occurs as a result of right carotid artery ligation.[110,113–118] Schumacher et al.[113] in 1988 reported on eight children with evidence of right hemispheric brain injury on neurologic examination or neuroimaging study. The number of infants with bilateral or right-sided lesions was not reported. A larger study by Taylor et al.[110] in 1989 of 207 infants found intracranial abnormalities in 95; 21 were right-sided,

16 were left-sided, and 58 were bilateral. They concluded that unilateral right-sided and left-sided lesions were seen with similar frequency and that there was no increased injury in the distribution of the right middle cerebral artery. Other evidence for right-sided injury is the increased incidence of left vs right focal seizures (nine left-sided versus two right-sided) seen following ECMO documented by Campbell et al.[116] A later study of the same children with seizures failed to find lateralization of motor findings; left hemiparesis was present in three and right hemiparesis in three.[116] Electroencephalographic studies of ECMO infants have had conflicting findings.[119,120] Streletz et al.[120] found no consistently lateralized electroencephalographic abnormalities during or after ECMO when compared to tracings obtained before cannulation of the right carotid artery. Hahn et al.[119] found more repetitive or periodic discharges arising from the right hemisphere in ECMO patients when compared with conventionally treated infants. Further investigation will be necessary to clarify the long-term effect of right carotid artery ligation.

Due to the patient's critical status, dependence on heart–lung bypass, and the inherent complexity of the ECMO equipment, the patients are at risk for both equipment failure and user error, which can result in significant morbidity and mortality. The overall incidence of mechanical complications on ECMO reported to the Extracorporeal Life Support Organization (ELSO) Registry is 81.2%.[108]

ECMO survivors have been identified as being at high risk for neurodevelopmental sequelae due to multiple factors. One major issue that remains is whether the neurologic sequelae seen in ECMO survivors are more indicative of the primary disease process, pre-ECMO therapy, or as a result of ECMO. There have been 14 ECMO follow-up studies reported in the literature and their results are summarized below and in Table 32.2.

ECMO follow-up studies

Krummel et al.[121] published the first study of six ECMO survivors. Five of the six were functioning normally with normal neurologic, neurodevelopmental, and neuroimaging examinations. One infant experienced an air embolus and had significant developmental delay and bilateral cortical atrophy. The authors concluded that the early results with ECMO were encouraging considering the degree of illness of the ECMO candidate.

A study by Towne et al.[122] investigated the outcome of children 4–11 years following ECMO. These children were among the first cohort of patients treated by Dr. R. Bartlett between 1973 and 1980. This study is one of the few performed on the ECMO population outside infancy. Towne et al. found that 10 of 16 had normal neurologic outcomes, three had minor mental or motor problems, and five had moderate-to-severe handicap. Mean McCarthy GCI scores were in the normal range for the nine children tested. Five children were found to have specific language problems. Two children were found to have a discrepancy between verbal and perceptual scores and this was thought to reflect differences in the function of the two hemispheres.

Andrews et al.[123] reported on the outcome of 14 survivors of ECMO evaluated between the ages of 1 and 3 years using the Bayley scales. Ten children (71%) had a normal MDI and nine (64%) had a normal PDI. The remaining children had scores less than 60. In addition, the incidence of cerebral palsy was 21%, microcephaly 29%, seizure disorder 7%, and chronic lung disease 28%. They concluded that the majority of these critically ill infants treated with ECMO have normal or near-normal outcomes.

Glass et al.[124] examined 42 infants at 1 year of age. Using the Bayley exam, 59% were found to be functioning in the normal range (MDI and PDI >90) with 20% suspect and 20% delayed. Sepsis, CLD, and neuroimaging abnormalities were associated with a poor outcome. No lateralizing signs consistent with a right hemispheric injury were found on neurologic or neuroimaging studies.

Adolph et al.[125] used the Bayley and McCarthy scales to evaluate ECMO survivors between the ages of 6 and 48 months. Twenty-four children were evaluated with the Bayley scales and 71% were classified as normal, 21% as suspect, and 8% as delayed.

Table 32.2. Outcome following extracorporeal membrane oxygenation (ECMO) therapy

Study	Description	Age	*n*	Neurologic outcome	*n*	Cognitive outcome	
Krummel et al. 1984[121]	ECMO	15–21 months	6	Normal: 83% Abnormal: 17%	5	Bayley MDI and PDI Range: 98–100	
Towne et al. 1985[122]	ECMO	4–11 years	16	Normal: 63% Abnormal: 37%	9	McCarthy GCI 99 (range 78–122)	
Andrews et al. 1986[123]	ECMO	1–3 years	14	CP: 21% Microcephaly: 29% Seizures: 7%	14	Bayley MDI ≥85: 71% <85: 29%	Bayley PDI 64% 36%
Glass et al. 1989[124]	ECMO	1 year	42	Normal: 75% Minor abnormality: 19% Definite abnormality: 5%	42	Bayley MDI and PDI MDI and PDI >90:59% MDI or PDI <90:20% MDI and PDI <90:11% MDI and PDI <70:10%	
Adolph et al. 1990[125]	ECMO	6–48 months	57	Normal: 98% Abnormal: 2%	36	Bayley MDI 105 McCarthy GCI 95	Bayley PDI 99
Schumacher et al. 1991[126]	ECMO	1–7 years	80	Seizures: 3.7% Hearing loss: 3.7% Microcephaly: 6%	74	Bayley MDI 109 (1 year) 103 (2 years) McCarthy GCI 96 (3 years) 115 (4 years) 93 (≥ 5 years)	Bayley PDI 99 (1 year) 102 (2 years)
Campbell et al. 1991[127]	ECMO Seizures	1–2 years	12	Seizures: 50% normal 50% abnormal No seizures: 100% normal	 12 15	Cattel DQ 89 105	
Hofkosh et al. 1991[128]	ECMO	6 months to 10 years	67	Normal: 81% Abnormal: 19%	67	Bayley MDI 101 Preschool IQ 91	Bayley PDI 98 School age IQ 109
Flusser et al. 1993[129]	ECMO	1 year	30	Normal: 63% Suspect: 13% Abnormal: 13%	30	Bayley MDI >85: 83% 70–85: 7% <70: 10%	Bayley PDI >85: 80% 70–85: 7% <70: 13%[3]
Van Meurs et al. 1994[118]	ECMO VV VA	4–24 months	40	 Normal: 100% Normal: 100%	40	Bayley MDI 111 112	Bayley PDI 111 102
Wildin et al. 1994[130]	ECMO	6–24 months	22	Normal: 87% Abnormal: 23%	22	Bayley MDI 108 (6 months) 106 (1 year) 100 (2 years)	Bayley PDI 110 (6 months) 106 (1 year) 100 (2 years)
	Controls		29	Not reported	29	Bayley MDI 126 (6 months) 112 (1 year) 115 (2 years)	Bayley PDI 122 (6 months) 106 (1 year) 112 (2 years)
Glass et al. 1995[131]	ECMO	5 years	102	Seizures: 2% Hearing loss: 3% CP: 6% Visual problem: 2%	102	WIPPSI-R Full Scale IQ 96	
	Controls		37		37	115	

Table 32.2. (*cont.*)

Study	Description	Age	*n*	Neurologic outcome	*n*	Cognitive outcome	
Kornhauser et al. 1998[132]	ECMO-BPD	2 years	17	Normal: 18% Mild: 34% Severe: 4%	17	Bayley MDI 76	Bayley PDI 103
	No BPD		47	Normal: 62% Mild: 34% Severe: 4%	47	74	97
Desai et al. 1999[133]	ECMO-	5 years				WIPPSI-R Full Scale IQ	
	RCA ligation		28	CP: 0%	28	95	
	No RCA ligation		35	CP: 14%	35	96	

Notes:

Unless otherwise noted, all scores are mean values. CP, cerebral palsy; MDI, Mental Developmental Index; PDI, Psychomotor Developmental Index; GCI, General Cognitive Index; DQ, developmental quotient; IQ, Intelligence quotient; BPD, bronchopulmonary dysplasia; RCA, right carotid artery; WIPPSI-R, Wechsler Preschool and Primary Scale of Intelligence – Revised; VV, venovenous; VA, venoarterial

Twelve patients were evaluated using the McCarthy scales with a mean score of 95, with 75% obtaining normal scores. Neurologic examination was normal in all but one child. No lateralizing findings were identified on physical examination or neuroimaging. An abnormal outcome was found to be associated with the presence of CLD.

A large study of 80 ECMO survivors between the ages of 1 and 7 years by Schumacher et al.[126] found 20% to be handicapped. "Handicapped" was defined as having moderate-to-severe neurologic abnormality requiring therapy or resulting in functional impairment, an MDI or IQ score more than 2 SD below the mean or SNHL requiring amplification. The oldest group of ECMO survivors had the highest incidence of handicap (45%), and this was felt to be due to a learning curve effect. Improvements in patient selection criteria and ECMO management were felt to result in a subsequent lower rate of handicap. Thirty-one percent were rehospitalized during the first year of life for respiratory illness. Speech and language abnormalities were identified in 15% of the ECMO survivors, with SNHL in 4%. Six children were found to have lateralizing injury: four had left-sided, and two right-sided weakness. The authors concluded that the outcome post-ECMO was similar to that reported in PPHN survivors treated with conventional medical therapy.

Campbell et al.[127] compared the neurologic and neurodevelopmental outcome of ECMO survivors with and without seizures in the neonatal period. Twelve of 41 ECMO survivors (29%) had neonatal seizures. The neurologic examination was abnormal in 50% of the children who had seizures. There was no predominance of left motor abnormalities and no association between the side of neonatal seizures and the lateralization of disability. None of the children without seizures had an abnormal neurologic examination. The Cattell DQ scales were significantly lower for ECMO survivors with seizures than for those ECMO survivors without seizures. The authors concluded that carotid artery ligation was not responsible for lateralizing findings in ECMO survivors, but that seizures were associated with a higher risk for cerebral palsy and developmental delay.

Hofkosh et al.[128] reported on the neurodevelopmental outcome of 67 ECMO survivors between the ages of 6 months and 10 years. Using the Bayley scales and the Stanford–Binet, mean scores were within the normal range for all ages, with 64% normal, 25% suspect, and 11% delayed. The 10 school-age ECMO survivors were compared with normal controls using the Stanford–Binet and no statistically significant differences were noted. Two children in the ECMO group were found to have behavioral concerns noted by classroom teachers, consisting of immaturity in one and impulsivity, distractibility, and hyperactivity in the second. Of the 33 children who had hearing evaluations, 21% were found to have SNHL. The authors noted that an abnormal outcome was significantly associated with chronic lung disease, seizures, and cerebral infarction, but not with other perinatal variables.

In a study by Flusser el al.[129] 30 children treated with ECMO received medical, neurologic, and developmental evaluations at 1 year of age. Seventeen percent had CLD with a need for supplemental oxygen, tracheostomy, or mechanical ventilation. Neurologic examination was normal in 63% of the population. Bayley MDI and PDI were normal in 83% and 80%, respectively. No relationship was found between neurodevelopmental outcome and perinatal factors such as Apgar scores, diagnosis, length of time on ECMO, neuroimaging abnormalities, seizures, or electroencephalographic findings. Ten infants in their study had congenital anomalies; CDH (5), cystic malformation of the lung (2), myotonic dystrophy (1), gastroschisis (1), and pulmonary atresia (1). They found that adverse outcomes were associated with the presence of congenital anomalies.

Van Meurs et al.[118] reported on the neurodevelopmental and neuroimaging findings in 24 VV ECMO survivors and 24 VA ECMO survivors matched by diagnosis, gestational age, sex, and Apgar scores. Comparison of the Bayley scores and neuroimaging results for VA and VV survivors found no statistically significant differences. The authors concluded that no differences attributable to carotid artery ligation were identified with either short-term neurodevelopmental evaluation or neuroimaging.

A study by Wildin et al.[130] reported on 20 ECMO survivors and 29 healthy control infants matched by race, sex, maternal age, maternal education, and socioeconomic status. Bayley scales were performed at 6, 12, and 24 months. Healthy term infants scored significantly better than ECMO infants at 6 and 24 months, although mean Bayley scores for the ECMO infants were within the normal range. Fifteen percent of the ECMO survivors had abnormal audiologic studies. A statistically significant difference was also found on the Sequenced Inventory of Communication Development between ECMO and control infants. The authors concluded that the overall rate of developmental delay found in this study (23%) was comparable to that reported in prior studies.

A large and comprehensive study by Glass et al.[131] of the neuropsychological outcome and educational adjustment of 102 ECMO survivors at age 5 and 37 age-matched controls found lower full-scale IQ scores and a higher incidence of neuropsychological deficits and behavioral problems in ECMO survivors. Although the mean full-scale IQ for the ECMO survivors was average, 77% were found to have one or more deficits in the following areas: language, fine motor efficiency/planning, visual/motor integration, lateralization, academic risk, verbal memory, or attention/impulse control. Major handicapping conditions were identified in 17%. Glass et al. concluded that, although the IQ scores are average and the incidence of major disability is similar to that in other high-risk populations, there exists an increased rate of behavioral problems and neuropsychological deficits putting ECMO survivors at increased risk for school failure.

Kornhauser et al.[132] examined the impact of bronchopulmonary dysplasia (BPD) on the outcome of the ECMO survivor. Complete follow-up data were available for 64 of 145 ECMO-treated survivors; BPD occurred in 17 (27%). The diagnosis of respiratory distress syndrome was significantly more common in the BPD group (53% vs 13%, $P<0.01$). In addition, the mean age of initiation of ECMO was later and the length of ECMO treatment longer for the BPD group. At both 2 years and 4 years the developmental testing revealed significantly lower scores for the BPD group. The rate of disability was also significantly higher in the BPD group (72% vs 38%). The reason that BPD is a marker for poor neurodevelopmental outcome is unknown.

A study by Desai et al.[133] sought to determine if

reconstruction of the right common carotid artery (RCCA) following ECMO resulted in improved neurodevelopmental outcome. Thirty-four children who had RCCA reconstruction were compared to 35 children who had permanent ligation of the RCCA. RCCA reconstruction was successful in 76%, with success defined as less than 50% stenosis. Both neuroimaging abnormalities and cerebral palsy were seen less frequently in the children who received RCCA reconstruction. No differences in neurodevelopmental test scores performed both at ages >30 months and at 5–6 years were noted. The authors suggest that RCCA reconstruction may result in improved cerebral circulation, but the long-term risks and benefits of this procedure remain undetermined.

Comparing the outcome of ECMO patients with congenital diaphragmatic hernia to other diagnoses

Infants with CDH treated with ECMO have significantly lower survival rates than infants with other diagnoses. The reason is felt to be related to the severity of the pulmonary hypoplasia and pulmonary hypertension seen in the more severely affected infants with CDH. Several authors have sought to compare the outcome of CDH infants with those of other diagnoses. These studies are reviewed and the results presented in Table 32.3.

Van Meurs et al.[134] found that the 18 CDH survivors had a longer time on ECMO, time to extubation and length of hospitalization when compared to other ECMO survivors. In addition, a higher percentage were discharged home on oxygen. An extremely high rate of gastroesophageal reflux (GER) and failure to thrive was noted. At both 1 and 2 years, 50% were less than the 5th percentile weight-to-length ratio. Eighty-nine percent had clinical evidence of GER and 44% were discharged home on nasogastric feedings. The authors suggested that more aggressive nutritional intervention was needed for CDH survivors. In this study, the neurodevelopmental outcome, as measured by the Bayley scales or Stanford–Binet scale at 1–4 years, was not different from other ECMO-treated survivors.

Stolar et al.[135] reported on the neurocognitive outcome of 25 CDH infants who were treated with ECMO and compared them to 26 ECMO-treated infants with other diagnoses. The age at follow-up ranged from 2 months to 7 years. The neurologic outcomes did not differ significantly, but the cognitive outcome was noted to be poorer in the CDH children. Male sex and limited maternal education were found to be additional risk factors for poor outcome. In this CDH cohort, none were discharged home on oxygen or had SNHL, but GER and nutritional problems were common. The authors speculate that the outcome reflects the severity of illness rather than the consequences of therapy.

A study by Bernbaum et al.[136] also found a longer ECMO duration and more complicated hospital course for CDH infants when compared to infants with meconium aspiration syndrome. At hospital discharge, there was a higher rate of chronic lung disease, GER, and hypotonia. During the first year of life, no differences in growth rate were seen, but 36% of CDH infants required nasogastric feedings. In addition, a higher percentage of CDH infants had CLD (50% vs 17%). At 1 year 79% of CDH infants remained hypotonic compared with 8% of the comparison group. On the Bayley scales at 1 year, CDH infants had lower MDI and significantly lower PDI.

The neurodevelopmental outcome at 3½ years of age was analyzed for 130 ECMO survivors with six different diagnoses. Nield et al.[137] found no significant differences between diagnostic groups in functional status or neurologic sequelae. Length of hospitalization was the only outcome variable found to have an influence on neurodevelopmental testing, functional status, and major neurologic sequelae. They noted that the neurodevelopmental test results in the CDH population done between 1 and 2 years are more worrisome than later testing, possibly due to the early medical condition of this group.

Outcome studies comparing conventional medical therapy and ECMO

There have been several studies directly comparing the outcomes of conventional medical therapy and

Table 32.3. Comparison of outcomes following extracorporeal membrane oxygenation (ECMO) or conventional medical therapy for infants with congenital diaphragmatic hernia

Study	Description	Age	*n*	Neurologic outcome	*n*	Cognitive outcome
						Bayley or Stanford–Binet
Van Meurs et al. 1993[134]	CDH	1–4 years	18	Not reported	15	MDI and PDI >90: 47%
						MDI or PDI <90: 40%
						MDI and PDI <90: 13%
						MDI and PDI <70: 0%
	Other diagnoses					MDI and PDI >90: 59%
						MDI or PDI <90: 19%
						MDI and PDI <90: 12%
						MDI or PDI<70: 10%
				Normal Suspect Abnormal		Normal Suspect Abnormal
Stolar et al. 1995[135]	CDH	2 months–	25	56% 24% 20%	25	60% 16% 24%
	Other diagnosis	7 years	26	50% 35% 15%	26	88% 4% 8%
						Bayley MDI Bayley PDI
Bernbaum et al. 1995[136]	CDH	1 year	14	Hypotonia: 79%	14	87 75
	MAS		12	Hypotonia: 8%	12	98 99
						Mean test score
Nield et al. 2000[137]	CDH	3.5 years	17	Not different	17	96
	MAS		67		67	89
	Sepsis		29		29	93

Notes:

Unless otherwise noted, all scores are mean values. CDH, congenital diaphragmatic hernia; MDI, Mental Developmental Index; PDI, Psychomotor Developmental Index; MAS, meconium aspiration syndrome.

ECMO. The five studies are discussed below and summarized in Table 32.4.

A comparison of the morbidity, mortality, and outcome of survivors treated with conventional medical management and ECMO was performed by Walsh-Sukys et al.[138] Survival in the conventionally treated group was 69% when compared to a survival of 90% in the ECMO group. The reasons for not initiating ECMO therapy in survivors of the conventionally treated group included improvement with additional treatment (89%) and suspected neurologic injury (11%). CLD occurred in 35% of the conventionally treated patients and in 16% of the ECMO-treated patients. Abnormal neurologic status was identified in 12% of the conventionally treated patients and 18% of the ECMO-treated patients. Developmental testing using the Bayley examination at 20 months of age found similar mean MDI scores, but lower PDI scores for the conventionally treated children. The authors concluded that infants treated with and without ECMO have similar neurodevelopmental outcomes, but there is a worse pulmonary outcome in conventionally treated patients, despite the ECMO patients having higher $AaDO_2$ values and being assessed to be more critically ill.

A second small study by Gratny et al.[139] compared the neurodevelopmental outcome and incidence of significant morbidity in 10 ECMO and 10 CMT survivors at 18 months of age. No statistically significant differences in the incidence of intracranial hemorrhage, motor impairment, sensorineural hearing deficit, or developmental delay were identified.

Table 32.4. Outcome following extracorporeal membrane oxygenation (ECMO) when compared to conventional medical therapy

Study	Description	Age	*n*	Neurologic outcome	*n*	Cognitive Outcome	
						Bayley MDI	Bayley PDI
Gratny et al. 1992[139]	CMT	18 months	10	Normal: 90% Abnormal: 10%	7	97	101
	ECMO		10	Normal: 80% Abnormal: 20%	10	104	94
						Bayley MDI	Bayley PDI
Walsh-Sukys et al. 1994[138]	CMT	20 months	17	Normal: 88% Abnormal: 12%	12	95	83
	ECMO		38	Normal: 82% Abnormal: 18%	32	96	83
						Bayley MDI	Bayley PDI
Robertson et al. 1995[140]	CMT	2 years	38	Disabled: 4% CP: 4%	38	100.5	96.4
	ECMO		26	Disabled: 16% CP: 5%	26	91.0	87.2
						Bayley MDI	Bayley PDI
Vaucher et al. 1996[141]	CMT	12–30 months	20	Normal: 61% Major disability: 25%		92	92
	ECMO		95	Normal: 74% Major disability: 11%		100	99
UK Collaborative ECMO Trial Group 1996[142]	CMT	1 year	24	Normal: 28%		Not reported	
	ECMO		43	Normal: 51%		Not reported	

Notes:
Unless otherwise noted, all scores are mean values. CMT, conventional medical therapy; MDI, Mental Developmental Index; PDI, Psychomotor Developmental Index; CP, cerebral palsy

Robertson et al.[140] examined the outcome of 38 ECMO-treated and 26 conventional medical therapy survivors. The conventional medical therapy group were described as near-miss ECMO patients who had lower severity of illness as measured by oxygenation index. The underlying diagnoses were similar, except for a higher percentage with a diagnosis of respiratory distress syndrome in the conventional medical therapy group. The reported outcomes, including the percent with disability, cerebral palsy, and hearing loss, were not statistically different. The mean MDI and PDI scores were lower in the ECMO-treated group, but again the difference was not statistically significant. Further analysis of their results suggested that an underlying diagnosis of sepsis identified the infants most likely to have lower Bayley scores. The distance transported and socioeconomic status were not found to be good predictors of neurodevelopmental outcome.

A large study by Vaucher et al.[141] compared the outcome of ECMO survivors to a group of ECMO-eligible infants who did not receive ECMO because they improved with continued convention mechanical ventilation, surfactant therapy, or HFV. Ninety-

Table 32.5. Outcome following inhaled nitric oxide therapy

Study	Description	Age	*n*	Neurologic outcome	*n*	Cognitive Outcome	
						Bayley MDI	Bayley PDI
Rosenberg et al. 1997[145]	iNO	2 years	33	Mild disability: 9.1% Severe disability: 12.1%	33	107	109
						Bayley MDI	Bayley PDI
Neonatal Inhaled Nitric Oxide Study Group 2000	iNO	18–24 months	85	Normal: 77.6% CP: 11.8%	79	85	85.7
	Controls		87	Normal: 79.3% CP: 10.3%	75	87	93.6
						Development quotient	
Ellington 2001	iNO	1–4 years	35	Disability: 9%	33	102	
	Controls		25	Disability: 20%		99	

Notes:
Unless otherwise noted, all scores are mean values. iNO, inhaled nitric oxide; CP, cerebral palsy; MDI, Mental Developmental Index; PDI, Psychomotor Developmental Index.

five ECMO survivors and 20 CMT survivors were seen between 12 and 30 months of age for neurologic and developmental evaluation. The follow-up rate for the conventional medical therapy group was lower (39% vs 69%). Cerebral palsy occurred in 6% of ECMO survivors vs 22% of conventional medical therapy survivors ($P=0.06$). CLD was seen more frequently in the conventional medical therapy group (25% vs 12%, $P=0.04$) and it independently increased the risk of neurodevelopmental delay at 12–30 months after adjusting for other perinatal and neonatal variables. Moderate-to-severe neuroimaging abnormalities also identified infants with abnormal neurodevelopmental outcome. The authors found that the assumption that ECMO-treated infants had higher rates of disability was incorrect. In this study, the ECMO survivors had lower rates of major disability and higher Bayley scores.

The UK collaborative randomized trial of ECMO also included a neurodevelopmental assessment at 1 year of age.[142] The manuscript reports on 42 ECMO survivors and 24 conventional medical therapy survivors. Children receiving anticonvulsant therapy, tube feeding, or supplemental oxygen were included in the disabled group. The overall rate of impairment with or without disability was found to be similar (26% ECMO vs 29% CMT).

Outcome for PPHN survivors treated with inhaled nitric oxide

iNO has been used in the treatment of PPHN following the initial reports by Roberts et al. and Kinsella et al. in 1992.[143,144] Two large multicenter randomized controlled trials demonstrated that iNO decreased the need for ECMO or death in newborns with hypoxemic respiratory failure.[50,51] Three studies have reported on the neurologic and neurodevelopmental outcome and are summarized below and in Table 32.5.

NO follow-up studies

Rosenberg et al.[145] first documented the medical and neurodevelopmental outcome of PPHN patients treated with iNO at 1 and 2 years of age. The notable findings were that 25% were <5th percentile for weight, 17.6% had gastrostomy feeds or a diagnosis of GER, and 27.5% had reactive airway disease. They found that 12.1% had a severe neurologic disability at 2 years defined as MDI or PDI <68, abnormal findings on the neurologic exam, or both. Comparison of children tested at both 1 and 2 years showed significant improvement in Bayley MDI and PDI scores and fewer children on supplemental oxygen (6.1% vs 15.7%).

The Neonatal Inhaled Nitric Oxide Study (NINOS) Group[54] reported on the outcome of the infants enrolled in the randomized controlled trial of iNO for hypoxemic respiratory failure. Comprehensive neurodevelopmental assessment of the survivors was performed at 18–24 months with a follow-up rate of 86.9%. The rates of neurologic abnormality, cerebral palsy, and low Bayley scores were not significantly different between the two groups. The overall rate of cerebral palsy (11%) was similar to the Rosenberg study. The rate of disability was not affected by the need for ECMO. The authors concluded that the timing of injury most likely is before ECMO or before birth.

A similar study was performed by Ellington et al.[146] who reported on the health and neurodevelopmental outcome of 60 of 83 survivors of another randomized controlled trial of iNO for PPHN. All results reported in this study were obtained by telephone interview. A 20% rate of disability was found in the control group compared to 9% in the iNO group. Disability was defined as having a seizure disorder, cerebral palsy, or DQ<70. This difference was not statistically significant given the sample size. The authors concluded that iNO did not increase the rate of adverse outcome.

Conclusions

Analysis of the outcome studies performed during infancy in PPHN survivors treated with conventional medical therapy, iNO, and ECMO yield grossly equivalent morbidities and outcomes. These findings suggest that the neurodevelopmental outcome is more related to the underlying illness than to the therapeutic intervention utilized.

Limitations imposed by some of these studies are the types of neurodevelopmental examinations performed, small sample sizes, the absence of an appropriate control population, and the length of follow-up. The most frequently performed neurodevelopmental assessment performed was the Bayley Scales of Infant Development, which is known not to be predictive of long-term outcome. In addition, many of these studies have been small with no control populations, which limited the conclusions which could be made. Some of the more recent randomized controlled studies have had large sample sizes with appropriate control groups. These studies have significantly improved our information. Without systematic longitudinal comparison of these two groups it is difficult to draw conclusions about the relative morbidities and outcomes and also the etiology of the neurologic and neurodevelopmental sequelae associated with PPHN. The continuation of these outcome studies into school age is critical. Few of the outcome studies have included the school-age child. Information from the few studies done in the ECMO-treated school-age child have yielded important findings; Glass et al. noted significantly lower scores on 13 of 15 neuropsychologic subtests for ECMO survivors when compared to control children despite average IQ scores and a low incidence of major handicaps in the ECMO group.[131] These deficits make ECMO survivors vulnerable to academic and psychosocial difficulties. Further research is needed to understand the full impact of the varying therapies for PPHN so that developmental and educational services can be developed to serve the needs of PPHN survivors.

REFERENCES

1 Levin DL, Heymann MA, Kitterman JA, et al. (1976). Persistent pulmonary hypertension of the newborn infant. *J Pediatr*, **89**, 626–630.

2 Drummond WH, Peckham GJ and Fox WW. (1977). The clinical profile of the newborn with persistent pulmonary hypertension. Observations in 19 affected neonates. *Clin Pediatr*, **16**, 335–341.

3 Benitz WE and Stevenson DK. (1988). Refractory neonatal hypoxemia diagnostic evaluation and pharmacologic management. *Resuscitation*, **16**, 49–64.

4 Gersony WM. (1984). Neonatal pulmonary hypertension:

pathophysiology, classification, and etiology. *Clin Perinatol*, **11**, 517–524.
5 Hagema JR, Adams MA and Gardner TH. (1984). Persistent pulmonary hypertension of the newborn. Trends in incidence, diagnosis, and management. *Am J Dis Child*, **138**, 592–595.
6 Morin FC and Stenmark KR. (1995). Persistent pulmonary hypertension of the newborn. *Am J Respir Crit Care Med*, **151**, 2010–2032.
7 Kinsella JP and Abman SH. (1995). Recent developments in the pathophysiology and treatment of persistent pulmonary hypertension of the newborn. *J Pediatr*, **126**, 853–864.
8 Long WA. (1984). Structural cardiovascular abnormalities presenting as persistent pulmonary hypertension of the newborn. *Clin Perinatol*, **11**, 601–626.
9 Geggel RL and Reid LM. (1981). The structural basis of PPHN. *Clin Perinatol*, **11**, 525–549.
10 Peckham G and Fox W. (1978). Physiologic factors affecting pulmonary artery pressure in infants with persistent pulmonary hypertension. *J Pediatr*, **93**, 1005–1010.
11 Murphy JD, Rabinovitch M, Goldstein JD, et al. (1981). The structural basis of persistent pulmonary hypertension of the newborn infant. *J Pediatr*, **98**, 962–967.
12 Fox WW and Duara S. (1983). Persistent pulmonary hypertension in the neonate: diagnosis and management. *J Pediatr*, **103**, 505–514.
13 Gersony WM, Morishima HO, Daniel SS, et al. (1976). The hemodynamic effects of intrauterine hypoxia: an experimental model in newborn lambs. *J Pediatr*, **89**, 631–635.
14 Drummond WH and Bissonnette JM. (1978). Persistent pulmonary hypertension in the neonate: development of an animal model. *Am J Obstet Gynecol*, **131**, 761–763.
15 Soifer SJ, Kaslow D, Roman C, et al. (1987). Umbilical cord compression produces pulmonary hypertension in newborn lambs: a model to study the pathophysiology of persistent pulmonary hypertension in the newborn. *J Dev Physiol*, **9**, 239–252.
16 Morin FC. (1989). Ligating the ductus arteriosus before birth causes persistent pulmonary hypertension in the newborn lamb. *Pediatr Res*, **25**, 245–250.
17 Wild LM, Nickerson PA and Morin FC. (1989). Ligating the ductus arteriosus before birth remodels the pulmonary vasculature of the lamb. *Pediatr Res*, **25**, 251–257.
18 Morin FC and Egan EA. (1989). The effect of closing the ductus arteriosus on the pulmonary circulation of the fetal sheep. *J Dev Physiol*, **11**, 283–287.
19 Abman SH, Shanley PF and Accurso FJ. (1989). Failure of postnatal adaptation of the pulmonary hypertension in fetal lambs. *J Clin Invest*, **83**, 1849–1858.
20 Walsh-Sukys MC, Cornell DJ, Houston LN, et al. (1994). Treatment of persistent pulmonary hypertension of the newborn without hyperventilation: an assessment of diffusion of innovation. *Pediatrics*, **94**, 303–306.
21 Walsh-Sukys MC. (1993). Persistent pulmonary hypertension of the newborn. The black box revisited. *Clin Perinatol*, **20**, 127–143.
22 Roberts JD Jr and Shaul PW. (1993). Advances in the treatment of persistent pulmonary hypertension of the newborn. *Pediatr Clin North Am*, **40**, 983–1004.
23 Walsh-Sukys MC, Tyson JE, Wright LL, et al. (2000). Persistent pulmonary hypertension of the newborn in the era before nitric oxide: practice variation and outcomes. *Pediatrics*, **105**, 14–20.
24 Wu TJ, Teng RJ and Tsou KI. (1995). Persistent pulmonary hypertension of the newborn treated with magnesium sulfate in premature neonates. *Pediatrics*, **96**, 472–474.
25 Tolsa JF, Cotting J, Sekarski N, et al. (1995). Magnesium sulphate as an alternative and safe treatment for severe persistent pulmonary hypertension of the newborn. *Arch Dis Child Fetal Neonatal Edn*, **72**, 184–187.
26 Abu-Osba YK, Galal O, Manasra K, et al. (1992). Treatment of severe persistent pulmonary hypertension of the newborn with magnesium sulphate. *Arch Dis Child*, **67**, 31–35.
27 Ryan CA, Finer NN and Barrington KJ. (1994). Effects of magnesium sulphate and nitric oxide in pulmonary hypertension induced by hypoxia in newborn piglets. *Arch Dis Child Fetal Neonatal Edn*, **71**, F151–F155.
28 Fineman JR, Wong J and Soifer SJ. (1993). Hyperoxia and alkalosis produce pulmonary vasodilation independent of endothelium-derived nitric oxide in newborn lambs. *Pediatr Res*, **33**, 341–346.
29 Lou H, Skov H and Pedersen H. (1979). Low cerebral blood flow: a risk factor in the neonate. *J Pediatr*, **95**, 606–609.
30 Wung JT, James LS, Kilchevsky E, et al. (1985). Management of infants with severe respiratory failure and persistence of the fetal circulation, without hyperventilation. *Pediatrics*, **76**, 488–494.
31 Dworetz AR, Moya FR, Sabo B, et al. (1989). Survival of infants with persistent pulmonary hypertension without extracorporeal membrane oxygenation. *Pediatrics*, **84**, 1–6.
32 Marron MJ, Crisafi MA, Driscoll JM Jr, et al. (1992). Hearing and neurodevelopmental outcome in survivors of persistent pulmonary hypertension of the newborn. *Pediatrics*, **90**, 392–396.
33 Lotze A, Stroud CY and Soldin SJ. (1995). Serial lecithin/sphingomyelin ratios and surfactant/albumin ratios in tracheal aspirates from term infants with respiratory

failure receiving extracorporeal membrane oxygenation. *Clin Chem*, **41**, 1182–1188.

34 Lotze A, Knight GR, Anderson KD, et al. (1994). Surfactant (beractant) therapy for infants with congenital diaphragmatic hernia on ECMO: evidence of persistent surfactant deficiency. *J Pediatr Surg*, **29**, 407–412.

35 Karamanoukian HL, Glick PL, Wilcox DT, et al. (1995). Pathophysiology of congenital diaphragmatic hernia. VIII: Inhaled nitric oxide requires exogenous surfactant therapy in the lamb model of congenital diaphragmatic hernia. *J Pediatr Surg*, **30**, 1–4.

36 Lotze A, Knight GR, Martin GR, et al. (1993). Improved pulmonary outcome after exogenous surfactant therapy for respiratory failure in term infants requiring extracorporeal membrane oxygenation. *J Pediatr*, **122**, 261–268.

37 Martin LD. (1995). New approaches to ventilation in infants and children. *Curr Opin Pediatr*, **7**, 250–261.

38 Ring JC and Stidham GL. (1994). Novel therapies for acute respiratory failure. *Pediatr Clin North Am*, **41**, 1325–1363.

39 Clark RH. (1994). High-frequency ventilation. *J Pediatr*, **124**, 661–670.

40 Frantz IDD. (1993). High-frequency ventilation. *Crit Care Med*, **21**, (suppl. 9), S370.

41 deLemos R, Yoder B, McCurnin D, et al. (1992). The use of high-frequency oscillatory ventilation (HFOV) and extracorporeal membrane oxygenation (ECMO) in the management of the term/near term infant with respiratory failure. *Early Hum Dev*, **29**, 299–303.

42 Ito Y, Kawano T, Miyasaka K, et al. (1994). Alternative treatment may lower the need for use of extracorporeal membrane oxygenation. *Acta Paediatr Jpn*, **36**, 673–677.

43 Varnholt V, Lasch P, Suske G, et al. (1992). High frequency oscillatory ventilation and extracorporeal membrane oxygenation in severe persistent pulmonary hypertension of the newborn. *Eur J Pediatr*, **151**, 769–774.

44 Waffarn F, Turbo R, Yang L, et al. (1995). Treatment of PPHN: a randomized trial comparing intermittent mandatory ventilation and HFOV for delivering NO. *Pediatr Res*, **37**, 243A.

45 Johns RA. (1991). EDRF/nitric oxide. The endogenous nitrovasodilator and a new cellular messenger. *Anesthesiology*, **75**, 927–931.

46 Fratacci MD, Frostell CG, Chen TY, et al. (1991). Inhaled nitric oxide. A selective pulmonary vasodilator of heparin-protamine vasoconstriction in sheep. *Anesthesiology*, **75**, 990–999.

47 Pepke-Zaba J, Higenbottam TW, Dinh-Xuan A, et al. (1991). Inhaled nitric oxide as a cause of selective pulmonary vasodilatation in pulmonary hypertension. *Lancet*, **338**, 1173–1174.

48 Kinsella JP and Abman SH. (1994). Efficacy of inhalational nitric oxide therapy in the clinical management of persistent pulmonary hypertension of the newborn. *Chest*, **105** (suppl.), 92S–94S.

49 Finer NN, Etches PC, Kamstra B, et al. (1994). Inhaled nitric oxide in infants referred for extracorporeal membrane oxygenation: dose response. *J Pediatr*, **124**, 302–308.

50 The Neonatal Nitric Oxide Study Group (NINOS). (1997). Inhaled nitric oxide and hypoxic respiratory failure in infants with congenital diaphragmatic hernia. *Pediatrics*, **99**, 838–845.

51 Clark RH, Kueser TJ, Walker MW, et al. (2000). Low-dose nitric oxide therapy for persistent pulmonary hypertension of the newborn. *N Engl J Med*, **342**, 469–474.

52 Hogman M, Frostell C, Arnberg H, et al. (1993). Bleeding time prolongation and NO inhalation (letter). *Lancet*, **341**, 1664–1665.

53 Samama CM, Diaby M, Fellahi JL, et al. (1995). Inhibition of platelet aggregation by inhaled nitric oxide in patients with acute respiratory distress syndrome. *Anesthesiology*, **83**, 56–65.

54 The Neonatal Inhaled Nitric Oxide Study Group. (2000). Inhaled nitric oxide in term and near-term infants: neurodevelopmental follow-up of the neonatal nitric oxide study group (NINOS). *J Pediatr*, **136**, 611–617.

55 Kinsella JP, Walsh WF, Bose CL, et al. (1999). Inhaled nitric oxide in premature neonates with severe hypoxaemic respiratory failure: a randomized controlled trial. *Lancet*, **354**, 1061–1065.

56 Bennett AJ, Shaw NJ, Gregg JE, et al. (2001). Neurodevelopmental outcome in high-risk preterm infants treated with inhaled nitric oxide. *Acta Paediatr*, **90**, 573–576.

57 Curtis J, O'Neill JT and Pettett G. (1993). Endotracheal administration of tolazoline in hypoxia-induced pulmonary hypertension. *Pediatrics*, **92**, 403–408.

58 Welch JC, Bridson JM and Gibbs JL. (1995). Endotracheal tolazoline for severe persistent pulmonary hypertension of the newborn. *Br Heart J*, **73**, 99–100.

59 Parida SK, Baker S, Kuhn R, et al. (1997). Endotracheal tolazoline administration in neonates with persistent pulmonary hypertension. *J Perinatol*, **17**, 461–464.

60 Crowley MR. (1997). Oxygen-induced pulmonary vasodilation is mediated by adenosine triphosphate in newborn lambs. *J Cardiovasc Pharmacol*, **30**, 102–109.

61 Patole S, Lee J, Buettner P, et al. (1998). Improved oxygenation following adenosine infusion in persistent pulmonary hypertension of the newborn. *Biol Neonate*, **74**, 345–350.

62 Aranda M, Bradford KK and Pearl RG. (1999). Combined

therapy with inhaled nitric oxide and intravenous vasodilators during acute and chronic experimental pulmonary hypertension. *Anesth Analg*, **89**, 152–158.

63 McCaffrey MJ, Bose CL, Reiter PD, et al. (1995). Effect of L-arginine infusion on infants with persistent pulmonary hypertension of the newborn. *Biol Neonate*, **67**, 240–243.

64 Thebaud B, Saizou C, Farnoux C, et al. (1999). Dipyridamole, a cGMP phosphodiesterase inhibitor, transiently improves the response to inhaled nitric oxide in two newborns with congenital diaphragmatic hernia. *Intensive Care Med*, **25**, 300–303.

65 Dukarm RC, Russell JA, Morin FC, et al. (1999). The cGMP-specific phosphodiesterase inhibitor E4021 dilates the pulmonary circulation. *Am J Respir Crit Care Med*, **160**, 858–865.

66 Nagamine J, Hill LL and Pearl RG. (2000). Combined therapy with zaprinast and inhaled nitric oxide abolishes hypoxic pulmonary hypertension. *Crit Care Med*, **28**, 2420–2424.

67 Steinhorn RH, Gordon JB and Todd ML. (2000). Site-specific effect of guanosine 3',5-cyclic monophosphate phosphodiesterase inhibition in isolated lamb lungs. *Crit Care Med*, **28**, 490–495.

68 Arensman RM and Cornish JD. (1993). *Extracorporeal Life Support*. Oxford: Blackwell.

69 Upp JR Jr, Bush PE and Zwischenberger JB. (1994). Complications of neonatal extracorporeal membrane oxygenation. *Perfusion*, **9**, 241–256.

70 Radack DM, Baumgart S and Gross GW. (1994). Subependymal (grade 1) intracranial hemorrhage in neonates on extracorporeal membrane oxygenation. Frequency and patterns of evolution. *Clin Pediatr*, **33**, 583–587.

71 O'Connor TA, Haney BM, Grist GE, et al. (1993). Decreased incidence of intracranial hemorrhage using cephalic jugular venous drainage during neonatal extracorporeal membrane oxygenation. *J Pediatr Surg*, **28**, 1332–1335.

72 Wilson JM, Bower LK, Fackler JC, et al. (1993). Aminocaproic acid decreases the incidence of intracranial hemorrhage and other hemorrhagic complications of ECMO. *J Pediatr Surg*, **28**, 536–541.

73 Bartlett RH. (1997). Extracorporeal life support registry report 1995. *ASAIO J*, **43**, 104–107.

74 Hirschl RB, Tooley R, Parent AC, et al. (1995). Improvement of gas exchange, pulmonary function, and lung injury with partial liquid ventilation. A study model in a setting of severe respiratory failure. *Chest*, **108**, 500–508.

75 Leach CL, Holm B, Morin FCR, et al. (1995). Partial liquid ventilation in premature lambs with respiratory distress syndrome: efficacy and compatibility with exogenous surfactant. *J Pediatr*, **126**, 412–420.

76 Jackson JC, Standaert TA, Trong WE, et al. (1994). Full-tidal liquid ventilation with perfluorocarbon for prevention of lung injury in newborn non-human primates. *Artif Cells Blood Substit Immobil Biotechnol*, **22**, 1121–1132.

77 Hirschl RB, Parent A, Tooley R, et al. (1995). Liquid ventilation improves pulmonary function, gas exchange, and lung injury in a model of respiratory failure. *Ann Surg*, **221**, 79–88.

78 Nesti FD, Fuhrman BP, Steinhorn DM, et al. (1994). Perfluorocarbon-associated gas exchange in gastric aspiration. *Crit Care Med*, **22**, 1445–1452.

79 Curtis SE, Peek JT and Kelly DR. (1993). Partial liquid breathing with perflubron improves arterial oxygenation in acute canine lung injury. *J Appl Physiol*, **75**, 2696–2702.

80 Tutuncu AS, Akpir K, Mulder P, et al. (1993). Intratracheal perfluorocarbon administration as an aid in the ventilatory management of respiratory distress syndrome. *Anesthesiology*, **79**, 1083–1093.

81 Barrington KJ, Singh AJ, Etches PC, et al. (1999). Partial liquid ventilation with and without inhaled nitric oxide in a newborn piglet model of meconium aspiration. *Am J Respir Crit Care Med*, **160**, 1922–1927.

82 Bifano EM and Pfannenstiel A. (1988). Duration of hyperventilation and outcome in infants with persistent pulmonary hypertension. *Pediatrics*, **81**, 657–661.

83 Landry S, Chapieski L and Fletcher J. (1988). Three year outcomes for low birthweight infants: differential effects of early medical complications. *J Pediatr Psychol*, **13**, 317–327.

84 Kennealy J, McLennan J, Loudon R, et al. (1980). Hyperventilation-induced cerebral hypoxia. *Am Rev Respir Dis*, **122**, 407–412.

85 Kety S and Schmidt C. (1946). The effects of active and passive hyperventilation on cerebral blood follow, cerebral oxygen consumption, cardiac output and blood pressure in normal young men. *J Clin Invest*, **25**, 107–119.

86 Cohen RS, Stevenson DK, Malachowski N, et al. (1980). Late morbidity among survivors of respiratory failure treated with tolazoline. *J Pediatr*, **97**, 644–647.

87 Brett C, Dekle M, Leonard CH, et al. (1981). Developmental follow-up of hyperventilated neonates: preliminary observations. *Pediatrics*, **68**, 588–591.

88 Bernbaum J, Russell P, Sheridan PH, et al. (1984). Long-term follow-up of newborns with persistent pulmonary hypertension. *Crit Care Med*, **12**, 579–588.

89 Ballard R and Leonard C. (1984). Developmental follow-up of infants with persistent pulmonary hypertension of the newborn. *Clin Perinatol*, **11**, 737–744.

90 Ferrara B, Johnson D, Chang, P-N, et al. (1984). Efficacy and neurologic outcome of profound hypocapneic alkalosis for the treatment of persistent pulmonary hypertension in infancy. *J Pediatr*, **105**, 457–461.

91 Sell EJ, Gaines JA, Gluckman C, et al. (1985). Persistent fetal circulation. Neurodevelopmental outcome. *Am J Dis Child*, **139**, 25–28.

92 Naulty CM, Weiss IP and Herer GR. (1986). Progressive sensorineural hearing loss in survivors of persistent fetal circulation. *Ear Hear*, **7**, 74–77.

93 Hendricks-Munoz KD and Walton JP. (1988). Hearing loss in infants with persistent fetal circulation. *Pediatrics*, **81**, 650–656.

94 Leavitt AM, Watchko JF, Bennett FC, et al. (1987). Neurodevelopmental outcome following persistent pulmonary hypertension of the neonate. *J Perinatol*, **7**, 288–291.

95 Cheung P-Y, Tyebkhan JM, Peliowski A, et al. (1999). Prolonged use of pancuronium bromide and sensorineural hearing loss in childhood survivors of congenital diaphragmatic hernia. *J Pediatr*, **135**, 233–239.

96 Hutchin ME, Gilmer C, Yarbrough, et al. (2000). Delayed-onset sensorineural hearing loss in a 3-year-old survivor of persistent pulmonary hypertension of the newborn. *Arch Otolaryngol Head Neck Surg*, **126**, 1014–1017.

97 Desai S, Hollros PR, Graziani LJ, et al. (1997). Sensitivity and specificity of the neonatal brain-stem auditory evoked potential for hearing and language deficits in survivors of extracorporeal membrane oxygenation. *J Pediatr*, **131**, 233–239.

98 Hageman JR, Dusik J, Kenler H, et al. (1988). Outcome of persistent pulmonary hypertension in relation to severity of presentation. *Am J Dis Child*, **142**, 293–296.

99 Kennedy C, Sakurada O, Shinohara M, et al. (1982). Local cerebral glucose utilization in the newborn macaque monkey. *Ann Neurol*, **12**, 333–340.

100 Pickles J. (1982). *An Introduction to the Physiology of Hearing*, pp. 48–69. New York: Academic Press.

101 Bulas DI, Taylor GA, Fitz CR, et al. (1991). Posterior fossa intracranial hemorrhage in infants treated with extracorporeal membrane oxygenation: sonographic findings. *Am J Roentgenol*, **156**, 571–575.

102 Cilley RE, Zwischenberger JB, Andrews AF, et al. (1986). Intracranial hemorrhage during extracorporeal membrane oxygenation in neonates. *Pediatrics*, **78**, 699–704.

103 Lazar EL, Abramso, SJ, Weinstein S, et al. (1994). Neuroimaging of brain injury in neonates treated with extracorporeal membrane oxygenation: lessons learned from serial examinations. *J Pediatr Surg*, **29**, 186–191.

104 Babcock DS, Han BK, Weiss RG, et al. (1989). Brain abnormalities in infants on extracorporeal membrane oxygenation: sonographic and CT findings. *Am J Roentgenol*, **153**, 571–576.

105 Luisiri A, Graviss ER, Weber T, et al. (1988). Neurosonographic changes in newborns treated with extracorporeal membrane oxygenation. *J Ultrasound Med*, **7**, 429–438.

106 Matamoros A, Anderson JC, McConnell J, et al. (1989). Neurosonographic findings in infants treated by extracorporeal membrane oxygenation (ECMO). *J Child Neurol*, **4**, S52–S61.

107 Taylor GA, Fitz CR, Miller MK, et al. (1987). Intracranial abnormalities in infants treated with extracorporeal membrane oxygenation: imaging with US and CT. *Radiology*, **165**, 675–678.

108 Extracorporeal Life Support Organization (ELSO). (2001). *Neonatal ECMO Registry*. Ann Arbor, Michigan: ELSO.

109 Taylor GA, Glass P, Fitz CR, et al. (1987). Neurologic status in infants treated with extracorporeal membrane oxygenation: correlation of imaging findings with developmental outcome. *Radiology*, **165**, 679–682.

110 Taylor GA, Fitz CR, Glass P, et al. (1989). CT of cerebrovascular injury after neonatal extracorporeal membrane oxygenation: implications for neurodevelopmental outcome. *Am J Roentgenol*, **153**, 121–126.

111 Taylor G, Short B and Fitz C. (1989). Imaging of cerebrovascular injury in infants treated with extracorporeal membrane oxygenation. *J Pediatr*, **114**, 635–639.

112 Wiznitzer M, Masaryk TJ, Lewin J, et al. (1990). Parenchymal and vascular magnetic resonance imaging of the brain after extracorporeal membrane oxygenation. *Am J Dis Child*, **144**, 1323–1326.

113 Schumacher RE, Barks JD, Johnston MV, et al. (1988). Right-sided brain lesions in infants following extracorporeal membrane oxygenation. *Pediatrics*, **82**, 155–161.

114 Schumacher RE, Spak C and Kileny PR. (1990). Asymmetric brain stem auditory evoked responses in infants treated with extracorporeal membrane oxygenation. *Ear Hear*, **11**, 359–362.

115 Raju TN, Kim SY, Meller JL, et al. (1989). Circle of Willis blood velocity and flow direction after common carotid artery ligation for neonatal extracorporeal membrane oxygenation. *Pediatrics*, **83**, 343–347.

116 Campbell LR, Bunyapen C, Holmes GL, et al. (1988). Right common carotid artery ligation in extracorporeal membrane oxygenation. *J Pediatr*, **113**, 110–113.

117 Mendoza JC, Shearer LL and Cook LN. (1991). Lateralization of brain lesions following extracorporeal membrane oxygenation. *Pediatrics*, **88**, 1004–1009.

118 Van Meurs K, Nguyen H, Rhine W, et al. (1994). Intracranial

abnormalities and neurodevelopmental status after venovenous extracorporeal membrane oxygenation. *J Pediatr*, **125**, 3007.

119 Hahn JS, Vaucher Y, Bejar R, et al. (1993). Electroencephalographic and neuroimaging findings in neonates undergoing extracorporeal membrane oxygenation. *Neuropediatrics*, **24**, 19–24.

120 Streletz LJ, Bej MD, Graziani LJ, et al. (1992). Utility of serial EEGs in neonates during extracorporeal membrane oxygenation. *Pediatr Neurol*, **8**, 190–196.

121 Krummel TM, Greenfield LJ, Kirkpatrick BV, et al. (1984). The early evaluation of survivors after extracorporeal membrane oxygenation for neonatal pulmonary failure. *J Pediatr Surg*, **19**, 585–590.

122 Towne BH, Lott IT, Hicks DA, et al. (1985). Long-term follow-up of infants and children treated with extracorporeal membrane oxygenation (ECMO): a preliminary report. *J Pediatr Surg*, **20**, 410–414.

123 Andrews A, Nixon C, Cilley R, et al. (1986). One to three year outcome for 14 survivors of extracorporeal membrane oxygenation. *Pediatrics*, **78**, 692–698.

124 Glass P, Miller M and Short B. (1989). Morbidity for survivors of extracorporeal membrane oxygenation: neurodevelopmental outcome at 1 year of age. *Pediatrics*, **83**, 72–78.

125 Adolph V, Ekelund C, Smith C, et al. (1990). Developmental outcome of neonates treated with extracorporeal membrane oxygenation. *J Pediatr Surg*, **25**, 43–46.

126 Schumacher RE, Palmer TW, Roloff DW, et al. (1991). Follow-up of infants treated with extracorporeal membrane oxygenation for newborn respiratory failure. *Pediatrics*, **87**, 451–457.

127 Campbell LR, Bunyapen C, Gangarosa ME, et al. (1991). Significance of seizures associated with extracorporeal membrane oxygenation. *Pediatrics*, **119**, 789–792.

128 Hofkosh D, Thompson AE, Nozza RJ, et al. (1991) Ten years of extracorporeal membrane oxygenation: neurodevelopmental outcome. *Pediatrics*, **87**, 549–555.

129 Flusser H, Dodge NN, Engle WE, et al. (1993). Neurodevelopmental outcome and respiratory morbidity for extracorporeal membrane oxygenation survivors at 1 year of age. *J Perinatol*, **13**, 266–271.

130 Wildin SR, Landry SH and Zwischenberger JB. (1994). Prospective, controlled study of developmental outcome in survivors of extracorporeal membrane oxygenation: the first 24 months. *Pediatrics*, **93**, 404–408.

131 Glass P, Wagner AE, Papero PH, et al. (1995). Neurodevelopmental status at age five years of neonates treated with extracorporeal membrane oxygenation. *J Pediatr*, **127**, 447–457.

132 Kornhauser MS, Baumgart S, Desai SA, et al. (1998). Adverse neurodevelopmental outcome after extracorporeal membrane oxygenation among neonates with bronchopulmonary dysplasia. *J Pediatr*, **132**, 307–311.

133 Desai SA, Stanley C, Gringlas M, et al. (1999). Five-year follow-up of neonates with reconstructed right common carotid arteries after extracorporeal membrane oxygenation. *J Pediatr*, **134**, 428–433.

134 Van Meurs KP, Robbins ST, Reed VL, et al. (1993). Congenital diaphragmatic hernia: long-term outcome in neonates treated with extracorporeal membrane oxygenation. *J Pediatr*, **122**, 893–899.

135 Stolar CJ, Crisafi MA and Driscoll YT. (1995). Neurocognitive outcome for neonates treated with extracorporeal membrane oxygenation: are infants with congenital diaphragmatic hernia different? *J Pediatr Surg*, **30**, 355–371.

136 Bernbaum J, Schwartz IP, Gerdes M, et al. (1995). Survivors of extracorporeal membrane oxygenation at 1 year of age: the relationship of primary diagnosis with health and neurodevelopmental sequelae. *Pediatrics*, **96**, 907–913.

137 Nield RA, Langenbacher D, Pulsen MK, et al. (2000). Neurodevelopmental outcome at 3.5 years of age in children treated with extracorporeal life support: relationship to primary diagnosis. *J Pediatr*, **136**, 338–344.

138 Walsh-Sukys M, Bauer R, Cornell D, et al. (1994). Severe respiratory failure in neonates: mortality and morbidity rates and developmental outcomes. *J Pediatr*, **125**, 104–110.

139 Gratny L, Haney B, Hustead V, et al. (1992). Morbidity and developmental outcome of ECMO survivors compared to concurrent control group. *Soc Pediatr Res*, **31**, 248A.

140 Robertson CMT, Finer NN, Suave RS, et al. (1995). Neurodevelopmental outcome after neonatal extracorporeal membrane oxygenation. *Can Med Assoc J*, **152**, 1981–1988.

141 Vaucher YE, Dudell GG, Bejar R, et al. (1996). Predictors of early childhood outcome in candidates for extracorporeal membrane oxygenation. *J Pediatr*, **128**, 109–117.

142 UK Collaborative ECMO Trial Group. (1996). UK collaborative randomized trial of neonatal extracorporeal membrane oxygenation. *Lancet*, **348**, 75–82.

143 Roberts J, Polaner D, Lang P, et al. (1992). Inhaled nitric oxide in persistent pulmonary hypertension of the newborn. *Lancet*, **340**, 818–819.

144 Kinsella J, Neish S, Shaffer E, et al. (1992). Low-dose inhalational nitric oxide in persistent pulmonary hypertension of the newborn. *Lancet*, **340**, 819–820.

145 Rosenberg AA, Hennaugh JM, Moreland SG, et al. (1997). Longitudinal follow-up of a cohort of newborn infants

treated with inhaled nitric oxide for persistent pulmonary hypertension. *J Pediatr*, **131**, 70–75.

146 Ellington M, O'Reilly D, Allred EN, et al. (2001). Child health status, neurodevelopmental outcome and parental satisfaction in a randomized, controlled trial of nitric oxide for persistent pulmonary hypertension of the newborn. *Pediatrics*, **107**, 1351–1356.

33

Pediatric cardiac surgery: relevance to fetal and neonatal brain injury

Michael D. Black

Stanford University School of Medicine, Stanford, CA, USA

Although the morbidity and mortality rates associated with cardiac surgery have drastically declined within the past decade, reduced to 5% in many centers, the concomitant recognition and treatment of significant neurological dysfunction in children have lagged far behind. Neurological dysfunction (either congenital and/or related to perioperative period) remains a serious comorbidity that significantly precludes successful long-term outcomes in children afflicted with congenital heart disease.[1] The mechanisms of injury remain multifactorial with up to 25% of children having residual neurological sequelae postcardiac surgery.[1–3] This chapter will exclusively deal with the perioperative sources of injury occurring around or at the time of the cardiac intervention.

A deliberate attempt to optimize neurological outcomes using selective cerebral perfusion techniques was initiated by the author in 1996 based upon previous institutional experiences as well as the body of international literature utilizing deep hypothermia and circulatory arrest (DHCA). Selective cerebral perfusion (SCAP) in theory allows for the continuous delivery of blood flow without the concomitant need for profound hypothermia and its deleterious effects on a multitude of organ systems, including the brain. Maintaining an adequate cerebral oxygen supply is a serious problem during aortic arch reconstruction in neonates with conditions such as hypoplastic left heart syndrome, interrupted aortic arch, and others. DHCA remains the most common method used for cerebral protection during cardiac surgery, allowing an extremely limited and a somewhat ill-defined period of up to 60 min as the maximum "safe" interval. Unfortunately, as one induces moderate-to-deep hypothermic temperatures, there is an unexpected uncoupling of the relationship between cerebral blood flow (CBF) and oxygen consumption. The autoregulatory properties of the cerebral vasculature are lost, with the end result being an unpredictable period of cerebral protection and the false sense of security.

All phases of care (pre-, intra-, and postoperative) must be attended to with an equal and judicious neurological protective strategy if an optimal outcome is to be obtained.

Preoperative period

The recognition of a significant cardiac malformation should set in motion a battery of investigations, frequently including cerebral ultrasonography, magnetic resonance imaging (MRI), computed tomography (CT) scan and/or an electroencephalography (EEG). The neonatologist, geneticist, neurologist, and critical care nurse must remain clear and unified with the proposed medical plan for both the child and family. Mixed messages or differences of opinions can be disastrous during this critical time of planning. A prolonged period of hypoxemia and/or hypotension frequently accompanies a history of a delayed recognition of a significant cardiac ailment with preferential pulmonary circulation which jeopardizes systemic perfusion including the brain (most frequently, single ventricle physiology). The association of neurological malformation as part of a well-defined chromosomal abnormality, or simply isolated, demands that the physician and paramedical team fully investigate the integrity of the brain prior to any planned cardiac surgical procedure. Frequently, deterioration in neurological function follows a period of cardiopulmonary bypass (CPB), especially when the neurological baseline is identified as being abnormal. An intracranial hemorrhage may preclude the use of systemic anticoagulants, i.e., heparin sulfate, for a period of 4–6 weeks. Occasionally, a palliative procedure may need to be performed in order to delay the utilization of CPB.

Neurological function in children with congenital heart disease

Infants with congenital heart disease are at an increased risk for associated dysgenetic lesions of the brain, or, less frequently, combined cardiac–cerebral manifestations of recognized genetic syndromes or inherited metabolic conditions.[1] Combined cardiac and neurologic manifestations are prevalent, particularly with certain chromosomal disorders, such as trisomies 21, 11, and 18. Dysgenetic brain lesions are common in trisomy 13 and are often severe, i.e., holoprosencephaly and agenesis of the corpus callosum. Trisomy 18 is frequently associated with neuronal migration defects while trisomy 21 is associated with milder structural and clinical findings, such as global hypotonia and the development of late cognitive dysfunction.[1]

The prevalence at autopsy of recognized cerebral dysgenesis in infants with congenital heart disease ranges from 10 to 29%.[4–6] As such, complete preoperative evaluation of children born with congenital heart disease is warranted. Cranial ultrasonography, being noninvasive, can be easily performed and remains excellent in identifying both cerebral atrophy and linear echodensities in the basal ganglia and thalamus, lesions which are more commonly found in children with congenital heart disease.[7,8] Certain cardiac lesions appear to be at particular risk as having an associated genetic and/or structural neurological defect, e.g., hypoplastic left heart syndrome.[4] Take, for example the latter condition, which until recently was uniformly fatal. With increasing success (decreased mortality and morbidity) with first-stage procedures, more infants are now able to complete all three phases of the reconstructive strategy. Children are living longer and are thus able to be more thoroughly investigated for neurological outcome. There is now an increased recognition of genetic disorder and other major extracardiac anomalies (28%) with hypoplastic left heart syndrome, emphasizing the need for a more thorough genetic preevaluation process prior to any surgical intervention.[4,9]

Intraoperative period

Circulatory arrest

Since its introduction in the early 1960s, circulatory arrest has been ubiquitous in centers with an expertise in pediatric cardiac surgery. The great advantage of this CPB strategy is the "bloodless" surgical field obtained. However, not even the surgical risks of the procedure provoke as much parental concern as the thought of the complete termination of CBF to their loved one for "whatever length of time".

The continued use of DHCA is based on the premise that there is a "safe" duration of total absence of organ perfusion, which is inversely related to body temperature. The cerebral metabolic rate remains significantly higher in children than in the adult counterpart and hypothermia remains the most frequently practiced form of neurological protection in order to reduce neurological cellular metabolism and the oxygen requirement. A decrease in the cerebral metabolic rate with cooling has been demonstrated in infants, neonates, and children as an exponential relationship between temperature and cerebral metabolic rate.[10,11] In addition, hypothermia has recently been suggested to be advantageous in the protection from reperfusion injury as well.[12]

The brain remains the organ most susceptible to cessation of the circulation. Conflicting reports of transient and permanent neurological dysfunction and also the presence of late developmental problems after DHCA have generated considerable controversies within the past 10 years.[13] The principal drawback is a defined and somewhat unpredictable safe period of cerebral ischemia and multiorgan dysfunction, i.e., coagulative, renal, and pulmonary complications related to low body temperatures and prolonged CPB time.[14] The relationships between the various mechanisms of cerebral injury continue to be poorly understood. Factors felt to have a crucial role in cerebral homeostasis include acid–base management, hematocrit, perfusion techniques, and surgical choices. Uneven or inadequate cerebral cooling may occur during CPB or at the time of circulatory arrest.[10] Recent data suggest that a reduction in cerebral morbidity might be associated with better monitoring of brain temperature in an attempt to minimize cerebral hyperthermia.[15]

In 1987, Ferry[16] reported strokes, diffuse hypoxic–ischemic lesions, intracranial hemorrhages, delayed choreoathetoid syndrome, and spinal cord lesions as sequelae of cardiac surgery in children. From 1988 to 1989, in a survey of six major pediatric cardiac surgical units in the USA and Canada, Ferry[2] attempted to estimate the prevalence and nature of neurological injury postoperatively. Based upon these observations, the reported prevalence of acute neurological morbidity varied between 1 and 25%.

Newburger et al. reported that infants subjected to a CPB strategy consisting of predominantly DHCA as compared to a low-flow strategy were associated with a significantly higher incidence of neurological abnormalities (11%); this percentage increased to 30% when continuous EEG recording was performed.[13] The same authors also reported that these infants had a prolonged recovery time and a greater release of the brain isoenzyme creatine phosphokinase over the first 6 postoperative hours.[13] The recent identification of a critical closing and opening pressure on the cerebral vasculature may place a nadir value on the rate of CPB flow during hypothermia.[17] After all, "ultra-low-flow" could be "no-flow" or a circulatory arrest equivalent.[18]

Several studies have tried to assess the clinical effects of DHCA on brain physiology.[18–26] CBF was measured with a xenon clearance technique during moderate hypothermia (25–32 °C), deep hypothermia (18–22 °C), or total DHCA (18 °C). While CBF decreases with hypothermia, it returns to baseline with rewarming, even exceeding it in the first two groups. Patients exposed to DHCA did not recover their initial CBF upon rewarming or even after weaning from CPB, demonstrating an uncoupling of CBF and the cerebral metabolic rate for oxygen.[26] Corroborating these latter studies, Filgueiras et al., using histopathology and magnetic resonance spectroscopy,[27] demonstrated the complete preservation of high-energy substrates with continuous low-flow (50 ml/kg/per min) versus decreased brain energetics with DHCA.

Hypothermia

Hypothermia remains the most commonly used technique for cerebral protection during cardiac surgery. However the method remains imperfect.

Although hypothermia contributes to reducing the cerebral metabolic rate for oxygen ($CMRO_2$) and increased cellular protection during cardiac surgery, the process is not complete. The $CMRO_2$ of the gray matter can be entirely inhibited by a temperature of 17 °C, whereas the corresponding $CMRO_2$ of the supportive cells (e.g., astrocytes) can only be reduced by 92%.[28] Therefore, even at 15 °C, substrate delivery (O_2 and glucose) of the remaining 8% of cerebral activity may not be met.

A recent investigation of 17 neonates, aged 4–21 days, measured oxygen saturation and total hemoglobin concentration in the cerebral circulation and showed that, during the first 45 min of deep DHCA, cerebral oxygen levels decreased, suggesting that oxygen extraction continued during this period.[29] The rapidity at which cooling and rewarming are performed during CPB may also be involved in the process of cellular disturbances and death.[30,31] Deep hypothermia, although cerebral-protective, affects the cerebrovascular reactivity and normal cerebral physiology which persists postoperatively in small infants and children.[32] These observations have been confirmed by other groups of investigators.[30,33] Cerebral perfusion and metabolism decrease with the introduction of hypothermia to a variable degree depending on the depth of hypothermia used.[17] During light (30 °C) and moderate (26 °C) hypothermia, the normal flow–metabolism relationship is preserved.[18] However, the coupling between CBF and oxygen consumption is lost during exposure to severe or deep hypothermic (15–17 °C) temperature[18] and this loss is presumed to be related to a cold-induced vasoparesis.[17,32]

The presence of cerebral autoregulation (CAU) is essential to the maintenance of a homogeneous distribution of CBF. The loss of CAU may lead to unevenly perfused and cooled regions of the brain during CPB, even with sufficient time to allow for "proper" cerebral cooling leading to cerebral injury.[23] During deep hypothermia (15 °C) and low-flow CPB, the temperature of some portions of the brain can rewarm to 35 °C within 15 min[33] and the cerebral arteriovenous difference in lactate (obtained from the right internal jugular bulb) can be significantly increased.[18] Furthermore, following rewarming from CPB, the CBF of infants subjected intraoperatively to DHCA did not return to preoperative values up to 6 h postoperatively.[34] Thus, detrimental effects on the cerebrum may occur both during and after DHCA.

To assess the effects of DHCA on brain physiology, the use of lactate has been previously suggested. Van der Linden et al.,[35] in a study of 17 patients undergoing congenital heart surgery during profound hypothermia, demonstrated that, following total circulatory arrest, lactate levels in the jugular venous blood were higher than the arterial levels from the beginning of rewarming until 3 h after the end of CPB. The release of lactate from the brain cannot be explained by inadequate CBF during the reperfusion period since, using transcranial Doppler sonography, these authors have demonstrated the presence of increased blood flow velocity in the middle cerebral artery during and after rewarming. The authors suggested that cerebral aerobic metabolism of glucose may have been disturbed following profound hypothermic circulatory arrest, resulting in anaerobic cerebral metabolism and lactate release.

Postoperative (reperfusion injury)

Recent evidence suggests that CBF in infants and children remains critically reduced during the postoperative period[36] and that a period of concomitant cerebral hyperthermia could be extremely detrimental during this period of cerebral hypoperfusion.

Experiments have shown that the nervous system remains exquisitely sensitive to heat.[37] Cerebral hyperthermia is associated with persistent deterioration of neurobehavioral outcome.[38,39] Pathological changes in the human brain can be demonstrated within 6 h of the hyperthermic insult,[37] despite optimal cerebral perfusion pressure.[34] Previous studies on focal ischemia in animals showed a direct correlation between elevated intracerebral temperature and worse clinical outcome.[40,41] Wass et al.[40] demonstrated in a canine model of cerebral ischemia that temperature increases of a mere 1 or 2 °C resulted in a significant deterioration of neurologic function, which correlated with histopathological lesions. Burrows et al. studied 21 neonates and infants undergoing CPB with DHCA and reported significant increases in anterior fontanel pressure at the end of rewarming.[42] These authors correlated this increase in intracranial pressure with the delayed return of cerebral electrical activity and showed that the duration of the increase correlated with the time taken for the visual evoked potentials to reappear. The association of decreased CBF and increased intracranial pressure in these patients might be of importance in the presence of cerebral hyperthermia, i.e., bidirectional cavopulmonary anastomosis and Fontan procedure. It has been demonstrated that brain temperature increases after cerebral ischemia despite normal ambient and core body temperature.[43]

Cerebral hyperthermia has been shown to increase extracellular glutamate concentration in rats.[44] Excitatory amino acid receptors are present at birth and their concentrations increase drastically during the first few weeks of life.[45–47] The level of neurotransmitter in a 3-month-old infant approximates the adult concentration. The occurrence of seizures in infants following cardiac surgery has been suggested to be due to excitotoxic mechanisms via neuronal injury and the release of excitatory amino acid.[3] Although the temperature of the brain was not reported in the latter study, it does not exclude the possibility that cerebral hyperthermia could have contributed to the effect of these neuromediators. In a recent paper, using astrocyte cell cultures during and after rewarming with sustained moderate hyperthermia (38.5 °C), the authors reported a continuous and significant increase in extracellular glutamate.[48] This astrocytic dysfunction and the resultant accumulation of extracellular glutamate may account for the observed neurological dysfunction seen in infants following repair of congenital heart disease. Marked cerebral swelling, which was mainly cortical in origin, was visible on magnetic resonance images immediately after hypothermic (28 °C) and normothermic CPB.[49,50] These authors were unable to explain the mechanism involved but it does not exclude the possibility that cerebral hyperthermia was present during the immediate postoperative period. In an editorial on brain protection during anesthesia, Drummond raised concerns about the occasional use of hyperthermic perfusate during rewarming and suggested that iatrogenic hyperthermia contributes to the substantial incidence of neuropsychiatric dysfunction observed after CPB in adults.[51] In a recent study, cerebral hyperthermia was found independent of the perfusate temperature.[52]

It has been suggested that temperatures recorded deep within the esophagus could equally well indicate brain temperature.[53,54] However our recent study demonstrated that temperatures taken deep within the esophagus failed to reflect cerebral temperatures, especially after 3 h.[52] Confounding variables are always present, i.e., mechanical ventilation, which can greatly affect temperature recordings within the esophagus.[52] The addition of such extraneous variables remains a poor correlation between esophageal and cerebral temperatures. Not surprisingly, tympanic membrane temperature demonstrates no relationship with jugular bulb temperatures (JBT).[52]

The importance of maintaining normothermia has been a fundamental premise in the neonatal and cardiac intensive care unit for many years.[38] This has led to the application of aggressive rewarming techniques for even modest degrees of hypothermia such as occur frequently after CPB.[38] Our study demonstrated that infants and children have significant cerebral hyperthermia during the first 6 h of recovery for congenital heart disease repaired using CPB. Whether cerebral hyperthermia accounts for apparent differences in outcome after CPB remains invalidated but it may well be causative![15] Obviously, no matter what the etiology of neurological injury following repair of CHD, there is ample evidence in animal studies to suggest that hyperthermia worsens neurological outcome.

The cerebral metabolic rate of the brain is one of the highest in the body and, as a result of this, heat is produced.[53,54] The normal brain temperature is on average 0.5 °C warmer than the core temperature.[55–57] The increase in JBT observed[52] could not be explained only on the basis of higher physiological cerebral metabolism. Cardiac surgery and CPB activate a systemic inflammatory response characterized clinically by systemic vasodilatation, hyperthermia, postoperative bleeding, and reperfusion injury, which can result in permanent or transient dysfunction.[58,59] It has been shown in a study of 20 children undergoing CPB that removing inflammatory mediators using zero-balanced hemofiltration resulted in lower maximum body temperature in the first 24 h postoperatively.[60] Although they did not measure the brain temperature, these observations correlate with the present study and may reflect the contribution of endogenous cerebral pyrogens such as cytokines in the rise in brain temperature.

Selective cerebral perfusion

The significant decrease in lactate concentration reported in one study might suggest that selective cerebral antegrade perfusion preserves better oxygenation, by ensuring proper cerebral aerobic metabolism and improved systemic substrate delivery.[52] The avoidance of DHCA, prolonged cerebral rewarming,[52] and the continuous delivery of CBF have been clinically associated with a lower incidence of seizures and gross neurological deficits in our group of infants and neonates.[61–63] Although the use of neurological markers in this study was nonspecific, similar postoperative surveillance strategies have demonstrated a statistically significant increase in neurological dysfunction in a similar population of infants at the same institution using conventional CPB techniques with DHCA.[64]

Conclusions

Injury to the neonatal and fetal brain can occur from a myriad of sources. Associated with improvements in the antenatal diagnosis of significant cardiac disease, we should expect a lower incidence of preoperative hypoxic–ischemic encephalopathy. As such, a judicious preoperative workup allowing for the identification of isolated or concomitant neurological defects should allow improvements in the perioperative course of most neonates born with cardiac disease. All phases (pre-, intra-, and postoperative) remain equally important if we are to discharge children with their fullest neurological potential.

REFERENCES

1 du Plessis A. (1997). Neurologic complications of cardiac disease in the newborn. *Clin Perinatol*, **24**, 807–826.

2 Ferry PC. (1990). Neurologic sequelae of open-heart surgery in children. An 'irritating question.' *Am J Dis Child*, **144**, 369–373.

3 Newburger JW, Jonas RA, Wernovsky G, et al. (1993). A comparison of the perioperative neurologic effects of hypothermic circulatory arrest versus low-flow cardiopulmonary bypass in infant heart surgery. *N Engl J Med*, **329**, 1057–1064.

4 Glauser T, Rorke L, Weinberg P, et al. (1990). Congenital brain anomalies associated with the hypoplastic left heart syndrome. *Pediatrics*, **85**, 984–990.

5 Jones M. (1991). Anomalies of the brain and congenital heart disease: a study of 52 necropsy cases. *Pediatr Pathol*, **11**, 721–736.

6 Terplan K. (1976). Brain changes in newborns, infants and children with congenital heart disease in association with cardiac surgery. Additional observations. *J Neurosurg*, **212**, 225.

7 Van Houten JP, Rothman A and Bejar R. (1996). High incidence of cranial ultrasound abnormalities in full-term infants with congenital heart disease. *Am J Perinatol*, **13**, 47–53.

8 Drull F, Latta K, Hoyer PF, et al. (1994). Cerebral ultrasonography before and after cardiac surgery in infants. *Pediatr Cardiol*, **15**, 159–162.

9 Natowicz M, Chatten J, Clancey R, et al. (1998). Genetic disorder and major extracardiac anomalies associated with the hypoplastic left heart syndrome. *Pediatrics*, **82**, 698–706.

10 Greeley WJ, Kern FH, Ungerleider RM, et al. (1991). The effect of hypothermic cardiopulmonary bypass and total circulatory arrest on cerebral metabolism in neonates, infants, and children. *J Thorac Cardiovasc Surg*, **101**, 783–794.

11 Hillier SC, Burrows FA, Bissonnette B, et al. (1991). Cerebral hemodynamics in neonates and infants undergoing cardiopulmonary bypass and profound hypothermic circulatory arrest: assessment by transcranial Doppler sonography. *Anesth Analg*, **72**, 723–728.

12 du Plessis A. (1997). Cerebral hemodynamics and metabolism during infant cardiac surgery. Mechanisms of injury and strategies for protection. *J Child Neurol*, **12**, 285–300.

13 Newburger JW, Jonas RA, Wernovsky G, et al. (1993). A comparison of the peri-operative neurologic effects of hypothermic circulatory arrest versus low-flow cardiopulmonary bypass in infant heart surgery. *N Engl J Med*, **329**, 1057–1064.

14 Testolin L, Roques X, Laborde MN, et al. (1998). Moderately hypothermic cardiopulmonary bypass and selective cerebral perfusion in ascending aorta and aortic arch surgery. Preliminary experience in twenty-two patients. *Cardiovasc Surg*, **6**, 398–405.

15 Murkin JM. (1995). Hypothermic cardiopulmonary bypass – time for a more temperate approach. *Can J Anaesth*, **42**, 663–668.

16 Ferry PC. (1987). Neurologic sequelae of cardiac surgery in children. *Am J Dis Child*, **141**, 309–312.

17 Burrows FA, Bissonnette B. (1993). Cerebral blood flow

velocity patterns during cardiac surgery utilizing profound hypothermia with low-flow cardiopulmonary bypass or circulatory arrest in neonates and infants. *Can J Anaesth*, **40**, 298–307.

18 Burrows FA and Bissonnette B. (1993). Monitoring the adequacy of cerebral perfusion during cardiopulmonary bypass in children using transcranial Doppler technology. *J Neurosurg Anesthesiol*, **5**, 209–212.

19 van der Linden J, Priddy R, Ekroth R, et al. (1991). Cerebral perfusion and metabolism during profound hypothermia in children. A study of middle cerebral artery ultrasonic variables and cerebral extraction of oxygen. *J Thorac Cardiovasc Surg*, **102**, 103–104.

20 Ekroth R, Rossi RF, Tsang V, et al. (1986). Serial measurement of arterial and internal jugular venous creatine kinase isoenzyme BB (CK-BB) after deep hypothermic total circulatory arrest in pediatric cardiac surgery. *J Thorac Cardiovasc Surg*, **34**, 223–225.

21 Rossi R, Ekroth R, Lincoln C, et al. (1986). Detection of cerebral injury after total circulatory arrest and profound hypothermia by estimation of specific creatine kinase isoenzyme levels using monoclonal antibody techniques (published erratum appears in *Am J Cardiol* 1987; 59, a12). *Am J Cardiol*, **58**, 1236–1241.

22 Greeley WJ, Ungerleider RM, Smith LR, et al. (1989). The effects of deep hypothermic cardiopulmonary bypass and total circulatory arrest on cerebral blood flow in infants and children. *J Thorac Cardiovasc Surg*, **97**, 737–745.

23 Greeley WJ. (1991). Con: Deep hypothermic circulatory arrest must be used selectively and discreetly. *J Cardiothorac Vasc Anesth*, **5**, 638–640.

24 Greeley WJ, Kern FH, Ungerleider RM, et al. (1991). The effect of hypothermic cardiopulmonary bypass and total circulatory arrest on cerebral metabolism in neonates, infants and children. *J Thorac Cardiovasc Surg*, **101**, 83–94.

25 Greeley WJ, Kern FH, Meliones JN, et al. (1993). Effect of deep hypothermia and circulatory arrest on cerebral blood flow and metabolism. *Ann Thorac Surg*, **56**, 1464–1466.

26 Mault JR, Ohtake S, Klingensmith ME, et al. (1993). Cerebral metabolism and circulatory arrest: effects of duration and strategies for protection. *Ann Thorac Surg*, **55**, 57–63.

27 Filgueiras C, Ryner L, Ye J, et al. (1996). Cerebral protection during moderate hypothermic circulatory arrest. Histopathology and magnetic resonance spectroscopy of brain energetics and intracellular pH in pigs. *J Thorac Cardiovasc Surg*, **112**, 1073–1080.

28 Michaenfelder JD, Milde JH, Katusic ZS. (1991). Postischemic canine cerebral blood flow is coupled to cerebral metabolic rate. *J Cereb Blood Flow Metab*, **11**, 611–616.

29 Kurth CD, Steven JM, Nicolson SC, et al. (1992). Kinetics of cerebral deoxygenation during deep hypothermic circulatory arrest in neonates. *Anesthesiology*, **77**, 656–661.

30 Wong PC, Barlow CF, Hickey PR, et al. (1992). Factors associated with choreoathetosis after cardiopulmonary bypass in children with congenital heart disease. *Circulation*, **86**(suppl. 5), II18– II26.

31 Bellinger DC, Wernovsky G, Rappaport LA, et al. (1991). Cognitive development of children following early repair of transposition of the great arteries using deep hypothermic circulatory arrest. *Pediatrics*, **87**, 701–707.

32 Greeley WJ, Bushman GA, Kong DL, et al. (1988). Effects of cardiopulmonary bypass on eicosanoid metabolism during pediatric cardiovascular surgery. *J Thorac Cardiovasc Surg*, **95**, 842–849.

33 Foster J, Burrows F and Bissonnette B. (1993). Does the brain cool evenly during hypothermic cardiopulmonary bypass? *Can J Anaesth*, **40**, A67.

34 O'Hare B, Bissonnette B, Bohn D, et al. (1995). Persistent low cerebral blood flow velocity following profound hypothermic circulatory arrest in infants. *Can J Anaesth*, **42**, 1–8.

35 van der Linden J, Astudillo R, Ekroth R, et al. (1993). Cerebral lactate release after circulatory arrest but not after low flow in pediatric heart operations. *Ann Thorac Surg*, **56**, 1485–1489.

36 O'Hare B, Bissonnette B, Bohn D, et al. (1995). Persistent low cerebral blood flow velocity following profound hypothermic circulatory arrest in infants. *Can J Anaesth*, **42**, 964–971.

37 Sminia P, van der Zee J, Wondergem J, et al. (1994). Effect of hyperthermia on the central nervous system: a review. *Int J Hyperthermia*, **10**, 1–30.

38 Shum-Tim D, Nagashima M, Shinoka T, et al. (1998). Postischemic hyperthermia exacerbates neurologic injury after deep hypothermic circulatory arrest. *J Thorac Cardiovasc Surg*, **116**, 780–792.

39 Kuroiwa T, Bonnekoh P and Hossmann KA. (1990). Prevention of postischemic hyperthermia prevents ischemic injury of CA1 neurons in gerbils. *J Cereb Blood Flow Metab*, **10**, 550–556.

40 Wass CT, Lanier WL, Hofer RE, et al. (1995). Temperature changes of >or = 1 degree C alter functional neurologic outcome and histopathology in a canine model of complete cerebral ischemia. *Anesthesiology*, **83**, 325–335.

41 Dietrich WD. (1992). The importance of brain temperature in cerebral injury. *J Neurotrauma*, **2**, S475–S485.

42 Burrows FA, Hillier SC, McLeod ME, et al. (1990). Anterior fontanel pressure and visual evoked potentials in neonates and infants undergoing profound hypothermic circulatory arrest. *Anesthesiology*, **73**, 632–636.

43 Colbourne F, Nurse SM and Corbett D. (1993). Spontaneous postischemic hyperthermia is not required for severe CA1 ischemic damage in gerbils. *Brain Res*, **623**, 1–5.

44 Tagushi J, Graf R, Wegener C, et al. (1995). Hyperthermia augments glutamate accumulation and infarct size in cat focal ischemia. *J Cereb Blood Flow Metab*, **15**, S321.

45 Insel TR, Miller LP and Gelhard RE. (1990). The ontogeny of excitatory amino acid receptors in rat forebrain – I. *N*-methyl-D-aspartate and quisqualate receptors. *Neuroscience*, **35**, 31–43.

46 Miller LP, Johnson AE, Gelhard RE, et al. (1990). The ontogeny of excitatory amino acid receptors in the rat forebrain – II. Kainic acid receptors. *Neuroscience*, **35**, 45–51.

47 McDonald JW and Johnston MV. (1990). Physiological and pathophysiological roles of excitatory amino acids during central nervous system development. *Brain Res Rev*, **15**, 41–70.

48 Bissonnette B, Pellerin L, Ravussin P, et al. (1999). Deep hypothermia and rewarming alters glutamate levels and glycogen content in cultured astrocytes. *Anesthesiology*, **91**, 1763–1769.

49 Harris DN, Bailey SM, Smith PL, et al. (1993). Brain swelling in first hour after coronary artery bypass surgery. *Lancet*, **342**, 586–587.

50 Harris DN, Oatridge A, Dob D, et al. (1998). Cerebral swelling after normothermic cardiopulmonary bypass. *Anesthesiology*, **88**, 340–345.

51 Drummond JC. (1993). Brain protection during anesthesia. A reader's guide. *Anesthesiology*, **79**, 877–880.

52 Bissonnette B, Holtby HM, Davis AJ, et al. (2000). Cerebral hyperthermia in children after cardiopulmonary bypass. *Anesthesiology*, **93**, 611–618.

53 Shiraki K, Sagawa S, Tajima F, et al. (1988). Independence of brain and tympanic temperatures in an unanesthetized human. *J Appl Physiol*, **65**, 482–486.

54 Wass CT, Cable DG, Schaff HV, et al. (1998). Anesthetic technique influences brain temperature during cardiopulmonary bypass in dogs. *Ann Thorac Surg*, **65**, 454–460.

55 Baker MA, Stocking RA and Meehan JP. (1972). Thermal relationship between tympanic membrane and hypothalamus in conscious cat and monkey. *J Appl Physiol*, **32**, 739–742.

56 Whitby JD and Dunkin LJ. (1971). Cerebral, oesophageal and nasopharyngeal temperatures. *Br J Anaesth*, **43**, 673–676.

57 Hayward JN and Baker MA. (1968). Role of cerebral arterial blood in the regulation of brain temperature in the monkey. *Am J Physiol*, **215**, 389–403.

58 Herskowitz A and Mangano DT. (1996). Inflammatory cascade. A final common pathway for perioperative injury? *Anesthesiology*, **85**, 957–960.

59 Hall RI, Smith MS and Rocker G. (1997). The systemic inflammatory response to cardiopulmonary bypass: pathophysiological, therapeutic, and pharmacological considerations. *Anesth Analg*, **85**, 766–782.

60 Journois D, Israel BD, Pouard P, et al. (1996). High-volume, zero-balanced hemofiltration to reduce delayed inflammatory response to cardiopulmonary bypass in children (see comments). *Anesthesiology*, **85**, 965–976.

61 Black MD and Pike N. (2001). Pediatric cardiac surgery: surgical considerations. In *Principles and Practice of Pediatric Anesthesia*, 1st edn. Bissonnette B and Dalens B (eds). New York: McGraw-Hill.

62 Black MD, Pike N, Koransky M, et al. (2001). Innovations and future directions in pediatric cardiac surgery. *Semin Cardiothor Vasc Anesthes*, **5**, 113–116.

63 Black MD and Bissonnette B. (1998). Selective cerebral perfusion: an alternative approach to cerebral protection in neonates/infants with complex cardiac procedures requiring aortic arch reconstruction. Canadian Cardiovascular Society, 51st annual meeting, Ottawa, Ontario, Oct 21st. *Can J Cardiol*, **14** (suppl. F), 87F.

64 Poirier NC, Van Arsdell GS, Brindle M, et al. (1999). Surgical treatment of aortic arch hypoplasia in children with biventricular hearts. *Ann Thorac Surg*, **68**, 2293–2298.

PART V

Management of the Depressed or Neurologically Dysfunctional Neonate

Neonatal resuscitation: immediate management

William E. Benitz, David K. Stevenson, Susan R. Hintz, and Philip Sunshine

Stanford University Medical Center, Palo Alto, CA, USA

Management of the infant during the immediate postpartum period is often subject to rigorous scrutiny by malpractice attorneys and their medical consultants. Although recent studies suggest that postpartum events account for only a fraction of untoward outcomes, such as cerebral palsy, mental retardation, and chronic seizure disorders (see Chapter 1), the potential for cerebral injury during the intrapartum period is real, and there is no doubt that skillful resuscitation can spare many distressed infants from exposure to potentially injurious circumstances. The approach to diagnosis and immediate management of the distressed neonate should reflect practical and well-coordinated procedures for facilitating the transition from fetal to neonatal cardiorespiratory function, as outlined in a review by Stevenson and Benitz.[1] Although extended intensive care may not be possible in level I or even level II nurseries, the current standard of care for any hospital that provides obstetrical delivery services requires availability of personnel who can provide competent resuscitation, emergency stabilization, and preparation for transport by a highly trained neonatal team to the nearest level III facility, if necessary.

Over the past two decades a concerted effort has been made to improve the approach of providing optimal care for the newly born infant. In September 2000, the international guidelines for neonatal resuscitation were published[2] and these comprehensively updated the recommendations that were published in 1992[3] and 1994[4] after the Fifth National Conference on Cardiopulmonary Resuscitation (CPR) and Emergency Cardiac Care (ECC). The new recommendations used a series of evidence-based data to accomplish their goals.[2,5,6] The recommendations were based upon the "current research, knowledge and experience, and could serve as a foundation for educational programs and national, regional and local processes which establish standards of practice".[2]

Objectives of neonatal resuscitation

The objectives of neonatal resuscitation must include not only survival of the distressed infant, but also mitigation of prepartum or intrapartum injuries and prevention of subsequent cerebral injury. The latter objectives, even more so than the first, require careful attention to each of the factors that affect utilization of metabolic substrates by the brain, especially oxygen and glucose. Optimal substrate utilization depends on adequate delivery of these materials to the brain, and cannot occur if the infant is hypoxemic or hypoglycemic or if cerebral perfusion is inadequate.

Even with normal substrate delivery, utilization may be compromised by metabolic disturbances. For example, severe acidosis may impair anaerobic glucose utilization by inhibiting the activity of phosphofructokinase. The practical goals for neonatal resuscitation as they relate to cerebral protection may therefore be summarized as follows: insure adequate cerebral perfusion, primarily by promoting sufficiency of cardiac output; insure adequate blood levels of oxygen and glucose; and correct conditions that may impair substrate utilization, such as acidosis or hypothermia.

Effective pursuit of these goals requires recognition of several circumstances that are unique to the fetus who suddenly has become a newborn infant. In utero, the placenta serves as the primary organ of gas exchange and the major source of glucose and other nutrients. The establishment of independent respiration, which becomes essential for survival immediately upon separation from the placenta, constitutes the most abrupt and dramatic set of physiologic adjustments required at any stage of life. Adequate gas exchange requires stable gaseous distension of the lungs, markedly increased pulmonary perfusion, and regular and effective respiratory effort. Delay or impairment of these processes represents the most common maladaptation requiring immediate management by a physician or other health-care personnel. In addition, the apparently "paradoxical" pressor response of the neonate's pulmonary vasculature to hypoxemia, hypercarbia, and acidosis (the handmaidens of asphyxia) may confound resuscitation attempts. This seemingly "maladaptive" response of the pulmonary vasculature to these stimuli is best understood by reference to the immediately previous fetal state of the neonate.

In the fetus, pulmonary vasoconstriction in response to hypoxemia, hypercarbia, or acidosis results in diversion of a greater proportion of the right ventricular output across the ductus arteriosus into the descending aorta, and thence back to the placenta for gas exchange.

A unique system of preferential streaming and shunting allows the most highly oxygenated blood from the placenta via the umbilical vein to be directed across the foramen ovale to the left atrium. The blood with the highest hemoglobin oxygen saturation is thereby available for perfusion of the heart and brain. The neonate, who no longer has access to a placenta but does have potentially patent fetal circulatory pathways (the foramen ovale and the ductus arteriosus), may exhibit similar vascular responses to asphyxia, resulting in the shunting of blood through fetal pathways (toward umbilical arteries that are no longer connected to a placenta), which may lead paradoxically to serious injury or death rather than correction of the metabolic crisis.[7] For the neonate the "appropriate" response of the fetus becomes an "inappropriate" response, contributing further to hypoxemia, hypercarbia, and acidosis.

This "vicious cycle" of physiologic responses often does not break spontaneously until injury has occurred or even until death approaches. Fortunately, correction of the "handmaidens of asphyxia" can usually be achieved with the appropriate use of assisted ventilation, improvement in oxygenation, and fluid resuscitation. Similarly, because the responsibility for maintenance of normoglycemia must be assumed by the neonatal liver immediately after birth, the distressed infant may be at risk for hypoglycemia if hepatic glycogen stores are inadequate or cannot be mobilized. Removal of the infant from the protected thermal environment of the uterus also mandates markedly increased thermogenesis, which poses a particular challenge for the small, wet infant in a cool delivery room. Superimposition of these dramatic physiologic adaptations on any pathologic processes leading to neonatal distress dictates that neonatal resuscitation must incorporate facilitation of the transition from fetus to neonate, as well as restoration of the prior state of homeostasis, which is the predominant feature of resuscitation efforts in older children and adults.

Anticipation of the need of resuscitation

This is one of the most important aspects of care that leads to a successful resuscitation. Communication among the health-care providers is paramount to this process. The details of maternal acute or chronic illness as well as complications of pregnancy and labor should be readily available to those providing care to the newborn infant.

Traditional methods of obstetrical assessment during pregnancy and labor allow diagnosis of many conditions for which neonatal resuscitation may be indicated, including prematurity, placental abruption, vasa or placenta previa, polyhydramnios, and possible sepsis. Recent advances in obstetrical practice have allowed both antenatal detection of fetal distress and antenatal diagnosis of specific fetal anomalies. Whenever these assessment tools provide evidence of any maternal or fetal abnormality that potentially compromises the adaptive response of the newly born infant, a resuscitation team should be in attendance at the delivery.[8] Some maternal complications, such as preeclampsia or vaginal bleeding, may place the infant at risk for prepartum or intrapartum asphyxia. Others, such as polyhydramnios, oligohydramnios, or poor fetal growth, may suggest intrinsic fetal abnormalities. Meconium staining of the amniotic fluid, aberrant fetal heart rate patterns, or a depressed pH of the fetal blood (obtained from the scalp) may indicate that fetal homeostasis is compromised; these changes may reflect underlying disease, such as congenital infection, which cause the infant to be intolerant to the stress of normal labor. Intercurrent problems, such as cord compression or impaired placental perfusion, may accentuate this stress. Prenatal screening of isoimmunization, elevated maternal alpha-fetoprotein levels, and glucose intolerance may reveal fetal diseases or conditions that are likely to result in fetal malformations or maladaptation. The increasing use of fetal ultrasonography, both routinely and in evaluation of other risk factors, has substantially increased the number of fetal abnormalities diagnosed early in gestation. More extensive discussion of these methods is provided elsewhere in the volume (see Chapters 10 and 11).

If delivery is not impending and the infant is not in acute distress, referral to a tertiary center should be considered when significant fetal abnormalities are diagnosed. Ideally, detection of one of these conditions should also lead to a concerted effort to identify its underlying cause, which often requires collaboration between the obstetrician (or perinatologist) and the pediatrician (or neonatologist). Thus, polyhydramnios should prompt examination for evidence of abnormalities of the fetal gastrointestinal tract or nervous system (by ultrasonography, for example). Preterm labor should prompt evaluation for fetal infection, especially if the membranes are ruptured.

These findings often provide specific diagnostic information that allows initiation of specific treatment by those responsible for resuscitation that can be initiated immediately after delivery; in many situations this can be of critical importance. For instance, if hydramnios is found, prompt diagnosis of a tracheoesophageal fistula or a duodenal atresia can be made readily, and prevention of aspiration can be instituted. In the infant with edema, anasarca, pleural effusions or ascites, prompt drainage of these fluid spaces can be carried out which otherwise might thwart resuscitation efforts. Responsibility for the exchange of information relating to fetal distress or fetal abnormalities, which should be a routine part of preparation for neonatal resuscitation, is shared by the obstetrical and pediatric staff.

Preparation

Personnel

Personnel trained to resuscitate distressed newborn infants must be readily available 24 h a day, in any hospital that offers obstetrical services.[8] Training and supervision of these personnel should be the responsibility of a physician or group of physicians, who are designated to prepare, review, and periodically revise protocols for resuscitation of infants in the delivery rooms. The composition of the resuscitation team may vary, depending on the personnel available in each hospital. In general, this team must have at least two members, one of whom is skilled in immediate assessment, initiation of resuscitation, and stabilization of the infant prior to transport to the nursery. He or she must be able to provide endotracheal intubation, assisted ventilation, umbilical catheter placement, and drug administration, as required. These tasks are often assigned to an anesthesiologist, pediatrician, or another physician. If a physician is not always available, these responsibilities may be assumed by a nurse or respiratory therapist. In teaching hospitals they may be shared by the house staff and/or neonatal nurse practitioners, but should be delegated only to those who have learned the techniques and principles of resuscitation under appropriate supervision. It is never appropriate to expect an inexperienced individual to resuscitate a potentially sick neonate.

When delivery of a distressed infant is anticipated, responsibility for various aspects of the resuscitation should be delegated to each team member prior to delivery. These tasks depend on the problems anticipated. One team member should attend to the airway and assist breathing, if necessary. Another should palpate the cord or ausculate the heart to assess the heart rate, provide this information to the team, and initiate chest compressions, if required. A third should be responsible for other procedures, such as umbilical vessel cannulation or thoracentesis. If necessary, others should prepare and administer drugs and record the progress of the resuscitation. Ideally the individual directing the resuscitation should not be responsible for any of these tasks so that he or she can provide full attention and direction to the entire team. Also, in an ideal situation, documentation of the techniques used, timing, the use and dosage of medications and the response of the infant to these procedures, should be delegated to someone not involved in the resuscitation. In situations where such documentation is not recorded immediately and is based on recall of events, many incorrect responses are charted and these can lead to serious medical–legal malfeasance.

Equipment

In many situations, the need for an infant to require resuscitative measures can be predicted, and appropriate personnel and equipment are readily available. However, Peliowski and Finer noted that as many as 50% of neonates requiring some form of assistance have no identifiable risk factors.[9] Thus an identifiable environment in close proximity to the birth of the infant, which is clean, warm, and has all of the resuscitation equipment necessary, must be available. Items that are required for resuscitation are listed in Table 34.1. This equipment must be checked periodically to insure that all items are readily available and are in working order. If the nursery is not adjacent to the delivery room, additional equipment may be needed in the delivery room or resuscitation room to allow more thorough stabilization of the infant prior to transfer to the nursery, as indicated in Table 34.1. Ready access to equipment for blood gas, hematocrit, and glucose determinations is also essential. In addition to these items, which should be routinely available, there are often occasions when additional materials are required. For example, blood products (preferably cross-matched against maternal blood) should be available for infants with severe isoimmune hemolytic disease or blood loss due to placenta or vasa previa, and large-bore intravenous catheters should be available to drain large pleural or pericardial effusions.

Universal precautions should be observed by all personnel in the delivery suite, and these individuals should be gloved and use other protective devices as necessary. Direct suctioning of the airway by tubing connected to the care giver's mouth should be avoided.

Immediate assessment

Immediate assessment of the distressed infant by experienced personnel is of critical importance. This process should begin with immediate observation of the infant's tone, color, heart rate, respiratory effort, and response to the stimulation of being dried with a towel or warm blanket for 10–20 s. Continuous observation of these physiologic parameters throughout the resuscitation should allow continuing evaluation of the efficacy of the resuscitation measures and the need for continued or more vigorous resuscitation. The traditional use of these criteria for assignment of the Apgar score at 1 and 5 min should not discourage earlier assessment of the infant's condition. Similarly, if the neonate does not respond promptly to resuscitation, Apgar scores should be assigned and recorded every 5 min up to 20 min of age or until the infant achieves two consecutive scores of 7 or more.

Most neonates respond quickly to standard resuscitative maneuvers and various algorithms have

Table 34.1. Equipment required for neonatal resuscitation

General	*Intubation equipment*
A firm padded resuscitation table with a source of radiant heat	Laryngoscopes with infant blades (Miller 0 and 1)
Overhead illumination (1000 lux minimum)	Extra bulbs and batteries
Wall clock with a sweep second hand	Endotracheal tubes sizes 2.5, 3.0, 3.5, and 4.0 mm ID (stylets optional)
Sources of compressed air and oxygen	*Umbilical vessel catheterization supplies*
Gas blender and heated humidifiers	Sterile umbilical catheter tray with instruments, umbilical tape, toweling, sutures, and stopcocks
Infant stethoscope	Betadine swabs
Warmed linens	Umbilical catheters 3.5 and 5.0 French
Gloves and other protective devices	Additional three-way stopcocks
Tape	Sterile syringes and needles
Alcohol sponges	*Fluids and medications*
Scissors	Isotonic saline 30- or 50-ml vials
Suction equipment	Isotonic saline or Ringer's lactate 100 or 250 ml
Bulb syringes	10% dextrose, 250 ml
Mechanical suction device and tubing	Epinephrine 1:10 000 (0.1 mg/ml) 3- or 10-ml ampules
Meconium aspiration device	Sodium bicarbonate 4.2% (5-mmol/10-ml) 10-ml ampules
Suction catheters 5, 8, 10, 12 French	Naloxone hydrochloride 0.4 mg/ml 1-ml ampules
Nasogastric feeding tubes 5 and 8 French	Infusion sets and tubing
Bag-and-mask equipment	*Additional equipment for extended resuscitation and stabilization*
Face masks (cushioned rims are preferable)	Pressure transducers and monitors
Bird or Bennett sizes 1–4 or Ambu sizes O and OA	Transcutaneous oxygen tension or saturation monitors
Anesthesia–ventilation bags, 500 ml, with adjustable pop-off valves and pressure manometers (nonself-inflating type preferred)	Thoracostomy trays and tubes (10 and 12 French)

Table 34.2. The ABCD of neonatal resuscitation

Airway
Breathing
Circulation
Drugs and fluids

been developed to assist the caretakers in developing an approach to this process regardless of the setting or cause of distress (Figure 34.1). After the initial rapid assessment of the infants' condition, during which time drying, wiping, and placing the infant on prewarmed dry linens in a warm environment is taking place, the ABCD approach to resuscitation should be carried out (Table 34.2). The infant should be kept warm during the process in order to decrease oxygen consumption.[10] Hypothermia and hyperthermia should be avoided. Newer data regarding the use of hypothermia as an adjunct in the treatment of asphyxia is an exciting approach in the treatment of the asphyxiated infant, and is discussed in Chapter 36 by Dr. Gunn and his coworkers. However, in the immediate newborn resuscitation, it is recommended that the infant be maintained in a neutral thermal environment.

Airway clearing and positioning of the infant

Several techniques have been utilized to clean the upper airway. A bulb syringe is often used to clear the mouth and nose after the head is delivered in an

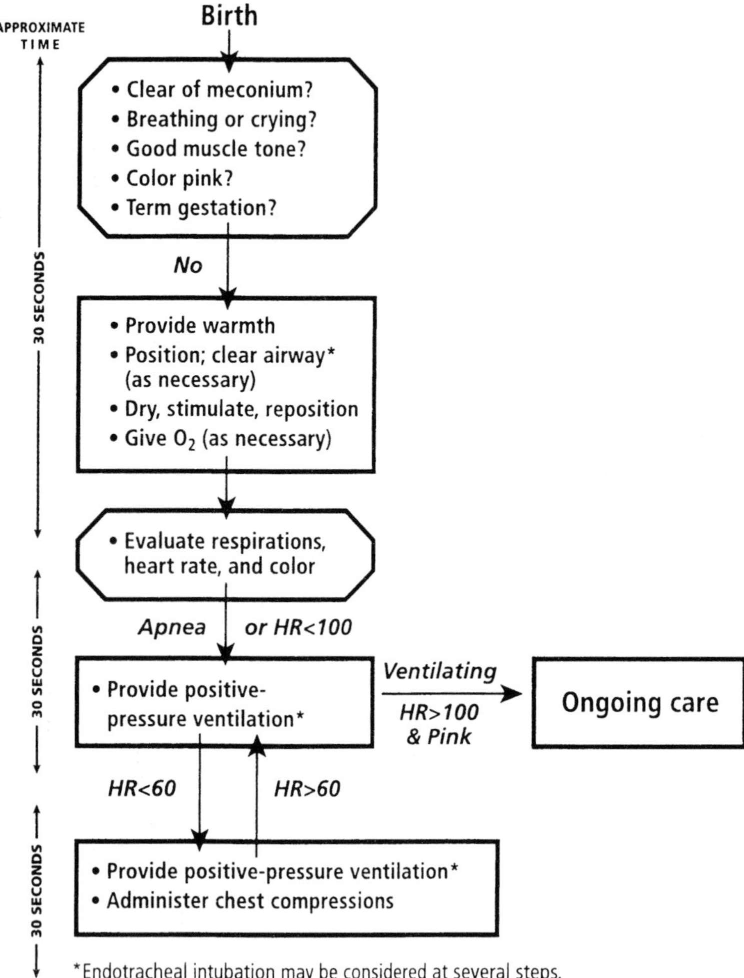

Figure 34.1 The resuscitation flow diagram. HR, heart rate. Used with permission of the American Academy of Pediatrics, *Neonatal Resuscitation Textbook*, 4th edn, © American Academy of Pediatrics, 2000.

infant in a vertex presentation. Continuing to suction the airway as the rest of the infant's body is delivered is also recommended. In breech deliveries this is difficult to accomplish and suctioning has to be instituted when the baby is placed on the resuscitation bed. Secretions can also be wiped away with a towel or gauze pad. One must be aware of various physiologic reflexes that exist in the neonate[11] and vigorous and aggressive suctioning of the pharyngeal area can cause laryngeal spasm and vagally induced bradycardia. The approach to the infant delivered in a meconium-stained environment is discussed later on in this chapter.

The infant should be placed supine with the head and neck in a "sniffing" position so that either bag-mask ventilation or endotracheal intubation can be accomplished. Often blow-by oxygen is all that is required for an infant who is cyanotic and/or bradycardic and this can be used while evaluating the need for additional support.

Breathing (ventilation)

Many infants who require assisted ventilation can be managed with the bag-mask technique. This is a very rapid approach and is much quicker than waiting for the baby to be intubated and then ventilated.[9] The face mask should have a cushioned rim and should provide a seal around the mouth and nose to prevent leakage. A small dead space of 5 ml or less is preferred. The pressure required to establish ventilation varies, but the peak inspiratory pressure and duration of inspirations should be sufficient to achieve good chest excursion and readily audible breath sounds upon auscultation of the chest. For the initial breaths, pressures of 40 cm of H_2O or more and inspiratory times of 1 s may be required in order to "move the chest wall."[12] These ventilation parameters can be reduced quickly as a normal functional residual capacity is established. Respiratory rates of 40–60 breaths/min should be used.

The two types of resuscitation bags include the self-inflation bags and the anesthesia bags. Although more training is required for using the latter, it provides better pressure regulation and oxygen delivery.

The infant should be reassessed after 30–60 s, and if spontaneous breathing is present and the heart rate is greater than 100 beats/min, then the bag-mask ventilations can be gradually eased and eventually discontinued. Gastric distension is one of the drawbacks of bag-mask ventilation, but it can be treated readily by inserting either a 5 or 8 French orogastric tube to decompress the stomach. In some situations, gastric distension can often protect the lungs from being overdistended during the resuscitation process.

If, however, the infant has not responded readily with this type of resuscitation, the infant should be intubated with an appropriate-sized endotracheal tube and ventilated appropriately. Endotracheal intubation provides definitive control of the airway and is easy to maintain during chest compression, suctioning to remove meconium, or instillation of cardiotonic drugs. It also avoids gastric distension. The position of the endotracheal tube can be ascertained by noting equal chest wall excursion, auscultating equal breath sounds in the auxillae with an appropriate-sized stethoscope, and by noting absence of air entry into the stomach. There should also be improvement in the infant's color, heart rate, and tone. Exhaled CO_2 monitors which change color in the presence of CO_2 have also been used to verify endotracheal intubation,[13] but these may be of limited value in small preterm infants.

Management of the infant with meconium staining of the amniotic fluid

This aspect of neonatal management is discussed at length in Chapter 31 by Dr. Wiswell. The current recommendations for the management of these infants[2,5,6,14] are somewhat different from those used previously.[3,4,15–17] The new recommendations change the basis for intervention from the consistency of the meconium (thick vs thin particulate matter) to that of the condition of the infant at birth. The newborn with meconium staining should have his or her mouth and nose suctioned while the head is on the perineum, and suction continued as the baby is being delivered.[18] If the infant is active, has a heart rate of greater than 100 beats/min and has effective spontaneous respirations, endotracheal intubation and suctioning are neither required nor recommended. The infant should be monitored carefully, and if evidence of respiratory distress or insufficiency or apnea develops, endotracheal intubation and suctioning should be initiated.

If, however, the infant is depressed, hypotonic, or bradycardic, direct laryngoscopy and suctioning with an appropriate-sized tube should be performed without delay. After the initial suctioning, the infant should be reintubated and ventilated. Repeated attempts at intubation and suctioning to remove particulate matter in an infant who has a low heart rate and no respiratory effort should be avoided. Such infants require positive pressure ventilation, and at times, cardiac compression, even though particulate matter is still present in the airway.

Improvement in cardiac output

While the literature previously recommended instituting cardiac compression if the infant's heart rate was less than 100 beats/min[3,4] more recent publications state that if the heart rate remains less than 60 beats/min despite adequate ventilation with 100% oxygen for at least 30 s, then cardiac compression should be initiated.[2,5,6] Although two-finger compression of the sternum is an accepted technique for cardiac compression, the two-thumb–encircling-hands technique placed on the lower third of the sternum may be preferred. The compression depth varies depending upon the size of the infant, but should be one-third to one-half of the anterior–posterior diameter of the chest. There should be a coordinated ratio of 3:1 with 90 compressions and 30 breaths/min.[2,5,6] The heart rate should be reassessed every 30–60 s, and compressions continued until the heart rate is greater than 60 beats/min.

In most situations, adequate ventilation with 100% oxygen and appropriate chest compressions will be all that most infants require. But if the heart rate remains less than 60 beats/min even with chest compressions, then the use of drug and fluid therapy should be considered. Identification and treatment of underlying disorders, such as pneumothoraces, congenital heart disease, or pulmonary malformations, also become critically important at this time.

Medications and fluid resuscitation

Drugs used in neonatal resuscitation may be classified as agents that restore or maintain metabolic homeostasis, increase cardiac output, alter the distribution of the circulation, alter pulmonary function or gas exchange, or treat the underlying condition.[19,20] Those in the first two categories are discussed in this chapter; the remaining three groups are addressed in Chapter 35.

Routes of drug administration

Drugs such as epinephrine (adrenaline) and atropine can be administered into the endotracheal tube prior to the establishment of vascular access.[21] However, vascular access is virtually always possible within minutes by cannulation of the umbilical vein.[22] Only the presence of an omphalocele or another major anomaly involving the umbilical anatomy precludes easy access. Although passage of a catheter through the ductus venous into the vena cava or right atrium is usually easy during the transitional period immediately after birth, it may not be possible after a very short time and generally is difficult after 12 h of age. Under emergency conditions the catheter can be inserted 3–5 cm until blood can be withdrawn freely. Although this is not optimal placement, fluids and drugs may be administered through the catheter in this position. If the catheter tip is in the portal venous system, there is a risk of hepatic or intestinal injury, but such injury is uncommon and the danger is outweighed by the risks of cardiopulmonary dysfunction necessitating the drug therapy. If a low umbilical venous catheter has been placed emergently, it should be removed and a new catheter placed under sterile conditions if central venous access continues to be required. Radiographic documentation is necessary to confirm appropriate placement of the catheter before it can be used for drug administration after the emergency has resolved. Insertion of the umbilical arterial catheter requires greater skill and usually should not be attempted during the first few minutes of a resuscitation, unless the resuscitation team is prepared for this procedure with designated personnel assigned to the task.

These measures ultimately provide access for measuring the blood pressure and sampling for blood gas determinations. However, intense splanchnic, renal, and peripheral vasoconstriction may occur after administration of catecholamines into arterial catheters, and must be avoided. Thus, the early placement of an umbilical venous catheter into a central position is advisable for the administration of vasopressor drugs, both early in resuscitation and in the extended care of the distressed infant. The distressed infant often has poor peripheral perfusion, making percutaneous venous cannulation for peripheral infusions or placement of a central venous catheter very difficult. Under extreme emergency conditions in which no access is available, an interosseous needle can be placed into the tibia or femoral marrow cavity for the administration of fluids and drugs.[23] This technique is not recommended in small preterm infants who have fragile bones and small interosseus spaces. As a last resort, drugs can be given directly into the heart, but this poses serious hazards, including intramyocardial infarction with necrosis, pneumopericardium, hemopericardium or pneumo- or hematothorax.

Epinephrine is the drug most frequently used during resuscitation when the heart rate remains below 60 beats/min. It can be given both endotracheally or intravenously and is indicated when there is asystole.

The use, indications, and effects of these drugs are discussed later in this chapter.

Restoration of metabolic homeostasis

Drug therapy in neonatal resuscitation is directed primarily at correction of metabolic abnormalities. Glucose, oxygen, and bicarbonate can restore or maintain metabolic homeostasis by providing substrates for cellular metabolism or by correcting abnormalities that impair the capacity of cells to utilize substrate. Naloxone reverses the effects of an endogenous agent.

Glucose

The infant depends on glucose as a major energy substrate during the transitional period. The cessation of glucose delivery via the placenta at the time of birth predisposes the neonate to hypoglycemia. Under normal circumstances the term neonate can easily mobilize hepatic glycogen stores as well as begin gluconeogenesis to maintain blood glucose levels. This transitional period is characterized by a transient fall of blood glucose levels, often to less than 30 mg/dl, achieving a nadir at about 1 h of age, followed by recovery to 40–60 mg/dl (0.4–0.6 mg/ml) by 2 h of age, even without feeding or other intervention[24] (see Chapter 26). Premature infants and intrauterine growth-retarded infants may have minimal glycogen stores and sometimes impaired gluconeogenesis, making them more vulnerable to hypoglycemia. Infants of diabetic mothers have abnormal metabolism, with inability to mobilize hepatic glycogen, impaired gluconeogenesis, and increased glucose utilization. Some premature infants who have been exposed to beta-mimetic drugs may have exhausted hepatic glycogen stores as well as enhanced insulin release. Moreover, glucose consumption may be increased by such conditions as hypoxia, hypothermia, hyperthermia, or infection (see Chapter 26). These factors account for the occurrence of hypoglycemia in many cases.

Hypoglycemia can be rapidly documented in the neonate by using any of several bedside colorimetric methods and should be confirmed by measurement of the blood glucose level by the glucose oxidase method. During resuscitation, therapy for suspected hypoglycemia often has to be initiated without the benefit of these diagnostic tests. If the clinical circumstances suggest hypoglycemia or if the blood glucose level is less than 40 mg/dl, intravenous administration of glucose (100–200 mg/kg or 1–2 ml/kg of 10% dextrose solution in water) should be followed by a continuous infusion of glucose at 6–8 mg/kg per min. Except when glucose utilization is increased, as in the infant of a diabetic mother or a premature infant exposed prenatally to beta-mimetic drugs, the administration of glucose at that rate is usually sufficient to maintain euglycemia. Infants of diabetic mothers, and sometimes infants with hypoxia, hypothermia, hyperthermia, or sepsis, may require infusions exceeding this rate, and therapy should be started at a rate of 8–10 mg/kg per min. Infants with adequate hepatic glycogen stores, such as infants of diabetic mothers, can be treated with glucagon (300 μg/kg, up to a total of 1 mg), administered intramuscularly, in order to correct hypoglycemia transiently while venous access is established. Although serious cerebral injury may

Table 34.3. Physiologic classification of hypoxic conditions

Physiological category	Group I Hypotonic hypoxemia	Group II Normotonic hypoxemia	Group III Hypodynamic hypoxia	Group IV Histotoxic hypoxia
Arterial O_2 tension	↓	↔	↔	↔
Arterial O_2 content	↓	↓	↔	↔
Arterial O_2 saturation	↓	↔	↔	↔
O_2-carrying capacity	↔	↓	↔	↔
Mixed venous O_2 saturation	↓	↓	↓	↑↓
Cardiac output	↔, ↓	↑↓	↓	↔, ↓↑
Tissue O_2 use	↓,↔	↓,↔	↓,↔	↓

not result from periods of hypoglycemia even in excess of 1 h, hypoglycemia represents a medical emergency which should be corrected expeditiously. Frequent measurement of the blood glucose level and repeated administration of glucose boluses until stable euglycemia is documented are required (see Chapter 28).

Oxygen

A physiologic classification of hypoxic conditions is presented in Table 34.3. The administration of oxygen is the most straightforward approach to correcting tissue hypoxia in many of these conditions. Hypotonic hypoxemia (group I, Table 34.3) is most likely to be responsive. Ventilation–perfusion mismatching, due to pneumonia or aspiration, or impaired oxygen diffusion, due to retained fluid or the respiratory distress syndrome, is likely to respond to supplemental oxygen alone. Other conditions usually require more specific therapies, such as assisted ventilation for hypoventilation. If there is fixed right-to-left shunting, as in cyanotic congenital heart disease, the administration of oxygen will not correct hypoxemia, but the lack of response may be of diagnostic importance.

During resuscitation in the delivery room, the administered oxygen concentration should be 100%. Until the nature of the hypoxia is delineated, it is appropriate to administer oxygen to any infant with cyanosis or respiratory distress. As the infant responds to resuscitation, the fractional inspired oxygen (FiO_2) value may be decreased but should be maintained at levels sufficient to relieve distress and keep the infant pink. As soon as possible, arterial blood gas measurements should be carried out to guide further adjustments of the FiO_2 level. In the premature infant a PaO_2 level of 50–60 mmHg (6.7–8.0 kPa) is usually adequate, but a PO_2 of 100–120 mm Hg (13–16 kPa) is more desirable in an infant with persistent pulmonary hypertension. Whether oxygenation is adequate depends on other factors, including oxygen-carrying capacity and cardiac output (see below). Failure to respond to oxygen administration should initiate a search for mechanical problems in the delivery system, such as kinked tubing, air entrainment, or disconnection of the oxygen source.

Oxygen is a drug, and it has potentially toxic as well as therapeutic actions. Inappropriate use of oxygen has been associated with the development of bronchopulmonary dysplasia, acute lung injury, and retinopathy of prematurity.

While most centers utilize 100% oxygen for resuscitation, recent studies have indicated that the use of room air is as effective as resuscitation with 100% oxygen.[25–28] Saugstad et al. reported on a prospective, international controlled multicenter study of

609 infants who weighed greater that 999 g at birth.[27] The study involved infants in both developed and developing countries, and had 288 infants in the room air group and 321 in the 100% oxygen group. Hypoxic–ischemic encephalopathy (HIE) grade II or III was not different between the groups, but the room air-resuscitated infants seemed to recover more quickly than those resuscitated with 100% oxygen. The long-term evaluation of these infants at 18 and 24 months of age is currently being conducted. Vento et al. confirmed these results in a smaller study, but also showed that the oxidative stress, as measured by the ratio of reduced glutathione to oxidized glutathione, was much lower in the infants resuscitated with 100% oxygen.[28] These data suggest that oxygen-free radical formation is reduced in the group resuscitated with room air.

Until more data are accumulated, the American Academy of Pediatrics and the American Heart Association still recommend resuscitation with 100% oxygen, but as the infant's oxygenation improves, the concentration of oxygen should be decreased as indicated by clinical and laboratory evaluations.[2]

Naloxone

Naloxone is a pure opiate antagonist that is useful for the reversal of respiratory depression resulting from maternal narcotic administration during the last 4 h prior to delivery. Initiation of assisted ventilation should not be delayed pending administration of or awaiting a response to naloxone. It must also be recognized that opiate intoxication does not produce cardiovascular impairment unresponsive to respiratory support, so naloxone is not indicated in that circumstance. The recommended concentration of the drug is the 0.1 mg/ml solution, and the current recommended dose is 0.1 mg/kg, preferably given by intravenous or endotracheal routes. Intramuscular administration is effective in infants with good peripheral perfusion. The previously recommended dose of 0.01 mg/kg and the neonatal formulation of 0.4 mg/ml should be abandoned. Naloxone should not be given to any neonate whose mother is, or is suspected of being, a narcotic abuser or is on a methadone maintenance program. The drug may precipitate seizures in these infants.

Bicarbonate

Correction of acidemia can result in improved cardiac output, tissue perfusion, and substrate utilization by reversing numerous detrimental effects, including impaired myocardial function, increased systemic and pulmonary vascular resistance, reduced response to catecholamines, and inhibition of oxidative glucose metabolism. During cardiorespiratory arrest or following severe asphyxia, bicarbonate may be given empirically at a dose of 1 mmol/kg followed by additional doses of 0.5–1 mmol/kg about every 10 min. In many situations appropriate ventilation and fluid resuscitation have decreased the need for bicarbonate in the resuscitative process. Arterial blood gas measurements should be used to guide the bicarbonate dosage as soon as possible. Unless the pH is less than 7.2, bicarbonate administration is usually unnecessary.

Metabolic acidosis caused by the accumulation of lactic acid after a short period of asphyxia usually corrects spontaneously, as lactate is converted in the liver to pyruvate and oxidative metabolism is reestablished. Persistent metabolic acidosis, resulting from the accumulation of organic acids, suggests inadequate delivery of substrate to tissues (decreased cardiac output, severe anemia), toxic hypoxia (sepsis, severe asphyxia), localized tissue infarction (necrotizing enterocolitis, intracranial hemorrhage, pulmonary hemorrhage), or inborn errors of metabolism. In these conditions bicarbonate administration is only useful as a transitional measure to allow survival until the underlying problem can be corrected.

Expeditious documentation of adequate alveolar ventilation is essential, because bicarbonate administration is contraindicated by inadequate ventilation.[29] In fact, the blood pH does not increase and the cerebrospinal fluid pH decreases after bicarbonate administration unless adequate alveolar ventilation insures excretion of the carbon dioxide generated by the buffer reaction.[30] Overcorrection of the pH early in resuscitation may also be detrimental, because subsequent metabolism of endogenous acids may lead to significant metabolic alkalosis, which impairs the dissociation of oxygen from hemoglobin and may impede oxygen delivery. Rapid infusion of hypertonic solutions should also be avoided.[31,32] The drug should be infused over 5–10 min, and the concentration should not exceed 0.5 mmol/ml (1000 mosmol/l). Catecholamines are inactivated by bicarbonate and calcium salts cause precipitation.

Enhancement of cardiac output

Clinical signs of decreased cardiac output include pallor, mottling, prolonged capillary filling times (more than 3–4 s), and cool or cyanotic extremities. Because of immature autonomic regulation of vascular tone, these findings are variably observed in very-low-birth-weight infants of less than 28 weeks' gestation, even when cardiac output is severely compromised. Hypotension and tachycardia may be manifestations of decreased cardiac output, but the absence of these findings does not rule out impaired cardiac output; sick newborn infants may not mount an adequate sympathetic response (and thus no tachycardia), and the blood pressure may be maintained by increased systemic vascular resistance, even with a substantially impaired systemic blood flow. Thus, the arterial blood pressure in the neonate should be measured immediately upon admission to the nursery, if not in the delivery room, because a low systemic blood pressure can be the sole cause of persistent cyanosis and imposes a clear risk of inadequate perfusion of vital tissues. If a low arterial blood pressure persists despite initiation of cardiorespiratory support with 100% oxygen and assisted ventilation, supportive therapy should be undertaken immediately. Urine output, although useless early in resuscitation, later becomes another indicator of adequacy of cardiac output. A urine output of less than 1 ml/kg per h, a urine sodium concentration of less than 10–15 mmol/l (20 mmol/l in the premature infant), or a fractional sodium excretion of less than 1% suggests that renal perfusion or intravascular volume is inadequate. Unfortunately, urine flow and sodium excretion may be maintained in the immature infant because of immature renal function even in the face of hypovolemia. Inappropriate diuresis can also result from acute renal failure. Metabolic acidosis (see above) is a late sign of severely compromised cardiac output. Doppler echocardiography may provide semiquantitative information in a given individual[33] but more classic techniques such as thermodilution are unreliable because of shunting through fetal pathways.[34] Assessment of the cardiac output in the neonate therefore still depends primarily on the physical examination and clinical evaluation.

In general, the drugs that affect cardiac output exert their action through the following effects on the primary determinants of cardiac output: improvement of cardiac rate and rhythm (chronotropy), increasing ventricular end-diastolic volume (preload), enhancement of myocardial contractility (inotropy), and reduction of vascular resistance (afterload). Drugs that primarily affect heart rate and preload are discussed in the following sections; those used for their inotropic or vasodilatory effects are discussed in Chapter 35.

Methods of increasing the heart rate

Unlike the adult, the newborn infant does not respond to bradycardia with an increased stroke volume, because the volume of the relatively noncompliant ventricles in the neonate is not significantly increased by increased end-diastolic pressures resulting from longer diastolic intervals.[35] Cardiac output in the infant is therefore virtually a linear function of heart rate, and is substantially compromised by even modest bradycardia.[34,35] A heart rate between 120 and 160 beats/min in term infants or 140–180 beats/min in preterm infants is usually sufficient to sustain an adequate cardiac output.

Although the heart rate generally responds to the administration of 100% oxygen and assisted ventilation, there are other causes of bradycardia in the neonate. The correction of bradycardia is generally nonspecific, although there may be specific causes, including increased vagal tone (often because of visceral distension), central nervous system dysfunction (associated with the postasphyxial state), congenital heart block (which may be associated with maternal systemic lupus erythematosus), and maternal medication (such as propranolol). Low-birth-weight infants occasionally may have low heart rates because of hypocalcemia. Besides decompression of a distended organ, such as the intestine or bladder, persistent bradycardia can be treated with atropine, calcium administration in the low-birth-weight infant, or chronotropic drug support.

Epinephrine and isoproterenol

Epinephrine can be administered in infants with bradycardia or asystole and may help restore myocardial contractility in infants with electromechanical dissociation. The dose (0.1 ml/kg of a 1/10000 solution intravenously) may be repeated every 3–5 min until an adequate cardiac rhythm is obtained. Endotracheal administration is also effective, but larger doses (up to 0.3 ml/kg) may be required.[21] High-dose epinephrine (1–2 ml/kg) has been advocated, but favorable effects in animal models have not been followed by demonstration of improved outcomes in infants, children and even adults using this strategy.[36] The drug has both β-and α-adrenergic effects and remains the primary choice for managing bradycardia in the neonate.[37] If repeated doses are required to maintain a heart rate of greater than 120 beats/min, an isoproterenol infusion (50–250 ng/kg per min, titrated to achieve the desired heart rate) can be started. If α-adrenergic effects are desirable, epinephrine can be infused continuously (50–250 ng/kg per min). The latter drug is better for maintaining systemic arterial pressure, as hypotension commonly complicates infusion of isoproterenol at higher doses. Isoproterenol is a pure β-adrenergic agonist. Notably, epinephrine is ineffective if the systemic pH is less than 7.1 and is inactivated by admixture with alkaline solutions. Tachycardia can occur, and excessive doses may impair renal, splanchnic, or peripheral perfusion. Extravasation of the drug peripherally or intramyocardial injection may cause local tissue necrosis.

Atropine

The dosage of atropine is 0.01–0.04 mg/kg every 2–5 min, as indicated for bradycardia with compromised cardiac output or for second- or third-degree heart block. It may also be effective for asystole refractory to epinephrine and calcium, but this circumstance is encountered infrequently. Because the response is dependent on vagolytic effects mediated by peripheral blockade of the muscarinic effects of acetylcholine, the degree of vagal tone is an important determinant of the efficacy of atropine. Vagal blockade is usually complete after cumulative doses of 0.1 mg/kg; thus, doses in excess of this amount are unlikely to be beneficial. A minimum dose of 0.1 mg has been recommended since an insufficient dose may stimulate medullary vagal nuclei and cause paradoxic bradycardia, but even this dose may be toxic in small infants. Atropine can cause tachyarrhythmias and increases myocardial oxygen consumption at therapeutic doses.

Cardioversion and defibrillation

Electrical stimulation of the heart is rarely indicated during neonatal resuscitation in the delivery room, because infants who might require this therapy usually have already sustained an overwhelming injury. The dose is 1–2 W/s per kg using pediatric paddles, which may occasionally restore a normal cardiac rhythm in infants with ventricular fibrillation, ventricular tachycardia, or asystole.

Drugs that increase preload

Fluid resuscitation

Because the cardiac ventricles of the neonate are less compliant than those of adults, increased cardiac output does not result from expansion of an already adequate vascular volume.[35] None the less, inadequate end-diastolic pressure due to decreased intravascular volume is one of the most common correctable causes of decreased cardiac output in the neonate, and hypovolemia should always be suspected in an infant who appears to be poorly perfused in spite of an adequate heart rate and assisted ventilation. This condition should also be expected in several clinical circumstances, such as placenta or vasa previa and severe hydrops fetalis. Hypovolemia may masquerade as respiratory distress, presenting with grunting respiration in the absence of apparent pulmonary disease, arterial spasm associated with an umbilical artery catheter, or refractory hypoxemia in an infant who is easily ventilated (Table 34.4).

If hypovolemia is suspected, the best diagnostic procedure is also therapeutic: administration of 10–20 ml/kg of isotonic saline. In the acute resuscitation situation, the clinical response (improved color and perfusion) may be the only indicator of efficacy. Later, invasive measurement of the central venous pressure, which is most readily achieved by catheterization of the umbilical vein, may serve as a guide to the adequacy of the intravascular volume. Positioning of the catheter tip must be documented, because crossing into the left atrium is not uncommon. Central venous pressures as high as 8–10 mmHg (1.1–1.3 kPa) or left atrial pressures of 12–15 mmHg (1.6–2.0 kPa) may be required to achieve an optimal cardiac output in a sick infant. End-diastolic pressures are slightly lower. However, isolated measurement of the central venous pressure is of little value unless considered in a clinical context; no reliance should be placed on absolute numbers without establishing their relationship to the clinical condition of the neonate. The intravascular volume may be adequate or excessive with a high central venous pressure, which may simply reflect a reduced capacity of the ventricles to accommodate and pump the quantity of blood returning to the heart (heart failure). If the central venous pressure is subnormal, the effects of transfusion of blood or plasma should be assessed. If blood or colloid solution is not available, the administration of crystalloid solution will temporarily increase the intravascular volume and cardiac output. If the infusions result in a sustained increase in the central venous or left atrial pressure, it can be assumed that the intravascular volume is adequate, especially if blood pressure and peripheral perfusion also improve. If filling pressures are not increased after volume administration, or rapidly decline to preinfusion levels, the infant is hypovolemic, and additional volume expansion is indicated. A single infusion may not be adequate for sustaining the blood pressure, necessitating continuous monitoring and repeated small infusions as indicated by the clinical condition of the neonate. In septic or severely asphyxiated infants, in whom significant capillary leak may be in evidence, surprisingly large quantities of volume expanders may be required to achieve an intravascular volume sufficient to maintain a cardiac output adequate for vital organ metabolism. Occasionally the fluid needed to maintain the intravascular volume may exceed the infant's blood volume.

Table 34.4. Signs of hypovolemia in the neonate

Poor capillary filling, pallor, mottling
Respiratory insufficiency in the absence of apparent lung disease
Arterial spasm secondary to the presence of an arterial catheter
Decreased mean arterial pressure
Persistently poor oxygenation in an infant who is readily ventilated
Persistent metabolic acidosis
Decreased venous pressure
Decreased urinary output

Crystalloid and colloid solutions

Isotonic saline and lactated Ringer's solutions are always readily available, inexpensive, and well tolerated when used empirically. The dosage is 20 ml/kg, which may be given in two doses of 10 ml/kg. After administration, complications such as hyponatremia, hypervolemia, and metabolic acidosis are highly unlikely. Albumin or plasma protein fractions are also readily available and easily stored. The dosage is 10 ml/kg. Although these drugs are distributed primarily into the vascular space, these effects are short-lived, and the protein may be distributed extravascularly into the periphery or pulmonary tissues, exacerbating anasarca and pulmonary edema. These products are also expensive.

Several studies have evaluated the benefits of crystalloid solutions in comparison to infusion of albumin in preterm infants.[38–46] In the study by So et al.[42] there were no differences in blood pressure, oxygenation states, need for ionotropic support, or incidence of chronic lung disease when the two were compared. Greenough[44] studied 30 preterm infants with albumin concentrations equal to or less than 3 g/dl. There were no differences in ventilation settings or oxygenation, but later follow-up data showed a greater mortality rate in the group recovering albumin as compared to the recovery crystalloids.[44]

A metaanalysis by the Cochrane group found an increased mortality rate with the use of albumin compared to no treatment or use of crystalloids in patients who required fluid resuscitation.[43] There were numerous drawbacks to these data, especially that few infants were included in the analysis and none were resuscitated in the delivery room. Nevertheless, in most situations crystalloid appears to be as effective as albumin when fluid resuscitation is required.

If colloid is required, the preferred solution is fresh frozen plasma, which appears to be more effective than albumin in many situations, but this apparent advantage has not been demonstrated by controlled clinical trials.[39,41] The mainstay of volume expansion, particularly when blood loss is suspected, is packed erythrocytes diluted to the desired hematocrit level with isotonic saline. Cytomegalovirus-seronegative, type-specific or type O, Rh-negative blood cross-matched against the mother's blood is ideal and should be available if delivery of a severely ill infant is anticipated. Uncross-matched type O, Rh-negative blood can also be used in emergencies, but transfusion reactions sometimes occur. The hematocrit level should be measured within 4 h of administration of the blood to determine whether additional transfusions may be required.

Inotropic drugs

Impaired myocardial function can result from many conditions that require specific treatment, such as sepsis (especially due to group B streptococcus, which produces a cardiotoxin), metabolic derangements, including acidemia, hypoglycemia, and hypocalcemia, and intrinsic disorders of the myocardium, such as hypertrophic cardiomyopathy (infants of diabetic mothers) or myocardial edema (hydrops fetalis). Cardiotonic therapy is only indicated after correction of the heart rate and intravascular volume (combined with exclusion of anatomic heart disease and cardiogenic persistent pulmonary hypertension of the newborn) has failed to correct systemic hypotension and other signs of poor cardiac output, including poor peripheral perfusion, low urine output, and hypoxemia. During acute resuscitation, inotropic therapy consists primarily of calcium administration (see below). As the infant is stabilized, administration of catecholamines (dopamine or dobutamine) may also be required; these drugs are discussed in Chapter 35. Such cardiotonic therapy should be undertaken by the primary care physician only in preparation for transport of the infant to a level III nursery, in consultation with the neonatologist who will be caring for the infant in the level III facility.

Calcium

Calcium has been shown to increase the heart rate, cardiac contractility, and blood pressure in premature infants with hypocalcemia[47,48] and may be useful in infants with low ionized calcium levels, as may occur after massive transfusions. During resuscitation, calcium chloride (20 mg/kg per dose, given intravenously over several minutes) is the preferred salt. It may be useful in the management of cardiac arrest or electromechanical dissociation. The dose can be repeated every 10 min as required.

Extravasation of calcium results in rapid tissue necrosis. For nonemergency situations calcium gluconate (50–100 mg/kg every 4–6 h) is a better choice, because it is less toxic to tissues. The use of calcium in the delivery suite is becoming a rare occurrence. It is mainly used in the neonatal unit when an infant has a sudden arrest due to a number of problems, such as hypocalcemia, hyperkalemia, or electromyocardial dissociation.

Delivery room decision making

Although the primary focus of this chapter has been on the approach to diagnosis and immediate management of the distressed neonate, ethical dilemmas in the delivery room often complicate further early decision making, which impacts long-term outcome. The controversial and emotionally laden decision to forgo, initiate, or withdraw intensive care in infants of borderline viability or with catastrophic unrecoverable injury to the brain is fraught with difficulty and uncertainty for those who practice and those who review the practices of others. A recent editorial by Saigal on the limits of viability[49] points out the critical issues regarding decision making at the edge of viablity (20–25 weeks' gestational age), emphasizing the fact that predicting survival is intrinsically inaccurate when applied to an individual. Further, the likelihood of impairment in individual infants is even less predictable.[50–54] The same critical issues apply to all infants who have birth injuries and uncertain prognoses. Thus, parental influence is paramount.[55–57]

Stevenson and Goldworth point out that the emotionally exhausting decision to withhold or withdraw life support in the early transitional period after birth is common but should never be routine.[58] The potential for development of functional status in the fetus or newborn is the single most important factor affecting immediate intervention and long-term outcome. The dilemma is that, although there is a threshold of maturity or extent of brain injury beyond which survival or survival without devastating sequelae is not possible, the exact threshold for a particular individual is not known prior to the attempt to assist the person. Although the proportion of individuals who must face an ultimate threshold increases dramatically below 25 weeks' gestation, there is considerable variation in performance by infants provided with appropriate technical assistance. Even successful resuscitation may only lead to protracted dying with some later lethal organ failure, which is typically lung but may be other vital organ systems as well.

It is also important to understand that, for the very immature person, vulnerability is equatable with survivability in the delivery room. Near the limits of viability, all infants are vulnerable and totally dependent upon the caretakers in attendance and the environments into which they are admitted. Lack of attention to detail in terms of resuscitation, or lack of anticipation of the particular needs for certain levels of assistance, may doom an infant in terms of chance of survival or avoidance of injury. Although the emphasis is often on presentation of the infant, it is important to understand that the way in which the infant is received in the world may have a tremendous impact on survivability and long-term outcome. None the less, in the case of extreme immaturity or an injured infant, informed anticipation and perfect technical assistance may still not yield an individual who can survive or survive without injury. No two 24-week gestation infants are alike and they may vary considerably with respect to their incapacities and their need for assistance. No two asphyxiated infants are alike because no two mechanisms of injury are exactly the same.

However, the parental voice must be a loud one at the limits of viability and the extremes of injury. While the resuscitative reception of the neonate is obviously an essential ingredient of outcome, a simple selfish perspective, ascribed to "the best interest of the infant," would be better couched in a parental context, where issues related to quality of life and the interests of the family members and society are also considered. There is great complexity of decision making at the edge of viability and in the presence of devastating brain injury, because depending upon the judgments made by the care givers and guardians of the infant, a fatal or injurious event may ensue from that decision. Futility is contextual, and what is futile must be considered in the larger arena which includes not just the infant at the limits of viability and recovery, but what is technically possible in the delivery room, intensive care nursery, and what is available to support the person in a particular familial societal setting. Stated in another way, parental decisions should not be based on the self-interest of the parents alone, because that may wrong the infant. However, it is equally egregious to ignore the fact that the life of the infant is entwined with the lives of the parents and with society and it is unrealistic to support that the parents can choose for the infant without choosing for themselves. It is not the physician but the parents who are the appropriate surrogates for their children, modified by education as to what is possible or not possible, likely or not likely, and the societal perspective represented by court precedents.

The simplest recommendation might be to argue that, when there is doubt, infants should be resuscitated. However, a legal defense is not always the best moral defense. Rather than insist blindly that resuscitation should occur regardless of the immaturity or anticipated incapacities of the person, it would be best to consider that, if the physician's doubt is great, the physician should defer to the parents.

Summary

Neonatal resuscitation is among the most frequently criticized medical activities in medicolegal litigation. The practitioner is both obligated and well advised to insure that resuscitation of the neonate is consistently performed skillfully and expeditiously. Optimal resuscitation requires anticipation and preparation, which demand collaboration between the obstetrician and pediatrician. Resuscitation should begin as soon as possible after delivery and should follow a specific and well-designed protocol for infant assessment and intervention. The practitioner responsible for resuscitation must be prepared to secure the airway, by endotracheal intubation if necessary, provide positive-pressure breathing with a ventilation bag, cannulate umbilical vessels, and administer appropriate resuscitation drugs. Measures to address underlying conditions must not be neglected. Most important, this individual must take charge of the situation and direct the activities of the other health-care personnel assisting in the resuscitation, to insure that it is carried out well. Skillful resuscitation should minimize postnatal cerebral injury, by insuring adequate delivery of substrate to the brain, but cannot be expected to alter the nature or severity of injury that has occurred prior to delivery.

REFERENCES

1 Stevenson, D.K. and Benitz, W.E. (1987). A practical approach to diagnosis and immediate care of the cyanotic neonate. *Clin Pediatr*, **26**, 325–331.

2 Niermeyer, S., Kattwinkel, J., Van Reempts, P. et al. (2000). International guidelines for neonatal resuscitation: an exerpt from guidelines 2000 for cardiopulmonary resuscitation and emergency cardiovascular care: international consensus in science. *Pediatrics*, **106**, e 29.

3 Emergency cardiac care committee and subcommittees, American Heart Association. (1992). Part VII, neonatal resuscitation. *JAMA*, **268**, 2276–2281.

4 Bloom, R.S., Cropley, C. and the AHA/AAP Neonatal Resuscitation Program Steering Committee (1994). *Textbook of Neonatal Resuscitation*. American Academy of Pediatric/American Heart Association.

5 Kattwinkel, J., Niermeyer, S., Nadkarni, V. et al. (1999). Resuscitation of the newly born infant. An advisory statement from the pediatric working group of the International Liaison Committee on Resuscitation. *Circulation*, **99**, 1927–1938.

6 Niermeyer, S., Van Reempts, P., Kattwinkel, J. et al. (2001). Resuscitation of newborns. *Ann Emerg Med*, **37**, 5110–5125.

7 Smith, C.A. and Nelson, N.M. (1976). *The Physiology of the Newborn*, 4th edn, pp. 61–62. Springfield, IL: Thomas.

8 Neonatal resuscitation. (1997). In *Guidelines for Perinatal care*, eds. J.C. Hauth and G.B. Merenstein, 4th edn, pp. 115–125. ElkGrove: AAP, and Washington, DC: ACOG.

9 Peliowski, A. and Finer, N.W. (1992). Birth asphyxia in the term infant. In *Effective Care of the Newborn Infant*, ed. J.C.

Sinclair and M.B. Bracken, pp. 249–279. Oxford: Oxford University Press.

10 Gandy, G.M., Adamson, S.K. Jr, Cunningham, N. et al. (1964). Thermal environment and acid base homeostasis in human infants during the first few hours of life. *J Clin Invest*, **43**, 751–758.

11 Halbower, A.C. and Jones, M.D. Jr. (1999). Physiologic reflexes and their impact on resuscitation of the newborn. *Clin Perinatol*, **26**, 621–627.

12 Milner, A.D. (1991). Resuscitation of the newborn. *Arch Dis Child*, **66**, 66–70.

13 Aziz, H.F., Martin, J.B. and Moore, J.J. (1999). The pediatric end tidal carbon dioxide detector role in endotracheal intubation in newborns. *J Perinatol*, **19**, 110–113.

14 Wiswell, T.E., Gannon, C.M., Jacob, J. et al. (2000). Delivery room management of the apparently vigorous meconium-stained neonate: results of the multicenter, international collaboration trial. *Pediatrics*, **105**, 1–7.

15 Gregory, G.A., Gooding, C.A., Phibbs, R.H. et al. (1974). Meconium aspiration in infants: a prospective study. *J Pediatr*, **85**, 715–721.

16 Ting, P. and Brady, J.P. (1975). Tracheal suction in meconium aspiration. *Am J Obstet Gynecol*, **122**, 767–771.

17 Wiswell, T.E. and Henley, M.A. (1992). Intratracheal suctioning, systemic infection, and the meconium aspiration syndrome. *Pediatrics*, **89**, 203–206.

18 Carson, B.S., Losey, R.W., Bowes, W.A. et al. (1976). Combined obstetric and pediatric approach to prevent meconium aspiration syndrome. *Am J Obstet Gynecol*, **126**, 712–714.

19 Benitz, W.E., Frankel, L.R. and Stevenson, D.K. (1986). The pharmacology of neonatal resuscitation and cardiopulmonary intensive care. Part I. Immediate resuscitation. *West J Med*, **144**, 704–709.

20 Benitz, W.E., Frankel, L.R. and Stevenson, D.K. (1986). The pharmacology of neonatal resuscitation and cardiopulmonary intensive care. Part II. Extended intensive care. *West J Med*, **145**, 47–51.

21 Polin, K., Brown, D.H. and Leikin, J.B. (1986). Endotracheal administration of epinephrine and atropine. *Pediatr Emerg Care*, **2**, 168–169.

22 Kitterman, J.A., Phibbs, R.H. and Tooley, W.H. (1970). Catheterization of umbilical vessels in newborn infants. *Pediatr Clin North Am*, **17**, 895–912.

23 Ellemunter, H., Simma, B., Trawoyer, R. et al. (1999). Intraosseous lines in preterm and full term neonates. *Arch Dis Child Fetal Neonatal Edn*, **80**, F74–F75.

24 Srinivasan, M.D., Pildes, R.S., Cuttamanchi, G. et al. (1986). Plasma glucose values in normal neonates. *J Pediatr*, **109**, 114–117.

25 Saugstad, O.D. (1998). Practical aspects of resuscitating asphyxiated newborn infants. *Eur J Pediatr* **157** (suppl. 1), S11–S515.

26 Saugstad, O.D. (1998). Resuscitation with room-air or oxygen supplementation. *Clin Perinatol*, **25**, 741–756.

27 Saugstad, O.D., Rootwelt, T. and Aalen, O. (1998). Resuscitation of asphyxiated newborn infants with room air or oxygen: an international controlled trial: the Resair 2 study. *Pediatrics*, **102**, e1.

28 Vento, M., Asensi, M., Sastre, J. et al. (2001). Six years of experience with the room air for the resuscitation of asphyxiated newly born term infants. *Biol Neonate*, **79**, 261–267.

29 Bishop, R.L. and Weisfeldt, M.L. (1976). Sodium bicarbonate administration during cardiac arrest – effect on arterial pH, pco_2 and osmolality. *JAMA*, **235**, 506–509.

30 Berenyi, K.J., Wolk, M. and Killip, T. (1975). Cerebrospinal fluid acidosis complicating therapy of experimental cardiopulomnary arrest. *Circulation*, **52**, 319–324.

31 Simmons, M.A., Adcock, E.W. III, Bard, H. et al. (1974). Hypernatremia and intracranial hemorrhages in neonates. *N Engl J Med*, **291**, 6–10.

32 Papile, L., Burnstein, J., Burnstein, R. et al. (1978). Relationship of intravenous sodium bicarbonate infusions and cerebral intraventricular hemorrhage. *J Pediatr*, **93**, 834–836.

33 Alverson, D.C., Eldridge, M., Dillon, T. et al. (1982). Noninvasive pulsed Doppler determination of cardiac output in neonates and children. *J Pediatr*, **101**, 46–50.

34 Rudolph, A.M. and Heymann, M.A. (1970). Circulatory changes during growth in the fetal lamb. *Circ Res*, **26**, 289–299.

35 Romero, T. and Friedman, W.F. (1979). Limited left ventricular response to volume overload in the neonatal period: a comparative study with the adult animal. *Pediatr Res*, **13**, 910–915.

36 Gedeborg, R., Silander, H.C., Ronne-Engstrom, E. et al. (2000). Adverse effects of high-dose epinephrine on cerebral blood flow during experimental cardiopulmonary resuscitation. *Crit Care Med*, **28**, 1423–1430.

37 Zartisky, A. and Chernow, B. (1984). Use of catecholamines in pediatrics. *J Pediatr*, **105**, 341–350.

38 Emery, E.F., Greenough, A. and Gamsu, H.R. (1992). Randomized controlled trial of colloid infusions in hypotensive preterm infants. *Arch Dis Child*, **67**, 1185–1188.

39 The Northern Neonatal Nursing Initiative Trial Group. (1996). A randomized trial comparing the effect of prophylactic intravenous fresh frozen plasma, gelatin or glucose on early mortality and morbidity in preterm babies. *Eur J Pediatr*, **155**, 580–588.

40 Roberton, N.R.C. (1997). Use of albumin in neonatal resuscitation. *Eur J Pediatr*, **156**, 428–431.

41 The Northern Neonatal Nursing Initiative Trial Group. (1996). Randomized trial of prophylactic early fresh frozen plasma or gelatin or glucose in preterm babies; outcome at 2 years. *Lancet*, **348**, 229–332.

42 So, K.W., Fok, T.F., Ng, P.C. et al. (1997). Randomized controlled trial of colloid or crystalloid in hypotensive preterm infants. *Arch Dis Child*, **76**, F43–F46.

43 Cochrane Injuries Group Albumin Reviewers. (1998). Human albumin administration in critically ill patients: systematic review of randomized controlled trials. *Br Med J*, **317**, 235–240.

44 Greenough, A. (1998). Use and misuse of albumin infusion in neonatal care. *Eur J Pediatr*, **157**, 699–702.

45 Kavvadia, V., Greenough, A., Dimitrioce, G. et al. (2000). Randomized trial of fluid restriction in ventilated very low birth weight infants. *Arch Dis Child Fetal Monabaul Gd*, **83**, F91–F96.

46 Finer, M.N., Hobar, J.D. and Carpenter, J.H. (1999). Cardiopulmonary resuscitation in the very low birth weight infant: the Vermont Oxford Network experience. *Pediatrics*, **104**, 428–434.

47 Salsburey, D.J. and Brown, D.R. (1982). Effect of parenteral calcium treatment on blood pressure and heart rate in neonatal hypocalcemia. *Pediatrics*, **69**, 605–609.

48 Mirro, R. and Brown D.J. (1984). Parenteral calcium treatment shortens the left ventricular systolic time intervals of hyopcalcemic neonates. *Pediatr Res*, **18**, 71–73.

49 Saigal S. (2001). The limits of viability. *Pediatr Res*, **49**, 451.

50 Wood, N.S., Marlow N., Costeloe, K. et al. (2000). Neurologic and developmental disability after extremely preterm birth. EPICure Study Group. *N Engl J Med*, **343**, 378–384.

51 Costeloe, K., Hennessy, E., Gibson, A.T. et al. (2000). The EPICure Study: outcomes to discharge from hospital for infants born at the threshold of viability. *Pediatrics*, **106**, 659–671.

52 deLeeuw, R., Cuttini, M., Nadai, M. et al. (2000). Treatment choices for extremely preterm infants: an international perspective. *J Pediatr*, **137**, 608–615.

53 Vohr, B.R., Wright, L.L., Dusick, A.M. et al. (2000). Neurodevelopment and functional outcomes of extremely low birth weight infants in the National Institute of Child Health and Human Development Neonatal Research Network, 1993–1994. *Pediatrics*, **1105**, 1216–1226.

54 El-Metwally, D., Vohr, B. and Tucker R. (2000). Survival and neonatal morbidity at the limits of viability in the mid 1900s: 22 to 25 weeks. *J Pediatr*, **137**, 616–622.

55 Watts, J. and Saigal, S. (1995). Replies to malcontent. Fumes from the spleen. *Pediatr Perinat Epidemiol*, **9**, 375–379.

56 Saigal, S., Stoskopf, B.L., Feeny, D. et al. (1999). Differences in preferences for neonatal outcomes among health care professionals, parents and adolescents. *JAMA*, **281**, 1991–1997.

57 Lorenz, J.M. and Paneth, N. (2000). Treatment decisions for the extremely premature infant. *J Pediatr*, **137**, 593–595.

58 Stevenson, D.K. and Goldworth, A. (1998). Ethical dilemmas in the delivery room. *Semin Perinatol*, **22**, 198–206.

35

Extended management

William E. Benitz, Susan R. Hintz, David K. Stevenson, and Philip Sunshine

Stanford University Medical Center, Palo Alto, CA, USA

The events that comprise the period of extended intensive care of the depressed neonate are subject to medicolegal challenge less frequently than are those of the immediate resuscitation and prenatal periods. In part, this may be the case because infants requiring extended intensive care are among the most critically ill and usually are transferred to level III intensive care nurseries where their management can be supervised by board-certified neonatologists. The range of therapies that can be undertaken in these well-equipped facilities, with subspecialist consultants and specifically trained nurses and other personnel, is quite broad and encompasses a variety of treatments that address specifically identified disabilities or dysfunctions. Within this spectrum of medical practice are many different management schemes that may be acceptable. It is not the intent in this chapter to review all the management protocols used for the numerous conditions encountered in neonatal intensive care. Rather we focus on the early transitional period following birth and resuscitation, during which the condition of a depressed infant can be substantially improved by expert care.

Failure to provide competent care, optimizing the opportunity for cerebral recovery, while the infant is prepared for referral to a level III intensive care nursery, is frequently the basis for litigation in the USA. As is the case with the initial resuscitation, the condition of the infant during this period may have been determined by factors whose effects were incurred prior to or during the delivery and initial resuscitation, many of which are beyond the control of the obstetrician and neonatologist. It is also important to recognize that significant neurologic or physiologic compromise is not always evident in poor Apgar scores; thus significant problems may become apparent only after an infant with good initial Apgar scores has left the intensive care environment. None the less, it is possible to identify many infants who require continuing intensive care after the initial resuscitation, including all those who remain depressed, require vigorous resuscitation, or remain dependent on supplemental oxygen, assisted ventilation, or drug administration. The roles of pharmacologic therapy in extended intensive care and in the management of refractory neonatal hypoxemia have been reviewed in detail.[1] In this chapter we provide an overview of the aspects of extended intensive care that address maintenance of cerebral integrity and preparation for transfer to a level III facility, and provide recommendations for the implementation of these interventions by the primary care practitioner.[2] These interventions consist of sustaining ventilation, supporting cardiac output, correcting anemia, and evaluating and initiating therapy for hypoxemia.

Supporting ventilation

Assisted ventilation should be provided for any infant who is not able to maintain acceptable arterial blood gas levels without such assistance, or who does so only with extreme effort. The range of desired arterial oxygen tensions depends on the clinical circumstances, as indicated in Chapter 34. In the premature infant a $Pa\text{o}_2$ of 50–60 mmHg (6.7–8.0 kPa) is usually adequate, but a $Pa\text{o}_2$ of 100–120 mmHg (13–16 kPa) may be more desirable in an infant with persistent pulmonary hypertension. In some situations extremely vigorous support (with a concomitant risk of adverse effects, such as pneumothorax, adult respiratory distress syndrome, or bronchopulmonary dysplasia) may be required to achieve these "ideal" arterial oxygen tensions. In this setting it may be preferable to accept lower oxygen tensions (35–50 mmHg or 4.7–6.7 kPa) if this allows less vigorous utilization of positive pressure ventilation or greatly reduced inspired oxygen concentrations, as long as both the oxygen-carrying capacity of the blood and the cardiac output are good. These compromises should be made only after consultation with a neonatologist at a level III nursery.

Similarly, the target range for the $Pa\text{co}_2$ level depends on the diagnosis. Although the "normal" range is 35–45 mmHg (4.7–6.0 kPa), higher values are often accepted as long as the arterial pH level is not excessively depressed because these values may be achieved with less aggressive mandatory ventilation, especially in patients with pulmonary parenchymal disease such as hyaline membrane disease. Hyperventilation to achieve elevated pH values has been utilized in the treatment of persistent pulmonary hypertension.[3,4] However, extreme hyperventilation results in alkalosis which shifts the hemoglobin–oxygen dissociation curve to the left, which is unfavorable to tissues. The effects of hyperventilation on cerebral metabolism are not fully understood, but cerebral blood flow may be compromised by this maneuver.[5] Cerebral vascular autoregulation may also be impaired in critically ill neonates and blood flow patterns may change after hypocapnia.[6–8] Retrospective clinical studies have also suggested an association of hyperventilation, as part of a therapeutic approach to persistent pulmonary hypertension, with later sensorineural hearing loss and poorer neurodevelopmental outcome.[9–11] Moreover, attempts to hyperventilate the infant with pulmonary disease using conventional mechanical ventilation entail significant risks of pulmonary injury, including pneumothorax and pulmonary interstitial emphysema. Cognizant of the potential short- and long-term complications associated with hyperventilation, and with the assistance of improved adjuvant therapies (see below), some tertiary care centers now employ more conservative ventilation strategies in the management of persistent pulmonary hypertension.[12,13] The decision to implement either ventilatory regimen, however, is severely limited by the paucity of randomized controlled trials. In any case, the primary care physician should not undertake any advanced respiratory treatment procedures during stabilization in preparation for transport.

Recent advances in our understanding of the mechanisms of lung injury have suggested that changes in lung volume rather than changes in applied proximal airway pressures may be most important in the development of chronic lung disease in ventilated infants. These observations, along with availability of several devices that can deliver small tidal volumes at rapid rates, has permitted adoption of high-frequency ventilation (HFV) as a strategy for supporting gas exchange while minimizing pulmonary injury.[14,15] There are several kinds of HFV; high-frequency oscillatory ventilation, HFOV; high-frequency jet ventilation, HFJV; high-frequency flow interruption, HFFI; and high-frequency positive-pressure ventilation, HFPPV. Each kind of HFV and the device used for its provision has its own specific indications and methods of application, and it remains unclear to what extent observations made using one type of HFV or HFV device may be applicable to others. In general, the strategy for use of these devices is to maintain the lung volume above functional residual capacity using a constant distending pressure and delivering small tidal volumes at rates between 2 and 20 Hz. HFV appears to be at least as effective as conventional positive-pressure ventilation for management of premature infants with respiratory distress syndrome (RDS), and may be the preferred mode of ventilation in infants with pulmonary interstitial emphysema or other airleak syndromes. Both HFOV and HFJV have been studied as methods for rescue of infants with severe respiratory failure who qualify for extracorporeal membrane oxygenation (ECMO) while on conventional ventilation.[14–17] Such HFV rescue has been shown to be most likely to succeed in infants with severe RDS and less so for those with meconium aspiration or congenital diaphragmatic hernia. However, there are very few randomized controlled trials in this area,[18] making establishment of clear recommendations difficult. Plans for further trials of ventilatory strategies alone will be complicated by use of other adjuvant interventions, as well as by dissimilar diagnoses and responses among infants with pulmonary failure. Increasing utilization of HFV in combination with other therapies is likely responsible for a dramatic decrease in need for ECMO in neonates with persistent pulmonary hypertension.[19]

Occasionally, large vigorous infants cannot be helped sufficiently by mechanically assisted ventilation. Asynchrony between the infant's respiratory effort and cycling of the mechanical ventilator or a large contribution of chest wall muscle tone to the total pulmonary resistance may make it virtually impossible to achieve adequate gas exchange safely. To facilitate safe and effective ventilatory management, pharmacologic neuromuscular blockade may be required. The administration of pancuronium bromide (0.1 mg/kg per dose) or vecuronium iodide (0.1–0.2 mg/kg per dose) every 2–4 h may allow maintenance of neuromuscular relaxation, produce significant improvement in gas exchange, and reduce the risk of barotraumas.[20,21] Both these drugs have weak atropine-like and histamine-releasing effects, which may cause a reduction in blood pressure, tachycardia, and an apparent increase in skin perfusion. It is also possible that these drugs may increase the risk of intracranial hemorrhage. Sedation with morphine sulfate (0.05–0.1 mg/kg every 1–4 h), fentanyl (1–2 µg/kg per h), or midazolam (0.1–0.2 mg/kg per h), is recommended during neuromuscular blockade.

A major advance in the management of respiratory insufficiency in preterm infants occurred with the introduction of surfactant replacement therapy. Investigational use of surfactants became widespread by 1989, and commercial products were introduced in 1990 (Exosurf, an entirely synthetic surfactant) and 1991 (Survanta, a bovine surfactant-based product). Other exogenous surfactant preparations such as Infasurf and Curosurf have since been marketed in the USA and Europe. Administration of one of these products to preterm infants with RDS has rapidly become the standard of care, and has resulted in reduced mortality, fewer pneumothoraces, and lower oxygen requirements and ventilatory settings in these patients.[22–24] Weight-specific mortality has been substantially reduced, especially in infants less than 28 weeks' gestation, and the effective threshold of viability has been reduced from 25–26 to 23–24 weeks' gestations. This single therapeutic innovation reduced the total neonatal mortality rate in the USA by 10% in the year it was introduced. Unfortunately, the prevalence of bronchopulmonary dysplasia (BPD) appears not to have changed significantly. This is most likely explained by improved survival among the sickest premature infants since the implementation of surfactant therapy, and a concomitant change in the pathophysiology of BPD.[25] However, a recent metaanalysis of randomized controlled trials of synthetic surfactant treatment in preterm infants does suggest a decrease in the risk of BPD as well as neonatal mortality.[24] The dose of surfactant is 5 ml/kg per dose (Exosurf), 4 ml/kg per dose (Survanta), 3 ml/kg per dose (Infasurf), or 2.5 ml/kg per dose (Curosurf). Recommended dosing schedules also vary for each surfactant preparation. For small infants, "prophylactic" administration as soon as possible after delivery is preferred, but it does not appear essential to give surfactant as a "preventilatory" immediate bolus in the delivery room.[23] With larger infants, it is recommended that the infant demonstrate respiratory insufficiency, by having an arterial oxygen tension ≤80 mmHg (10.6 kPa) with an $Fio_2 \geq 40\%$ or an alveolar–arterial oxygen tension ratio <0.22, for example, before the surfactant replacement is given. This "rescue" therapy appears to be most effective if initiated within the first 4 h of life. In spite of extensive data from well-organized clinical trials, the optimal timing and numbers of doses of surfactants have not been clearly defined. Some analyses suggest that there is little benefit from use of more than two doses, but there may be infants with severe disease who benefit from additional treatment.

Term infants with severe respiratory failure have also been shown to benefit from surfactant therapy. Meconium, blood, and infection may inactivate or wash out endogenously produced surfactant; thus, replacement with exogenous surfactant has been added to the armamentarium of treatments for severe respiratory failure in newborns.[26] A multicenter, randomized, double-blind, placebo controlled trial recently demonstrated that a four-dose regimen of beractant (Survanta) decreases the need for ECMO without increasing complications in critically ill term and near-term infants with meconium aspiration, sepsis, or persistent pulmonary hypertension, especially if the treatment was administered early in the course.[27] In term infants, surfactant treatment is most often utilized in combination with other advanced ventilatory and therapeutic modalities. Administration of surfactant occasionally results in desaturation episodes, which could prove life-threatening for the patient with severe pulmonary hypertension. Therefore, prudence and safety dictate that surfactant treatment of critically ill and unstable neonates be initiated in a tertiary care facility where other therapies such as inhaled nitric oxide (iNO) and ECMO may be offered.

Surfactant use has not been associated with significant adverse effects. Neither the incidence of intraventricular hemorrhage nor that of patency of the ductus arteriosus has been consistently increased in clinical trials. Some trials have suggested an increased frequency of pulmonary hemorrhage, but this appears to result from increased recognition rather than a true increase in the incidence of this complication. The major hazards of surfactant use relate to hypoxic episodes if the agent is given too rapidly and air leak complications if ventilatory support is not reduced appropriately as lung mechanics improve after surfactant administration. Finally, although the course of illness is much less severe in treated infants, the time to recovery is not greatly reduced, and infants with significant RDS can still be expected to require assisted ventilation and careful monitoring for the first 4 or 5 days of life. For these reasons, it is important that all infants who are treated with exogenous surfactant receive their care in level III nurseries that are appropriately equipped and staffed to provide this ongoing care.

iNO has dramatically impacted the way in which term and near-term infants with respiratory failure are managed. The Neonatal Inhaled Nitric Oxide Study Group demonstrated that iNO significantly reduced the need for ECMO in term infants with hypoxic respiratory failure other than congenital diaphragmatic hernia, but did not reduce mortality.[28,29] Food and Drug Administration approval of iNO for specific use in term and near-term newborns with hypoxic respiratory failure was obtained in 1999. Investigations of applications of iNO therapy for other indications, such as severe respiratory failure in premature infants, are ongoing. A multicenter randomized controlled trial of early administration of iNO in term and near-term infants with respiratory failure has recently closed and results are pending. Many centers have also now made iNO available for transport, allowing stabilization of extremely critical neonates who may otherwise not survive transfer to a level III nursery. Complacency as to the reliable effectiveness of iNO therapy in avoiding ECMO may be developing however, and a temptation to use iNO routinely at non-ECMO centers has followed. The potential danger in this scenario should not be underestimated. The appropriate and safe use of iNO requires an integrated team comprised of respiratory therapists, nurses, and physicians, and is best carried out through an approach to initiation, weaning, and discontinuation of the drug following a protocol, at a center where ECMO is readily available.

Sustaining cardiac output

If the cardiac output remains impaired after correction of bradycardia (by assisted ventilation or the administration of epinephrine, isoproterenol, or atropine), hypovolemia, and metabolic disorders (acidemia, hypoglycemia, and hypocalcemia), as described in Chapter 34, inotropic or vasodilator drug therapy may be required.

Inotropic drugs

It is important for the clinician to remember that the absence of bradycardia by auscultation does not necessarily insure an adequate cardiac output because inotropy has an important role in this context. Some infants may have myocardial injury and dysfunction because of sepsis or severe asphyxia. Less commonly, myocardial edema, as with hydrops, may compromise myocardial contractility. Administration of beta-mimetic catecholamines may increase the stroke volume and cardiac output under such conditions. Such drugs may not increase the cardiac output in infants with structural abnormalities of the heart, such as endocardial fibroblastosis or congenital cardiac malformations (especially ventricular hypoplasia). Infants of poorly controlled diabetic mothers may have a temporary congenital defect characterized by hypertrophic cardiomyopathy. These infants may have a reduced cardiac output when treated with such drugs because of narrowing of the right ventricular infundibulum.[30] Knowledge of this condition would contraindicate the use of such drugs, or at least require weighing the risks and benefits in the context of a particular case. Finally, administration of these drugs is also unlikely to result in beneficial changes in the circulation if the heart rate or diastolic ventricular volume is inadequate, the pH is below 7.1, or they are inactivated by admixture with alkaline solutions for infusion. Tissue necrosis, because of severe local ischemia following extravasation, can be prevented by prompt infiltration with phentolamine mesylate (0.5–1 mg) into the affected area. In general, peripheral intravenous administration of the drug should be avoided, but this can be done for short periods in larger full-term or near-term infants. Intraarterial infusions or catecholamines are contraindicated.

Dopamine

Dopamine is the cardiotonic drug most frequently used in the level III nursery. Its effects are dose-dependent and similar to those seen in adult patients. Measurable beneficial effects may occur at doses as low as 0.8 μg/kg per min. Typically, however, the initial dose is 2–5 μg/kg per min. At this rate of administration the effect is predominantly dopaminergic receptor-mediated dilation of renal and splanchnic vessels, causing an increase in the glomerular filtration rate, urine output, and urinary sodium excretion. β-Adrenergic effects result in improved cardiac contractility, a moderate increase in the heart rate, and mild peripheral vasodilation, all contributing to an increased cardiac output.[31] Such effects are observed with doses up to 15 μg/kg per min, but any increases above the 5 μg/kg per min range may be associated with increasing α-adrenergic effects. These effects may result in increased systemic vascular resistance and arterial blood pressures, with a reduction in cardiac output and renal perfusion. The effects on the pulmonary vascular resistance and pulmonary artery pressure may be less pronounced under some conditions, and the α-adrenergic effects of dopamine may be useful in establishing a favorable ratio of systemic to pulmonary vascular resistance, leading to decreased right-to-left shunting in infants with hypoxemia refractory to mechanical ventilation. This differential systemic vasoconstriction may be observed at doses between 10 and 25 μg/kg per min, particularly when combined with vasodilator infusion. A rapid method of preparing and calculating infusion rates is to dilute 30 mg of dopamine per kilogram of body with up to 50 ml in 5 or 10% dextrose in water. This provides a solution for which the dose in micrograms per kilogram per minute equals the 10-times rate of infusion in millimeters per hour.

Despite its frequent use in newborn intensive care, dopamine is not a harmless medicine. It should only be used for appropriate indications, and its use requires continued monitoring. Even when used properly, it can increase myocardial oxygen demands and sometimes causes tachyarrhythmias. In unusual infants it can also cause intensive vasoconstriction and hypertension at doses that would be considered dopaminergic. This phenomenon is most common with excessive doses.

Dobutamine

This selective β-adrenergic drug can increase cardiac contractility and cardiac output but has minimal effects on heart rate and vascular tone.[31] It has been used primarily for cardiac shock refractory to dopamine infusion and is often used in conjunction with dopamine. It should be administered at a dose between 2.5 and 15 µg/kg per min, titrated to achieve the desired improvement in cardiac performance. In the context of sepsis it must be used with great caution, because hypotension can occur. There is generally less experience with the use of dobutamine in infants younger than 12 months, and it must be used with caution, particularly if used alone.

Epinephrine (adrenaline)

For cardiogenic shock unresponsive to other catecholamines, epinephrine infusion (50–250 ng/kg per min) may have to be used.[31] However, the benefits of increased contractility are often balanced against the adverse effects of increased vascular resistance.

Afterload reduction

Another strategy for the management of severely compromised myocardial function is to decrease the systemic vascular resistance (afterload). This should be attempted only after aggressive management of the heart rate, preload, and inotropic therapy have been optimized to improve the cardiac output. Administration of a vasodilator may improve the Frank–Starling relationship between cardiac output and end-diastolic ventricular volumes, moving the curve upward and to the left,[32] without affecting myocardial function itself. Dilation of arterioles and precapillary sphincters may reduce the systemic vascular resistance, resulting in increased cardiac output. However, cardiac output may decrease because of reduced preload which is due to increased venous capacitance; or it may be unchanged if these effects are balanced. Therefore, use of these drugs requires frequent assessment of cardiac output and continuous invasive monitoring of systemic arterial and central venous pressures. The intravascular volume must be at least normal and supported by judicious expansion of the vascular volume in preparation for vasodilator therapy. Blood or plasma should always be immediately available when vasodilator infusion is initiated.

Nitroprusside

Infusion of this vasodilator should begin at a dose of 0.25–0.5 µg/kg per min and this can be doubled every 15–20 min until the cardiac output and systemic perfusion improve, hypotension or excessive tachycardia supervenes, or the dose reaches 6 µg/kg per min.[33] After 12–24 h of hemodynamic stability, the dose can be decreased as tolerated, in decrements of 15–25% at intervals of 4–6 h, until it is reduced to 0.25–0.5 µg/kg per min, when the infusion can be discontinued. Occasionally rebound hypertension during weaning may necessitate moving in small decrements at more frequent intervals. Nitroprusside in combination with dopamine and intravascular volume replacement was previously used in the management of persistent pulmonary hypertension of the newborn to achieve a balance of circulatory resistances favoring pulmonary perfusion.[33] With the availability of iNO, use of this therapeutic regimen is no longer required or recommended for term and near-term infants.[28]

Management of anemia

The oxygen-carrying capacity of the blood is especially important for the newborn infant. Hemoglobin F interacts less well with 2,3-diphosphoglycerate, thus limiting any compensatory response to hypoxia by a shift in the hemoglobin–oxygen dissociation curve.[34] Practically, oxygen-carrying capacity of at least 16 ml of oxygen per deciliter may provide a margin of safety for oxygenation in the asphyxiated infant with a normal cardiac output. This translates to a hemoglobin concentration of 12 mg/dl, because 1 g of hemoglobin can bind 1.34 ml of oxygen. The "magic" number of 40% for a minimal desirable hematocrit level in a distressed neonate is thus derived. In infants in whom optimal oxygen tensions cannot be achieved, the increased oxygen-carrying capacity imparted by elevation of the hematocrit level to 50% may insure adequate tissue oxygen delivery, allowing marginal oxygen tensions to be better tolerated. These objectives can be realized by transfusion of packed erythrocytes, as described in Chapter 34; several transfusions may be necessary, depending on the hematocrit level prior to treatment.

Evaluation and management of refractory hypoxemia

The infant who remains hypoxemic in spite of ventilation with 100% oxygen is at risk for cerebral injury, depending on the severity and duration of the hypoxemic episode. Although the metabolic hallmark of severe hypoxemia is metabolic acidosis, it is better to suspect hypoxemia and initiate therapy than to identify its late consequences. A physiologic classification of hypoxemic conditions is given in Table 34.3. The practitioner should recognize that hypoxemia may be present despite a normal arterial oxygen tension (Pao_2 level greater than 50 mmHg or 6.7 kPa) or hemoglobin saturation (greater than 90%). In particular, severe anemia (physiologic group II) is a common and easily correctable problem, which may have consequences as serious as those created by a low oxygen tension. In fact, infants with severe anemia may present with respiratory distress despite having normal arterial oxygen tensions and oxygen saturations. A normal Pao_2 value with an arterial blood gas sample may be falsely reassuring in the presence of pallor caused by anemia or acidosis. Thus, the practitioner should remember that cyanosis may not always be observed with clinically significant hypoxemia. Conversely, a Pao_2 level as low as 40 mmHg (5 kPa) may be associated with an oxygen saturation exceeding 90% and adequate oxygen delivery to tissues, especially if hemoglobin F is the predominant hemoglobin and the oxygen-carrying capacity (red cell mass) is normal. Conditions included in group II (methemoglobinemia, hemoglobinopathies) are uncommon causes of hypoxemia in the newborn. From a practical perspective most infants with reduced arterial oxygen contents have arterial oxygen tensions below 50 mmHg (6.9 kPa) and present with respiratory difficulties. The physiologic processes contributing to this syndrome include alveolar hypoventilation, impaired diffusion of oxygen from alveoli into blood, ventilation–perfusion mismatching, and right-to-left shunting. Studies useful in evaluation of the neonate with hypotonic hypoxemia (Pao_2 less than 50 mmHg or 6.7 kPa), listed in Table 35.1, will be discussed later. In addition, the medical record should include a careful history and physical examination, which may contribute to the diagnosis suggested by those studies. Metabolic disorders (acidosis, hypoglycemia, hypocalcemia) and rheologic abnormalities (hyperviscosity) should always be ruled out before this evaluation is initiated.

Hyperoxia test

By definition, infants with refractory hypoxemia have already been subjected to the hyperoxia test, which consists simply of determining the Pao_2 level during the administration of 100% oxygen. Most infants who have low arterial oxygen tensions under these conditions have right-to-left shunting as a result of congenital heart disease or pulmonary vascular disease. However, some infants with severe pulmonary parenchymal disease may have persistently low Pao_2 levels owing to diffusion block or ventilation–perfusion mismatching. Those with the latter conditions often respond well to administration of continuous positive airway pressure at 5–6 cm of water (0.5–0.6 kPa), with a significant increment in the Pao_2 value. Contrarily, infants with pulmonary hypertension or congenital heart disease usually do less well during such administration and require additional evaluation.

Detection of ductal shunting

Simultaneous measurement of preductal (temporal or right radial artery) and postductal (umbilical, dor-

Table 35.1. Evaluation of the neonate with hypotonic hypoxemia

Test	Result	Probable diagnosis	Potential causes of error	Additional studies
Hyperoxia	*Pa*o_2 < 150 mmHg (20 kPa)	Pulmonary parenchymal disease	Reactive pulmonary hypertension	Consider pre- and postductal *Pa*O_2 or echocardiography
	Pao_2 100–150 mmHg (13–20 kPa)		All diagnoses possible	Compare pre- and postductal *Pa*O_2; consider trial of continuous positive airway pressure
Preductal and postductal *Pa*o_2	*Pa*o_2 > 100 mmHg (13 kPa)	Right-to-left shunting	Severe pulmonary parenchymal disease	
	Preductal < postductal	Transposition of great arteries	Venous preductal sample	Echocardiogram
	Preductal = postductal	Intracardiac or intrapulmonary right-to-left shunting	May result from cardiac disease, severe parenchymal disease, or severe pulmonary hypertension	Hyperventilation–hyperoxia test, echocardiogram, electrocardiogram
	Preductal > postductal	Ductal right-to-left shunting	Must distinguish pulmonary from reduced left ventricular output	Hyperventilation–hyperoxia test, assess systemic blood pressure and cardiac output
Hyperventilation–hyperoxia test	*Pa*o_2 > 100 mmHg (13 kPa)	Pulmonary hypertension	Hypoplastic left heart, interrupted aortic arch with ventricular septal defect, total anomalous pulmonary venous return	Consider echocardiogram
	Pao_2 < 100 mmHg (13 kPa)	Fixed right-to-left shunting	Must distinguish heart disease from intrapulmonary shunting	Echocardiogram, electrocardiogram

Source: From Stevenson and Benitz.[2]

salis pedis, or posterior tibial artery) oxygen tensions can be performed by the clinician while the infant is breathing 100% oxygen. If the postductal *Pa*o_2 level exceeds the preductal value, transposition of the great arteries can be suspected clinically. Right-to-left ductal shunting is present if the preductal *Pa*o_2 level exceeds the postductal value by more than 15–20 mmHg (2–3 kPa). If both the preductal and postductal *Pa*o_2 values are low, the absence of such a difference does not exclude ductal shunting. Shunting at other levels (foramen ovale, intrapulmonary) cannot be either excluded or detected by this test. Measurement of the systemic blood pressure and assessment of the systemic cardiac output are essential in interpreting this observation, because right-to-left shunting may result from a decrease in the systemic arterial pressure or cardiac output, as well as increased pulmonary arterial pressures. These hemodynamic abnormalities must be corrected before evaluation of the cause of

Table 35.2. Pathophysiologic categories of refractory hypoxemia

Category	Characteristics
Reduced systemic pressure	Ductal or intracardiac right-to-left shunting
	Usually no improvement in Pao_2 during hyperventilation
	Reduced systemic blood pressure or cardiac output
Pulmonary hypertension	Ductal or intracardiac right-to-left shunting
	Hyperventilation produces $Pao_2 > 100$ mmHg (13 kPa) in those conditions associated with partially reversible pulmonary arterial constriction
	If the cause of pulmonary hypertension is not associated with reversible arterial constriction of the pulmonary vasculature, the diagnosis depends upon recognition of prolonged right ventricular systolic time intervals and exclusion of intrapulmonary right-to-left shunting, cardiac malformations, and systemic hypotension
Congenital heart disease	Ductal or intracardiac right-to-left shunting
	No improvement in Pao_2 during hyperventilation
	Echocardiogram usually diagnostic
Intrapulmonary shunting	No demonstrable ductal shunt
	Modest or no improvement in Pao_2 during hyperventilation
	Usually no evidence for pulmonary hypertension

Source: From Stevenson and Benitz.[2]

refractory hypoxemia can be completed, using the studies described below.

In current practice, measurement of pre- and postductal arterial oxygen tensions to detect right-to-left ductal shunting has been replaced by color Doppler echocardiography. This technology permits detection of cardiac structural abnormalities, as well as shunt flows in either (or both) directions at the foramen ovale or ductus arteriosus, and should be readily available in all level III nurseries.

Hyperoxia–hyperventilation test

This test consists of measurement of the Pao_2 level during manual hyperventilation with 100% oxygen to achieve alkalosis. There is little evidence that hyperventilation, when applied for a short period as a diagnostic procedure, is deleterious to the neonatal brain.[3] However, if adequate oxygenation (Pao_2 greater than 80 mmHg or 10 kPa) can be achieved with moderate hypocarbia, this is preferable. If the arterial oxygen tension increases to a value greater than 100 mmHg in response to hyperventilation, the diagnosis of pulmonary arterial vasoconstriction can be made. Unfortunately, the absence of a response does not exclude this diagnosis, and other diagnoses, including hypoplastic left heart syndrome, aortic arch interruption hypoplastic left heart syndrome, and anomalous pulmonary venous return, cannot be excluded by this test alone. If pulmonary venous obstruction is present, hyperventilation usually does not improve oxygenation. Similarly, infants with complex and lethal diagnoses, such as alveolar capillary dysplasia[35] and surfactant protein B deficiency,[36] may have brief and incomplete responses to testing. Patients with these irreversible disease processes are often mistakenly diagnosed with uncomplicated severe pulmonary hypertension and frequently progress to treatment with ECMO, usually with definitive diagnosis made only on autopsy. It is therefore important for the clinician to be alert to progressively ominous indicators of more severe diagnoses, and respond accordingly.

Information obtained from these diagnostic maneuvers must be combined with that obtained from other studies, including chest radiography and echocardiography. These data often do not correspond precisely to a description of a typical infant with any of the conditions listed in Table 35.2 and

Table 35.3. Priorities in management of neonatal hypoxemia[a]

Promote oxygenation by administering 100% oxygen and assisted ventilation
Correct hypotension and/or anemia by correcting bradycardia and administering plasma and/or blood
Correct metabolic acidosis by administering bicarbonate (after adequate alveolar ventilation is confirmed by arterial blood gas analysis)
Correct hypoglycemia with intravenous glucose
Correct hypocalcemia with intravenous calcium gluconate
Correct polycythemia by partial exchange transfusion
Obtain cultures and treat potential infection with antibiotics
Request consultation from the neonatologist at a tertiary care nursery for any infant who does not improve promptly in response to these interventions

Note:
[a] Although these interventions are listed sequentially, it is imperative that they be carried out as expeditiously as possible; it is not appropriate to delay subsequent items while observing the response to initial measures.
Source: From Stevenson and Benitz.[2]

may appear to be contradictory or confusing. Thoughtful synthesis of all available information, including that from the history, physical examination, and laboratory studies, is required. All diagnostic information must be reevaluated frequently if it becomes apparent that the infant's condition has changed or that the initial diagnostic impression was incorrect or incomplete.

The primary care physician should have a clear understanding of the priorities in the management of neonatal hypoxemia. These priorities are summarized in Table 35.3. However, the ventilatory approaches and the pharmacologic management of infants with this syndrome surpass the capabilities of the facilities in which most primary care physicians practice, and it is invariably necessary to refer these infants to the regional level III nursery. The management of any infant with the syndrome of refractory hypoxemia should be discussed with the neonatologist at the regional level III nursery while transport is being arranged. The details of this management depend on the diagnosis, the facilities available, and the preferences of the consulting neonatologist. Most of these infants require attention to maintenance of the cardiac output, using volume expansion and inotropic drugs, as already described. A comprehensive discussion of the management of conditions that cause refractory hypoxemia is beyond the scope of this work; a brief review of three common categories of disease is given in the following sections.

Severe pulmonary parenchymal disease

Pulmonary parenchymal disease, such as bacterial pneumonia or severe hyaline membrane disease, that is refractory to surfactant therapy, administration of 100% oxygen, and assisted ventilation at low-to-moderate pressures and rates is most commonly treated by increasingly aggressive mechanical ventilation. This can be achieved in a variety of ways, including the use of an increased end-expiratory pressure, longer inspiratory times, higher gas flow rates, or higher rates of ventilation. In some instances these maneuvers succeed in improving arterial oxygenation. They must be used with caution, however, because they increase the risk of air leaks (e.g., pneumothorax, pneumopericardium, interstitial emphysema). In addition, excessive distending pressures may compromise pulmonary perfusion, resulting in increased extrapulmonary right-to-left shunting and exacerbation of hypoxemia. Neuromuscular blocking drugs may be useful in improving ventilator management in large vigorous infants, as discussed previously.

Diuretic therapy may help improve pulmonary gas exchange, especially if there is significant pulmonary edema. Diuretics are most effective in patients with hypervolemia or pulmonary overperfusion, but should be used with great caution in infants with pulmonary edema due to increased capillary permeability (e.g., in postasphyxial or septic infants), in whom intravascular volumes may already be diminished. The effects of diuretics result primarily from the decrease in vascular volume achieved by diuresis, but furosemide (frusemide) also increases venous capacitance, allowing translocation of pulmonary interstitial fluid into the venous system. Prolonged use of furosemide may lead to hyopkalemia, hyponatremia, hypochloremia, and metabolic alkalosis. Moreover, long-term furosemide use may be associated with renal calculi, related to hypercalciuria.[37] Thus, the use of other diuretics, such as chlorothiazide, may be preferable.

Persistent patency of the ductus arteriosus beyond the first 48 h of life is often associated with the shunting of blood from the aorta into the pulmonary artery (left to right), causing pulmonary congestion, increased interstitial lung fluid, and congestive heart failure. Such patency can exacerbate pulmonary disease in premature infants, leading to a requirement for increased mechanical ventilatory support and consequent complications. This complication is managed most effectively by closure of the ductus arteriosus. There is no uniform agreement regarding the optimal approach in selection of infants for therapy, choice of medical vs surgical intervention, or the protocol for medical management. In most centers active intervention is reserved for selected infants with demonstrable respiratory compromise due to left-to-right shunting through the ductus arteriosus. In most cases initial management can consist of fluid restriction and diuretic therapy. Such procedures can eliminate the ductus arteriosus as an important clinical factor in 25% of infants with hemodynamic abnormalities.

If ductal patency and significant pulmonary hyperperfusion persist, attempted closure of the ductus with indometacin is appropriate, if there are no contraindications to administration of the drug. Indomethacin is most effective if given in the first few days of life and soon after ductal patency becomes clinically apparent. Closure is achieved most consistently in premature infants with birth weight greater than 1000 g. Indometacin is used at a dose of 0.2–0.25 mg/kg, given intravenously two to three times at 12–24-h intervals. Other dose schedules may be preferable if drug levels can be monitored. A recent multicenter randomized trial demonstrated that ibuprofen may be as effective as indometacin in the pharmacological treatment of patent ductus arteriosus in preterm infants.[38] Surgical ligation is often required in infants who do not improve after treatment with indometacin. The effect of prophylactic treatment with indometacin on short-term outcome in preterm infants has also been studied by a number of groups, and is routinely used in some institutions. Dosage regimens have varied enormously, from 0.2 mg/kg given as a single dose to 0.1 mg/kg given every 24 h for 6 days. A recent metaanalysis of randomized controlled trials concluded that prophylactic treatment with intravenous indometacin results in significant reductions in symptomatic patent ductus arteriosus and severe intraventricular hemorrhage.[39] Available long-term follow-up studies suggest that such therapy is not associated with adverse neurodevelopmental outcome at 36 or 54 months' corrected age.[40,41] The incidence of clinically significant ductus arteriosus, in fact, varies greatly among institutions, reflecting differences in fluid management and ventilator management.

Glomerular filtration, urinary sodium excretion, and urine output can be affected adversely (decreased) after treatment with indometacin, especially in infants who already have compromised renal function because of large ductus arteriosus.[42] Administration of furosemide concurrently with indometacin may ameliorate these adverse effects, but theoretically also may reduce the efficacy of indometacin in blocking prostaglandin synthesis. Indometacin should not be given to an infant with impaired renal function (a blood urea nitrogen level more than 30 mg/dl (0.3 mg/ml) or a creatinine level greater than 1.8 mg/dl (0.018 mg/ml) or oliguria (urine output less than 0.5 ml/kg per h in the preceding 8 h). Because platelet function may also be compromised (decreased aggregability), indometacin should not be used in infants with a bleeding diathesis or a platelet count less than 60 000 per microliter. Because necrotizing enterocolitis and focal gastrointestinal perforation have been associated with oral indometacin use, the drug should not be used in infants with clinical or radiographic evidence of gastrointestinal dysfunction. Intracranial hemorrhage, detected by echoencephalography, may also be a relative contraindication to treatment with indometacin.

Refractory hypoxemia secondary to severe RDS has become much less common since the widespread introduction of surfactant replacement therapy. This treatment significantly reduces the incidence of RDS and markedly reduces its severity in infants who develop RDS in spite of surfactant therapy. Numerous studies of differing design evaluating the potential benefit of elective or rescue HFV in the management of RDS have arrived at different conclusions. Recent reviews and metaanalyses of available studies were unable to recommend conclusively any particular ventilatory strategy.[43–45] A multicenter, randomized, double-masked controlled clinical trial of iNO for preterm infants with severe respiratory failure sponsored by the National Institute of Child Health and Human Development (NICHD) Neonatal Research Network is currently underway.

Pulmonary arterial disease

Intrinsic disease of the pulmonary arteries is encountered most frequently in cases of persistent pulmonary hypertension of the newborn, which is often associated with meconium aspiration. Pulmonary vascular disease is also a common correlate of disorders which produce an imbalance between pulmonary blood flow and the ability of the pulmonary vascular bed to accommodate flow in utero, such as may occur with pulmonary hypoplasia (e.g., with congenital diaphragmatic hernia), premature (intrauterine) closure of the ductus arteriosus, and cardiac malformations associated with increased pulmonary blood flow or pulmonary venous obstruction. Infants with these disorders have both structural and functional abnormalities of the pulmonary arteries, typified by excessive muscularity and hyperreactivity to a variety of stimuli, including hypoxia and acidemia. These conditions are characterized by increased pulmonary arterial and right heart pressures, and right-to-left shunting via the ductus arteriosus and foramen ovale. The diagnosis and management of these disorders are addressed in greater detail in Chapter 32.

Table 35.4. Patent ductus arteriosus-dependent cardiac malformations

Right-sided heart obstruction
Tricuspid atresia
Pulmonary atresia or severe stenosis
Truncus arteriosus with ductus-dependent pulmonary arteries
Tetralogy of Fallot
Left-sided heart obstruction
Coarctation of the aorta (preductal or juxtaductal)
Interruption of the aortic arch
Severe aortic stenosis
Mixing dependent lesions
Transposition of the great arteries with an intact ventricular septum

Source: From Benitz et al.[1]

Cyanotic congenital heart disease

In a variety of congenital cardiac malformations, including those in which pulmonary blood flow must be derived from the aorta via the ductus arteriosus (because of obstruction of the right heart), those in which systemic perfusion is dependent on blood flow from the pulmonary artery to the aorta via the ductus arteriosus (due to left-sided heart obstruction), and those in which admixture of blood from the systemic and pulmonary circulations is essential for maintaining systemic arterial oxygen content (Table 35.4), maintaining patency of the ductus arteriosus may be life-saving. This can be accomplished with the infusion of 50–100 ng/kg per min of prostaglandin E. Once patency of the ductus is established, the dose can usually be gradually decreased to 10–30 ng/kg per min.[46] Infusion at higher doses may cause pulmonary and systemic vasodilation, but other drugs (see above) may be more desirable for these purposes. Higher doses of prostaglandin E_1 can be associated with diarrhea, fever, tachyarrhythmias, and systemic hypertension. Apnea can also be life-threatening, especially if the patient is not intubated. Because most community hospitals are not equipped to undertake definitive diagnostic (echocardiography, cardiac catheterization) or therapeutic (cardiac or vascular surgery) procedures for the newborn infant, this treatment should be initiated only in consultation with the neonatologist at a center capable of providing these services, where the infant should be transferred as soon as possible.

Management of cerebral edema

The management of cerebral edema in infants with hypoxic–ischemic encephalopathy (HIE) remains a controversial issue. Although data in human adults and in intrauterinely asphyxiated fetal monkeys demonstrated that cerebral edema is a major complication of HIE and begins soon after the asphyxic episode, extrapolation of these observations to the human infant is speculative at best.[47–49] Studies in neonatal rats[50] and dogs[51] suggest that the immature brain is relatively resistant to the development and severity of the edema that is seen in the mature animal. Based upon studies by Myers[47–49] and Brann and Myers in fetal monkeys,[48] it has been postulated that intrauterine asphyxia leads to intracellular edema, followed by generalized cerebral edema and increased intracranial pressure (ICP). This in turn leads to decreased cerebral blood flow and necrosis of brain tissue. Excellent reviews by Volpe,[52] Lupton and coworkers,[53] and Hill[54] suggest an alternate theory. That is, following the asphyxial episode there is loss of vascular autoregulation of cerebral blood flow. This, coupled with systemic hypotension, leads to brain injury and brain necrosis, which are then followed by the development of cerebral edema.

Not only is there controversy regarding the mechanisms by which cerebral edema occurs, but the incidence and severity of the brain swelling following HIE have not been clearly elucidated. Lupton and coworkers evaluated 32 asphyxiated term infants during their first week of life with serial ICP measurements, using the Ladd ICP monitor; and 26 of the 32 infants had correlative CT scans performed as well.[53] They found that 22% of the infants had increased ICP and that the pressure reached maximum levels between 36 and 72 h rather than within the first few hours of life. Levene and Evans, using catheters placed in the subarachnoid space to measure ICP, found that 70% of severely asphyxiated newborns had a sustained increase in ICP of greater than 10 mmHg, for at least 60 min.[55] In 23 severely asphyxiated infants, nine infants did not have increased ICP at any time, nine had marked and sustained ICP that was resistant to medical therapy consisting of hyperventilation and infusions of mannitol, and five infants had sustained but mild elevations of ICP which did not respond to infusions of mannitol. Of these five infants, three died but two infants survived and were subsequently found to be normal. In their series, intracranial monitoring of the 23 infants was of benefit to two infants who responded to mannitol and survived. (See further discussion of mannitol, below.) In later reviews, Levene noted that "there is no evidence that routine monitoring of ICP and appropriate management of the elevation of ICP makes any improvement in outcome" in the severely asphyxiated newborn.[56,57]

Table 35.5. Methods of treatment for increased intracranial pressure

Fluid restriction
Hyperventilation
Corticosteroids
Mannitol

Methods of decreasing cerebral edema

Since many infants with HIE have inappropriate secretion of antidiuretic hormone, fluid restriction and the avoidance of fluid overload are of primary concern. Careful monitoring of fluid intake and output as well as serum electrolytes is indicated in the asphyxiated infant. Other methods of decreasing cerebral edema are listed in Table 35.5.

Hyperventilation

Infants have variable respiratory responses to HIE. Some will hyperventilate, some will have a normal respiratory rate, and some will hypoventilate and be unresponsive to hypercarbia. By hyperventilating to hypocarbic ranges, cerebral blood flow can be reduced significantly. By decreasing the $Pa\text{CO}_2$ by 1 mmHg, the cerebral blood flow will be decreased by 3% over the physiological $Pa\text{CO}_2$ range.[6,58] The response is lessened when the $Pa\text{CO}_2$ is decreased to 20 mmHg or less.[6] Hyperventilation has been used extensively in the treatment of neonates with persistent pulmonary hypertension of the newborn, and this form of therapy has been associated with significant pulmonary vasodilatation and an increase in the $Pa\text{O}_2$ in many of the infants. The initial follow-up of infants treated in this fashion suggested that hypocarbia was safe and did not result in brain damage.[3] However, follow-up studies of infants with persistent pulmonary hypertension of the newborn by Bernbaum et al. noted that infants who had abnormal neurological findings had longer periods of hypotension and longer periods of hypocarbia ($Pa\text{CO}_2$ of less than 25 mmHg) than did infants without neurological sequelae.[59]

Bifano and Pfannenstiel also demonstrated that the surviving infants with persistent pulmonary hypertension of the newborn who had adverse neurological sequelae had longer periods of hypocarbia than did survivors without neurological impairment.[10] Similar to the data of Bernbaum et al.,[59] the infants who were treated with prolonged hyperventilation were most likely those infants who were most severely affected with persistent pulmonary hypertension of the newborn.

Gleason and coworkers, studying paralyzed and sedated newborn lambs, evaluated the effects of 6 h of hypocarbia with $Pa\text{CO}_2$ levels down to 15 ± 2 mmHg on cerebral blood flow. Although the cerebral blood flow was decreased by 35% initially, it returned to baseline levels by 6 h. Abrupt termination of the hyperventilation resulted in a marked increase in cerebral blood flow within 30 min.[6] These authors cautioned that if hypocarbia that occurs after hyperventilation is stopped, this could possibly increase the incidence of intracranial hemorrhage. Such situations occur clinically in neonates who fail to respond to hyperventilation and then require treatment with iNO or with ECMO.

Wiswell and coworkers studied a group of prematurely born infants of 33 weeks' gestation or less who were treated with HFJV during the first 72 h of life.[60] They found that the incidence of cystic periventricular leukomalacia (cPVL) was much greater in infants whose periods of hypocarbia during the first 24 h of life were greater that those infants in whom cPVL did not develop. Other factors, such as degree of hypertension, acidosis, or hypoxemia, did not increase the incidence of cPVL.

A recent study of 790 infants who were less than or equal to 28 weeks' gestation who had hypocarbia during their first day of life also reported an increased incidence of echo lucency when a univariable analysis was performed. This association was diminished when a multivariate analysis was performed.[61] Nevertheless, it is apparent that hypocarbia should be avoided in the infant if at all possible.

Studies by Vannucci et al., using an asphyxiated neonatal model, demonstrated a protective effect of mild-to-moderate hypercarbia in animals with asphyxia.[62] Severe hypocarbia did not offer this protective effect.[63]

To date, there have been no reported clinical studies evaluating hyperventilation and subsequent hypocarbia as an adjunct in the therapy of infants with HIE. Recommendations that hyperventilation be used to prevent or treat cerebral edema must be viewed with caution. It is currently recommended that normocarbic levels be maintained in these infants, and hyper- or hypocarbia be avoided.

Corticosteroids

Corticosteroids have been used effectively in reducing vasogenic cerebral edema, but they have had little, if any, effect in edema secondary to HIE, meningitis, or edema following trauma to the cranium.[64–66] Controlled studies in comatose adults secondary to trauma failed to alleviate the increased ICP or to mitigate neurological sequelae.[64] Similar results have been reported using corticosteroids following strokes in mature laboratory animals.[67] Svenningsen et al., in their evaluation of the protective effect of phenobarbital in the treatment of severe neurological asphyxia, used betamethasone and furosemide as adjuncts to their therapy, but did not specifically study the effects of either of these two agents.[68] Levene and Evans found no improvement of cerebral perfusion pressure when using dexamethasone in the treatment of infants with HIE.[69] Since there are numerous side-effects of steroids, including hypertension, hyperglycemia, and electrolyte aberrations, the use of these agents in an already fragile patient is not recommended.

Interestingly, Barks et al.[70] and Tuor et al.[71] have shown that, when neonatal rats are pretreated 24 h or more with dexamethasone, even at low doses, they were protected from subsequent episodes of cerebral damage due to asphyxia. Treatment with dexamethasone, even in large amounts, had no protective effects if given less than 24 h prior to or within 24 h of the asphyxic event. These data are interesting in light of the fact that preterm infants of mothers who had been pretreated with betamethasone and dexamethasone had a decreased incidence and severity of intraventricular hemorrhage in the neonatal period.[72] A recent metaanalysis of available studies has confirmed the significant reduction in intraventricular hemorrhage afforded by prophylactic antenatal corticosteroid treatment.[73]

Mannitol

Mannitol and other hyperosmolar agents have been used to reduce the amount of cerebral edema following brain injury.[74] Mujsce et al., studying brain injury due to HIE in immature rats, infused mannitol immediately after the event and every 12 h thereafter for a total of four infusions.[50] Although mannitol reduced the amount of edema and brain water, it did not alter the severity of the brain damage when compared to control animals.

Adhikari and coworkers treated 12 severely asphyxiated infants with a single infusion of 1 g/kg of mannitol and compared them with 13 similarly affected infants who were not given mannitol.[74] No differences were found in the mortality rate, the severity of cerebral edema as measured ultrasonographically, or in short-term outcome.

In an uncontrolled study, Marchal and coworkers treated over 200 asphyxiated infants with intravenous mannitol either before or after 2 h of age.[75] There were fewer deaths and better neurological outcome in those infants who were treated early than in those treated after 2 h. Unfortunately the types of infants treated and the variability in the severity of disease processes make the interpretation of these data difficult.

Although some investigators recognize the efficacy of intravenous mannitol in lowering ICP in treating asphyxiated newborns with cerebral edema, most authorities do not recommend its use as an adjunct in the treatment of infants with HIE.[52,63]

Other potential strategies as adjuncts in the management of infants with hypoxic-ischemic encephalopathy (Table 35.6)

Barbiturates

While barbiturates are readily used to control seizures that often accompany severe HIE (see Chapter 37), their use to prevent further brain damage after an asphyxic episode has also been recommended. Since the early 1970s, investigators have demonstrated that barbiturates decrease the rates of cerebral metabolism, decrease intracranial pressure, and reduce cellular injury due to the elaboration of free radicals.

Svenningsen et al. evaluated 35 term infants with neonatal asphyxia in two separate time periods. During the first 3 years of the study, 1973–1976, affected infants received what was considered conservative management. During the second 3-year period, infants were ventilated early and effectively, had aggressive plasma and blood transfusions, and were given 10 mg/kg of phenobarbital within 60 min after birth and then daily thereafter.[68] Betamethasone and furosemide were also added to this regime. Both the mortality rates and the incidence of neurodevelopmental handicaps were reduced significantly during this latter aggressive period.

Goldberg et al. studied 32 consecutively admitted

Table 35.6. Potential strategies that have been used as adjuncts in the management of infants with hypoxic–ischemic encephalopathy

Barbiturates
Excitatory amino acid receptor inhibitors
Magnesium sulfate
Calcium-channel blockers
Oxygen free radical inhibitors
Monosialgangliosides
Lazaroids
Growth factors
Hypothermia

term neonates with severe asphyxia, all of whom required supportive ventilation.[76] Half of the group was given thiopental infusions beginning 1 and 3 h after birth. Sustained elevation of ICP was encountered infrequently in all patients, and the outcome was the same in the two groups. Those infants receiving thiopental required pressor support more frequently than did the control group (14/16 vs 7/15). These authors could not recommend thiopental as an adjunct to therapy in term asphyxiated neonates. Similar data were obtained in adult patients who received thiopental following cardiac arrest.[77]

Hall et al. studied the effects of phenobarbital given to term infants with severe asphyxia in a randomized controlled prospective trial.[78] After the infant's blood pressure, ventilation, and acid–base status were stabilized, the infants were given 40 mg/kg of the drug. Seizures occurred in nine of 15 study infants and 14 of 16 infants in the control group. A follow-up evaluation 3 years later revealed that 11 of 15 infants in the treatment group had a normal outcome, but only three of 16 in the control group were normal.[78] There were a few drawbacks to the study in that a placebo was not used; after the babies were randomized, the caretakers were not blinded to the type of treatment; and five infants were lost to follow-up, two in the treatment group and three in the control group. Nevertheless, this was an important study in that no adverse effects were encountered with a drug that is often used in an intensive care nursery, and that it appeared to result in a significant decrease in neurological damage. As the authors note, more comprehensive studies using continuous electroencephalographic monitoring, magnetic resonance spectroscopy, and monitoring of cerebral blood flow would enhance the study of a much larger group of patients in a randomized, blinded, and prospectively carried out trial.

Excitatory amino acids (EAA) receptor inhibitors

EAA, especially glutamate and aspartate, are the major neurotransmitters found in mammalian brain. The EAA also have a trophic effect on differentiating neurons and are involved in the regulation of neuroendocrine function as well.[79] When hypoxic–ischemic insults occur, there is increased release of these EAAs up to 100-fold in the brains of adult animals and to a much lesser extent in fetal and neonatal brain tissues.[80] These EAAs activate postsynaptic receptors which in turn are coupled to channels that regulate the flow of sodium and calcium ions into the cell. There are two major types of receptors, metabotropic and ionotropic, the latter of which has been extensively studied. The major subtypes of the ionotropic receptors are *N*-methyl-D-aspartate (NMDA) and α-amino-3-hydroxy-5-methyl-4-isoxazole propionic acid (AMPA). This latter receptor also mediates the effects of kainic acid and is referred to as the AMPA/kainic acid (KA) receptor.[81]

Antagonists to these receptors have been studied and utilized, and have also been divided into the subtypes competitive and noncompetitive antagonists. The competitive antagonists block the glutamate site directly, but because they are polar substances, do not cross the blood–brain barrier readily. The noncompetitive antagonists to NMDA are utilized more frequently as they do cross the blood–brain barrier readily. These compounds include ketamine, phencyclidine (PCP or angel dust), dizocilpine (MK-801), aptiganel hydrochloride (CNS 112, Cerestat) and dextrorotary opioid derivatives, such as dextrorphan and dextromethorphan.[81,82]

MK-801, which has the highest affinity for the ion-channel site, has demonstrated significant neuroprotective effects in both adult and newborn animals. This agent is effective when given prior to or following the asphyxic event in decreasing, but not abolishing the neuronal damage. However, the toxicity of the agent is profound, even when used in low dosage, and neurobehavioral changes in the surviving animals have been noted as well.[82]

Dextromethorphan is another noncompetitive NMDA antagonist and has demonstrated neuroprotective effects in a rabbit model of transient ischemia.[83,84] The use of this agent as an adjunct to prophylactic therapy in patients undergoing neurosurgical procedures has also demonstrated beneficial effects with modest and reversible side-effects.[81] Whether this agent will prove to have neuroprotective effects without inducing other abnormalities following an asphyxic insult remains to be seen.

A competitive NMDA receptor antagonist, selfotel, which binds directly to the NMDA site of the glutamate receptor had been shown to limit neuronal damage in several animal stroke studies. It was used as a single 1.5 mg/kg dose in humans to evaluate whether it could reduce mortality from acute ischemic stroke. Unfortunately, it was shown not to be an effective form of therapy for acute ischemic stroke, and even exhibited neurotoxic effects in brain ischemia patients.[85]

The magnesium ion also acts as a noncompetitive NMDA antagonist,[86] and has improved survival following myocardial infarctions and has been associated with decreased neurological damage following traumatic brain injury and strokes in adults.[87] Magnesium sulfate ($MgSO_4$) has been used as a tocolytic agent, an antihypertensive agent, and as protection against the development of seizures in women with preeclampsia.[88]

$MgSO_4$ has reduced the severity of asphyxiated brain damage in immature rats[89] and mice,[90] but when studied in near-term fetal lambs[91] and piglets,[92] it did not reduce injury to the cerebral cortex.

Levene et al. evaluated two different doses of $MgSO_4$ in a group of infants when 10-min Apgar scores were less than 6, or a 5-min Apgar score of less than 6 with other clinical and laboratory evidence of fetal distress.[93] The infants received either 250 or 400 mg/kg intravenously. All of the infants receiving 400 mg/kg had cessation of respiratory function for 3–6 h, but since the infants had already been intubated and ventilated, no harm was encountered. The electroencephalogram did not change, but muscle tone and activity were diminished. The infants also had significant lowering of blood pressure. The lower dose did not cause hypotension but did cause some respiratory depression. These authors have advised against using the higher dose of $MgSO_4$, and also cautioned that respiratory failure can occur even with the lower dose. A multicenter study to evaluate $MgSO_4$ as a neuroprotector has been suspended.[94]

Calcium-channel blockers

Because of the toxicity of increased intracellular calcium accumulation that occurs when a cell is damaged, various drugs have been developed to prevent the influx of the ion into neurons. Investigators from New Zealand demonstrated a neuroprotective effect of one of these blockers, flunarizine, in immature rats,[95] as well as in fetal sheep.[96] However, when Levene et al. used nicardipine, another calcium-channel blocker, in four severely asphyxiated neonates, they had severe complications.[97] The mean arterial blood pressure decreased in three infants and two developed sudden and dramatic hypotension. They strongly cautioned against the use of this drug in infants with HIE.

Oxygen free radical inhibitors

The mechanisms by which oxygen free radicals initiate and perpetuate cellular damage are clearly evaluated in Chapter 3 by Vannucci and Palmer. Although the body produces naturally occurring antioxidants such as catalase, superoxide dismutase, endoperoxidases, glutathione, and cholesterol, as well as using vitamins C and E in such situations, the elaboration of the oxygen free radicals following an asphyxial event may exceed the infant's ability to generate adequate protection.[98] Drugs such as allopurinol and oxypurinol have been utilized to treat such infants.[98–102] Superoxide dismutase and catalase, when conjugated with polyethylene glycol in order to prolong their effects and allow intracellular penetration, have been used as well, especially in laboratory animals. Van Bel et al. studied 22 infants who were equal to or older than 35 weeks' gestation and who had severe HIE.[101] Eleven infants were given a single 40 mg/kg intravenous injection of allopurinol, with the remaining 11 serving as controls. Six control infants died, one survivor had speech and language delay, and four were normal at 2 years of age.[103] In the allopurinol-treated group, two infants died, one had disabling mental retardation, cerebral palsy and epilepsy, one had speech and language delay, and seven were normal.[103] Although this study suggested a potential beneficial effect of allopurinol, a much larger study will have to be carried out to verify these results.

Monosialgangliosides

These glycosphingolipids, found throughout the body, are found in high concentrations in the nervous system and are important components of cell membranes. Monosialoganglioside (GMI) crosses the placenta and blood–brain barriers and can be incorporated into neural cell membranes. Tan et al., in elegant studies using a fetal sheep model, showed that GMI given prior to and following repeated episodes of asphyxial damage protected the animals from neurological sequelae that would have ordinarily taken place.[104,105] They demonstrated that "systemic treatment with GMI reduced morphologic, biochemical, neurophysiological and behavioral manifestation of hypoxic–ischemic brain damage."[105] The agent did not cause hypotension or metabolic disturbances in the animals. To date, this form of therapy has not been reported in human neonates.

Lazaroids (21-aminosteroids)

Methylprednisone has been used for many years to diminish the severity of sequelae following brain and spinal cord injury.[106] When given in high doses, some beneficial effect was noted in a few patients. Subsequent studies demonstrated that the therapeutic effect was not related to the glucocorticoid or mineralocorticoid actions of the drug, but to its effect of limiting lipid peroxidation.[107] Thus, 21-aminosteroids were developed as inhibitors of lipid peroxidation. These agents have neither glucocorticoid nor mineralocorticoid activity and are essentially nontoxic. The 21-aminosteroid that has been selected for the acute treatment of brain and spinal injury, ischemic stroke, and subarachnoid hemorrhage is tirilazad mesylate, which is a potent inhibitor of oxygen radical-induced, ion-catalyzed lipid peroxidation. It appears to exert its effect by a radical scavenging activity and by stabilization of the cellular membrane. This agent also prevents the posttraumatic permeability of the blood–brain barrier, reduces the extent of cerebral edema, and maintains and preserves endogenous vitamin E levels in tissue.[108]

The vast majority of studies with the lazaroids have been accomplished in laboratory animals, including subhuman primates, and phase I trials in humans showed that tirilazad mesylate did not affect cardiovascular parameters, nor did it have any adverse interaction with the calcium-channel blocker nimodipine. In phase II studies of 245 patients with aneurysmal subarachnoid hemorrhage, symptomatic vasospasm was reduced and the Glasgow outcome score was improved in the lazaroid-treated patients compared to controls.[108] Further studies utilizing this agent in acute head and spinal injury, aneurysmal subarachnoid hemorrhage, and ischemic stroke should be forthcoming; and if the drugs have beneficial effects in these patients, use in neonates with HIE may prove beneficial as well. To date, no reports of the use of lazeroids in human neonates have been published.

Growth factors and hypothermia

The use of these modalities as adjuncts in the therapy of infants with HIE is the most exciting new approach that has occurred in the past 20 years.[109–112] These are described in detail in Chapter

36 by Dr. Gunn et al. There is also an excellent review of the neuroprotective effects of cerebral hypothermia by Gunn and Gunn, outlining in greater detail the use and benefits of this form of neuroprotection.[110]

Consultation and referral

Attempts to manage critically ill neonates beyond the initial stabilization (in preparation for transfer to level III facilities) may contribute to unnecessary additional risk and possible compromise of the neonate. Even though a physician has been appropriately trained to do so, the temptation to care for such neonates in a level I or II nursery should be resisted because these facilities rarely include all appropriate equipment and sufficient specially trained personnel to support the diagnostic and therapeutic undertakings required to confirm the diagnosis of cyanotic congenital heart disease or treat persistent pulmonary hypertension of the newborn. Thus, consultation should always be obtained with an experienced neonatologist, usually from the regional level III facility to which the infant will be transported, if special procedures are judged to be necessary immediately, such as the use of prostaglandin in an infant suspected of having a ductus-dependent congenital cardiac defect. However, encountering the syndrome of hypoxemia (Pao_2 level less than 50 mmHg or 6.7 kPa) refractory to 100% oxygen and assisted ventilation mandates the physical attendance by the primary care physician until the arrival of the transport team.

Because of the high medicolegal hazard to all physicians involved in the care of a depressed infant in the USA, all easily treated conditions contributing to the infant's disorder should be addressed immediately after birth by the physician in attendance. At a minimum, the practitioner should be able to insert an umbilical venous catheter providing administration of crystalloid, colloid, or drugs to support the blood pressure and ideally should also be able to insert an umbilical arterial catheter for direct measurement of the blood pressure and monitoring blood gases. In consultation with the neonatologist, the practitioner should initiate specific therapies to correct cardiac dysfunction in the context of hypoxemia refractory to assisted ventilation. In addition, there may be correctable problems that can contribute to the syndrome of hypoxemia. Such treatment should also constitute preparation of the infant for transport to the nearest level III facility, if necessary. None the less, complete characterization of and appropriate treatment for cyanotic congenital heart disease are not expected of the primary care physician at a level I or II nursery. Clearly, what is expected of the practitioner at such a nursery is different from what is expected of the neonatologist at a level III facility, where a variety of special diagnostic and therapeutic procedures might be attempted to correct or ameliorate the problem after the patient's arrival.

When the problem is considered in the medicolegal context, generalization about the extended intensive care of depressed infants should be considered a disservice to the legal as well as the medical community. With the presentation of certain clinical facts in retrospect, some comments can be made about therapeutic options and the application of therapies. However, it is inappropriate to guess about the reasoned decision making of a physician involved with the care of such an infant without that physician's supplying the context in which the decision was made. Moreover, it undermines the trust of the public in the health-care professionals who have dedicated their lives to caring for such infants. Most important, the clinical determinant of standard of care must remain the response of the patient to therapies selected and should be independent of individual preferences.

REFERENCES

1 Benitz, W.E., Frankel, L.R. and Stevenson, D.K. (1986). The pharmacology of neonatal resuscitation and cardiopulmonary intensive care. Part II. Extended intensive care. *West J Med*, **145**, 47–51.

2 Stevenson, D.K. and Benitz, W.E. (1987). A practical approach to diagnosis and immediate care of the cyanotic infant. *Clin Pediatr*, **26**, 325–331.

3 Bruce, D.A. (1984). Effects of hyperventilation on cerebral blood flow and metabolism. *Clin Perinatol*, **11**, 673–680.

4 Walsh-Sukys, M.C., Tyson D.E., Wright, L.L., et al. (2000). Persistent pulmonary hypertension of the newborn in the era before nitric oxide: practice evaluation and outcome. *Pediatrics*, **105**, 14–20.

5 Kusuda, S., Shishida, W., Miyagi, N., et al. (1999). Cerebral blood flow during treatment for pulmonary hypertension. *Arch Dis Child Neonatal Edn.*, **80**, F30–F33.

6 Gleason, C.A., Short, B.L. and Jones, M.D. Jr. (1989). Cerebral blood flow and metabolism during and after prolonged hypocapnia in newborn lambs. *J Pediatr*, **115**, 309–314.

7 Liem, K.D., Hopman, J.C.W., Oeseburg B., et al. (1995). Cerebral oxygenation and hemodynamics during induction of extracorporeal membrane oxygenation as investigated by near infrared spectrophotometry. *Pediatrics*, **95**, 555–561.

8 Toft, P.M., Leth, H., Lou, H.C., et al. (1995). Local vascular CO_2 reactivity in the brain assessed by functional MRI. *Pediatr Radiol*, **25**, 420–424.

9 Leavitt, A.M., Watchko, J.F., Bennett, F.C., et al. (1987). Neurodevelopmental outcome following persistent pulmonary hypertension of the neonate. *J Perinatol*, **7**, 288–291.

10 Bifano, E.M. and Pfannenstiel, A. (1988). Duration of hyperventilation and outcome in infants with persistent pulmonary hypertension. *Pediatrics*, **81**, 657–661.

11 Hendricks-Munoz, K.D. and Walton, J.P. (1988). Hearing loss in infants with persistent fetal circulation. *Pediatrics*, **81**, 650–656.

12 Wung, J.T., James, L.S., Kilchevsky, E., et al. (1985). Management of infants with severe respiratory failure and persistence of the fetal circulation, without hyperventilation. *Pediatrics*, **76**, 488–494.

13 Walsh-Sukys, M.C., Cornell, D.J., Houston, L.N., et al. (1994). Treatment of persistent pulmonary hypertension of the newborn without hyperventilation: an assessment of diffusion of innovation. *Pediatrics*, **94**, 303–306.

14 Clark, R.H., Yoder, B.A. and Sell, M.S. (1994). Prospective, randomized comparison of high frequency oscillation and conventional ventilation in candidates for extracorporeal membrane oxygenation. *J Pediatr*, **124**, 447–454.

15 Clark, R.H. (1994). High frequency ventilation. *J Pediatr*, **124**, 661–670.

16 deLemos, R., Yoder, B., McCurnin, D., et al. (1992). The use of high frequency oscillatory ventilation and extracorporeal membrane oxygenation in the management of the term/near term infant with respiratory failure. *Early Hum Dev*, **29**, 299–303.

17 Baumgart, S., Hirschel, R.B., Butler, S.Z., et al. (1992). Diagnosis-related criteria in the consideration of extracorporeal membrane oxygenation in neonates previously treated with high frequency jet ventilation. *Pediatrics*, **89**, 491–494.

18 Bhuta, T., Clark, R.H. and Henderson-Smart, D.J. (2000). Rescue high frequency oscillatory ventilation vs. conventional ventilation in infants with severe pulmonary dysfunction born at or near term. *Cochrane Database Syst Rev*, **1**, CD002974.

19 Hintz, S.R., Suttner, D.M., Sheehan, A.M., et al. (2000). Decreased use of neonatal extracorporeal membrane oxygenation (ECMO): how new treatment modalities have affected ECMO utilization. *Pediatrics*, **106**, 1339–1343.

20 Goudsouzian, N.G., Liu, M.P.L. and Savarese, J.J. (1978). Metocurine in infants and children: neuromuscular and clinical effects. *Anesthesiology*, **49**, 266–269.

21 Crone, R.K. and Favorito, J. (1980). The effects of pancuronium bromide on infants with hyaline membrane disease. *J Pediatr*, **97**, 991–993.

22 Jobe, A.H. (1993). Pulmonary surfactant therapy. *N Engl J Med*, **328**, 861–868.

23 Kendig, J.W., Ryan, R.M., Sinkin, R.A., et al. (1998). Comparison of two strategies for surfactant prophylaxis in very premature infants: a multicenter randomized trial. *Pediatrics*, **101**, 1006–1012.

24 Soll, R.F. (2000). Synthetic surfactant for respiratory distress syndrome in preterm infants. *Cochrane Database Syst Rev*, **2**, CD001149.

25 Bancalari, E. and del Moral, T. (2001). Bronchopulmonary dysplasia and surfactant. *Biol Neonate*, **80**, 7–13.

26 Greenough, A. (2000). Expanded use of surfactant replacement therapy. *Eur J Pediatr*, **159**, 635–640.

27 Lotze, A., Mitchell, B.R., Bulas, D.I., et al. (1998). Multicenter study of surfactant (beractant) use in the treatment of term infants with severe respiratory failure. Survanta in term infant study group. *J Pediatr*, **132**, 40–47.

28 The Neonatal Inhaled Nitric Oxide Study Group. (1997). Inhaled nitric oxide in full term and nearly full term infants with hypoxic respiratory failure. *N Engl J Med*, **336**, 597–604.

29 The Neonatal Inhaled Nitric Oxide Study Group. (1997). Inhaled nitric oxide and hypoxic respiratory failure in infants with congenital diaphragmatic hernia. *Pediatrics*, **99**, 838–845.

30 Breitweser, J.A., Meyer, R.A., Sperling, M.A., et al. (1980). Cardiac septal hypertrophy in hyperinsulinemic infants. *J Pediatr*, **96**, 535–539.

31 Zaritsky, A. and Chernow, B. (1984). Use of catecholamines in pediatrics. *J Pediatr*, **105**, 341–350.

32 Friedman, W.F. and George, B.L. (1985). Treatment of congestive heart failure by altering loading conditions of the heart. *J Pediatr*, **106**, 697–706.

33 Benitz, W.E., Malachowski, N., Cohen, R.S., et al. (1985). Use of sodium nitroprusside in neonates: efficacy and safety. *J Pediatr*, **105**, 102–110.

34 Bard, H. (2000). Hemoglobin synthesis and metabolism during the neonatal period. In *Hematologic Problems of the Neonate*, ed. R.D. Christensen, pp. 374–377. Philadelphia: Saunders.

35 Kane, T.D., Greenberg, J.M., Bove, K.E., et al. (1998). Alveolar capillary dysplasia with misalignment of the pulmonary veins: a rare but fatal cause of neonatal respiratory failure. *Pediatr Surg Int*, **14**, 89–91.

36 Nogee, L.M. (1997). Surfactant protein B deficiency. *Chest*, **111**, 1295–1355.

37 Yeh, T.F., Shibli, A., Leu, S.T., et al. (1984). Early furosemide therapy in premature infants (≤ 2000 gm) with respiratory distress syndrome: a randomized controlled trial. *J Pediatr*, **105**, 603–609.

38 Van Overmeire, B., Smets, K., Lecoutere, K., et al. (2000). A comparison of ibuprofen and indomethacin for closure of patent ductus arteriosus. *N Engl J Med*, **343**, 674–681.

39 Fowlie, P.W. (2000). Intravenous indomethacin for preventing mortality and morbidity in very low birthweight infants. *Cochrane Database Syst Rev*, **2**, CD000174.

40 Couser, R.J., Hoekstra, R.E., Ferrara, T.B., et al. (2000). Neurodevelopmental follow-up at 26 months corrected age of preterm infants treated with prophylactic indomethacin. *Arch Pediatr Adolesc Med*, **154**, 598–602.

41 Ment, L.R., Vohr, B., Allan, W., et al. (2000). Outcome of children in the indomethacin intraventricular hemorrhage prevention trial. *Pediatrics*, **105**, 485–491.

42 Clyman, R.I. (1996). Recommendations for the postnatal use of indomethacin: an analysis of four separate strategies. *J Pediatr*, **128**, 601–607.

43 Cools, F. and Offrinya, M. (1999). Meta-analysis of elective high frequency ventilation in preterm infants with respiratory distress syndrome. *Arch Dis Child Fetal Neonatal Edn*, **80**, F15–F20.

44 Thome, U.H. and Carlo, W.A. (2000). High-frequency ventilation in neonates. *Am J Perinatol*, **17**, 1–9.

45 Henderson-Smart, D.J., Bhuta, T., Cools, F., et al. (2000). Elective high frequency oscillatory ventilation versus conventional ventilation from acute pulmonary dysfunction in preterm infants. *Cochrane Database Syst Rev*, **2**, CD000104.

46 Heymann, M.A. (1981). Pharmacologic use of prostaglandin E_1 in infants with congenital heart disease. *Am Heart J*, **101**, 837–843.

47 Myers, R.E. (1972). Two patterns of perinatal brain damage and their conditions of occurrence. *Am J Obstet Gynecol*, **112**, 246–276.

48 Brann, A.W. and Myers, R.E. (1975). Central nervous system findings in the newborn monkey following severe in utero partial asphyxia. *Neurology*, **25**, 327–338.

49 Myers, R.E. (1977). Experimental models of perinatal brain damage: relevance to human pathology. In *Intrauterine Asphyxia and the Developing Fetal Brain*, ed. L. Gluck, pp. 37–97. Chicago: Year-Book.

50 Mujsce, D.J., Christensen, M.A. and Vannucci, R.C. (1990). Cerebral blood flow and edema in perinatal hypoxic ischemic brain damage. *Pediatr Res*, **27**, 450–453.

51 Young, R.S.K. and Yagel, S.K. (1984). Cerebral physiological and metabolic effects of hyperventilation in the neonatal dog. *Ann Neurol*, **16**, 337–342.

52 Volpe, J.J. (2001). *Hypoxic–Ischemic Encephalopathy in Neurology of the Newborn*, 4th edn. Philadelphia: W.B. Saunders.

53 Lupton, B.A., Hill, A., Roland, E.H., et al. (1988). Brain swelling in the asphyxiated term newborn: pathogenesis and outcome. *Pediatrics*, **82**, 139–146.

54 Hill, A. (1991). Current concepts of hypoxic ischemic cerebral injury in the term infant newborn. *Pediatr Neurol*, **7**, 317–325.

55 Levene, M.I. and Evans, D.H. (1983). Continuous measurement of subarachnoid pressure in the severely asphyxiated newborn. *Arch Dis Child*, **58**, 1013–1015.

56 Levene, M.I., Evans, D.H., Forde, A., et al. (1987). Value of intracranial pressure monitoring of asphyxiated newborn patients. *Dev Med Child Neurol*, **29**, 311–319.

57 Levene, M.I. (1995). Management and outcome of birth asphyxia. In *Fetal and Neonatal Neurology and Neurosurgery*, 2nd edn, ed. M.I. Levene and R.J. Lilforde, pp. 427–442. Edinburgh: Churchill Livingston.

58 Rosenberg, A.A., Jones, M.D. Jr, Traysman, R.J., et al. (1982). Response of cerebral blood flow to changes in $P\text{CO}_2$ in fetal, newborn and adult sleep. *Am J Physiol*, **242**, H862–H868.

59 Bernbaum, J.D., Russell, P., Sheridan, P.H., et al. (1984). Long term follow-up of newborns with persistent pulmonary hypertension. *Crit Care Med*, **121**, 579–583.

60 Wiswell, T.E., Graziani, L.J., Kornhauser, M.S., et al. (1996). Effects of hypocarbia on the development of cystic periventricular leukomalacia in premature infants treated with high-frequency jet ventilation. *Pediatrics*, **98**, 918–924.

61 Damman, D., Allred, E.N., Kuban, K.C.K., et al. (2001). Hypocarbia during the first 24 post natal hours and white matter echolucencies in newborns ≤28 weeks gestation. *Pediatr Res*, **49**, 388–393.

62 Vannucci, R.C., Towfighi, J., Heitjan, D.F., et al. (1995). Carbon dioxide protects the perinatal brain from hypoxic–ischemic damage: an experimental study in the immature rat. *Pediatrics*, **95**, 868–874.

63 Vannucci, R.C., Towfighi, J., Brucklacher, R.M., et al. (2001). Effect of extreme hypercapnia on hypoxic–ischemic brain damage in the immature rat. *Pediatr Res*, **49**, 799–803.

64 Cooper, P.R., Moody, S., Clark, W.K., et al. (1979). Dexamethasone and severe head injury: a prospective double-blind study. *J Neurosurg*, **51**, 307–316.

65 Gudeman, S.K., Miller, J.D. and Becker, D.P. (1979). Failure of high-dose steroid therapy to influence intracranial pressure in patients with severe head injury. *J Neurosurg*, **51**, 301–306.

66 Dearden, N.M., Gibson, J.S., McDowell, D.C., et al. (1986). Effect of high-dose dexamethasone on outcome from severe head injury. *J Neurosurg*, **64**, 81–88.

67 Lee, M.C., Mastri, R.A., Waltz, A.G., et al. (1974). Ineffectiveness of dexamethasone for treatment of experimental cerebral infarction. *Stroke*, **5**, 216–218.

68 Svenningsen, N.W., Blennow, G., Lindroth, M., et al. (1982). Brain oriented intensive care treatment in severe neonatal asphyxia. Effects of phenobarbitone protection. *Arch Dis Child*, **57**, 176–183.

69 Levene, M.I. and Evans D.H. (1985). Medical management of raised intracranial pressure after severe birth asphyxia. *Arch Dis Child*, **60**, 12–16.

70 Barks, J.D., Post, M. and Tuor, U.I. (1991). Dexamethasone prevents hypoxic–ischemic brain damage in the neonatal rat. *Pediatr Res*, **29**, 558–563.

71 Tuor, U.I., Simone C.S., Barks, J.D.E., et al. (1993). Dexamethasone prevents cerebral infarction without affecting cerebral blood flow in neonatal rats. *Stroke*, **24**, 452–457.

72 National Institutes of Health Consensus Development Panel on the Effect of Corticosteroids for Fetal Maturation of Perinatal Outcomes. (1994). Effect of corticosteroids for fetal maturation on perinatal outcomes *JAMA*, **273**, 413–418.

73 Crowley, P. (2000). Prophylactic corticosteroids for preterm birth. *Cochrane Database Syst Rev*, **2**, CD000065.

74 Adhikari, M., Moodley M. and Desai, P.K. (1990). Mannitol in neonatal cerebral oedema. *Brain Dev*, **12**, 349–351.

75 Marchal, C., Costagliolu, P., Leveau, P., et al. (1974). Treatment de la souffrance cerebrale neonatale d'orisivie auoxique par le mannitol. *Rev Pediatr*, **9**, 581–589.

76 Goldberg, R.N., Moscoso, P., Bauer, C.R., et al. (1986). Use of barbiturate therapy in severe perinatal asphyxia: a randomized controlled trial. *J Pediatr*, **109**, 851–856.

77 Brain Resuscitation Clinical Trial I Study Group. (1986). Randomized clinical study of thiopental loading in comatose survivors of cardiac arrest. *N Engl J Med*, **314**, 397–403.

78 Hall, R.T., Hall, F.K. and Daily, D.K. (1998). High-dose phenobarbital therapy in term newborn infants with severe perinatal asphyxia: a randomized, prospective study with three-year follow-up. *J Pediatr*, **132**, 345–348.

79 Giacom, G.P. (1993). Asphyxial brain damage in the newborn: new insights into pathophysiology and possible pharmacologic intervention. *South Med J*, **86**, 676–682.

80 Kjellmer, I. (1991). Mechanisms of perinatal brain damage. *Ann Med*, **23**, 675–679.

81 Muir, K.W. and Lees, K.R. (1995). Clinical experience with excitatory amino acid antagonist drugs. *Stroke*, **26**, 503–513.

82 Levene, M. (1992). Role of excitatory amino acid antagonists in the management of birth asphyxia. *Biol Neonate*, **62**, 248–251.

83 Steinberg, G.K., Kunis, D., DeLaPaz, R., et al. (1993.) Neuroprotection following focal cerebral ischemia with the NMDA antagonist dextromethorphan has a favorable dose response profile. *Neurol Res*, **15**, 174–180.

84 Steinberg, G.K., Bell, T.E. and Yenari, M.A. (1996). Dose escalation safety and tolerance study of the *N*-methyl-D-aspartate antagonist dextromethorphan in neurosurgery patients. *J Neurosurg*, **84**, 883–887.

85 Davis, S.M., Lees, K.R., Albers, G.W., et al. (2000). Selfotel in acute ischemic stroke: possible neurotoxic effects of an NMDA antagonist. *Stroke*, **31**, 347–354.

86 Parikka, H., Toivonen, L., Naukkarinen, V., et al. (1999). Decreases by magnesium of QT dispersion and ventricular arrhythmias in patients with acute myocardial infarction. *Eur Heart J*, **20**, 111–120.

87 Lampl, Y., Gilad, R., Geva, D., et al. (2001). Intravenous administration of magnesium sulfate in acute stroke: a randomized double-blind study. *Clin Neuropharmacol*, **24**, 11–15.

88 Lucas, M.J., Leveno, K.J. and Cunningham, F.G. (1995). A comparison of magnesium sulfate with phenytoin for the prevention of eclampsia. *N Engl J Med*, **333**, 201–205.

89 McDonald, J.W., Silverstein, F.S. and Johnston, M.V. (1990). Magnesium reduces *N*-methyl-D-aspartate (NMDA)-mediated brain injury in perinatal rats. *Neurosci Lett*, **109**, 234–238.

90 Marret, S., Gressens, P., Gadisseux, J.F., et al. (1995). Prevention by magnesium of excitotoxic neuronal death in the developing brain: an animal model for clinical intervention studies. *Dev Med Child Neurol*, **37**, 473–484.

91 de Haan, H.H., Gunn, A.J., Williams, C.E., et al. (1997).

Magnesium sulfate therapy during asphyxia in near-term fetal lambs does not compromise the fetus but does not reduce cerebral injury. *Am J Obstet Gynecol*, **176**, 18–27.

92 Penrice, J., Amess, P.N., Punwani, S., et al. (1997). Magnesium sulfate after transient hypoxia–ischemia fails to prevent delayed cerebral energy failure in the newborn piglet. *Pediatr Res*, **41**, 443–447.

93 Levene, M., Blennow, M., Whitelaw, A., et al. (1995). Acute effects of two different doses of magnesium sulphate in infants with birth asphyxia. Arch Dis *Child Fetal Neonatal Edn*, **73**, F174–F177.

94 Robertson, N.J. and Edwards, A.D. (1998). Recent advances in developing neuroprotective strategies for perinatal asphyxia. *Curr Opin Pediatr*, **10**, 575–580.

95 Gunn, A.J., Mydlar, T., Bennet, L., et al. (1989). The neuroprotective actions of a calcium channel antagonist, flunarizine, in the infant rat. *Pediatr Res*, **25**, 573–576.

96 Gunn, A.J., Williams, C.E., Mallard, E.C., et al. (1994). Flunarizine, a calcium channel antagonist, is partially prophylactically neuroprotective in hypoxic-ischemic encephalopathy in the fetal sheep. *Pediatr Res*, **35**, 657–663.

97 Levene, M.I., Gibson, N.A., Fenton, A.C., et al. (1990). The use of a calcium-channel blocker, nicardipine, for severely asphyxiated newborn infants. *Dev Med Child Neurol*, **32**, 567–574.

98 Buonocore, G., Perrone, S. and Bracci, R. (2001). Free radicals and brain damage in the newborn. *Biol Neonate*, **79**, 180–186.

99 Saugstad, O.D. (1996). Role of xanthine oxidase and its inhibitor in hypoxia: reoxygenation injury. *Pediatrics*, **98**, 103–107.

100 Shadid, M., Moison, R., Steendijk, P., et al. (1998). The effect of antioxidative combination therapy on post hypoxic–ischemic perfusion, metabolism, and electrical activity of the newborn brain. *Pediatr Res*, **44**, 119–124.

101 Van Bel, F., Shadid, M., Moison, R.M., et al. (1998). Effect of allopurinol on postasphyxial free radical formation, cerebral hemodynamics, and electrical brain activity. *Pediatrics*, **101**, 185–193.

102 Peeters, C. and van Bel, F. (2001). Pharmacotherapeutical reduction of post-hypoxic–ischemic brain injury in the newborn. *Biol Neonate*, **79**, 274–280.

103 Veen, S., De Haan, M.J.J., Martens, S.E., et al. (1999). Allopurinol (ALLO) treatment following severe asphyxia: follow-up at 2-years of age. *Pediatr Res*, **45**, 230A.

104 Tan, W.K., Williams, C.E., Gunn, A.J., et al. (1993). Pretreatment with monosialoganglioside GM1 protects the brain of fetal sheep against hypoxic–ischemic injury without causing systemic compromise. *Pediatr Res*, **34**, 18–22.

105 Tan, W.K., Williams, C.E., Mallard, C.E., et al. (1994). Monosialoganglioside GM1 treatment after a hypoxic–ischemic episode reduces the vulnerability of the fetal sheep brain to subsequent injuries. *Am J Obstet Gynecol*, **170**, 663–669.

106 Hall, E.D. (1992). The neuroprotective pharmacology of methylprednisolone. *J Neurosurg*, **76**, 13–22.

107 Amar, A.P. and Levy, M.L. (1999). Pathogenesis and pharmacological strategies for mitigating secondary damage in acute spinal cord injury. *Neurosurgery*, **44**, 1027–1040.

108 Hall, E.D., McCall, J.M. and Means, E.D. (1994). Therapeutic potential of the lazaroids (21-aminosteroids) in acute central nervous system trauma, ischemia and subarachnoid hemorrhage. *Adv Pharmacol*, **28**, 221–268.

109 Trescher, W.H., Ishiwa, S. and Johnston, M.V. (1997). Brief post-hypoxic–ischemic hypothermia markedly delays neonatal brain injury. *Brain Dev*, **19**, 326–338.

110 Gunn, A.J. and Gunn, T.R. (1998). The 'pharmacology' of neuronal rescue with cerebral hypothermia. *Early Hum Dev*, **53**, 19–35.

111 Thoresen, M. (2001). Cooling the newborn after asphyxia. Physiological and experimental background and its clinical use. *Semin Neonatol*, **5**, 61–73.

112 Battin, M.R., Dezoete, J.A., Gunn, T.R., et al. (2001). Neurodevelopmental outcome of infants treated with head cooling and mild hypothermia after perinatal asphyxia. *Pediatrics*, **107**, 480–484.

36

Neuroprotective mechanisms after hypoxic–ischemic injury

Alistair J. Gunn, Jian Guan, and Laura Bennet

Liggins Institute and Dept of Paediatrics, University of Auckland, Auckland, New Zealand

Introduction

As discussed in Chapter 4, exposure to acutely compromised gas exchange is very common, and yet only a small minority of newborns develop evidence of hypoxic–ischemic encephalopathy (HIE). Indeed, even severe metabolic acidosis at birth is associated with HIE in less than half of cases.[1] Similarly, experimental studies typically report that cerebral injury occurs only in a very narrow temporal window between survival with complete recovery and death.[2] Partly this is a reflection of the efficiency of the fetal adaptations that maintain perfusion to the essential organs. In addition, an acute event activates protective endogenous cellular responses, many mediated by glia, that help limit neural injury. These processes may be modified, raising the possibility of treating acute encephalopathy.

Biphasic cell death after hypoxic–ischemic injury

The seminal observation derived from both experimental studies in vivo and in vitro and clinical observations has been that HIE is not a single event but is rather an evolving process. Although neurons may die during the actual ischemic or asphyxial event (primary cell death), many neurons initially recover at least partially from the primary insult, only to die hours or even days later (secondary or delayed cell death). Using magnetic resonance spectroscopy, Azzopardi and coworkers showed that infants with evidence of moderate-to-severe asphyxia often have normal cerebral oxidative metabolism shortly after birth, but many then go on to develop delayed energy failure 6–15 h later.[3] This phenomenon is associated with a severe mortality. In survivors, the degree of secondary energy failure after 24–48 h was closely associated with neurodevelopmental outcome at 18 months and 4 years of age.[4] An identical pattern of secondary energy failure was seen after hypoxia–ischemia in the piglet[5] and the severity of energy failure was closely correlated with the severity of cell death in the cortex.[6]

Figure 36.1 illustrates the pathophysiological defined phases of injury observed in near-term fetal lambs subject to 30 min of cerebral ischemia induced by bilateral carotid occlusion. This paradigm leads to a watershed pattern of injury to the cortex, hippocampus, and striatum (as shown in Figure 36.2).[7–9] The phases of injury include the immediate reperfusion period lasting approximately 30 min, during which cellular energy metabolism is restored, with resolution of the acute hypoxic–depolarization and cell swelling. This is followed by a latent phase starting approximately 30–45 min after reperfusion, lasting for up to 6–15 h, in which oxidative cerebral energy metabolism normalizes but electroencephalogram (EEG) activity remains depressed, often with a delayed period of reduced cerebral blood flow (CBF).[7] The latent phase appears to correspond with the initiation of the intracytoplasmic components of the delayed cell

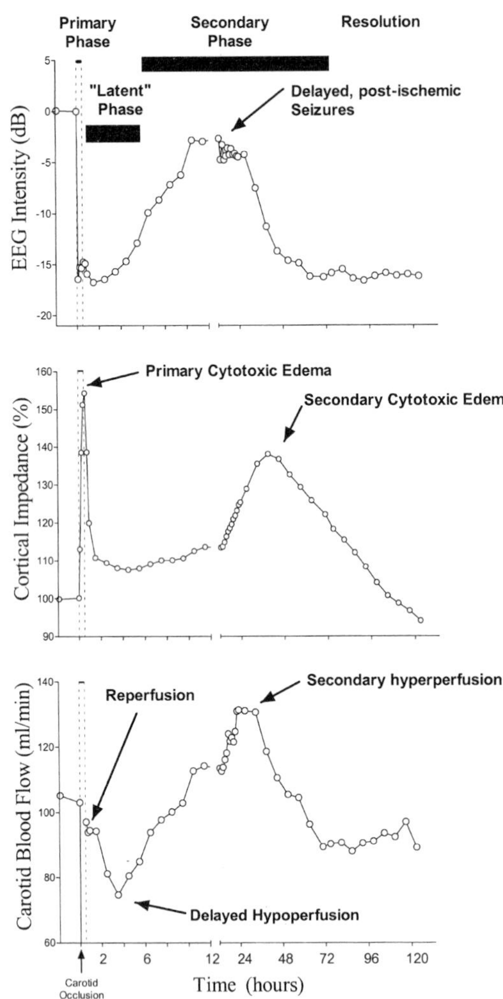

Figure 36.1 An illustration of the pathophysiological phases of injury after 30 min of global cerebral ischemia in fetal sheep ($n = 7$). data derived from Gunn et al.[7] See text for details.

death cascade.[10] Following the latent phase there is secondary deterioration with delayed seizures and cytotoxic edema,[7] increased blood flow,[11] extracellular accumulation of potential cytotoxins (such as the excitatory neurotransmitters),[12] and approximately 6–15h after the asphyxia, failure of oxidative metabolism and damage.[13] The acute changes in this phase may take 3 days or more to resolve. There is no secondary energy failure after lesser insults that do not produce encephalopathy.[14]

Mechanisms of delayed cell loss

The precise events which initiate the cascade leading to delayed cell death after hypoxia–ischemia (HI) are poorly understood, but are undoubtedly multifactorial. It may be partially related to loss of trophic support by growth factors,[15] to the action of cytotoxins such as free radicals during hypoxia and early reperfusion,[16] and/or to cytokines released by activated microglia which are activated following asphyxial injury.[17] Disordered calcium homeostasis during and after HI appears to have a critical role in triggering delayed cell death.[18] Excessive entry of calcium into cells occurs, both passively through depolarization-mediated activation of the L-type calcium channels and reversal of the energy-dependent Na^{+}–Ca^{2+} exchange pump, and actively through channels linked to excitatory neurotransmitters such as glutamate. Strong data suggest that this intracellular calcium influx leads to inappropriate activation of key enzyme systems.[19]

Two morphological patterns of delayed cell death have been described, necrosis and apoptosis. Necrosis is defined by loss of plasma membrane integrity associated with a random pattern of DNA degradation. Typically there is swelling of the cytoplasm and organelles, with little change initially to the nucleus. Apoptosis is defined morphologically by the development of karyohexis. Karyohexis is the classic microscopic picture of condensation of chromatin (i.e., a dark shrunken nucleus) with loss of the reticular formation in the cytoplasm (leading to eosinophilia on light microscopy); ultimately, the shrunken cell breaks into small fragments.[20] By analogy with the active process of developmental loss of excess cells (including neurons),[21] it was suggested that an apoptotic morphology reflected active or programmed cell death.[22-25] In contrast, necrosis was suggested to reflect biophysical damage to the cell (cell membrane instability, ion shifts, etc.), particularly lysis in the primary phase.[22,26] Both patterns are clearly described in infants dying after perinatal asphyxia.[25,26]

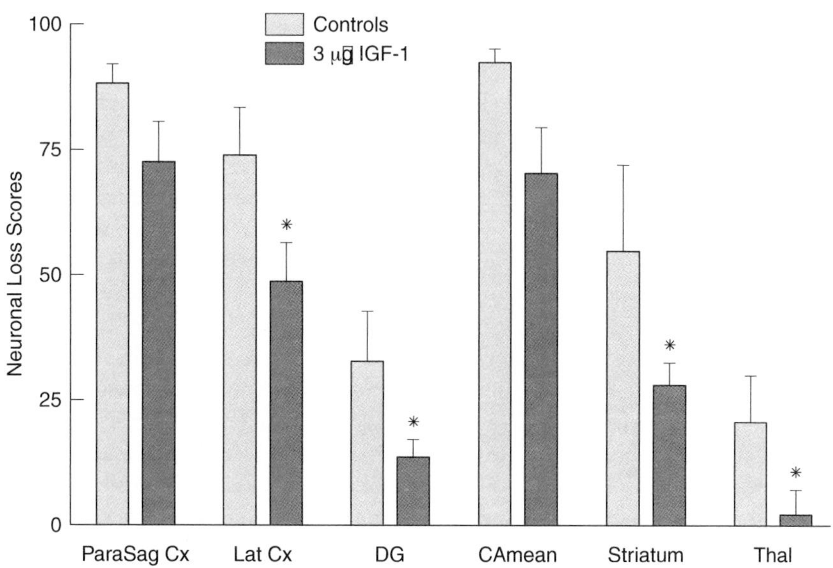

Figure 36.2 Improvement in histological injury with insulin-like growth factor-1 (IGF-1) therapy given intracerebroventricularly 2 h after 30 min of cerebral ischemia in the fetal sheep, assessed after 96 h recovery. This insult leads to a watershed pattern of neuronal loss, greatest in the parasagittal cortex (ParaSag Cx) and dorsal cornu ammonis (CA) of the hippocampus (CAmean is the average for CA regions 1–4). Note the significant improvement in the lateral or temporal cortex (Lat Cx) and subcortical structures, including the dentate gyrus (DG) of the dorsal hippocampus, striatum and thalamus (Thal). *, Significant differences. Data derived in part from Guan et al.[9]

The intracytoplasmic stage of apoptosis involves alterations in the ratio of various intracellular factors such as the protooncogene *Bcl-2*, which inhibits apoptosis,[27] and *Bax*, which promotes apoptosis,[27,28] leading to activation of the cysteine proteases (caspases) which mediate the subsequent self-amplifying cascade of events.[29,30] The final, irreversible execution phase of apoptosis is intranuclear, involving endonuclease-mediated DNA fragmentation.[10,22]

Recently, it has become clear that the precise morphology of delayed cell death is not as informative as originally thought. Posthypoxic cell death in vitro includes elements of both apoptotic and necrotic processes, with one or the other being most prominent depending on factors such as maturity.[31–33] Consistent with this, there is evidence that mitochondrial calcium overload is a critical event in both apoptotic and necrotic cell death,[34] while antiapoptotic proteins such as Bcl may also inhibit necrotic cell death.[35] The concept remains an important one, since if neuronal and glia cell death is an active response (preprogrammed or functionally mediated by secondary mechanisms such as cytotoxin exposure), then it should logically be possible to interrupt these events.

Endogenous neuroprotective responses

The brain has a range of endogenous protective responses that act to limit injury. These responses include release of neuromodulators and inhibitory neurotransmitters, induction of neurotrophic factors and intracellular antiapoptotic systems, and, postnatally, spontaneous cerebral hypothermia. An illustration of the potential protective effects of endogenous cellular responses is that a single subthreshold insult that does not cause damage may markedly increase resistance to a subsequent more severe insult.[36,37] Several hours must elapse for preconditioning to be seen, and its effect then attenuates after several days. This is consistent with the time course of induction of a wide range of inhibitory neurotransmitters and stress gene responses to ischemia.[37,38]

Inhibitory neuromodulators

Ischemia and asphyxia are typically associated with a large increase in inhibitory neuromodulators such as gamma-aminobutyric acid (GABA), adenosine, and cerebral opioids.[39] Microdialysis studies in the fetal lamb suggest that, unlike postnatal studies, there is a disproportionately large release of GABA relative to that of the excitotoxins during ischemia.[12] Interestingly, adult species such as the turtle that are very tolerant to hypoxia also show a very similar dramatic elevation in GABA during anoxia.[40] After reperfusion in the fetal lamb, there is a rapid fall in cerebral GABA levels,[12] with no elevation of GABA during the secondary phase. This loss of GABA release during the secondary phase may be one contributor to the development of very intense and difficult-to-manage seizures in neonatal HIE, and suggests that increasing cerebral inhibition after ischemia may be a logical treatment.[39] In support of this concept, GABA agonists such as muscimol have consistently been shown to be protective in adult models of cerebral ischemia.[41] However, as recently reviewed, benzodiazepines which also act through the GABA(A) receptor show less consistent effects, suggesting that efficacy is highly dependent on specific activation of particular subtypes of the GABA(A) receptor.[42]

Similarly, adenosine plays a significant role in reducing the cerebral metabolic rate for oxygen and increasing CBF during hypoxia.[43] The initial depression of synaptic transmission during hypoxia has been shown to be due to endogenous adenosine acting at neuronal adenosine A(1) receptors.[44] Nevertheless, although protection has been reported with selective adenosine agonists, it is striking that protection has also been found with adenosine receptor antagonists.[39,45] This discrepancy may be related in part to the very wide range of different cerebral effects caused by the multiple subtypes of adenosine receptor, and in part to the confounding effect of systemic vasodilatation and hypotension mediated by the cardiovascular adenosine receptors.[46]

Cellular factors

Biochemical responses within cells may also help reduce damage. Increased expression of antiapoptotic proteins such as Bcl-2 following mild ischemia may act to limit neuronal loss.[47] A further potential modality is the transient increase in the expression of the calcium binding protein calbindin D28k after ischemia.[48] This response is postulated to buffer the increased intracellular free calcium after ischemia. A significant protective role for calbindin is supported by the differential expression of calbindin across different neuronal populations. Cell populations such as mature granule cells in the dentate gyrus of the hippocampus, and elsewhere, that are very resistant to ischemic injury, express high levels of calbindin.[49,50] In their immature state these cells do not express calbindin, and are as susceptible to ischemia as other populations.[49] Furthermore, the neuroprotective actions of some neurotrophic factors have been related to induction of calbindin expression, supporting the concept that part of their action is mediated by stabilizing calcium homeostasis.[51–53]

Cerebrovascular responses in the delayed phase

A delayed period of hyperperfusion or "luxury perfusion" is well described after perinatal asphyxia.[54] There is some evidence that this late hyperperfusion may help, in part, to protect marginally viable tissue.[11] Putatively neuroprotective agents such as the calcium antagonists which depress blood pressure and thus impair CBF in the postasphyxial period are reported to aggravate brain injury.[8,55]

Factors which may mediate the hyperperfusion involved include nitric oxide (NO),[55] and prostacyclin.[56] NO is a volatile, rapidly regulated neuromodulator which can be produced by NO synthases (NOS) in endothelial cells (eNOS), neurons (nNOS) and neutrophils or microglia (inducible NOS, or iNOS). Citrulline, a degradation product of NO, is induced in extracellular brain fluid in the secondary phase after ischemia, consistent with induction of NO playing a role in delayed hyperperfusion.[12]

It is vital to take into consideration these multiple roles of NO in order to interpret its effects on neural injury. The endothelial NO is a vasodilator which under physiological conditions plays an important role in the regulation of CBF, cerebral autoregulation, blood flow–metabolism coupling, and the control of platelet aggregation and adhesion.[57] NO has also been shown to play a role in regulating fetal CBF.[58] Thus, it is perhaps not surprising that since most NO production derives from induction of endothelial NOS, nonspecific inhibition of NO production following ischemia has been associated with increased cerebral injury, probably due to impairment of cerebral perfusion.[55]

In contrast, selective inhibition of nNOS or iNOS may be more consistently neuroprotective.[59] nNOS is Ca^{2+}-dependent and thus activated by intracellular calcium accumulation during ischemia, and nNOS expression in the developing brain correlates with regions of selective neuronal loss in the developing rat brain. iNOS is inducible by cytokines and released by activated macrophages in very highly concentrated killing bursts. Macrophage activation occurs late in the delayed phase of injury, and thus is a likely mediator of cytotoxicity in that phase. However, much more work is required to dissect the direct contribution of macrophages to brain damage, as opposed to their role in removing already dying cells.

Endogenous neurotrophic factors

It has been known for some time that the injured brain can release neurotrophic growth factors, but they have only recently been characterized. Nieto-Sampedro and colleagues showed that neurotrophic activity was dramatically increased after wounding of the rat cortex and that this response was considerably greater in the juvenile compared to the adult brain.[60] Extensive studies have been performed after unilateral HI injury in the immature rat. These studies show that shortly after the end of hypoxia there is minimal induction of mRNAs coding for members of the nerve growth factor family (nerve growth factor beta, brain-derived neurotrophic factor; neurotrophin 3). Such induction is restricted to the hippocampus of the noninjured side and has been shown to be induced by postasphyxial seizures.[61,62]

The strong induction of other classes of endogenous growth factors after HI is extended over a much longer period. Much recent attention has focused on insulin-like growth factor 1 (IGF-1) because of its potent and very broadly based antiapoptotic actions. Based on these observations, it was hypothesized that these growth factors might act as endogenous neuroprotective factors, limiting neural injury.[63] This has lead to numerous studies of their use as therapeutic agents to protect neural cells after brain injury.

Insulin-like growth factors

The IGF axis is made up of two biologically active peptides, IGF-1 and IGF-2, six known binding proteins (IGFBP 1–6), and two known receptors, IGF type 1 receptor (IGF-R) and the IGF type 2/mannose-6-phosphate receptor (IGF-2/M6P-R). It is thought that the actions of IGF-1 are mediated mainly by the IGF-R.[64] At high ligand concentrations the insulin receptor is also activated. The IGFBPs are thought to act as modulators of the actions of the IGFs, although some of the IGFBPs have actions independent of IGF-1. In the central nervous system there are two variants of IGF-R: one with an apparent altered molecular weight of the alpha subunit,[65] and another with an altered beta subunit.[66] The actions of IGFs on cells are generally anabolic in nature, including stimulation of mitosis, DNA synthesis, proliferation, and differentiation, as well as increased glucose uptake and protein production.

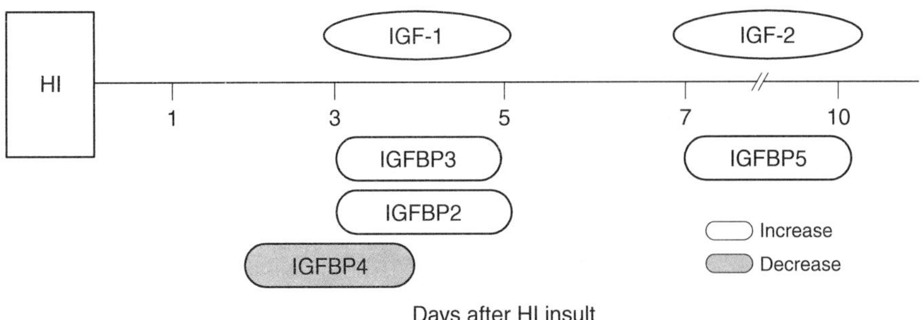

Figure 36.3 The time-course of induction of insulin-like growth factor-1 (IGF-1) and temporal relation to the IGF-2 and IGF binding proteins (IGFBPs) after hypoxia–ischemia (HI) in the infant rat. IGF-1 mRNA is coexpressed with the IGFBP-2 and 3 at 3 days after the HI injury, while IGFBP-4 expression is rapidly reduced. The later induction of IGF-2 is parallel to the IGFBP-5 expression.[63]

In the central nervous system IGF-1 activity occurs across a variety of neuronal and glial phenotypes, including the promotion of neuronal survival, neurite outgrowth, and protein synthesis in vitro on sympathetic, sensory, cortical, and motor neurons;[67–69] enhancing mitosis, differentiation, and maturation of neurons in vitro;[70] the promotion of thymidine incorporation in astrocytes[71] and the promotion of the proliferation, maturation, and myelination of oligodendrocytes.[72] IGF-1 is strongly antiapoptotic, and has been shown to block developmental apoptosis in vivo,[73] and experimental apoptosis in vitro.[74,75]

IGFs in the injured central nervous system

The induction of IGF-1 and related factors after hypoxic–ischemic injury has been extensively characterized post-natally, particularly in the 21-day-old rat, as outlined in Figure 36.3. IGF-1 mRNA is induced in injured glia in a dose-related manner 3–5 days after injury.[76] Similarly, after electrolytic damage, enhanced IGF-1 protein release has been found in microdialysate several days later.[77] Immunohistochemically, the IGF-1 protein can be shown to be largely associated with reactive microglia and with astrocytes juxtaposed to surviving neurons surrounding the area of infarction.[78] The induction is specific to IGF-1 as IGF-2 is not induced until much later.[79]

IGFBP-2 and IGFBP-3 are also induced in parallel with IGF-1, peaking 3 days after injury.[78,80] In contrast, IGF-2 and IGFBP-5 are not induced until 3–10 days after injury, presumably as part of a wound repair mechanism.[79] IGFBP-2 mRNA was strongly induced in reactive astrocytes throughout the injured hemisphere, whereas IGFBP-3 and IGFBP-5 mRNA were moderately induced in association with reactive microglia and neurons respectively within the injured hippocampus. Survival of neurons and the induction of IGFBP-2 in supporting cells in the injured hemisphere are closely related. With neuronal death there is no induction of IGFBP-2. These findings suggest that IGF-1 produced by microglia after injury is transferred to perineuronal reactive astrocytes expressing IGFBP-2.[78] The presence of the binding protein may enable targeting of IGF-1 to the injured neurons.

Studies evaluating the transportation of IGF-1 have shown that within 30 min of intracerebroventricular administration, a significantly higher accumulation of IGF-1 was found in the hemisphere ipsilateral to the HI injury, suggesting that injury increases the permeability of the ependyma of the ventricles.[81] The early intracerebral transportation of IGF-1 from the cerebrospinal fluid was closely related to the white-matter tracts and the perivascular space.[82] ^{3}H-labeled IGF-1 was associated with both neurons and glia by 6 h after administration. This binding was specific as it could be displaced by administration of unlabeled IGF-1.[82]

Neuronal rescue with IGF-1

The first demonstration of neuronal rescue activity of IGF-1 was in 1992.[76] IGF-1 administered 2 h after severe unilateral HI injury in adult rats reduced cortical infarction from 84 to 27%.[76,83] Further, IGF-1 also reduced selective neuronal loss in a dose-dependent fashion in the pyriform cortex, lateral cortex, striatum, and the hippocampus.[83] As well as histological improvement, functional improvement has been demonstrated in this model, with improvement in a bilateral tactile test (unpublished observation). In contrast to the effect of postinsult therapy, IGF-1 given 1 h prior to HI was not neuroprotective.[83] A critical role for IGF BP, particular IGFBP-2, in mediating IGF-1 uptake and distribution from the lateral ventricles has been strongly suggested by comparison of the neuroprotective effects and uptake of IGF-1 (which is strongly linked to IGFBP-2), with the very limited effects of des-IGF-1 which does not bind IGFBP-2. Furthermore, coadministration of IGF-2, which has 100 times greater affinity for the IGFBPs than IGF-1, blocked the neuroprotective effects of IGF-1, probably by displacing IGF-1 from IGFBP-2.[84]

A similar neuroprotective effect of IGF-1 has also been demonstrated in the sheep fetus after cerebral ischemia by reversible carotid artery occlusion which causes laminar necrosis of the parasagittal cortex and widespread neuronal loss throughout the cerebrum.[14] IGF-1, administered intracerebroventricularly within 2 h of ischemia, significantly improved overall neurohistological outcome, in particular, in the lateral cerebral cortex, striatum, and the dentate gyrus of the dorsal horn of the hippocampus[9,85] (Figure 36.2). IGF-1 also reduced the incidence of postasphyxial seizures and attenuated the secondary rise in cytotoxic edema, showing that IGF-1 is acting by suppressing the evolution of delayed neuronal death.[85]

Insulin-like growth factors and white-matter injury

The studies presented so far have focused on neuronal injury. Although injury of immature white matter is well known to be the dominant cause of neural handicap in very premature infants,[86] white-matter damage later in life has been relatively neglected.[87] This is at least in part because white matter was believed to be less vulnerable to injury than gray matter.[88] Recent imaging data show that cerebral white-matter injury also contributes to developmental disability after perinatal HI injury at term.[89,90] Experimentally, it is increasingly recognized that differentiated oligodendrocytes and myelinated axons are at least as vulnerable to ischemic injury as neurons.[91–95] For example, after focal ischemia in the adult rat, oligodendrocyte loss is reported to develop earlier than neuronal injury.[91] Similarly, the mildest lesion seen after asphyxia in the near-term fetal sheep was vacuolation and loss of myelin in white matter, rather than neuronal death.[95]

The pathogenesis of demyelination after injury may be due to primary death of mature oligodendrocytes,[92,96] or to secondary loss, related to either microglial activation or to loss of trophic support after axonal degeneration.[96] A number of lines of evidence suggest that IGF-1 may have a particular role in limiting both primary and secondary post-ischemic white-matter injury. IGF-1 promotes the proliferation and differentiation of oligodendroglia, and upregulates myelin production in vitro.[72,97–100] It has broad, receptor-mediated antiapoptotic effects in vitro and in vivo,[73–75] and specifically inhibited the primary, apoptotic loss of oligodendrocytes associated with cytokine toxicity and metabolic insults.[100,101] Experimental demyelination is associated with distinctive patterns of induction of IGF-1 in astrocytes and of the IGF-1 receptor in oligodendrocytes during regeneration,[102,103] suggesting that endogenous IGF-1 may play a key role in remyelination. Similarly, as discussed above IGF-1 is also intensely induced in reactive glia 3–5 days after HI injury.[63]

Recent data have now shown that postischemic

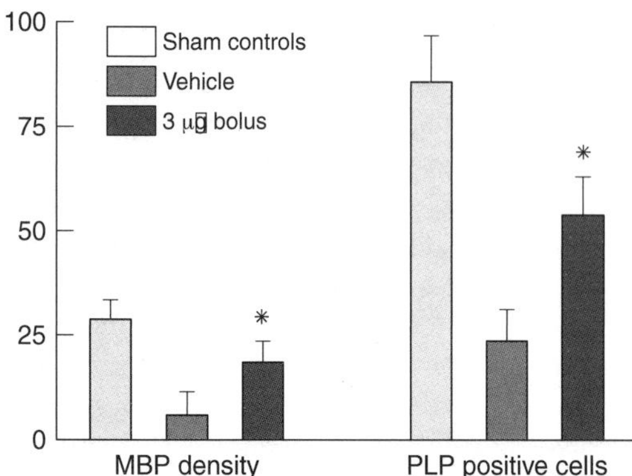

Figure 36.4 The effect of insulin-like growth factor-1 (IGF-1) treatment 90 min after reperfusion from dense ischemia in the fetal sheep on myelin basic protein (MBP) density and survival of oligodendrocytes, identified by labeling for proteolipid protein (PLP) mRNA (PLP, a major component of myelin, is expressed in the brain only in mature oligodendrocytes) in the parasagittal cortex, after 4 days' recovery. Ischemic injury resulted in a marked loss in average density of MBP ($P<0.05$), and a massive loss of PLP mRNA-positive cells in the intragyral white-matter tracts ($P<0.001$), compared with sham occlusion. IGF-1 treatment given 90 min after reperfusion from global cerebral ischemia significantly improved the postischemic reduction in intragyral MBP density and numbers of PLP-positive cells. * $P<0.05$ vs vehicle-treated fetuses. Data derived from Euan et al.[104]

administration of exogenous IGF-1 can prevent the severe delayed postischemic oligodendrocyte cell loss and associated demyelination that occur after 30 min of cerebral ischemia in the near-term fetal sheep (Figure 36.4).[104] Intriguingly, white-matter protection with IGF-1 was associated with increased gliosis, with greater numbers of both reactive astrocytes and microglia. These data, combined with the close colocalization of PLP-expressing cells with nonmyelinating cell types during recovery from ischemic injury,[92] suggest that reactive glia may have a secondary role either in preventing demyelination or promoting remyelination. Although reactive astrocytes and microglia have been considered to play opposing roles, promoting and impairing neuronal survival in vitro respectively,[17,105] astrocytes and microglia secrete factors that contribute to each other's survival.[106] Furthermore, induction of mRNA for IGF-1 after brain injury has been found in microglia as well as in reactive astrocytes, suggesting that both cell types may make a contribution to white-matter recovery.[76,78]

Derivative molecules

The actions of IGF-1 may be mediated at least in part by derivative molecules. Evidence has accumulated suggesting that IGF-1 is proteolytically cleaved in tissues into des(1–3) IGF-1 and the *N*-terminal tripeptide glycine-proline-glutamate (GPE).[107] The biological role of GPE in the central nervous system has been shown to be different from des-(1–3) IGF-1[108,109] as it does not bind to the IGF-1 receptors.[110] The biological effects of GPE can be altered by IGF BP. However, there is no direct evidence that GPE is present endogenously in tissues,[111] and a specific receptor for GPE has not yet been identified, although there is some evidence that GPE may act as an endogenous antagonist at glutamate receptors.[112,113]

GPE (in a dose equimolar to the maximally neuroprotective dose of IGF-1) administered intracerebroventricularly to adult rats 2 h after HI was neuroprotective in the cortex, hippocampus, and striatum.[114] The regional neuroprotective effects of GPE appeared to be different from those of both native and des-(1–3) IGF-1. GPE administration selectively prevented the loss of choline acetyltransferase, glutamate acid decarboxylase, and somatostatin neurons, but not neuropeptide Y and nNOS containing neurons in the striatum. Interestingly, an increase in the numbers of nNOS containing neurons in the hemisphere contralateral to the injury was observed, suggesting that GPE can also influence neuronal activity after HI injury. Similarly, GPE administration also prevents the loss of dopaminergic neurons and upregulates neurotransmission in the substantia nigra after 6-hydroxydopamine administration in the middle forebrain bundle.[115]

Activin and transforming growth factor-β

Many other growth factors are induced in the brain after injury, including transforming growth factor-β (TGF-β) and activin. TGF-β_1 mRNA is induced in injured areas of the brain after a severe insult, from 5 h to 3 days.[116] TGF-β_1 is involved in a number of cellular processes that include regulation of inflammation and wound repair.[117] Thus, TGF-β_1 may function as a neuroprotective molecule by suppressing the release of cytotoxins by macrophages[118] and microglia.[119] In the infant rat model of HI injury treatment with 10 ng of recombinant human TGF-β_1 reduces the microglia response within 48 h of insult. This microglial suppression was accompanied by reduced cortical infarction and neuronal loss in the piriform cortex, lateral cortex, dentate gyrus, thalamus, and striatum, but with no effect on cell loss in the cornu ammonis (CA)1–4 region of the hippocampus.[120]

Activin is a member of the TGF-β superfamily of growth and differentiation factors, that is known to promote the survival of neurons in culture,[121,122] and protect neurons against toxicity.[123] Similarly to TGF-β, its mRNA is strongly induced in neurons and glia following HI injury,[124] with an increase in mRNA between 5 and 10 h after HI.[125] Subsequently we have shown that after HI in the infant rat, 1 mg activin A reduces selective neuronal loss in the CA1/2 region of the hippocampus and in the dorsolateral striatum.[125] The pattern of neuroprotection is consistent with the distribution of the activin receptor type II subunit.[125,126]

Postnatal hypothermia

The concept that temperature could affect the outcome of resuscitation from severe perinatal asphyxia is not new. At birth there is a physiological fall in temperature, of approximately 0.5–0.7°C, which is further augmented by greater cooling of the surface of the brain postnatally by thermal radiation, compared with the core temperature.[127,128] This physiological fall is greatly exaggerated by exposure to hypoxia, leading to the concept that mild hypothermia may indeed be a natural adaptive response to hypoxia. Early experimental studies, mainly in precocial species such as kittens, demonstrated that hypothermia greatly extended the "time to last gasp." This led to a series of small uncontrolled studies in the 1950s and 1960s where infants not breathing spontaneously at 5 min were immersed in cold water until respiration resumed.[129–131]

Although outcomes after hypothermia were said to be better than in historical controls, this experimental approach was overtaken by two important developments: the introduction of active ventilation and resuscitation of such infants, and the recognition that even mild hypothermia is associated with a wide range of potential adverse systemic effects,[132] including increased oxygen requirements, reduced cardiac contractility, reduced surfactant production, and greater mortality in the premature newborn.[133] Thus modern resuscitation guidelines have until very recently simply emphasized keeping the newly born warm, i.e., avoiding hypothermia.[134] Recent systematic studies have now shown that changes in cerebral temperature during and after HI can significantly affect brain injury.

Temperature and experimental hypoxia–ischemia

Hypothermia during experimental cerebral ischemia is consistently associated with potent, dose-related,[135] long-lasting neuroprotection.[136–138] Conversely, hyperthermia of even 1–2°C extends and markedly worsens damage,[135,139–145] and particularly tends to promote pannecrosis of glia as well as neurons.[135,140] Although the majority of studies of hyperthermia involved ischemia in adult rodents, similar results have been reported from studies of ischemia or HI in the newborn piglet and 7-day-old rat respectively.[146,147]

The impact of cerebral cooling or warming the brain by only a few degrees is disproportionate to the known changes in brain metabolism (approximately a 5% change in oxidative metabolism per °C,[148] suggesting that hypothermia is acting to suppress many of the factors mediating ischemic injury.[135,149]

Mechanisms that may be involved include reduced release of oxygen free radicals and excitatory neurotransmitters such as glutamate, reduced toxicity of glutamate on neurons,[150] reduced dysfunction of the blood–brain barrier,[151] and prevention of cytoskeletal proteolysis.[152]

Effect of temperature during resuscitation/reperfusion

In most cases of perinatal HIE reperfusion (return of cerebral circulation) corresponds with clinical resuscitation at birth. The distinctive feature of this phase is the rapid increase in oxygen levels. There is experimental evidence that this leads to a transient burst of oxygen free radical production (in the perinatal rat and fetal sheep) with damaging peroxidation of structural cell membrane lipids.[16,153] Cooling during this brief phase reduced NO release in the piglet,[154] and suppressed oxygen free radical release and lipid peroxidation in the young adult dog and gerbil.[155,156]

In practice, however, brief (0.5–3h) mild-to-moderate hypothermia immediately after HI injury has had inconsistent effects on neuronal loss in studies in the 7-day-old rat[147,157,158] the piglet[159–161] and the adult rodent,[138,162–164] cat[165] and dog.[166] On balance the effects of brief, early hypothermia appear to be relatively modest, to be increased by longer durations of cooling, usually an hour or more, and to be exquisitely sensitive to delay in initiation. For example, after 15 min of reversible ischemia in the piglet, mild hypothermia (2–3 °C) for 1 h significantly improved recovery and partially reduced neuronal loss 3 days later.[160] However, this effect was lost if hypothermia was delayed until 30 min after ischemia.[161] This is consistent with reports in adult species showing that protection was lost if brief hypothermia was delayed by as little as 15–45 min after ischemia.[163,164,166]

Studies of hyperthermia lead to very similar conclusions. In adult rodents mild hyperthermia (increases of 1.5–3 °C), for up to an hour, started no more than 15 min after ischemia increased neural injury.[141,167] However, when hyperthermia was delayed by 45 min or more after ischemia, the deleterious effects of hyperthermia were greatly attenuated.[167]

It is important to appreciate that the majority of these studies evaluated neural outcome after relatively short periods of 3–7 days' recovery. There is some evidence in adult and neonatal rodents that a major part of the effect of early but short periods of hypothermia is to delay, and of hyperthermia to accelerate, the evolution of damage,[138,158,168] with progressive attenuation of the effect over time.[158]

Cooling in the secondary phase

A more recent approach has been to continue hypothermia for 6–72h, into the latent and secondary phases of injury. Such prolonged cooling has been associated with more consistent protection. For example, in contrast to the transient effect of moderate hypothermia for 3h after HI in the 7-day-old rat,[158] 6h of moderate (32°C) hypothermia was associated with a persistent reduction in infarct volume, and behavioral improvement after 6 weeks.[169] However, in these studies hypothermia was still started immediately after the end of hypoxia.

Even more prolonged periods of hypothermia may offer protection despite delayed initiation of hypothermia.[170] The effects of such prolonged hypothermia have been systematically examined in a model of 30 min of cerebral ischemia induced by bilateral carotid artery occlusion in the fetal sheep. This insult leads to delayed seizures and cytotoxic cell swelling between 6 and 72h after reperfusion, and severe cerebral injury in a watershed distribution.[7,171,172] Moderate hypothermia begun 90 min after reperfusion, and continued until 72h after ischemia, prevented secondary cytotoxic edema, and improved EEG recovery.[7] There was a concomitant substantial reduction in parasagittal cortical infarction and improvement in neuronal loss scores in all regions assessed (Figure 36.5). When the start of hypothermia was delayed until just before the onset of secondary seizures in this paradigm, 5.5h after reperfusion, partial

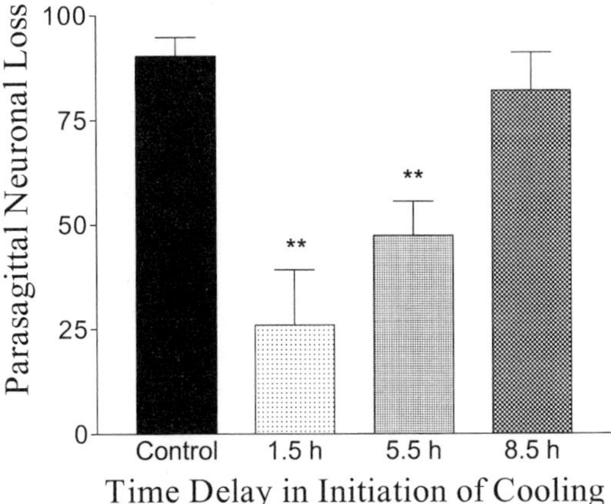

Figure 36.5 The effect of delaying the initiation of cerebral cooling on neuroprotection of the parasagittal parietal cortex. Near-term fetal sheep were exposed to 30 min of cerebral ischemia and allowed to recover for 5 days. Hypothermia was started at different times after reperfusion and continued until 72 h. Compared with the sham cooled group ($n=13$), cooling which was started 90 min after reperfusion ($n=7$) or just before the end of the latent phase (5.5 h after reperfusion, $n=11$) was protective, whereas cooling that was started shortly after the start of the secondary phase (8.5 h after reperfusion, $n=5$) was not. Only cooled fetuses in which the extradural temperature was successfully maintained below 34 °C have been included. Data derived from Gunn et al.[7,171,172] $^{**}P<0.005$ compared with sham-cooled (control) fetuses, Mann–Whitney U test. Mean ± SEM.

neuroprotection was seen.[171] With further delay until after seizures were established (8.5 h after reperfusion), there was no electrophysiological or overall histological protection with cooling, as shown in Figure 36.5.[172] These data strongly suggest that hypothermia is acting by suppressing prolonged encephalopathic processes that begin in the latent phase. However encouraging, the parameters of timing and depth of hypothermia required for successful clinical neuroprotection are simply not known in humans, and remain to be established in systematic randomized trials of postresuscitative hypothermia; the first such studies are now in progress.[173]

Hypothermia and the window of opportunity for other therapies

A number of studies in adult and newborn animals have reported that short periods of active postinsult cerebral cooling can substantially delay the evolution of neuronal death.[138,158,174] Thus, even if hypothermia alone proves not to be practical, this delay of injury may be of considerable importance. The timely selection and enrollment of patients for therapeutic trials of acute encephalopathy present formidable logistic difficulties. Despite the proven efficacy of anticoagulation after acute ischemic stroke, for example, the majority of patients are not able to be enrolled within its known, narrow therapeutic window.[175] Recent studies have confirmed that such early but mild cooling can critically extend the window of opportunity for neuronal rescue with IGF-1 from 2 h after HI up to as long as 6 h, as shown in Figure 36.6.[168] This approach may increase the number of patients with an HI insult who may be able to be enrolled for therapeutic trials, while minimizing the known side-effects associated with prolonged moderate hypothermia, including impaired immunocompetence and delayed coagulation.[132]

Conclusions

Experimental studies of HI have shown that neural injury is an evolving process, characterized by an early latent phase, followed by the ultimate development of delayed neuronal death. The latent phase may be viewed as the foundation period during which the processes that ultimately mediate injury develop. Thus the latent phase appears to represent the critical window of opportunity for rescue therapy. Moderate cerebral hypothermia initiated during the latent phase and continued for a sufficient period to allow resolution of secondary processes is protective across a wide range of species and experimental models. Similarly, we have shown that the IGF system and other endogenous growth factors are induced in response to injury and may act in part to help limit injury. Exogenous administration of IGF-1 and other broadly active neurotrophic factors during the latent phase greatly attenuated delayed neuronal loss, indicating the potential of these to act as neuronal rescue therapeutic agents.

While experimental studies to date are very promising, many questions remain before they can be considered for clinical evaluation.[176] In particular, the rate of progression of the "latent phase" of programmed cell death, during which intervention is most likely to be effective, is very unclear in clinical HIE and, because of the potential for prenatal evolution, may well be substantially shorter than seen in many experimental models. Even if the tempo is comparable, substantial time often elapses between the apparent start of the typically intermittent insult in labor, and birth.[177] Nevertheless, the knowledge gained over the last decade suggests that effective therapies will ultimately be developed. We may predict that an effective strategy will probably combine multiple modalities for optimal effectiveness, for example a combination of early hypothermia and antiapoptotic agents.

Acknowledgments

The authors' work reported in this review has been supported by National Institutes of Health grant RO-1 HD32752, and by grants from the Health Research Council of New Zealand, the Lottery Health Board of New Zealand, and the Auckland Medical Research Foundation.

REFERENCES

1 Low, J.A., Lindsay, B.G., Derrick, E.J. (1997). Threshold of metabolic acidosis associated with newborn complications. *Am J Obstet Gynecol* **177**: 1391–1394.

2 Gunn, A.J., Parer, J.T., Mallard, E.C. et al. (1992). Cerebral histologic and electrocorticographic changes after asphyxia in fetal sheep. *Pediatr Res* **31**: 486–491.

3 Azzopardi, D., Wyatt, J.S., Cady, E.B. et al. (1989). Prognosis of newborn infants with hypoxic–ischemic brain injury assessed by phosphorus magnetic resonance spectroscopy. *Pediatr Res* **25**: 445–451.

4 Roth, S.C., Baudin, J., Cady, E. et al. (1997). Relation of deranged neonatal cerebral oxidative metabolism with neurodevelopmental outcome and head circumference at 4 years. *Dev Med Child Neurol* **39**: 718–725.

5 Lorek, A., Takei, Y., Cady, E.B. et al. (1994). Delayed ("secondary") cerebral energy failure after acute hypoxia–ischemia in the newborn piglet: continuous 48-hour studies by phosphorus magnetic resonance spectroscopy. *Pediatr Res* **36**: 699–706.

6 Mehmet, H., Yue, X., Penrice, J. et al. (1998). Relation of impaired energy metabolism to apoptosis and necrosis following transient cerebral hypoxia–ischaemia. *Cell Death Differentiation* **5**: 321–329.

7 Gunn, A.J., Gunn, T.R., de Haan, H.H. et al. (1997). Dramatic neuronal rescue with prolonged selective head cooling after ischemia in fetal lambs. *J Clin Invest* **99**: 248–256.

8 Gunn, A.J., Williams, C.E., Mallard, E.C. et al. (1994). Flunarizine, a calcium channel antagonist, is partially prophylactically neuroprotective in hypoxic–ischemic encephalopathy in the fetal sheep. *Pediatr Res* **35**: 657–663.

9 Guan, J., Bennet, L., George, S. et al. (1999). Selective neuroprotective effects with insulin-like growth factor-1 in phenotypic striatal neurons following ischemic brain injury in fetal sheep. *Neuroscience* **95**: 831–839.

10 Samejima, K., Tone, S., Kottke, T.J. et al. (1998). Transition from caspase-dependent to caspase-independent mechanisms at the onset of apoptotic execution. *J Cell Biol* **143**: 225–239.

11 Abi Raad, R., Tan, W.K., Bennet, L. et al. (1999). Role of the cerebrovascular and metabolic responses in the delayed phases of injury after transient cerebral ischemia in fetal sheep. *Stroke* **30**: 2735–2742.

12 Tan, W.K., Williams, C.E., During, M.J. et al. (1996). Accumulation of cytotoxins during the development of seizures and edema after hypoxic–ischemic injury in late gestation fetal sheep. *Pediatr Res* **39**: 791–797.

13 Marks, K.A., Mallard, E.C., Roberts, I. et al. (1996). Delayed

Figure 36.6 (*Right*) Effect of early, very mild cerebral cooling on the window of opportunity for neuroprotection with insulin-like growth factor-1 (IGF-1) in the 21-day-old rat. (*a*) IGF-1 significantly reduced the percentage of cortical damage when administered centrally at 2 h, but not 6 h posthypoxia–ischemia (HI) in rats exposed to a warm recovery environment (an air temperature of 31°C) for 2 h after HI. $^{*}P<0.05$ compared to vehicle controls. (*b*) In contrast, IGF-1 significantly reduced cortical damage when given 6 h post-HI to rats exposed to a cool environment (23 °C) for the first 2 h after hypoxia. Data derived from Guan et al.[168]

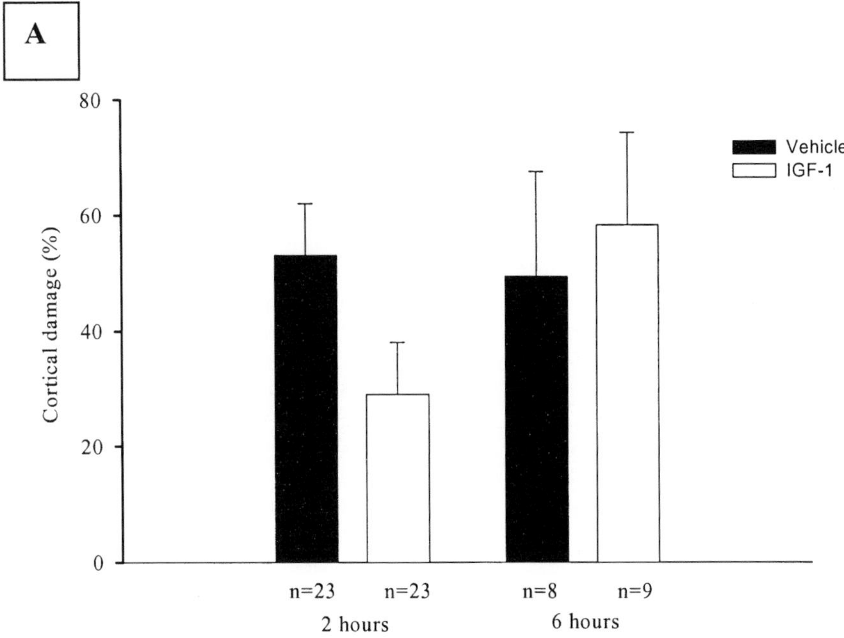
A
80
60
40
20
0
Cortical damage (%)
Vehicle
IGF-1
n=23 n=23 n=8 n=9
2 hours
6 hours

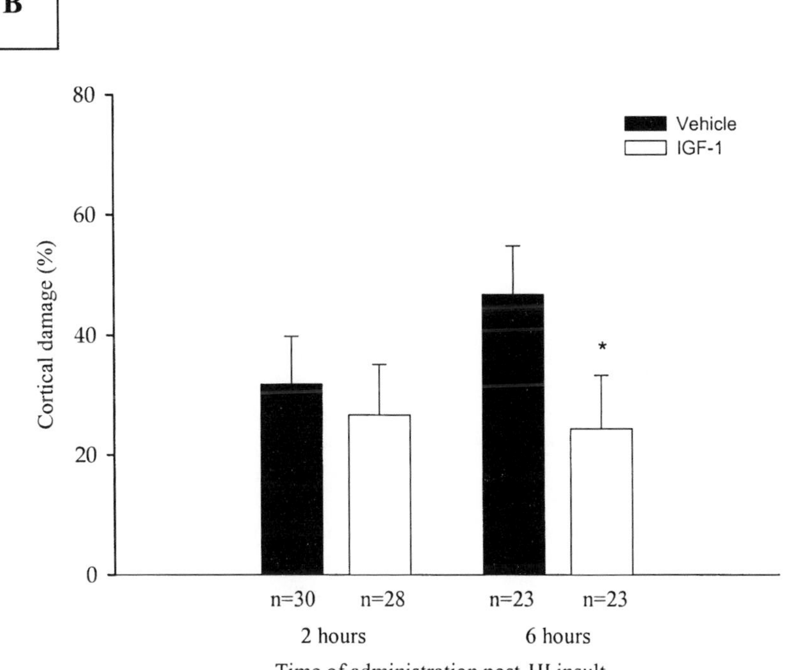
B
80
60
40
20
0
Cortical damage (%)
Vehicle
IGF-1
*
n=30 n=28 n=23 n=23
2 hours
6 hours
Time of administration post-HI insult

vasodilation and altered oxygenation following cerebral ischemia in fetal sheep. *Pediatr Res* **39**: 48–54.

14 Williams, C.E., Gunn, A.J., Gluckman, P.D. (1991). Time course of intracellular edema and epileptiform activity following prenatal cerebral ischemia in sheep. *Stroke* **22**: 516–521.

15 Clawson, T.F., Vannucci, S.J., Wang, G.M. et al. (1999). Hypoxic–ischemic-induced apoptotic cell death correlates with IGF-1 mRNA decrease in neonatal rat brain. *Biol Signals Recept* **8**: 281–293.

16 Bagenholm, R., Nilsson, U.A., Gotborg, C.W. et al. (1998). Free radicals are formed in the brain of fetal sheep during reperfusion after cerebral ischemia. *Pediatr Res* **43**: 271–275.

17 Giulian, D., Vaca, K. (1993). Inflammatory glia mediate delayed neuronal damage after ischemia in the central nervous system. *Stroke* **24**: I84–I90.

18 Trump, B.F., Berezesky, I.K. (1995). Calcium-mediated cell injury and cell death. *FASEB J* **9**: 219–228.

19 Zipfel, G.J., Lee, J.M., Choi, D.W. (1999). Reducing calcium overload in the ischemic brain. *N Engl J Med* **341**: 1543–1544.

20 Wyllie, A.H. (1980). Glucocorticoid-induced thymocyte apoptosis is associated with endogenous endonuclease activation. *Nature* **284**: 555–556.

21 Raff, M.C. (1992). Social controls on cell survival and cell death. *Nature* **356**: 397–400.

22 Beilharz, E.J., Williams, C.E., Dragunow, M. et al. (1995). Mechanisms of delayed cell death following hypoxic–ischemic injury in the immature rat: evidence for apoptosis during selective neuronal loss. *Brain Res* **29**: 1–14.

23 Yue, X., Mehmet, H., Penrice, J. et al. (1997). Apoptosis and necrosis in the newborn piglet brain following transient cerebral hypoxia–ischaemia. *Neuropathol Appl Neurobiol* **23**: 16–25.

24 Dell'Anna, E., Chen, Y., Engidawork, E. et al. (1997). Delayed neuronal death following perinatal asphyxia in rat. *Exp. Brain Res* **115**: 105–115.

25 Edwards, A.D., Cox, P., Hope, P.L. et al. (1997). Apoptosis in the brains of infants suffering intrauterine cerebral injury. *Pediatr Res* **42**: 684–689.

26 Scott, R.J., Hegyi, L. (1997). Cell death in perinatal hypoxic–ischaemic brain injury. *Neuropathol Appl Neurobiol* **23**: 307–314.

27 Larsen, C.J. (1994). The BCL2 gene is the prototype of a gene family that controls programmed cell death (apoptosis). *Ann Genet Paris* **37**: 121–134.

28 MacGibbon, G.A., Lawlor, P.A., Sirimanne, E.S. et al. (1997). Bax expression in mammalian neurons undergoing apoptosis, and in Alzheimer's disease hippocampus. *Brain Res* **750**: 223–234.

29 Zhu, C., Wang, X., Hagberg, H. et al. (2000). Correlation between caspase-3 activation and three different markers of DNA damage in neonatal cerebral hypoxia–ischemia. *J Neurochem* **75**: 819–829.

30 Troy, C.M., Stefanis, L., Prochiantz, A. et al. (1996). The contrasting roles of ICE family proteases and interleukin-1beta in apoptosis induced by trophic factor withdrawal and by copper/zinc superoxide dismutase down-regulation. *Proc Natl Acad Sci USA* **93**: 5635–5640.

31 Porteracailliau, C., Price, D.L., Martin, L.J. (1997). Excitotoxic neuronal death in the immature brain is an apoptosis–necrosis morphological continuum. *J Comp Neurol* **378**: 70–87.

32 Gottron, F.J., Ying, H.S., Choi, D.W. (1997). Caspase inhibition selectively reduces the apoptotic component of oxygen–glucose deprivation-induced cortical neuronal cell death. *Mol Cell Neurosci* **9**: 159–169.

33 Colbourne, F., Sutherland, G.R., Auer, R.N. (1999). Electron microscopic evidence against apoptosis as the mechanism of neuronal death in global ischemia. *J Neurosci* **19**: 4200–4210.

34 Beck, K.D., Powell-Braxton, L., Widmer, H.R. et al. (1995). IGF1 gene disruption results in reduced brain size, CNS hypomyelination, and loss of hippocampal granule and striatal parvalbumin-containing neurons. *Neuron* **14**: 717–730.

35 Kane, D.J., Ord, T., Anton, R. et al. (1995). Expression of bcl-2 inhibits necrotic neural cell death. *J Neurosci Res* **40**: 269–275.

36 Vannucci, R.C., Towfighi, J., Vannucci, S.J. (1998). Hypoxic preconditioning and hypoxic–ischemic brain damage in the immature rat: pathologic and metabolic correlates. *J Neurochem* **71**: 1215–1220.

37 Heurteaux, C., Lauritzen, I., Widmann, C. et al. (1995). Essential role of adenosine, adenosine A1 receptors, and ATP-sensitive K^+ channels in cerebral ischemic preconditioning. *Proc Natl Acad Sci USA* **92**: 4666–4670.

38 Massa, S.M., Swanson, R.A., Sharp, F.R. (1996). The stress gene response in brain. *Cerebrovasc Brain Metab Rev* **8**: 95–158.

39 Shuaib, A., Kanthan, R. (1997). Amplification of inhibitory mechanisms in cerebral ischemia: an alternative approach to neuronal protection. *Histol Histopathol* **12**: 185–194.

40 Nilsson, G.E., Lutz, P.L. (1991). Release of inhibitory neurotransmitters in response to anoxia in turtle brain. *Am J Physiol* **261**: R32–R37.

41 Shuaib, A., Mazagri, R., Ijaz, S. (1993). GABA agonist "muscimol" is neuroprotective in repetitive transient forebrain ischemia in gerbils. *Exp Neurol* **123**: 284–288.

42 Green, A.R., Hainsworth, A.H., Jackson, D.M. (2000). GABA potentiation: a logical pharmacological approach for the treatment of acute ischaemic stroke. *Neuropharmacology* **39**: 1483–1494.

43 Bell, M.J., Robertson, C.S., Kochanek, P.M. et al. (2001). Interstitial brain adenosine and xanthine increase during jugular venous oxygen desaturations in humans after traumatic brain injury. *Crit Care Med* **29**: 399–404.

44 Gervitz, L.M., Lutherer, L.O., Davies, D.G. et al. (2001). Adenosine induces initial hypoxic–ischemic depression of synaptic transmission in the rat hippocampus in vivo. *Am J Physiol Regul Integr Comp Physiol* **280**: R639–R645.

45 Bona, E., Aden, U., Gilland, E. et al. (1997). Neonatal cerebral hypoxia–ischemia – the effect of adenosine receptor antagonists. *Neuropharmacology* **36**: 1327–1338.

46 Spalding, M.B., Ala-Kokko, T.I., Kiviluoma, K. et al. (2000). The hemodynamic effects of adenosine infusion after experimental right heart infarct in young swine. *J Cardiovasc Pharmacol* **35**: 93–99.

47 Shimazaki, K., Ishida, A., Kawai, N. (1994). Increase in bcl-2 oncoprotein and the tolerance to ischemia-induced neuronal death in the gerbil hippocampus. *Neurosci Res* **20**: 95–99.

48 Lowenstein, D.H., Gwinn, R.P., Seren, M.S. et al. (1994). Increased expression of mRNA encoding calbindin-D28K, the glucose-regulated proteins, or the 72 kDa heat-shock protein in three models of acute CNS injury. *Mol Brain Res* **22**: 299–308.

49 Goodman, J.H., Wasterlain, C.G., Massarweh, W.F. et al. (1993). Calbindin-D28k immunoreactivity and selective vulnerability to ischemia in the dentate gyrus of the developing rat. *Brain Res* **606**: 309–314.

50 Waldvogel, H.J., Faull, R.L.M., Dragunow, M. (1991). Differential sensitivity of calbindin and parvalbumin immunoreactive cells in the striatum to excitotoxins. *Brain Res* **546**: 329–335.

51 Nakao, N., Kokaia, Z., Odin, P. et al. (1995). Protective effects of BDNF and NT-3 but not PDGF against hypoglycemic injury to cultured striatal neurons. *Exp Neurol* **131**: 1–10.

52 Nietobona, M.P., Busiguina, S., Torresaleman, I. (1995). Insulin-like growth factor I is an afferent trophic signal that modulates calbindin-28kD in adult Purkinje cells. *J Neurosci Res* **42**: 371–376.

53 Yamaguchi, T., Keino, K., Fukuda, J. (1995). The effect of insulin and insulin-like growth factor-I on the expression of calretinin and calbindin D-28k in rat embryonic neurons in culture. *Neurochem Int* **26**: 255–262.

54 Ilves, P., Talvik, R., Talvik, T. (1998). Changes in Doppler ultrasonography in asphyxiated term infants with hypoxic–ischaemic encephalopathy. *Acta Paediatr Scand* **87**: 680–684.

55 Marks, K.A., Mallard, E.C., Roberts, I. et al. (1996). Nitric oxide synthase inhibition attenuates delayed vasodilation and increases injury following cerebral ischemia in fetal sheep. *Pediatr Res* **40**: 185–191.

56 Walton, M., Sirimanne, E., Williams, C. et al. (1997). Prostaglandin H synthase-2 and cytosolic phospholipase A_2 in the hypoxic–ischemic brain: role in neuronal death or survival? *Mol Brain Res* **50**: 165–170.

57 Faraci, F.M., Heistad, D.D. (1998). Regulation of the cerebral circulation: role of endothelium and potassium channels. *Physiol Rev* **78**: 53–97.

58 Green, L.R., Bennet, L., Hanson, M.A. (1996). The role of nitric oxide synthesis in cardiovascular responses to acute hypoxia in the late gestation sheep fetus. *J Physiol (Lond)* **497**: 271–277.

59 Bolanos, J.P., Almeida, A. (1999). Roles of nitric oxide in brain hypoxia–ischemia. *Biochim Biophys Acta* **1411**: 415–436.

60 Nieto-Sampedro, M., Lewis, E.R., Cotman, C.W. et al. (1982). Brain injury causes a time-dependent increase in neurotrophic activity at the lesion site. *Science* **217**: 860–861.

61 Gunn, A.J., Dragunow, M., Faull, R.L. et al. (1990). Effects of hypoxia–ischemia and seizures on neuronal and glial- like c-fos protein levels in the infant rat. *Brain Res* **531**: 105–116.

62 Dragunow, M., Beilharz, E., Sirimanne, E. et al. (1994). Immediate-early gene protein expression in neurons undergoing delayed death, but not necrosis, following hypoxic–ischaemic injury to the young rat brain. *Mol Brain Res* **25**: 19–33.

63 Hughes, P.E., Alexi, T., Walton, M. et al. (1999). Activity and injury-dependent expression of inducible transcription factors, growth factors and apoptosis-related genes within the central nervous system. *Prog Neurobiol* **57**: 421–450.

64 Czech, M.P. (1989). Signal transmission by the insulin-like growth factors. *Cell* **59**: 235–238.

65 Ocrant, I., Valentino, K.L., Eng, L.F. et al. (1988). Structural and immunohistochemical characterization of insulin-like growth factor I and II receptors in the murine central nervous system. *Endocrinology* **123**: 1023.

66 Mascotti, F., Caceres, A., Pfenninger, K.H. et al. (1997). Expression and distribution of IGF-1 receptors containing a beta-subunit variant (betagc) in developing neurons. *J Neurosci* **17**: 1447–1459.

67 Aizenman, Y., De Vellis, J. (1987). Brain neurons develop in a serum and glial free environment: effects of transferrin, insulin, insulin-like growth factor-I and thyroid hormone on neuronal survival, growth and differentiation. *Brain Res* **406**: 32–42.

68 Caroni, P., Grandes, P. (1990). Nerve sprouting in innervated adult muscle induced by exposure to elevated levels of insulin-like growth factors. *J Cell Biol* **110**: 1307–1317.

69 Knusel, B., Hefti, F. (1991). Trophic actions of IGF-I, IGF-II and insulin on cholinergic and dopaminergic brain neurons. *Adv Exp Med Biol* **293**: 351–360.

70 Pahlman, S., Meyerson, G., Lindgren, E. et al. (1991). Insulin-like growth factor I shifts from promoting cell division to potentiating maturation during neuronal differentiation. *Proc Natl Acad Sci USA* **88**: 9994–9998.

71 Ballotti, R., Nielsen, F.C., Pringle, N. et al. (1987). Insulin-like growth factor I in cultured rat astrocytes: expression of the gene, and receptor tyrosine kinase. *EMBO J* **6**: 3633–3639.

72 McMorris, F.A., Mckinnon, R.D. (1996). Regulation of oligodendrocyte development and CNS myelination by growth factors: prospects for therapy of demyelinating disease. *Brain Pathol* **6**: 313–329.

73 Yin, Q.W., Johnson, J., Prevette, D. et al. (1994). Cell death of spinal motoneurons in the chick embryo following deafferentation: rescue effects of tissue extracts, soluble proteins, and neurotrophic agents. *J Neurosci* **14**: 7629–7640.

74 Galli, C., Meucci, O., Scorziello, A. et al. (1995). Apoptosis in cerebellar granule cells is blocked by high KCl, forskolin, and IGF-1 through distinct mechanisms of action: The involvement of intracellular calcium and RNA synthesis. *J Neurosci* **15**: 1172–1179.

75 Parrizas, M., Saltiel, A.R., LeRoith, D. (1997). Insulin-like growth factor 1 inhibits apoptosis using the phosphatidylinositol 3′-kinase and mitogen-activated protein kinase pathways. *J Biol Chem* **272**: 154–161.

76 Gluckman, P., Klempt, N., Guan, J. et al. (1992). A role for IGF-1 in the rescue of CNS neurons following hypoxic–ischemic injury. *Biochem Biophys Res Commun* **182** : 593–599.

77 Yamaguchi, F., Itano, T., Miyamoto, O. et al. (1991). Increase of extracellular insulin-like growth factor I (IGF-I) concentration following electrolytical lesion in rat hippocampus. *Neurosci Lett* **128**: 273–276.

78 Beilharz, E.J., Russo, V.C., Butler, G. et al. (1998). Co-ordinated and cellular specific induction of the components of the IGF/IGFBP axis in the rat brain following hypoxic–ischemic injury. *Mol Brain Res* **59**: 119–134.

79 Beilharz, E.J., Bassett, N.S., Sirimanne, E.S. et al. (1995). Insulin-like growth factor II is induced during wound repair following hypoxic–ischemic injury in the developing rat brain. *Mol Brain Res* **29**: 81–91.

80 Klempt, N.D., Klempt, M., Gunn, A.J. et al. (1992). Expression of insulin-like growth factor binding protein-2 (IGFBP-2) following transient hypoxia–ischemia in the infant rat brain. *Brain Res* **15**: 55–61.

81 Guan, J., Skinner, S.J., Beilharz, E.J. et al. (1996). The movement of IGF-I into the brain parenchyma after hypoxic–ischaemic injury. *NeuroReport* **7**: 632–636.

82 Guan, J., Beilharz, E.J., Skinner, S.J.M. et al. (2000). Intracerebral transportation and cellular localisation of insulin-like growth factor-1 following central administration to rats with hypoxic–ischemic brain injury. *Brain Res* **853**: 163–173.

83 Guan, J., Williams, C.E., Gunning, M. et al. (1993). The effects of IGF-1 treatment after hypoxic–ischemic brain injury in adult rats. *J Cereb Blood Flow Metab* **13**: 609–616.

84 Guan, J., Williams, C.E., Skinner, S.J.M. et al. (1996). The effects of insulin-like growth factor (IGF)-1, IGF-2, and Des-IGF-1 on neuronal loss after hypoxic–ischemic brain injury in adult rats – evidence for a role for IGF binding proteins. *Endocrinology* **137**: 893–898.

85 Johnston, B.M., Mallard, E.C., Williams, C.E. et al. (1996). Insulin-like growth factor-1 is a potent neuronal rescue agent after hypoxic–ischemic injury in fetal lambs. *J Clin Invest* **97**: 300–308.

86 Inder, T.E., Huppi, P.S., Warfield, S. et al. (1999). Periventricular white matter injury in the premature infant is followed by reduced cerebral cortical gray matter volume at term. *Ann Neurol* **46**: 755–760.

87 Petty, A.M., Wettstein, J.G. (2000). White matter ischaemia. *Brain Res Brain Res Rev* **31**: 58–64.

88 Marcoux, F.W., Morawetz, R.B., Crowell, R.M. et al. (1982). Differential regional vulnerability in transient focal cerebral ischemia. *Stroke* **13**: 339–346.

89 Mercuri, E., Guzzetta, A., Haataja, L. et al. (1999). Neonatal neurological examination in infants with hypoxic ischaemic encephalopathy: correlation with MRI findings. *Neuropediatrics* **30**: 83–89.

90 Okumura, A., Hayakawa, F., Kato, T. et al. (1997). MRI findings in patients with spastic cerebral palsy. I: Correlation with gestational age at birth. *Dev Med Child Neurol* **39**: 363–368.

91 Pantoni, L., Garcia, J.H., Gutierrez, J.A. (1996). Cerebral white matter is highly vulnerable to ischemia. *Stroke* **27**: 1641–1646.

92 Mandai, K., Matsumoto, M., Kitagawa, K. et al. (1997). Ischemic damage and subsequent proliferation of oligodendrocytes in focal cerebral ischemia. *Neuroscience* **77**: 849–861.

93 Petito, C.K., Olarte, J.P., Roberts, B. et al. (1998). Selective glial vulnerability following transient global ischemia in rat brain. *J Neuropathol Exp Neurol* **57**: 231–238.

94 Jelinski, S.E., Yager, J.Y., Juurlink, B.H. (1999). Preferential injury of oligodendroblasts by a short hypoxic–ischemic insult. *Brain Res* **815**: 150–153.

95 Ikeda, T., Murata, Y., Quilligan, E.J. et al. (1998). Physiologic and histologic changes in near-term fetal lambs exposed to asphyxia by partial umbilical cord occlusion. *Am J Obstet Gynecol* **178**: 24–32.

96 Shuman, S.L., Bresnahan, J.C., Beattie, M.S. (1997). Apoptosis of microglia and oligodendrocytes after apinal cord contusion in rats. *J Neurosci Res* **50**: 798–808.

97 D'Ercole, A.J., Ye, P., Calikoglu, A.S. et al. (1996). The role of the insulin-like growth factors in the central nervous system. *Mol Neurobiol* **13**: 227–255.

98 Shinar, Y., McMorris, F.A. (1995). Developing oligodendroglia express mRNA for insulin-like growth factor-I, a regulator of oligodendrocyte development. *J Neurosci Res* **42**: 516–527.

99 Wilczak, N., Keyser, J.D. (1997). Insulin-like growth factor-1 receptors in normal appearing white matter and chronic plaques in multiple sclerosis. *Brain Res* **772**: 243–246.

100 Ye, P., D'Ercole, A.J. (1999). Insulin-like growth factor 1 protects oligodendrocytes from tumor necrosis factor-alpha-induced injury. *Endocrinology* **140**: 3063–3072.

101 Mason, J.L., Ye, P., Suzuki, K. et al. (2000). Insulin-like growth factor-1 inhibits mature oligodendrocyte apoptosis during primary demyelination. *J Neurosci* **20**: 5703–5708.

102 Hinks, G.L., Franklin, R.J. (1999). Distinctive patterns of PDGF-A, FGF-2, IGF-1 and TGF-beta 1 gene expression during remyelination of experimentally-induced spinal cord demyelination. *Mol Cell Neurosci* **14**: 153–168.

103 Komoly, S., Hudson, L.D., Webster, H.D. et al. (1992). Insulin-like growth factor I gene expression is induced in astrocytes during experimental demyelination. *Proc Natl Acad Sci USA* **89**: 1894–1898.

104 Guan, J., Bennet, L., Wu, D. et al. (2001). Insulin-like growth factor-1 reduces white matter damage following ischemic brain injury in fetal sheep. *J Cereb Blood Flow Metab* **21**: 493–502.

105 Vaca, K., Wendt, E. (1992). Divergent effects of astroglial and microglial secretions on neuron growth and survival. *Exp Neurol* **118**: 62–72.

106 Giulian, D., Li, J., Leara, B. et al. (1994). Phagocytic microglia release cytokines and cytotoxins that regulate the survival of astrocytes and neurons in culture. *Neurochem Int* **25**: 227–233.

107 Yamamoto, H., Murphy, L.J. (1995). Enzymatic conversion of IGF-I to des(1–3)IGF-I in rat serum and tissues: a further potential site of growth hormone regulation of IGF-I action. *J Endocrinol* **146**: 141–148.

108 Bourguignon, J.P., Alvarez Gonzalez, M.L., Gerard, A. et al. (1994). Gonadotropin releasing hormone inhibitory autofeedback by subproducts antagonist at *N*-methyl-D-aspartate receptors: a model of autocrine regulation of peptide secretion. *Endocrinology* **134**: 1589–1592.

109 Ikeda, T., Waldbillig, R.J., Puro, D.G. (1995). Truncation of IGF-I yields two mitogens for retinal Muller glial cells. *Brain Res* **686**: 87–92.

110 Tomas, F.M., Knowles, S.E., Owens, P.C. et al. (1991). Effects of full-length and truncated insulin-like growth factor-I on nitrogen balance and muscle protein metabolism in nitrogen-restricted rats. *J Endocrinol* **128**: 97–105.

111 Bourguignon, J.P., Gerard, A. (1999). Role of insulin-like growth factor binding proteins in limitation of IGF-1 degradation into the *N*-methyl-D-aspartate receptor antagonist GPE: evidence from gonadotrophin-releasing hormone secretion in vitro at two developmental stages. *Brain Res* **847**: 247–252.

112 Saura, J., Curatolo, L., Williams, C.E. et al. (1999). Neuroprotective effects of Gly-Pro-Glu, the N-terminal tripeptide of IGF-1, in the hippocampus in vitro. *Neuroreport* **10**: 161–164.

113 Alexi, T., Hughes, P.E., van Roon-Mom, W.M. et al. (1999). The IGF-I amino-terminal tripeptide glycine-proline-glutamate (GPE) is neuroprotective to striatum in the quinolinic acid lesion animal model of Huntington's disease. *Exp Neurol* **159**: 84–97.

114 Guan, J., Waldvogel, H.J., Faull, R.L.M. et al. (1999). The effects of the N-terminal tripeptide of insulin-like growth factor-1, glycine-proline-glutamate in different regions following hypoxic–ischemic brain injury in adult rats. *Neuroscience* **89**: 649–659.

115 Guan, J., Krishnamurthi, R.V., Waldvogel, H.J. et al. (2000). N-terminal tripeptide of IGF-1 (GPE) prevents the loss of TH positive neurons after 6–OHDA induced nigral lesion in rats. *Brain Res* **859**: 286–292.

116 Klempt, N.D., Sirimanne, E., Gunn, A.J. et al. (1992). Hypoxia–ischemia induces transforming growth factor beta 1 mRNA in the infant rat brain. *Mol Brain Res* **13**: 93–101.

117 Amento, E.P., Beck, L.S. (1991). *Clinical Applications of TGF-beta*, 1st edn. West Sussex, England: John Wiley.

118 Tsunawaki, S., Sporn, M., Ding, A. et al. (1988). Deactivation of macrophages by transforming growth factor-beta. *Nature* **334**: 260–262.

119 Suzumura, A., Sawada, M., Yamamoto, H. et al. (1993).

Transforming growth factor-β1 suppresses activation and proliferation of microglia in vitro. *J Immunol* **151**: 2150–2158.

120 McNeill, H., Williams, C.E., Guan, J. et al. (1994). Neuronal rescue with transforming growth factor-beta(1) after hypoxic–ischaemic brain injury. *NeuroReport* **5**: 901–904.

121 Schubert, D., Kimura, H., LaCorbiere, M. et al. (1990). Activin is a nerve cell survival molecule. *Nature* **344**: 868–870.

122 Iwahori, Y., Saito, H., Torii, K. et al. (1997). Activin exerts a neurotrophic effect on cultured hippocampal neurons. *Brain Res* **760**: 52–58.

113 Krieglstein, K., Suter Crazzolara, C., Fischer, W.H. et al. (1995). TGF-beta superfamily members promote survival of midbrain dopaminergic neurons and protect them against MPP+ toxicity. *EMBO J* **14**: 736–742.

124 Lai, M., Sirimanne, E., Williams, C.E. et al. (1996). Sequential patterns of inhibin subunit gene expression following hypoxic–ischemic injury in the rat brain. *Neuroscience* **70**: 1013–1024.

125 Wu, D.D., Lai, M., Hughes, P.E. et al. (1999). Expression of the activin axis and neuronal rescue effects of recombinant activin A following hypoxic–ischemic brain injury in the infant rat. *Brain Res* **835**: 369–378.

126 Funaba, M., Murata, T., Fujimura, H. et al. (1997). Immunolocalization of type I or type II activin receptors in the rat brain. *J Neuroendocrinol* **9**: 105–111.

127 Simbruner, G., Nanz, S., Fleischhacker, E. et al. (1994). Brain temperature discriminates between neonates with damaged, hypoperfused, and normal brains. *Am J Perinatol* **11**: 137–143.

128 Gunn, A.J., Gunn, T.R. (1996). Effect of radiant heat on head temperature gradient in term infants. *Arch Dis Child Fetal Neonat Edn* **74**: F200–F203.

129 Westin, B., Miller, J.A., Nyberg, R. et al. (1959). Neonatal asphyxia pallida treated with hypothermia alone or with hypothermia and transfusion of oxygenated blood. *Surgery* **45**: 868–879.

130 Miller, J.A., Miller, F.S., Westin, B. (1964). Hypothermia in the treatment of asphyxia neonatorum. *Biol Neonate* **6**: 148–163.

131 Cordey, R. (1964). Hypothermia in resuscitating newborns in white asphyxia. A report of 14 cases. *Obstet Gynecol* **24**: 760–767.

132 Schubert, A. (1995). Side effects of mild hypothermia. *J Neurosurg Anesthesiol* **7**: 139–147.

133 Silverman, W.A., Fertig, J.W., Berger, P.A. (1958). The influence of the thermal environment upon the survival of newly born premature infants. *Pediatrics* **31**: 876–885.

134 Niermeyer, S., Kattwinkel, J., Van Reempts, P. et al. (2000). International guidelines for neonatal resuscitation: an excerpt from the Guidelines 2000 for Cardiopulmonary Resuscitation and Emergency Cardiovascular Care: International Consensus on Science. *Pediatrics* **106**: E29.

135 Busto, R., Dietrich, W.D., Globus, M.Y. et al. (1987). Small differences in intraischemic brain temperature critically determine the extent of ischemic neuronal injury. *J Cereb Blood Flow Metab* **7**: 729–738.

136 Green, E.J., Dietrich, W.D., Van Dijk, F. et al. (1992). Protective effects of brain hypothermia on behavior and histopathology following global cerebral ischemia in rats. *Brain Res* **580**: 197–204.

137 Nurse, S., Corbett, D. (1994). Direct measurement of brain temperature during and after intraischemic hypothermia: correlation with behavioral, physiological, and histological endpoints. *J Neurosci* **14**: 7726–7734.

138 Dietrich, W.D., Busto, R., Alonso, O. et al. (1993). Intraischemic but not postischemic brain hypothermia protects chronically following global forebrain ischemia in rats. *J Cereb Blood Flow Metab* **13**: 541–549.

139 Dietrich, W.D., Busto, R., Valdes, I. et al. (1990). Effects of normothermic versus mild hyperthermic forebrain ischemia in rats. *Stroke* **21**: 1318–1325.

140 Minamisawa, H., Smith, M.L., Siesjo, B.K. (1990). The effect of mild hyperthermia and hypothermia on brain damage following 5, 10, and 15 minutes of forebrain ischemia. *Ann Neurol* **28**: 26–33.

141 Chen, H., Chopp, M., Welch, K.M. (1991). Effect of mild hyperthermia on the ischemic infarct volume after middle cerebral artery occlusion in the rat. *Neurology* **41**: 1133–1135.

142 Chen, Q., Chopp, M., Bodzin, G. et al. (1993). Temperature modulation of cerebral depolarization during focal cerebral ischemia in rats: correlation with ischemic injury. *J Cereb Blood Flow Metab* **13**: 389–394.

143 Haraldseth, O., Gronas, T., Southon, T. et al. (1992). The effects of brain temperature on temporary global ischaemia in rat brain. A 31-phosphorous NMR spectroscopy study. *Acta Anaesthesiol Scand* **36**: 393–399.

144 Wass, C.T., Lanier, W.L., Hofer, R.E. et al. (1995). Temperature changes of >or = 1 degree C alter functional neurologic outcome and histopathology in a canine model of complete cerebral ischemia. *Anesthesiology* **83**: 325–335.

145 Thornhill, J., Asselin, J. (1998). Increased neural damage to global hemispheric hypoxic ischemia (GHHI) in febrile but not nonfebrile lipopolysaccharide *Escherichia coli* injected rats. *Can J Physiol Pharmacol* **76**: 1008–1016.

146 Laptook, A.R., Corbett, R.J., Sterett, R. et al. (1994). Modest

hypothermia provides partial neuroprotection for ischemic neonatal brain. *Pediatr Res* **35**: 436–442.

147 Yager, J., Towfighi, J., Vannucci, R.C. (1993). Influence of mild hypothermia on hypoxic–ischemic brain damage in the immature rat. *Pediatr Res* **34**: 525–529.

148 Laptook, A.R., Corbett, R.J.T., Sterett, R. et al. (1995). Quantitative relationship between brain temperature and energy utilization rate measured in vivo using ^{31}P and ^{1}H magnetic resonance spectroscopy. *Pediatr Res* **38**: 919–925.

149 Towfighi, J., Housman, C., Heitjan, D.F. et al. (1994). The effect of focal cerebral cooling on perinatal hypoxic–ischemic brain damage. *Acta Neuropathol Berl* **87**: 598–604.

150 Suehiro, E., Fujisawa, H., Ito, H. et al. (1999). Brain temperature modifies glutamate neurotoxicity in vivo. *J Neurotrauma* **16**: 285–297.

151 Dietrich, W.D., Busto, R., Halley, M. et al. (1990). The importance of brain temperature in alterations of the blood–brain barrier following cerebral ischemia. *J Neuropathol Exp Neurol* **49**: 486–497.

152 Ginsberg, M.D., Busto, R. (1998). Combating hyperthermia in acute stroke: a significant clinical concern. *Stroke* **29**: 529–534.

153 Bagenholm, R., Nilsson, U.A., Kjellmer, I. (1997). Formation of free radicals in hypoxic ischemic brain damage in the neonatal rat, assessed by an endogenous spin trap and lipid peroxidation. *Brain Res* **773**: 132–138.

154 Thoresen, M., Satas, S., Puka-Sundvall, M. et al. (1997). Post-hypoxic hypothermia reduces cerebrocortical release of NO and excitotoxins. *NeuroReport* **8**: 3359–3362.

155 Lei, B., Tan, X., Cai, H. et al. (1994). Effect of moderate hypothermia on lipid peroxidation in canine brain tissue after cardiac arrest and resuscitation. *Stroke* **25**: 147–152.

156 Zhao, W., Richardson, J.S., Mombourquette, M.J. et al. (1996). Neuroprotective effects of hypothermia and U-78517f in cerebral ischemia are due to reducing oxygen-based free radicals – an electron paramagnetic resonance study with gerbils. *J Neurosci Res* **45**: 282–288.

157 Thoresen, M., Bagenholm, R., Loberg, E.M. et al. (1996). Posthypoxic cooling of neonatal rats provides protection against brain injury. *Arch Dis Child Fetal Neonatal Edn* **74**: F3–F9.

158 Trescher, W.H., Ishiwa, S., Johnston, M.V. (1997). Brief post-hypoxic–ischemic hypothermia markedly delays neonatal brain injury. *Brain Dev* **19**: 326–338.

159 Haaland, K., Loberg, E.M., Steen, P.A. et al. (1997). Posthypoxic hypothermia in newborn piglets. *Pediatr Res* **41**: 505–512.

160 Laptook, A.R., Corbett, R.J., Sterett, R. et al. (1997). Modest hypothermia provides partial neuroprotection when used for immediate resuscitation after brain ischemia. *Pediatr Res* **42**: 17–23.

161 Laptook, A.R., Corbett, R.J., Burns, D.K. et al. (1999). A limited interval of delayed modest hypothermia for ischemic brain resuscitation is not beneficial in neonatal swine. *Pediatr Res* **46**: 383–389.

162 Iwai, T., Niwa, M., Yamada, H. et al. (1993). Hypothermic prevention of the hippocampal damage following ischemia in Mongolian gerbils: comparison between intra-ischemic and brief postischemic hypothermia. *Life Sci* **52**: 1031–1038.

163 Busto, R., Dietrich, W.D., Globus, M.Y. et al. (1989). Postischemic moderate hypothermia inhibits CA1 hippocampal ischemic neuronal injury. *Neurosci Lett* **101**: 299–304.

164 Shuaib, A., Trulove, D., Ijaz, M.S. et al. (1995). The effect of post-ischemic hypothermia following repetitive cerebral ischemia in gerbils. *Neurosci Lett* **186**: 165–168.

165 Horn, M., Schlote, W., Henrich, H.A. (1991). Global cerebral ischemia and subsequent selective hypothermia. A neuropathological and morphometrical study on ischemic neuronal damage in cat. *Acta Neuropathol Berl* **81**: 443–449.

166 Kuboyama, K., Safar, P., Radovsky, A. et al. (1993). Delay in cooling negates the beneficial effect of mild resuscitative cerebral hypothermia after cardiac arrest in dogs: a prospective, randomized study. *Crit Care Med* **21**: 1348–1358.

167 Kuroiwa, T., Bonnekoh, P., Hossmann, K.A. (1990). Prevention of postischemic hyperthermia prevents ischemic injury of CA1 neurons in gerbils. *J Cereb Blood Flow Metab* **10**: 550–556.

168 Guan, J., Gunn, A.J., Sirimanne, E.S. et al. (2000). The window of opportunity for neuronal rescue with insulin-like growth factor-1 after hypoxia–ischemia in rats is critically modulated by cerebral temperature during recovery. *J Cereb Blood Flow Metab* **20**: 513–519.

169 Bona, E., Hagberg, H., Loberg, E.M. et al. (1998). Protective effects of moderate hypothermia after neonatal hypoxia–ischemia: short- and long-term outcome. *Pediatr Res* **43**: 738–745.

170 Gunn, A.J., Gunn, T.R. (1998). The 'pharmacology' of neuronal rescue with cerebral hypothermia. *Early Hum Dev* **53**: 19–35.

171 Gunn, A.J., Gunn, T.R., Gunning, M.I. et al. (1998). Neuroprotection with prolonged head cooling started before postischemic seizures in fetal sheep. *Pediatrics* **102**: 1098–1106.

172 Gunn, A.J., Bennet, L., Gunning, M.I. et al. (1999). Cerebral hypothermia is not neuroprotective when started after

postischemic seizures in fetal sheep. *Pediatr Res* **46**: 274–280.

173 Battin, M.R., Dezoete, J.A., Gunn, T.R. et al. (2001). Neurodevelopmental outcome of infants treated with head cooling and mild hypothermia after perinatal asphyxia. *Pediatrics* **107**: 480–484.

174 Coimbra, C., Drake, M., Boris-Moller, F. et al. (1996). Long-lasting neuroprotective effect of postischemic hypothermia and treatment with an anti-inflammatory/antipyretic drug. Evidence for chronic encephalopathic processes following ischemia. *Stroke* **27**: 1578–1585.

175 Famularo, G., Polchi, S., Panegrossi, A. (1998). Thrombolysis enters the race: a new era for acute ischaemic stroke? *Eur J Emerg Med* **5**: 249–252.

176 Gluckman, P.D., Williams, C.E. (1992). Is the cure worse than the disease? Caveats in the move from the laboratory to clinic. *Dev Med Child Neurol* **34**: 1015–1018.

177 Westgate, J.A., Gunn, A.J., Gunn, T.R. (1999). Antecedents of neonatal encephalopathy with fetal acidaemia at term. *Br J Obstet Gynaecol* **106**: 774–782.

37

Neonatal seizures: an expression of fetal or neonatal brain disorders

Mark S. Scher

Rainbow Babies and Children's Hospital, Case Western Reserve University, Cleveland, OH, USA

Neonatal seizures are one of the few neonatal neurological conditions that require immediate medical attention. While prompt diagnostic and therapeutic plans are needed, multiple challenges impede the physician's evaluation of the newborn with suspected seizures (Box 37.1).[1–3] Clinical and electroencephalographic (EEG) manifestations of neonatal seizures vary dramatically from older children, and recognition of the seizure state remains the foremost challenge to overcome. This dilemma is underscored by the brevity and subtlety of the clinical repertoire of the neonatal neurological examination. Environmental restrictions in an intensive care setting of the sick infant, who may be confined to an isolette, intubated, and attached to multiple catheters limit accessibility. Medications alter arousal and muscle tone and limit the clinician's ability to distinguish clinical neurologic signs reflective of the underlying disease state. Brain injury from antepartum factors may precipitate neonatal seizures as part of an encephalopathic clinical picture during the intrapartum and neonatal periods,[4] well beyond when brain injury occurred. Overlapping medical conditions from fetal through neonatal periods must be factored into the most appropriate etiologic algorithm to explain seizure expression before applying the most accurate prognosis. Medication options to treat seizures effectively remain elusive, and may need to be applied on a specific etiologic basis. This review discusses issues regarding recognition, differential diagnosis, prognosis, and treatment of neonatal seizures, in the context of current neurobiologic and pathophysiologic explanations of the causes for neonatal seizures and the consequences leading to brain injury. Potential neuroresuscitative strategies proposed for the encephalopathic neonate with seizures must consider maternal, placental/cord, and fetal disease conditions which cause or contribute to neonatal seizure expression and potential brain injury as part of both fetal and neonatal brain disorders of varying etiologies.[5]

Box 37.1 Dilemmas regarding neonatal seizures

1. Diagnostic choices – reliance on clinical vs electroencephalographic criteria
2. Etiologic explanations – multiple prenatal/neonatal conditions as a function of time.
3. Treatment decisions – who, when, how, and for how long?
4. Prognostic questions – consider mechanisms of injury based on etiologies vs intrinsic vulnerability of the immature brain to prolonged seizures

Diagnostic dilemmas: reliance on clinical vs EEG criteria for seizures

Neonatal seizures are generally brief and subtle in clinical appearance, sometimes comprised of unusual behaviors which are difficult to recognize and classify. While some claim that seizures are relatively common events in neonates who are symptomatic by intercurrent medical conditions, medical personnel vary significantly in their ability to recognize suspicious behaviors, contributing to both overdiagnosis and underdiagnosis. The most common practice has been to classify clinical behaviors as seizures without EEG confirmation. However, abnormal motor or autonomic behaviors may represent age and state-specific behaviors in healthy infants, or nonepileptic paroxysmal conditions in symptomatic infants. For these reasons, confirmation of suspicious clinical events with coincident EEG recordings is now more widely recommended. While patients with few seizures may be missed as brief random events on routine EEG studies,[6] synchronized video/EEG/polygraphic recordings potentially establish a more reliable start and endpoint for electrically-confirmed seizures that require consideration for treatment[7] intervention. Rigorous physiologic monitoring will also better integrate the diagnosis of the seizure state with etiologic, treatment, and prognostic considerations.

Clinical seizure criteria

Neonatal seizures are presently listed separately from the traditional classification of seizures and epilepsy during childhood. The International League Against Epilepsy's classification adopted by the World Health Organization still considers neonatal seizures within an unclassified category.[8] A recent classification scheme now suggests a strict distinction of clinical seizure (nonepileptic) events from electrographically confirmed (epileptic) seizures, with respect to possible treatment interventions.[9] Continued refinements of such novel classifications are needed to reconcile the variable agreement between clinical and EEG criteria for establishing a seizure diagnosis,[10,11] in the context of nonepileptic movement disorders caused by acquired diseases, malformations, and/or medications.

Several caveats (Box 37.2) may be useful in the identification of suspected neonatal seizures, yet continue to raise questions regarding our diagnostic acumen.

Box 37.2 Caveats concerning recognition of neonatal seizures

1. Specific stereotypic behaviors occur in association with normal neonatal sleep or waking states, medication effects, and gestational maturity
2. Consider that any abnormal repetitive activity may be a clinical seizure if out of context for expected neonatal behavior
3. Attempt to document coincident electrographic seizures with the suspected clinical event
4. Abnormal behavioral phenomena may have inconsistent relationships with coincident electroencephalographic seizures, suggesting a subcortical seizure focus
5. Nonepileptic pathologic movement disorders are events that are independent of the seizure state, and may also be expressed by neonates

The clinical criteria for neonatal seizure diagnosis was historically subdivided into five clinical categories: focal clonic, multifocal or migratory clonic, tonic, myoclonic, and subtle seizures.[12] A more recent classification expands the clinical subtypes, adopting a strict temporal occurrence of specific clinical events with coincident electrographic seizures, to distinguish neonatal clinical "nonepileptic" seizures from "epileptic" seizures (Table 37.1 and 37.2).[9]

Subtle seizure activity

This is the most frequently observed category of neonatal seizures, which include repetitive buccolingual movements, orbital–ocular movements, unusual bicycling or peddling, and autonomic findings (Figure 37.1*a*). Any subtle paroxysmal event which interrupts the expected behavioral repertoire of the newborn infant, and appears stereotypic or repetitive, should heighten the clinician's level of suspicion for seizures. However, alterations in cardiorespiratory regularity, body movements, and other behaviors during active (rapid eye movement: REM), quiet (non-REM: NREM) sleep or waking segments must be recognized before proceeding to a seizure evaluation.[13,14] Within the subtle category of neonatal seizures are stereotypic changes in heart rate, blood pressure, oxygenation, or other

Table 37.1. Clinical characteristics, classification, and presumed pathophysiology of neonatal seizures

Classification	Characterization
Focal clonic	Repetitive, rhythmic contractions of muscle groups of the limbs, face, or trunk May be unifocal or multifocal May occur synchronously or asynchronously in muscle groups on one side of the body May occur simultaneously but asynchronously on both sides Cannot be suppressed by restraint Pathophysiology: epileptic
Focal tonic	Sustained posturing of single limbs Sustained asymmetrical posturing of the trunk Sustained eye deviation Cannot be provoked by stimulation or suppressed by restraint Pathophysiology: epileptic
Generalized tonic	Sustained symmetrical posturing of limbs, trunk and neck May be flexor, extensor, or mixed extensor/flexor May be provoked by stimulation May be suppressed by restraint or repositioning Presumed pathophysiology: nonepileptic
Myoclonic	Random single rapid contractions of muscle groups of the limbs, face, or trunk Typically not repetitive or may recur at a slow rate May be generalized, focal, or fragmentary May be provoked by stimulation Presumed pathophysiology: may be epileptic or nonepileptic
Spasms	May be flexor, extensor, or mixed extensor/flexor may occur in clusters Cannot be provoked by stimulation or suppressed by restraint Pathophysiology: epileptic
Motor automatisms Ocular signs	Random and roving eye movements or nystagmus (distinct from tonic eye deviation) May be provoked or intensified by tactile stimulation Presumed pathophysiology: nonepileptic
Oral–bucco–lingual Movements	Sucking, chewing, tongue protrusions May be provoked or intensified by stimulation Presumed pathophysiology: nonepileptic
Progression movements	Rowing or swimming movements Pedalling or bicycling movements of the legs May be provoked or intensified by stimulation May be suppressed by restraint or repositioning Presumed pathophysiology: nonepileptic
Complex purposeless movements	Sudden arousal with transient increased random activity of limbs May be provoked or intensified by stimulation Presumed pathophysiology: nonepileptic

Source: From Mizrahi EM and Kellaway P (1998). *Diagnosis and Management of Neonatal Seizures*, pp. 1–155, with permission from Lippincott-Raven.

Table 37.2. Classification of neonatal seizures based on electroclinical findings

Clinical seizures with a consistent electrocortical signature (pathophysiology: epileptic)
Focal clonic
Unifocal
Multifocal
Hemiconvulsive
Axial
Focal tonic
Asymmetrical truncal posturing
Limb posturing
Sustained eye deviation
Myoclonic
Generalized
Focal
Spasms
Flexor
Extensor
Mixed extensor/flexor
Clinical seizures without a consistent electrocortical signature (pathophysiology; presumed nonepileptic)
Myoclonic
Generalized
Local
Fragmentary
Generalized tonic
Flexor
Extensor
Mixed extensor/flexor
Motor automatisms
Oral–buccal–lingual movements
Ocular signs
Progression movements
Complex purposeless movements
Electrical seizures without clinical seizure activity

Source: From Mizrahi EM and Kellaway P (1998). *Diagnosis and Management of Neonatal Seizures*, pp. 1–155, with permission from Lippincott-Raven.

autonomic signs, particularly during pharmacological paralysis for ventilatory care. Other unusual autonomic events include penile erections, skin changes, salivation, tearing, etc. Autonomic expressions may be intermixed with motoric findings. Isolated autonomic signs such as apnea, unless accompanied by other clinical findings, are rarely associated with coincident electrographic seizures (Figure 37.1*b*).[15,16] Since subtle seizures are both clinically difficult to detect and only variably coincident with EEG seizures, synchronized video/EEG/polygraphic recordings are recommended to document temporal relationships between clinical behaviors and coincident electrographic events.[7,9,17,18] Despite the "subtle" expression of this seizure category, these children may have suffered significant brain injury.

Clonic seizures

Rhythmic movements of muscle groups in a focal distribution, which consist of a rapid phase followed by a slow return movement, are clonic seizures, to be distinguished from the symmetric "to-and-fro" movements of tremulousness or jitteriness.[2] Gentle flexion of the affected body part easily suppresses the tremor, while clonic seizures persist. Clonic movements can involve any body part, such as the face, arm, leg, and even diaphragmatic or pharyngeal muscles. Generalized clonic activities can occur in the newborn but rarely consist of a classical tonic followed by clonic phase, characteristic of the generalized motor seizure noted in older children and adults. Focal clonic and hemiclonic seizures have been described with localized brain injury, usually from cerebrovascular lesions[7,19–21] (Figure 37.2*a*) but can also be seen with generalized brain abnormalities. As with older patients, focal seizures in the neonate may be followed by transient motor weakness, historically referred to as a transient Todd's paresis or paralysis,[22] to be distinguished by a more persistent hemiparesis over multiple days to weeks. Clonic movements without EEG-confirmed seizures have been described in neonates with normal EEG backgrounds and their neurodevelopment outcome can be normal.[17]

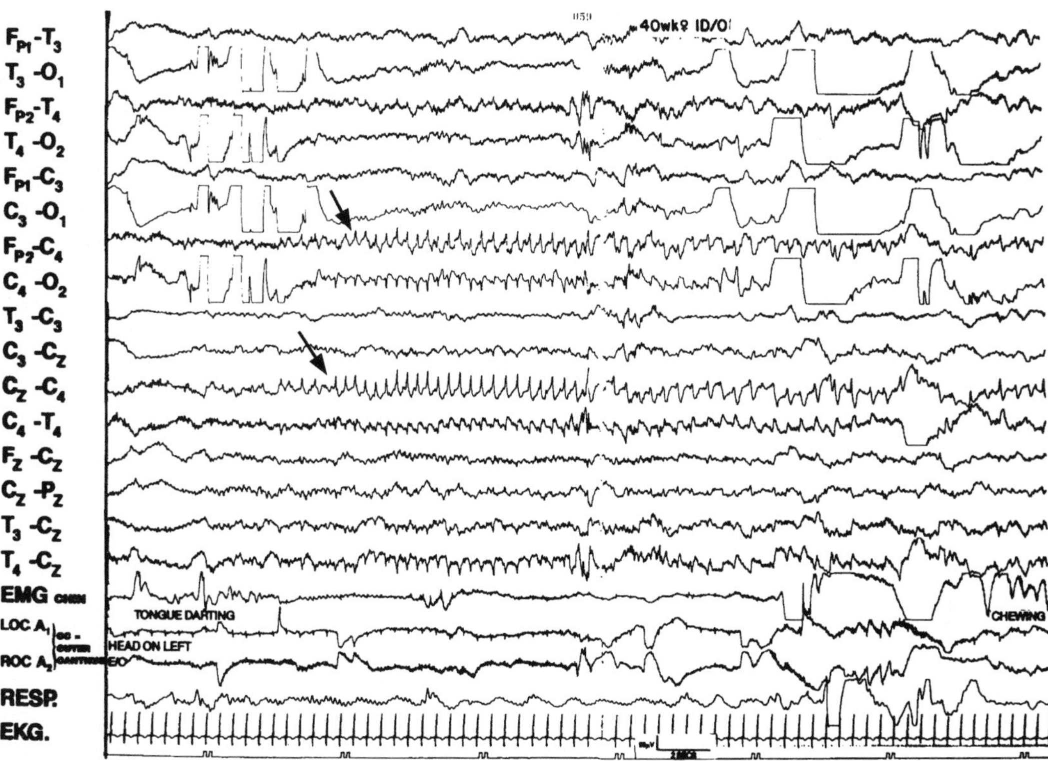

Figure 37.1*a* Electroencephalographic (EEG) segment of a 40-week 1-day-old female following severe asphyxia resulting from rupture of velamentous insertion of the umbilical cord during delivery. An electrical seizure in the right central/midline region is recorded (arrows), coincident with buccolingual and eye movements (see comments and eye channels on record). From Scher MS, Painter MJ (1990). Electrographic diagnosis of neonatal seizures. Issues of diagnostic accuracy, clinical correlation and survival. In: Wasterlain CG, Vert P (eds) *Neonatal Seizures*, p. 17. New York, NY: Raven Press, with permission.

Multifocal (fragmentary) clonic seizures

Multifocal or migratory clonic activities spread over body parts either in a random or anatomically appropriate fashion. Such seizure movements may alternate from side to side and appear asynchronously between the two halves of the child's body. The word "fragmentary" was historically applied to distinguish this event from the more classical generalized tonic-clonic seizure seen in the older child. Multifocal clonic seizures may also resemble myoclonic seizures which alternatively consist of brief shock-like muscle twitching of the midline and/or extremity musculature. Neonates with this seizure description suffer death or significant neurological morbidity.[23]

Tonic seizures

Tonic seizures refer to a sustained flexion or extension of axial or appendicular muscle groups. Tonic movements of a limb or sustained head or eye turning may also be noted. Tonic activity with coincident EEG needs to be carefully documented, since

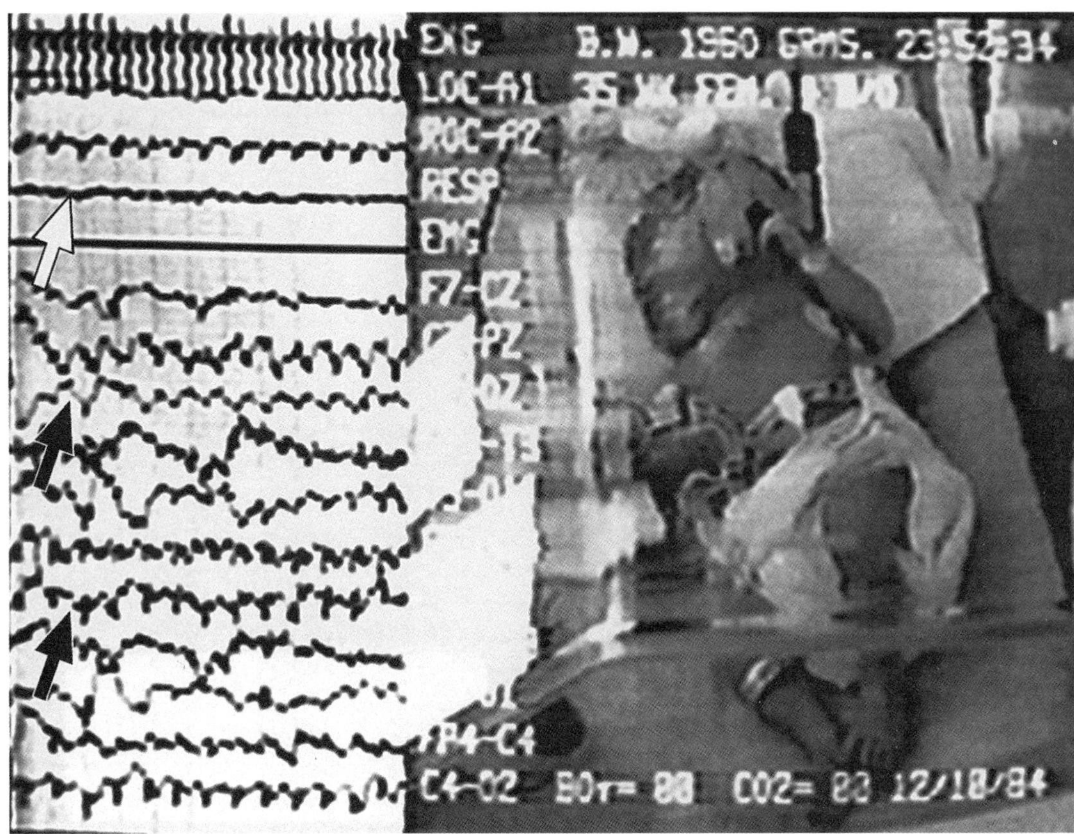

Figure 37.1*b* Synchronized video electroencephalographic (EEG) record of a 35-week-gestation 1-day-old female with *Escherichia coli* meningitis and cerebral abscesses. The open arrow notes apnea coincident with prominent right hemispheric and midline electrographic seizures (closed arrows). In addition to apnea, other motoric signs coincident to EEG seizures were noted at other times during the record. From Scher MS, Painter MJ (1989). Controversies concerning neonatal seizures. *Pediatr. Clin. North Am.* 36: 288, with permission.

30% of such movements lack a temporal correlation with electrographic seizures[24] (Figure 37.3). "Brainstem release" resulting from functional decortication after severe neocortical dysfunction or damage is one physiologic explanation for this nonepileptic activity, to be discussed below. Extensive neocortical damage or dysfunction results permits the emergence of uninhibited subcortical expressions of extensor movements.[25] Tonic seizures may also be misidentified, when the nonepileptic movement disorder of dystonia is the more appropriate behavioral description. Both tonic movements and dystonic posturing may also simultaneously occur.

Myoclonic seizures

Myoclonic movements are rapid, isolated jerks which can be generalized, multifocal, or focal in an axial or appendicular distribution. Myoclonus lacks the slow return phase of the clonic movement complex described above. Healthy preterm infants commonly exhibit myoclonic movements without

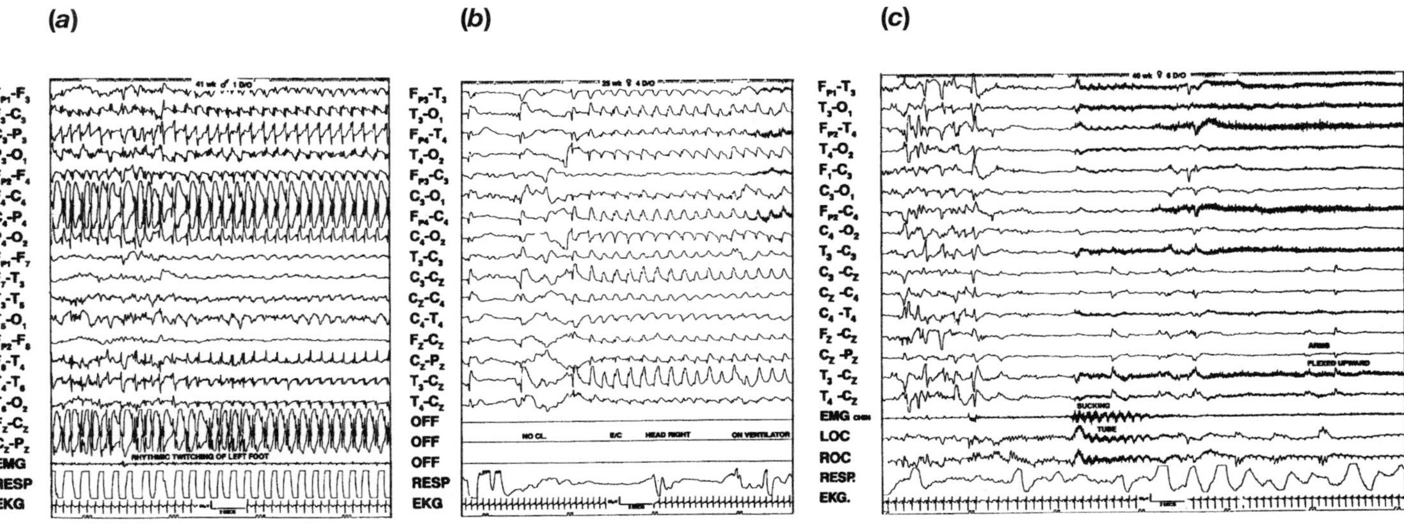

Figure 37.2 (*a*) Segment of encephalogram (EEG) of a 41-week 1-day-old male with an electroclinical seizure characterized by rhythmic clonic movements of the left foot coincident with bihemispheric electrographic discharges of higher amplitude in the right hemisphere. This seizure was documented prior to antiepileptic medication. (*b*) Segment of EEG of a 25-week, 4-day-old female with an electrographic seizure without clinical accompaniments. (*c*) Segment of an EEG of a 40-week-gestation, 6-day-old infant with stereotypic flexion posturing in the absence of electrographic seizures (note muscle artifact). From Scher MS (1999). Pediatric electroencephalography and evoked potentials. In: Swaiman KS (ed.) *Pediatric Neurology: Principles and Practice*, p. 164. St Louis, MO: CV Mosby, with permission.

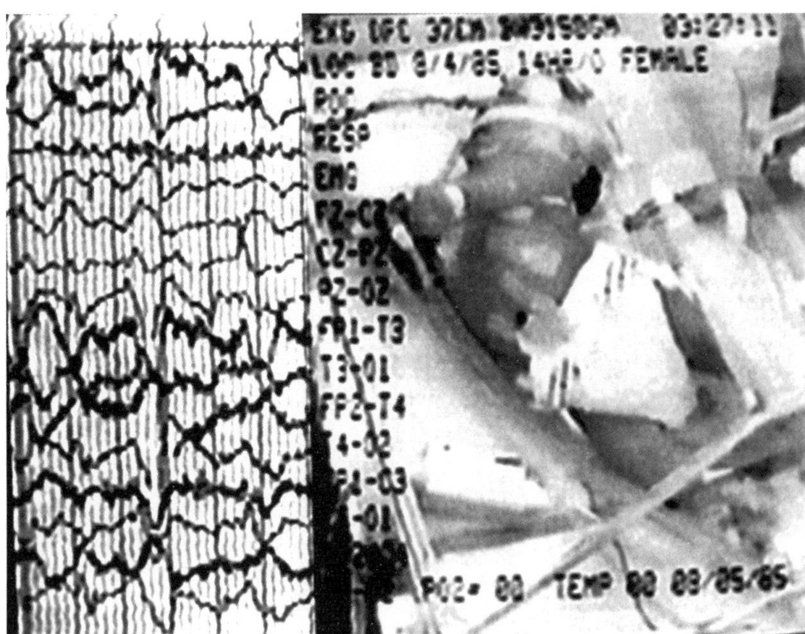

Figure 37.3*a* Segment of a synchronized video electroencephalographic recording of a 37-week-gestation, 1-day-old female who suffered asphyxia, demonstrating prominent opisthotonos with left arm extension in the absence of coincident electrographic seizure activity.

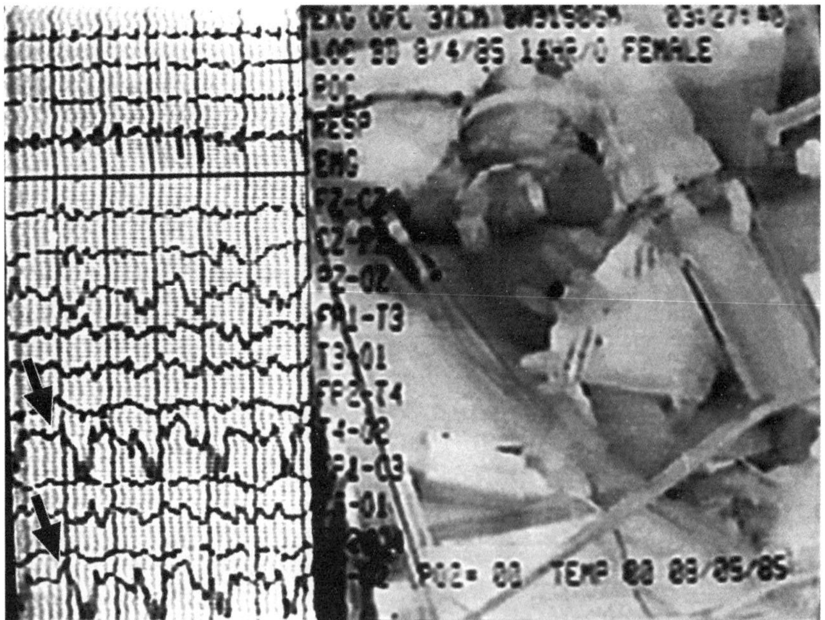

Figure 37.3*b* Synchronized video electroencephalographic recording of the same patient as in Figure 37.3*a*, documenting electrographic seizure in the right posterior quadrant (arrows), following cessation of left arm tonic movements and persistent opisthotonos. From Scher MS, Painter MJ (1989). Controversies concerning neonatal seizures. In: Pellock JM (ed.) *Seizure Disorders. Pediatric Clinics of North America*, vol. 36, p. 392. Philadelphia, PA: WB Saunders, with permission.

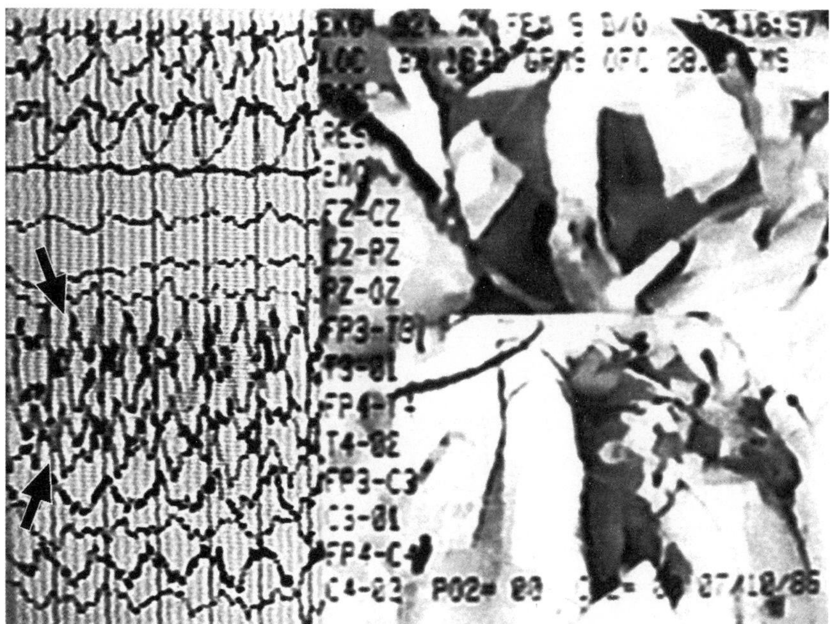

Figure 37.3*c* Segment of a video electroencephalographic recording documenting a fixed tonic neck reflex with coincident electrographic seizures in the temporal regions (arrows), described as a tonic seizure.

seizures or a brain disorder. EEG, therefore, is recommended to confirm the coincident appearance of electrographic discharges with these movements (Figure 37.4*a*). Pathologic myoclonus in the absence of EEG seizures can also occur in severely ill preterm or full-term infants after suffering severe brain dysfunction or damage.[26] As with older children and adults, myoclonus may reflect injury at multiple levels of the neuraxis from the spine and brainstem to cortical regions. Stimulus-evoked myoclonus with either single coincident spike discharges or sustained electrographic seizures have been reported[27] (Figure 37.4*a* and *b*). An extensive evaluation must be initiated to exclude metabolic, structural, and genetic causes. Rarely, healthy sleeping neonates exhibit abundant myoclonus which subsides with arousal to the waking state;[28,29] this is termed benign sleep myoclonus of the newborn.

Nonepileptic behaviors of neonates

Specific nonepileptic neonatal movement repertoires continually challenge the physician's attempt to reach an accurate diagnosis of seizures and avoid the unnecessary use of antiepileptic medications. Coincident paper or synchronized video/EEG/polygraphic recordings are now the suggested diagnostic tool to confirm the temporal relationship between the suspicious clinical phenomena and electrographic expression of seizures.[30] The following three examples of nonepileptic movement disorders incorporate a new classification scheme,[9] based on the absence of coincident EEG seizures.

Tremulousness or jitteriness without EEG correlates

Tremors are frequently misidentified as clonic activity. Unlike the unequal phases of clonic movements described above, the flexion and extension phases of tremor are equal in amplitude. Children are generally alert or hyperalert but may also appear somnolent. Passive flexion and repositioning of the affected tremulous body part diminish or eliminate the movement. Such movements are usually spontaneous but can be provoked by tactile stimulation. Metabolic or toxin-induced encephalopathies, including mild asphyxia, drug withdrawal,

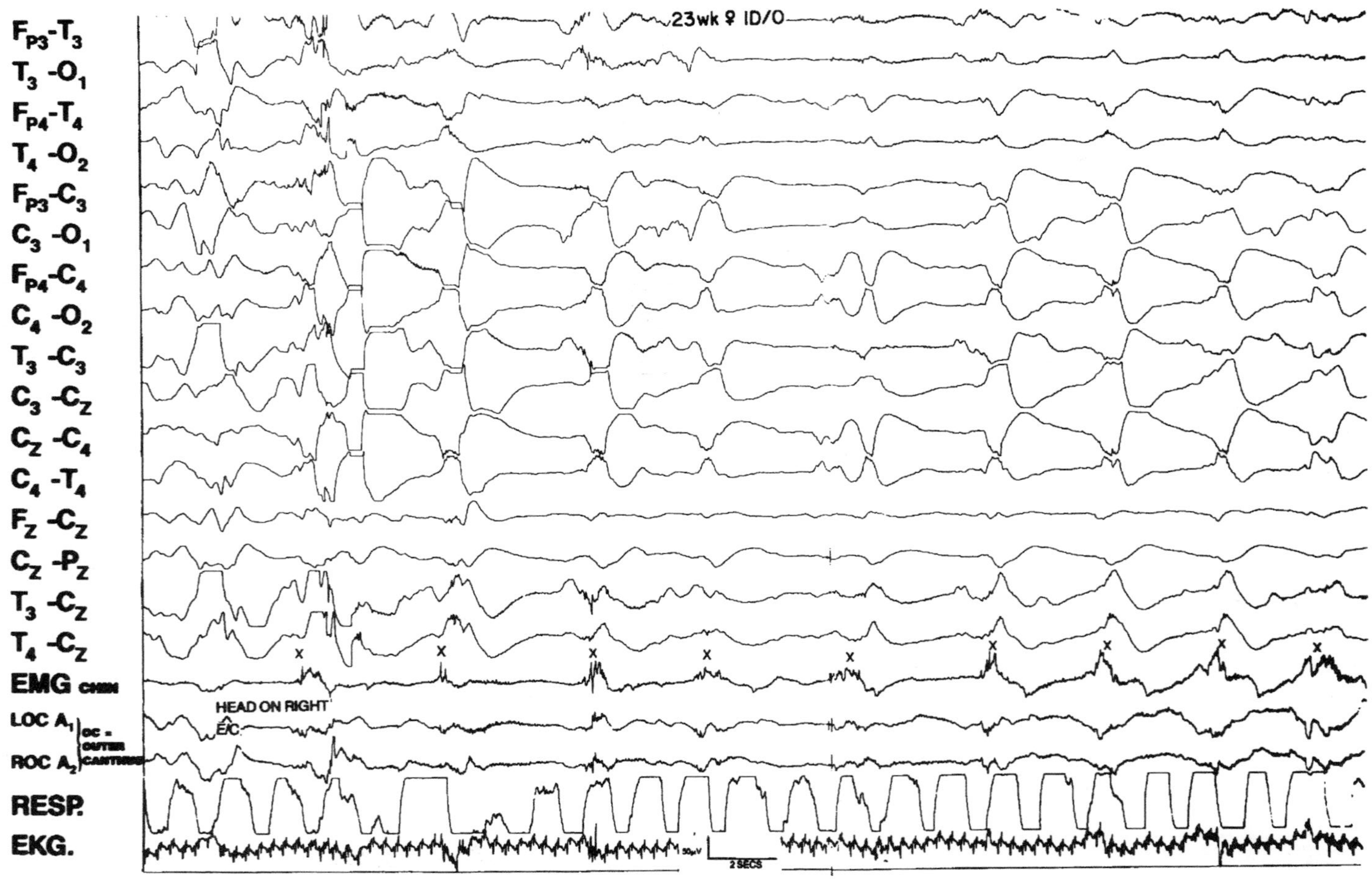

Figure 37.4*a* Electroencephalographic segment of a 23-week 1-day-old female with grade III intraventricular hemorrhage and progressive ventriculomegaly. An electroclinical seizure is noted coincident with myoclonic movements of the diaphragm (x marks). From Scher MS (1985). Pathological myoclonus of the newborn: electrographic and clinical correlations. *Pediatr Neurol* 1:342–348, with permission.

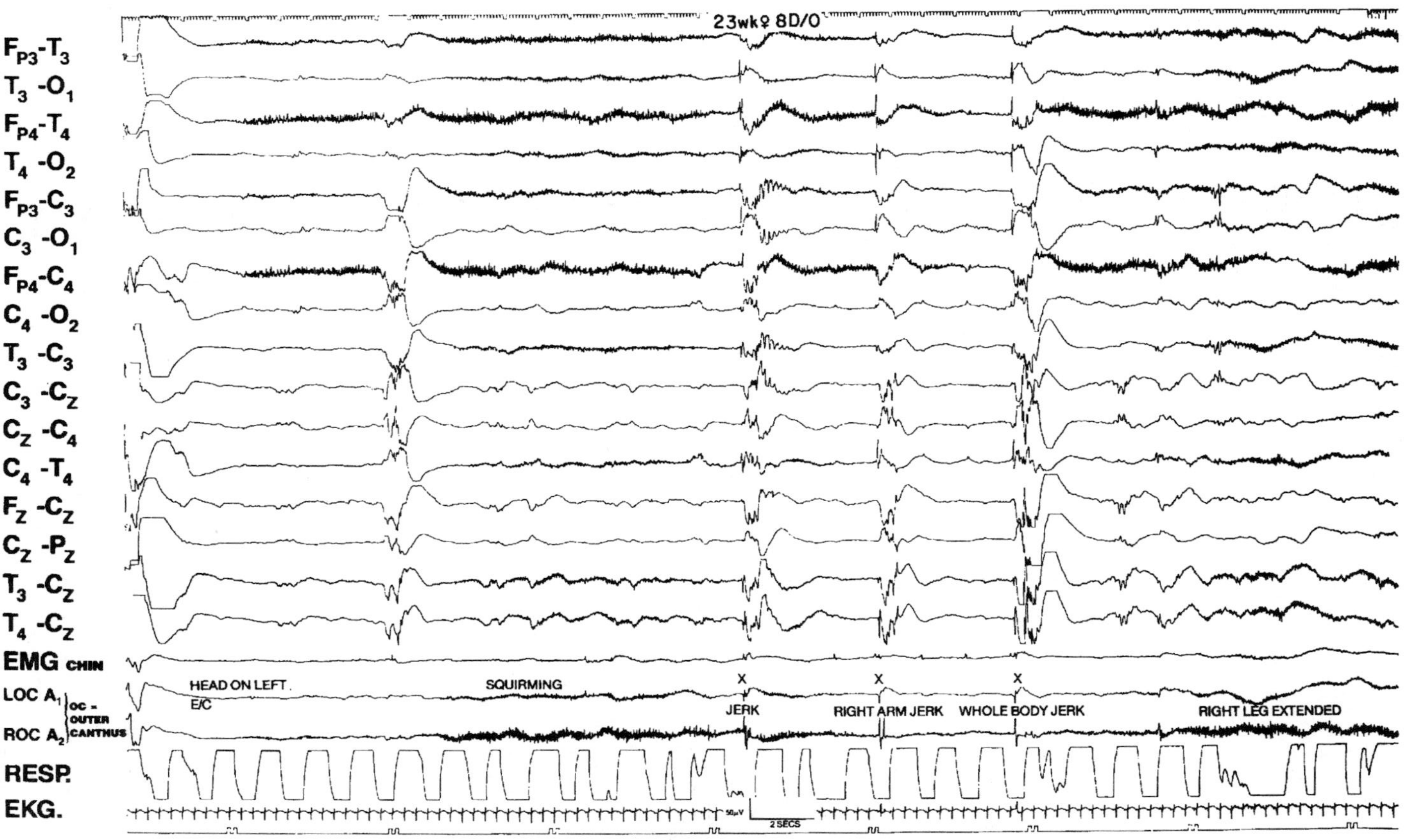

Figure 37.4*b* Segment of an electroencephalographic recording of an asymptomatic 23-week, 8-day-old female with spontaneous generalized focal myoclonus without electrographic discharges other than myogenic spike potentials.

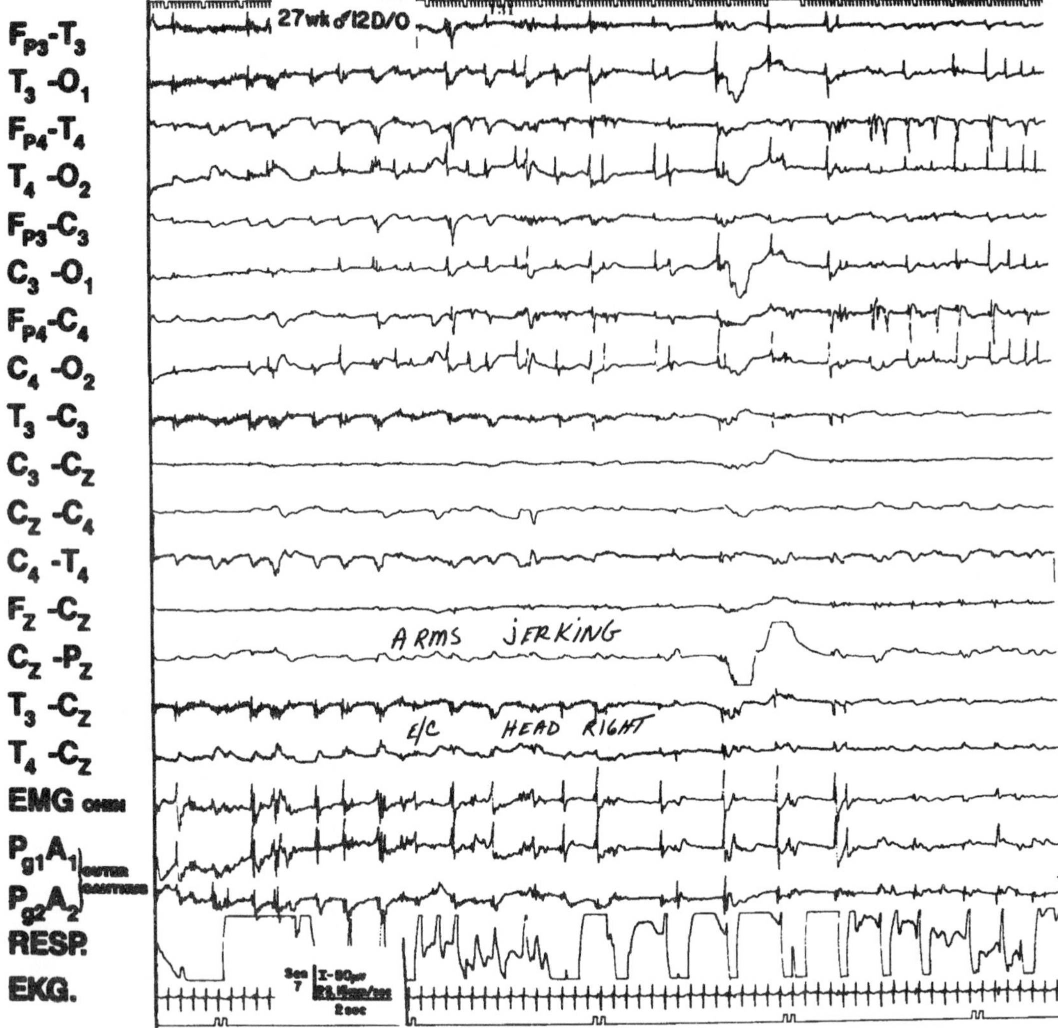

Figure 37.4*c* Segment of an electroencephalographic (EEG) recording of an encephalopathic 27-week, 12-day-old male with herpes encephalitis who exhibits nonepileptic multifocal myoclonus (myogenic potentials as EEG artifacts).

hypoglycemia–hypocalcemia, intracranial hemorrhage, hypothermia, and growth restriction are common clinical scenarios when such movements occur. Neonatal tremors generally decrease with age; for example, 38 full-term infants with excessive tremulousness resolved spontaneously over a 6-week period, with 92% neurologically normal at 3 years of age.[31] Medications are rarely considered to treat this particular movement disorder.[32]

Neonatal myoclonus without EEG seizures

Myoclonic movements are either bilateral and synchronous, or asymmetric and asynchronous in

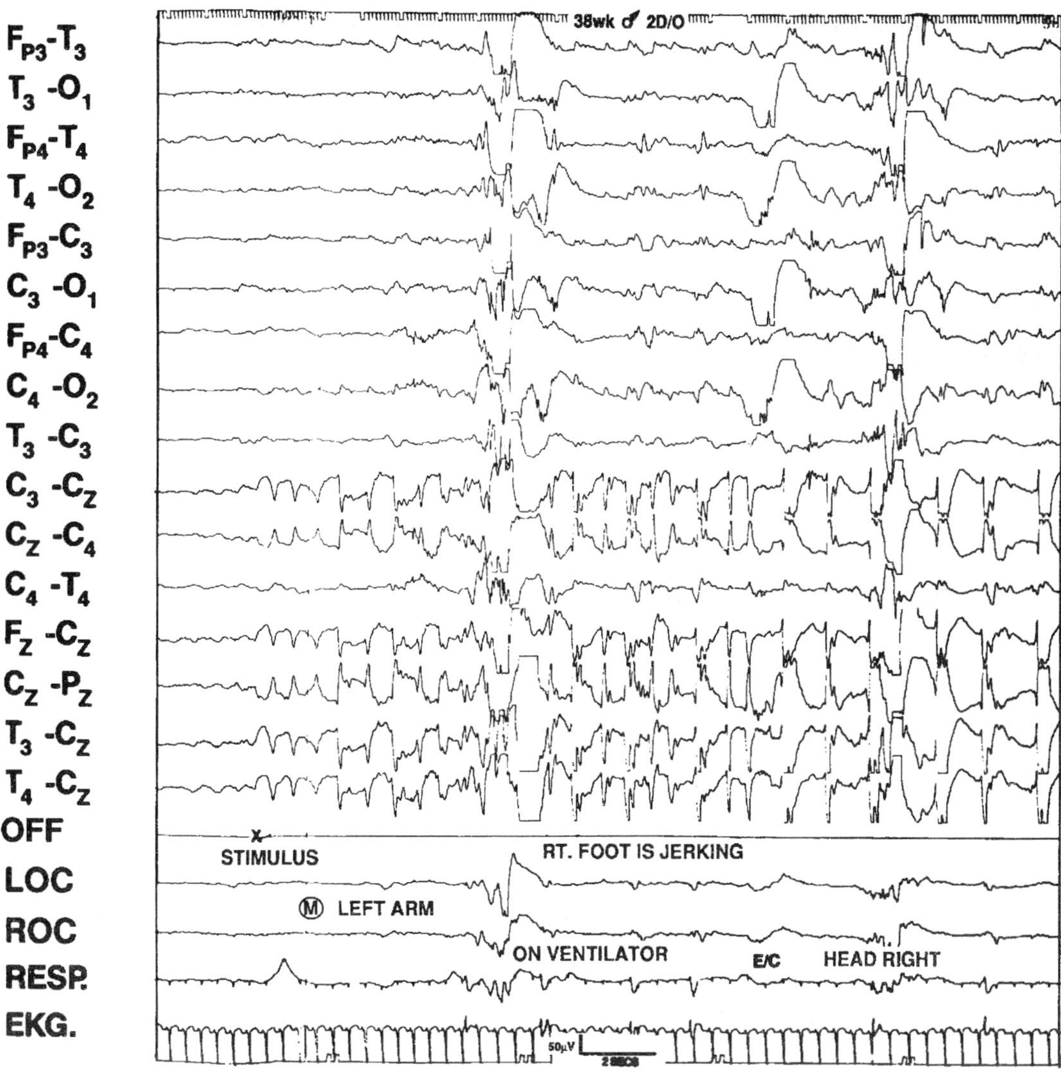

Figure 37.5*a* Segment of an electroencephalographic recording of a 38-week, 2-day-old male with glycine encephalopathy who has stimulus-sensitive generalized and multifocal myoclonus. Note the onset of a midline (C_z-onset) electrographic seizure with a painful stimulus, followed by right foot myoclonus.

appearance. Clusters of myoclonic activity occur more predominantly during active (REM) sleep, are more predominant in the preterm infant,[14,33] but also occur in healthy full-term infants. These benign movements are not stimulus-sensitive and have no coincident electrographic seizure activity or changes in the EEG background rhythms. When this movement occurs in the healthy full-term neonate it is usually suppressed during wakefulness. This clinical entity of benign neonatal sleep myoclonus is a diagnosis of exclusion after an extensive consideration of pathologic diagnoses.[28]

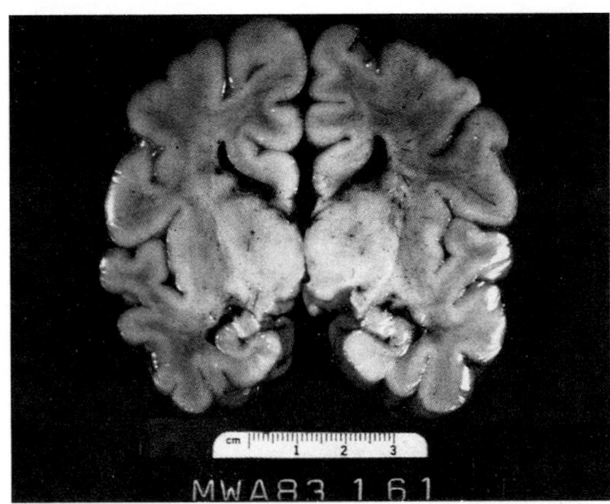

Figure 37.5*b* Coronal section of the brain for the patient shown in Figure 37.5*a*, with agenesis of the corpus callosum and bat-winged shape of lateral ventricles. Spongy myelinosis was noted on microscopic examination. From Scher MS (1985). Pathological myoclonus of the newborn: electrographic and clinical correlations. *Pediatr Neurol* 1:342–348, with permission.

There are also infants with severe central nervous system dysfunction who present with nonepileptic spontaneous or stimulus-evoked myoclonus. Metabolic encephalopathies (such as glycine encephalopathy), cerebrovascular lesions, brain infections, or congenital malformations may present with nonepileptic myoclonus (Figure 37.4*a,b*).[26,34] Encephalopathic neonates may respond to tactile or painful stimulation by isolated focal, segmental, or generalized myoclonic movements. Rarely, cortically generated spike or sharp-wave discharges as well as seizures may also be noted on the EEG coincident with these myoclonic movements (Figures 37.5).[26] Medication-induced myoclonus as well as stereotypic movements have also been described.[35]

A rare familial disorder has been described in the neonatal and early infancy periods, specifically termed hyperekplexia. These are usually misinterpreted as a hyperactive startle reflex. These infants are stiff with severe hypertonia which may lead to apnea and bradycardia. Forced flexion of the neck or hips sometimes alleviates these events. EEG background is generally age-appropriate. The postulated defect of these individuals pertains to regulation of brainstem centers facilitating myoclonic movements.[36] Occasionally benzodiazepines or valproic acid lessen the startling, stiffening, or falling events.[37] Neurologic prognosis is variable.

Neonatal dystonia without EEG seizures

Dystonia is a third commonly misdiagnosed movement disorder that is often misrepresented as tonic seizures, or may be expressed with nonepileptic tonic movements. Dystonia can be associated with either acute or chronic disease states involving basal ganglia structures or extrapyramidal pathways, commonly injured after antepartum or intrapartum severe asphyxia (i.e., termed status marmoratus)[12] or, rarely, with specific inherited metabolic diseases.[38,39] Alternatively, posturing reflects subcortical motor pathways that remain functionally unopposed because of a diseased or malformed neocortex[25] (Figures 37.2*c* and 37.6). Documentation of EEG seizures with coincident video/EEG/polygraphic recordings will help avoid misdiagnosis.

Electrographic seizure criteria

Over the last several decades electrographic/polysomnographic studies have become invaluable tools for the assessment of suspected seizures.[2,7,9,24,30,40,41] Technical and interpretative skills of normal and abnormal neonatal EEG sleep patterns must be mastered before one develops a confident visual analysis style for seizure recognition.[13,14,42–44]

Corroboration with the EEG technologist is always an essential part of the diagnostic process since physiologic and nonphysiologic artifacts can masquerade as EEG seizures. The physician must also anticipate expected behaviors for the child for a specific gestational maturity, medication use, and state of arousal, in the context of potential artifacts. Synchronized video EEG documentation permits careful offline analysis for more accurate documentation.

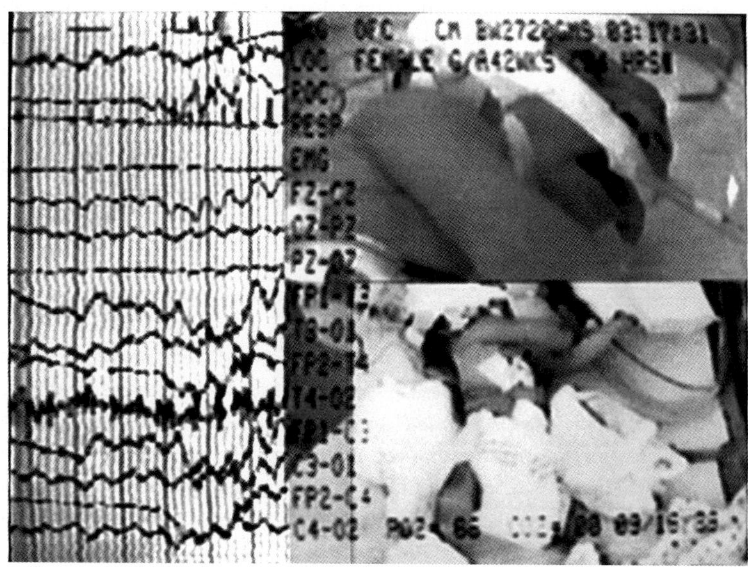

Figure 37.6 Segment of a video electroencephalogram (EEG) of a 42-week <24-hour-old growth-restricted female demonstrating stereotypic posturing and eye opening with no coincident electrographic seizure. The child presented with nonimmune hydrops fetalis with significant neocortical injury from a fetal time period. The EEG background is markedly slow and suppressed, representing a severe interictal electrographic abnormality. From Scher MS (1997). Seizures in the newborn infant. *Clin Perinatol* 24:74, with permission.

For the epileptic older child and adult, it is generally accepted that the epileptic seizure is a clinical paroxysm of altered brain function with the simultaneous presence of an electrographic event on an EEG recording. Therefore, when assessing the suspected clinical event in the neonate, synchronized video/EEG/polygraphic monitoring is a useful tool to distinguish an epileptic from a nonepileptic event. Some advocate the use of single-channel computerized devices for prolonged monitoring[45] given the multiple logistical problems using conventional multichannel recording devices. This specific device may consequentially not detect focal or regional seizures because recording from a single channel will not detect localized disease processes, distant from the channel.

Epilepsy monitoring services for older children and adults readily utilize intracerebral or surface electrocorticography to detect seizures. Such recording strategies, however, are not ethically appropriate or practical for the neonatal patient. Subcortical foci are consequentially difficult to eliminate definitively from consideration, as will be discussed below.

Ictal EEG patterns – a more reliable marker for seizure onset, duration, and severity

Neonatal EEG seizure patterns commonly consist of a repetitive sequence of waveforms which evolve in frequency, amplitude, electrical field, and morphology. Four types of ictal patterns have been described: focal ictal patterns with normal background, focal patterns with abnormal background, multifocal ictal patterns,[43] and focal monorhythmic periodic patterns of various frequencies. It is generally suggested that a minimal duration of 10 s with the evolution of discharges is required to distinguish electrographic seizures from repetitive but nonictal epileptiform discharges[7,46–48] (Figure 37.1*a* and 37.2*a* and *b*). Clinical neurophysiologists generally classify brief or prolonged repetitive discharges with a lack of evolution as nonictal patterns, but some argue that simply the presence of epileptiform discharges is confirmatory of seizures.[47] The specific features of electrographic seizure duration and topography are unique to the neonatal period.

Seizure duration and topography

Few studies have quantified minimal or maximal seizure durations in neonates.[7,46,48] Most notably, the definition of the most severe expression of seizures which potentially promotes brain injury, status epilepticus, can be problematic. For the older patient, status epilepticus is defined as at least 30 min of continuous seizures or two consecutive seizures with an interictal period during which the patient fails to return to full consciousness. This definition is not easily applied to the neonate for whom the level of arousal may be difficult to assess, particularly if sedative medications are given. One study arbitrarily defined neonatal status epilepticus as continuous seizure activity for at least 30 min, or 50% of the recording time;[48] 33% or 11 of 34 full-term infants had status epilepticus with a mean duration of 29.6 min prior to antiepileptic drug use, with another 9% or three out of the 34 preterm infants who also had status epilepticus with an average duration of 5.2 min per seizure (i.e., 50% of the recording time). The mean seizure duration was longer in the full-term infant (5 min) compared to the preterm infant (2.7 min). Given that more than 20% of this study group fit the criteria for status epilepticus based on EEG documentation, concerns must be raised regarding the underdiagnosis of the more severe form of seizures that potentially contribute to brain injury.

Uncoupling of the clinical and electrographic expressions of neonatal seizures after antiepileptic medication administration also contributes to an underestimation of the true seizure duration, including status epilepticus (Figure 37.7). One study estimated that 25% of neonates expressed persistent electrographic seizures despite resolution of their clinical seizure behaviors after receiving antiepileptic medications,[49] termed electroclinical uncoupling. Other pathophysiological mechanisms besides medication effect might also explain uncoupling.[10]

Most neonatal electrographic seizures arise focally from one brain region. Generalized synchronous and symmetrical repetitive discharges can also occur. In one study, 56% of seizures were seen in a single location at onset; specific sites included temporal–occipital (15%), temporal–central (15%), central (10%), frontotemporal central (6%), frontotemporal (5%), and vertex (5%). Multiple locations at the onset of the electrographic seizures were noted in 44%.[7] Electrographic discharges may be expressed as specific EEG frequency ranges from fast to slow, including beta, alpha, theta, or delta activities. Multiple electrographic seizures can also be expressed independently in anatomically unrelated brain regions.

Periodic discharges – prolonged repetitive discharges; ictal or interictal?

Clinical neurophysiologists distinguish periodic nonseizure EEG patterns from electrographic seizures for patient populations of varying ages. As with older patients, the neonate may express or sustain repetitive or periodic discharges which do not satisfy electrographic criteria for seizures (Figure 37.8*a*). Sustained periodic lateralized epileptiform discharges of 10 min or 20% of the recording time (defined as PLEDs on recordings of older children and adults) are rarely noted for the newborn.[50] This particular repetitive pattern of electrographic discharges in older patients is commonly associated with acute brain injuries from stroke, hemorrhage, or trauma, and may also follow or precede electrographic seizures. Periodic discharges are less commonly noted in neonates (i.e., 5% of the 1114 neonatal recordings), with PLEDs noted in only four of 34 infants. Most newborns with periodic discharges were expressed as shorter durations than classically defined PLEDs. However, nearly half of neonates with periodic discharges also expressed electrographic seizures at other times during the same EEG recording. Cerebrovascular lesions were

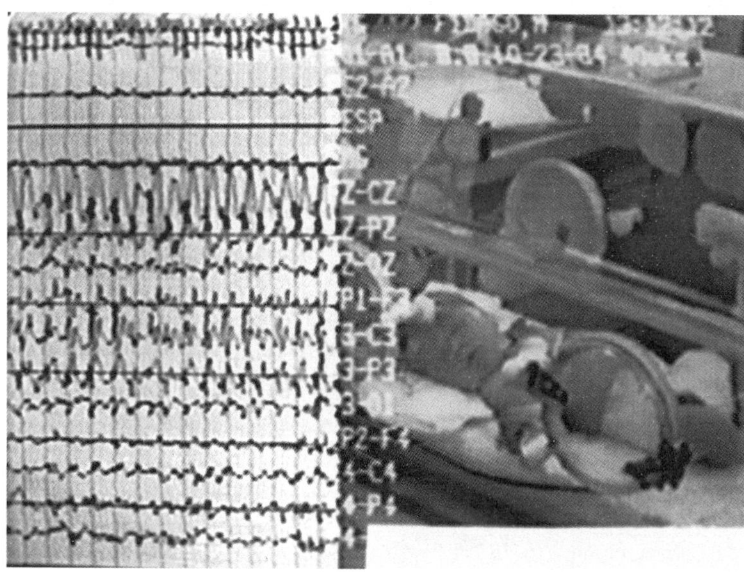

Figure 37.7 Segment of a synchronized video electroencephalogram of a 40-week, 1-day-old male with electrographic status epilepticus noted in the left central/midline regions, after antiepileptic medication administration. Focal right shoulder clonic activity was only intermittently noted, while continuous electrographic seizures were documented mostly without clinical expression. This phenomenon of uncoupling of electrical and clinical seizure activities is associated with antiepileptic drug administration use (see text). From Scher MS, Painter MJ (1989). Controversies concerning neonatal seizures. In: Pellock JM (ed.) *Seizure Disorders. Pediatric Clinics of North America*, vol. 36, p. 290. Philadelphia, PA: WB Saunders, with permission.

the most common brain lesion in 53% (18 of 34) of this group of newborns. Periodic EEG discharges for 26 preterm neonates lasted less than 60 s, and were located in the parasagittal regions, whereas discharges in eight term neonates were longer than a minute and located in the temporal regions. Forty-four percent of neonates died (15 of 34); 58% (11 of 19 infants) survived with neurological sequelae. Therefore, neonates with periodic discharges identified on EEG recordings require aggressive investigation for underlying brain injuries and prognostic considerations for neurologic sequelae, independent of the decision to treat with antiepileptic drugs.

Brief rhythmic discharges – ictal or interictal?

At the opposite end of the spectrum from periodic discharges, brief rhythmic discharges that are less than 10 s in duration have also been addressed with respect to an association with seizures and outcome (Figure 37.8*b*). Neonates with electrographic seizures may also exhibit these brief discharges; other neonates only express isolated discharges without seizures. Neonates with brief discharges can suffer from hypoglycemia or periventricular leukomalacia, which carries a higher risk for neurodevelopmental delay.[51]

Subcortical seizures vs nonictal functional decortication

Experimental animal models offer conflicting neuronal mechanisms to explain clinical events which do not have coincident EEG confirmation. Most clinical neurophysiologists require documentation of an ictal pattern by surface EEG electrodes. However, subcortical seizures with only intermittent propagation to the surface may occur. At the other end of the spectrum, nonictal "brainstem release" phenomena must be considered, particularly if EEG seizures are never expressed.[24] A more integrated electroclinical approach has been suggested to classify clinical events as seizures vs. nonepileptic movement disorders, based on documentation by synchronized video EEG monitoring.[9]

Brainstem release phenomena

Synchronized video EEG polygraphic monitoring provides the physician with documentation of a suspicious event with a concurrent electrographic pattern on surface recordings.[18] The temporal relationship between clinical and electrographic phenomena has been described, based on the synchronized video EEG polygraphic monitoring. Based on 415 clinical seizures in 71 babies, clonic seizure activity had the best correlation with coincident electrographic seizures. "Subtle" clinical events, on the other hand, had a more inconsistent relationship, with coincident EEG seizure activity suggesting a nonepileptic brainstem release phenomenon for at least a proportion of such events. Functional decortication resulting from neocortical damage without coincident EEG seizures[24] has therefore been suggested, such as with tonic posturing, as illustrated in Figure 37.3*a*. Newborns with nonseizure brainstem release activity may express a different functional pattern of metabolic dysfunction, detected as altered glucose uptake on single-photon emission tomography studies, than neonates with seizures.[52] A recent suggestion to document increased prolactin levels with clinical seizures has also been reported,[53] but such levels have not yet been correlated with electrographic seizures.

Electroclinical dissociation suggesting subcortical seizures

Experimental studies on immature animals also support the possibility that subcortical structures may initiate seizures, which subsequently, although intermittently, propagate to the cortical surface.[54–56]

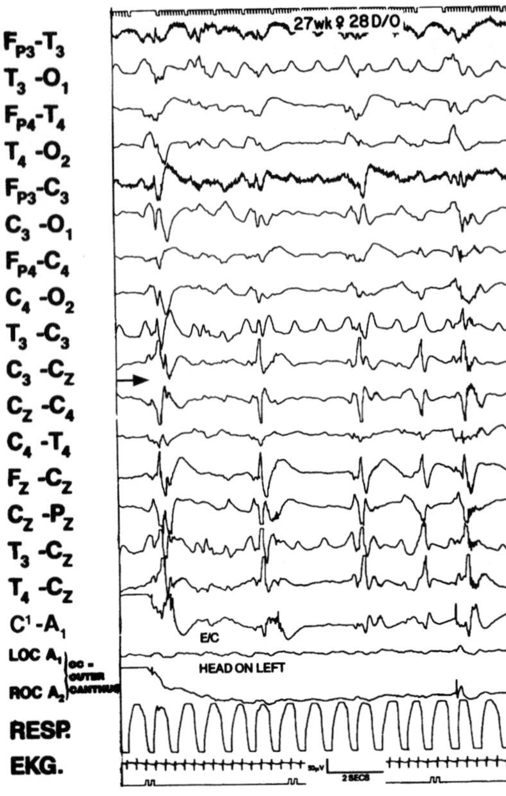

Figure 37.8*a* Electroencephalographic segment of a 27-week, 28-day-old female with intraventricular hemorrhage and periventricular leukomalacia. Continuous discharges in the midline region (C_z electrode, arrow) comprised of periodic positive sharp waves without an evolution of discharges were noted with seizures. From Scher MS (1997). Seizures in the newborn infant. *Clin Perinato* 24:247, with permission.

While EEG depth recordings in adults and adolescents help document subcortical seizures both with and without clinical expression, this technology is not applicable or appropriate to the neonate. Only one anecdotal report of a human infant documented seizures emanated from possible deep gray-matter structures.[57]

Electroclinical dissociation (ECD) is one proposed mechanism by which subcortical seizures may only intermittently appear on surface-recorded EEG studies.[11] ECD has been defined as a reproducible

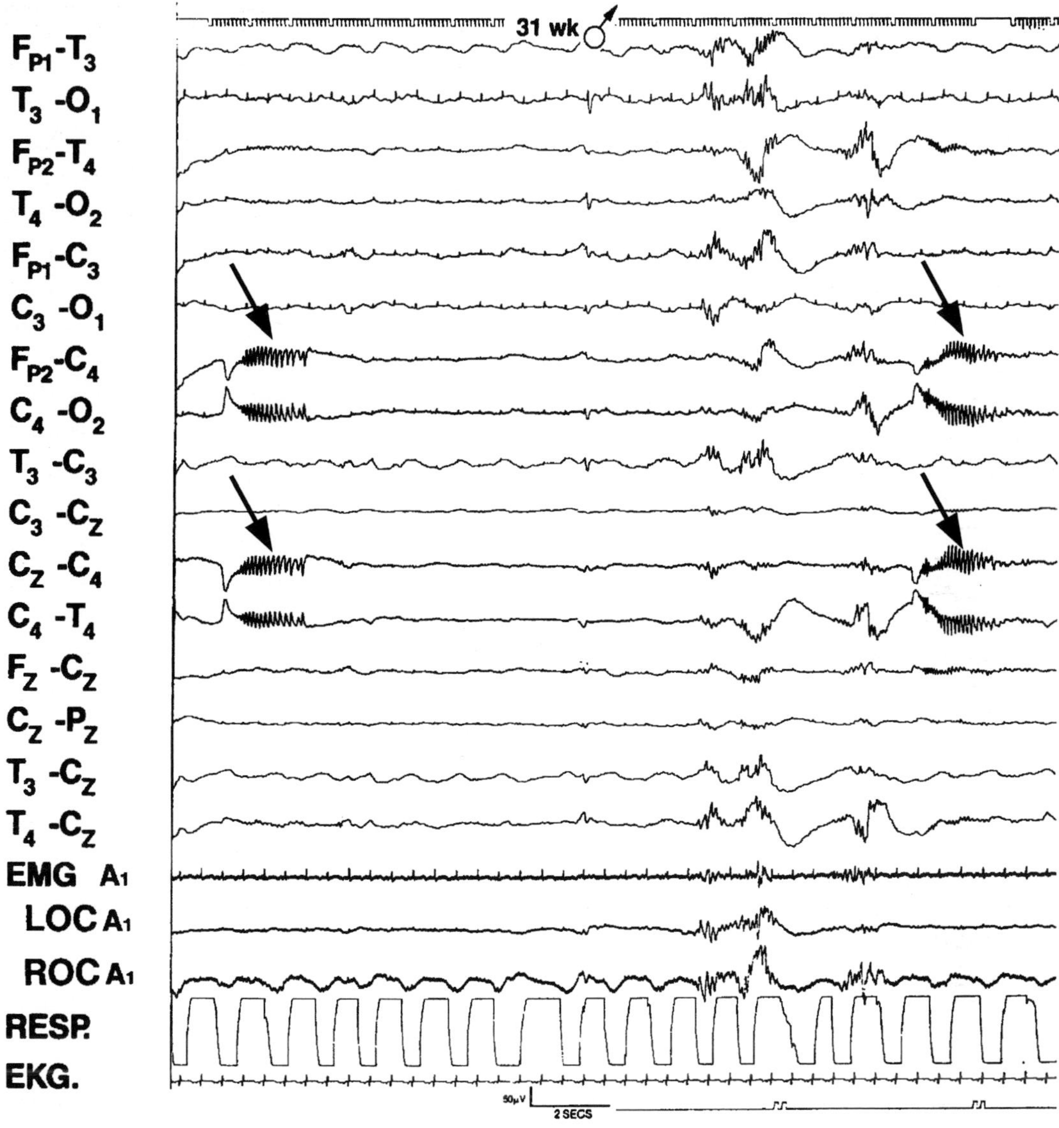

Figure 37.8*b* Electroencephalographic segment of a 31-week male with repetitive brief epileptiform discharges in the right central region (arrows) that are less than 10 s in duration, and do not qualify as an electrographic seizure.

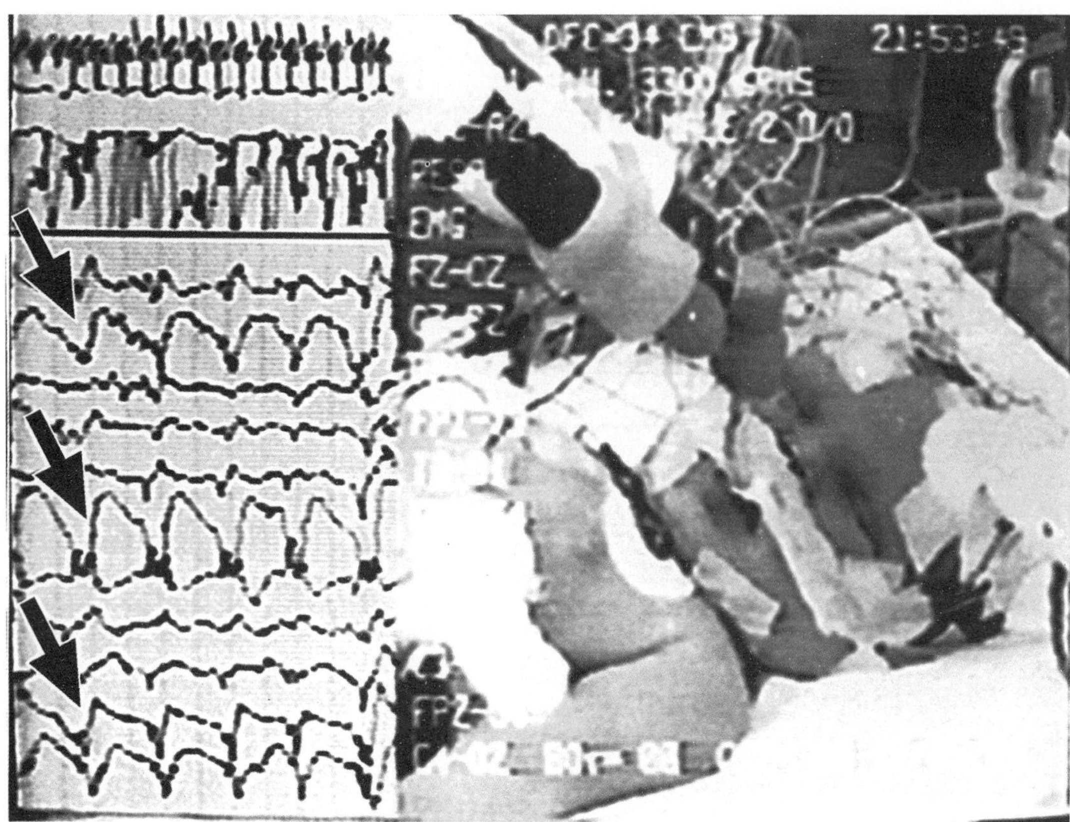

Figure 37.9*a* Segment of a synchronized video electroencephalographic record of a 38-week-gestation, 2-day-old male who is pharmacologically paralyzed for ventilatory care. A seizure is noted in the right posterior quadrant and midline (arrows). From Scher MS, Painter MJ (1989). Controversies concerning neonatal seizures. In: Pellock JM (ed.) *Seizure Disorders. Pediatric Clinics of North America*, vol. 36, p. 287. Philadelphia, PA: WB Saunders, with permission.

clinical event that occurs both with and without coincidental electrographic seizures. In one group of 51 infants with electroclinical seizures, 33 infants simultaneously expressed both electrical and clinical seizure phenomena. Extremity movements were more significantly associated with synchronized electroclinical seizures. However, a subset of 18 of 51 neonates, 35%, also expressed ECD on EEG recordings. For neonates who expressed ECD, the clinical seizure component always preceded the electrographic seizure expression, suggesting that a subcortical focus initiated the seizure state. Some of these children also expressed synchronized electroclinical seizures, even on the same EEG record.

Controversy remains whether subcortical seizures vs nonictal functional decortication best categorize suspicious clinical behaviors without coincident EEG documentation. This dilemma should encourage the clinician to use the EEG as a neurophysiologic yardstick by which more exact seizure start and endpoints can be assigned, before offering pharmacologic treatment with antiepileptic drugs.[30] Neonates certainly exhibit electrographic seizures that go undetected unless EEG is utilized.[58–63] Two examples are neonates who are pharmacologically paralyzed for ventilatory assistance (Figure 37.9*a*), or clinical seizures which are suppressed by the use of antiepileptic drugs (Figure 37.9*b*).[7,49,60–63] In one

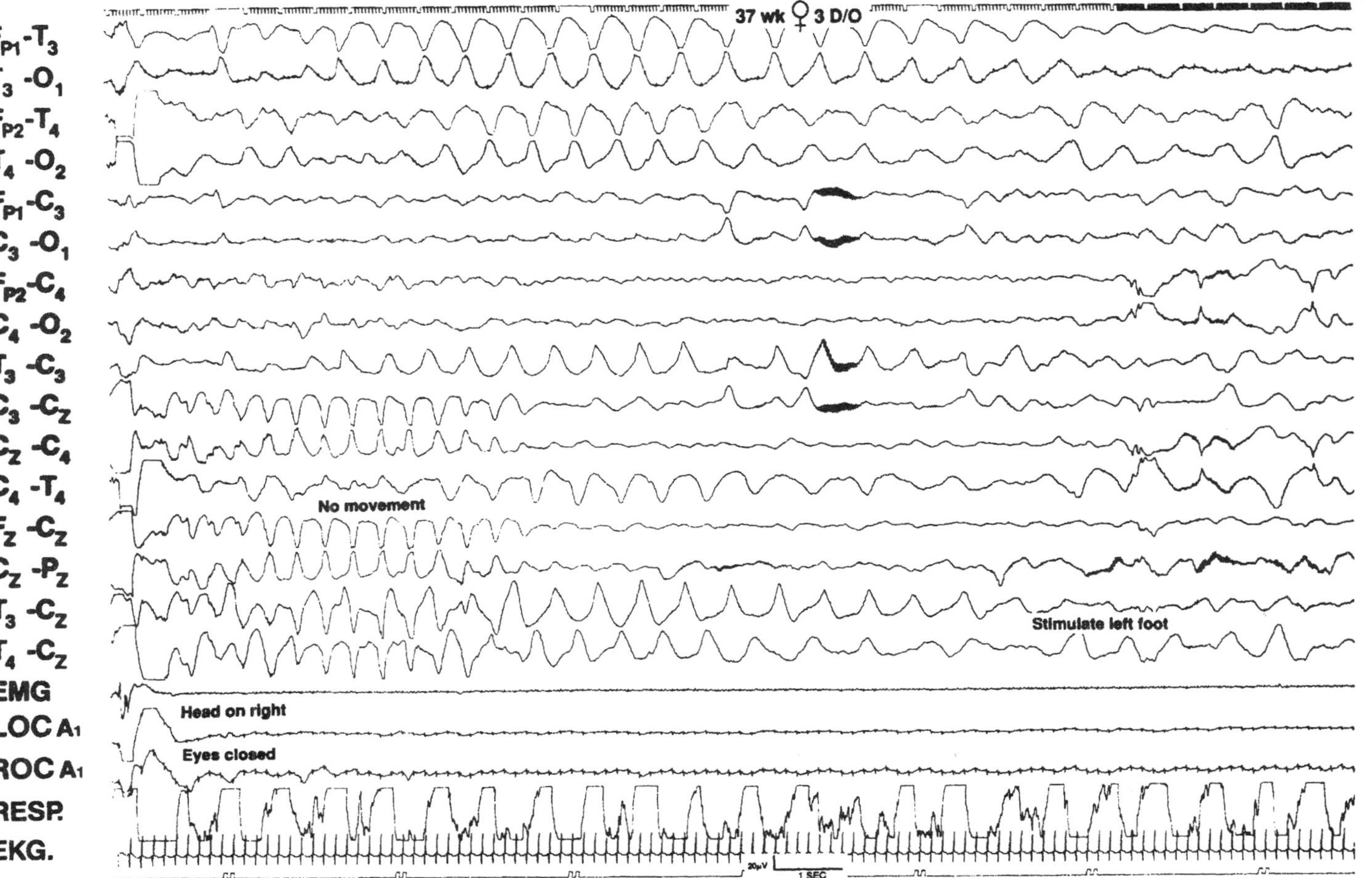

Figure 37.9*b* Electroencephalographic (EEG) segment for a 37-week, 3-day-old female after antiepileptic drug use with multifocal electrical seizures in the delta frequency range in the temporal and midline regions. Note the marked suppression of normal EEG background. From Scher MS (1997). Neonatal seizures. Seizures in special clinical settings. In: Wyllie E (ed.) *The Treatment of Epilepsy. Principles and Practice,* 2nd edn, p. 608. Baltimore, MD: Williams & Wilkins, with permission.

cohort of 92 infants, 60% of whom were pretreated with antiepileptic medications, 50% of neonates had electrographic seizures with no clinical accompaniment.[60] Both clinical and electrographic seizure criteria were noted for 45% of 62 preterms and 53% of 33 full-term infants. Seventeen infants were pharmacologically paralyzed when the EEG seizure was first documented. A later cohort of 60 infants, none of whom were pretreated with antiepileptic medications, included 7% of infants with only electrographic seizures prior to antiepileptic drug administration,[49] and 25% who expressed electroclinical uncoupling after antiepileptic drug use.

The underestimation of seizures in the newborn period may also result from inadequate monitoring for specific neurologic signs. Autonomic changes in respirations, blood pressure, oxygenation, heart rate, pupillary size, skin color, and salivation are examples of subtle ictal signs (Figure 37.10). In one study, autonomic seizures accompanied electrographic seizures in 37% of 19 preterm neonates.[60] Newer classifications of neonatal seizures emphasize documentation of autonomic findings on EEG recordings.[9]

Variation in the incidence of neonatal seizures based on clinical vs EEG criteria

Overestimation and underestimation of neonatal seizures are consequentially reported whether clinical or electrical criteria are used. Using clinical criteria, seizure incidences ranged from 0.5% in term infants to 22.2% in preterm neonates.[64–66] Discrepancies in incidence reflect not only varying postconceptional ages of the study populations chosen, but also poor interobserver reliability[67] and the hospital setting in which the diagnosis was made. Hospital-based studies[60] which include high-risk deliveries generally report a higher seizure incidence. Population studies[68] which include less medically ill infants from general nurseries report lower percentages. Incidence figures based only on clinical criteria without EEG confirmation include "false positives", consisting of the neonates with either normal or nonepileptic pathologic neonatal behaviors. Conversely, the absence of scalp-generated EEG seizures may include a subset of "false negatives" who express seizures only from subcortical brain regions without expression on the cortical surface. Closer consensus between clinical and EEG criteria is still required.

Interictal EEG pattern abnormalities

Interictal EEG abnormalities (including nonictal repetitive epileptiform discharges) have important prognostic implications for both preterm and full-term infants.[69,70] Severely abnormal bihemispheric patterns include the suppression-burst (i.e., paroxysmal) pattern (Figure 37.11), electrocerebral inactivity, low-voltage invariant pattern (Figure 37.4*c*), persistently slow background pattern (Figure 37.6), multifocal sharp waves, and marked asynchrony.[71] For infants with hypoxic–ischemic encephalopathy, subclassifications of specific EEG patterns such as burst-suppression with or without reactivity may give a more accurate prediction of outcome.[72] Dysmaturity of the EEG sleep background for child's corrected age has also been an important feature to recognize; discordance between cerebral and non-cerebral components of sleep state, or immaturity of EEG patterns for the given postconceptional age of the infant predict a higher risk for neurological sequela.[4,73–75] Even focal or regional patterns have prognostic significance such as with preterm infants who express repetitive positive sharp waves at the midline or central regions (Figure 37.8*a*), often noted with intraventricular hemorrhage and periventricular leukomalacia.[13]

Screening infants at risk for neonatal seizures with a routine EEG soon after birth allows identification of more severe interictal EEG background abnormalities which more likely predict seizure occurrence on subsequent neonatal records.[76]

Interictal EEG findings are not pathognomonic for particular etiologies, pathophysiologic mechanisms, or timing.[4] Historical, physical examination and laboratory findings need to be integrated with the electrographic interpretation of both ictal and interictal pattern abnormalities for the particular

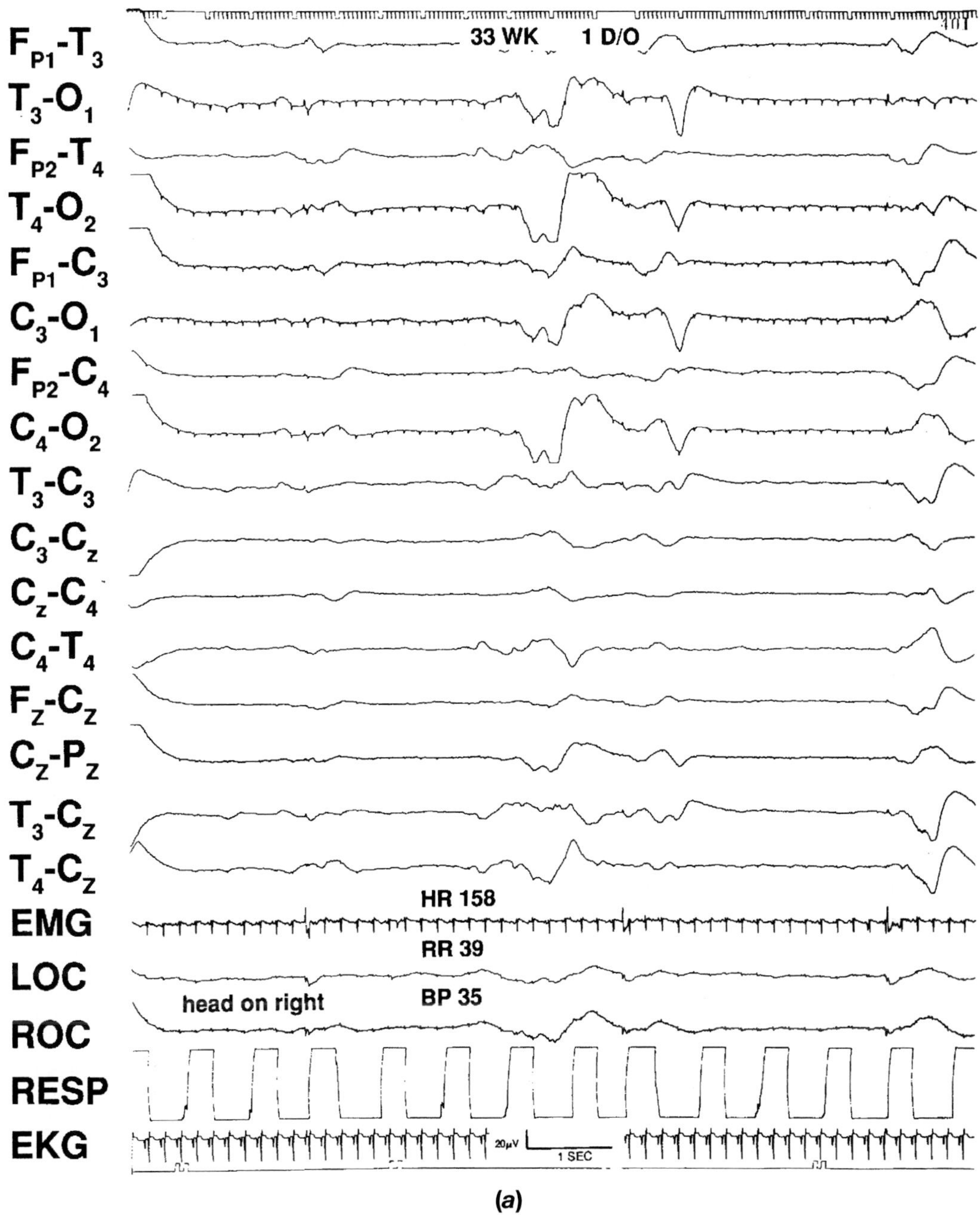

(*a*)

Figure 37.10 (*a* and *b*) Electroencephalographic (EEG) segments of a 31-week, 1-day-old male documenting drops in heart rate and blood pressure measurements after the onset of an electrographic seizure.

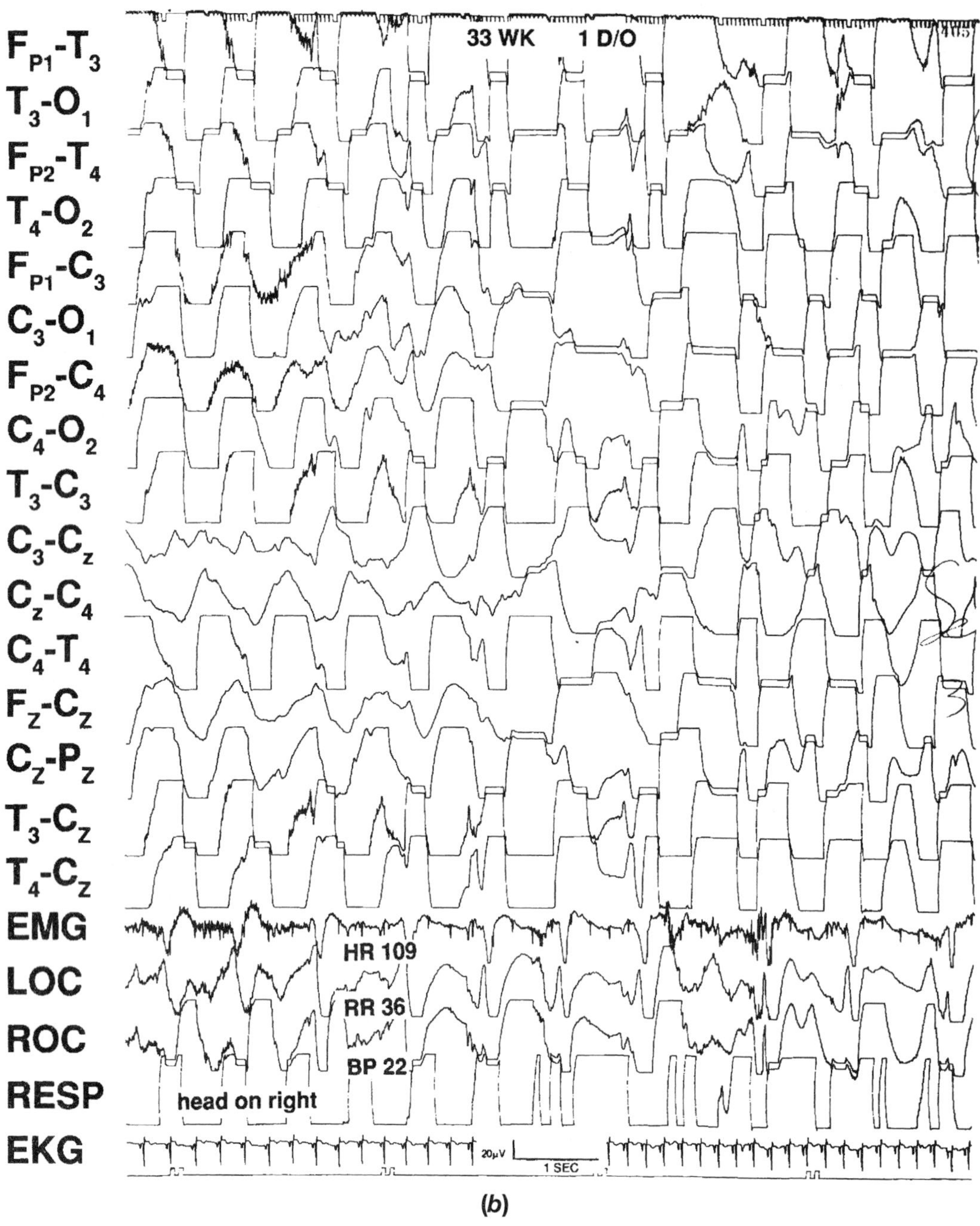

Figure 37.10 (*cont.*)

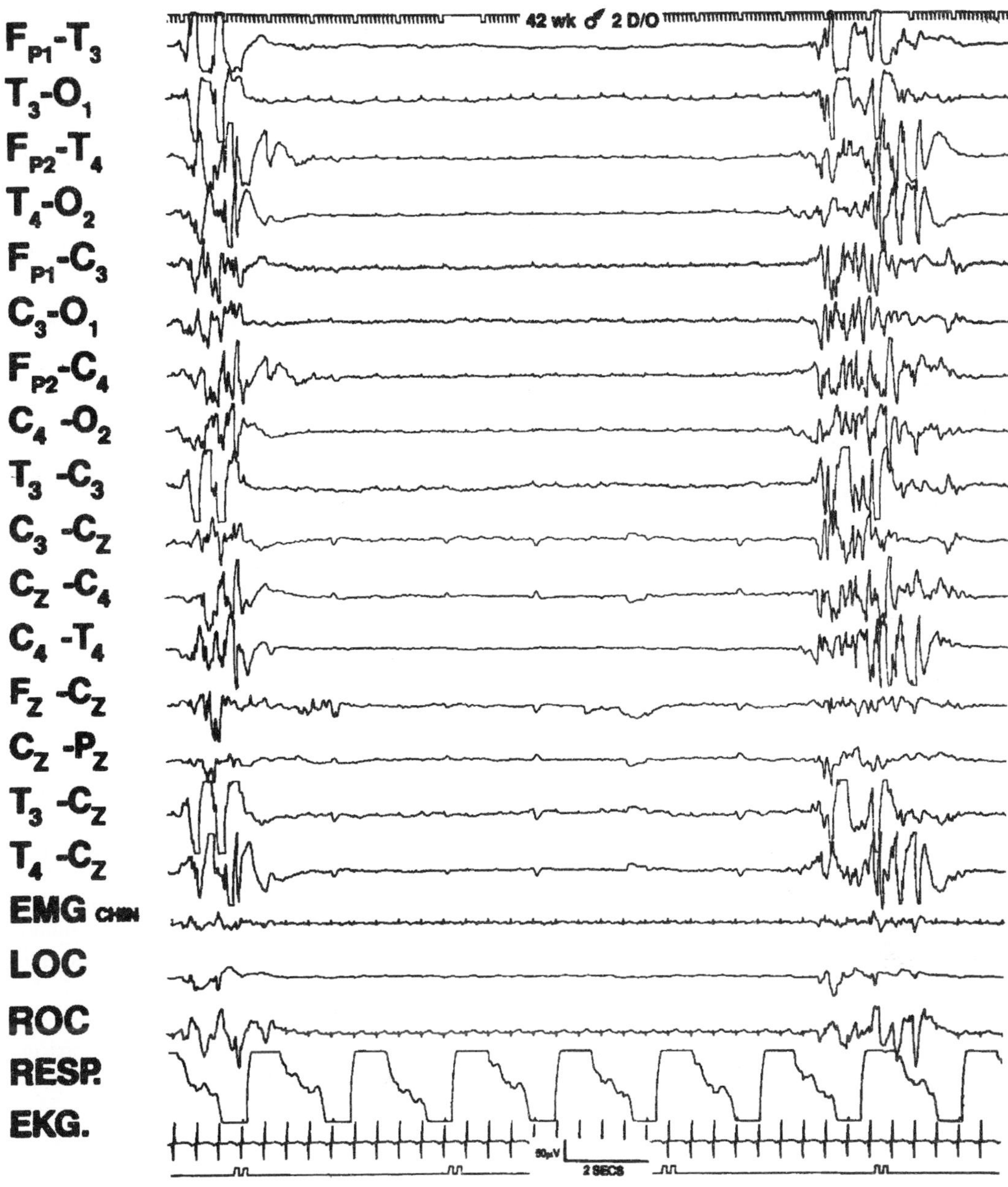

Figure 37.11 Electroencephalographic (EEG) segment of a 42-week, 2-day-old male expressing a severely abnormal interictal EEG background abnormality, termed a burst-suppression or paroxysmal pattern.

child. Serial EEG studies better assist the clinician in diagnostic and prognostic interpretations.[69,70] As with abnormal examination findings into the second week of life, the persistence of electrographic abnormalities also raises prognostic concerns. For example, the newborn who expresses severe EEG abnormalities into the second week of life implies a greater likelihood for neurologic impairment, even despite the resolution of clinical dysfunction. Conversely, the child who rapidly recovers from a significant brain disorder, with the reemergence of normal EEG features during the first few days after birth, may suffer comparatively fewer neurologic sequelae. Interictal EEG pattern abnormalities also reflect fetal brain disorders that preceded labor and delivery. The depth and severity of the neonatal brain disorder (defined by clinical and electrographic criteria) therefore may reflect chronic injury to the fetus who subsequently becomes symptomatic after a stressful intrapartum period, with or without more recent injury.

Diagnostic dilemmas: clinical scenarios of neonates with suspected seizures

Diverse medical conditions of the newborn can be associated with seizure activity[2,77] (Table 37.3). However, neonatal brain disorders may also result from these same conditions without seizure expression, leading to diagnostic and/or therapeutic approaches which do not require antiepileptic drug administration. In one prospective study of 157 infants screened by EEG for possible seizures, prior to antiepileptic drug use, based on seven clinical inclusion criteria, only 60 of 157 neonates or 38% had EEG confirmation of seizures,[78] despite the clinical concern for a brain disorder. Suspicious clinical behavior for seizures in 88 (56%) of the children was the most frequent screening criteria. Twenty-seven percent were based on asphyxia; 9 and 6% respectively were obtained from prenatal drug exposure or central nervous system infection, and 2% from central nervous system malformation; none of these latter three groups included suspicious behaviors. No neonates who were initially screened experienced cerebral trauma or were pharmacologically paralyzed for ventilatory management. For the segment of the cohort with suspicious behavior, only 49% (43/88) had EEG confirmation of seizures, 30% of whom required multiple EEG studies before EEG seizures were documented. Specifically, for the group with asphyxia, only 29% (12 of 41) had EEG confirmation of seizures; 50% (six of 12) were diagnosed on subsequent EEG studies after an initially negative study. Surprisingly, for the 60 neonates with EEG-confirmed seizures, 45% had no clinical signs of a brain disorder at delivery. Eighteen were transferred to the neonatal intensive care unit from well-child nurseries because of isolated seizures without encephalopathy. Nine asymptomatic newborns with isolated seizures later expressed postnatal illnesses from central nervous system infection, sepsis, or severe pulmonary disease.

Similarly, in a study of 40 neonates with clinical seizures, only 37.5% were associated with asphyxia, while the majority of these term infants had early-onset seizures that were not preventable from antepartum or intrapartum time periods, due to malformation, infarction, infection, or intracranial hemorrhage.[79]

Major etiologies for seizures – multiple overlapping conditions along a variable timeline

Neonatal seizures are not disease-specific, and can be associated with a variety of medical conditions which occur before or after parturition. Documentation of asphyxia is one frequently diagnosed entity when seizures occur: this illustrates the dilemma of overlapping medical conditions over multiple time points. Seizures may occur as part of an asphyxial injury during and/or after birth (termed hypoxic–ischemic encephalopathy), or alternatively occur with other etiologies for neonatal encephalopathy besides asphyxia or as an isolated clinical sign from a remote antepartum asphyxial stress without other signs of a postnatal encephalopathy. A logistic model to predict seizures emphasizes the accumulation of both antepartum and intrapartum factors to increase the likelihood of

Table 37.3. Selected differential diagnosis of neonatal seizures[a]

Metabolic	*Infections*
Hypoxia–ischemia (i.e., asphyxia)	Bacterial meningitis
Hypoglycemia	Viral-induced encephalitis
Hypocalcemia	Congenital infections
Hypomagnesemia	Herpes
Hypoglycemia	Cytomegalovirus
Intrauterine growth retardation	Toxoplasmosis
Infant of a diabetic mother	Syphilis
Glycogen storage disease	Coxsackie meningoencephalitis
Galactosemia	Acquired immune deficiency syndrome (AIDS)
Idiopathic	Brain abscess
Hypocalcemia	*Brain anomalies (i.e., cerebral dysgenesis from either congenital or acquired causes)*
Hypomagnesemia	
Infant of a diabetic mother	
Neonatal hypoparathyroidism	*Drug withdrawal or toxins*
Maternal hyperparathyroidism	Prenatal substance – methadone, heroin, barbiturate, cocaine, etc.
High phosphate load	
Other electrolyte imbalances	Prescribed medications – propoxyphene, isoniazid
Hypernatremia	Local anesthetics
Hyponatremia	*Hypertensive encephalopathy*
Intracranial hemorrhage	*Amino acid metabolism*
Subarachnoid hemorrhage	Branched-chain amino acidopathies
Subdural/epidural hematoma	Urea-cycle abnormalities
Intraventricular hemorrhage	Nonketotic hyperglycinemia
Cerebrovascular lesions (other than trauma)	Ketotic hyperglycinemia
Cerebral infarction	*Familial seizures*
Thrombotic vs. embolic	Neurocutaneous syndromes
Ischemic vs. hemorrhagic	Tuberous sclerosis
Cortical vein thrombosis	Incontinentia pigmenti
Circulatory disturbances from hypoperfusion	Autosomal dominant neonatal seizures
Trauma	*Selected genetic syndromes*
	Zellweger's syndrome
	Neonatal adrenoleukodystrophy
	Smith–Lemli–Opitz syndrome

Note:

[a] Etiology independent of timing from fetal to neonatal periods.

Source: Adapted from Scher.[77]

neonatal seizure occurrence.[80] While separately these same factors had low positive predictive values, a significant cumulative risk profile included antepartum maternal anemia, bleeding, and asthma, meconium-stained amniotic fluid, abnormal fetal presentation, fetal distress, and shoulder dystocia.

Neonatal encephalopathy was not caused by intrapartum hypoxia in a matched-case-control study of 89 full-term infants.[81] While these newborns appeared encephalopathic with seizures, had altered arousal and tone abnormalities, and exhibited feeding or central apnea, logistic regression analysis identified antepartum etiologies which better explained the neonatal encephalopathy.

Hypoxia–ischemia (i.e., asphyxia) is traditionally considered the most common cause associated with neonatal seizures.[12,41,82–85] However, children suffer asphyxia either before or during parturition; and only 10% of asphyxia results from postnatal causes.[12] When asphyxia is suspected during the labor and delivery process, biochemical confirmation must be attempted. However, only a minority with asphyxia at birth are associated with seizures, as part of a neonatal brain disorder known as hypoxic–ischemic encephalopathy. For example, only 29% in one cohort who fulfilled an arbitrary biochemical definition of intrapartum asphyxia (i.e., pH$\leq$7.2 and a base deficit of ≤ -10) were later diagnosed with seizures confirmed by EEG.[78]

Intrauterine factors prior to labor can result in fetal asphyxia without later documentation of acidosis at birth. Maternal illnesses such as thrombophilia or preeclampsia or specific uteroplacental abnormalities such as abruptio placentae or cord compression may contribute to fetal asphyxial stress without the opportunity to document in utero acidosis. Antepartum maternal trauma and chorioamnionitis are acquired conditions which also contribute to the intrauterine asphyxia secondary to uteroplacental insufficiency without availability for biochemical testing prior to labor and delivery. Intravascular placental thromboses and infarction of the placenta or umbilical cord noted on placental examinations are additional surrogates for possible fetal asphyxia. Meconium passage into the amniotic fluid also promotes an inflammatory response within the placental membranes, causing vasoconstriction and either de novo or additional asphyxia.[86] Neuroimaging may later define the destructive brain lesions that resulted from in utero asphyxia, even without hypoxic–ischemic encephalopathy expressed at birth.[87,88] Therefore, asphyxial-induced brain injury may result from in utero maternal–fetal–placental diseases which are later expressed as neonatal seizures, independent of the biochemical marker of acidosis at birth, as well as the evolving hypoxic–ischemic encephalopathy syndrome in the days after birth.

Postnatal medical illnesses also cause or contribute to asphyxial-induced brain injury and seizures without hypoxic–ischemic encephalopathy from labor and delivery events. Persistent pulmonary hypertension of the newborn, cyanotic congenital heart disease, sepsis, and meningitis are principal diagnoses. In one hospital-based study over a 14-year period, 62 of 247 infants presented with EEG-confirmed seizures after an uneventful delivery without fetal distress during labor or neonatal depression at birth. Twenty of these 62 infants, or 32%, later presented with postnatal onset of pulmonary disease, sepsis, or meningitis.[2]

A recent case-control study of term infants with clinical seizures reported a fourfold increase in the risk of unexplained early-onset seizures after intrapartum fever. All known causes of seizures were eliminated, including meningitis or sepsis. These 38 newborns, compared to 152 controls, experienced intrapartum fever as an independent risk factor on logistic regression and this predicted seizures. The authors speculated on the role of circulating maternal cytokines which triggered "physiologic events" contributing to seizures.[89]

The American College of Obstetricians and Gynecologists published guidelines that suggest criteria to define postasphyxial neonatal encephalopathy, i.e., hypoxic–ischemic encephalopathy,[90] after significant clinical depression noted at birth. These guidelines include the following:

1 profound umbilical metabolic or mixed acidemia with a pH less than 7.00

2 persistence of an Apgar score of 0–3 for longer than 5 min
3 neonatal neurological sequelae (seizures, coma, and hypotonia)
4 multiorgan system dysfunction (significant cardiovascular, gastrointestinal, hematologic, pulmonary, and renal involvement)

Postasphyxial encephalopathy refers to an evolving clinical syndrome over days after birth depression during which neonatal seizures may occur, usually in children who also exhibit severe early metabolic acidosis, hypoglycemia, or hypocalcemia, and multiorgan dysfunction.[12,85] Yet, other epiphenomena around asphyxia may contribute to seizures. Eighty of 142 infants with seizures after asphyxia[83,84] also had trauma or intracranial hemorrhage; the remaining 62 with seizures were assessed as having brain damage based on other neurological diagnoses besides asphyxia.

The physical examination of the infant with hypoxic–ischemic encephalopathy and seizures includes coma, hypotonia, brainstem abnormalities, and loss of fetal reflexes. Postasphyxial seizures generally occur within the first 3 days of life depending on the length and degree of asphyxial stress during the intrapartum period.[12] An early occurrence of seizures, within several hours after delivery, sometimes suggests an antepartum occurrence of a fetal brain disorder, when compared with specific fetal heart rate patterns.[91] Although in and of itself seizure onset is not a reliable indicator of timing of fetal brain injury. Earlier seizure onset, within 4 h of birth in encephalopathic newborns, may predict severe adverse outcome, independent of etiology for asphyxia.[92]

Asphyxia is conventionally diagnosed, based on the association of several metabolic parameters on an umbilical or serum blood gas; a reduced Po_2 level usually 40 mmHg or less indicates a severe disturbance of oxygen exchange, associated with acidosis. The duration of asphyxia, however, will be difficult to assess based on either single or even multiple Po_2 values. Scalp and/or umbilical cord artery pH levels of less than 7.2 are considered of greater clinical concern for predicting hypoxic–ischemic encephalopathy, although the suggested guideline of a pH of <7.0 is one criterion by which the clinical entity of hypoxic–ischemic encephalopathy might be better predicted.[90] A metabolic definition of asphyxia should also include at least a base deficit of ≤ -10. More recently, a base deficit of ≤ -16 has been suggested because of the higher prediction for the emergence of the hypoxic–ischemic encephalopathy syndrome including clinical seizures.[93] One caveat should always be remembered before assigning a relative risk to a pH value; elevated Pco_2 values introduce a superimposed respiratory acidosis secondary to hypercarbia. Elevated Pco_2 with respiratory acidosis is comparatively less harmful to brain tissue and is more rapidly corrected by aggressive ventilatory support. Alternatively, metabolic acidosis suggests a more profound alteration of intracellular function that better predicts an evolving brain disorder, which may include seizures as part of hypoxic–ischemic encephalopathy.

Low Apgar scores are traditionally associated with infants with suspected neurological depression after delivery, with possible evolution to hypoxic–ischemic encephalopathy and seizures. Low 1-min and 5-min Apgar scores indicate the continued need for resuscitation but only low scores at 10, 15, and 20 min carry a more accurate prediction for sequelae.[94] Normal Apgar scores, however, do not eliminate the possibility of severe antepartum brain injury, from either asphyxia or other causes. As many as two-thirds of neonates who exhibit cerebral palsy at older ages had normal Apgars at birth without hypoxic–ischemic encephalopathy.[95] In one hospital-based study, only 13% (25 out of 193 neonates) with EEG-confirmed seizures within the first 120 h of life met the four suggested criteria for hypoxic–ischemic encephalopathy.[2]

Placental findings may reflect disease states at any time point before birth either with or without metabolic acidosis and evolving hypoxic–ischemic encephalopathy after birth.[86] While in utero meconium passage commonly occurs in otherwise healthy newborns, meconium staining of the child's skin may be correlated with meconium-laden macrophages within placental membranes in a depressed newborn. Meconium staining through the chorionic layer to the amnion suggests a longer-standing asphyxial stress, such as over 4–6 h.

Placental weights below the 10th or above the 90th percentile suggest chronic perfusion abnormalities to the fetus. Microscopic evidence of lymphocytic infiltration, altered villous maturation, chorangiosis, and erythroblastic proliferation of villi of the placenta all support chronic asphyxial stresses to the fetus.[86] Gross and microscopic samples of chronic placental lesions are described in Chapter 24. In a study of preterm and full-term neonates (23–42 weeks' conceptional age) with electrically confirmed seizures, a significant association between seizures and chronic (with or without acute) placental lesions was noted, increasing to a factor of 12.1 ($P < 0.003$) by term age. Odds ratios were not significant for infants with seizures and exclusively acute placental lesions, presumably from events closer to labor and delivery.[96]

Specific clinical examination findings in the depressed neonate with suspected hypoxic–ischemic encephalopathy may reflect antepartum disease states.[5,97] Intrauterine growth restriction, hydrops fetalis, or joint contractures (including arthrogryposis) are exam findings that suggest in utero diseases which may have been associated with antepartum asphyxia, and that was later expressed as intrapartum fetal distress and/or neonatal depression. Hypertonicity, often with cortical thumbs, in a depressed child who rapidly recovers after a successful resuscitative effort also commonly reflects longer-standing fetal neurological dysfunction. Sustained hypotonia and unresponsiveness for 3–7 days are the expected signs of hypoxic–ischemic encephalopathy after an intrapartum asphyxial stress, with or without brain injury. Encephalopathic newborns with depressed arousal and hypotonia, none the less, may paradoxically reflect an antepartum disease process with neonatal dysfunction or superimposed injury as a result of a problematic intrapartum period. For example, this was described in 10 of 20 neurologically depressed infants with EEG seizures and isoelectric interictal EEG pattern abnormalities who were comatose and flaccid for days, requiring ventilator assistance after difficult deliveries.[98] All children appeared neurologically depressed after asphyxial stress during the intrapartum period (i.e., depressed Apgars and metabolic acidosis). Evidence of fetal brain injury was supported by preexisting maternal disease, placental lesions, neuroimaging findings, and/or neuropathological postmortem findings. While intrapartum asphyxial stress may have worsened brain injury in these children, it was impossible to differentiate their neonatal encephalopathy from preexisting antepartum brain injury.

Hypoglycemia

Hypoglycemia is generally defined as glucose levels of ≤20 mg/dl in preterm infants and ≤30 mg/dl in term infants.[99,100] No clear consensus exists concerning a direct cause and effect of hypoglycemia with seizure occurrence.[101] Methods of glucose determination (dextrose stick versus serum sampling) will affect the accuracy of the value. Also, associated disturbances may coexist, such as hypocalcemia, craniocerebral trauma, cerebrovascular lesions, and asphyxia, and these may also contribute to lowering the infant's threshold for seizures. Infants born of diabetic or toxemic mothers, particularly those who were small-for-gestational-age, are also at risk for hypoglycemia. Jitteriness, apnea, and altered tone are clinical signs which may appear in children with hypoglycemia, but are not representative of a seizure state. Cerebrovascular lesions in posterior brain regions have been reported in children who suffer hypoglycemia.[102] Vulnerability of brain to ischemic insults is enhanced by concomitant hypoglycemia, as reported in mature animals[103] and neonatal infants.[102,104]

Hypocalcemia

Total serum calcium levels lower than 7.5 mg/dl in preterm and 8 mg/dl in term infants generally define hypocalcemia. The ionized fraction is a more sensitive indicator of seizure vulnerability. As with hypoglycemia, the exact level of hypocalcemia at which seizures occur is debatable. An ionized fraction of 0.6 or less may have a more predictable association with the presence of seizures. Late-onset hypocalcemic-induced seizures have been previously cited as a common cause of seizures[23,105,106] due to high phosphate-containing infant formula. However, hypocalcemia now more commonly occurs with infants with trauma, hemolytic disease, or asphyxia, and may coexist with hypoglycemia or hypomagnesemia. Rarely, congenital hypoparathyroidism in association with other genetic abnormalities, such as DiGeorge syndrome (i.e., velocardiofacial syndrome, or 22q11 deletion with cardiac and brain anomalies) must be considered. These infants may have severe congenital heart disease, as well as hypoparathyroid state with hypocalcemia and hypomagnesemia, which precipitates seizures.[104,107] Infants with hypocalcemia of unknown etiology may also be the result of maternal hypercalcemia. Ascertainment of the mother's calcium status should be considered since maternal hypercalcemia can suppress fetal parathyroid development.

Hyponatremia and hypernatremia

Hyponatremia is a metabolic disturbance that may result from inappropriate secretion of antidiuretic hormone following severe brain trauma, infection, or asphyxia,[12] but is an uncommon isolated cause of neonatal seizures. Hypernatremia also is a rare cause of seizures, usually associated with congenital adrenal abnormalities or iatrogenic disturbance of serum sodium balance, by the use of intravenous fluids with high concentrations of sodium.

Cerebrovascular lesions

Hemorrhagic or ischemic cerebrovascular lesions are associated with neonatal seizures, on either an arterial or venous basis.[19–21,34,108–111] Intraventricular or periventricular hemorrhage (IVH/PVH) is the most common intracranial hemorrhage of the preterm infant, and has been associated with seizures in as many as 45% of a preterm population with EEG-confirmed seizures.[60,112] In a cohort of newborns with clinical seizures, IVH was the most predominant cause of seizures in preterm infants less than 30 weeks' gestational age[113] (Figure 37.12). Intracranial hemorrhage is usually expected within the first 72 hours of life of the preterm infant. While IVH/PVH may occur in otherwise asymptomatic infants, the neonate with a catastrophic deterioration of clinical status will include signs of apnea, bulging fontanel, hypertonia, and seizures.[12] Seventeen percent of preterm infants with IVH may have acute seizures during the first month of life, or suffered remote seizures (after discharge) in 10% of one cohort.[114] Full-term infants present less commonly with IVH, usually originating from the choroid plexus or thalamus.

Other sites of intracranial hemorrhage include the subarachnoid space, which may cause seizures, but this is generally associated with a more favorable outcome. Subdural hematoma, whether spontaneous or with craniocerebral trauma, should always be considered, particularly when focal trauma to the face, scalp, or head has occurred; simultaneous occurrences of cerebral contusion and infarction should also be considered.

Cerebral infarction has been described in neonates with seizures and can result from events during the antepartum, intrapartum, or neonatal periods. Either preterm or term neonates with infarction may also present without seizure expression.[115] Seizures can also occur in otherwise healthy infants, suggesting an antepartum time period when cerebral infarction occurred (Figure 37.13).[34,116] Aggressive use of neuroimaging during the antepartum period or within the first days after birth by fetal sonography or magnetic resonance imaging (MRI) may document remote brain lesions.[5] In a group of 62 healthy infants with EEG seizures after an uneventful delivery, 23 (37%) had cerebrovascular lesions, 18 of whom had ischemic brain lesions.[78] Destructive lesions such as porencephaly require approximately 5–7 days before appearing radiographically demonstrable (Figure 37.9). More recent intrapartum or neonatal time periods during which injury occurred can be supported by the presence of early cerebral edema using diffusion-weighted MRI

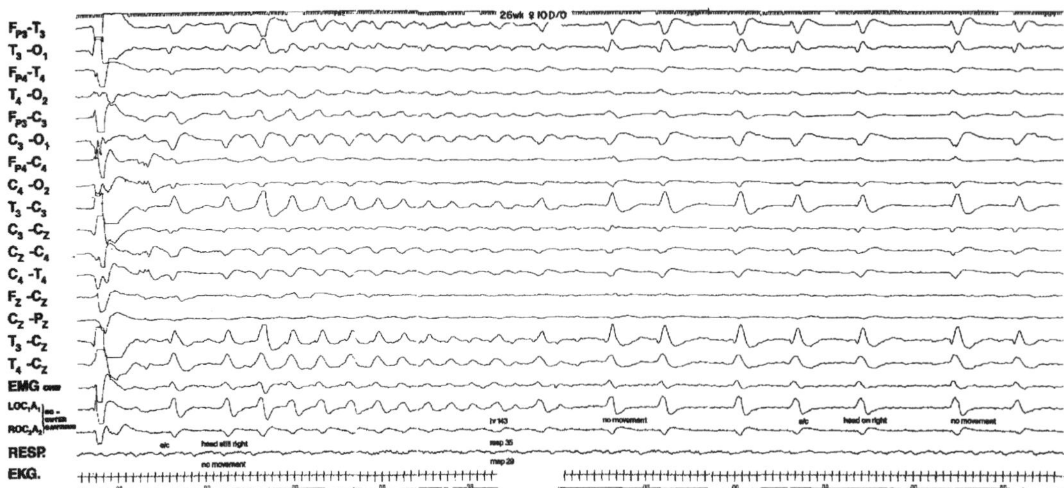

Figure 37.12*a* Segment of electroencephalographic record of a 26-week, 10-day-old female with sepsis and disseminated intravascular coagulation who expresses an electrographic seizure prominently in the left hemisphere and midline regions.

images.[117] Cerebral infarction may also occur during the postnatal period from asphyxia, polycythemia, dehydration, or coagulopathy (Figure 37.10).

Persistent pulmonary hypertension of the newborn with severe and recurrent hypoxia can also be associated with cerebrovascular lesions and seizures (Figure 37.14).[21] Certain infants with persistent pulmonary hypertension of the newborn will require extracorporeal membrane oxygenation to treat severe forms of this pulmonary disease as it does not respond to traditional ventilatory therapy. Radiographic documentation of brain lesions needs to be diagnosed before beginning extracorporeal membrane oxygenation, because the anticoagulation required for extracorporeal membrane oxygenation may convert "bland" or ischemic infarctions to hemorrhagic forms, with greater risk for cerebral edema and herniation. While meconium aspiration syndrome has historically been identified with an intrapartum/neonatal presentation of persistent pulmonary hypertension of the newborn, most children with this lung disease generally reflect antepartum maternal/fetal or placental conditions which predispose the fetus to thickening of the muscular layers of the pulmonary arteries while in utero, with

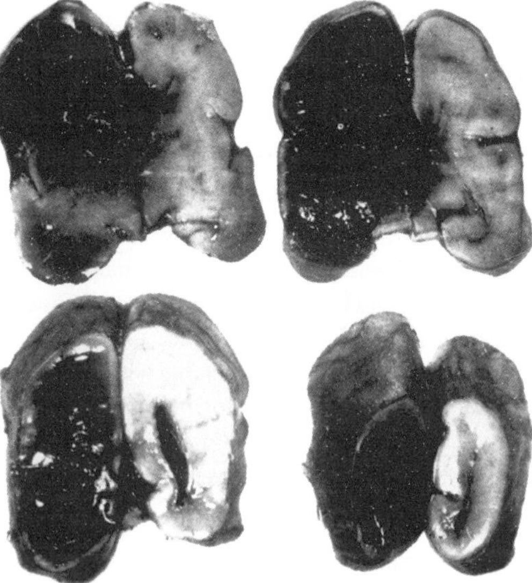

Figure 37.12*b* Postmortem coronal slices of brain of the preterm infant shown in Figure 37.12*a* with prominent hemorrhagic infarction of the left hemisphere as well as intraventricular hemorrhage.

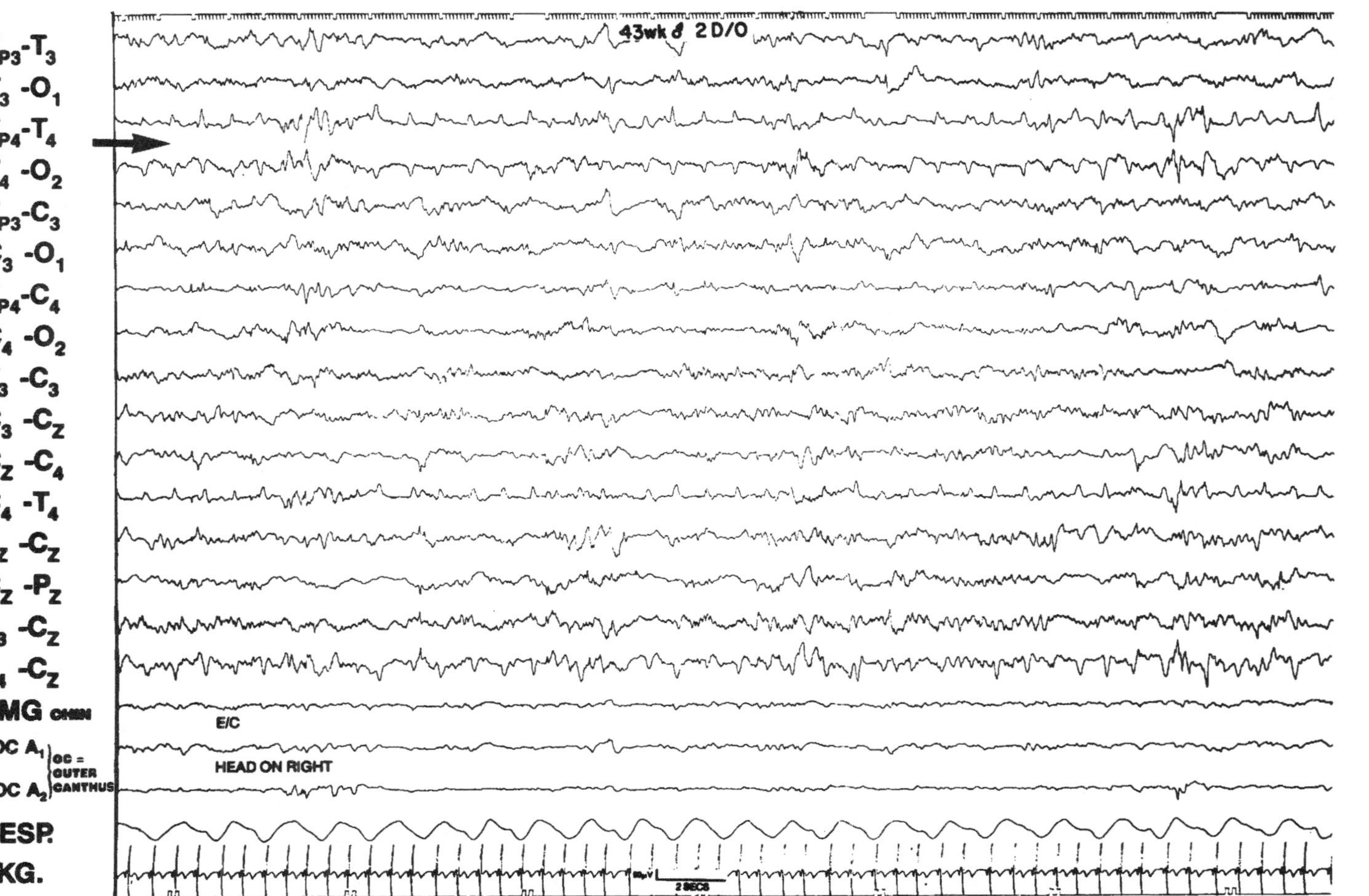

Figure 37.13*a* Electroencephalographic segment of a 43-week, 2-day-old male with focal electrographic seizures in the right temporal region (arrow).

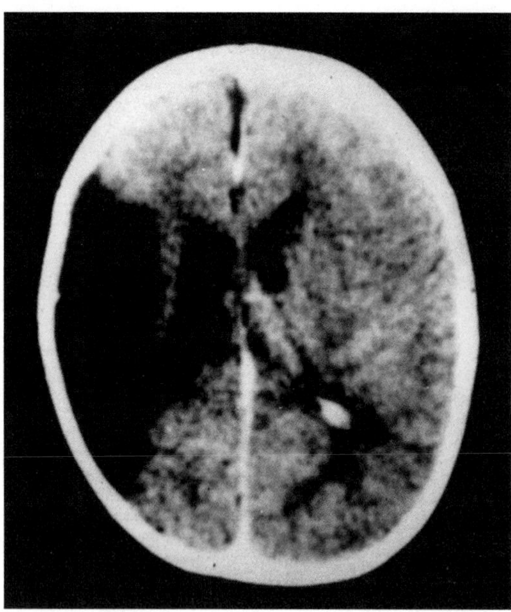

Figure 37.13*b* Computed tomography scan on day 1 of life for the child shown in Figure 37.13*a*, documenting a right middle cerebral artery infarction that occurred in the antepartum period.

resultant sustained increased pulmonary vascular resistance after birth.[118]

Cerebral infarction in the venous distribution of the brain may also lead to neonatal seizures.[109,111] Lateral or sagittal sinus thromboses after coagulopathy can occur secondary to systemic infection, polycythemia, or dehydration. Venous infarction within the deep white matter of the preterm brain also occurs in association with IVH.

Infection

Central nervous system infections during the antepartum or postnatal periods can be associated with neonatal seizures.[119] Congenital infections, commonly referred to by the acronym TORCH, (i.e., toxoplasmosis, rubella, cytomegalic inclusion disease, and herpes; Figure 37.4*c*) can produce severe encephalopathic damage which results in seizures, as well as more diffuse brain disorders. Other congenital infections include enteroviruses and parvoviruses. Specific infections, for instance neonatal herpes encephalitis, have been associated with severe EEG pattern abnormalities.[120] Rubella, toxoplasmosis, and cytomegalic inclusion disease can also lead to devastating encephalitis, usually presenting with microcephaly, jaundice, body rash, hepatosplenomegaly, and/or chorioretinitis. Increasing lethargy and obtundation with or without seizures may suggest the subacute presentation of encephalitis during the postnatal period. Serial spinal fluid analyses document progressively increasing protein and/or pleocytosis.

Acquired in utero or postnatal bacterial infections from either Gram-negative or Gram-positive organisms are also associated with neonatal seizures. Some organisms, such as *Escherichia coli*, group B streptococci, *Listeria monocytogenes*, and *Mycoplasma* infections, may produce severe leptomeningeal infiltration, with possible abscess formation and cerebrovascular occlusions (Figure 37.1*b*). A high percentage of survivors suffer significant neurological sequelae.

Central nervous system malformations

Disorders of induction, segmentation, proliferation, migration, myelination, and synaptogenesis of neuronal components can contribute to varying degrees of malformation. Seizures may result for the newborn with malformations who experiences stress around the time of birth,[121] presumably lowering seizure thresholds. Brain anomalies may occur as a result of either genetic causes from conception and/or acquired defects during the first half of gestation. Specific dysgenesis syndromes, such as holoprosencephaly and lissencephaly, are often associated with characteristic facial or body anomalies. Cytogenetic studies may document trisomies or deletion defects. Unfortunately, infants may also lack physical clues to the presence of a brain malformation. The clinician's high index of suspicion is then warranted to evaluate neonates with persistent seizures. Nine percent of 356 infants presenting with neonatal seizures had brain malformations.[113]

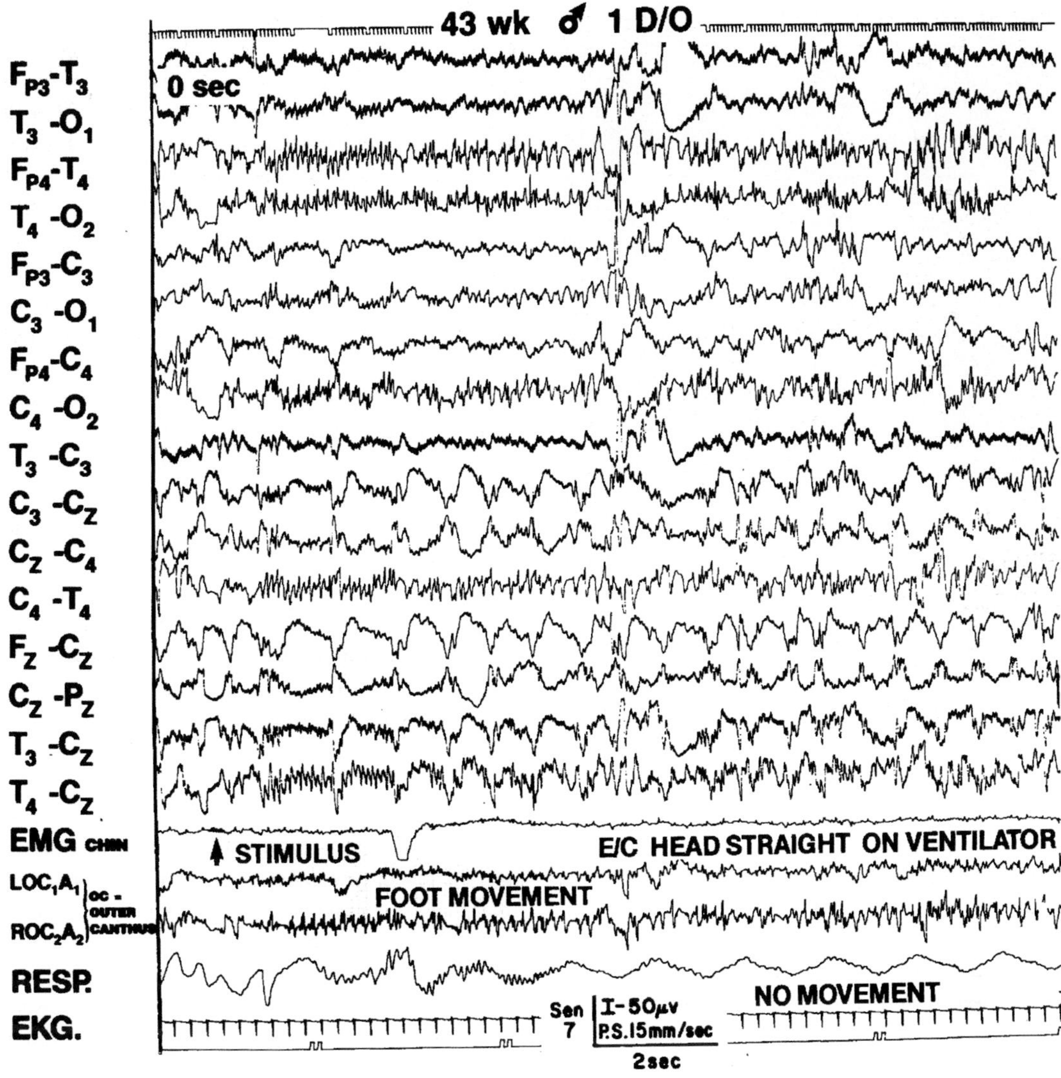

Figure 37.14*a* Electroencephalographic segment of record of a 43-week, 1-day-old male with a stimulus-evoked electrographic seizure (arrow) without clinical accompaniments in the right temporal region. The child required ventilatory care for persistent pulmonary hypertension of the newborn (see text).

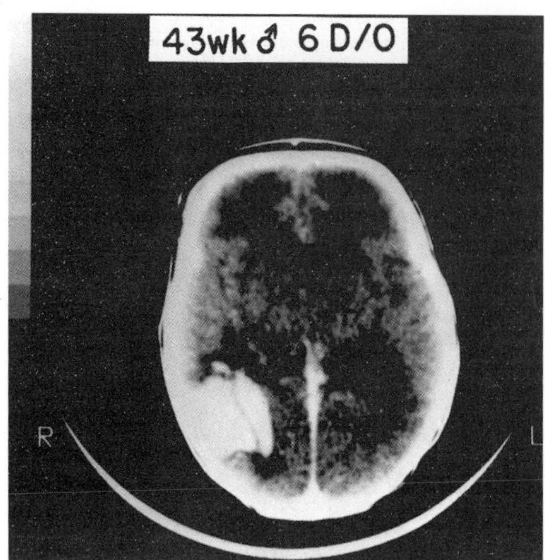

Figure 37.14*b* Computed tomography scan on day 6 for the patient shown in Figure 37.14*a*, documenting a hemorrhagic infarction in the right posterior quadrant with surrounding edema. From Scher MS, Klesh KW, Murphy TF, Guthrie RD (1986). Seizures and infarction in neonates with persistent pulmonary hypertension. *Pediatr Neurol* 2:332–339, with permission.

Neuroimaging, preferably magnetic resonance techniques, documents brain dysgenesis in children who may also express severe electrographic EEG disturbances including seizures (Figure 37.15). Focal or regional brain malformations are rare causes of early-onset epilepsy in neonates and young infants;[122,123] functional imaging studies such as positron emission tomography scans[124] may identify localized areas of altered brain metabolism, which can assist in a neurosurgical approach to seizure management, even in young children who fail to respond to antiepileptic drug maintenance.[125]

Inborn errors of metabolism

Inherited biochemical abnormalities are rare causes of neonatal seizures.[39] Intractable seizures associated with elevated lactate and pyruvate levels in blood and spinal fluid may reflect specific inborn errors of metabolism. Dysplastic or destructive brain lesions, as documented on neuroimaging, may be associated with specific biochemical defects, such as glycine encephalopathy or branched-chain aminoacidopathies (Figure 37.5). Pregnancy, labor, and delivery histories for these infants are commonly uneventful. The emergence of food intolerance, as well as increasing lethargy, stupor, coma, and seizures, are early indications of an inborn metabolic disturbance during the first few days of life. The newborn with an inherited metabolic disorder may initially present as a neurologically depressed and hypotonic child with asphyxia and seizures.[38] Some children respond to specific dietary therapies, including vitamin supplementation,[126] depending on the enzymatic defect. Specific urea-cycle defects, such as carbamoylphosphate synthetase deficiency, may present with coma and seizures during the first 2 days of life, with marked elevations in plasma ammonia levels. These infants may respond to aggressive treatment with an exchange transfusion, dialysis, and appropriate dietary adjustments.

Vitamin B_6 or pyridoxine dependence is a rare cause of neonatal seizures.[127,128] Pyridoxine acts as a cofactor in gamma-aminobutyric acid synthesis, and its absence or paucity promotes seizures. The mother occasionally reports paroxysmal fetal movements.[129] The infant who is unresponsive to conventional antiepileptic medications should promptly receive an intravenous injection of 50–500 mg pyridoxine, preferably with concomitant EEG monitoring. Termination of the seizure within minutes to hours as well as resolution of EEG background disturbances suggests a pyridoxine-dependent seizure state. Prophylactic doses of pyridoxine may be needed to achieve and maintain seizure control.

Other rare causes of seizures include disorders of carbohydrate metabolism with coincident hypoglycemia,[39] as well as peroxisomal disorders, such as neonatal adrenoleukodystrophy or Zellweger's syndrome. A defect in a glucose transporter protein necessary to move glucose across the blood–brain barrier has also been reported; this results in

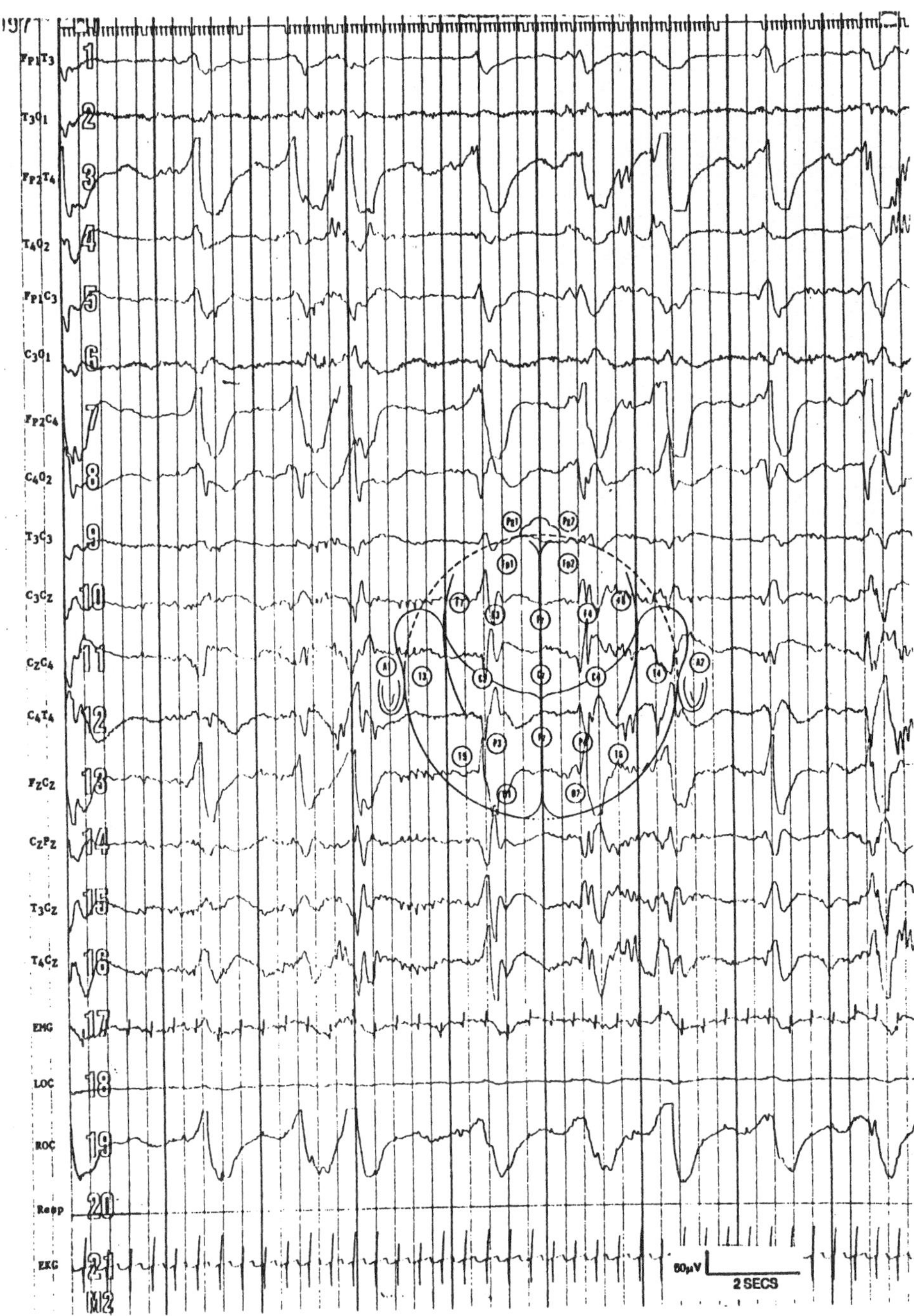

Figure 37.15*a* Electroencephalographic segment of 38-week, 1-day-old infant with right hemisphere predominant generalized electrographic seizures without clinical signs.

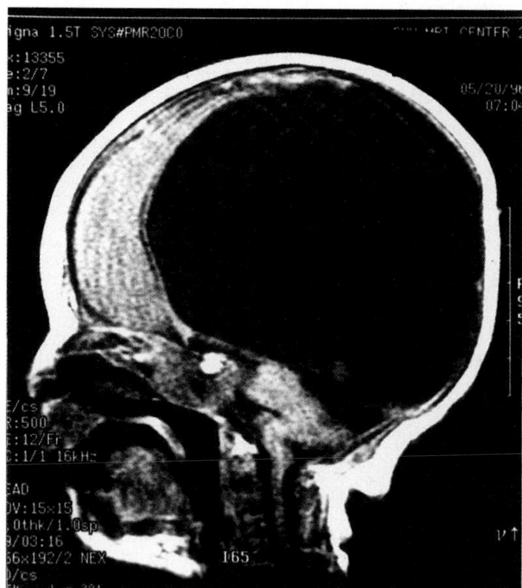

Figure 37.15*b* Magnetic resonance imaging scan for the patient shown in Figure 37.15*a*, demonstrating severe cerebral dysgenesis, including lissencephaly, holoprosencephaly, and a small atrophic cerebellum and brainstem. From Scher MS (1997). Seizures in the newborn infant. *Clin Perinatol* 24:763, with permission.

hypoglycorrhachia and seizures.[130] Such children may achieve seizure control with a ketogenic diet, but none the less suffer delayed development.

Molybdenum-cofactor deficiency and isolated sulfite oxidase deficiences are other rare metabolic defects that cause neonatal seizures and associated destructive changes on neuroimaging, and which may resemble cerebrovascular disease or asphyxia.[131]

Drug withdrawal and intoxication

Newborns born to mothers with prenatal substance use may have an increased risk for neonatal seizures.[132,133] Exposure to barbiturates, alcohol, heroin, cocaine, or methadone commonly presents with neurologic findings which include tremors and irritability. Withdrawal symptoms, in addition to seizures, may occur as long as 4–6 weeks after birth;[134] EEG studies are useful to corroborate such movements with coincident electrographic seizures. Certain drugs may be associated with seizures within the first several days of life, such as short-acting barbiturates.[135] Seizures may occur directly after substance withdrawal, or associated with longer-standing uteroplacental insufficiency, promoted by chronic substance use and poor prenatal health maintenance by the mother. Careful review of placental/cord specimens may reveal chronic or acute pathologic lesions that will contribute to antepartum or intrauterine asphyxia.

Inadvertent fetal injection with a local anesthetic agent during delivery may induce intoxication, and this is a rare cause of seizures.[136,137] Patients present during the first 6–8 h of life with apnea, bradycardia, and hypotonia, and are comatose, without brainstem reflexes. If the obstetrical history indicates that pudendal administration of an anesthetic was given to the mother, a careful examination of the child's scalp or body for puncture marks is indicated. Determination of plasma levels of the suspected anesthetic agent will establish the diagnosis. Treatment consists of ventilatory support and removing the drug by therapeutic diuresis, acidification of the urine, or exchange transfusion. Antiepileptic medications are rarely indicated.

Progressive neonatal epileptic syndromes

Progressive epileptic syndromes rarely present during the first month of life.[138] These children usually exhibit myoclonic or migratory seizures that are poorly controlled by antiepileptic medications, with brain malformations often demonstrable on brain imaging.[92,123] These neonatal epileptic syndromes are termed early myoclonic encephalopathy and early infantile epileptic encephalopathy (Ohtahara syndrome), and the EEG commonly documents burst-suppression or markedly disorganized background rhythms. Rarely, an idiopathic group of neonates with localization-related or partial seizures without neuroimaging abnormalities present with intractable epilepsy.[139]

Neurocutaneous syndromes, such as incontinentia pigmenti and tuberous sclerosis, may also present as symptomatic epilepsy during the neonatal period, as one clinical manifestation of these genetic disorders. Incontinentia pigmenti is accompanied by a vesicular crusting rash, which initially mimics a herpetic infection. Seizures may or may not be present. The skin lesions evolve into lightly pigmented raised sebaceous lesions in older infants and children. Tuberous sclerosis also rarely presents with skin lesions in the newborn period. Hypopigmented lesions, initially noted under ultraviolet light, usually appear later during infancy. Two common fetal presentations of tuberous sclerosis are a cardiac tumor, usually a rhabdomyoma, or, rarely, a connatal brain tumor, both noted on fetal sonography. Neonatal seizures may also be the presenting feature,[140] with documentation of intracranial lesions on postnatal neuroimaging.

Benign familial neonatal seizures

The autosomal dominant form of neonatal seizures is a rare genetic epilepsy that should be considered in the context of a positive family history.[141–143] Exclusion of infectious, metabolic, toxic, or structural causes needs to be completed before considering this entity. The genetic defect was first described on chromosome 20q,[143] specifically at the D20S19 and D20S20 loci, as well as a locus EBN2 on chromosome 8q24. By positional cloning, a potassium channel gene (KCNQ[2]) located on 20q13.3 was first isolated and found to be expressed in brain.[141] A second potassium channel (KCNQ3) has also been described, and may explain the varied phenotypic expression of seizures and outcome.[144] Mutations in ion channels have also recently been implicated in Jervell and Lange–Nielsen syndromes: symptoms include congenital deafness and cardiac arrhythmias.[145] Infant outcomes range from excellent to guarded, depending on the persistence of seizures beyond the neonatal period. Response to antiepileptic medication is generally good, although some authors describe variable success. Further studies are needed to clarify the relationship between phenotypic and genotypic expressions of this disorder.

Seizures in the clinical context of maternal–fetal–placental diseases following a diagnostic algorithm

Once seizures are confirmed by EEG, the neurologist must place these events into the context of clinical, historical, and laboratory findings to determine the pathogenesis and timing of an encephalopathic process in the symptomatic neonate. Seizures associated with neonates after asphyxia support either acute intrapartum events and/or antepartum disease processes. Does the child with seizures also express clinical and laboratory signs of evolving cerebral edema? The presence of a bulging fontanel with neuroimaging evidence of increased intracranial pressure and cerebral edema (obliterated ventricular outline and abnormal diffusion-weighted MRI images) strongly suggests a more recent asphyxial disease process, in or around the intrapartum period. Hyponatremia and increased urine osmolality suggest the syndrome of inappropriate secretion of antidiuretic hormone accompanying acute or subacute cerebral edema.

Alternatively, failure to document evolving cerebral edema during the first 3 days after asphyxia, or documentation of encephalomalacia or cystic brain lesions on neuroimaging shortly after birth (even in the encephalopathic newborn), suggests a more chronic disease process and remote antepartum brain injury. Liquefaction necrosis requires 2 weeks or longer after the presumed in utero asphyxial event to produce a cystic cavity,[146] which is then visible on neuroimaging.

Isolated seizures in an otherwise asymptomatic neonate also suggest a disease process that occurs during either the postnatal or antepartum periods. Neonates present with seizures as a result of postnatal illnesses from intracranial infection, cardiovascular lesions, drug toxicity, or inherited metabolic diseases. Children with antepartum injury may express isolated seizures after in utero cerebrovascular injury on the basis of thrombolytic and/or embolic disease of the mother, placenta, or fetus. Fetal injury alternatively may occur after ischemic–hypoperfusion events from circulatory disturbances, such as maternal shock, chorioamnionitis, or placental fetal vasculopathy.[147]

Only a percentage of neonates with in utero cerebrovascular disease present with neonatal seizures.[115] Why others remain asymptomatic until later during childhood is unknown. Neonatal expression of seizures may reflect recent physiologic stress during parturition which lowers seizure threshold in susceptible brain regions that have been previously damaged.

Following a careful review of the medical histories of the mother, fetus, and newborn, determination of serum glucose, electrolytes, ammonia, lactate, pyruvate, magnesium, calcium, and phosphorus levels may diagnose correctable metabolic conditions in newborns with seizures who will not require antiepileptic medications. Spinal fluid analyses include cell count, protein, glucose, lactate, pyruvate, amino acids, and culture studies to consider central nervous system infection, intracranial hemorrhage, and metabolic disease. Metabolic acidosis on serial arterial blood gas determinations may alternatively suggest an inherited metabolic disease, particularly if intrapartum asphyxia was not judged to be severe. Absence of multiorgan dysfunction may alert the clinician to other etiologies for seizures besides intrapartum asphyxia. Signs of chronic in utero stress, such as growth restriction, early hypertonicity after neonatal depression, joint contractures, or elevated nucleated red blood cell values, all suggest longer-standing antepartum stress to the fetus. Identification of genetic or syndromic conditions can contribute to the expression of neonatal encephalopathies independent of asphyxial injury.[148] Careful review of placental and cord specimens can also be extremely useful. Neuroimaging, preferably using MRI, can help locate, grade the severity, and possibly time an insult.[149] Ancillary studies may also include long-chain fatty acids and chromosomal/DNA analyses, as deemed necessary by family and clinical histories. Finally, serum and urine organic acid and amino acid determinations may be needed to delineate a specific biochemical disorder for the child with a persistent metabolic acidosis. Lysosomal enzyme studies are also occasionally considered to diagnose specific enzymatic deficiencies in children with neonatal seizures.

Prognosis

Mortality of infants who present with clinical neonatal seizures has been reported to decline from 40 to 15%.[3] Studies of EEG-confirmed seizures documented 50% mortality in preterm and 40% in full-term infants during the 1980s.[60,150] During the 1990s in the same institution, this mortality dropped below 20%.[2] Adverse neurologic sequelae, however, remain high for approximately two-thirds of survivors. Even if major neurodevelopmental sequelae such as motor deficits and mental retardation were avoided in survivors after neonatal seizures, subtle neurodevelopmental vulnerability may manifest in late teenage years as specific learning difficulties or poor social adjustment,[151] underscoring more recent experimental findings of long-term deficits in animal populations.[152]

Prediction of outcome should also consider the etiology for seizures, such as severe asphyxia, significant craniocerebral trauma, and brain infections. More accurate imaging procedures have heightened our awareness of destructive as well as congenital brain lesions, with a higher risk for compromised outcome.

Interictal EEG pattern abnormalities are extremely helpful in predicting neurologic outcome in the neonate with seizures.[69,70] Major background disturbances such as burst-suppression (Figure 37.11) are highly predictive of poor outcome, particularly when persistently abnormal findings are still present on serial EEG studies into the second week of life. Ictal patterns alone may not be as accurate to predict outcome, unless quantified to high numbers, long durations and multifocal distribution.[153] Normal findings on interictal EEG were associated with an 86% chance of normal development at 4 years of age in 139 neonates with seizures;[23] by contrast, neonates with markedly abnormal EEG background disturbances had only a 7% chance for normal outcome. Another study[154] reported outcome in term and preterm infants with seizures, concluding that the EEG background was more predictive of outcome than the presence of isolated sharp-wave discharges. Even the interpretation of severe EEG abnormalities by single-channel spectral EEG recordings after asphyxia carries a higher risk for sequelae.[45]

Neonates with seizures have a risk for epilepsy during childhood.[41] Based on clinical seizure criteria, 20–25% of neonates with seizures later develop epilepsy.[155] Excluding febrile seizures, the prevalence of epilepsy by 6–7 years of age is also estimated to be between 15 and 30%; based on EEG-confirmed seizures for an inborn hospital population, two-thirds of this cohort were preterm neonates.[60] This is contrasted with an incidence of 56% with epilepsy for an exclusively outborn neonatal population of primarily full-term newborns with seizures.[156] Epilepsy risk therefore reflects selection bias of specific study groups, as well as referral patterns in different hospital settings.

Diagnostic dilemmas regarding treatment

Rapid infusion of glucose or other supplemental electrolytes should be initiated before antiepileptic medications are considered. Hypoglycemia can be readily corrected by intravenous administration of 5–10 mg/kg of a 10–15% dextrose solution, followed by an infusion of 8–10 mg/kg per min. Persistent hypoglycemia may require more hypertonic glucose solutions. Rarely, prednisone 2 mg/kg per day may be needed to establish a glucose level within the normal range.[2]

Hypocalcemic-induced seizures should be treated with an intravenous infusion of 200 mg/kg of calcium gluconate. This dosage should be repeated every 5–6 h over the first 24 h. Serum magnesium concentrations should also be measured, since hypomagnesemia may accompany hypocalcemia; 0.2 mg/kg magnesium sulfate should be given by intramuscular injection.[2]

Disorders of serum sodium are rare causes of neonatal seizures. Either fluid restriction or replacement with hypotonic solutions is generally the mode of therapy for correcting sodium dysmetabolism.[2]

Pyridoxine dependence requires the injection of 50–500 mg pyridoxine during a seizure with coincident EEG monitoring. A beneficial pyridoxine effect occurs either immediately or over the first several hours. A daily dose of 50–100 mg pyridoxine should then be administered.[2]

If the decision to treat neonates with antiepileptic medications is reached, important questions must be addressed with respect to who should be treated, when to begin treatment, which drug to use, and for how long should neonates be treated?[1,3] Some authors suggest that only neonates with clinical seizures should receive medications; brief electrographic seizures need not be treated. Others suggest more aggressive treatment of EEG seizures, since uncontrolled seizures potentially have an adverse effect on immature brain development.[157–161] An alternative observation suggests that early administration of an antiepileptic drug, such as phenobarbital, even before signs of hypoxic–ischemic encephalopathy, may have adverse effects on outcome in term infants.[162]

Phenobarbital and phenytoin, none the less, remain the most widely used antiepileptic medications; benzodiazepines, primidone, and valproic acid have been anecdotally reported.[126] The half-life of phenobarbital ranges from 45 to 173 h in the neonate;[163–165] the initial loading dose is recommended at 20 mg/kg, with a maintenance dose of 3–4 mg/kg per day. Therapeutic levels are generally suggested to be between 16 and 40 μg/ml; however, there is no consensus with respect to drug maintenance.

The preferred loading dose of phenytoin is 15–20 mg/kg.[164,165] Serum levels of phenytoin are difficult to maintain because this drug is rapidly redistributed to body tissues. Blood levels cannot be well maintained using an oral preparation.

Benzodiazepines may also be used to control neonatal seizures. The drug most widely used is diazepam. One study suggests a half-life of 54 h in preterm infants to 18 h in full-term infants.[166] Intravenous administration is recommended since it is slowly absorbed after an intramuscular injection. Diazepam is highly protein-bound; alteration of bilirubin binding is low. Recommended intravenous doses for acute management should begin at 0.5 mg/kg. Deposition into muscle precludes its use as a maintenance antiepileptic medication, since profound hypotonia and respiratory depression may result, particularly if barbiturates have also been administered.

Efficacy of treatment

Conflicting studies report varying efficacy with phenobarbital or phenytoin. Most studies only apply a clinical endpoint to seizure cessation. One study[164] found that only 36% of neonates with clinical seizures responded to phenobarbital, while another study noted cessation of clinical seizures with phenobarbital in only 32% of neonates.[163] With doses as high as 40 mg/kg,[167] seizure control was reported to be 85%. A more recent study reported that the earlier administration of high-dose phenobarbital in a group of asphyxiated infants was associated with a 27% reduction in clinical seizures and better outcome than a group who did not receive high dosages.[168] However, coincident EEG studies are now suggested to verify the resolution of electrographic seizures. One report suggests that 30% of neonates have persistent electrographic seizures after suppression of clinical seizure behaviors following drug administration.[49] With EEG as an endpoint to judge cessation of seizures, neither phenobarbital nor phenytoin was effective to control seizure activity.[169]

The use of free or drug-bound fractions of antiepileptic drugs has been suggested to assess better both efficacy and potential toxicity of antiepileptic drugs in pediatric populations.[170] Drug binding in neonates with seizures has only recently been reported, and can be altered in a sick neonate with organ dysfunction. Toxic side-effects may result from elevated free fractions of a drug which adversely affect cardiovascular and respiratory function. To guard against untoward effects, evaluation of treatment and efficacy must take into account both total and free antiepileptic drug fractions, in the context of the newborn's progression or resolution of systemic illness.

New anticonvulsant alternatives to treat seizures are being suggested with *N*-methyl-D-aspartate antagonists such as topiramate,[171] developed from experimental models of hypoxia-induced seizure activity in immature brain. Such models provide data regarding pharmacological and physiological characteristics of neuronal responses after an asphyxial stress which causes excessive release of excitotoxic neurotransmitters,[172] such as glutamate. Specific cell membrane receptors, termed metabotropic glutamate receptors (MGluRs), are sensitive to extracellular glutamate release and may play a role in epileptogenesis and seizure-induced brain damage.[173] Subclasses of MGluRs will lead to investigations of novel drugs which block these membrane receptors as the mode of treatment for neonatal seizures.[174]

Discontinuation of drug use

The clinician's decision to maintain or discontinue antiepileptic drug use is also uncertain.[1,3] Discontinuation of drugs before discharge from the neonatal unit is generally recommended, since clinical assessments of arousal, tone, and behavior will not be hampered by medication effect. However, newborns with congenital or destructive brain lesions on neuroimaging, or those with persistently abnormal neurologic examinations at the time of discharge, may suggest to the clinician that a slower taper-off medication is required over several weeks or months. Most children with neonatal seizures rarely have a recurrence during the first 2 years of life, and prophylactic antiepileptic drug administration need not be maintained past 3 months of age, even in the child at risk. This is supported by a study suggesting a low risk of seizure recurrence after early withdrawal of antiepileptic drug therapy in the neonatal period.[175] Also, older infants who present with specific epileptic syndromes, such as infantile spasms, will not respond to the conventional antiepileptic drugs that were initially begun during the neonatal period. This honeymoon period without seizures commonly persists for many years in most children before isolated or recurrent seizures appear.

The potential damage of the developing central nervous system by antiepileptic drugs also emphasizes the need to consider early discontinuation of these agents in the newborn period. Adverse effects on the morphology and metabolism of neuronal cells have been extensively reported from collective research performed over the last several decades.[176]

Consequences of neonatal seizures on brain development

Embedded in the controversy surrounding the diagnosis of neonatal seizures is the association with altered brain development and poor neurologic outcome. The clinician must first appreciate the diverse neuropathologic processes associated with specific etiologies which are responsible for neonatal seizures and neurological sequelae, independent of the seizure process.[176] Definable factors such as central nervous system infections or severe asphyxia contribute to our limited understanding of the underlying mechanisms responsible for brain damage in neonates with seizures.

Direct effects of the seizure state may also have adverse effects on the developing brain.[152] Seizures can disrupt a cascade of biochemical/molecular pathways which are normally responsible for the plasticity or activity-dependent development of the maturing nervous system. Seizures may disrupt the processes of cell division, migration, sequential expression of receptor formation, and stabilization of synapses which contribute to neurologic sequelae.[177]

Experimental models of seizures in immature animals suggest less vulnerability to seizure-induced brain injury than mature animals.[178] In adult animals, seizures alter the growth of hippocampal granule cells, axonal and mossy fiber growth, resulting in long-term deficits in learning, memory, and behavior. A single prolonged seizure in an immature animal, on the other hand, results in less cell loss or fiber sprouting, and consequentially fewer deficits in learning, memory, and behavior. Resistance to brain damage from prolonged seizure activity, however, is age-specific, as evidenced by increased cell damage after only 2 weeks of age.[179]

Repetitive or prolonged neonatal seizures increase the susceptibility of the developing brain to suffer subsequent seizure-induced brain injury during adolescence or early adulthood from altered neuronal connectivity rather than increased cell death.[152,177,180,181] Neonatal animals subjected to status epilepticus have reduced seizure thresholds at later ages and impairments of learning, memory, and activity levels when stressed with seizures as adults. Proposed mechanisms of injury also include reduced neurogenesis in the hippocampus, for example, possibly because of both ischemic-induced apoptosis and necrotic pathways.[182] Other suggested mechanisms of injury include effects of nitric oxide synthetase inhibition on cerebral circulation which then contributes to ischemic injury.[183] Neonatal seizures therefore may initiate a cascade of diverse changes in brain development that become maladaptive at older ages, and increase the risk of damage after subsequent insults. Destructive mechanisms, such as mossy fiber sprouting in the hippocampus or increased neuronal apoptosis, may explain mutually exclusive pathways by which the immature brain suffers altered connectivity and reduced cell number and is "primed" for later seizure-induced cell loss at older ages.

A lack of well-designed clinical investigations of outcome after neonatal seizures unfortunately fails to support these experimental findings.[176] Better definitions of neonatal seizures of epileptic origin as well as the critical seizure duration required to injure brain remain controversial. Overlapping effects of underlying central nervous system injury or dysgenesis from specific etiologies vs seizure-induced brain damage make it difficult to differentiate preexisting brain lesions from the direct injurious effects of seizures themselves. The use of microdialysis probes in white and gray matter of piglet brains subjected to hypoxia indicates elevated lactate/pyruvate ratios after hypoxia but no direct association with seizure activity.[184] These findings support the conclusion that seizures themselves may not be injurious to metabolic function.

Aggressive use of antiepileptic medications also

contributes to both the inaccurate estimate of seizure severity in neonates and possible medication-induced brain injury. Intractable seizures generally require the use of multiple antiepileptic medications. Such drugs impede the clinician's observations to recognize prolonged seizures because of the uncoupling phenomenon in which the clinical expression may be suppressed while the electrical expression of seizures continues. Clinical definitions of seizure occurrence and duration consequently underestimate seizure severity, which appears to be associated with increased risk for damage. Antiepileptic drug use also has secondary harmful effects on cardiac and respiratory function, with resultant circulatory disturbances that contribute to brain injury.[176] Finally, antiepileptic drug use may have teratogenetic effects on brain development with exposure over long periods of time.

Summary

The recognition and classification of seizures remain problematic. The clinician should rely on synchronized video/EEG/polygraphic recordings to correlate suspicious behaviors with electrographic seizures. This practice must be integrated with an appreciation of the pathophysiologic mechanisms responsible for brain injury and which implicate maternal–fetal–placental diseases with expression of brain disorders during the antepartum, intrapartum, or neonatal periods.

REFERENCES

1 Camfield PR, Camfield CS (1987). Neonatal seizures: a commentary on selected aspects. *J. Child Neurol.* 2:244–251.

2 Scher MS (1997). Seizures in the newborn infant. Diagnosis, treatment and outcome. *Clin. Perinatol.* 24:735–772.

3 Scher MS, Painter MJ (1989). Controversies concerning neonatal seizures. In: Pellock JM (ed). *Seizure Disorders. The Pediatric Clinics of North America*, pp. 281–310. Philadelphia, PA: WB Saunders.

4 Scher MS (1994). Neonatal encephalopathies as classified by EEG-sleep criteria. Severity and timing based on clinical/pathologic correlations. *Pediatr. Neurol.* 11:189–200.

5 Scher MS (2001). Perinatal asphyxia: timing and mechanisms of injury relative to the diagnosis and treatment of neonatal encephalopathy. *Curr. Neurol. Neurosci. Repts.* 1:175–184.

6 Glauser TA, Clancy RR (1992). Adequacy of routine EEG examinations in neonates with clinically suspected seizures. *J. Child Neurol.* 7:215–220.

7 Bye AME, Flanagan D (1995). Spatial and temporal characteristics of neonatal seizures. *Epilepsia* 36:1009–1016.

8 Commission on Classification and Terminology of the International League Against Epilepsy (1981). Proposal for revised clinical and electroencephalographic classification of epileptic seizures. *Epilepsia* 22:489–501.

9 Mizrahi EM, Kellaway P (1998). *Diagnosis and Management of Neonatal Seizures*, pp. 1–155. Philadelphia: Lippincott-Raven.

10 Biagioni E, Ferrari F, Boldrini A, et al. (1998). Electroclinical correlation in neonatal seizures. *Eur. J. Paediatr. Neurol.* 2:117–125.

11 Weiner SP, Painter MJ, Scher MS (1991). Neonatal seizures: electroclinical disassociation. *Pediatr. Neurol.* 7:363–8.

12 Volpe JJ (2001). *Neurology of the Newborn*, 4th edn, pp. 178–214. Philadelphia, PA: WB Saunders.

13 Scher MS (1999). Electroencephalography of the newborn: normal and abnormal features. In: Niedermeyer E, Da Silva L (eds) *Electroencephalography*, 4th edn, pp. 869–946. Baltimore, MD: Williams and Wilkins.

14 Scher MS (1996). Normal electrographic-polysomnographic patterns in preterm and fullterm infants. *Semin. Pediatr. Neurol.* 3:12.

15 DaSilva O, Guzman GMC, Young GB (1998). The value of standard electroencephalograms in the evaluation of the newborn with recurrent apneas. *J. Perinatol.* 18:377–380.

16 Fenichel GM, Olson BJ, Fitzpatrick JE (1979). Heart rate changes in convulsive and nonconvulsive apnea. *Ann. Neurol.* 7:577–582.

17 Boylan GB, Pressler RM, Rennie JM, et al. (1999). Outcome of electroclinical, electrographic, and clinical seizures in the newborn infant. *Dev. Med. Child Neurol.* 41:819–825.

18 Mizrahi EM, Kellaway P (1987). Characterization and classification of neonatal seizures. *Neurology* 37:1837–1844.

19 Clancy R, Malin S, Laraque D, et al. (1985). Focal motor seizures heralding a stroke in full-term neonates. *Am. J. Dis. Child.* 139:601–606.

20 Levy SR, Abroms IF, Marshall PC, et al. (1985). Seizures and cerebral infarction in the full-term newborn. *Ann. Neurol.* 17:366–370.

21 Scher MS, Klesh KW, Murphy TF, et al. (1986). Seizures and infarction in neonates with persistent pulmonary hypertension. *Pediatr. Neurol.* 2:332–339.

22 Holmes G (1987). Diagnosis and management of seizures in childhood. In: Markowitz M (ed.) *Major Problems in Clinical Pediatrics, XXX*, pp. 237–261. Philadelphia, PA: WB Saunders.

23 Rose AL, Lombroso CT (1970). A study of clinical, pathological, and electroencephalographic features in 137 full-term babies with a long-term follow-up. *Pediatrics* 45:404–425.

24 Kellaway P, Hrachovy RA (1983). Status epilepticus in newborns: a perspective on neonatal seizures. In: Delgado-Escueta AV, Wasterlain CG, Treiman DM, Porter RJ (eds) *Status Epilepticus: Mechanisms of Brain Damage and Treatment*, pp. 93–99. New York, NY: Raven Press.

25 Sarnat HB (1984). Anatomic and physiologic correlates of neurologic development in prematurity. In: Sarnat HB (ed.) *Topics in Neonatal Neurology*, pp. 1–25. Orlando: Grune and Stratton.

26 Scher MS (1985). Pathological myoclonus of the newborn: electrographic and clinical correlations. *Pediatr. Neurol.* 1:342–348.

27 Scher MS (1997). Stimulus-evoked electrographic patterns in neonates: abnormal form of reactivity. *Electroenceph. Clin. Neurophysiol.* 103:679–691.

28 Coulter DL, Allen RJ (1982). Benign neonatal sleep myoclonus. *Arch. Neurol.* 39:191–192.

29 Resnick TJ, Moshé SL, Perotta L, et al. (1986). Benign neonatal sleep myoclonus: relationship to sleep states. *Arch. Neurol.* 43:266–268.

30 Clancy RR (1996). The contribution of EEG to the understanding of neonatal seizures. *Epilepsia* 37:S52–S59.

31 Shuper A, Zalzberg J, Weitz R et al. (1991). Jitteriness beyond the neonatal period: a benign pattern of movement in infancy. *J. Child Neurol.* 6:243–245.

32 Parker S, Zuckerman B, Bauchner H, et al. (1990). Jitteriness in full-term neonates: prevalence and correlates. *Pediatrics* 85:17–23.

33 Hakamada S, Watanabe K, Hara K, et al. (1981). Development of motor behavior during sleep in newborn infants. *Brain Dev.* 3:345–350.

34 Scher MS, Belfar H, Martin J, et al. (1991). Destructive brain lesions of presumed fetal onset: antepartum causes of cerebral palsy. *Pediatrics* 88:898–906.

35 Sexson WR, Thigpen J, Stajich GV. (1995). Stereotypic movements after lorazepam administration in premature neonates: a series and review of the literature. *J. Perinatol.* 15:146–199.

36 Brown P, Rothwell JC, Thompson PD, et al. (1991). The hyperekplexias and their relationship to the normal startle reflex. *Brain* 114:1903–1928.

37 Andermann F, Andermann E (1988). Startle disorders of man: hyperekplexia, jumping, and startle epilepsy. *Brain Dev.* 10:213–222.

38 Barth PJ (1992). Inherited progressive disorders of the fetal brain: a field in need of recognition. In: Fukuyama Y, Suzuki Y, Kamoshita S, et al. (eds) *Fetal and Perinatal Neurology*, pp. 299–313. Basel: Karger.

39 Lyon G, Adams RD, Kolodny EH (1996). *Neurology of Hereditary Metabolic Diseases of Children*, 2nd edn, pp. 6–44. New York: McGraw-Hill.

40 Oliveira AJ, Nunes ML, da Costa JC (2000). Polysomnography in neonatal seizures. *Clin. Neurophysiol.* 111:S74–S80.

41 Watanabe K, Kuroyanagi M, Hara K, et al. (1982). Neonatal seizures and subsequent epilepsy. *Brain Dev.* 4:341–346.

42 Hrachovy RA, Mizrahi EM, Kellaway P (1990). Electroencephalography of the newborn. In: Daly DD, Pedley TA (eds) *Current Practice of Clinical Electroencephalography*, 2nd edn, pp. 201–242. New York, NY: Raven Press.

43 Lombroso CT (1985). Neonatal polygraphy in full-term and preterm infants: a review of normal and abnormal findings. *J. Clin. Neurophysiol.* 2:105–115.

44 Pope SS, Stockard JE, Bickford RG (1992). *Atlas of Neonatal Electroencephalography*. New York, NY: Raven Press.

45 Hellström-Westas L (1992). Comparison between tape recorded and amplitude integrated EEG monitoring in sick newborn infants. *Acta Pediatr.* 81:812–819.

46 Clancy R, Legido A (1987). The exact ictal and interictal duration of electroencephalographic neonatal seizures. *Epilepsia* 28:537–541.

47 Sheth RD (1999). Electroencephalogram confirmatory rate in neonatal seizures. *Pediatr. Neurol.* 20:27–30.

48 Scher MS, Hamid MY, Steppe DA, et al. (1993). Ictal and interictal durations in preterm and term neonates. *Epilepsia* 34:284–288.

49 Scher MS, Alvin J, Gaus L, et al. (1994). Uncoupling of electrical and clinical expression of neonatal seizures after antiepileptic drug administration. *Pediatr. Neurol.* 11:83.

50 Scher MS, Beggarly M (1989). Clinical significance of focal periodic patterns in the newborn. *J. Child. Neurol.* 4:175–185.

51 Oliveira AJ, Nunes ML, Haertel LM, et al. (2000). Duration of rhythmic EEG patterns in neonates: new evidence for clinical and prognostic significance of brief rhythmic discharges. *Clin. Neurophysiol.* 111:1646–1653.

52 Alfonso I, Papazian O, Litt R, et al. (2000). Single photon

emission computed tomographic evaluation of brainstem release phenomenon and seizure in neonates. *J. Child Neurol.* 15:56–58.

53 Kilic S, Tarim Ö, Eralp Ö (1999). Serum prolactin in neonatal seizures. *Pediatr. Int.* 41:61–64.

54 Browning RA (1985). Role of the brainstem reticular formation in tonic–clonic seizures: lesion and pharmacological studies. *Fed. Proc.* 44:2425–2431.

55 Caveness WF, Kato M, Malamut BL, et al. (1980). Propagation of focal motor seizures in the pubescent monkey. *Ann. Neurol.* 7:213–221.

56 Hosokawa S, Iguchi T, Caveness WF, et al. (1980). Effects of manipulation of sensorimotor system on focal motor seizures in the monkey. *Ann. Neurol.* 7:222–237.

57 Danner R, Shewmon DA, Sherman MP (1985). Seizures in an atelencephalic infant. Is the cortex essential for neonatal seizures? *Arch. Neurol.* 42:1014–1016.

58 Coen RW, McCutchen CB, Wermer D, et al. (1982). Continuous monitoring of electroencephalogram following perinatal asphyxia. *J. Pediatr.* 100:628–630.

59 O'Meara WM, Bye AME, Flanagan D (1995). Clinical features of neonatal seizures. *J. Pediatr. Child. Health* 31:237–240.

60 Scher MS, Aso K, Beggarly ME, et al. (1993). Electrographic seizures in preterm and full-term neonates: clinical correlates, associated brain lesions, and risk for neurological sequelae. *Pediatrics* 91:128–134.

61 Staudt F, Roth G, Engel RC (1981). The usefulness of electroencephalography in curarized newborns. *Electroencephalogr. Clin. Neurophysiol.* 51:205–208.

62 Eyre P, Oozen RC, Wilkinson AR (1983). Continuous electroencephalographic recording to detect seizures in paralyzed newborns. *Br. Med. J.* 286:1017–1018.

63 Goldberg RN, Goldman SL, Ramsay RE, et al. (1982). Detection of seizure activity in the paralyzed neonate using continuous monitoring. *Pediatrics* 69:583–586.

64 Ericksson M, Zetterstrom R (1979). Neonatal convulsions. Incidence and causes in the Stockholm area. *Acta Pediatr. Scand.* 68:807–811.

65 Seay AR, Bray PF (1977). Significance of seizures in infants weighing less than 2500 grams. *Arch. Neurol.* 34:381–382.

66 Ronen GM, Penney S, Andrews W (1999). The epidemiology of clinical neonatal seizures in Newfoundland: a population-based study. *J. Pediatr.* 134:71–75.

67 Lanska MJ, Lanska DJ, Baumann RJ, et al. (1996). Interobserver variability in the classification of neonatal seizures based on medical record data. *Pediatr. Neurol.* 15:120–123.

68 Lanska MJ, Lanska DJ, Baumann RJ, et al. (1995). A population-based study of neonatal seizures in Fayette County, Kentucky. *Neurology* 45:724–732.

69 Monod N, Pajot N, Guidasci S (1972). The neonatal EEG: statistical studies and prognostic value in full-term and preterm babies. *Electroencephalogr. Clin. Neurophysiol.* 32:529–544.

70 Tharp BR, Cukier F, Monod N (1981). The prognostic value of the electroencephalogram in premature infants. *Electroencephalogr. Clin. Neurophysiol.* 51:219.

71 Bye AME, Cunningham CA, Chee KY, et al. (1997). Outcome of neonates with electrographically identified seizures, or at risk of seizures. *Pediatr. Neurol.* 16:225–231.

72 Sinclair DB, Campbell M, Byrne P, et al. (1999). EEG and long-term outcome of term infants with neonatal hypoxic–ischemic encephalopathy. *Clin. Neurophysiol.* 110:655–659.

73 Scher MS (1997). Neurophysiological assessment of brain function and maturation. I. A measure of brain adaptation in high risk infants. *Pediatr. Neurol.* 16:191–198.

74 Scher MS (1997). Neurophysiological assessment of brain function and maturation. II. A measure of brain dysmaturity in healthy preterm neonates. *Pediatr. Neurol.* 16:287–295.

75 Tharp BR, Scher MS, Clancy RR (1989). Serial EEGs in normal and abnormal infants with birth weights less than 1200 grams – a prospective study with long term follow-up. *Neuropediatrics* 20:64–72.

76 Laroia N, Guillet R, Burchfiel J, et al. (1998). EEG background as predictor of electrographic seizures in high-risk neonates. *Epilepsia* 39:545–551.

77 Scher MS (2000). Neonatal seizures. Seizures in special clinical settings. In: Wyllie E (ed.) *The Treatment Of Epilepsy. Principles and Practice*, 3rd edn. Baltimore: Williams & Wilkins.

78 Scher MS, Alvin J, Minnigh MB, et al. (1995). EEG screening for seizures in an inborn neonatal population prior to antiepileptic drug administration. *Pediatr. Res.* 37:385A.

79 Lien JM, Towers CV, Quilligan EJ, et al. (1995). Term early-onset neonatal seizures: obstetric characteristics, etiologic classifications, and perinatal care. *Obstet. Gynecol.* 85:163–169.

80 Patterson CA, Graves WL, Bugg G, et al. (1989). Antenatal and intrapartum factors associated with the occurrence of seizures in the term infant. *Obstet. Gynecol.* 74:361–365.

81 Adamson SJ, Alessandri LM, Badawi N, et al. (1995). Predictors of neonatal encephalopathy in full term infants. *Br. Med. J.* 311:598–602.

82 Bergman I, Painter MJ, Hirsh RP, et al. (1983). Outcome in neonates with convulsions treated in an intensive care unit. *Ann. Neurol.* 14:642–647.

83 Brown JK, Cockburn F, Forfar JO (1972). Clinical and chemical correlates in convulsions of the newborn. *Lancet* 1:135–139.

84 Brown JK, Previce RJF, Forfar JO, et al. (1974). Neurological aspects of perinatal asphyxia. *Dev. Med. Child. Neurol.* 16:567–580.

85 Sarnat HB, Sarnat MS (1976). Neonatal encephalography following fetal distress. A clinical and encephalographic study. *Arch. Neurol.* 33:696–705.

86 Autschuler G (1997). Chapter 34: The relationship of placental pathology to causation of detrimental pregnancy outcome. In: Stevenson D, Sunshine P (eds) *Fetal and Neonatal Brain Injury*, pp. 585–601. New York, NY: BC Decker.

87 Bejar R, Wozniak P, Allard M, et al. (1988). Antenatal origin of neurologic damage in newborn infants. *Am. J. Obstet. Gynecol.* 159:357–363.

88 Evrard P, Kadhim HJ, de Saint-George P, et al. (1989). Abnormal development and destructive processes of the human brain during the second half of gestation. In: Evans P, Minkowski A (eds) *Developmental Neurobiology*, pp. 21–39. New York, NY: Raven Press.

89 Lieberman E, Eichenwald E, Mathur G, et al. (2000). Intrapartum fever and unexplained seizures in term infants. *Pediatrics* 106:983–988.

90 ACOG. (1993). Fetal and neonatal neurologic injury. ACOG Technical Bulletin 163, January 1992, pp 1–6. *Int. J. Gynaecol. Obstet.* 41:97–101.

91 Ahn MO, Korst LM, Phelan JP, et al. (1998). Does the onset of neonatal seizures correlate with the timing of fetal neurologic injury? *Clin. Pediatr.* 37:673–676.

92 Ekert P, Perlman M, Steinlin M, et al. (1997). Predicting the outcome of postasphyxial hypoxic–ischemic encephalopathy within 4 hours of birth. *J. Pediatr.* 131:613–617.

93 Low JA, Panagiotopoulos L, Derrick EJ (1994). Newborn complications after intrapartum asphyxia with metabolic acidosis at term. *Am. J. Obstet. Gynecol.* 170:1081–1087.

94 Nelson KB, Ellenberg JH (1981). Apgar scores as predictors of chronic neurologic disability. *Pediatrics* 68:36–44.

95 Nelson KB, Leviton A (1991). How much of neonatal encephalopathy is due to birth asphyxia? *Am. J. Dis. Child.* 145:1325–1331.

96 Scher MS, Trucco J, Beggarly ME, et al. (1998). Neonates with electrically- confirmed seizures and possible placental associations. *Pediatr. Neurol.* 19:37–41.

97 McIntire DD, Bloom SL, Casey BM, et al. (1999). Birth weight in relation to morbidity and mortality among newborn infants. *N. Engl. J. Med.* 340:1234–1238.

98 Barabas RE, Barmada MA, Scher MS (1993). Timing of brain insults in severe neonatal encephalopathies with an isoelectric EEG. *Pediatr. Neurol.* 9:39–44.

99 Cornblath M, Schwartz R (1967). *Disorders of Carbohydrate Metabolism in Infancy*, pp. 33–54. Philadelphia, PA: WB Saunders.

100 Milner RDG (1972). Neonatal hypoglycemia: a critical reappraisal. *Arch. Neurol.* 47:679–682.

101 Senior B (1973). Neonatal hypoglycemia. *N. Engl. J. Med.* 289:790–793.

102 Griffiths AD, Laurence KM (1974). The effect of hypoxia and hypoglycemia on the brain of the newborn human infant. *Dev. Med. Child Neurol* 16:308–319.

103 Siemkowicz E, Hansen AJ (1978). Clinical restitution following cerebral ischemia in hypo-normo, and hyperglycemic rats. *Acta Neurol. Scand.* 58:1–9.

104 Glauser TA, Rorke LB, Weinberg PM, et al. (1990). Acquired neuropathologic lesions associated with the hypoplastic left heart syndrome. *Pediatrics* 85:991–1000.

105 Keen JH, Lee D (1973). Sequelae of neonatal convulsions. Study of 112 infants. *Arch. Dis. Child.* 48:541–542.

106 McInterny JK, Schubert WK (1969). Prognosis of neonatal seizures. *Am. J. Dis. Child.* 117:261–264.

107 Lynch BJ, Rust RS (1994). Natural history and outcome of neonatal hypocalcemic and hypomagnesemic seizures. *Pediatr. Neurol.* 11:23–27.

108 Ment LR, Duncan CC, Ehrenkranz RA (1984). Perinatal cerebral infarction. *Ann. Neurol.* 16:559–568.

109 Rivkin MJ, Anderson ML, Kaye EM (1992). Neonatal idiopathic cerebral venous thrombosis: an unrecognized cause of transient seizures or lethargy. *Ann. Neurol.* 32:51–56.

110 Scher MS, Tharp B (1982). Significance of focal abnormalities in neonatal EEG – radiologic correlation and outcome. *Ann. Neurol.* 12:217.

111 Shevell MI, Silver K, O'Gorman AM et al. (1989). Neonatal dural sinus thrombosis. *Pediatr. Neurol.* 5:161–165.

112 Hill A, Volpe JJ (1981). Seizures, hypoxic–ischemic brain injury and intraventricular hemorrhage in the newborn. *Ann. Neurol.* 10:109–121.

113 Sheth RD, Hobbs GR, Mullett M (1999). Neonatal seizures: incidence, onset, and etiology by gestational age. *J. Perinatol.* 19:40–43.

114 Strober JB, Bienkowski RS, Maytal J (1997). The incidence of acute and remote seizures in children with intraventricular hemorrhage. *Clin. Pediatr.* 36:643–648.

115 De Vries LS, Groenendaal F, Eken P, et al. (1997). Infarcts in the vascular distribution of the middle cerebral artery in preterm and fullterm infants. *Neuropediatrics* 28:88–96.

116 Mercuri E, Cowan F, Rutherford M, et al. (1995). Ischaemic

and haemorrhagic brain lesions in newborns with seizures and normal apgar scores. *Arch. Dis. Child.* 73:F67–F74.

117 Forbes KPN, Pipe JG, Byrd R (2000). Neonatal hypoxic–ischemic encephalopathy. detection with diffusion-weighted MRI imaging. *Am. J. Neuroradiol.* 21:1490–1496.

118 Benitz WE, Rhine WD, VanMeurs KP (1997). Persistent pulmonary hypertension of the newborn. In: Stephenson DK and Sunshine P (eds) *Fetal and Neonatal Brain Injury*, pp. 564–582. Oxford: Oxford Medical Publications.

119 Kairam R, DeVivo DC (1981). Neurologic manifestations of congenital infection. *Clin. Perinatol.* 8:455–465.

120 Mizrahi EM, Tharp BR (1982). Characteristic EEG pattern in neonatal herpes simplex encephalitis. *Neurology* 32:1215–1220.

121 Palmini A, Andermann E, Andermann F (1994). Prenatal events and genetic factors in epileptic patients with neuronal migration disorders. *Epilepsia* 35:965–973.

122 Aicardi J (1985). Early myoclonic encephalopathy. In: Roger J, Dravet C, Office M, et al. (eds) *Epileptic Syndromes in Infancy, Childhood, and Adolescence*, pp. 12–22. London, England: J Libbey Eurotext.

123 Ohtahara S (1978). Clinico-electrical delineation of epileptic encephalopathies in childhood. *Asian Med. J.* 21:7–17.

124 Chugani HT, Rintahaka PJ, Shewmon DA (1994). Ictal patterns of cerebral glucose utilization in children with epilepsy. *Epilepsia* 35:813–822.

125 Pedespan JM, Loiseau H, Vital A, et al. (1995). Surgical treatment of an early epileptic encephalopathy with suppression-bursts and focal cortical dysplasia. *Epilepsia* 36:37–40.

126 Painter MJ, Bergman I, Crumrine PK (1984). Neonatal seizures. In: Pellock MJ, Myer EC (eds) *Neurologic Emergencies in Infancy and Childhood*, pp. 17–35. New York, NY: Harper & Row.

127 Bejsovec M, Kulenda Z, Ponca E (1967). Familial intrauterine convulsions in pyridoxine dependency. *Arch. Dis. Child.* 42:201–207.

128 Clarke TA, Saunders BS, Feldman B (1979). Pyridoxine-dependent seizures requiring high doses of pyridoxine for control. *Am. J. Dis. Child.* 133:963–965.

129 Osiovich H, Barrington K (1996). Prenatal ultrasound diagnosis of seizures. *Am. J. Perinatol.* 13:499–501.

130 DeVivo DC, Trifiletti RR, Jacobson RI, et al. (1991). Defective glucose transport across the blood–brain barrier as a cause of persistent hypoglycorrhachia, seizures, and developmental delay. *N. Engl. J. Med.* 325: 703–709.

131 Slot HMJ, Overweg-Plandsoen WC, Bakker HD, et al. (1993). Molybdenum-cofactor deficiency: an easily missed cause of neonatal convulsions. *Neuropediatrics* 24:139–142.

132 Herzlinger RA, Kandall SR, Vaughn HG (1977). Neonatal seizures associated with narcotic withdrawal. *J. Pediatr.* 92:638–641.

133 Zelson C, Rubio E, Wasserman E (1971). Neonatal narcotic addiction: 10 year observation. *Pediatrics* 48:178–189.

134 Kandall SR, Garner LM (1974). Late presentation of drug withdrawal symptoms in newborns. *Am. J. Dis. Child.* 127:58–61.

135 Bleyer WA, Marshall RE (1972). Barbiturate withdrawal syndrome in a passively addicted infant. *JAMA* 221:185–186.

136 Dodson WE (1976). Neonatal drug intoxication: local anesthetics. *Pediatr. Clin. North Am.* 23:399–411.

137 Hillman LS, Hillman RE, Dodson WE (1979). Diagnosis, treatment, and follow- up of neonatal mepivacaine intoxication secondary to paracervical and pudendal blocks during labor. *J. Pediatr.* 94:472–477.

138 Mizrahi EM, Clancy RR (2000). Neonatal seizures: early-onset seizure syndromes and their consequences for development. *MRDD Res. Rev.* 6:229–241.

139 Natsume J, Watanabe K, Negoro T, et al. (1996). Cryptogenic localization-related epilepsy of neonatal onset. *Seizure* 5:317–319.

140 Miller SP, Tasch T, Sylvain M, et al. (1998). Tuberous sclerosis complex and neonatal seizures. *J. Child Neurol.* 13:619–623.

141 Bjerre I, Corelius E (1978). Benign familial neonatal convulsions. *Acta Paediatr. Scand.* 57:557–561.

142 Petit RE, Fenichel GM (1980). Benign familial neonatal seizures. *Arch. Neurol.* 37:47–48.

143 Ryan SG, Wiznitzer M, Hollman C, et al. (1991). Benign familial neonatal convulsions: evidence for clinical and genetic heterogeneity. *Ann. Neurol.* 29:469–473.

144 Leppert M, Singh N (1999). Benign familial neonatal epilepsy with mutations in two potassium channel genes. *Curr. Opin. Neurol.* 12:143–147.

145 Jentsch TJ, Schroeder BC, Kubisch C, et al. (2000). Pathophysiology of KCNQ channels: neonatal epilepsy and progressive deafness. *Epilepsia* 41:1068–1069.

146 Friede RL (1975). Porencephaly, hydranencephaly, multilocular cystic encephalopathy. In: Friede RL (ed.) *Developmental Neuropathology*, pp. 102–113. New York: Springer-Verlag.

147 Miller V (2000). Neonatal cerebral infarction. In: Roach ES and DeVeber G (eds) *Cerebrovascular Diseases in Childhood*. In: *Sem. Pediatr. Neurol.* 7:278–288.

148 Felix JF, Badaw N, Kuringzuk JJ, et al. (2000). Birth defects in children with newborn encephalopathy. *Dev. Med. Child. Neurol.* 42:803–808.

149 Leth H, Toft PB, Herning M, et al. (1997). Neonatal seizures

associated with cerebral lesions shown by magnetic resonance imaging. *Arch. Dis. Child. Fetal Neonatal Edn.* 77:F105–F110.

150 Scher MS, Painter MJ (1990). Electrographic diagnosis of neonatal seizures. Issues of diagnostic accuracy, clinical correlation and survival. In: Wasterlain CG, Vert P (eds) *Neonatal Seizures.* New York, NY: Raven Press.

151 Temple CM, Dennis J, Carney R, et al. (1995). Neonatal seizures: long-term outcome and cognitive development among 'normal' survivors. *Dev. Med. Child Neurol.* 37:109–118.

152 Holmes GL, Ben-Ari Y (2001). The neurobiology and consequences of epilepsy in the developing brain. *Pediatr. Res.* 49:320–325.

153 McBride M, Laroia N, Guillet R (2000). Electrographic seizures in neonates correlate with poor neurodevelopmental outcome. *Neurology* 55:506–513.

154 Rowe RJ, Holmes GL, Hafford J, et al. (1985). Prognostic value of electroencephalogram in term and preterm infants following neonatal seizures. *Electroencephalogr. Clin. Neurophysiol.* 60:183–196.

155 Holden KR, Mellits ED, Freeman JM (1982). Neonatal seizures, I: Correlation of prenatal and perinatal events with outcomes. *Pediatrics* 70:165–176.

156 Clancy RR, Legido A (1991). Postnatal epilepsy after EEG-confirmed neonatal seizures. *Epilepsia* 32:69–76.

157 Dwyer BE, Wasterlain CG (1982). Electroconvulsive seizures in the immature rate adversely affect myelin accumulation. *Exp. Neurol.* 78:616–628.

158 Wasterlain CG, Plum F (1973). The vulnerability of developing rat brain to electroconvulsive seizures. *Arch. Neurol.* 19:38–45.

159 Wasterlain CG (1997). Controversies in epilepsy. Recurrent seizures in the developing brain are harmful. *Epilepsia* 38:728–734.

160 Wasterlain CG (1976). Effects of neonatal status epilepticus on rat brain. *Dev. Neurol.* 26:975–986.

161 Wasterlain CG (1978). Neonatal seizures in brain growth. *Neuropediatrics* 9:213–228.

162 Ajayi OA, Oyaniyi OT, Chike-Obi UD, et al. (1998). Adverse effects of early phenobarbital administration in term newborns with perinatal asphyxia. *Trop. Med. Int. Health* 3:592–595.

163 Lockman LA, Kriel R, Zaske D, et al. (1979). Phenobarbital dosage for control of neonatal seizures. *Neurology* 29:1445–1449.

164 Painter MJ, Pippenger C, McDonald H, et al. (1978). Phenobarbital and diphenylhydantoin levels in neonates with seizures. *J. Pediatr.* 9:315–319.

165 Painter MJ, Pippenger C, Wasterlain C, et al. (1981). Phenobarbital and phenytoin in neonatal seizures, metabolism, and tissue distribution. *Neurology* 31:1107–1112.

166 Smith BI, Misoh RE (1971). Intravenous diazepam in the treatment of prolonged seizure activity in neonates and infants. *Dev. Med. Child. Neurol.* 13:630–634.

167 Gal P, Toback J, Boer HR, et al. (1982). Efficacy of phenobarbital monotherapy in treatment of neonatal seizures. Relationship of blood levels. *Neurology* 32:1401–1404.

168 Hall RT, Hall FK, Daily DK (1998). High-dose phenobarbital therapy in term newborn infants with severe perinatal asphyxia: a randomized, prospective study with three-year follow-up. *J. Pediatr.* 132:345–348.

169 Painter MJ, Scher MS, Alvin J, et al. (1999). A comparison of the efficacy of phenobarbital and phenytoin in the treatment of neonatal seizures. *N. Engl. J. Med.* 341:485–489.

170 Painter MJ, Minnigh B, Mollica L, et al. (1987). Binding profiles of anticonvulsants in neonates with seizures. *Ann. Neurol.* 22:413–420.

171 Jensen FE (1999). Acute and chronic effects of seizures in the developing brain: experimental models. *Epilepsia* 40:S51–S58.

172 Jensen FE, Wang C (1996). Hypoxia-induced hyperexcitability in vivo and in vitro in the immature hippocampus. *Epilepsy Res.* 26:131–140.

173 Aronica EM, Gorter JA, Paupard M-C, et al. (1997). Status epilepticus-induced alterations in metabotropic glutamate receptor expression in young and adult rats. *J. Neurosci.* 17:8588–8595.

174 Lie AA, Becker A, Behle K, et al. (2000). Up-regulation of the metabotropic glutamate receptor mGluR4 in hippocampal neurons with reduced seizure vulnerability. *Ann. Neurol.* 47:26–35.

175 Hellström-Westas L, Blennow G, Lindroth M, et al. (1995). Low risk of seizure recurrence after early withdrawal of antiepileptic treatment in the neonatal period. *Arch. Dis. Child.* 72:F97–F101.

176 Mizrahi EM (1999). Acute and chronic effects of seizures in the developing brain: lessons from clinical experience. *Epilepsia* 40:S42–S50.

177 Holmes GL, Gairsa JL, Chevassus-Au-Louis N, et al. (1998). Consequences of neonatal seizures in the rat: morphological and behavioral effects. *Ann. Neurol.* 44:845–857.

178 Huang L-T, Cilio MR, Silveira DC, et al. (1999). Long-term effects of neonatal seizures: a behavioral electrophysiological, and histological study. *Dev. Brain Res.* 118:99–107.

179 Sankar R, Shin D, Mazarati AM, et al. (2000). Epileptogenesis after status epilepticus reflects age- and model-dependent plasticity. *Ann. Neurol.* 48:580–589.

180 Koh S, Storey TW, Santos TC, et al. (1999). Early-life seizures in rats increase susceptibility to seizure-induced brain injury in adulthood. *Neurology* 53:915–921.

181 Schmid R, Tandon P, Stafstrom CE, et al. (1999). Effects of neonatal seizures on subsequent seizure-induced brain injury. *Neurology* 53:1754–1761.

182 McCabe BK, Silveira DC, Cilio MR, et al. (2001). Reduced neurogenesis after neonatal seizures. *J. Neurosci.* 21:2094–2103.

183 Takei Y, Takashima S, Ohyu J, et al. (1999). Effects of nitric oxide synthase inhibition on the cerebral circulation and brain damage during kainic acid-induced seizures in newborn rabbits. *Brain Dev.* 21:253–259.

184 Thoresen M, Hallström ASA, Whitelaw A, et al. (1998). Lactate and pyruvate changes in the cerebral gray and white matter during posthypoxic seizures in newborn pigs. *Pediatr. Res.* 44:746–754.

38

Improving performance, reducing error, and minimizing risk in the delivery room

Louis P. Halamek

Stanford University Medical School, Palo Alto, CA, USA

Introduction

In 1999 the Institute of Medicine published *To Err is Human: Building a Safer Health System*, a report on human error and patient safety in the USA.[1] In this report the authors estimate that between 44 000 and 98 000 Americans die each year as a result of medical errors. Although this figure has been highly debated, it is based on extrapolation of the data contained in published studies out of Colorado, Utah, and New York.[2–4] This figure is the equivalent of a large commercial airliner falling out of the sky every day. If the airline industry experienced that degree of failure, all flights would be voluntarily grounded until a thorough investigation revealed the causes and solutions were put into place. Yet medicine has yet to examine adequately the complex relationship among medical training, human performance, and medical errors.

While many factors influence the incidence of medical error in the USA today, this chapter will focus on training and education. Similarly, while medical errors occur across every medical specialty and affect all patients, this chapter will center on the newborn in the first minutes of life in the delivery room. First, the history of medical training will be reviewed. Next, new methodologies designed to improve the performance of professionals working in dynamic environments will be reviewed. Finally, the impediments to future enhancements of medical training and potential solutions to these will be discussed.

Historical perspective

Traditional medical training is essentially a two-step process. First, trainees read about the many different aspects of medical practice. This begins in the first 2 years of medical school when much time is spent either studying and working from textbooks or listening to lectures describing the basic science underlying modern medical practice. Second, trainees then begin to care for real human patients. Caring for patients typically begins with trainees observing senior colleagues in the practice of medicine followed by trainees' efforts to mimic the performance of their colleagues while under varying degrees of supervision. This has historically been described as "see one, do one, teach one;" while that phrase is an unfair criticism of medical training in many respects, certain elements continue to ring true.[5]

Several assumptions underlie the traditional two-step model of medical training. First, this model assumes that current methodologies in medical education are optimal for all adult learners. Second, there exists an assumption that the close of a training period implies that the trainee is competent to practice all aspects of medicine in his or her specialty. Yet the limitations to these assumptions are obvious. Adults learn best via active participation; passive training exercises such as reading or observing others tend to be less effective than active immersion on the part of the trainee. Adults also have different strengths and weaknesses. Training models that more or less offer the same content in the same fashion to all adult learners in essence demand that these learners accommodate the training model. This failure to recognize the inherent differences in trainees impairs their ability to succeed and suppresses unique contributions from trainees with different life experiences.

In a similar fashion, acquisition of skills occurs at different rates for different trainees and retention of skills is not uniform across trainees. Training programs that assume that exposure of the trainee to a particular environment for a defined period of time is adequate preparation for the practice of medicine fail to recognize that all training programs are by definition limited in time and depth. As an example, the Residency Review Committee for Residency Training Programs in General Pediatrics in the USA recently revised the requirements for residency training and reduced the amount of time that residents spend in intensive care environments.[6] Yet there are few objective data in the medical literature regarding the time required for skill acquisition and retention in intensive care domains. Therefore it is not currently known whether the decrease in time spent in intensive care units by pediatric residents as directed by the Residency Review Committee goes too far or not far enough. In addition, there appear to be no objective measures in place for monitoring the effects of this change over time.

Other limitations to the traditional model include the relative lack of a systematic approach to clinical training due to the very random nature of patient care experiences. This model of training, based upon whatever patients are admitted to the hospital or seen in the clinic is accurately termed "education by random opportunity"[7] (Krummel, personal communication). Because common things are common, such a model usually provides adequate training in the management of common medical conditions. However, this model is sorely deficient in preparing trainees to handle rare but potentially devastating events. Another weakness of the traditional training model is its focus on the individual trainee as the one solely responsible for patient care. In reality many medical domains are characterized by a need for communication among and coordination of multidisciplinary teams of professionals. Individuals trained in different specialties typically in isolation from one another are often forced in emergencies to function as an integrated team despite any real experience in doing so.

New methodologies

How can the limitations of the traditional medical training model be overcome? In looking for answers to this question it is useful to examine other dynamic domains where the risk to human life is high and where similar limitations have been successfully surmounted. Both aerospace and dynamic medical domains like the delivery room are characterized by an inherent risk to human life. Action/feedback loops are marked by short time constants and time pressure is intense in each. There is a direct relationship between actions and outcomes and technical skills are vital, be it in the cockpit or the delivery room. Communication in these domains is primarily verbal and immediate, involves multiple personnel, and is characterized by changes in pitch, intensity, and word compression as well as nonverbal cues including eye movement and body language. Effective human interface with technology is critical in both flying aircraft and resuscitating neonates in the delivery room. The tradition of pilot as commander-in-chief of the aircraft is similar to that of the physician bearing ultimate responsibility for the care of the newborn. Thus medicine shares many characteristics with aerospace and stands to benefit from adopting similar training methodologies.

Flying large aircraft has been described as "hours and hours of boredom interspersed by moments of terror" (this is also a reasonable description of working in a busy delivery room!). The downing of a commercial aircraft is devastating, both in terms of loss of human life and destruction of expensive technology. Because of this, the aerospace industry long ago recognized the need to develop a better understanding of why planes crash in an effort to reduce the incidence of such events. One of the first steps in this effort was to equip the cockpits of commercial aircraft with devices that record the communications of the crew and the readings of the plane's instruments. These devices provide an objective, time-coded record of the events as they occur during flight. Analysis of the data from these "black boxes" indicated that approximately two-thirds of airline accidents occurred not because of major mechanical failures or lack of technical knowledge on the part of the crew but rather because of suboptimal communication and teamwork by those responsible for flying the plane.[7] This information was surprising in that the pilots, copilots, and flight engineers flying these large commercial aircraft were some of the most experienced in the industry, having logged thousands of hours of flight time in a variety of aircraft under a wide array of conditions, yet were unable to utilize and integrate their collective skills during in-flight crises.

In response to these findings the aerospace industry developed a training program known as Crew Resource Management (CRM).[8] In CRM crews are taught the appropriate technical responses to in-flight crises. In addition, heavy emphasis is placed upon the necessary behavioral responses (effective teamwork and communication) vital to optimal crew performance. The key to effective CRM training is creating a "suspension of disbelief" in those participating in the exercise; this is greatly enhanced by creating a training environment that simulates a cockpit with high fidelity. Flight simulators are designed to be identical to the physical layout of a real cockpit and provide realistic visual, auditory, and kinesthetic cues to those training within the simulator. The simulator contains working controls, alarms, and other devices; these must be operated as in real life or the desired responses by the simulated aircraft will not occur. It is not possible simply to talk one's way out of a problem, nor pick the correct solution from a list of multiple-choice options, in a flight simulator. If the crew does not exhibit the correct technical and behavioral responses to the events in the simulator exactly as would be necessary in the real cockpit during actual flight, the scenario cannot be successfully completed and the simulator "crashes."

The aerospace industry has succeeded in overcoming many of the barriers to effective error detection, analysis, and prevention. Error detection is enhanced by a system that encourages crews to report near-miss and adverse events to a national agency, the Federal Aviation Administration (FAA), without risk of liability. The FAA database serves as a valuable resource to flight crews and the industry in general and allows for early recognition of systematic problems. The industry's experience with error analysis is unsurpassed; this experience includes recognition of good decisions on the part of crews in addition to detailed analysis of suboptimal aspects of performance. The FAA and other agencies, such as the National Aeronautics and Space Administration (NASA), provide ongoing support of human performance research, including efforts to study optimal modes of communication, effects of sleep deprivation, and other human factors. Ultimately, the goal of these efforts is to prevent errors and improve the safety of passengers and crew. Evaluation of the effects of simulation-based flight training indicates that the experience gained in realistic simulators improves crew performance; although confounded by concomitant advances in technology, passenger safety has improved since the initiation of mandatory annual CRM training by all flight crews of major commercial airlines.

Given the similarities between these high-risk domains, what has been done in medicine to mimic the successes in training (as in CRM) experienced by aerospace? Videotape has been used to record the actions and words of physicians and nurses in emergency rooms and trauma centers.[9–12] This video record of events augments the written record and memories of team members and is used in debriefing the teams after major events. Anesthesiologists have combined videotape with human patient simulators in creating the medical equivalent of a flight simulator. Their course, anesthesia crisis resource management (ACRM), was the first high-fidelity simulation-based medical training program.[13]

The delivery room possesses many similarities to the operating room. It is characterized by high risk, intense time pressure, and reliance upon technical skills and verbal communication. Unlike the operating room, there are at least two (and occasionally three or more) patients present, demanding coordinated team action between groups of physicians and nurses who in many institutions spend most of their time working in isolation from one another on separate adult and pediatric units. Recently the use of videotape to record the actions of delivery room resuscitation teams as a quality assurance instrument has been reported.[14] This study found that the videotape record provides a useful quality assurance tool for monitoring the conduct of newborn resuscitation and providing constructive feedback.

NeoSim is a simulation-based training program, based upon the CRM program in aerospace, that is focused on the individuals responsible for resuscitation of the neonate.[15] The objectives of this program are to recognize the collective responsibility of delivery room personnel to the health of mothers and babies, identify the technical and behavioral skills necessary for optimal human performance, and practice these skills in a realistic and safe environment. Each program begins with a general introduction to the principles of simulation-based training followed by review of videotapes depicting simulation-based training in aerospace and medicine. Review of these videotapes is meant to stimulate the trainees to think about the technical and behavioral skills (or lack thereof) exhibited by those captured on these "trigger" videos. Trainees are then oriented to the equipment, supplies (including medications and fluids), patients, and colleagues in the simulated delivery room. Once this familiarization is complete, trainees are immersed in multiple realistic, challenging clinical scenarios involving problems with patients, devices, colleagues, and multisystem failures. The details of these scenarios are captured on time-coded videotape and each scenario is immediately followed by a debriefing facilitated by simulator faculty. Typically conduct of a thorough debriefing requires twice the length of time required for the conduct of the scenario itself.

Sim DR is a team training program directed at all of the individuals caring for both the mother (obstetrician/perinatologist, anesthesiologist/obstetric anesthesiologist, scrub nurse, circulating nurse) and the baby (pediatrician/neonatologist, neonatal nurse practitioner, nursery nurse) in the delivery room. The success of this program demonstrates that it is possible to overcome the difficulties inherent in simultaneous training and debriefing of multiple groups of medical professionals.

There are many aspects of simulation-based training that intuitively appear to be significant advantages over traditional training methodologies. The ability to create specific scenarios eliminates the dependence on "education by random opportunity" described earlier. The ability to conduct numerous scenarios during the conduct of a single training program provides for a very intense experience in a relatively short period of time, maximizing time, money, and other resources. Scenarios can be scaled to challenge both the novice and the experienced clinician. Videotape provides an unbiased, objective, detailed, time-coded record of the actions of the trainees, reducing dependence on more subjective records such as human memory as occurs in reviewing the events during a real medical emergency. Debriefings are conducted immediately after each scenario; rarely is constructive feedback provided in such quantity and quality and so expeditiously in the real world after a crisis situation. Finally, simulation-based medical training presents no risk to patients and very minimal risk to trainees (a small risk of injury to users is present whenever real working medical equipment is used, as in the simulator).

The future

What will it take to improve human performance in medicine in general, and perinatal medicine (maternal–fetal medicine and neonatology) in particular? There is no doubt that significant barriers to progress exist. These barriers are technical, financial, legal, and psychological in nature. Human birth is a complex process, characterized by numerous continuous changes in the physiology, anatomy, and spatial relationships among various physical structures in both mother and baby. These technical barriers to high-fidelity simulation of birth are daunting at first glance. However, suspension of disbelief can be achieved with far less than 100% fidelity. Close collaboration among physicians, computer scientists, biomedical engineers, medical artists, and others will be vital in overcoming these technical challenges in a timely and cost-efficient manner.

Medicine is currently faced with tremendous financial pressures to improve efficiency and lower cost, ostensibly to deliver more care to more people. This means that it will not be adequate simply to develop and implement simulation- and virtual reality-based training programs. Validation of new training programs and devices will be necessary to insure that the skills learned in medical simulators can be effectively transferred to the real medical domain and result in improved human performance, reduced medical error rates, and better patient outcomes. This will require randomized, prospective trials that include appropriate control groups in order to evaluate and standardize these new methodologies. Any improvements over historically accepted training models should be weighed against the costs of these newer methodologies averaged over time. Financial resources to conduct this research and development must be made available.

There is much about the legal climate within the USA that discourages recognition of, detailed open discussion about, and widespread dissemination of information regarding medical errors. The threat of loss of reputation, current income, and long-term financial security thwarts any substantive effort to examine systematically the issue of patient safety. There is no method by which medical errors are logged and this database made universally accessible to practicing physicians, nurses, and allied health-care personnel. In the absence of this shared knowledge, the same errors, many of which are preventable, continue to occur repeatedly in the hospitals, clinics, and other health-care delivery sites throughout this country. Until a system that encourages responsible, blameless reporting of "medical near-misses" and adverse patient outcomes exists, medicine will never begin to approach the safety record of high-risk industries such as aerospace.

Medicine must also shoulder the blame for the current lack of patient safety initiatives; in many ways medicine has done little to alter its "culture of blame." Whenever an adverse event occurs, the question typically asked is "Who is responsible?" in order to assign blame to an individual rather than closely examine the system for the inherent flaws that set up these individuals for failure. The burden of error prevention must shift from the shoulders of individual practitioners to the health-care system as a whole. Only then will the promise of new training methodologies, physician order entry, and other technologies designed to enhance the safety of patients be fulfilled.

Conclusion

Improvement in the safety of newborns and their mothers will require a new paradigm of education and training. Faster microprocessors, advanced algorithms, and sophisticated haptic interfaces will lead to the development of sophisticated fetal, neonatal, and maternal patient simulators based on realistic physiologic models. Regional centers that utilize the tremendous potential of these simulation- and virtual reality-based technologies in their curricula will be established to serve as resources for the physicians and nurses seeking training and accreditation. The traditional two-step model of medical education will evolve. This new model will consist of four steps, and will be more in line with the successful training models found in aerospace and other industries like nuclear power where the risk to human life is high:

1. Read about health and disease in textbooks and journals.
2. Interact with virtual patients (computer-generated renderings).
3. Practice on simulated patients (sophisticated physical manikins).
4. Care for real patients.

Rather than asking "Can we afford to do this?" the proper question to be asked is "Can we afford *not* to do this?" The Institute of Medicine, in its 1999 report, states: "The status quo is not acceptable and cannot be tolerated any longer. Despite the cost pressures, liability constraints, resistance to change and other seemingly insurmountable barriers, it is simply not acceptable for patients to be harmed by the same health care system that is supposed to offer healing and comfort . . . A comprehensive approach to improving patient safety is needed."[16] Adopting a new paradigm of training and education in delivery room medicine, one that incorporates the use of simulation- and virtual reality-based technologies, should be a major component of this comprehensive approach to improving the care and safety of babies and their mothers.

REFERENCES

1 Kohn LT, Corrigan JM, and Donaldson MS, eds. (1999) To err is human: building a safer health system. Washington, D.C.: National Academy Press.

2 Thomas EJ, Studdert DM, Burstin HR, et al. (2000) Incidence and types of adverse events and negligent care in Utah and Colorado. *Med Care*, 38; 261–71.

3 Brennan TA, Leape LL, Laird NM, et al. (1991) Incidence of adverse events and negligence in hospitalized patients. Results of the Harvard Medical Practice Study I. *N Engl J Med*, 324; 370–6.

4 Leape LL, Brennan TA, Laird NM, et al. (1991) The nature of adverse events in hospitalized patients. Results of the Harvard Medical Practice Study II. *N Engl J Med*, 324; 377–84.

5 Hall JG. (1991) See one, do one, teach one. *Pediatrics*, 103; 155–6.

6 Program Requirements for Residency Education in Pediatrics. Residency Review Committee for Pediatrics. (2001). Accreditation Council for Graduate Medical Education. *http://www.acgme.org/rrc/peds.htm*

7 Billings CE and Reynard WD. (1984) Human factors in aircraft incidents: results of a 7-year study. *Aviat Space Environ Med*, 55; 960–5.

8 Weiner EL, Kanki BG, Helmreich RL, eds. (1993) *Cockpit Resource Management*. San Diego, CA: Academic Press.

9 Ellis DG, Lerner EB, Jehle D, et al. (1999) A multi-state survey of videotaping practices for major trauma resuscitations. *J Emerg Med*, 17; 597–604.

10 Ritchie PT and Cameron PA. (1999) An evaluation of trauma team leader performance by video recording. *Aust NZ J Surg*, 69; 183–6.

11 Mann CJ and Heyworth J. (1996) Comparison of cardiopulmonary resuscitation techniques using video camera recordings. *J Accid Emerg Med*, 13; 198–9.

12 Weston C, Richmond P, McCabe MJ, et al. (1992) Video recording of cardiac arrest management: an aid to training and audit. *Resuscitation*, 24; 13–15.

13 Howard SK, Gaba DM, Fish KJ, et al. (1992) Anesthesia crisis resource management training: teaching anesthesiologists to handle critical incidents. *Aviat Space Environ Med*, 63; 763–70.

14 Carbine DN, Finer NN, Knodel E, et al. (2000) Video recording as a means of evaluating neonatal resuscitation performance. *Pediatrics*, 106; 654–8.

15 Halamek LP, Kaegi DM, Gaba DM, et al. (2000) Time for a new paradigm in pediatric medical education: teaching neonatal resuscitation in a simulated delivery room environment. *Pediatrics*, 106; e45. URL: http://www.pediatrics.org/cgi/content/full/106/4/e45.

16 Kohn LT, Corrigan JM, Donaldson MS, eds. (1999) *To Err is Human: Building a Safer Health System*, vol. 3, Washington, D.C.: National Academy Press.

39

Nutritional support of the asphyxiated infant

John A. Kerner, Jr

Stanford University Medical Center, Palo Alto, CA, USA

Routine nutritional support of the premature infant

Optimal nutritional support is critical in helping to obtain a successful outcome for the ever-increasing number of surviving small premature infants.[1] Although it is paramount to insure that the infant receives an adequate caloric intake, the ability of the very-low-birth-weight (VLBW) infant to digest, absorb, and metabolize enteral nutrients is limited. In addition, complications of prematurity, such as respiratory distress, cardiovascular instability, hemorrhagic diatheses, and an immature renal system, create a challenge to the provision of proper nutritional support.

To provide nutrition to the premature infant appropriately, one must have an understanding of the biochemical and physiologic processes that occur during the development of the gastrointestinal tract. By 28 weeks of gestation the anatomic development of the gastrointestinal tract in humans is nearly complete. Yet, as an organ of nutrition, the gut is functionally immature. Details of gastrointestinal tract development have been described previously,[2–4] and have been summarized in tabular form (Table 39.1). Further, complications due to the incomplete development of gastrointestinal tract in the low-birth-weight infant have been well delineated by Sunshine (Table 39.2).

Enteral feeding

Gastric feeding: intermittent gavage or continuous infusion

Nasogastric (NG) feeds may be given continuously or intermittently. Intermittent feeding, also known as gavage feeding, is easy to administer, and it is possible to evaluate the gastric emptying time by checking the gastric residual before each meal. The stomach takes less time to empty with human milk than with formula[5] and when in the prone or lateral position.[6]

Premature infants are predisposed to develop gastroesophageal (GE) reflux due to their incompetent lower esophageal sphincter, small stomach capacity, and delayed gastric emptying. Hence, to prevent this GE reflux and subsequent risk of aspiration and apnea, it is necessary to feed these infants smaller volumes on a more frequent basis.[7] Also, gastric distension may interfere with respiratory function.[8] For these reasons premature infants may benefit from continuous NG feeds.

Toce et al. demonstrated that infants whose birth weight was between 1000 and 1249 g had better weight gain when fed via continuous NG infusion rather than via gavage feeds.[9] A reduction in stool weight was also reported. Both observations were presumed to be secondary to less stimulation of the gastrocolic reflex with a resulting longer transit time, allowing for better absorption.

Table 39.1. Development of the human gastrointestinal tract

Age (weeks)	Crown–rump length (mm)	Stage of development
2.5	1.5	Gut not distinct from yolk sac
3.5	2.5	Foregut and hindgut present
		Yolk sac broadly attached at midgut
		Liver bud present
		Mesenteries forming
4	5.0	Intestine present as a single tube from mouth to cloaca
		Esophagus and stomach distinct
		Liver cords, ducts, and gallbladder forming
		Omental bursa forming
		Pancreatic buds appear as outpouching of gut
5.6	8.0–12.0	Intestine elongates into a loop and duodenum begins to rotate under superior mesenteric artery
		Stomach rotates
		Parotid and submandibular buds appear
		Cloaca elongates and septum forms to divide cloaca
7	17.0	Circular muscle layer present
		Duodenum temporarily occluded
		Intestinal loops herniated into cord
		Villi begin to develop
		Pancreatic anlagen fuse
8	23	Villi lined by single layer of cells
		Small intestine coiling within cord
		Taste buds appear
		Microvilli short, thick, and irregularly spaced
		Lysosomal enzymes detected
		Cloacal membrane which sealed the rectum begins to disappear
9–10	30–40	Auerbach's plexus appears
		Intestine reenters abdominal cavity
		Crypts of Lieberkühn develop
		Active transport of glucose appears aerobically and anaerobically
		Dipeptidases present
		Microvilli of enterocytes more regular and glycocalyx present
		Mitochondria numerous below microvilli
12	56	Parietal cells present in stomach
		Muscular layers of intestine present
		Alkaline phosphatase and disaccharidases detectable
		Active transport of amino acids present
		Mature taste buds present
		Enterochromaffin cells appear
		Pancreatic islet cells appear
		Bile secretions begin
		Colonic haustra appear
		Coelomic extension into umbilical cord obliterated
		Meconium first detected in ileum

Table 39.1. (*cont.*)

Age (weeks)	Crown–rump length (mm)	Stage of development
13–14	78–90	Meissner's plexus appears
		Circular folds appear
		Peristalsis detected
		Lysosomes detected ultrastructurally
16	112	Pancreatic lipase and tryptic activity detected
		Lymphopoiesis present
		Peptic activity present
		Swallowing evident – 2–7 ml/24 h
20	160	Peyer's patches present
		Muscularis mucosa present
		Mesenteric attachments complete
		Zymogen granules present and well developed in pancreas (22 weeks)
		Intestine has lost ability to transport glucose anaerobically
24	200	Paneth's cells appear
		Maltase and sucrase and alkaline phosphatase very active
		Ganglion cells detected throughout small and large intestine and in the rectum
		Amylase activity present in intestine
28	240	Enterokinase activity increases
		Esophageal glands present
		Frequency and intensity of duodenal peristaltic contractions increasing
32	270	Lactase activity increases
		Hydrochloric acid found in stomach
34	290–300	Sucking and swallowing become coordinated
		Esophageal peristalsis rapid, nonsegmental contraction occurs
		Small intestinal motility becomes coordinated
36–38	320–350	Maturity of gastrointestinal tract achieved

Source: Reproduced with permission from Sunshine.[53]

Continuous feeding is not without disadvantages. Nutrients, especially fat, may be lost within the tubing during continuous infusion of breast milk.[10] Preterm formulas with a high mineral content may precipitate and clog the tubing.[11] Further, intermittent feeding may be important in the induction of metabolic and endocrine changes which occur in early postnatal life.[12]

Transpyloric feeding

Transpyloric feeding is defined as instilling the nutrients directly into the small intestine. The advantages of this method are: minimal gastric distension, lower risk of aspiration, and, at least during the first 10 days of life, potentially greater volume tolerance with less initial weight loss than with NG feeding.[13] Two prospective studies compared continuous NG and transpyloric feeding,[14,15] but only one[14] concluded there was an advantage to transpyloric feeding during the first 2-3 weeks of life. Roy et al. compared every-2-hour bolus NG feeds versus nasojejunal (NJ) feeds in healthy low-birth-weight infants and found no difference in growth or weight gain in the two groups.[16] Since the stomach was bypassed in the NJ group and fat digestion starts in the stomach, more fat malabsorption occurred in the NJ-fed babies. The fat malabsorption may be

Table 39.2. Complications due to the incomplete development of the gastrointestinal tract in the low-birth-weight infant

Incomplete development of motility	*Inadequate digestion of nutrients*
Poor coordination of sucking and swallowing	Decreased digestion of protein
Aberrant esophageal motility	Decreased activity of enterokinase
Biphasic esophageal peristalsis	Trypsin activity low prior to 28 weeks
Decreased or absent lower esophageal sphincter pressure	Decreased concentration of gastric hydrochloric acid and pepsinogen
Delayed gastric emptying time	Decreased digestion of carbohydrates
Poorly coordinated motility of the small and large intestine	Decreased hydrolysis of lactose
Stasis	Decreased ability to transport glucose actively
Dilation	Decreased activity of pancreatic amylase
Impaired blood supply	Decreased digestion of lipids
Functional obstruction	Decreased production and reabsorption of bile acids
Delayed ability to regenerate new epithelial cells	Decreased activity of pancreatic lipase
Decreased rates of proliferation	*Increased incidence of other problems that may indirectly lead to poor gastrointestinal function*
Decreased cellular migration rates	Hyaline membrane disease
Shallow crypts	Intraventricular hemorrhage
Shortened villi	Patent ductus arteriosus
Decreased mitotic indices	Hypoxemic–ischemic states
Inadequate host resistance factors	
Decreased gastric acidity	
Decreased concentrations of immunoglobulins in lamina propria and intestinal secretions	
Impaired humoral and cellular response to infection	

Note:
Reproduced with permission from Sunshine.[53]

minimized by duodenal placement of the feeding tube.[14]

Further, in two studies, transpyloric feeding was not recommended in infants requiring either ventilatory support via a face mask or nasopharyngeal suctioning,[17,18] due to the risk of dislodgement and subsequent aspiration. Lucas evaluated seven randomized trials comparing transpyloric (nasoduodenal or NJ) with intragastric feeding.[19] None of the trials were large or conclusive, but collectively they argue against transpyloric feeding. Lucas stated, "There is no convincing evidence that transpyloric feeding improves enteral feed tolerance and growth, or reduces aspiration pneumonia."[19]

Polyvinyl chloride tubes were used initially as they are relatively stiff and easily positioned. However, if left in the duodenum for several days, they harden and may perforate the intestine.[20] Silastic tubes are now commonly used, but they are more flexible and, hence, difficult to position. They are usually weighted at the tip and placed with the help of gravity. Being more flexible, they can curl back into the stomach. Perforation even with the Silastic tubes has been reported.[21]

A change in the microbial flora of the upper intestine of infants fed via transpyloric feeds has been reported. The upper intestine of the normal infant is sterile or contains sparse Gram-positive flora. However, Dellagrammaticus et al.[22] have shown that the presence of a tube facilitates colonization with "fecal-type" flora, of which *Streptococcus faecalis* and Gram-negative bacteria predominate. Theoretically, a heavy resident flora of the upper intestine could lead to poorer assimilation of feeds. Conflicting data exist on the relationship of necrotizing enterocolitis (NEC) to transpyloric feeds.[17,23] As detailed later in this chapter, it is not the route of feeding that was responsible in the above studies for the NEC, but rather the increased osmolality of the formula used. In controlled studies, NEC was proven not to be more frequent during transpyloric feeds compared to NG feeds.[14,17,24]

The European Society of Paediatric Gastroenterology and Nutrition (ESPGN) issued guidelines for feeding the preterm infant.[13]

ESPGN guidelines

Enteral feeding should be introduced as soon as it is safe to do so.

1 Intermittent gastric tube feeding seems more physiological than transpyloric feeding and whenever possible should be preferred.
2 When there are feeding difficulties such as regurgitation, poor gastric emptying, or gastric distension, continuous gastric feeding or even transpyloric feeding may be necessary, as they are useful alternatives either to reduced oral feeding or total parenteral nutrition.
3 The success of any feeding technique is at least partly the result of the skill of the staff of the unit in following their own practiced routines.
4 Nursery routines should encourage the mother to play an active role in feeding. This will help her to become confident in the care of her baby.[13]

Schanler and colleagues, in an elegant randomized trial in 171 premature infants, showed that bolus tube feeding was associated with significantly less feeding intolerance and greater rate of weight gain than the continuous feeding method.[25] More importantly, his group demonstrated the benefit of early gastrointestinal priming.[25]

Gastrointestinal priming is a practice with sound scientific rationale. Also known as "minimal feedings," "gut stimulation," "trophic feedings," or "hypocaloric feedings," this practice attempts to enable the premature infant's intestine to adapt to later advancement of full enteral feedings while preventing the known mucosal atrophy and unphysiologic gut hormone status noted in animals and humans kept NPO.[26–28] Schanler et al. were congratulated by Kliegman[29] for their large randomized controlled trial that confirmed the overall safety of gastrointestinal priming (no increased incidence of NEC) while clearly demonstrating the positive effects of this novel feeding practice – better calcium and phosphorus retention, improved feeding tolerance, reduced risk of physiologic jaundice, cholestasis, metabolic bone disease, and glucose intolerance.[25] Kliegman went on to state that "gastrointestinal priming must now become the standard of care for very low birthweight infants."[29] In Schanler's study the gastrointestinal priming group (prime continuous, prime bolus) received 20 ml/kg per day of milk (either formula or breast milk) from day 4 through day 14.[25]

Early feeding of the preterm infant has been shown to decrease intestinal permeability[30] and increase lactase activity.[31] Trophic feeding has been shown to:[32]

1. shorten time to regain birth weight;
2. improve feeding tolerance;
3. reduce the duration of phototherapy;
4. reduce duration of parenteral nutrition;
5. lower the incidence of cholestasis;
6. reduce metabolic bone disease;
7. improve gastrointestinal maturation, motility, and hormone responses;
8. improve mineral absorption;
9. enhance enzyme maturation;
10. reduce intestinal permeability;
11. be safe (the practice does not increase the incidence of NEC).

Parenteral feeding

Since sick and premature newborns are often not fed enterally, the alternative is parenteral nutrition (PN). In a review by Moyer-Mileur and Chan, parenteral feeds in VLBW infants requiring assisted ventilation for more than 6 days led to a decrease in the percentage of weight loss from birth weight and a lesser amount of time required for recovery of birth weight than in those fed enterally or by a combination of enteral and parenteral feeds.[33] A delay in enteral feeds increased the tolerance to subsequent enteral feeds in the infants. Tolerance was defined as absence of residuals, abdominal distension, or guaiac-positive, reducing substance-positive stools.[33] Another retrospective study presented inconclusive data regarding the benefits and risks of PN.[34]

Limited data exist on the potential benefit of PN in the treatment of preterm infants. A controlled study[35] of peripheral total parenteral nutrition (TPN) composed of casein hydrolysate, dextrose, and soybean emulsion in 40 premature infants with respiratory distress syndrome (RDS) showed that TPN neither favorably altered the clinical course of the syndrome nor worsened an infant's pulmonary status. Among infants weighing less than 1500 g, those who received TPN had a greater survival rate when compared with a control group (71% vs 37%).

Yu and coworkers performed a controlled trial of TPN on 34 preterm infants with birth weights of less than 1200 g.[36] Infants in the TPN group had a greater mean daily weight gain in the second week of life and regained birth weight sooner than did control infants. Four in the milk-fed control group developed NEC whereas none did in the TPN group. The results of a more recent study conducted by Kerner et al.[37] of 40 infants who weighed less than1500 g at birth were in agreement with the two mentioned controlled studies.[35,36] No increased risk in using peripheral PN as compared with conventional feeding techniques was found. Also, comparable growth was reported in the two groups.

Fifty-nine infants weighing less than 1500 g were randomly assigned either to a PN regimen via central catheter or to a transpyloric feeding regimen (mother's milk or SMA Gold Cap (Wyeth Laboratories, Philadelphia)) via a Silastic nasoduodenal tube.[38] The authors postulated that some of the problems of enteral feeding in VLBW infants might be overcome if enteral nutrients were delivered beyond the pylorus.[39] The PN group had a higher incidence of bacterial sepsis. Conjugated hyperbilirubinemia occurred only in the PN group. In spite of the observations that 34% (10 of 29) of the infants in the transpyloric group failed to establish full enteral feeding patterns by the end of the first week of life and, therefore, had achieved lower protein-energy intake than the PN group, no beneficial effect on growth or mortality was found in the PN group.

The authors concluded that "Parenteral nutrition does not confer any appreciable benefit and because of greater complexity and higher risk of complications should be reserved for those infants in whom enteral nutrition is impossible."[38] Zlotkin and coworkers disagreed with this conclusion: "Had peripheral-vein feeding been used rather than central venous alimentation, or had nasogastric gavage feeding been used in preference to transpyloric feeding, the morbidity and mortality would have declined and the results comparing TPN with enteral feeds would have been quite different."[40]

A study that remains a model for nutritional support in the VLBW infant was performed by Cashore and associates.[41] They described 23 infants who weighed less than 1500 g in whom peripheral PN was begun on day 2 of life to supplement enteral feedings, thus allowing for adequate nutrition while avoiding overtaxing the immature gastrointestinal tract. These infants regained their birth weight by the age of 8–12 days and achieved growth rates that approximated intrauterine rates of growth. Interestingly, infants weighing less than 1000 g were still not taking all their nutrients enterally by 25 days of age.

Premature infants, especially those who have RDS and are incapable of full oral feeds, often receive PN because of their extremely limited substrate reserve, very rapid growth rate, and perceived susceptibility to irreversible brain damage secondary to malnutrition.[40] A survey of 269 neonatal intensive care units showed that TPN was used exclusively during the first week of life in 80% of infants weighing 1000 g or less at birth.[42] The others received a combination of parenteral and enteral feedings in the first week. Adamkin begins PN by 72 h of age in neonates with a birth weight of less than 1000 g in whom respiratory disease and intestinal hypomotility limit the safety of feedings in the first 1–2 weeks of life.[43]

In some nurseries umbilical arterial catheters are used for infusing PN. Few studies exist regarding the safety of this practice. Yu et al. studied 34 infants with birth weight <1200 g and randomly assigned them to TPN via umbilical arterial catheters or enteral feeds.[36] The TPN group had better nitrogen balance, weight gain, less NEC, and unchanged mortality compared with the enterally fed group. No data on catheter-related complications were presented, although bacterial or fungal septicemia did not occur in either group in the study period.[36] Higgs and coworkers[44] described a controlled trial of TPN versus formula feeding by continuous NG drip. The study included 86 infants weighing from 500 to 1500 g. The TPN, including glucose, amino acids, and fat emulsion, was administered by umbilical artery catheter for the first 2 weeks of life. There was no difference in neonatal morbidity or mortality between the two groups. Specifically, there was no difference in septicemia, although four of the 43 TPN babies had "catheter problems," described in the text only as "blockage" of the catheter.

As in the study of Higgs et al., Hall and Rhodes found that morbidity, mortality, and common complications, such as infection and thrombosis, were similar in infants receiving umbilical lines for TPN compared to infants receiving tunneled jugular catheters for TPN.[45] They concluded that TPN by indwelling umbilical catheters presents no greater risk than infusion through tunneled jugular catheters. However, careful analysis of the authors' data raises questions about their conclusions. According to the authors, "Six deaths may have been catheter-related."[45] Five of those deaths occurred in the umbilical artery catheter group; death resulted from thrombosis of the aorta in one patient, candidal septicemia in two, streptococcal septicemia in one, and enterococcal septicemia in one. One death occurred in the jugular venous catheter group, with right atrial thrombosis, superior vena cava syndrome, and *Staphylococcus epidermidis* on blood culture.

Merritt cautions against the use of umbilical arterial catheters for TPN as this practice is associated with a high incidence of arterial thrombosis.[46] Coran, a pediatric surgeon, strongly recommends that PN not be given through either umbilical arteries or umbilical veins.[47] PN through umbilical veins causes phlebitis, which may lead to venous thrombosis and portal hypertension. He is especially concerned about infusing PN solutions into an umbilical arterial line, since this practice can lead to thrombosis of the aorta or iliac vessels. Severe damage, such as thrombosis of the aorta, may occur to an artery without being recognized. Only over a period of time will the side-effects of umbilical arterial catheter use, such as inappropriate growth of one limb,[47] become clinically evident. Even the use of 12.5% dextrose infused through an umbilical arterial line has increased osmolality that has been shown to cause thrombophlebitis.[47] Although the first three studies described earlier all claimed there were no short-term complications, they did not address the problem of long-term complications.[48]

Coran states that if PN is required and peripheral veins are not usable or if peripheral vein delivery is inadequate to provide necessary calories, he would consider percutaneous subclavian vein catheterization, which he can perform successfully even in a 900 g infant.[47] In a study by Sadig,[49] central venous line-associated complications were compared in VLBW infants vs older infants ($n=48$). Sixty-nine percent of catheter-associated infections occurred in VLBW infants and only 20% in infants weighing more than 1500 g. Seventy-eight percent (14/18) of these infections were successfully treated with antibiotics without catheter removal. The rate of thrombosis was also higher in VLBW infants. A retrospective review compared TPN via umbilical catheters vs central lines in 48 neonates (birth weight 1.7 ± 0.58 kg).[50] There was no difference in infection rate between the two groups when adjustment was made for the number of days of catheter life. Transient hypertension occurred in two (4%) of the umbilical arterial catheter group and in one (3.8%) of the central catheter group. There was one aortic thrombus noted on autopsy in the umbilical arterial catheter group. There was one vegetation on the tricuspid valve in the central catheter group. They concluded that umbilical arterial catheters are a reasonable route for PN solutions.

As nurseries become more comfortable with percutaneous central lines,[51,52] hopefully umbilical arterial catheters will be used less frequently to provide nutrition.

Nutritional support of the asphyxiated infant

Asphyxia may cause significant injury to the gastrointestinal tract. This injury may predispose an infant to develop NEC. During acute episodes of shock or hypoxemia the "vital structures," which include the heart, brain, and adrenal glands, are preferentially perfused. Perfusion of the "nonvital" organs, including the skin, muscle, lungs, kidney, and gastrointestinal tract, is decreased significantly. With limited periods of hypoxia, the newborn has some autoregulatory capabilities of maintaining blood flow to the intestine. However, if the period of ischemia is maintained for a prolonged period, perforation and significant mucosal hemorrhage may occur.[53] Coupled with asphyxia, feeding the premature infant heightens the risk for the development of neonatal NEC.

Most centers do not enterally feed an asphyxiated infant for the first 5 days to 2 weeks. This practice is extrapolated from animal data on cellular proliferation and migration. The intestinal mucosa of newborn and suckling rats has a very slow rate of cellular proliferation and migration compared to adult animals.[54] While the turnover of intestinal epithelia in the adult jejunum is 48–72 h, the rate in the 10-day-old animal is at least twice that long and in the 2–3-day-old animal it may be even longer.[55] In a study by Sunshine and colleagues[56] in the adult animal, labeled cells reached the tips of the villi within 48 h. During the same period of time the labeled cells had migrated only one-eighth to one-fourth of the length of the villi in the suckling animal. There are indications that this same slower rate of turnover of intestinal epithelia exists in the newborn human.[57]

Necrotizing enterocolitis

NEC is a well-described and extensively investigated affliction of the high-risk newborn. The etiology of this multifactorial disorder remains elusive, and currently, there is no universally accepted theory of pathogenesis.[58,59]

Epidemiology

The incidence varies widely, with some centers reporting rare isolated cases,[60] while others report an incidence of 3–5% of all neonatal admissions.[61] Among patients in whom NEC develops, the average birth weight is 1400–1500 g and the mean gestational age is 30–32 weeks.[62] In one study by Stoll and coworkers[63] the overall incidence was three per 1000 live births, but increased to 66 per 1000 live births for infants less than 1500 g. Similarly, the mortality was 0% for infants greater than 2500 g and increased to 40% for infants less than 1500 g. The age at diagnosis ranged from 2 to 44 days and was inversely related to gestational age. All babies >35 weeks' gestational age were diagnosed by 1 week of age. Stoll et al. felt there may be two populations who develop NEC – an early population consisting of term and preterm infants, and a later group of solely preterm babies who are smaller and sicker, who presumably have ongoing insults to their gastrointestinal tracts and are, therefore, at continued risk to develop the disease. These babies must be closely monitored for the possible development of NEC later in their hospital course.[63] It is important to appreciate that approximately 10% of all NEC cases occur in full-term neonates.[58]

There are two distinct patterns of NEC: endemic and epidemic.[64] Superimposed on an endemic rate, epidemics (which refer to cases clustered in location and time) may be observed. No seasonal pattern of occurrence of these epidemics has been demonstrated. Patient characteristics appear to differ during epidemics – they are more mature with fewer antecedent neonatal illnesses, acquire NEC later, and have been fed for a longer period than those patients who develop NEC during nonepidemic times.

Clinical picture

NEC may assume a broad spectrum of clinical severity. Some infants have little in the way of signs and symptoms with a benign course and others have fulminant disease characterized by extensive gangrene, perforation, shock, and death.

The diagnosis of NEC is suspected when two or more typical gastrointestinal signs and symptoms occur simultaneously with nonspecific signs.[62] The initial signs and symptoms of 123 consecutive patients are presented in Table 39.3, as found by Walsh and Kliegman in a 9-year study.[65] Not all patients will have every symptom and the signs will vary chronologically in their appearance depending on the severity of the illness (Table 39.4).

Because the initial symptoms of NEC are nonspecific and the findings on physical examination may be deceptively benign, radiographic findings are used to support the diagnosis of NEC. Radiographic examinations of the abdomen may show nonspecific findings of distension, ileus, and ascites.[66] The two diagnostic radiologic signs are pneumatosis intestinalis (intramural intestinal gas) and intrahepatic portal venous gas. One of these is essential to confirm the diagnosis. More severe disease will result in perforation and pneumoperitoneum. However, pneumatosis intestinalis may be subtle and fleeting. It is typically first seen in the ileocecal area but may be seen anywhere from the stomach to rectum. Two patterns are described: a curvilinear intramural radiolucency probably representing subserosal gas, and a cystic form assuming a foamy or bubbly appearance probably representing submucosal gas. Gas mixed with stool in the bowel, however, can be difficult to distinguish from pneumatosis intestinalis.[63] Pneumatosis may also be present in other clinical situations – intestinal gangrene secondary to vascular occlusion, Hirschsprung's disease with enterocolitis, obstruction at the site of bowel atresia, pyloric stenosis, and meconium ileus.

Investigators have developed screening tests for NEC such as breath hydrogen analysis,[67,68] urine analysis for D-lactate[69] (produced by enteric flora when fed excess carbohydrate), and, more recently, serum D-lactic acid (a bacterial fermentation product of unabsorbed carbohydrates) levels,[70] but these tests have not become routine in clinical monitoring up to the present.

Table 39.3. Initial signs and symptoms of necrotizing enterocolitis

Signs	Percentage of Patients[a]
Abdominal distention	73
Bloody stool	28
Apnea, bradycardia	26
Abdominal tenderness	21
Retained gastric contents	18
Guaiac-positive stool	17
"Septic appearance"	12
Shock	11
Bilious emesis	11
Acidosis	10
Lethargy	9
Diarrhea	6
Cellulitis of abdominal wall	6
Right lower quadrant mass	2

Note:
[a] Total exceeds 100%, as many patients had more than one sign.
Source: Reproduced with permission from Walsh and Kliegman.[65]

Table 39.4. Unusual manifestations of necrotizing enterocolitis

10% occur in term infants
10–12% occur in infants who have never been fed
10–15% will not have pneumatosis intestinalis
10–15% will have no blood in stools
10–15% will develop intestinal strictures

Source: Reproduced with permission from Sunshine.[53]

Treatment

Since NEC can manifest within a wide range of severity along a continuum of various stages of bowel disease, the true nature or clinical course that NEC will follow is usually not known until 48 h of onset.

Bell and associates[71] proposed important clinical staging criteria for NEC, which allowed accurate comparisons of patients with disease of similar severity. Kliegman and associates modified Bell's staging criteria to include systemic, intestinal, and radiographic signs and suggested treatment regimens based on the stages[72] (Table 39.5).

In addition to the recommendations in Table 39.5, a large-bore, double-lumen NG tube should also be placed to decompress the stomach. The length of time the bowel is allowed to "rest" will depend on the progression or lack of progression of the disease and on the philosophy of the institution. PN is recommended in patients with documented NEC during the period of intestinal recovery. When prolonged parenteral feedings are required, a central venous line may need to be placed. PN allows for a slow return to enteral feedings – it is common for this transition to take 1–3 weeks to reestablish full enteral feedings. Infants requiring surgical resection of the bowel will have a more protracted course, especially with extensive resections, and may develop "short-bowel syndrome." The specifics of such management are described elsewhere.[73] Immediate surgical management of NEC has been recently reviewed.[74–76] The preferred operation for VLBW infants is currently being investigated in a randomized clinical trial.[75]

Pathogenesis

There is no universal acceptance of a unifying theory regarding the pathogenesis of NEC. Numerous controlled studies have been performed in order to delineate the neonate at risk. Stoll et al. determined that affected infants were quite similar to controls and identified no risk factors.[63] Kliegman et al. failed to delineate any important risk factor. They therefore concluded that perinatal problems which precede NEC are equally common to all high-risk infants.[72]

A unifying theory must explain the development of NEC in the enterally fed or fasted high-risk neonate and in the healthy term newborn.[62] It seems likely that NEC represents the final response of the immature gastrointestinal tract to one or more unrelated stresses. Because there are many stressful factors, there may be a wide range in the severity of bowel injury and, therefore, a continuous spectrum of clinical disease. Perhaps in the mildly affected infant the stresses are not as injurious, and in the severely affected infant, multiple stresses act synergistically to produce more severe damage.[62]

Enteral feeding

Conflicting opinions exist regarding the relationship of enteral feeding practices and the development of NEC.

It is important to bear in mind that 5–10% of patients who develop NEC have never been fed.[58] Controlled studies comparing feeding techniques in infants with and without NEC fail to consistently support feeding as an important precursor, though controversy certainly persists.

There are numerous ways by which feedings might contribute to the pathogenesis or progression of NEC:

1. direct mucosal injury by hypertonic feedings;
2. alteration of intestinal flora;
3. structural immaturity of the premature infant's intestine;
4. absence of breast milk's immunologically protective effect in formula-fed infants;
5. the effect of early or large volume feedings on an alimentary tract compromised by an adverse perinatal event.

The pragmatic issues, such as timing of feedings, the rate and volume of feedings, and the osmolarity of feedings have been evaluated.

Timing of enteral feeding

There is a definite trend to delay enteral feedings in the sick premature infant. In a survey of 269 neona-

Table 39.5. Modified Bell's staging criteria for necrotizing enterocolitis (NEC)

Stage	Systemic signs	Intestinal signs	Radiologic signs	Treatment
IA Suspected NEC	Temperature instability, apnea, bradycardia, lethargy	Elevated pregavage residuals, mild abdominal distension, emesis, guaiac-positive stool	Normal or intestinal dilation, mild ileus	NPO, antibiotics × 3 days pending culture
IB Suspected NEC	Same as above	Bright red blood from rectum	Same as above	Same as above
IIA Definite NEC: Mildly ill	Same as above	Same as above, plus absent bowel sounds, ± abdominal tenderness	Intestinal dilation, ileus, pneumatosis intestinalis	NPO, antibiotics × 7–10 days if exam is normal in 24–48 h
IIB Definite NEC: Moderately ill	Same as above, plus mild metabolic acidosis, mild thrombocytopenia	Same as above, plus absent bowel sounds, definite abdominal tenderness, ± abdominal cellulitis or right lower quadrant mass	Same as IIA, plus portal vein gas, ± ascites	NPO, antibiotics × 14 days, $NaHCO_3$ for acidosis
IIIA Advanced NEC: severely ill, bowel intact	Same as IIB, plus hypotension, bradycardia, severe apnea, combined respiratory and metabolic acidosis, disseminated intravascular coagulation, neutropenia	Same as above, plus signs of generalized peritonitis marked tenderness, distension of abdomen, abdominal wall erythema	Same as IIB, plus definite ascites	Same as above, plus as much as 200 ml/kg fluids, fresh frozen plasma, inotropic agents, ventilation therapy, paracentesis
IIIB Advanced NEC: severely ill, bowel perforated	Same as IIIA, sudden deterioration	Same as IIIA, sudden increased distension	Same as IIB, plus pneumoperitoneum	Same as above, plus surgical intervention

Source: Reproduced with permission from Walsh and Kliegman.[65]

tal intensive care units by Churella et al.[42] (described previously) most units (80%) gave parenteral feedings during the first week of life to infants weighing <1000 g at birth. None started enteral feeds alone and 20% used a combination of enteral and parenteral feeds. Sixty-nine percent of those weighing between 1001 and 2399 g received a combination of parenteral and enteral feeds. The first enteral feed was begun at a mean of 7 days after birth for infants <1000 g birth weight, 5 days after birth for those with a birth weight 1001–1500 g, and 3 days after birth for those infants weighing more than 1500 g.[42]

In a prospective study by Eyal et al.,[77] delaying feedings in VLBW infants (<1500 g) from 2–3 days to 2–3 weeks decreased the incidence of NEC from 18 to 3%. It is interesting to note that in those patients (3%) who developed NEC after delayed onset of enteral feeds, the time of the first symptoms ranged from 23 to 60 days compared to 7–23 days in those infants fed enterally within the first week of life. Hence, those infants in whom enteral feeds are delayed must be observed for a longer period for the development of NEC.

Brown and Sweet[60] felt that NEC was virtually eliminated from their nursery with the initiation of an extremely cautious feeding protocol which fostered late initiation of enteral feeds, slow advancement to reach full feeds after 2 weeks of onset of feeds, and prompt discontinuance of feeds when untoward signs suggesting hypoxia, hypoperfusion, or gastrointestinal dysfunction developed (i.e., distension, guaiac-positive stools, or apnea).

On the other hand, Ostertag et al. in a prospective study of 34 low-birth-weight infants (<1500 g) who were fed on day 1 or day 7 did not show any significant increase in the incidence of NEC – 29% of those enterally fed on day 1 compared to 35% fed enterally on day 7 developed NEC. There were no differences in the perinatal risk factors in the two groups.[78] In a study by Unger and coworkers,[34] delayed initiation of enteral feedings was associated with a decreased incidence of NEC only among male infants with birth weight <775 g; hence their study did not support elective withholding of enteral feeds in other groups of low-birth-weight infants.[34]

Rate and volume of enteral feeds

Aggressive feeding practices were found to be associated with NEC by Krousop.[79] In his case material, infants who developed NEC received an average of 43 ml/kg during the initial day of enteral feeds and 72 ml/kg during the second day.[79]

Book and associates,[80] in a small prospective study comparing fast and slow feeding rates (increase of 20 vs 10 ml/day) designed to attain complete enteral feedings at 7 and 14 days, respectively, did not find any difference in the incidence of NEC. Goldman, however, in a retrospective uncontrolled study found an increased incidence of NEC when feedings were advanced by large volumes (>40–60 ml/kg per day).[81] He also found a higher percentage of disease in infants receiving volumes greater than 150 ml/kg per day. Anderson et al.[82] noted an increased incidence of NEC among those low-birth-weight infants fed aggressively – advanced at a rate exceeding 20 ml/kg per day.

The mechanism by which excessive feeding predisposes to NEC is uncertain. There may be relative mucosal ischemia due to an imbalance between mucosal blood flow and oxygen extraction due to an excessive load.[62] Alternatively, the already low concentration of lactase in preterm infants may be overwhelmed by the excessive lactose load. The excess lactose is then fermented by the microflora, resulting in H_2 production, initiating NEC.[62] Reducing substances are also a byproduct of this bacterial fermentation. Book and coworkers[83] found that 75% of infants who developed NEC had 3–4 plus reducing substances in their stools from 1 to 4 days prior to clinical manifestations of disease.

Walsh and coworkers[62] recommended starting enteral feeds at 1 ml every 1–2 h and advancing feeds slowly, no greater than 20 ml/kg per day. They successfully feed 1-kg infants who require ventilatory support. However, the infant is continuously monitored for intolerance – increased residuals, distension, guaiac-positive stools, or reducing substances in the stool.

Sweet recommended holding feeds if there are significant residuals in the stomach prior to a feed.[84] If residue persists, then the bowel is rested for 5–7 days. If abdominal distension develops during feeds, appropriate cultures and radiographs are obtained. Even if they are inconclusive, he will not feed the infant for 1–2 weeks. In his conservative approach, infants who develop sudden episodes of apnea, pallor, bradycardia, or poor skin perfusion are not fed for 1 week or more. They have had only one episode of NEC in 5 years out of 300 infants (89 infants weighing <1000 g and 211 weighing between 1000 and 2500 g).

Osmolality of feeds

Both animal studies and clinical data have implicated hypertonic feeds in causing mucosal injury. DeLemos et al. produced enterocolitis in goats fed hypertonic formula.[85] Book et al. found that feeding infants <1200 g an elemental formula with an osmolarity of 650 mosmol/l resulted in an 87% incidence of NEC, in comparison to 25% of neonates fed standard cow's milk-based formula (359 mosmol/1).[86] Willis et al. noted a higher frequency of NEC among infants fed undiluted hypertonic calcium lactate than among those unsupplemented or supplemented with diluted calcium lactate.[87] The American Academy of Pediatrics has recommended that infant feedings have an osmolarity of less than 400 mosmol/l (equivalent to an osmolality of approximately 450 mosmol/kg H_2O).[88]

Hypertonic formulas may be the result of added oral medications. In an excellent review by White and Harkavy,[89] the osmolalities of five oral preparations were studied: theophylline, calcium glubionate, digoxin, phenobarbital, and dexamethasone. The osmolalities of all five were >3000 mosmol/kg H_2O and hence should be given undiluted orally with extreme caution. When mixed with formula, theophylline, calcium glubionate, and digoxin had acceptable osmolalities (<400 mosmol/kg H_2O) but dexamethasone and phenobarbital elixirs still had osmolalities of approximately 1000 mosmol/l, when 3.8 and 1 ml respectively were mixed with 15 ml of formula.[89] Ernst et al. showed that 1 ml of Polyvisol added to 30 ml of a standard formula increased the osmolality from 375 to 744 mosmol/kg H_2O.[90] If an intravenous line is required for other reasons, then the intravenous route of drug administration may be preferred over the oral route.

Immunologic considerations

The newborn protects its mucosa by secretory immunoglobulin A (SIgA). SIgA inhibits bacterial adherence to mucosal cells in addition to preventing other toxins and antigenic material from binding to the epithelial cells. However, in term infants SIgA is not demonstrable in intestinal fluids until 1 week of age and adult values are not reached until 1 month of age.[91] However, nature has its way of protecting the newborn. SIgA-producing plasma cells in the maternal gut are antigenically stimulated and migrate to the breast where specific antibodies are secreted into the colostrum. Thus, the breast-fed newborn receives some passive protection against the bacteria he or she is most likely to harbor (i.e., his or her mother's).

The possibility of improving gut defenses has been explored extensively.[92] Eibl and coworkers[93] reported their results using an oral immunoglobulin preparation (73% IgA and 26% IgG) in reducing the incidence of NEC in low-birth-weight infants (800–2000 g). These were infants for whom breast milk was not available. In 88 infants fed the oral IgA-IgG, there were no cases of NEC compared with six cases among the 91 control infants. The IgA-lgG preparation was made from human serum. Although the study's results were very promising, additional confirmation of their results should occur before such immunoglobulin use becomes common practice.[93]

Benefits of human milk

The possibility that breast milk (containing IgA) offers similar immunoprotective benefit has also been studied. In the nonbreast-fed premature infant, whose intestine is already immature, there is no protection against bacteria when microbial colonization occurs. Hence, maternal milk has potential importance in protecting the newborn. The work of Barlow et al. in rats substantiates the importance of breast milk in preventing NEC.[94] They consistently produced a disease similar to NEC by producing a hypoxic insult in those rats fed artificial formula. All breast-fed asphyxiated rats were protected from disease. In the rat model, live milk leukocytes appeared to be prophylactic. They concluded that breast milk induced protective enteric immunity for newborn rats, and it may similarly protect premature infants.[94] However, NEC has been reported in neonates exclusively fed fresh, frozen, or pasteurized human milk.[95]

In the past, many nurseries fed premature infants pooled frozen human milk. Kliegman et al. found that there was no difference in the incidence of NEC among these infants and those fed commercial formula.[96] The reason for this, despite the theoretical advantages of breast milk, could include the adverse affects of storage on the viability and functional integrity of the cellular components of milk in addition to the possibility of contamination. In a study by Stevenson et al.,[97] there was no difference in the intestinal flora of preterm hospitalized infants fed stored frozen breast milk and a proprietary formula. However, all the infants fed breast milk had been treated with parenteral antibiotics.[97]

Lucas and Cole reported a large prospective multicenter study of 926 preterm infants formally assigned to their early diet.[98] The results argue strongly for a highly protective effect of human milk on the subsequent development of NEC. In exclusively formula-fed babies, confirmed NEC was six to 10 times more common than in those fed breast milk alone and three times more common than in those who received formula plus breast milk. Among babies born at more than 30 weeks' gestation, confirmed NEC was rare in those whose diet included human milk; it was 20 times more common in those fed formula only. Pasteurized donor milk seemed to be as protective as raw maternal milk. In formula-fed but not breast-fed infants, delayed feeding was associated with a lower frequency of NEC. In babies fed breast milk (alone or with formula) there was a sharp decline in incidence of NEC with length of gestation. Beyond 30 weeks' gestation there was only one confirmed case of NEC among 376 babies receiving human milk. The authors concluded that early introduction of breast milk into the diets of preterm infants could make NEC beyond 30 weeks' gestation a rarity.[98]

Schanler et al. in their recent randomized trial[25] confirmed the value of feeding human milk to VLBW infants. In their study, independent of treatment group assignment, those infants receiving the most human milk had a significantly lower incidence of NEC.[25] Further, Schulman et al.[30] showed that the feeding of human milk (vs formula) was associated with decreased intestinal permeability at 28 days of age ($P=0.02$). Fresh human milk is composed of numerous immunoprotective factors including: neonatal antigen-specific antibodies (IgA, IgM, and IgG), macrophages, lymphocytes, neutrophils, enzymes, lactoferrin, lysozyme, growth factors (e.g., epidermal growth factor (EGF)) hormones, oligosaccharides, polyunsaturated fatty acids, nucleotides, and specific glycoproteins. Another potential beneficial component of human milk that was recently discovered is platelet-activating factor (PAF) acetyl hydrolase (PAF-AH). This enzyme inhibits the activity of PAF, which is likely to be a significant mediator in the pathophysiologic cascade of NEC.[99]

Ischemia and hypoxia

Ischemia and subsequent damage to the intestinal mucosa have been hypothesized in the pathogenesis of NEC. Investigators developed an ischemic model of NEC in piglets and postulated a "diving reflex." This is a well-documented reflex in marine animals when there is arterial constriction in the vascular beds of the skin, kidney, and gastrointestinal tract in an attempt to preserve cardiac and cerebral blood flow during prolonged diving. Premature infants may respond in a similar manner to repeated episodes of gut ischemia. Factors implicated in the "ischemia–hypoxia" pathogenesis of NEC include prenatal asphyxia, hypotension, hypothermia, umbilical vessel catheterization, patent ductus arteriosus (PDA), polycythemia, and exchange transfusion. None the less, NEC does not develop in the majority of infants with these risk factors,[61,63] and NEC has been reported in premature infants with no risk factors.[100]

Umbilical vessel catheterization has been widely implicated in the pathogenesis of mucosal ischemia; 80% of infants with umbilical artery catheters have been found to have distinct arterial thrombosis.[101] Plasticizer levels in tissues of neonates with NEC were found to be significantly higher than those without catheters.[102] A significant increase in portal venous pressure was noted in newborn piglets undergoing exchange transfusion via umbilical venous catheter. The authors concluded that alterations in mucosal vascular pressures produced ischemia secondary to vascular congestion and hemorrhage.[103]

The presence of a low umbilical catheter has been reported to increase the risk of NEC, especially if the infant is fed during the period of catheterization. However, a prospective randomized clinical trial did not support this association.[104] Kliegman's own experience reinforces the safety and value of feeding infants as small as 600 g who are on a ventilator while an umbilical catheter is in place.[29] In the study of Schanler et al.,[25] there was no association between the use of umbilical catheters, concomitant feeding, and either feeding intolerance or NEC.

Role of vitamin E

Premature infants weighing <1500 g maintained at high serum levels of vitamin E for retinopathy of prematurity (ROP) prophylaxis have been found to have a higher incidence of NEC.

Johnson et al.[105] found that premature infants weighing <1500 g who received prophylactic vitamin E had a higher incidence of NEC and sepsis if maintained at pharmacologic levels (>3.0 mg/dl or 0.03 mg/ml) for more than 1 week. Hence, they recommend serum vitamin E levels be kept between 1.0 and 3.0 mg/dl.[105] In a recent study high serum vitamin E levels (>3.5 mg/dl) were found in premature infants weighing <1500 g when receiving the recommended dosage of MVI Pediatric;[106] hence, they recommend weekly serum vitamin E in those infants weighing between 1 and 3 kg. Further, infants with elevated vitamin E levels should have multivitamins held until serum vitamin E levels normalize; infants <3 kg should receive 2 ml/kg (maximum 5 ml) of MVI Pediatric daily to avoid elevations in serum vitamin E and the increased NEC risk.

The most likely reason for the increased incidence of NEC is that pharmacologic serum vitamin E levels result in a decrease in oxygen-dependent intracellular killing ability, which leads to an increased susceptibility to infection in preterm infants.

Role of infectious agents

Many consider NEC to be an infectious disease as many infants are colonized with a resistant and invasive organism. These organisms are capable of producing hydrogen gas, which leads to pneumatosis. The most commonly encountered organisms have been *Escherichia coli, Klebsiella, Clostridium,* and more recently, *Staphylococcus epidermidis* has been implicated in a number of patients.[53] The premature infant has decreased resistance; and coupled with the inability to mount an appropriate immune response, these infections can be overwhelming.

Prophylactic use of oral aminoglycosides was initially hailed as a means of either prevention of NEC altogether or prevention of perforation if NEC had already developed. Prospective studies have demonstrated that oral gentamicin does not prevent intestinal perforation or alter the course of the disease. Further, oral aminoglycosides can be absorbed across the damaged intestine and increase serum levels, possibly leading to drug toxicity.[62] In addition, Neu and coworkers showed that in animals who had been asphyxiated, the use of gentamicin significantly decreased jejunal lactase levels.[107]

Maternal cocaine use

Maternal cocaine use has recently been implicated in NEC in infants.[76] Cocaine compromises the uterine blood flow and fetal oxygenation in pregnant ewes, thus potentially impairing fetal gut development.[108] Lopez[109] studied 1284 neonatal intensive care unit admissions and found that 12% of exposed infants vs 3% of nonexposed infants developed NEC. In low-birth-weight or premature infants, the risk is two to three times higher during the first 2 weeks in the exposed babies but rises to five times higher after 2 weeks, particularly in those infants smaller than 1500 g.

Role of corticosteroids

In a large multicenter collaborative trial using antenatal corticosteroids to prevent RDS, a significantly decreased incidence of NEC was noted in infants treated with steroids.[110] Similar results have been shown prospectively in infants treated prenatally, with a trend in reduction of NEC even with postnatal treatment.[111] Additionally, corticosteroids stimulate PAF-AH and inhibit the PAF synthesis pathway.[112] In the study of Schulman et al.,[30] antenatal steroid administration was associated with decreased intestinal permeability at 28 days of age ($P=0.017$). Corticosteroids are one of the growth factors implicated in the physiologic maturation of the intestinal barrier, and in animal studies they help to mature many components of the microvillous surface and enhance the intestinal barrier to the uptake of antigens.[76] Postnatal glucocorticoids are clearly not the ultimate answer to decrease NEC, since their use is associated with a number of significant adverse effects, including growth retardation, hyperglycemia, hypertension, infections, hypertrophic cardiomyopathy, gastrointestinal bleeding, and intestinal perforation.[113]

Newer thoughts on etiology

Enteral feeding, bacterial infection, and mesenteric ischemia appear to play significant roles in the pathogenesis of NEC, but are likely secondary to the basic underlying defects of intestinal barrier immaturity. Contributing to this barrier of young (compared to more mature) intestine may be:[114]

1. decreased mucus production or immature mucin composition;
2. increased susceptibility to disruption of the epithelial cell layer at the cell membrane and/or the basement membrane level;
3. decreased repair capacity of the epithelial cell layer;
4. decreased tissue antioxidant activity;
5. decreased ability to maintain tissue oxygenation secondary to immature regulation of blood flow and oxygenation;
6. increased susceptibility to inflammatory mediators;
7. dysfunctional immune response; and
8. abnormal motility.

One – or, more likely, several – of these factors contributing to gut immaturity may then result in mucosal injury that progresses to NEC.[115,116]

NEC seems to involve a final common pathway that includes the endogenous production of inflammatory mediators involved in the development of intestinal injury. Endotoxin lipopolysaccharide, PAF, tumor necrosis factor (TNF), and other cytokines together with prostaglandins and leukotrienes are thought to be involved in the final common pathway of NEC pathogenesis.[99]

PAF has emerged as a primary mediator of pathogenesis of NEC.[117,118] PAF exerts local paracrine effects, and is rapidly hydrolyzed by PAF-AH. PAF binds to a specific receptor, leading to hypotension, increased vascular permeability, hemoconcentration, lysosomal enzyme release, and platelet and neutrophil aggregation.[118] Gonzalez-Crussi and Hsueh have shown that intraaortic injection of PAF resulted in experimental bowel necrosis in the adult rat that is similar to NEC.[119] Plasma levels of PAF-AH, the PAF-degrading enzyme, have been shown to be significantly lower in preterm neonates, and PAF levels in stools increase after the initiation of enteral feeding.[117]

PAF receptor antagonists or PAF-AH mixed in the formula prevented the development of experimental NEC.[117] The bowel necrosis can be exacerbated by a nitric oxide synthase inhibitor.[99]

Epithelial cells of the intestinal mucosa turn over naturally by the removal of some cells via programmed cell death (apoptosis) and by replacement of the dying cells with proliferating cells in the crypts. Abundant apoptosis might lead to a breach in the mucosal barrier, allowing bacterial translocation into the submucosa and triggering an inflammatory cascade. PAF is a potent stimulator of apoptosis in cultured intestinal epithelial cells.[119]

Intestinal trefoil factor (ITF) is a cytoprotective peptide secreted by the intestinal goblet cells which has been shown to protect the gut mucosa against damage induced by several injurious agents. In an experimental rat model of NEC, ITF protected against PAF-mediated injury.[120] A proposed schematic of the etiology of NEC is show in Figure 39.1.

Nitrous oxide is synthesized from arginine and is critical for intestinal barrier function. Inhibition of nitrous oxide synthesis increases intestinal damage. Glutamine and arginine serum levels have both been shown to be significantly lower in premature infants with NEC compared to controls.[121]

Salivary EGF has been shown to be decreased in NEC infants compared to controls. There is a ques-

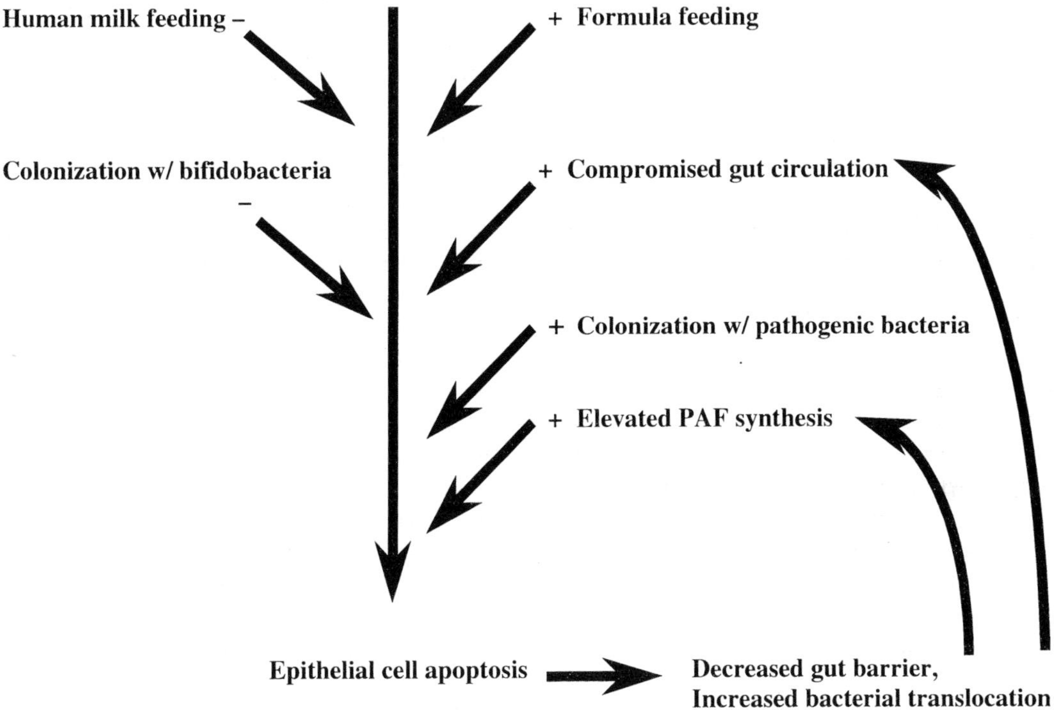

Figure 39.1 Proposed schematic of the etiology of necrotizing enterocolitis. PAF, platelet-activating factor. – protective effect; + damaging effect. Modified with permission from Caplan and Jilling.[117]

tion of whether a fall in EGF predicts the onset of NEC. If EGF were low, EGF supplementation could possibly be given.[114]

Early colonization of the gut might have an important role in developing susceptibility to NEC. Therefore, the supplementation of infant formula with probiotics might be a feasible prevention strategy to reduce the incidence of NEC in high-risk populations. Bifidobacterial supplementation reduced the incidence of NEC in a neonatal rat model.[122] Supplementation of formula with live bifidobacteria prevented the development of NEC in a quail model.[123] Recent work from the laboratory of Butel et al. has focused on the contribution of the prebiotic, oligofructose, to the protective role of bifidobacteria.[124] Thus the combination of a probiotic and prebiotic may offer a new therapeutic way of preventing NEC.

If human milk is not available, altered premature formulas may lower the incidence of NEC. Delipidated formula (formula without fat) has been shown not to alter intestinal permeability, while premature formulas increase intestinal permeability.[114] Recently, Carlson et al. studied preterm infants fed on experimental formula with egg phospholipids (one or more of which may have enhanced immature intestinal function) in a randomized, double-blind clinical study. Those infants fed the experimental formula developed significantly less stage II and stage III NEC compared to controls.[125]

Outcome of NEC

In addition to post-NEC strictures, the most common complication is short-bowel syndrome – estimated to be 25% in one review.[75] Since patients with short-bowel syndrome are dependent on PN for varied periods of time, some patients progress to TPN-associated cholestasis, with subsequent cirrhosis and liver failure.[75]

Neurodevelopmental outcome has also been studied in babies surviving NEC. Sonntag studied 20 of 22 surviving VLBW infants diagnosed with NEC between 1992 and 1996. Severe developmental delay was especially frequent in the NEC group: it was found in 55% of the infants after NEC but only 22.5% of the infants without NEC at 20 months' corrected age.[126] In an additional study of 1151 extremely-low-birth-weight infants, factors significantly associated with increased neurodevelopmental morbidity included chronic lung disease, grades 3–4 intraventricular hemorrhage/periventricular leukomalacia, steroids for chronic lung disease, NEC, and male gender.[127]

Prevention of NEC

Given the multitude of known beneficial effects of breast milk for feeding premature infants, administration of fresh breast milk should be given top priority as the most natural and safe way of lowering the risk of NEC.[114] Early gastrointestinal priming with human milk, using the bolus tube-feeding method, "may provide the best advantage for the premature infant."[25]

Since there will continue to be infants for whom breast milk feeding is not an option, investigation into the ideal nutrient composition for infant formulas and the administration of formula additives should be actively pursued.[114] Premature formulas must be altered to minimize adverse effects on intestinal barrier function. Omega-3 fatty acids and egg phospholipid-containing diets have been used in both animal and human studies.[125,128] These lipids seem to have an antiinflammatory effect, with reduction of the levels of PAF and leukotrienes in the intestinal mucosa and a significant decrease in the incidence of stage III NEC in less-than-32-week premature infants.[76]

In a recent study,[129] increasing the volume of feedings at a slow vs fast rate was not shown to result in a difference in incidence in NEC. The study was a randomized, controlled prospective trial. One hundred and eighty-five preterm infants, <1500 g, were randomized to receive either "slow" feeding advancement of 15 ml/kg per day or "fast" advancement at 35 ml/kg per day. The authors found no difference in the incidence of NEC between the groups (13% with the slow regimen vs 9% with the fast regimen). The group randomized to the fast regimen regained their birth weight more rapidly.[129] These unexpected findings suggest that VLBW infants may not require as much caution in their feeding regimens as previously suggested, but few neonatologists currently advance feedings rapidly in preterm infants.[117] Experience dictates a very slow regimen for increases in feeding, beginning early.[130,131]

Future therapies potentially beneficial in preventing NEC include:

1. supplementation of feedings with probiotics (e.g., bifidobacteria) and, possibly, prebiotics (e.g., oligofructose);
2. PAF antagonists or recombinant PAF-AH;
3. dietary supplements with growth factors (e.g., EGF, glutamine);
4. arginine supplementation of the preterm infant's diet – an amino acid essential to intestinal integrity;
5. promotion of intestinal mucus production and addition of mucin to commercially prepared infant formula;
6. antioxidant administration, especially glutathione and vitamin E.[114]

Our knowledge of optimal nutrition in the premature infant is in a continuing state of evolution. Current recommendations for providing nutrition in the asphyxiated premature infant appear below.

Recommendations for nutritional management of asphyxiated infants

Several preventive measures can be proposed for at-risk infants. At-risk infants are those who are suspected to have had an intrauterine or neonatal episode of asphyxia or shock leading to poor bowel perfusion.

Late introduction of feedings

At-risk infants should receive nothing enterally for the first 5 days to 2 weeks of life; they should receive TPN. Enteral feedings are then initiated slowly, but at the first sign of abdominal distension, increasing gastric residuals, regurgitation, guaiac-positive or clinitest-positive (anhydrous Benedict's reagent) stools, enteral feedings should be stopped and not reintroduced for several days to weeks.

Slow advancement of feedings

At the end of 5 days to 2 weeks, or if feedings are to be initiated earlier than stated above (e.g., in tiny newborns on ventilators), one should begin with 1 ml every 1–2 h and advance slowly to increase the total feedings by no more than 20 ml/kg per day.

Human milk

While early studies suggested that human milk would be protective against NEC, NEC has been described even in infants receiving fresh human milk. However, the immune protection from fresh human milk is thought by many to be very important to the preterm infant and the large study of 926 preterm infants by Lucas and Cole[98] argues strongly for the protective effects of human milk. The recent study of Schanler et al.[25] also supported the use of human milk – the greater the quantity of human milk fed, the lower the morbidity. Since human milk may not meet calcium, phosphorus, caloric, and protein needs of low-birth-weight infants, it can be supplemented with a human milk fortifier. In our laboratory, we have shown that such supplementation has no adverse effects on key antiinfective factors in human milk.[132]

Route of feeding

Intermittent gavage tube feeding appears more physiologic than transpyloric feeding, and, wherever possible, is preferred. Schanler and coworkers recently confirmed the advantage of such bolus feedings.[25] Enteral nutrition may be the critical element that triggers postnatal gut maturation through release of gut peptide hormones.[133] If the patient has regurgitation, poor gastric emptying, or gastric distension, continuous NG feeding or even transpyloric feeding may be required.[13]

Observe for early signs of NEC

Carefully monitor all high-risk infants for any early signs of NEC. These signs may occur up to 60 days of life in infants whose first feed is delayed beyond the first week of life. If the diagnosis of NEC is suspected, feedings are stopped, and the infant receives nutrition by the parenteral route for several days to 2 weeks depending on the severity of symptoms.

Summary: asphyxia and necrotizing enterocolitis

Asphyxiated infants may have experienced a significant insult to the gut, predisposing them to NEC. Enteral feedings are usually withheld for the first 5 days to 2 weeks after the insult, then advanced slowly. Prolonged bowel rest may arrest gut maturation, but maturation will resume when intraluminal nutrients are reintroduced.[134] Gut atrophy in the chronically parenterally fed infant may lead to increased intestinal permeability of bacteria.[135,136]

REFERENCES

1 Committee on Nutrition. (1985). Nutritional needs of low birthweight infants. *Pediatrics*, 75, 976–986.
2 Grand RJ, Watkins JB and Torti FM. (1976). Development of

the human gastrointestinal tract. *Gastroenterology,* **70**, 790–810.

3 Lebenthal E and Le PC. (1983). Interactions of determinants in the ontogeny of the gastrointestinal tract: a unified concept. *Pediatr Res,* **17**, 19–24.

4 Milla PJ. (1984). Development of intestinal structure and function. In *Neonatal Gastroenterology – Contemporary Issues,* eds. MS Tanner and RJ Stocks, pp. 1–20. Newcastle upon Tyne: Scholium International.

5 Cavell B. (1979). Gastric emptying in preterm infants. *Acta Paediatr Scand,* **68**, 725–730.

6 Yu VYH. (1975). Effect of body position on gastric emptying in the neonate. *Arch Dis Child,* **50**, 500–504.

7 Herbst JJ, Minton SD and Book LS. (1979). Gastroesophageal reflux causing respiratory distress and apnea in newborn infants. *J Pediatr,* **95**, 763–768.

8 Pitcher-Wilmott R, Shurack JG and Fox WW. (1979). Decreased lung volume after nasogastric feeding of neonates recovering from respiratory distress. *J Pediatr,* **96**, 914–916.

9 Toce SS, Keenan WJ and Homan SM. (1987). Enteral feeding in very low-birth-weight infants – a comparison of two nasogastric methods. *Am J Dis Child,* **141**, 439–444.

10 Narayanan I, Singh B and Harvey D. (1984). Fat loss during feeding of human milk. *Arch Dis Child,* **59**, 475–477.

11 Moyer L and Chan GM. (1982). Clotted feeding tubes with transpyloric feeding of premature infant formula. *J Pediatr Gastroenterol Nutr,* **1**, 55–57.

12 Lucas A, Bloom SR and Aynsley-Green A. (1978). Metabolic and endocrine events at the time of the first feed of human milk in preterm and term infants. *Arch Dis Child,* **53**, 731–736.

13 Bremer HJ, Brooke OG, Orzalesi M, et al. (1987). *Nutrition and Feeding of Preterm Infants,* pp. 197–198. Oxford: Blackwell.

14 Van Caillie M and Powell GK. (1975). Nasoduodenal versus nasogastric feeding in the very low birth weight infant. *Pediatrics,* **56**, 1065–1072.

15 Whitfield MF. (1982). Poor weight gain of the low birthweight infant fed nasojejunally. *Arch Dis Child,* **57**, 597–601.

16 Roy RN, Polluitz RP, Hamilton JR, et al. (1977). Impaired assimilation of nasojejunal feeds in healthy low-birth weight infants. *J Pediatr,* **90**, 431–434.

17 Beddis I and McKenzie S. (1979). Transpyloric feeding in the very low birthweight (1500 gm and below) infant. *Arch Dis Child,* **54**, 213–217.

18 Whittfield MF. (1980). Transpyloric feeding in infants undergoing intensive care. *Arch Dis Child,* **55**, 571.

19 Lucas A. (1993). Enteral nutrition. In *Nutritional Needs of the Premature Infant,* eds. RC Tsang, A Lucas, R Uauy, et al., pp. 209–223. Baltimore: Williams and Wilkins.

20 Hayhurst EG and Wyman M. (1975). Morbidity associated with prolonged use of polyvinyl feeding tubes. *Am J Dis Child,* **129**, 72–74.

21 Rodriguez JP, Guero J, Frias EG, et al. (1978). Duodenorenal perforation in a neonate by a tube of silicone rubber during transpyloric feeding. *J Pediatr,* **92**, 113–116.

22 Dellagrammaticus HD, Duerden BI and Milner RDG. (1983). Upper intestinal bacterial flora during transpyloric feeding. *Arch Dis Child,* **58**, 115–119.

23 Vazquez C, Arroyos A and Valls A. (1980). Necrotizing enterocolitis: increased incidence in infants receiving nasoduodenal feeding. *Arch Dis Child,* **55**, 826.

24 Pereira GR and Lemons JA. (1981). Controlled study of transpyloric and intermittent gavage feeding in the small preterm infant. *Pediatrics,* **67**, 68–72.

25 Schanler RJ, Schulman RJ, Lau C, et al. (1999). Feeding strategies for premature infants: randomized trial of gastrointestinal priming and tube-feeding method. *Pediatrics,* **103**, 434–439.

26 Lucas A, Bloom SR and Aynsley-Green A. (1986). Gut hormones and "minimal enteral feeding." *Acta Paediatr Scand,* **75**, 719–723.

27 Dunn L, Hulman S, Weiner J, et al. (1988). Beneficial effects of early hypocaloric enteral feeding on neonatal gastrointestinal function: preliminary report of a randomized trial. *J Pediatr,* **112**, 622–629.

28 Slagle TA and Gross SJ. (1988). Effect of early low-volume enteral substrate on subsequent feeding tolerance in very low birth weight infants. *J Pediatr,* **113**, 526–531.

29 Kliegman RM. (1999). Experimental validation of neonatal feeding practices. *Pediatrics,* **103**, 492–493.

30 Schulman RJ, Schanler RJ, Lau C, et al. (1998). Early feeding, antenatal glucocorticoids, and human milk decrease intestinal permeability in preterm infants. *Pediatr Res,* **44**, 519–523.

31 Schulman RJ, Schanler RJ, Laue C, et al. (1998). Early feeding, feeding tolerance, and lactase activity in premature infants. *J Pediatr,* **133**, 645–649.

32 Schanler RJ. (1999). Feeding strategies in premature infants.Presented as a lecture at Advances in Perinatal and Pediatric Nutrition Conference, Stanford University, July. Published in Course Syllabus, pp. 454–461.

33 Moyer-Mileur L and Chan GM. (1986). Nutritional support of very-low birth-weight infants requiring prolonged assisted ventilation. *Am J Dis Child,* **140**, 929–932.

34 Unger A, Goetzman BW, Chan C, et al. (1986). Nutritional

practices and outcome of extremely premature infants. *Am J Dis Child*, **140**, 1027–1033.

35 Gunn T, Reaman G, Outerbridge EW, et al. (1978). Peripheral total parenteral nutrition for premature infants with the respiratory distress syndrome: a controlled study. *J Pediatr*, **92**, 608–613.

36 Yu VYH, James B, Hendry P, et al. (1979). Total parenteral nutrition in very low birthweight infants: a controlled trial. *Arch Dis Child*, **54**, 653–661.

37 Kerner JA, Hattner JAT, Trautman MS, et al. (1988). Postnatal somatic growth in very low birth weight infants on peripheral parenteral nutrition. *J Pediatr Perinat Nutr*, **2**, 27–34.

38 Glass EJ, Hume R, Lang MA, et al. (1984). Parenteral nutrition compared with transpyloric feeding. *Arch Dis Child*, **59**, 131–135.

39 Dryburgh E. (1980). Transpyloric feeding in 49 infants undergoing intensive care. *Arch Dis Child*, **55**, 879–882.

40 Zlotkin SH, Stallings VA and Pencharz PB. (1985). Total parenteral nutrition in children. *Pediatr Clin North Am*, **32**, 381–400.

41 Cashore WJ, Sedaghatian MR and Usher RH. (1975). Nutritional supplements with intravenously administered lipid, protein hydrolysate, and glucose in small premature infants. *Pediatrics*, **56**, 8–16.

42 Churella HR, Bachhuber BS and MacLean WC. (1985). Survey: methods of feeding low-birth-weight infants. *Pediatrics*, **76**, 243–249.

43 Adamkin DA. (1986). Nutrition in very very low birth weight infants. *Clin Perinatol*, **13**, 419–443.

44 Higgs SC, Malan AF and Heese H DeV. (1974). A comparison of oral feeding and total parenteral nutrition in infants of very low birthweight. *S Afr Med J*, **48**, 2169–2173.

45 Hall RT and Rhodes PG. (1976). Total parenteral alimentation via indwelling umbilical catheters in the newborn period. *Arch Dis Child*, **51**, 929–934.

46 Merritt RJ. (1981). Neonatal nutritional support. *Clin Consult Nutr Support*, **1**, 10.

47 Coran AG. (1981). Parenteral nutritional support of the neonate. Tele Session (a group telephone workshop, August 17), Tele Session Corporation, New York.

48 Kerner JA. (1983). The use of umbilical catheters for parenteral nutrition. In *Manual of Pediatric Parenteral Nutntion*, ed. JA Kerner, pp. 303–306. New York: Wiley.

49 Sadig HF. (1987). Broviac catheterization in low birth weight infants: incidence and treatment of associated complications. *Crit Care Med*, **15**, 47–50.

50 Kanarek KS, Kuznicki MB and Blair RC. (1991). Infusion of total parenteral nutrition via the umbilical artery. *J Parenter Enteral Nutr*, **15**, 71–74.

51 Nakamura KT, Sato Y and Erenberg A. (1990). Evaluation of a percutaneously placed 27-gauge central venous catheter in neonates weighing less than 1200 grams. *J Parenter Enteral Nutr*, **14**, 295–299.

52 Abdulla F, Dietrich KA and Pramanik AK. (1990). Percutaneous femoral venous catheterization in preterm neonates. *J Pediatr*, **117**, 788–791.

53 Sunshine P. (1990). Fetal gastrointestinal physiology. In *Assessment and Care of the Fetus: Physiological, Clinical and Medicolegal Principles*, eds. RD Eden and FH Boehm, pp. 93–111. East Norwalk: Appleton & Lange.

54 Koldovsky O, Sunshine P and Kretchmer N. (1966). Cellular migration of intestinal epithelia in suckling and weaned rats. *Nature*, **212**, 1389–1390.

55 Herbst JJ and Sunshine P. (1969). Postnatal development of the small intestine of the rat. *Pediatr Res*, **3**, 27–33.

56 Sunshine P, Herbst JJ, Koldovsky O, et al. (1971). Adaptation of the gastrointestinal tract to extrauterine life. *Ann NY Acad Sci*, **176**, 16–29.

57 Herbst JJ, Sunshine P and Kretchmer N. (1969). Intestinal malabsorption in infancy and childhood. *Adv Pediatr*, **16**, 11–64.

58 Kliegman RM and Fanaroff AN. (1984). Necrotizing enterocolitis. *N Engl J Med*, **310**, 1093–1103.

59 Kosloske AM. (1984). Pathogenesis and prevention of necrotizing enterocolitis: a hypothesis based on personal observation and a review of the literature. *Pediatrics*, **74**, 1086–1092.

60 Brown E and Sweet AY. (1978). Preventing necrotizing enterocolitis in neonates. *JAMA*, **240**, 2452–2454.

61 Frantz ID, L'Heureux P, Engel RR, et al. (1975). Necrotizing enterocolitis. *J Pediatr*, **56**, 259–263.

62 Walsh MC, Kliegman R and Fanaroff A. (1988). Necrotizing enterocolitis: a practitioner's perspective. *Pediatr Rev*, **9**, 219–226.

63 Stoll BJ, Kanto WP Jr, Glass RI, et al. (1980). Epidemiology of necrotizing enterocolitis: a case control study. *J Pediatr*, **96**, 447–451.

64 Moonijian AS, Peckham G, Fox W, et al. (1978). Necrotizing enterocolitis: endemic vs. epidemic. *Pediatr Res*, **12**, 530.

65 Walsh MC and Kliegman RM. (1986). Necrotizing enterocolitis: treatment based on staging criteria. *Pediatr Clin North Am*, **33**, 179–200.

66 Mata AG and Rosenpart RM. (1980). Intraobserver variability in the radiographic diagnosis of necrotizing enterocolitis. *Pediatrics*, **66**, 68–71.

67 Kirschner B, Lahr C and Lahr D. (1980). Detection of increased breath hydrogen in infants with necrotizing enterocolitis. *Gastroenterology*, **72**, A57/1080.

68 Stevenson DK, Shahin SM, Ostrander CR, et al. (1982). Breath hydrogen in preterm infants: correlation with changes in bacterial colonization of the gastrointestinal tract. *J Pediatr*, **101**, 607–610.
69 Garcia J, Smith FR and Cucinelli SA. (1984). Urinary D-lactate in infants with necrotizing enterocolitis. *J Pediatr*, **104**, 268–270.
70 Rivas Y, Solans C and Spivak W. (2000). Serum D-lactic acid level, a new marker for necrotizing enterocolitis. *J Pediatr Gastroenterol Nutr*, **31** (suppl. 2), S236.
71 Bell MJ, Ternberg JL, Feigin RD, et al. (1978). Neonatal necrotizing enterocolitis: therapeutic decisions based upon clinical staging. *Ann Surg*, **187**, 1–7.
72 Kliegman RM, Hack M, Jones P, et al. (1982). Epidemiologic study of necrotizing enterocolitis among low-birth-weight infants: absence of identifiable risk factors. *J Pediatr*, **100**, 440–444.
73 Kerner JA Jr, Hartman GE and Sunshine P. (1985). The medical and surgical management of infants with the short bowel syndrome. *J Perinatol*, **5**, 517–521.
74 Raine PAM. (1995). Neonatal necrotizing enterocolitis. In *Diseases of the Fetus and Newborn*, 2nd edn., eds. GB Reed, AE Claireaux and F Cockburn, pp. 1485–1491. London: Chapman and Hall Medical.
75 Dimmitt RA and Moss RL. (2001). Clinical management of necrotizing enterocolitis. *Neo Rev*, **2**, e110–e117.
76 Israel EJ and Morera C. (2000). Necrotizing enterocolitis. In *Pediatric Gastrointestinal Disease*, 3rd edn., eds. Walker WA, Durie PR, Hamilton JR, et al., pp. 665–676. Ontario, Canada: BC Decker.
77 Eyal F, Sagi E and Avital A. (1982). Necrotizing enterocolitis in the very low birthweight infant: expressed breast milk feeding compared with parenteral feeding. *Arch Dis Child*, **57**, 274–276.
78 Ostertag SG, LaGamma EF, Reisen CE, et al. (1986). Early enteral feeding does not affect the incidence of necrotizing enterocolitis. *Pediatrics*, **77**, 275–280.
79 Krousop RW. (1980). The influences of feeding practices. In *Necrotizing Enterocolitis*, eds. EG Brown and AY Sweet, p. 57. New York: Grune and Stratton.
80 Book LS, Herbst JJ and Jung AL. (1976). Comparison of fast-and-slow feeding rate schedules to the development of necrotizing enterocolitis. *J Pediatr*, **89**, 463–466.
81 Goldman HI. (1980). Feeding and necrotizing enterocolitis. *Am J Dis Child*, **134**, 553–555.
82 Anderson DM, Rome ES and Kliegman RM. (1985). Relationship of endemic necrotizing enterocolitis to alimentation. *Pediatr Res*, **19**, 331A.
83 Book LS, Herbst JJ and Jung AL. (1976). Carbohydrate malabsorption in necrotizing enterocolitis. *Pediatrics*, **57**, 201–204.
84 Sweet AY. (1980). Necrotizing enterocolitis: feeding the neonate weighing less than 1500 grams – nutrition and beyond. In *Report of the 79th Ross Conference on Pediatnc Research*, ed. P Sunshine. Columbus, Ohio: Ross Products Division.
85 DeLemos RA, Rogers JH and McLaughlin GW. (1974). Experimental production of necrotizing enterocolitis in newborn goats. *Pediatr Res*, **8**, 380.
86 Book LS, Herbst JJ, Atherton SO, et al. (1975). Necrotizing enterocolitis in low-birth-weight infants fed an elemental formula. *J Pediatr*, **87**, 602–605.
87 Willis DM, Chabot J, Radde IC, et al. (1977). Unsuspected hyperosmolality of oral solutions contributing to necrotizing enterocolitis in very-low-birth weight infants. *Pediatrics*, **60**, 535–538.
88 AAP Committee on Nutrition. (1976). Commentary on breast feeding and infant formulas including proposed standards for formulas. *Pediatrics*, **57**, 278–285.
89 White KC and Harkavy KZ. (1982). Hypertonic formula resulting from added oral medications. *Am J Dis Child*, **136**, 931–933.
90 Ernst JA, Williams JM and Glick MR. (1983). Osmolality of substances used in the intensive care nursery. *Pediatrics*, **72**, 347–352.
91 Barnard J, Greene H and Cotton R. (1983). Necrotizing enterocolitis. In *Nutritional Adaptation of the Gastrointestinal Tract of the Newborn*, eds. N Kretchmer and A Minkowski, pp. 103–128. *Nestle Nutrition*, vol. 3. New York: Raven.
92 Udall JN. (1990). Gastrointestinal host defense and necrotizing enterocolitis. *J Pediatr*, **117**, 33–43.
93 Eibl MM, Wolf HM, Furnkranz H, et al. (1988). Prevention of necrotizing enterocolitis in lowbirth-weight infants by IgA-lgG feeding. *N Engl J Med*, **319**, 1–7.
94 Barlow B, Santulli TV, Heird WC, et al. (1974). An experimental study of acute neonatal necrotizing enterocolitis – the importance of breast milk. *J Pediatr Surg*, **9**, 587–595.
95 Reisner SH and Garty B. (1977). Necrotizing enterocolitis despite breast-feeding. *Lancet*, **ii**, 507.
96 Kliegman RM, Pittard WB and Fanaroff AA. (1979). Necrotizing enterocolitis in neonates fed human milk. *J Pediatr*, **95**, 450–453.
97 Stevenson DK, Yang C, Kerner JA, et al. (1985). Intestinal flora in the second week of life in hospitalized preterm infants fed stored frozen breast milk or a proprietary formula. *Clin Pediatr*, **24**, 338–341.
98 Lucas A and Cole TJ. (1990). Breast milk and neonatal necrotising enterocolitis. *Lancet*, **336**, 1519–1523.

99 Neu J. (1996). Necrotizing enterocolitis: the search for a unifying pathogenic theory leading to prevention. *Pediatr Clin North Am*, **43**, 409–432.

100 Kliegman RM and Fanaroff AA. (1981). Neonatal necrotizing enterocolitis: a nine-year experience: epidemiology and uncommon observations. *Am J Dis Child*, **135**, 603–614.

101 Lehmiller DH and Kanto WF. (1978). Relationship of mesenteric thromboembolism, oral feeding and necrotizing enterocolitis. *J Pediatr*, **92**, 96–100.

102 Hillman LS, Goodwin SL and Sherman WR. (1975). Identification and measurement of plasticiser in neonatal tissues after umbilical catheters and blood products. *N Engl J Med*, **292**, 381–386.

103 Touloukian RJ, Kadaw A and Spencer RP. (1973). The gastrointestinal complications of umbilical venous exchange transfusion: a clinical and experimental study. *Pediatrics*, **51**, 36–42.

104 Davey AM, Wagner CL, Cox C, et al. (1994). Feeding premature infants while low umbilical artery catheters are in place: a prospective, randomized trial. *J Pediatr*, **124**, 795–799.

105 Johnson L, Bowen FW, Abbasi S, et al. (1985). Relationship of prolonged pharmacologic serum levels of vitamin E to incidence of sepsis and necrotizing enterocolitis in infants with birth weight 1500 grams or less. *Pediatrics*, **75**, 619–638.

106 Kerner JA, Poole RL, Sunshine P, et al. (1987). High serum vitamin E levels in premature infants receiving MVI-Pediatric. *J Pediatr Perinat Nutr*, **1**, 75–82.

107 Neu J, Masi M, Stevenson DK, et al. (1981). Effects of asphyxia and oral gentamicin on intestinal lactase in the suckling rat. *Pediatr Pharmacol*, **1**, 215–220.

108 Czyrko C, Del Pin CA, O'Neill JA Jr, et al. (1991). Maternal cocaine abuse and necrotizing enterocolitis: outcome and survival. *J Pediatr Surg*, **26**, 414–418.

109 Lopez SL. (1995). Time of onset of necrotizing enterocolitis in newborn infants with known prenatal cocaine exposure. *Clin Pediatr*, **34**, 424.

110 Bauer CR, Morrison JC, Poole WK, et al. (1984). A decreased incidence of necrotizing enterocolitis after prenatal glucocorticoid therapy. *Pediatrics*, **73**, 682–688.

111 Halac E, Halac J, Begue EF, et al. (1990). Prenatal and postnatal corticosteroid therapy to prevent neonatal necrotizing enterocolitis: a controlled trial. *J Pediatr*, **117**, 132–138.

112 Muguruma K, Gray PW, Tjoelker LW, et al. (1997). The central role of PAF in necrotizing enterocolitis development. *Adv Exp Med Biol*, **407**, 379–382.

113 Thebaud B, Lacaze-Masmonteil T and Watterberg K. (2001). Postnatal glucocorticoids in very preterm infants: "the good, the bad, and the ugly." *Pediatrics*, **107**, 413–415.

114 Crissinger KD. (2001). Pathogenesis of necrotizing enterocolitis. Workshop presented at the 25th Clinical Congress of A.S.P.E.N. Program Book, pp. 203–204. Chicago, IL: Clinical Congress of the American Society for Parenteral and Enteral Nutrition.

115 Crissinger K. (1999). Understanding necrotizing enterocolitis – promising directions. *Pathophysiology*, **5**, 247–256.

116 Kliegman R, Walker W, Yolken R. (1993). Necrotizing enterocolitis research agenda for a disease of unknown etiology and pathogenesis. *Pediatr Res*, **34**, 701–708.

117 Caplan MS and Jilling T. (2001). The pathophysiology of necrotizing enterocolitis. *Neo Rev*, **2**, e103–e109.

118 Rabinowitz SS, Dzakpasu P, Piecuch S, et al. (2001). Platelet-activating factor in infants at risk for necrotizing enterocolitis. *J Pediatr*, **138**, 81–86.

119 Gonzalez-Crussi F and Hsueh W. (1983). Experimental model of ischemic bowel necrosis. The role of platelet activating factor and endotoxin. *Am J Pathol*, **112**, 127–135.

120 Chang H, Gonzalez-Crussi F, Hsueh W, et al. (2000). Prevention of experimental necrotizing enterocolitis with intestinal trefoil factor (ITF). *Gastroenterology*, **118**, A197.

121 Becker RM, Wue G, Galanko JA, et al. (2000). Reduced serum amino acid concentrations in infants with necrotizing enterocolitis. *J Pediatr*, **137**, 785–793.

122 Caplan MS, Miller-Catchpole R, Kaup S, et al. (1999). Bifidobacterial supplementation reduces the incidence of necrotizing enterocolitis in a neonatal rat model. *Gastroenterology*, **117**, 577–583.

123 Butel MJ, Roland N, Hilbert A, et al. (1998). Clostridial pathogenicity in experimental necrotizing enterocolitis in gnotobiotic quails and protective role of bifidobacteria. *J Med Microbiol*, **47**, 391–399.

124 Catala I, Butel MJ, Bensaada M, et al. (1999). Oligofructose contributes to the protective role of bifidobacteria in experimental necrotizing enterocolitis in quails. *J Med Microbiol*, **48**, 89–94.

125 Carlson SE, Montalto MB, Ponder DL, et al. (1998). Lower incidence of necrotizing enterocolitis in infants fed a preterm formula with egg phospholipids. *Pediatr Res*, **44**, 491–498.

126 Sonntag J, Grimmer I, Scholz T, et al. (2000). Growth and neurodevelopmental outcome of very low birthweight infants with necrotizing enterocolitis. *Acta Paediatr*, **89**, 528–532.

127 Vohr BR, Wright LL, Dusick AM, et al. (2000). Neurodevelopmental and functional outcomes of extremely low birthweight infants in the National Institute

of Child Health and Human Developmental Neonatal Research Network, 1993–1994. *Pediatrics,* **105**, 1216–1226.

128 Akisu M, Baka M, Coker I, et al. (1998). Effect of dietary *n*-3 fatty acids on hypoxia-induced necrotizing enterocolitis in young mice. *n*-3 fatty acids alter platelet-activating factor and leukotriene B_4 production in the intestine. *Biol Neonate,* **74**, 31–38.

129 Rayyis SF, Ambalavanan N, Wright L, et al. (1999). Randomized trial of "slow" versus "fast" feed advancements on the incidence of necrotizing enterocolitis in very low birth weight infants. *J Pediatr,* **134**, 293–297.

130 La Gamma E and Browne L. (1994). Feeding practices for infants less than 1500 grams at birth and the pathogenesis of necrotizing enterocolitis. *Clin Perinatol,* **21**, 271–306.

131 Brown E and Sweet A. (1982). Neonatal necrotizing enterocolitis. *Pediatr Clin North Am,* **29**, 114–170.

132 Quan R, Yang C, Rubinstein S, et al. (1994). The effect of nutritional additives on anti-infective factors in human milk. *Clin Pediatr,* **33**, 325–328.

133 Aynsley-Green A. (1985). Metabolic and endocrine interrelation in the human fetus and neonate. *Am J Clin Nutr,* **41**, 399–417.

134 Feng JJ, Kwong LK, Kerner JA, et al. (1987). Resumption of intestinal maturation upon reintroduction of intraluminal nutrients: functional and biochemical correlations. *Clin Res,* **35**, 228A.

135 Mascarenhas MR, Kerner JA Jr and Stallings VA. (2000). Parenteral and enteral nutrition. In *Pediatric Gastrointestinal Disease,* 3rd ed, eds. Walker WA, Durie PR, Hamilton JR, et al., pp. 1705–1752. Ontario, Canada: BC Decker.

136 Zenk KE, Sills JH and Koeppel RM. (2000). *Neonatal Medications and Nutrition: A Comprehensive Guide,* 2nd edn, pp. 527–528. Santa Rosa, CA: NICU Ink Book.

PART VI

Assessing the Outcome of the Asphyxiated Infant

Assessment of preterm infants' neurobehavioral functioning: reliability, validity, normative data, and prediction to age two

Anneliese F. Korner

Stanford University School of Medicine, Palo Alto, CA, USA

Back in 1977, we began to develop a neurobehavioral assessment for preterm infants that would allow us to measure the effects of a longitudinal, randomized, controlled intervention study[1] with preterm infants. In designing our assessment procedure we started from the premise that the most relevant and important goal of any intervention would be to facilitate the normality of the infants' developmental course so that their maturity and ultimate development would not be too discrepant from that of full-term newborns within the normal range.[2] Therefore, to assess the effects of our intervention, our prime objective was to use an instrument that could measure the differential maturity of functioning of randomly assigned experimental and control groups of preterm infants.

At the time, only very few assessments existed that measured the neurobehavioral maturity of premature newborns. Most of the ones available were techniques that measured gestational age and they were applicable only to infants within the first week after birth (e.g., Robinson,[3] Dubowitz et al.,[4] and Finnström[5]). The only assessments available in 1977 for measuring longitudinally the maturity of functioning of preterm infants were those by Amiel-Tison[6] and Saint-Anne Dargassies.[7]

Although these French neonatal neurologists systematically assessed and documented the maturational course of neural functions of preterm infants aged 28 weeks postconception to term, they illustrated and scored the age differences in infant functioning only in 2-week increments. Since it was unrealistic to expect gains of 2 weeks or more in the performance of the experimental group as a result of our intervention, we decided we needed to develop a more sensitive and fine-grained procedure that could measure more subtle differences in functioning between the two groups.

The pilot version of the Neurobehavioral Assessment of the Preterm Infant

In developing our procedure we relied most heavily on test items from the Amiel-Tison examination.[6] Also included in the test were a few items from the Prechtl and Beintema[8] and the Brazelton[9] assessments. We devised a scoring system that potentially could discriminate the level of preterm performance in 1-week increments.

Results from the preliminary version of the Neurobehavioural Assessment of the Preterm Infant (NAPI) revealed that this assessment was sufficiently sensitive to discriminate between the experimental and control groups.[1] Randomly assigned infants raised on gently oscillating waterbeds, examined by a neurologically trained pediatrician who was blind to the infants' group status, demonstrated that infants in the experimental group performed significantly better in the following: motorically they were more mature, they were less irritable, they were twice as often in the visually alert, inactive state and were more able to attend and pursue visual and auditory stimuli than were controls.[1] The NAPI also had good test–retest reliability in a number of important functions, and interobserver reliability was readily established. These results prompted us further to develop the NAPI for general use.

To accomplish this task we decided to proceed with a unique approach that had never been tried before in developing neonatal assessment procedures. Most often, the reliability and validity of a procedure, if assessed at all, were evaluated only after the test development was completed. This after-the-fact approach has most frequently led to disappointing results. We chose instead to investigate the reliability and developmental validity of all items and clusters of items before we included them in the final version of the procedure.

Description of our approach to developing the NAPI

Conceptual framework

In revising the preliminary version of the NAPI, we limited our selection of test items to those that promised to show reliable developmental changes over time as suggested by prior studies (e.g., Amiel-Tison;[6] Brandt[10]). In line with our goal of developing a maturity assessment, we devised a numerical scoring system in which all item scores ranged from the least to the most mature responses. Also, rather than including in the procedure a collection of maneuvers commonly used, but whose developmental significance seemed unclear, we made it our first priority to include in the assessment only conceptually and clinically meaningful test items. Additionally, we excluded commonly used stressful maneuvers such as the Moro and pinprick and any item that required instrumentation or elaborate equipment. This was done to make sure that the assessment could be used widely in different clinical settings. Once the item selection was completed, they were grouped into conceptually and statistically cohesive clusters.

Statistical approach

We next established a priori guidelines for all statistical analyses which subsequently were adhered to at all times. These were used to explore the psychometric properties of the procedure. Thus, before incorporating any items or clusters into the procedure, their test–retest reliability, their redundance, and their developmental validity were assessed. Any of the test items or clusters failing to have a test–retest reliability of 0.60 on two consecutive days, or that were not showing significant developmental changes over several weeks were dropped from the procedure.

In the process of the test development of the NAPI, 179 preterm infants participated on whom 354 examinations were performed.[11]

Replication and validation study of the NAPI

For this study, an independent cohort of 290 preterm infants were recruited on whom 553 examinations were performed. For this sample, the test–retest reliability and the developmental validity were again assessed.[12]

Description of the NAPI

Following the methodological and statistical approach described above, we managed to develop a psychometrically reliable and developmentally valid assessment procedure for measuring the maturity of preterm infants.

Subjects

To recruit as representative a sample of preterm infants as was feasible, infants were picked from both tertiary and intermediate care nurseries from four Bay Area hospitals and one nursery in Portland, Oregon. Also, in order to generate results that would be representative of preterm infants in general, exclusion criteria for the subjects in the two independent cohorts were kept to an absolute minimum. Excluded were infants whose gestational age estimates were discrepant from each other by more than 2 weeks. The four gestational age estimates used were the mother's and obstetrician's estimated dates of confinement (EDC), the gestational age assessment by Ballard et al.,[13] the infant's head circumference[14] and, when available, an ultrasound examination. To reduce further potential errors in gestational age estimates, the most commonly available estimates (EDC and Ballard) of the eligible infants were averaged. The only other infants excluded were those who had diagnoses suggesting central nervous system damage, such as known grade III and IV intraventricular hemorrhages, persistent seizures, disseminated herpes, or severe asphyxia at birth. Data for the two independent cohorts were collected between 1983 and 1989. Informed consent for the infants' inclusion in the studies was obtained from one or both parents.

The examination

The NAPI is applicable to medically stable infants from 32 weeks postconceptional age to term, who are on room air and free of intravenous lines and gastric tubes. To obtain a reliable picture of the babies' performance, we made a rule that examiners should delay testing infants after stressful medical procedures such as circumcision, blood transfusions, or eye examinations. Since both low and high temperatures can be harmful to infants and also adversely affect their performance, they were examined in an appropriately heated incubator or under an overhead warmer. Scoring was done immediately after each item was presented, to facilitate the examiners' recall of the exact details of the infants' responses.

Because preterm infants have a relatively small neurobehavioral repertoire, most of the test items in the assessment necessarily overlap with those used in other neurobehavioral examinations. The NAPI differs primarily in the developmental rationale underlying the choice of the test items, in the scoring system, and in the statistical approach to establishing the test's reliability and developmental validity.

One of our most important decisions was to use a strictly invariant sequence of item presentation, a sequence that was designed to bring about the kinds of behavioral states that are most likely to elicit the best possible responses from preterm infants. Although we were keenly aware of the fact that infants' states strongly influence their responses,[15] we found empirically that, with young preterm infants, the requirement of a predetermined state before administering each item was not feasible. An attempt to achieve the appropriate predetermined state through various rousing or soothing maneuvers would have greatly prolonged the examination, fatigued the infant, or failed altogether. For this reason, we chose to build into the assessment a standard sequence of rousing, soothing, and alerting items that would maximize the chance of testing the various functions in appropriate states and would minimize the need to intervene with some infants more than with others.

To illustrate, we try to rouse the infants who, for the most part, are asleep when we begin the examination approximately 45 min before they are fed, by administering the scarf sign and the arm and leg recoil. Items like the popliteal angle, ventral suspension, head lift, and spontaneous crawling can then be tested in more awake states. All infants are then swaddled to calm those who have become irritable. The rotation test is then administered in preparation for modified Brazelton[9] orientation items, as we had found in earlier studies[16,17] that the vestibular-proprioceptive stimulation entailed in moving the infants predictably produced visual alertness. This approach of a standard sequence of item presentation prevents the examination from becoming a different procedure for each infant and guarantees that the examination is comparable from one infant to the next. This strategy also provided the opportunity to study systematically the age changes in the infants' states in response to a standard sequence of identical events.[18]

Table 40.1 shows the flow of the examination.

After completing the examination, summary ratings are made regarding the number and quality of the infant's spontaneous movements, irritability and vigor of crying, and quality and duration of

Table 40.1. Neurobehavioral Assessment of the Preterm Infant (NAPI) test items and the sequence of their presentation

State rating	Remove cover and clothing
State rating	Scarf sign
State rating	Leg resistance and recoil
State rating	Forearm resistance and recoil
State rating	Popliteal angle
State rating	Ventral suspension
Prone head raising	
Spontaneous crawling	
State rating	Dress infant, observe power of active movements
State rating	Swaddle infant
State rating	Rotation test
Response to:	
Inanimate auditory stimulation	
Inanimate auditory and visual stimulation	
Animate auditory stimulation	
Animate visual and auditory stimulation	
State rating	Ratings of quality and duration of visual alertness
Place infant on examining table	
State rating	Observe infant's movements for 1 minute
State rating	

Table 40.2. Test–retest reliability

Dimensions	Cohort I (n=30)	Cohort II (n=55)
Motor development and vigor	0.59	0.70
Scarf sign	0.86	0.85
Popliteal angle	0.90	0.85
Alertness and orientation	0.77	0.60
Vigor of crying	0.72	0.67
Irritability	0.60	0.63
Percent asleep ratings	0.69	0.51

Note: All correlations of test–retest reliabilities were significant at $P<0.0001$

Table 40.3. Interobserver reliabilities

Dimensions	Cohort I (n=30)	Cohort II (n=48)
Motor development and vigor	0.95	0.84
Scarf sign	0.74	0.93
Popliteal angle	0.97	0.83
Alertness and orientation	0.97	0.98
Vigor of crying	0.89	0.64
Irritability	0.76	0.82
Percent asleep ratings	0.96	0.92

Note: Interobserver reliabilities of all original and replicated dimensions were significantly different from 0 at $P<0.0001$

alertness during the entire assessment. Also rated is the degree of arousal with which the infant responded to the stimulation provided by the assessment. All test item scores are then converted to scores ranging from 0 to 100, with 0 representing the least and 100 representing the most mature responses. The process of numerically summing up the test results takes less than 10 min.

Our methodological and statistical approach resulted in a relatively brief and gentle instrument consisting of seven reliable and developmentally valid clusters or single-item neurobehavioral dimensions that represent a conceptually and clinically meaningful spectrum of preterm functions.[19] These dimensions, which contain 27 subitems, are:

- Motor development and vigor
- Scarf sign
- Popliteal angle
- Alertness and orientation
- Vigor of crying
- Irritability
- Percent asleep ratings

Table 40.2 shows the test–retest Spearman correlations of the seven neurobehavioral dimensions in the two independent cohorts.

On an ongoing basis, the interobserver reliabilities were also assessed in the two independent cohorts. The Spearman correlations obtained are displayed in Table 40.3.

In exploring the developmental validity of the NAPI, we longitudinally assessed 52 infants from cohort I and 79 infants from cohort II (Table 40.4).

Table 40.4. Developmental validity of the seven neurobehavioral dimensions

Dimensions	Cohort I (n=52) Effect size	Cohort II (n=79) Effect size
Motor development and vigor	7.57****	9.15****
Scarf sign	6.69****	13.7****
Popliteal angle	5.44****	9.49****
Alertness and orientation	2.35*	2.98***
Vigor of crying	5.72****	4.80****
Irritability	7.76****	2.85**
Percent asleep ratings	−3.94*	−2.78**

Notes: * $P<0.05$; ** $P<0.01$; *** $P<0.005$; **** $P<0.0001$.

Testing was done in weekly intervals over a period of 3 weeks or more. We found that the average performance on each of the seven dimensions improved significantly with age. The scores of each variable increased with age except for the percent asleep ratings during the examination, which decreased.[12]

Additionally, and in consultation with Professor Lee Cronbach, we were able to establish normative guidelines for preterm infants spanning from 32 through 37 week postconceptional age. As we had hoped, the means and medians of the converted scores for each function showed week-to-week age changes in the expected direction. The normative guidelines also included standard deviations of infant performance in each of the seven neurobehavioral dimensions at each age. This information can be used to identify consistent lags in performance over time. The normative data also permit developing a profile of the infant's performance at each age, reflecting special strengths and weaknesses of different functions and how these change over time.

Clearly, these normative guidelines must be used judiciously, particularly in clinical contexts. Preterm infants are a very heterogeneous group whose performance is readily influenced by variability in infant health status. It is therefore important to use the normative guidelines primarily to identify infants who, on repeated examinations, show developmental lags, so that appropriate follow-up and remedial intervention can be instituted.

The clinical validity of the NAPI

Even though we had established the test–retest and interobserver reliabilities and the developmental validity of the NAPI, we did not as yet know whether or not this instrument was sufficiently sensitive to detect the impact of adverse perinatal and/or postnatal medical complications on infant performance. To find out, we developed the Neonatal Medical Index (NMI).[20] Because severe illness usually weakens an organism, we hypothesized that test items requiring infant vigor and strength would be affected by prior medical complications, whereas other functions might be unaffected. Based on the data from 471 infants, the results of this study clearly supported this hypothesis. Infants' scores in motor development and vigor, irritability, and vigor of crying were significantly reduced in infants with a history of severe illness. The results of this study, as displayed in Table 40.5, thus clearly confirmed the clinical validity of the NAPI.

The discriminatory power of the NMI was not only seen in this study, but it was confirmed in a predictive external validation study.[21] In this study, we had the opportunity to use the preexisting data from the eight-site Infant Health and Development Program.[22] The data from this study indicated that the NMI predicted later Bayley cognitive and motor development, and that in infants born at less than 1500 g, the effects of neonatal medical complications persisted at least until the subjects were 3 years old.

Since the time we had used the NMI for our clinical validity study of the NAPI and for predicting later development in the Infant Health and Development Program,[22] other investigators have begun to use the NMI for different purposes. Brown et al.[23] have used it to describe the characteristics of their study population. It has also been used as an outcome measure in an intervention study by Anand et al.[24] Randomly

Table 40.5. Effect of Neonatal Medical Index on neurobehavioral dimensions[a]

Neurobehavioral dimensions	t-test[b]	Expected differences in scores between NMI = V and NMI = I
Motor development and vigor	−3.74**	−10.15
Scarf sign	1.20	3.55
Popliteal angle	−0.64	−2.94
Alertness and orientation	0.20	0.78
Vigor of crying	−5.02***	−26.90
Irritability	−3.63*	−13.32
Percent asleep ratings	−0.79	−4.15

Notes:

[a] Based on the regression coefficient for each dimension (as percent from lowest to higher possible score) regression Neonatal Medical Index (NMI) score (I–V) with conceptional age as a second independent variable.

[b] *t*-test from the linear regression of each specific dimension on NMI and conceptional age; degrees of freedom for error ranged from 392 to 468, varying due to missing values for some dimension; r^2 varied from 0.06 to 0.16, $P<0.001$, for the analysis of each dimension.

* $P<0.0003$; ** $P<0.0002$; *** $P<0.0001$.

Source: Reproduced from Korner et al.[20] with permission.

assigned infants in the experimental group who had not differed in health status at birth from the control group showed significantly better NMIs at hospital discharge after being sedated during ventilatory care. A 15-site replication study of the results of Anand et al. is now in progress.

Description of the NMI

In developing the NMI, we sought to produce a simple classification system that, at the time of hospital discharge, would summarize in bold strokes the medical course of preterm infants. The NMI was designed to measure how ill the infants were during their hospital stay and was not intended to provide a complete inventory of all the different complications and symptoms the infants had experienced. The few components of the NMI were selected because of their clinical salience and their ready availability on brief chart reviews.

NMI classifications range from I to V, with I describing preterm infants free of significant past medical problems and V characterizing infants with the most serious complications. NMI classification is based on two overarching principles:

1. infants with birth weights more than 1000 g who experienced no major medical complications are assigned NMI classifications of I or II. Infants born at less than 1000 g or heavier babies who had experienced major medical complications receive NMI classifications of III, IV, or V.
2. the need and duration of mechanically assisted ventilation required (ventilatory care or intubation on continuous positive airway pressure (CPAP), or mask or nasal CPAP).

The choice of the assisted ventilation classification principle was based on the rationale that, with a few exceptions, the duration of assisted ventilation would be dictated by the length and severity of illness and/or complications.

The following are the criteria for classifying the NMI:

I. Birth weight greater than 1000 g; free of respiratory distress and other major medical complications; no oxygen required; absence of apnea or bradycardia; allowable complications are benign heart murmur and need for phototherapy.

II. Birth weight more than 1000 g; assisted ventilation for 48 hours or less and/or oxygen required for 1 day or more; no periventricular hemorrhage–intraventricular hemorrhage (PVH–IVH); allowable complications are occasional apnea and/or bradycardia not requiring theophylline or related drugs; patent ductus arteriosus (PDA) not requiring medication such as indometacin.

III. Assisted ventilation for 3–14 days and/or any conditions listed under III below.

IV. Assisted ventilation for 15–28 days and/or any conditions listed under IV below.

V. Assisted ventilation for 29 days or more and/or any conditions listed under V below.

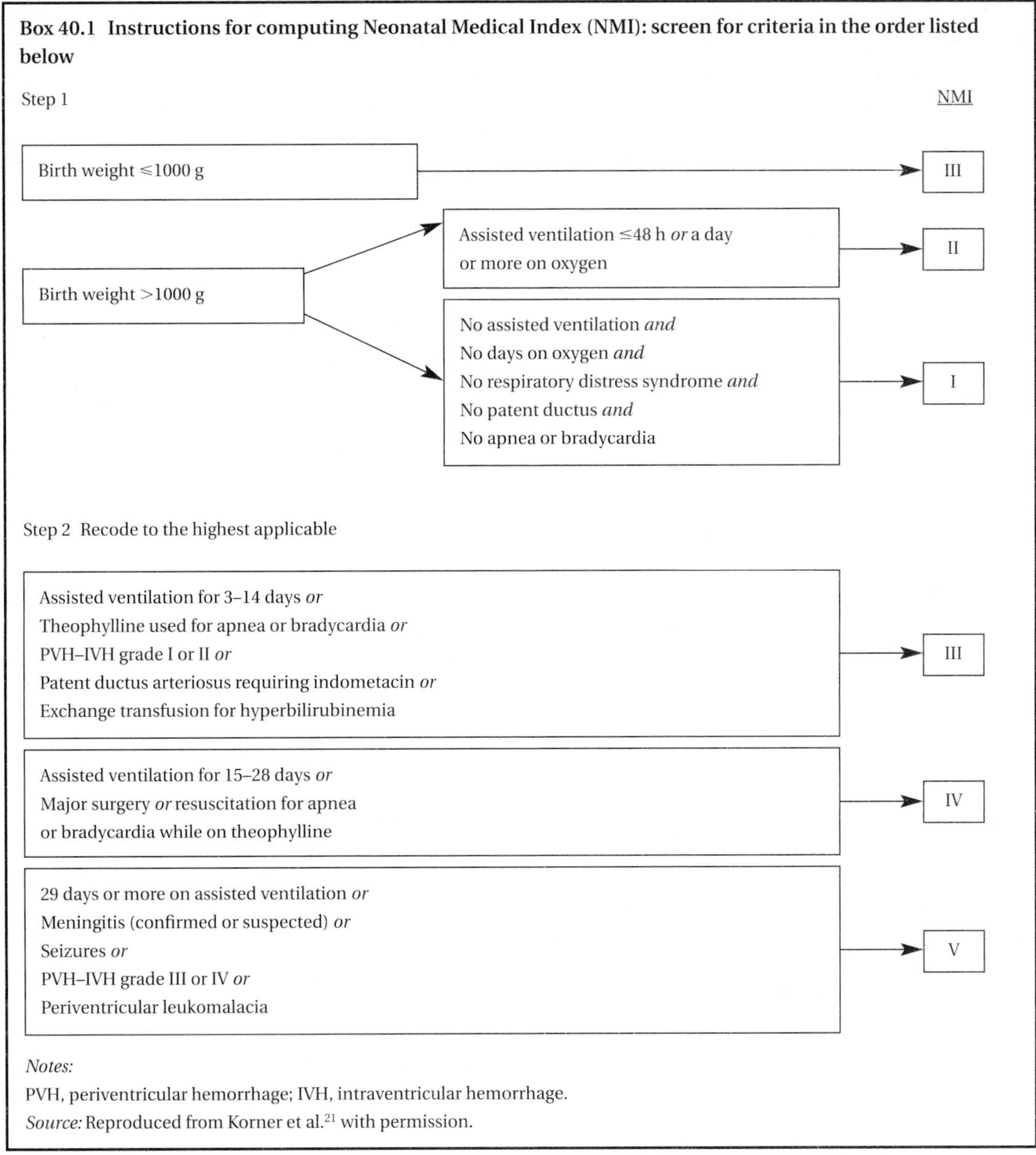

Box 40.1 Instructions for computing Neonatal Medical Index (NMI): screen for criteria in the order listed below

Notes:
PVH, periventricular hemorrhage; IVH, intraventricular hemorrhage.
Source: Reproduced from Korner et al.[21] with permission.

Conditions requiring a classification of III, IV, or V, regardless of length of time on assisted ventilation

III. Birth weight less than 1000 g; PVH-IVH grade I or II; apnea and/or bradycardia requiring theophylline; PDA requiring indometacin; hyperbilirubinemia requiring exchange transfusion.

IV. Resuscitation needed for apnea or bradycardia while on theophylline; major surgery including PDA (exclude hernias, testicular torsion).

V. Meningitis confirmed or suspected; seizures; PVH–IVH grade III or IV; periventricular leukomalacia.

All of the above criteria for NMI classifications apply to appropriate, small- and large-for-gestational-age infants. Box 40.1 displays the algorithm with a set of instructions to compute the NMI.

The predictive validity of the NAPI

When we developed the NAPI, our only goal was to test the differential maturity of preterm infants who, in an intervention study, had been randomly assigned to experimental and control groups. Although we hoped that the NAPI would identify infants at special risk for developmental delays, we did not expect to find any predictive validity of the test. We held this view because the functions assessed at early ages differ from those tested later. Also, we knew that the different socioeconomic and familial circumstances in which children are raised would strongly impact on their development.[25,26] We were therefore surprised when a number of investigators using the NAPI discovered both the short- and longer-term predictive validity of the test.

Dittrichová et al.[27] found that NAPI scores at 36 weeks postconceptional age correlated significantly with Bayley score[28] and a neurological examination at 3 months corrected age. Constantinou et al.[29] reported significant Spearman correlations between the NAPI administered at 36 weeks postconception and 2-year Bayley score[28] ranging from 0.53 to 0.75. A longitudinal study with over 100 infants is now in progress that will test whether or not the predictive validity of the NAPI found in the pilot study can be replicated. Also, Constantinou et al.[30] predicted to the Bayley Infant Neurodevelopmental Screener[31] from the NAPI administered at 36 weeks postconception. Furthermore, in her current longitudinal study of very-low-birth-weight preterm infants, Constantinou is finding that the NAPI administered at 36 weeks postconception predicts well to 18 months cognitive and motor development – far better, in fact, than does a magnetic resonance imaging scan taken at the same age (personal communication, 22 December 2000).

Using the NAPI, Sampers and Caldwell[32] did a study that identified early predictors of poor motor outcome in extremely premature infants. These investigators are now testing the hypothesis that these early indicators may predict later cerebral palsy.

And finally, Newham,[33] in her Australian longitudinal study, predicted cognitive and temperamental characteristics at 1 and 2 years of age from preterm NAPI performance.

The question arises: why does the NAPI predict later behavioral development, particularly since most neonatal assessments predict poorly subsequent childhood functioning? Why is the NAPI predictive, even though early age-specific functions are not necessarily related to those tested at a later time?

Four possible explanations come to mind:

1. The NAPI may tap into basic biological givens which may persist, expressing themselves in later development despite the attenuating impact of the different socioeconomic and familial circumstances in which children are raised.
2. The NAPI does not contain any items or cluster of items that do not have high day-to-day stability. Without an adequate test–retest reliability, any examination may generate scores that are little more than random numbers.
3. By using a strictly invariant sequence of item presentation containing standard rousing, soothing, and alerting maneuvers, we managed to avoid having to intervene with some infants more than with others, thus making the examination comparable from one baby to the next. In this way each infant was exposed to a standard sequence of identical events.
4. We did not examine our subjects before they were 1 week old. This decision was made for two reasons. Clinically, preterm infants in the first week of life are often medically too precarious to be tested. Developmentally, neonates, during the first few days after birth, must make more numerous and more radical adaptations than at any other time in their lives in the transition from intrauterine to extrauterine functioning. Such dramatic changes surely must create behavioral instability immediately after birth.

Any or all of the above strategies may have enhanced the predictive power of the NAPI.

External validation of the NAPI norms

When we established the normative guidelines in 1989, we were concerned about whether or not they would hold up over time. With neonatal medical care evolving, we feared that our norms would no longer apply. Also, even though we collected our data in four different Bay Area hospital nurseries and at one site in Portland, Oregon, there was always a chance that our data were not representative of preterm infants in general. Furthermore, reports from multi-site studies usually indicate significant site effects which diminish the clarity of the results. Because of these concerns, we were surprised to find that the performance of Czech preterm infants tested at 36 weeks postconception did not differ significantly and was, in fact, almost identical to that of our American samples.[27]

Brown et al.[23] also externally validated our norms. No significant differences were found between the performance of northern Californian and Oregon babies and black preterm infants in Atlanta, Georgia.

As a result of these findings, an international collaboration is now in progress to determine whether or not our norms will hold up in additional sites.

Limitations of the NAPI

The most important constraint shared by all investigators of developmental processes is the common uncertainty of their subjects' gestational age at birth. Not infrequently, gestational age estimates vary by 3 weeks or more. In our studies we have tried to cope with this problem by excluding all infants whose gestational age estimates varied by more than 2 weeks. This resulted in a great loss of eligible subjects.

Another very serious constraint that is also shared by anyone assessing the performance of neonates is that the result from one examination alone may not be fully representative of an infant's capabilities. It is highly desirable therefore to assess infants more than once, but this is not always feasible in clinical or research contexts.

While the NAPI can highlight gross neurological deficits, it is not primarily a neurological assessment. Any neurologically suspect evidence from the NAPI examination should, however, be used to refer an infant for a complete neurological workup.

Although the NAPI was standardized on preterm infants, several investigators have begun to use it with full-term neonates. Hopefully, normative guidelines will eventually be established for these babies.

NAPI training

Potentially, any professional caring for or studying preterm infants in an intensive or intermediary care nursery is eligible to become a NAPI examiner. The training consists of two major and equally important components: achieving reliability of administering the examination and achieving reliability of scoring. Prior experience in handling young preterm infants and knowing about the medical problems and physiological stress reactions commonly seen in preterms is essential.

The NAPI kit contains, among other things, a manual of instructions and a training video tape. To become a qualified examiner, it is essential to view the training tape repeatedly to learn exactly how the examination should be administered. It is especially important to learn the sequence and flow of the examination as well as the standard, slowly paced, gentle method of handling an infant, a method that differs in certain respects from that used in other assessments. Adherence to the standard examination technique is essential, not only to minimize infant stress but also to elicit infant responses within the range of those obtained during the standardization of the assessment.

The training period includes practice in administering and scoring the examination of approximately 20 preterm infants of various postconceptional ages, with reviewing the training tape, and rereading the manual between assessments as needed. To complete the training, the reliability of administration and scoring should be evaluated by a qualified teacher of the assessment.

Diverse uses of the NAPI

Having established a reliable and developmentally and clinically valid neonatal assessment procedure, this instrument can be and has been used to address a wide variety of research and clinical issues. Examples are:

- Evaluating the effects of intervention, clinical trials, or changes in medical care.[1,34]
- Studying the behavioral differences between addicted babies and controls.[23,35–37]
- Assessing the development of small-for-gestational-age babies, and infants of diabetic mothers.
- Identifying persistent lags in the development of specific infant functions.
- Monitoring the developmental progress of individual infants.
- Generating normative data that describe the gradual unfolding of the behavioral repertoire of preterm infants as they grow to term.[19,38]
- Studying basic questions about the development of preterm infants.[18]
- Assessing the stability of individual differences in developmentally changing preterm infants.[39]
- Studying the antecedents of later temperament.[33,40]
- Showing the NAPI to parents to enhance their understanding of their infant's behavioral cues.[41,42]
- Using the NAPI as a therapeutic tool by demonstrating to concerned parents that their infant is making steady progress over weekly examinations.

Acknowledgments

The author's research reported in this chapter was supported by grant MH 36884 from the National Institute of Mental Health, Prevention Research Branch, Division of Clinical Research, and by grant RR-81 from General Clinical Research Center of the Division of Human Resources, National Institute of Health.

REFERENCES

1 Korner, A.F., Schneider, P. and Forrest, T. (1983). Effects of vestibular-proprioceptive stimulation on the neurobehavioral development of preterm infants: a pilot study. *Neuropediatrics*, 14, 170–175.

2 Korner, A.F. (1987). Preventive intervention with high-risk newborns: theoretical, conceptual and methodological perspectives. In: J.D.Osofsky (ed.) *Handbook of Infant Development*, 2nd edn, pp. 1006–1036. New York: Wiley-Interscience.

3 Robinson, R.J. (1966). Assessment of gestational age by neurological examination. *Archive of Diseases in Childhood*, 41, 437–447.

4 Dubowitz, L.M.S., Dubowitz, V. and Goldberg, C. (1970). Clinical assessment of gestational age in the newborn infant. *Journal of Pediatrics*, 77, 1–10.

5 Finnström, O. (1971). Studies in the maturity in newborn infants. III Neurological examination. *Neuropaeditrie*, 3, 72–96.

6 Amiel-Tison, C. (1968). Neurological evaluation of the maturity of newborn infants. *Archives of Diseases of Childhood*, 43, 89–93.

7 Saint-Anne Dargassies, S. (1966). Neurological maturation of the premature infant of 28 to 41 weeks gestational age. In: F. Falkner (ed.) *Human Development*, pp. 306–325. Philadelphia: Saunders.

8 Prechtl, H.F.T. and Beintema, D. (1964). *The Neurological Examination of the Fullterm Newborn Infant. Little Club Clinics in Developmental Medicine*, no. 12. London: Heinemann Medical.

9 Brazelton, T.B. (1973). *Neonatal Behavioral Assessment Scale. Clinics in Developmental Medicine*, no. 50. Philadelphia: J.B. Lippincott.

10 Brandt, I. (1979). Patterns of early neurological development. In: Falkner F. and Tanner J.M. (eds) *Human Growth – Neurobiology and Nutrition*, vol. 3, pp. 243–304. New York: Plenum.

11 Korner, A.F., Kraemer, H.C., Reade, E.P., et al. (1987). A methodological approach to developing an assessment procedure for testing the neurobehavioral maturity of preterm infants. *Child Development*, 58, 1478–1487.

12 Korner, A.F., Constantinou, J., Dimiceli, S., Brown B.W. Jr and Thom, V.A. (1991). Establishing the reliability and developmental validity of a neurobehavioral assessment for preterm infants: a methodological process. *Child Development*, 62, 1200–1208.

13 Ballard, J.L., Novak, K.K. and Driver, M. (1979). A simplified score for assessment of fetal maturation of newly born infants. *Journal of Pediatrics*, 95, 769–774.

14 Usher, R. and McLean, E. (1969). Intrauterine growth of live-born Caucasian infants at sea level: standards obtained from measurements in 7 dimensions of infants born between 25 and 44 weeks of gestation. *Journal of Pediatrics*, 74, pp. 900–910.

15 Korner, A.F. (1972). State as variable, as obstacle and as mediator of stimulation in infant research. *Merrill-Palmer Quarterly*, 18, 77–94.

16 Korner, A.F. and Grobstein, R. (1966). Visual alertness as related to soothing in neonates: implications for maternal stimulation and early deprivation. *Child Development*, 37 (4), 867–876.

17 Korner, A.F. and Thoman, E.B. (1970). Visual alertness in neonates as evoked by maternal care. *Journal of Experimental Child Psychology*, 10, 67–78.

18 Korner, A.F., Brown, B.W. Jr, Reade, E.P., et al. (1988). State behavior of preterm infants as a function of development, individual and sex differences. *Infant Behavior and Development*, 11, 111–124.

19 Korner, A.F. and Thom, V.A. (1990). *Neurobehavioral Assessment of the Preterm Infant*. San Antonio, TX: The Psychological Corporation/Harcourt, Brace and Jovanovich.

20 Korner, A.F., Stevenson, D.K., Forrest, T., et al. (1994). Preterm medical complications differentially affect neuro-behavioral functions: results from a new neonatal medical index. *Infant Behavior and Development*, 17, 37–43.

21 Korner, A.F., Stevenson, D.K., Kraemer H.C., et al. (1993). Prediction of development of low birth weight preterm infants by a new neonatal medical index. *Developmental and Behavioral Pediatrics*, 14, 106–111.

22 Infant Health and Development Program. (1990). Enhancing the outcomes of low-birthweight premature infants. *Journal of the American Medical Association*, 263, 3035–3042.

23 Brown J.V., Bakeman R., Cole, C.C., Sexton R. and Demi, A.S. (1998). Maternal drug use during pregnancy: are preterm and full-term infants affected differently? *Developmental Psychology*, 34, 540–554.

24 Anand, K.J.S., McIntosh, N., Lagercrantz, H., et al. (1999). Analgesia and sedation in ventilated preterm neonates. *Archives of Pediatric and Adolescent Medicine*, 153, 331–338.

25 Samaroff, A. and Chandler, M. (1975). Reproductive risk and the continuum of care-taking casualty. In: F.D. Horowitz, M. Hetherington, S. Scarr–Salapatek and G. Siegel (eds) *Review of Child Development Research*, pp. 187–244. Chicago, IL: University of Chicago Press.

26 Samaroff, A.J., Seifer, R., Barochas, R., Zaks, M. and Greenspan, S. (1987). Intelligence quotient scores of 4-year-old children: social–environmental risk factors. *Pediatrics*, 79, 343–350.

27 Dittrichová, J.D., Sobotková, D., Procházková, E. and Vondriáĉek, J. (2000). Early development of preterm infants: use of the Neurobehavioral Assessment of the Preterm Infant (NAPI). *Prenatal and Perinatal Psychology and Medicine*, 12, 77–87.

28 Bayley, N. (1969). *Manual for the Bayley Scales of Infant Development*. New York: Psychological Corporation.

29 Constantinou, J.C., Adamson-Macedo, E.N., Korner, A.F. and Fleisher, B.E. (2000). Prediction of the Neurobehavioral Assessment of the Preterm Infant to the Bayley Infant Neurodevelopmental Screener. Presented at the *International Conference of Infant Studies*, Brighton, England, July 17. http://www.isisweb.org/

30 Constantinou, J.C., Fleisher, B.E., Korner, A.F. and Stevenson, D.K. (1997). Prediction from the Neurobehavioral Assessment of the Preterm Infant to the Bayley II at two years of age. *Journal of Investigative Medicine*, 45, 117A.

31 Aylward, G.P. (1995). *Infant Neurodevelopmental Screener*. San Antonio, TX: The Psychological Corporation/Harcourt, Brace & Jovanovich.

32 Sampers, J. and Caldwell, R. (2000). Early predictors of poor motor outcome in extremely premature infants. Presented at the *International Conference of Infant Studies*, Brighton England, July 17. http://www.isisweb.org/

33 Newham, C.A. (1999). The prediction of cognitive and temperamental characteristics from neonatal behaviour in preterm infants. Doctoral dissertation. La Trobe University, Bundoor, Victoria, Australia.

34 Ariagno, R.L., Thoman, E.B., Boediker, M.A., et al. (1997). Developmental care does not alter sleep and development. *Pediatrics*, 100, E91–E97.

35 Espy, K.A, Rise, M.L. and Francis, D.J. (1995). Neurobehavioral development in preterm infants prenatally exposed to cocaine. Poster presented, printed and distributed at *The Society for Research in Child Development*. Indianapolis, IN, March 30–April 2.

36 Espy, K.A., Rise, M.L. and Francis, D.J. (1997). Neurobehavior in preterm neonates exposed to cocaine, alcohol and tobacco. *Infant Behavior and Development*, 20, 297–309.

37 Espy, K.A., Francis, D.J. and Riese, M.L. (2000). Prenatal cocaine exposure and prematurity: neurodevelopmental growth. *Journal of Developmental and Behavioral Pediatrics*, 21, 262–270.

38 Korner, A.F., Brown, J.V., Thom, V.A., and Constantinou, J. (2000). *The Neurobehavioral Assessment of the Preterm*

Infant, 2nd edn. distributed by Child Development Media, 5632 Van Nuys Blvd., Suite 286, Van Nuys, CA 91401, U.S.A.

39 Korner, A.F., Brown, B.W. Jr., Dimiceli, S., et al. (1989). Stable individual differences in developmentally changing preterm infants. *Child Development*, 60, 501–513.

40 Korner, A.F. (1996). Reliable individual differences in preterm infants' excitation management. *Child Development*, 67, 1793–1805.

41 Constantinou, J. and Korner, A.F. (1993). Neurobehavioral Assessment of the Preterm Infant as an instrument to enhance parental awareness. *Childrens' Health Care*, 22, 39–46.

42. Sobotková, D., Dittrichová, J., Prochazková, E. and Vondrâĉek, J. (1996). Neurobehavioral Assessment of the Preterm Infant (NAPI) as a technique of early intervention. Presented and printed at the *XIV Biannual SSBD Conference*, Quebec City, August 12–16.

Long-term follow-up of term infants with perinatal asphyxia

Charlene M.T. Robertson

University of Alberta, Edmonton, Alberta, Canada

Introduction

Follow-up, longitudinal, and cohort studies play a unique role in the prediction of outcomes such as mortality, disability, growth, and child development within the science of pediatric epidemiology.[1] These studies are useful to generate and test hypotheses. To assess "the outcomes approach" in the study of perinatal asphyxia, the role, advantages, and disadvantages of long-term follow-up should be reviewed.

Central to long-term follow-up studies is the prospective definition of the reference population, tracking of individuals over time, and the consistent use of specific measurement tools to determine outcome.[2] Longitudinal studies in the narrow sense measure individuals at several well-defined occasions and usually every individual is measured on each occasion.[2] These studies are particularly important in demonstrating the accumulation of risk over time and in identifying latent effects.[1] They rely on variations that occur in risk factors, hence the degree of association can be quantified for different exposure levels. They also clarify the direction in which the associations are likely to operate, although they cannot provide "proof" of causality. A recent comparison of randomized controlled trials and observational (cohort and case-control) studies affirms the value of the latter.[3] Uniformity of outcome measures, with a focus on health and functional status, add to the value of long-term follow-up of at-risk neonates.[4] Overall, longitudinal studies are important in identifying long-term sequelae of physical disability, as well as intellectual and educational outcome,[1] and hence, they assist in providing information that can be used for the prediction of childhood developmental disorders.

Disadvantages of longitudinal studies include the expense and effort of establishing and maintaining contact with cohort members, sample attrition, and associated bias depending upon the characteristics of those lost to follow-up, and the time-lag to obtain results.[1] Specific biases in selection of cohorts for neonatal follow-up studies have been outlined by Saigal.[5] These may include selection bias based on referral patterns to tertiary centers from primary or secondary health-care facilities, and bias of management depending upon the expertise and orientation of care givers, including elective termination of treatment.[6] Bias in identification and recruitment may be a greater problem in the follow-up of term infants with low incidence events and a range of clinical presentations than for very preterm newborns identified by birth weight. Childhood death after discharge also introduces bias into long-term follow-up studies. Neonatal transport could produce selection bias; however, in a small outcome study on severely hypoxic newborns referred for extracorporeal membrane oxygenation (ECMO), modern neonatal transport did not adversely affect outcome.[7] Social demographic factors, parental educational levels, and language of assessment must always be considered in neonatal follow-up studies.[5] The care with which most follow-up programs record these confounding variables lessens their potential to distort results.

Follow-up of children thought to have perinatal asphyxia has added to our understanding of the proportionately small role intrapartum asphyxia plays in childhood cerebral palsy,[8] and has clarified the low risk of this developmental motor disability for asymptomatic newborns.[9] The value of the presence of and staging for hypoxic–ischemic encephalopathy (HIE) is widely accepted.[10,11] Outcome studies have documented that school-age children who have had mild HIE are similar to community peer children.[12] They are free from death, and disability, and the proportion of this group with academic delay is as expected for their peer group.[12] Those with moderate or severe HIE are at risk for adverse outcome.[12] Longitudinal studies have advanced the understanding of the natural history of what has been called HIE associated with perinatal asphyxia for the term infant. The value of long-term neurological and psychoeducational follow-up studies will be even greater and allow more accurate prediction of outcome in the future as asphyxia becomes better defined by newer investigative techniques, particularly those by cranial imaging.[13]

The use of longitudinal studies to determine the outcome of perinatal asphyxia presents some specific problems and limitations in two vital areas: diagnosis and outcome measurement. With regard to diagnosis, the strength of a good longitudinal study is the unbiased prospective collection of information from an inception cohort with suspected risk factors before outcome is determined. The greatest difficulty in "outcomes research" of birth asphyxia is with the diagnosis and the lack of its universal application.[14,15] In the study of perinatal asphyxia the diagnosis is often not uniform, the time of exposure to antepartum events may be unrecognized and undocumented, and the diagnosis of asphyxia related to intrapartum events is not universally accepted. In standard reproductive care terminology, perinatal refers to the period of 20 weeks' gestation until 1 week after birth; prenatal refers to the period before or after 20 weeks' gestation, but before labor. For the term infant with neonatal encephalopathy, perinatal asphyxia usually refers to hypoxic–ischemic events in the periods of late pregnancy but before labor, labor and delivery, postdelivery resuscitation, or in the early neonatal period often associated with respiratory failure. Where a hypoxic–ischemic event is thought to have occurred during pregnancy but where there has been in utero recovery and the term infant is without neonatal encephalopathy, the event is classed as prenatal. Generally, perinatal asphyxia refers to an acute total (or near-total) or partial prolonged hypoxic–ischemic event measured respectively in minutes or hours, unless the word chronic is mentioned, where weeks or months of adverse intrauterine environment may be present. The greatest difficulty in categorization or diagnosis appears to be for those infants with an apparent hypoxic–ischemic event in the late antepartum period who present without cord markers of metabolic acidosis but with imaging and clinical evidence of asphyxia, including neonatal encephalopathy. Until recently many outcome studies of perinatal asphyxia have relied upon the clinical triad of fetal distress (using a variety of measures), depression at birth (usually using the Apgar score) and the need for resuscitation, and abnormal newborn neurological examination, often termed neonatal encephalopathy, to diagnose asphyxia.[11] Reliance upon this triad for diagnosis has resulted in the inclusion in long-term follow-up studies of infants with late antepartum hypoxic–ischemic events as well as those with intrapartum asphyxia.

Lack of specificity and the many causes of neonatal encephalopathy raise serious questions about the use of the phrases HIE and perinatal asphyxia.[16] The debate is not whether birth asphyxia occurs and can cause brain damage, but rather what proportion of neurological impairment in children is due to perinatal hypoxia–ischemia, how many infants with asphyxia have predisposing factors for that asphyxia, and what nonasphyxial factors contribute to or determine unfavourable outcome.[16] The recent international consensus statement has attempted to define an acute intrapartum hypoxic event that is sufficient to play a causation role in cerebral palsy as evidence of a metabolic acidosis in intrapartum fetal, umbilical arterial cord, or very early neonatal blood samples (pH<7.00 and base deficit ≥12 mmol/l); early onset of severe or moderate neonatal encephalopathy in infants of >34 weeks' gestation; and cerebral palsy of the spastic quadriplegic or dyskinetic type.[17] These are supported by nonspecific evidence of a sentinel (single) hypoxic event occurring immediately before or during labor; a sudden, rapid, and sustained deterioration of the fetal heart rate pattern usually after the hypoxic sentinel event where the pattern was previously normal; Apgar scores of 0–6 for longer than 5 min; early evidence of multisystem involvement; and early imaging evidence of acute cerebral abnormality.[17] While this statement functions as a much needed operational definition of intrapartum asphyxia, it may retard the advancement of the understanding of the broader perinatal asphyxia. Responses to this template have challenged the need for metabolic acidemia to complete this diagnosis, citing the example of neonatal encephalopathy following placental abruption and acute asphyxia without time for the development of severe acidemia and with subsequent athetoid cerebral palsy.[18] Similarly, some individual case reports do not support the criteria of a pH <7.00.[19] A parallel challenge has pointed out the value of brain imaging and electroencephalography to determine when brain insults have occurred.[20] Also, the consensus does not consider "the hierarchy of metabolic needs" within the brain determined from animal models.[21] Pasternak and Gorey point out that in relatively brief, acute, near-total asphyxia the organs of highest metabolic rate are affected most with greater subcortical nuclear damage (basal ganglia and thalamus) than cerebral hemisphere damage and with relative sparing of the nonbrain organs.[22] This is in contrast to the prolonged partial asphyxia affecting the cerebral cortex and white matter beginning in parasagittal (watershed) regions that commonly precedes HIE.[22] Another statement to define operationally hypoxic–ischemic late antenatal insults where umbilical cord metabolic acidosis is absent but where there is no other cause of encephalopathy would help to improve the understanding of watershed injury not explained by birth asphyxia. The template includes intrapartum events, thus by definition excludes hypoxic–ischemic events occurring before labor or where no labor occurs.

We are coming into a new era of research in the diagnosis of perinatal asphyxia. Clinical studies are now taking into consideration the maturity of certain brain cells at the time of hypoxic–ischemic insults; the vulnerability to insult of specific brain cells related to metabolic function; autoregulation; blood shift protective mechanisms; time, degree, and duration of insult; and reoxygenation injury.[23,24] The impact of the insult on developmental neuropathology and its progression years later to acquired cortical dysplasia in the surrounding brain tissue are beginning to be documented.[25] This improved clarity of diagnosis and refining of the timing of hypoxic–ischemic insults will assist future longitudinal studies to provide more focused outcome information.

Longitudinal studies could become more valuable in the understanding of the natural history of perinatal asphyxia if greater attention was paid to the outcome measurements used and the duration of follow-up. The only outcomes of perinatal asphyxia generally considered are death or cerebral palsy with or without other impairment.[26,27] As stated by the 1985 National Institutes of Health Report, "only when associated with cerebral palsy is severe [mental] retardation possibly linked to asphyxia."[28] It is worthwhile exploring how this perception came about. In 1981, Nelson and Ellenburg,[29] while reporting on children enrolled in the Collaborative Perinatal Project of the National Institutes of Neurological and Communication Disorders and Stroke, concluded that "there was no statistically significant increase in mental retardation among children with very low late Apgar scores who did not also have CP". A 10-min or later Apgar score of 0–3 occurred in 86 7-year-old children without cerebral palsy. Of these 86, 30 were ≤2500 g birth weight. In this paper, cognitive-specific outcome is not separate for the term and preterm newborns. Five or 5.8%

of the 86 children without cerebral palsy had scores of less than 70 on the Wechsler Intelligence Scales for Children (WISC) and this was said not to exceed the proportion of mental retardation from all causes for the comparison race-adjusted population.[29] It should be noted that, by using a standardized intelligence scale with scores distributed on the bell-shaped curve, 2.27% of all births will be expected to have scores below 70 and this cognitive deficit will be due to all possible causes. Nelson and Ellenburg's paper reported a frequency of mental retardation of more than 2.5 times expected for a population where other causes were not given consideration. Without further evidence, Perlman restated the task force conclusion as "only when CP is associated with severe mental retardation can a possible link to a peripartum etiology be suggested."[26] Another analysis of the same Collaborative Perinatal Project Database concluded that there was an association between mental retardation and birth asphyxia.[30] Broman reported that among 7-year-old children the rate for controls of WISC intelligence quotient scores under 70 were 1% in whites and 5% in blacks.[30] She then compared the rate of mental retardation for 8192 selected control white children with white subjects with variously defined asphyxia as follows: 1-min Apgar score in 849 subjects of ≤3, 3.9% mental retardation ($P<0.01$); 5-min Apgar score in 117 of ≤3, 5.1% ($P<0.001$); apneic episodes in 60, 6.7% ($P<0.01$), and respiratory difficulty in 262, 6.9% ($P<0.001$).[30] Another reanalysis of 19117 children of the 56000 pregnancies of the Collaborative Perinatal Project reported no association between WISC scores of 50–70 found in 2% of 7-year-old survivors with acute hypoxia as measured by a 1-min Apgar score of ≤6.[31] In view of the age of this perinatal project, definitions of asphyxia based upon Apgar scores, and varying results, new long-term studies with broader outcome measures should be done to enhance our understanding of perinatal asphyxia.

The restriction of possible diverse neurodevelopmental consequences of asphyxia to developmental motor disability or death limits what can be learned to a narrow perinatal viewpoint.[32] The vitally important aspect of both trials and observational studies in perinatal medicine is the appropriate endpoint, such as motor or sensory impairment, behavioral or educational outcome, and this underlines the importance of long-term follow-up.[33] Recommendations for the timing and type of individual childhood follow-up after birth asphyxia have long been available emphasizing key times for documenting severe motor or sensory loss (first year), low developmental quotient (second year), fine and gross motor dysfunction and behavioral abnormalities (2–4 years), abnormalities in cognitive function (4–7 years), and learning disabilities (7–9 years).[34] While uncommon, longitudinal studies have a place in defining the outcome of perinatal asphyxia. In summarizing the sequential assessments of our first cohort of survivors of neonatal encephalopathy associated with birth asphyxia,[12,35,36] Levene has commented that cognitive impairment as measured by the intelligence quotient (IQ) appears to represent a continuum of disability reflecting the severity of the initial asphyxial insult.[37]

Further discussion on the diagnosis of asphyxia, limitation of the terms, pathophysiology, and imaging, electrophysiological, and laboratory assessment in perinatal asphyxia can be found elsewhere in this book. This chapter will focus on the long-term childhood outcomes of cerebral palsy, epilepsy, sensory deficit, growth, motor skills, cognitive and language ability, academic function, and learning abilities related to clinically diagnosed perinatal asphyxia of the term infant. This work refers to and expands similar previous reviews.[38,39]

Neonatal neurological examination in relation to early childhood outcome.

Overview

In the pediatric and adult-acquired brain injury literature, it is accepted that a cause-and-effect relationship with outcome is unlikely to occur unless the insult is closely followed by encephalopathy. For the term newborn free from congenital or genetic abnormality, adverse long-term outcome of birth asphyxia does not occur unless signs of neurological dysfunction are present in the newborn period.[9,11] Epidemiological studies show geographic differences in the birth prevalence of newborn encephalopathy of children born a decade ago: Western Australia, 3.8 per 1000;[40] and Sweden, 1.8 per 1000.[41] Sweden attributes decreasing rates of neonatal HIE to effective antenatal care.[41] Published neonatal encephalopathy systems of categorization have been reviewed and their limitations discussed.[42] Generally, neonatal encephalopathy associated with perinatal asphyxia has been described in three stages. The most common staging system is that of Sarnat and Sarnat:[43] stage 1 (mild), hyperalertness, hyperexcitability; stage 2 (moderate), lethargy, hypotonia, suppressed primitive reflexes; and stage 3 (severe), stupor, flaccidity, absent primitive reflexes. The early progressive nature of the encephalopathy has been well documented.[43–45] However the problem of staging severity is increased by ventilation and sedation of the newborn or with associated newborn respiratory, cardiac, or infectious diseases. Newborns with a predisposition to malpresentation due to fetal hypotonia as often seen in myotonic dystrophy or Prader–Willi syndrome may present with HIE and intrapartum asphyxia may complicate their neurodevelopmental prognosis; however, when diagnosed, such children are excluded from reports of HIE outcome.[35,44] When possible to assess, we have found the prognostic value of the stage of encephalopathy is greatest when the newborn neurological examination is staged according to the most severe signs seen between 1 h and 7 days of life.[35]

Overall, the classification of neonatal encephalopathy associated with perinatal asphyxia has been clinically useful and could be used further as an outcome tool for perinatal studies.[13,45] To be of value, the clinical assessment of HIE must be precise.[38] We have noted some common ways of categorizing neonatal encephalopathy that may lead to errors in prognosis:

1. Neonates with proximal hypotonia for the first few days of life may be categorized as having mild encephalopathy and the child's family given a good prognosis; however, subsequent disability and/or academic difficulties may occur. In such cases a categorization of moderate encephalopathy due to the presence of hypotonia would have been more appropriate.
2. Neonates with hypotonia and lethargy but not flaccidity or stupor have been classed as having severe encephalopathy and given a poor prognosis. As such a child has a good chance of being healthy, this prognosis leads to undue parental anxiety.
3. Neonates with difficult-to-control seizures have been classed as having severe encephalopathy even when they are hypotonic, not flaccid, and have present, albeit reduced, spontaneous movement and primitive reflexes. This may result in a very poor prognosis and consideration of termination of treatment for a child with moderate neonatal encephalopathy.
4. Application of the staging of HIE to preterm newborns. This is inappropriate due to their low tone.

The usefulness of HIE staging is greater when applied to newborns of 37 or more completed weeks' gestation. Due to the normal low muscle tone of preterm infants, the predictive ability of the categories of HIE to children ≥34 weeks' gestation but before 37 weeks, as included in the international consensus statement, is not clear. A variation of the Sarnat scoring system using a numerical score of 0–22 has been published with an overall sensitivity of 100% and specificity of 93% for 1-year outcome period.[46] This recent adaptation may improve the utility of the clinical scoring system of HIE. As serial imaging of the neonatal brain improves, there may be less reliance on HIE categories for prognosis.[47]

It is likely that the nonstatic encephalopathy seen in the neonatal period occurs in late pregnancy following fetal hypoxic–ischemic insults. The fetus probably shows postasphyxial stages similar to those of the neonate following intrapartum asphyxia. Application to the fetus of HIE categories similar to those used for neonatal encephalopathy and their prognosis may extend our understanding of perinatal asphyxia.

Categories of neonatal encephalopathy

Stage 1 (mild) neonatal hypoxic–ischemic encephalopathy

The mild category of neonatal encephalopathy, that is stage 1 as described by Sarnat and Sarnat,[43] includes hyperalertness, staring (decreased frequency of blinking without enhanced visual tracking), normal or decreased spontaneous motor activity, and a lower threshold for all stimuli including an easily elicited Moro reflex, all of which can be related to sympathomimetic manifestations. While all newborns of Sarnat and Sarnat's study[43] with stage 1 progressed to stage 2, usually this mild stage is reported as self-limiting and does not progress.[48,49] We have found that the signs of stage 1 may persist for several days.[35] Studies that have reported 8-year outcome of newborns with this mild category, regardless of its duration, and that have excluded all children with shoulder girdle or proximal upper-extremity hypotonia (or any transient hypotonia) have shown that all children in this category do well.[12] Studies that include children in the mild category who have, or develop, transient hypotonia and/or suppressed primitive reflexes report occasional adverse outcome within the group.[44,50–54] It should be remembered that mild HIE may resemble neonatal abstinence syndrome and if the former is diagnosed in error there may be an outcome less favorable than expected.

Stage 2 (moderate) neonatal hypoxic–ischemic encephalopathy

The moderate category of neonatal encephalopathy, that is stage 2 as described by Sarnat and Sarnat,[43] includes neonates with lethargy, increased stimuli threshold, decreased spontaneous movement accompanied by hypotonia, suppressed primitive reflexes, and predominantly parasympathetic responses. Localized hypotonia (shoulder girdle and proximal upper-extremity hypotonia) may improve within a few days, or may persist for several weeks. This pattern of hypotonia correlates with imaging that demonstrates parasagittal hypoxic–ischemic (watershed) injury[11] as found in partial prolonged asphyxia.[22] More severe and generalized hypotonia may be due to a greater severity of partial prolonged asphyxia or may be due to acute total intrapartum asphyxia.[22] Prolonged hypotonia or difficult-to-control seizures correlate with adverse outcomes.[35] Approximately 20% of children with previous moderate HIE are disabled.[12]

Stage 3 (severe) neonatal hypoxic–ischemic encephalopathy

The severe category of neonatal encephalopathy, that is stage 3 as described by Sarnat and Sarnat,[43] includes flaccidity with stupor and absent primitive reflexes at some time during the postasphyxial period. Surviving children who have had stage 3 HIE often have multiple disabilities, including two or more of severe spastic quadriparetic cerebral palsy, severe/profound cognitive deficit, cortical visual impairment, and/or epilepsy. Some authors have reported that normal children make up 30% of the survivors of those in the severe category of HIE;[48,50,54] in these reports encephalopathy staging criteria place less emphasis on flaccidity and absent primitive reflexes and categorize newborns with hypotonia, suppressed primitive reflexes, and severe neonatal seizures in stage 3. When staging is determined according to Sarnat and Sarnat[43] then later death or disability occurs in all survivors of severe encephalopathy.[12] Similar outcomes occur using Fenichel's categorization.[49,55] Asphyxial cord damage may occur with accompanying transiently absent deep tendon reflexes as is sometimes recorded for children with severe HIE. As children with severe HIE are usually multiply disabled, they often remained dependently handicapped and their life expectancy is shortened.[12,35,56]

Early childhood disability outcomes

Outcome measurements

Improved understanding of the selective vulnerability of specific areas of the developing brain,[24] revisitation of the classic animal studies by Myers,[21] new animal models of perinatal asphyxia,[57] the use of combinations of early asphyxial markers as predictors,[58] and an increasing openness of mind when assessing clinical situations[22,59] are improving our understanding of perinatal asphyxia. We must also give careful consideration to the outcome measurements used to study asphyxia and its treatments. Following perinatal asphyxia, spastic quadriplegic cerebral palsy with or without dyskinesia has been the outcome of greatest concern and the only outcome other than death used by some authors.[27,28,60] Although providing very early 1-year outcome results, some recent studies are combining a detailed neurological examination including muscle tone and reflex results with a developmental measure (usually the Griffiths Developmental Scales,[61] or the Bayley Scales of Infant Development[62]) and a record of sensory impairment.[63–67] Developmental concerns beyond cerebral palsy have been noted and longer follow-up is planned by these research groups. By age 4 years, accurate outcome measurements are available to evaluate specific neurodevelopment, including gross and fine motor skills, and speech, language, cognitive, and behavioral abilities.

Our source of outcome data

Over the past 25 years all surviving term newborns that received tertiary-level neonatal intensive care through the Northern Alberta Regional Perinatal Program and had abnormal neurological signs after 1 h of age with a history of abnormal fetal heart rate patterns, 1- or 5-min Apgar scores of <5, or immediate neonatal resuscitation, including bag-and-mask ventilation or intubation with ventilation, have been referred to the Neonatal and Infant Follow-up Clinic at the Glenrose Rehabilitation Hospital. Detailed audit tabulations of outcome have been maintained by this author and all examinations have been completed by one of four pediatricians experienced in neonatal follow-up. All physical disabilities have been confirmed by the same pediatric physiatrist. Data of all children with syndromes or congenital malformations associated with developmental delay are excluded from analyses. From this data, two inception cohorts of children with neonatal encephalopathy (cohort 1, born 1974–79; cohort 2, born 1982–86) were identified and followed until school age as specific studies.[12,35,36,38,39] The school-age childhood disability outcome of the two cohorts is similar (Tables 41.1 and 41.2). Early childhood outcome is available for other children with the same inclusion and exclusion criteria born in 1980, 1981, and 1987 to the present.[12,35,36,38]

Table 41.1. Overview of school-age death and disability outcome of two cohorts with neonatal moderate/severe neonatal hypoxic–ischemic encephalopathy[a]

	Cohort 1 (born 1974–79)	Cohort 2 (born 1982–86)
Discharged from neonatal intensive care unit	$n=130$	$n=123$
Postdischarge deaths	13 (10%)	10 (8%)
n (%) follow-up	89 (76%)	103 (91%)
n (%) disabled	23/89 (26%)	26/103 (25%)
n (%) multiply-disabled	12/89 (13%)	14/103 (14%)
n (%) nondisabled[b]	66/89 (74%)	77/103 (75%)

Notes:
[a] See Robertson et al.[12] and Robertson.[39]
[b] Includes children with unilateral or mild bilateral sensorineural hearing impairment
not requiring hearing aids (cohort 1, $n=3$; cohort 2, $n=6$).

Specific disabilities

Cerebral palsy

A 1994 study from Oxford shows that children with cerebral palsy who were born at term and had neonatal encephalopathy were more likely to have signs of intrapartum asphyxia and more likely to have a severe form of cerebral palsy than those without a history of neonatal encephalopathy.[68] Sixteen to 20%

Table 41.2. Disabilities of school-age survivors of neonatal moderate and severe hypoxic–ischemic encephalopathy by neonatal category and cohort[a]

	Cohort 1 (born 1974–79)		Cohort 2 (born 1982–86)	
Neonatal encephalopathy category	Moderate	Severe	Moderate	Severe
Total follow-up	84	5	97	6
n (%) disabled	18 (21%)	5 (100%)	20 (21%)	6 (100%)
With one or more of:				
Cerebral palsy	8	5	14	6
Spastic quadriplegia	1	5	4	6
Spastic-athetoid quadriplegia	2	0	3	0
Athetoid quadriplegia	2	0	2	0
Ataxia	1	0	1	0
Spastic hemiplegia	2	0	4	0
Cognitive deficit (severe/profound)	7	3	7	6
Epilepsy	2	5	2	3
Legal blindness	2	1	0	4
Severe neurosensory hearing loss (aided)	5	1	5	0
n (%) multiply-disabled	7 (8%)	5 (100%)	8 (8%)	6 (100%)

Note:
[a] See Robertson et al.[12] and Robertson.[39]

of singleton term children with cerebral palsy are considered to have had intrapartum asphyxia;[69,70] this drops to 10% when all children with cerebral palsy are considered.[68,70] About 12% of term children with cerebral palsy are considered to have a potentially preventable cerebral palsy.[69] Failure to respond to fetal distress and inadequate response after delivery are uncommon.[71]

For most children with cerebral palsy following perinatal asphyxia, the developmental motor diagnosis and subtype can be assured by 2 years of age. The subtype may change after 2 years in a few children usually due to the increasing prominence of athetosis.[72] Children with spastic quadriplegia following severe partial prolonged asphyxia with necrosis of the subcortical white matter and cortex,[22] or following acute total asphyxia that is sufficiently prolonged to cause extensive necrosis,[59] often have microcephaly and cognitive deficit. Acute near-total asphyxial insults of short duration resulting in moderate encephalopathy may give dyskinetic cerebral palsy with normal head growth and overall average cognitive abilities.[73,74] Delayed-onset dystonia associated with perinatal asphyxia has been reported.[75]

A population-based case-control retrospective study has reported that spastic hemiparetic cerebral palsy does not follow potentially asphyxiating conditions in infants of normal birth weight.[60] However, perinatal asphyxia has been reported to be the cause of hemiparetic cerebral palsy by other authors.[76–79] Hemiparetic cerebral palsy has been an outcome of neonates with moderate encephalopathy in our previous outcome studies,[35] as seen in Table 41.2. In our series of 46 tertiary-level neonatal intensive care unit survivors, born from 1983 to 1997 with neonatal stroke, 26 presented with neonatal encephalopathy associated with perinatal asphyxia.[77] Subtypes of perinatal cortical infarction within the middle cerebral artery trunks lead to a variety of clinical presentations.[76]

Ataxic cerebral palsy may follow neonatal encephalopathy (Table 41.2) and, in our opinion, requires further investigation.

Even after delivery at term, it is accepted that the likely origin of childhood spastic diplegia is a prenatal event. The specific brain vulnerability to insults of the periventricular white matter that lead to spastic diplegia occur before term.[24]

Variations in the reports of cerebral palsy in relation to perinatal asphyxia depend upon a number of variables that are difficult to control. The interobserver agreement and classification of the subtypes of cerebral palsy have been reported to be about 50% overall.[80] As well, the subtype diagnoses of cerebral palsy may change in early childhood.[72] Unexplained regional differences in the frequency of cerebral palsy have been found. The prevalence of cerebral palsy in singleton children of >2500 g birth weight in relation to live births in a study from England and Scotland shows a rate of 1.1 (confidence interval 1.1, 1.2).[81] In contrast, the prevalence of cerebral palsy in a similar population of children from our province of Alberta, Canada, is 1.7 (confidence interval 1.4, 2.1).[82]

Many authors are attempting to find the best early predictors of cerebral palsy following birth asphyxia. Although not early enough to instigate neuroprotective therapy, Prechtl has determined that qualitative assessment of spontaneous movement (abnormal fidgety movement) from 6 to 20 weeks of age is the best early predictor of cerebral palsy.[83,84] This is important for the initiation of early physical therapy. It is particularly important as therapy for children at risk for cerebral palsy as determined by cranial imaging, but not yet diagnosed with cerebral palsy, and has been found not to be beneficial in reversing signs and symptoms of cerebral palsy.[85]

There have been many attempts to move beyond classifying cerebral palsy by subtype diagnoses or by terms such as mild, moderate, and severe. Overall prognosis for ambulation in children with cerebral palsy depends on the type of cerebral palsy, persistence of primitive reflexes, and the absence of postural reactions.[86] Generally the ability to sit by 2 years of age unless the child has severe cognitive deficit or visual impairment implies at least community ambulation.[72] A system to classify reliably gross motor function in children with cerebral palsy has been developed giving a gradation range of level I–V.[87] The application of this functional classification system is useful in clinical practice, research, teaching, and administration.[87] Choices for the treatment of children with cerebral palsy are increasing and include physical therapy of various types, drug treatment for spasticity (for example, baclofen or botulism toxin), orthosis and other appliances, orthopedic surgery (for complications of spasticity, osteoporosis, or scoliosis) and neurosurgery (rhizotomy) preceded by gait analysis to determine the preciseness of the surgery.[88] Of increasing importance is the multidisciplinary team approach to insure that not only motor care, but appropriate growth, school performance, and adaptation to adult life, are considered.[88]

Cognitive deficit

Cognitive deficit labels vary according to country. In the USA, the terms moderate and severe mental retardation are similar to severe learning disability in the UK. Younger children tested with developmental measures are given a Mental Developmental index (MDI). After about 3 years of age and depending upon the measure used, cognitive ability is recorded as IQ. The predictive correlation of the MDI with childhood IQ is low for infants and improves when tests are done in the second year of life.[62] Today, the Wechsler Intelligence Scales are the "gold standard" for measuring reasoning, concept formation, and problem solving for children. The DSM IV-TR defines mental retardation as a disorder characterized by significant subaverage intellectual functioning (an IQ of approximately 70 or below, that is approximately 2 SD below the mean for the test used) with onset before age 18 years and with concurrent deficits or impairments in adaptive functioning.[89] Considering the standard error of tests used, mild mental retardation is an IQ level of 50–55 to approximately 70, moderate 35–40 to 50–55, and severe or profound below 35–40.[89] The mild category was previously called educable and the moderate, trainable. Borderline intellectual functioning refers to IQ ranges that are higher than those for mental retardation, generally 71–84. From the bell-shaped curve, we expect 2.27% of children to test at more than 2 SD below the mean on any given intelligence test. Community prevalence studies of level of functioning during school years suggest that 1.1–1.5% of all children function within this range.[90] Children with IQ scores more than 2 SD below the mean on standardized testing have significant cognitive challenges and require a modified school curriculum.

Mental retardation is well known as part of the complex of multiple disabilities that may follow perinatal asphyxia. However, for children with previous moderate HIE, mental retardation without cerebral palsy has been reported by a number of longitudinal studies.[12,35,91–93] Cowan has observed that neonates with intact basal ganglia despite widespread white-matter abnormality have fewer neonatal neurological abnormalities than those with basal ganglia involvement with relatively good motor outcome and good vision, but with cognitive deficits that become obvious with time.[13]

To clarify the issue of an increased prevalence of mental retardation without cerebral palsy following perinatal asphyxia, we undertook a secondary analysis of previously published data.[94] Subjects included term newborns with moderate HIE. Inclusion and exclusion criteria are documented above in the section on Our source of outcome data. There were 172 8-year-old survivors born from 1974 to 1979 and 1982 to 1986 and 235 18-month-old survivors born 1987 to 1996. Forty mentally delayed children with age-appropriate test results of 2 SD or more below the mean (<70) but without cerebral palsy, hearing or vision loss, or epilepsy were identified. Isolated cognitive deficit was found in 19 (11%) of the 172 8-year-old children and 21 (9%) of the 235 18-month-old children. Thus the prevalence of isolated mental retardation was 9.8% – 4.3 times more common than expected for mental retardation from all causes. The clinical history of these 40 children coincides with partial prolonged late antenatal or intrapartum asphyxia. For many of these children serial cranial imaging utilizing computed axial tomography shows early cerebral edema at 3–5 days of life, extensive subcortical white-matter damage at 3–4 weeks, and cerebral atrophy developing over subsequent months. The rate of head growth velocity decreased in the early months of life, leaving 12 of the 40 children with microcephaly. This outcome study demonstrates that isolated mental retardation without other disability and not associated with known syndromes or malformations does occur in children following perinatal asphyxia and moderate HIE. As cranial imaging and associated long-term follow-up studies improve, more information will become available on this outcome of perinatal asphyxia.

Epilepsy

Neonatal seizures are well known to be part of HIE. Birth asphyxia occurs in approximately half of children with neonatal seizures.[78,95] The outcome of perinatal asphyxia with HIE and neonatal seizures that has been reported over the last 20 years includes children treated with anticonvulsants. The role of anticonvulsants on long-term outcome is unknown. A recent review of the benefits and harm of administering anticonvulsants to infants of 37 weeks' gestation or more following perinatal asphyxia with the primary aim of prevention of death or subsequent severe neurodevelopmental disability and/or the prevention of seizures recommends not to use anticonvulsants for routine practice other than prolonged or frequent clinical seizures.[96] It will be many years before the outcome of such children not receiving antiepileptics is known.

Epilepsy following perinatal asphyxia occurs in 10% of survivors with moderate or severe HIE at 3.5

years[35] and 6% of survivors at 8 years,[39] with the decrease reflecting the increased death rate among those multiply disabled survivors with epilepsy. Seizures in childhood usually continue from the neonatal period or begin again in early infancy. Childhood onset of epilepsy in survivors without cerebral palsy or mental delay is rare. Survivors with spastic hemiplegia or mental retardation may have childhood-onset epilepsy.

Vision loss

Abnormal visual function in the absence of ocular abnormalities occurs following perinatal asphyxia.[97] The term "cortical visual impairment" has replaced that of "cortical blindness" and refers to damage of the posterior visual pathway, including the primary visual cortex. Evidence using magnetic resonance imaging suggests basal ganglia damage increases the likelihood of impairment of visual function.[98] The most common causes of cortical visual impairment is hypoxic–ischemia.[99]

Functional vision of infants after 5 months of age can be accurately assessed using the Atkinson Battery of Child Development for Examining Functional Vision.[100] This battery includes ocular movements, pupil responses, optokinetic nystagmus, acuity, visual fields, attention over distance, fixation shift, and orientation-reversal and phase-reversal visual evoked potentials.[101] Infants with moderate HIE have been shown to have abnormal visual function as measured by the battery[100] and supportive imaging evidence of insult to the optic radiation, occipital cortex, basal ganglia, and thalamus.[101] Visual functional assessment in infancy correlates well with 2-year outcome.[102]

Vision loss, defined as legal blindness or best corrected vision of <20/200, occurs with variable prevalence in children with moderate and severe HIE: 11 (10.9%) of 101 3.5-year-old children,[35] to six (25%) of 24 5-year-old children.[91] Ongoing ophthalmological assessments of survivors of moderate and severe HIE should evaluate children for visual field defects or homonymous hemianopsia, optic atrophy, roving eye movements, and amblyopia. Some improvement in cortical visual impairment may occur over time.[103]

Hearing loss

Following perinatal asphyxia, term neonates requiring neonatal intensive care are at risk for sensorineural hearing loss (SNHL).[12,35,91,104] There has been no suggestion that children with perinatal asphyxia are at increased risk for conductive hearing loss unless they require prolonged intubation. The Joint Committee on Infant Hearing risk criteria (1991)[105] lists markers of perinatal asphyxia as risks of SNHL, yet severely multiply disabled children with histories of HIE do not usually have hearing loss. We previously reported nine children with previous neonatal HIE and SNHL at school age (Tables 41.1 and 41.2), but only one was multiply disabled. The prevalence of hearing loss increased from 3.5 to 8 years and two further children of the same cohort developed SNHL at ages 12 and 14 years. Common viral causes of SNHL were ruled out and there were no family histories of SNHL among these patients. For children born in the mid-1970s with clinical perinatal asphyxia, SNHL was uncommon.[106] Among 26 such children followed through the preschool years only one (not the child with hearing loss) was ventilated to 24 h of age. D'Souza et al. concluded that most children had a favorable outcome with regard to SNHL difficulties and that neither gentamicin treatment nor incubator noise seemed to affect hearing.[106] The common pattern of hearing loss following perinatal asphyxia is bilateral sloping loss to a severe degree in the high frequencies requiring amplification to assist development.[38] Flat severe to profound SNHL has also been noted. The pathophysiology of hearing loss following perinatal asphyxia has not yet been fully determined. An overview suggests that birth asphyxia is not correlated with hearing loss in babies with complicated deliveries but that prolonged artificial ventilation in the presence of severe HIE or persistent pulmonary hypertension of the newborn are important factors.[107]

A late-onset, often progressive, sloping high-frequency SNHL has been described in a number of groups of term and near-term infants requiring neonatal intensive care, particularly those with respiratory failure requiring inhaled nitric oxide[108] and those needing ECMO.[109] A similar hearing loss pattern has been found among children with congenital diaphragmatic hernia and severe respiratory failure in the newborn where the prolonged use of pancuronium bromide has been linked to the hearing loss.[110] Because of the late onset of this type of hearing loss repeated testing is required following the neonatal period.

The relationship between auditory brainstem responses suggesting neural dysfunction and adverse neurodevelopment following perinatal asphyxia has been known for some time.[111] This pattern of a reduction of wave V amplitude followed by a decrease in the V/I amplitude ratio has been found to relate to the degree and duration of asphyxia as well as to the residual neurodevelopmental deficits but not to long-term effects of sound transmission.[112]

Microcephaly

Microcephaly is usually defined as head growth measuring below the third percentile or 2 SD below the mean for age and sex for children. Microcephaly is common among asphyxiated infants and results from cerebral atrophy associated with a loss of postnatal brain growth potential,[113] is related to deranged neonatal cerebral oxidative metabolism in the first week of life,[92] and found with neonatal magnetic resonance imaging of involvement of the white matter with or without involvement of the basal ganglia and thalamic lesions.[114] Microcephaly by 3 months of age predicts poor neurodevelopmental outcomes in survivors of perinatal asphyxia.[91] Of 24 such children, 10 had neuromotor sequelae and another five had intelligence quotients in the borderline range or below.[91] Various methods have been used to record the slower head growth in early life. A decrease of head circumference ratio of >3.1% between birth and 4 months of age has been found to be highly predictive of the development of microcephaly before age 18 months of age (sensitivity 90%, specificity 85%) and was associated with adverse outcome.[115] Suboptimal head growth as classified by a drop of >2 SD across the percentiles with or without the development of microcephaly has also been found to be predictive of abnormal neurodevelopmental outcome at 12 months of age with a sensitivity of 79% and a specificity of 78%, compared with microcephaly at 1 year of age, which had a sensitivity of 65% and a specificity of 73%.[114]

One of the difficulties with the studies relating early reduced head growth to adverse outcome is the timing of the first head circumference measurement. Early brain swelling is associated with perinatal asphyxia,[47,116] and begins early.[47] Because children with perinatal asphyxia are often very ill, head circumference measurements may not be taken within the first few days of life. The subsequent head circumference measurement on day 3 or 4 may be 1–2 cm larger than the measurement if taken immediately at birth. This increased measurement could result in errors for those using head circumference ratios to predict future microcephaly and adverse outcome. Should late antenatal asphyxia occur, brain swelling and, hence, an accelerated rate of increased head circumference may begin before birth.

Early childhood disabilities using a current operational definition of intrapartum asphyxia[17]

Discussions about metabolic acidosis at birth occur elsewhere in this book. Comments here relate only to long-term outcome. After a detailed follow-up at 4½ years of age of 1210 consecutive deliveries where 72 neonates had a pH of <7.10 and a base deficit of >12 mmol/l, Dennis et al. did not find metabolic acidosis alone to be predictive of long-term outcome.[117] However, where 21 of 29 neonates (eight lost to follow-up) with metabolic acidosis and encephalopathy were followed from 6 months to 4 years of age, both motor and cognitive abnormalities were found.[118] Clustering of perinatal markers of asphyxia to abnormal fetal heart rate patterns, acidemia, and encephalopathy limits severe adverse outcome among survivors.[119] In addition to early motor disability, differences in outcome of speech development have been noted in two preschool groups with acidosis at birth.[119,120] While underlining the importance of severe motor disability as an outcome, these studies do show that there is concern about other outcomes as well. There is concern that few neonates presenting with asphyxia will meet the current strict definition criteria.[121] Of 292 neonates with HIE, only 10 or 3.4% had profound acidemia (umbilical cord artery pH <7.00), an Apgar score of ≤3 for 5 min or longer, seizures within 24 h of birth, and multiorgan system dysfunction.[121]

In order to attempt to determine the outcome of children meeting the criteria for the 1999 International Consensus Statement,[17] we reviewed our database. A description of the data collection is found above under Our source of outcome data. Outcome was determined at 18 months of age or more using neurological and audiological examinations,[35] the Bayley Scales of Infant Development,[62] and a parent-report measure of receptive and expressive language.[122] Of 94 term neonates admitted to our tertiary-level neonatal intensive care units during 1997–99 with moderate or severe HIE, 41 had sufficient data to meet the consensus statement criteria other than the frequently missing variables of umbilical arterial base deficit. Of these 41 children, 10 (24%) died: four in hospital and six multiply disabled children after discharge. The remaining 31 survivors had complete multidisciplinary follow-up. Eight children had spastic quadriplegia or spastic-athetoid quadriplegia and cognitive deficit. One child had spastic-athetoid quadriplegia without cognitive deficit at this time. Five had mental retardation (MDI <70) without cerebral palsy, 14 others had borderline MDI (71–84), and three others had MDI ≥85. Language scores for children without cerebral palsy demonstrated that the receptive scores were commensurate with mental development; however 20 children had severely delayed expressive language scores. This pattern of delayed mental development and particularly delayed expressive language requires further study. One child without cognitive or language concerns presented with severe behavioural problems. None of the 31 survivors could be classed as having normal development at 18 months of age.

Long-term childhood outcome following perinatal asphyxia

Growth

One of the early longitudinal studies of the outcome of perinatal asphyxia reported anoxic study children to be taller and heavier than control children at 3 years of age and by 7 years of age these children had significantly larger chest circumference and height measurements;[123] they concluded that there was no evidence of subsequent decreased growth among anoxic newborns. In a 5-year follow-up study of term infants with perinatal asphyxia determined by multisystem involvement, Shankaran et al. demonstrated that height and weight growth curves matched standards.[91] The head circumference growth curve for nondisabled children was as expected; however, for children with neurodevelopmental deficits, there was failure of head growth by 3 months of age with subsequent plateau of head growth and microcephaly.[91] The reason for restricted somatic growth in height and weight of some of the disabled children who have had perinatal asphyxia is probably related to nutritional as well as nonnutritional factors, as it is for other children with similar degrees of cerebral palsy.[124,125]

Motor skills

Little has been published about the long-term motor abilities of nondisabled children, that is, those free from cerebral palsy, cognitive delay, sensory loss, epilepsy, and syndromes or malformations of known association with developmental delay who have had previous moderate HIE. Nondisabled kindergarten-age survivors have been shown to have poorer motor skills than community-matched children.[39] This study comprised 71 of 77 nondisabled survivors of moderate neonatal encephalopathy reported from this center (cohort 2, born 1982–86).[39] Motor skills were compared with 71 community children without newborn illness, born during the same time period, and matched for age (67 months), gender (58% boys), kindergarten attendance (6 months), mother's

Table 41.3. Percentage of achievement to age for motor tasks of nondisabled survivors of moderate neonatal hypoxic–ischemic encephalopathy and matched-comparison children at two ages, 5½ years and 9 years[a]

	Kindergarten-age groups		School-age groups	
Task domains	Study $n=71$	Comparison $n=71$	Study $n=64$	Comparison $n=64$
Everyday motor				
Walking	50 (70%)[b]	70 (99%)	58 (91%)[c]	64 (100%)
Running	39 (49%)[b]	67 (94%)	51 (80%)	59 (92%)
Stair climbing				
Up	33 (46%)[b]	65 (91%)	57 (89%)	61 (65%)
Down	22 (31%)[b]	61 (86%)	46 (72%)[b]	61 (95%)
Complex motor				
Straight-line walking (5½ years)	49 (69%)[b]	68 (96%)		
Tandem walking forward (9 years)			36 (56%)[b]	59 (92%)
Hopping dominant foot	45 (63%)	63 (89%)	62 (97%)	64 (100%)
Standing balance (5½ years)	26 (37%)[b]	65 (92%)		
Romberg (9 years)			17 (24%)[c]	51 (80%)
Fine motor				
Finger-nose dominant hand	43 (61%)[b]	66 (93%)	50 (78%)[b]	60 (94%)
Alternate fingers dominant hand	49 (69%)[b]	69 (97%)	29 (45%)[b]	43 (67%)

Notes:

[a] See Robertson.[39]

[b] Denotes significant difference ($P<0.001$) from matched-comparison group, (individual Cochran Q-test).

[c] Denotes significant difference ($P<0.01$) from matched-comparison group, (individual Cochran Q-test).

Achievement determined by age-referenced published data[127,128] with expectations greater for school-age children. "Non-disabled survivors" refers to children free from cerebral palsy, severe/profound cognitive deficit, vision or hearing loss, or epilepsy.

education (12.4 years), mother tongue (89% English), and socioeconomic level (Blishen index, 44).[126] Skills were tested by individual assessment by the same assessor, under the same conditions, with standards of proficiency for each motor task related to age.[127,128] Results show that more study than comparison children were delayed in motor task achievement (Table 41.3). Two-thirds of study children did not go downstairs using alternate feet without hand support but rather used two feet per step. Most of these same children had delayed standing balance.

As part of the longitudinal study of this cohort the kindergarten-age study and matched-comparison children were reassessed at 9 years of age. While the

Table 41.4. Means and standard deviations of standard scores of the Wechsler Intelligence Scale for Children – Revised[135] for school-age nondisabled survivors of moderate neonatal hypoxic–ischemic encephalopathy: two cohorts and their community comparison groups[a]

	Study 1 (born 1974–79)		Study 2 (born 1982–86)	
	Cohort 1 study (n=66)	Peer comparison (n=155)	Cohort 2 study (n=64)	Matched comparison (n=64)
Intelligence quotients				
Full-scale	102±17[b]	112±13	100 + 14[b]	109 + 11
Verbal	100±17[b]	110±13	99 + 14[b]	107 + 12
Performance	103±17[b]	113±13	101 + 15[b]	109 + 11

Notes:

[a] See Robertson et al.[12] and Robertson.[39]

Normative score for intelligence quotients, 100 + 15. "Nondisabled survivors" refers to children free from cerebral palsy, severe/profound cognitive deficit, vision or hearing loss, or epilepsy. Analyses: study 1, student t-test; study 2, correlated t-test.

[b] Denotes significant difference ($P<0.01$) from comparison group.

proportion of 64 school-aged study children achieving motor skills to age level[127,128] increased for some motor tasks, significantly more study children than comparison children continued to have motor delay, for example, difficulty going downstairs using alternate feet, and delayed tandem walking and standing balance skills (Table 41.3).

Documented delay in motor tasks of a proportion of nondisabled children who have had moderate encephalopathy associated with perinatal asphyxia is not unexpected. Children with lack of everyday motor skill proficiency may benefit from intervention and counseling.

Cognitive ability

In all follow-up studies the major predictors of cognitive outcome are measures of genetic potential and nurturing environment. Cognitive testing among nondisabled survivors of perinatal asphyxia diagnosed neonatally by various methods but not specifically by neonatal encephalopathy has not been found to be sensitive to subtle brain insult.[30,51,123,129–134] Reporting on 24 studies that took place before the early 1970s, Gottfried concluded that, in survivors without frank neuropathology, cognitive deficits were more prevalent in infants and preschoolers than in older children.[130] Similar results were found in the St Louis prospective study of anoxia (determined by respiratory delay and method used for resuscitation) where cognitive delay of 3-year-old survivors resolved by 7 years.[123]

The severity of perinatal asphyxia as measured by the category of encephalopathy has been demonstrated to be predictive of school-age cognitive outcome.[12,35] Robertson et al.[12] have shown that the mean full-scale IQ for the mild encephalopathy group (none had motor, sensory, or mental disability) was 106 ± 13 and scores were not different from that of a peer group selected by two-stage, stratified, random-sample method. Nondisabled survivors of moderate neonatal encephalopathy had scores significantly below the peer group (102 ± 17 vs 112 ± 13). Disabled survivors of moderate and severe neonatal encephalopathy had markedly decreased scores (68 ± 27 and 48 ± 21 respectively).[12] School-age results from this center[12] have been confirmed using data from a second cohort (born 1982–86)[39] from 64 nondisabled survivors of moderate HIE (Table 41.4). The mean full-scale, verbal, and

Table 41.5. Percentage of school-age nondisabled survivors of moderate neonatal hypoxic–ischemic encephalopathy with academic achievement >1 grade level below expected grade level: two cohorts and their community comparison groups[a]

	Study 1 (born 1974–79)		Study 2 (born 1982–86)	
	Cohort 1 study (n=66)	Peer comparison (n=155)	Cohort 2 study (n=64)	Matched comparison (n=64)
Mean age at testing	8 years	8 years	9 years	9 years
Reading delay	35%[b]	15%	41%[c]	13%
Arithmetic delay	20%[b]	12%	39%[c]	9%
Reading or arithmetic delay	36%[b]	19%	52%[c]	16%

Notes:

[a] See Robertson et al.[12] and Robertson.[39]

[b] Denotes significant difference ($P<0.01$) from comparison group (chi-square test).

[c] Denotes significant difference ($P<0.001$) from comparison group (Cochran Q-test).

Cohort 1:
Reading standard – McCracken.[136]
Arithmetic standard – Connolly et al.[137]

Cohort II:
Reading and arithmetic standards – Woodcock-Johnson: Woodcock and Mather.[138]

"Nondisabled survivors" refers to children free from cerebral palsy, severe/profound cognitive deficit, vision or hearing loss, or epilepsy.

performance IQs are similar to those of normative data but significantly lower than a comparison group of children of the same age, matched for gender, maternal education, and family economic status (Table 41.4). The history of the presence of neonatal seizures lowers cognitive preschool scores when encephalopathy groups with or without disability are combined.[35,36,126]

Academic function

Few longitudinal studies of outcome of perinatal asphyxia have assessed school-age academic performance. The St Louis study reported that 29% of 7-year-old children were nonreaders.[123] Six- to 9-year-old children who were grouped by fetal heart rate patterns did not demonstrate any difference in academic performance between the groups.[129] This center has studied the long-term academic achievement of two cohorts of nondisabled children with moderate neonatal encephalopathy associated with perinatal asphyxia.[12,39] Table 41.5 shows the consistency of proportion in delay of academic achievement of the two cohorts, with significantly more study than comparison children being delayed.

We have previously reported that the strongest predictor of academic achievement delay in survivors of neonatal encephalopathy is the category of encephalopathy.[12] Those with mild HIE perform in a manner similar to community peer children.[12] The newborn finding of moderate encephalopathy places nondisabled as well as disabled children at risk for low academic achievement. We suggest that early school surveillance of the preschool and school performance of these children may identify those with difficulty and make it possible to offer early intervention.

Psychoeducational ability

Reports of psychoeducational/neuropsychological testing of children who have had perinatal asphyxia are sparse.[38] As for cognitive abilities and academic functioning, scores for psychoeducational tasks in subjects following perinatal asphyxia are similar to comparison groups unless neonatal moderate or severe encephalopathy is present.[123,133,134]

Kindergarten-age skills

Focusing on the survivors of moderate neonatal encephalopathy free from cerebral palsy, sensory or cognitive deficit, or epilepsy, Robertson and Finer[36] found 42% of 71 nondisabled kindergarten-age children delayed on school-readiness tests.[36] Scores for visual–motor integration, letter recognition, vocabulary, qualitative language, detailed recognition, auditory attention for related syllables, auditory discrimination of similarities and differences in initial, middle, and final sounds, sound blending as part of sound discrimination, and auditory memory were delayed compared with three other nondisabled comparison groups – mild encephalopathy, term neonatal comparison without encephalopathy, and a peer group.[36] Low scores for vocabulary and visual–motor integration measures recovered by 8 years from their delay found at 5.5 years.[12] Forty-four percent of a second cohort (born 1982–86) of 71 nondisabled moderate encephalopathy children determined in exactly the same way as the first cohort (born 1974–79) were found to have school-readiness delay.[126]

School-age skills

A great deal of debate has occurred about a continuum of causality after intrapartum asphyxia. Handley-Derry et al. have clearly demonstrated that, of 43 term neonates with no ($n=35$) or mild ($n=8$) encephalopathy but with an umbilical artery base deficit of >12 mmol/l there is no adverse outcome up to 8 years of age on gross and fine motor, cognitive, attention, memory, family functioning, and life stress measures compared with controls.[134] Subjects did not include neonates with lethargy, abnormal tone, or seizures.[134] Handley-Derry's study clarifies a threshold of intrapartum asphyxia where long-term deficit does not occur. It does not address children without cerebral palsy but who have had moderate encephalopathy due to late antenatal hypoxic–ischemic events, intrapartum asphyxia, or early neonatal asphyxia. In part his study explains negative results found previously where the majority of children with intrapartum asphyxia recover without modern intensive care.[123,133] In addition, many earlier studies made the assumption that, if cerebral palsy did not occur after term perinatal asphyxia, then adverse outcome would likely affect global intelligence or visual–spatial skills, hence test measures attempted to rule out long-term complications with intelligence tests or the Bender-Gestalt Test,[139] where results were found to be within normal limits.

Our school-age psychoeducational assessments of survivors of HIE free from cerebral palsy, sensory deficit, epilepsy, or mental retardation suggest a continuum of disability,[12,35,38,39] with the greatest area of weakness in verbal and auditory processing areas. We analyzed the psychoeducational test results of 8-year-old nondisabled HIE survivors of the 1974–79 cohort (cohort 1)[12] to determine the strengths and weaknesses of both visually and verbally related test results and to determine whether a homogeneous subgroup could be found within the nondisabled, moderate encephalopathy group.[39] Test results of 56 nondisabled mild and 66 nondisabled moderate neonatal encephalopathy survivors were compared with community peer group children and 69 term neonatal comparison group children without neonatal encephalopathy or known syndromes or central nervous system malformations.[38,39] Neonatal comparison children were identified in the neonatal period from the same intensive care units as the study children.[12,38] Detailed test results show more study children than comparison children have difficulties with verbally presented material.[38] Some motor speed and visual attention difficulties were also seen.[38] Overall, visual–perceptual skills were not a weakness. Analysis of the

Table 41.6. Means and standard deviations of scores or percent delayed scores for auditory skills (as identified in ordered domains by factor analysis) for 64 9-year-old nondisabled survivors of moderate neonatal hypoxic–ischemic encephalopathy and their matched-comparison group[a]

Auditory skills	Moderate encephalopathy group (n=64)	Matched-comparison group (n=64)
Domain 1: auditory-language/selective auditory attention/binaural separation		
Phonological sensitivity,[149] sound categorization		
Initial position	8.4 (2)	8.6 (2)
Middle position	7.4 (3)	7.8 (2)
Last position	7.6 (3)	7.8 (3)
Phonemic segmentation[150]	9.3 (2)	9.8 (2)
Digit span, forward[135]	9.0 (3)	8.5 (3)
Competing sentences, better ear[148]	53%	37%
Domain 2: auditory learning/recall/memory		
CAVLT, level of learning[151]	98 (16)[b]	104 (15)
CAVLT, immediate recall[151]	96 (18)[b]	105 (15)
CAVLT, delayed recall[151]	95 (15)[b]	103 (16)
Domain 3: binaural integration/sequencing and linguistic labeling		
Dichotic digits[152,153]		
Better ear	26%[b]	8%
Poorer ear	44%[b]	19%
Pitch pattern sequences[154]		
Hummed	11%[b]	0%
Verbal	60%[b]	41%
Individual results (not loading on above domains)		
CAVLT, immediate attention[151]	97 (15)	100 (15)
Digit span, backward[135]	9.6 (3)	10.5 (3)
CAVLT, recognition accuracy[151]	22%	27%
CAVLT, total intrusions[151]	19%	20%

Notes:

[a] See Robertson.[39]

[b] Denotes significant difference ($P<0.01$) from comparison group (Cochran Q-test, correlated t-test).

CAVLT, Children's auditory verbal learning test[151] (subtests: immediate attention, level of learning, immediate recall, delayed recall – normative score, 100 + 15); (subtests: recognition accuracy, total intrusions – delay is below 17th percentile of normative values).

Auditory tests of competing sentences,[148] dichotic digits,[152,153] pitch pattern sequences[154] – delay is >2 SD below mean of normative data.

Phonological and phonemic test results[149,150] = raw scores.

Digit span (subtest of the Wechsler Intelligence Scale for Children – Revised[135]) – normative scores, 10 ± 3.

"Nondisabled survivors" refers to children free from cerebral palsy, severe/profound cognitive deficit, vision or hearing loss, or epilepsy.

verbally related results of the psychoeducational test battery suggests that the nondisabled moderate encephalopathy group performed significantly below that of the peer group for phonetics,[140] auditory discrimination,[141] auditory subtests of verbal absurdities (comprehension),[142] auditory memory for related syllables (sentences),[142] auditory memory for unrelated syllables (words),[142] auditory closure,[143] sound blending,[143] and sentence production.[144] The results of measures of recall[142] were lower in the study group than comparison groups.

Central auditory processing skills

Clinical observations of school-age nondisabled survivors with moderate neonatal encephalopathy suggest that auditory-related processing difficulties may occur within a significant subgroup of these children. Histories include distractibility in a noisy background, difficulty following long or complex messages/instructions, delayed responses to questions, poor auditory memory, difficulty with phonics and sound discrimination, and difficulty in sequencing auditory information. These observations and the psychoeducational test results[38] led us to further investigations of the central auditory function of this group. We expected that more children who had had nondisabled moderate HIE would have central auditory dysfunction compared with matched-comparison children and that this dysfunction could be linked to the known increase in proportion of these children with academic delay.[12] The central auditory processing test battery chosen was divided into audiological and psychophysical tests[145–148] and completed by two certified audiologists.[39] Normative data are available.[145–148] Assessors were unaware of the group assignment, study, or comparison. Age, gender, socioeconomic status, and mother's education were the same for the two groups. All audiological measures were carried out in a sound-controlled testing room with calibrated audiometric measurements.

Analyses show that the results of the psychoeducational central auditory battery of tests divide well into three factors or domains of auditory skills plus some individual results (Table 41.6). Measures of auditory attention and concentration as well as language and binaural separation did not differ between the nondisabled survivors or moderate neonatal encephalopathy and the comparison group (Table 41.6). The study group had significantly lower scores for the processing of auditory learning over several trials, immediate and delayed recall, as well as binaural integration, and sequencing and labeling (Table 41.6). Auditory skill test results correlated with reading and arithmetic levels (Table 41.7).

Language skills

The susceptibility of language function to hypoxic–ischemic insult is well known. In 1981, D'Souza et al. reported that, following perinatal asphyxia, one-third of children without serious mental or physical handicap had deficits in speech and language.[106] Early expressive language delay has been documented for more recent nondisabled survivors of moderate HIE with severe metabolic acidosis (see Early childhood disability outcomes, earlier in this chapter). While developmental dysarthria may play a role in late abnormal speech development in some of these children,[155] central expressive language delay must also be considered.[117,120] Using the Clinical Evaluation of Language Function[144] moderate HIE nondisabled school-age survivors had significantly lower scores than a peer group.[38] A recent article on possible roles of the insula in speech and language processing explores possible effects of early damage to this area.[156] This problem may be clarified with the ability to assess accurately the cerebral operculum with imaging.[157]

Expressive and/or receptive language delay has been reported following early localized, unilateral cerebral infarction in 14 infants, seven with abnormal intrapartum and neonatal histories.[158] The side of the hemiparesis did not correspond with the subsequent early language delay.[158] However, early language damage to the left cerebral hemisphere has been shown to result in subtle, select deficit in language abilities, particularly syntactic skills in older children.[159] In a detailed study of the rate of progress of

Table 41.7. Significant correlations[a] ($P<0.05$) of reading and arithmetic levels with auditory measure results for 64 9-year-old non-disabled survivors of moderate neonatal hypoxic–ischemic encephalopathy[b]

	Reading (*r*)	Arithmetic (*r*)
Dichotic digits[152,153]		
Better ear	0.35	0.31
Poorer ear	0.26	0.35
Pitch pattern sequences[154]		
Hummed	0.32	0.32
Verbal	0.39	0.28
Competing sequences[148]		
Better ear	0.21	0.26
Phonological sensitivity[149]		
Sound categorization		
Initial position	0.28	0.41
Middle position	0.47	0.42
Final position	0.44	0.37
Phonemic segmentation[150]	0.44	0.45
CAVLT[151]		
Immediate attention	NS	0.24
Level of learning	0.36	0.28
Immediate recall	0.29	NS
Delayed recall	0.33	0.24
Recognition accuracy	0.21	NS
Total intrusions	0.26	NS
Digit span[135]		
Forward	0.41	0.42
Backward	0.41	0.53

Notes:

[a] Pearson product moment correlations: correlations of ≥0.21 differ significantly from zero at the $P<0.05$ level; ≥0.39 at the $P<0.001$ level.

[b] See Robertson.[39]

CAVLT, Children's auditory verbal learning test;[151] NS, not significant.

"Nondisabled survivors" refers to children free from cerebral palsy, severe/profound cognitive deficit, vision or hearing loss, or epilepsy.

language development from 15 to 48 months in eight children with perinatal brain damage, individual growth trajectories followed an early delayed but normal pattern.[160] The developmental patterns suggest that both cerebral hemispheres may play critical roles in the very earliest of language acquisition.[160]

In our experience, autistic disorder is uncommon among survivors of perinatal asphyxia. In the follow-up of more than 500 survivors with moderate or severe HIE born in this region from 1974 to 1999, we have diagnosed one boy with higher-level autism. Autism is rarely mentioned as part of the outcome profile of these children in the literature.

Memory

In general, the testing of memory in childhood involves tests for explicit memory that measure the conscious recollection of materials learned in a previous episode. This so-called long-term memory is defined by the ability to retain, store, and retrieve information beyond the capacity of short-term memory which has a very limited capacity and a short time limit, as measured in seconds, unless rehearsed. Explicit or declarative memory includes episodic memory or memory for events such as reliable account of the day's events, messages, or stories read; and somatic memory or the ability to learn new facts or procedures.[161] This is in contrast to implicit or nondeclarative memory such as the ability to remember skills and habits.[161] Episodic memory relies on an intact hippocampal function of the mediotemporal lobe system, the diencephalon, and the frontal lobes of the cerebral cortex.[161]

Among term asphyxiated infants, neurons of the CA1 region of the hippocampus (Sommer's section), deeper layers of the cerebral cortex, putamen, thalamus, and cerebellar Purkinje's cells are injured most frequently by hypoxic–ischemic insult.[23] Such neonates with abnormalities of the hippocampus on early magnetic resonance imaging have also been found to have changes in the basal ganglia.[47] This corresponds with neuropathological studies where the hippocampus has been found to be susceptible to hypoxic–ischemic injury but rarely in isolation.[162]

However, quantitative magnetic resonance imaging investigations have shown severe bilateral hippocampal atrophy associated with bilateral reductions in the gray matter in the regions of the putamen and the ventral thalamus in three term infants with neonatal HIE but without cerebral palsy and cognitive deficit.[163] These children had severe impairment of memory for the following: 90-min delayed recall of stories, 40-min delayed copying of geometric design, and 20-min delayed recall of auditory verbal learning tasks.[163] We have found similar delayed results for auditory memory in nondisabled moderate HIE school-age survivors.[38,39]

A study of the follow-up of young adults with previously normal neurodevelopmental assessments who had neonatal seizures of intrapartum or neonatal origin may be helpful to investigate further this question of outcome of memory.[164] Of these 22 children, the 15 assessed at ages 17–19 years showed abnormal neuropsychological results with a scattering of the IQ test profile, socially disruptive behavior, and delayed spelling and memory.[164] Memory for late recall of a copied image scored below the fifth percentile for eight of the 15 subjects. This would be a score below that expected for average 10-year-old children. The pattern of memory loss was not specific. In addition, four of the 15 subjects obtained extremely low scores on facial and word recognition.[164]

Two case studies

The following case studies show significant adverse childhood outcome without cerebral palsy following perinatal asphyxia. Consider the timing of the hypoxic–ischemic event for these children from a prospective point of view, that is, whether it occurred in the late antenatal, natal, or neonatal period. Upon investigation, no causes other than perinatal asphyxia have been determined to explain the outcome of these children.

Case 1

This boy was born at a primary-level hospital and transported to our tertiary-level neonatal intensive care unit at 8 h of age. Serial follow-up assessments occurred until age 5 years. Mother, age 35, gravida two, married, and healthy with a low antenatal risk score, delivered at 41 weeks' gestation. She had had no fever and membranes ruptured spontaneously 30 min before delivery. Decreased fetal movement was reported 2 days prior to delivery and a nonstress test completed 30 h before delivery demonstrated no variability. A synthetic analog gel of prostaglandin E_2 induced labor. Throughout a labor of approximately 9 h, there was no variability to the fetal heart tracing other than late in the first stage of labor when bradycardia occurred. Meconium was present. A forceps vaginal delivery occurred in the vertex position. No birth trauma occurred. Umbilical artery gases were not available. The Apgar score at 1 min was 1 and at 5 min was 5. Intubation and ventilation occurred. The birth weight was 3700 g and the head circumference 37 cm. The neonatal course was complicated by persistent pulmonary hypertension requiring ventilation and inotropic support. The baby was in room air at 6 days of age. Recurrent subtle seizures began at 9 h of age and phenobarbital was used. On day 3, an electroencephalograph demonstrated a burst-suppression pattern. The neurological examination was abnormal and overall classed as moderate HIE. The most abnormal examination occurred on days 3 and 4. At this time there was some visual awareness, severe hypotonia, suppressed primitive reflexes, tongue fasciculation with constant tongue protrusion, transiently absent deep tendon reflexes, and an increase of head circumference of 1 cm above the birth head circumference. At 5 days of age a nerve conduction test suggested the presence of an electrical ankle jerk. An electromyography was done with good recruitment with no fibrillation or fasciculations, hence suggesting no anterior horn cell disease. Computed axial tomography was completed at 10 days of age and demonstrated decreased attenuation of the parietal–occipital white matter with smaller occipital ventricular horns and some gray-matter involvement. Brainstem audiological evoked response testing was completed at 6 and 10 days of age and showed normal peripheral hearing but prolonged wave III–V interpeak latencies, reduced wave V:I amplitude ratio, and a barely detectable wave V suggesting neurological dysfunction. Breast-feeding was established at 10 days of age. Neonatal seizures did not recur.

From birth to 4 months of age, this boy's head circumference ratio decreased by 11%. At 18 months of age the head circumference was 1.5 SD below the mean. The Mental Development Index[62] was 55. He was sociable and engaging with gross motor skills 3–4 months delayed, fine motor skills 6–8 months delayed, and expressive language 6 months below age. Seizures began at 3½ years of age with nocturnal vomiting and headaches. An electroencephalogram showed distinct epileptiform changes from the left central parietal region. These apparent seizures have been controlled with Tegretol. At almost 5 years of age he had above average somatic growth, head circumference 1.5 SD below the mean, a mild right homonymous hemianopsia as a manifestation of mild cortical visual impairment, reduced stereoacuity, and no hearing loss. A diagnosis of trainable mental retardation was made using standardized testing and an adaptive measure. Gross motor skills were low-normal, fine motor skills at the 3-year range, and language skills at the 3–3½ year range. Magnetic resonance imaging completed at almost 5 years showed no cranial malformation but marked white-matter atrophy of the occipital and posterior parietal lobes, greater on the left, with dilatation of adjacent occipital horns and decreased prominence of the overlying subarachnoid space with widening of the sulci.

Case 2

This boy was born at a secondary-level hospital and transferred to our tertiary-level neonatal intensive care unit at 10½h of age. Serial follow-up assessments occurred until 8 years of age. Mother, age 29, gravida one, married, was healthy with a low antenatal risk score. Seven days prior to delivery she presented with backache and a nonstress test was completed which was reactive. She presented for spontaneous vertex delivery at 39½ weeks gestation with the first stage of spontaneous labor lasting 3½h and the second stage of labor lasting 18 min. During labor the fetal heart rate tracing was initially reassuring, then showed loss of beat-to-beat variability, and bradycardia of 90 beats/min just before the second stage. Membranes ruptured at delivery and meconium was present. There was a tight nuchal cord. Umbilical cord gases were not available. The baby was stillborn. The birth weight was 3500g and the head circumference 35 cm. The Apgar score was zero at 1, 5, and 10 min. A pulse was obtained at 20 min of life and the first spontaneous gasp occurred at 1h of age. Intubation, ventilation, and complete cardiopulmonary resuscitation with epinephrine were used. At 20 min of age the arterial pH was 7.08, $P\text{CO}_2$ was 40mmHg, and the base deficit was 17mmol/l. Multifocal seizures began at 3h of age and phenobarbital was given. At 3½h of age the pH was 7.19, $P\text{CO}_2$ was 30mmHg, and base deficit 15mmol/l. Hypotension continued and a cardiac arrest occurred at 5h of age with a subsequent pH of 6.79, $P\text{CO}_2$ of 66mmHg, and base deficit 25mmol/l. After full consultation, aggressive treatment was withdrawn at 6½h of age followed by a cardiopulmonary arrest. Spontaneous gasps occurred within 10 min of this arrest. Compassionate care was given with no supplemental oxygen used thereafter. Between these episodes of arrest, the baby had periods of no muscle tone and no movement. While this could be considered severe encephalopathy, the baby was not stable enough to categorize the encephalopathy. Pleural effusions, thrombocytopenia, anuria, low serum sodium, and bloody stools occurred. After several days bottle-feeding began and at 12 days of age a cranial ultrasound was reported to be within normal limits.

From birth to 4 months of age this boy's head circumference ratio decreased by 1%. At 18 months of age the head circumference was 0.5 SD below the mean for age and the Mental Development Index[62] was 98. Gross motor, fine motor and language skills were within normal limits. A left esotropia was noted and a visual field defect suspected. Repeated assessments between 5½ and 8 years of age demonstrated above average somatic growth, average head circumference, average cognitive development with an increased verbal–performance split as measured by standardized testing, normal peripheral hearing, normal right vision, but limited depth perception with a severe left amblyopia. Academic performance was decreased for age and he had developed avoidance strategies when work was found to be difficult. He was easily distractable in class. Extensive specialized educational programs were given. No seizures occurred and an electroencephalogram was not done. Cranial magnetic resonance imaging carried out at age 6½ years of age showed no congenital developmental malformations. Cortical spinal tract gliosis was diagnosed with abnormality in the motor sensory cortex around the rolandic fissure. The rolandic gyri appeared slightly smaller than the gyri elsewhere. The periventricular white matter was not significantly decreased in thickness. The basal ganglia and thalami were normal. The visual radiation appeared abnormal and the visual cortex was slightly decreased in size.

Because of this boy's learning difficulties and distractability at school, central auditory processing testing was completed.[145–154] He demonstrated below-expected range for the dichotic digits test, significantly delayed competing sentences test with absent responses on the left, decreased speech in noise test, and well below expected range for the staggered spondaic word test. These test results suggest some difficulty with listening in noise and decreased short-term memory as well as difficulty accurately processing speech and lack of sequence and organization when recalling words. He became restless during testing and frustrated on more difficult tasks. Overall, this testing suggested moderate-to-severe central auditory processing difficulties. Counseling of the parents and teacher was done and a personal FM free-field system of amplification was recommended. While his clinical presentation on school tasks is that of a child with some attentional and listening problems, he does not fit a category of attentional deficit disorder because his difficulties are only present in the school setting.[89] No medication for attention deficit disorder has been prescribed to date. His classroom learning improved with the amplification system.

Life expectancy

After 8 years of follow-up we reported fewer than 25% of neonates with severe HIE to be alive.[12] When combining moderate and severe HIE, about 10% of children die before school age (Table 41.2). Recently we noted that 10 (24%) of 41 neonates with moderate/severe HIE and umbilical artery pH of <7.00 died before 18 months of age. Deaths occurred in children with multiple disabilities, primarily cerebral palsy, mental retardation, and epilepsy, and often associated with terminal pulmonary difficulties.

Children with cerebral palsy born at term and with neonatal encephalopathy are more likely to have a more severe form of cerebral palsy than those without neonatal encephalopathy.[68] Among children with cerebral palsy, survival is less with an increasing number of limbs involved.[165] Similarly, death rate is increased with spastic quadriplegia, severe-to-profound mental retardation, and epilepsy,[166] and increased functional disability.[167] However, in the 1990s, life expectancy for children with cerebral palsy improved over previous years.[167]

Summary

The value of long-term follow-up of term infants with perinatal asphyxia has been questioned because of the lack of a uniform accepted diagnosis to provide a definition for the reference population. The phrase "perinatal asphyxia of the term neonate" encompasses a variety of times of occurrence and degrees of hypoxic–ischemic insults as well as selective vulnerability of the neonatal brain as reflected in a wide range of clinical childhood outcomes. Restrictive operational definitions for intrapartum asphyxia and the limitation of outcome measures to death and quadriplegic cerebral palsy have value in focusing obstetrical preventive and neonatal neuroprotective measures. However, acknowledgment of broader perinatal asphyxial insults and consideration of a wider variety of childhood outcomes could improve the understanding of both of these areas. Neonatal brain imaging and clinical assessments suggest more research is needed to improve knowledge of hypoxic–ischemic events occurring in the late antepartum period when obstetrical intervention could take place. Longitudinal studies of such survivors could be useful to examine the spectrum of outcome of perinatal asphyxia.

To date, the presence of and categorization for the early outcome measure of neonatal encephalopathy associated with clinical hypoxic–ischemic events remains among the most useful single indicator of long-term outcome following any suspected perinatal asphyxia, regardless of the degree of other indicators such as metabolic acidosis. This clinical examination is simple, universally available, inexpensive, repeatable, and, when done properly, is a useful prognostic tool. The most useful aspect of this tool is that the presence of mild encephalopathy or the lack of encephalopathy following a presumed asphyxial insult indicates a good outcome. The exception to this statement may occur following cerebral infarction when no encephalopathy or any one of the stages of neonatal encephalopathy may be associated with sequelae. A clinical picture of moderate-to-severe neonatal HIE places the neonate at risk for death or disability. When the surviving child is free from cerebral palsy, cognitive deficit, sensory loss, or epilepsy, there continues to be a risk of motor and/or academic delay. Psychoeducational and psychophysical central auditory processing measures suggest that an increased proportion of these children have verbally and/or auditorily related learning problems. Major visual–perceptual difficulties have not been common. Further neuropsychological studies on the acquisition of new learning, memory, problem solving, and reasoning may be helpful to delineate further the learning profiles of these children. SNHL, when it occurs, tends to be a late-onset high-frequency loss of uncertain etiology and more common among children with associated neonatal respiratory failure. Further knowledge about the long-term outcome of neonatal encephalopathy associated with perinatal asphyxia could lead to enhanced, focused surveillance of these children and provide opportunity for early intervention.

Acknowledgments

Support for the database from which long-term follow-up outcome is derived is from the Northern Alberta Regional Perinatal Program and the Glenrose Rehabilitation Hospital, Edmonton, Alberta, Canada. It is with deep appreciation that we acknowledge the children and their parents who regularly attend our Neonatal and Infant Follow-up Clinic.

REFERENCES

1 Power C. (1994). The special role of longitudinal studies. In *The Epidemiology of Childhood Disorders*, ed. Pless IB, pp. 31–46. Oxford: Oxford University Press.

2 Goldstein H. (1979). *The Design and Analysis of Longitudinal Studies: Their Role in the Measurement of Change*, pp. 1–13. London: Academic Press.

3 Benson K and Hartz AJ. (2000). A comparison of observational studies and randomized, controlled trials. *N Engl J Med*, **342**, 1878–1886.

4 Johnson A. (1997). Follow-up studies: a case for a standard minimum data set. *Arch Dis Child*, **76**, F61–F63.

5 Saigal S. (1991). Follow-up of high risk infants: methodological issues, current status, and future trends. In *Reproductive and Perinatal Epidemiology*, ed. Kiely M, pp. 337–355. Boca Raton, USA: CRC Press.

6 Ryan CA, Byrne P, Kahn S, et al. (1993). Resuscitation and withdrawal of therapy in a neonatal and a pediatric intensive care unit in Canada. *J Pediatr*, **123**, 534–538.

7 Robertson CMT, Sauve RS, Whitfield MF, et al. (1995). Neurodevelopmental outcome after neonatal extracorporeal oxygenation. *Can Med Assoc J*, **152**, 1981–1988.

8 Blair E and Stanley FJ. (1988). Intrapartum asphyxia: a rare cause of cerebral palsy. *J Pediatr*, **112**, 115–119.

9 Nelson KB and Ellenberg JH. (1987). The asymptomatic newborn and risk of cerebral palsy. *Am J Dis Child*, **141**, 1333–1338.

10 Patel J and Edwards AD. (1997). Prediction of outcome after perinatal asphyxia. *Curr Opin Pediatr*, **9**, 128–132.

11 Volpe JJ. (1995). Hypoxic–ischemic encephalopathy: clinical aspects. In *Neurology of the Newborn*, ed. Volpe JJ, 3rd edn, pp. 314–369. Philadelphia: WB Saunders.

12 Robertson CMT, Finer NN and Grace MGA. (1989). School performance of survivors of neonatal encephalopathy associated with birth asphyxia at term. *J Pediatr*, **114**, 753–760.

13 Cowan F. (2000). Outcome after intrapartum asphyxia in term infants. *Semin Neonatol*, **5**, 127–140.
14 Bax M and Nelson KB. (1993). Birth asphyxia: a statement. *Dev Med Child Neurol*, **35**, 1015–1024.
15 Blair E. (1993). A research definition for 'birth asphyxia'. *Dev Med Child Neurol*, **35**, 449–455.
16 Edwards AD and Nelson KB. (1998). Neonatal encephalopathies. Time to reconsider the cause of encephalopathies. *Br Med J*, **317**, 1537–1538.
17 MacLennan A. (1999). A template for defining a causal relationship between acute intrapartum events and cerebral palsy: international consensus statement. *Br Med J*, **319**, 1054–1059.
18 Dear P and Newell S. (2000). Establishing probable cause in cerebral palsy. How much certainty is enough. *Br Med J*, **320**, 1075–1076.
19 Goodlin RC. (1995). Do concepts of causes and prevention of cerebral palsy require revision? *Am J Obstet Gynecol*, **172**, 1830–1836.
20 Rosenbloom K and Rennie JM. (2000). There are problems with the consensus statement. *Br Med J*, **320**, 1076.
21 Myers R. (1975). Four patterns of perinatal brain damage and their conditions of occurrence in primates. *Adv Neurol*, **10**, 223–234.
22 Pasternak JF and Gorey MT. (1998). The syndrome of acute near-total intrauterine asphyxia in the term infant. *Pediatr Neurol*, **18**, 391–398.
23 Inder TE and Volpe JJ. (2000). Mechanisms of perinatal brain injury. *Semin Neonatol*, **5**, 3–16.
24 Johnston MV. (1998). Selective vulnerability in neonatal brain. *Ann Neurol*, **44**, 155–156.
25 Marin-Padilla M. (1999). Developmental neuropathology and impact of perinatal brain damage. III: Gray matter lesions of the neocortex. *J Neuropathol Exp Neurol*, **58**, 407–429.
26 Perlman JM. (1997). Intrapartum hypoxic–ischemic cerebral palsy and subsequent cerebral palsy: medicolegal issues. *Pediatrics*, **99**, 851–858.
27 Nelson KB. (1999). The neurologically impaired child and alleged malpractice at birth. *Neurol Clin*, **17**, 283–293.
28 Task Force on Joint Assessment of Prenatal and Perinatal Factors Associated With Brain Disorders. (1985). National Institutes of Health report on causes of mental retardation and cerebral palsy. *Pediatrics*, **76**, 457–458.
29 Nelson KB and Ellenburg JH. (1981). Apgar scores as predictors of chronic neurologic disability. *Pediatrics*, **68**, 36–44.
30 Broman SH. (1979). Perinatal anoxia and cognitive development in early childhood. In *Infants Born at Risk*, eds. Broman SH, Field T, Sostek A, et al., pp. 29–52. New York: Spectrum Press.
31 Naeye RL and Peters EC. (1987). Antenatal hypoxia and low IQ value. *Am J Dis Child*, **141**, 50–54.
32 Bennett FC. (1997). Foreword. In *Fetal and Neonatal Brain Injury: Mechanisms, Management and the Risks of Practice*, 2nd edn, eds. Stevenson DK and Sunshine P, pp. v–xi. Oxford: Oxford Medical Publications.
33 Johnson A. (1997). Randomized controlled trials in perinatal medicine: 3. Identifying and measuring endpoints in randomized controlled trial. *Br J Obstet Gynaecol*, **104**, 768–771.
34 Amiel-Tison C and Ellison P. (1986). Birth asphyxia in the full term newborn: early assessment and outcome. *Dev Med Child Neurol*, **28**, 617–682.
35 Robertson CMT and Finer NN. (1985). Term infants with hypoxic–ischemic encephalopathy: outcome at 3.5 years. *Dev Med Child Neurol*, **27**, 473–484.
36 Robertson CMT and Finer NN. (1988). Educational readiness of survivors of neonatal encephalopathy associated with birth asphyxia at term. *J Dev Behav Pediatr*, **9**, 298–306.
37 Levene MI. (1995). Management and outcome of birth asphyxia. In *Fetal and Neonatal Neurology and Neurosurgery*, eds. Levene MI, Lilford RJ, Bennett MJ, et al., pp. 427–442. London: Churchill Livingstone.
38 Robertson CMT and Finer NN. (1993). Long-term follow-up of term neonates with perinatal asphyxia. *Clin Perinatol*, **20**, 483–500.
39 Robertson CMT. (1997). Long-term follow-up of term infants with perinatal asphyxia. In *Fetal and Neonatal Brain Injury: Mechanisms, Management and the Risks of Practice*, 2nd edn, eds. Stevenson DK and Sunshine P, pp. 615–630.Oxford: Oxford University Press.
40 Badawi N, Kurinczuk JJ, Keogh JM, et al. (1998). Intrapartum risk factors for newborn encephalopathy: the Western Australian case-control study. *Br Med J*, **317**, 1554–1558.
41 Thornberg E, Thiringer K, Odeback A, et al. (1995). Birth asphyxia: incidence, clinical course and outcome in a Swedish population. *Acta Paediatr*, **84**, 927–932.
42 Leviton A and Nelson KB. (1992). Problems with definitions and classifications of newborn encephalopathy. *Pediatr Neurol*, **8**, 85–90.
43 Sarnat HB and Sarnat MS. (1987). Neonatal encephalopathy following fetal distress, a clinical and electroencephalographic study. *Arch Neurol*, **33**, 696–705.
44 Levene MI, Sands C, Grindulis H, et al. (1986). Comparison of two methods of predicting outcome in perinatal asphyxia. *Lancet*, **1**, 67–69.

45 Barabas RE, Barmada MA and Scher MS. (1993). Timing of brain insults in severe neonatal encephalopathies with isoelectric EEG. *Pediatr Neurol*, **9**, 39–44.

46 Thompson CM, Paterman AS, Linley LL, et al. (1997). The value of a scoring system for hypoxic–ischemic encephalopathy. *Acta Paediatr*, **86**, 757–761.

47 Rutherford MA, Pennock JM, Schwieso JE, et al. (1995). Hypoxic ischemic encephalopathy: early magnetic resonance imaging findings and their evolution. *Neuropediatrics*, **26**, 183–191.

48 Levene MI, Kornberg J and Williams THC. (1985). The incidence and severity of post-asphyxial encephalopathy in full term infants. *Early Hum Dev*, **11**, 2125.

49 Fenichel GM. (1983). Hypoxic–ischemic encephalopathy in the newborn. *Arch Neurol*, **40**, 261–266.

50 Amiel-Tison C and Stewart A. (1989). Cerebral palsy Doppler ultrasonography for prediction of outcome after perinatal asphyxia. *Lancet*, suppl. **a**, 67–72.

51 Low JA, Galbraith RS, Muir DW, et al. (1988). Motor and cognitive deficits after intrapartum fetal hypoxia in the mature fetus. *Am J Obstet Gynecol*, **158**, 356–361.

52 Hull J and Dodd KL. (1992). Falling incidence of hypoxic–ischemic encephalopathy in term infants. *Br J Obstet Gynaecol*, **99**, 386–391.

53 Painter MJ. (1989). Fetal heart rate patterns, perinatal asphyxia, and brain injury. *Pediatr Neurol*, **5**, 137–144.

54 Whitelaw A. (1989). Intervention after birth asphyxia. *Arch Dis Child*, **64**, 66–71.

55 Gray P, Tudehope DJ, Masel JP, et al. (1993). Perinatal hypoxic–ischemic brain injury: prediction of outcome. *Dev Med Child Neurol*, **35**, 965–973.

56 Eyman RK, Grossman HJ and Chaney RH. (1990). The life expectancy of profoundly handicapped people with mental retardation. *N Engl J Med*, **323**, 584–588.

57 Martin JJ, Brombrink A, Kochler RC, et al. (1997). Primary sensory and forebrain motor systems in the newborn brain are preferentially damaged by hypoxic–ischemia. *J Comp Neurol*, **377**, 262–285.

58 Cheung P-Y and Robertson CMT. (2000). Predicting the outcome of term neonates with intrapartum asphyxia. *Acta Paediatr*, **80**, 262–271.

59 Roland EH, Poskitt K, Rodriguez E, et al. (1998). Perinatal hypoxic–ischemic thalamic injury: clinical features and neuroimaging. *Ann Neurol*, **44**, 161–166.

60 Nelson KB and Grether JK. (1998). Potentially asphyxiating conditions and spastic cerebral palsy in infants of normal birth weight. *Am J Obstet Gynecol*, **179**, 507–513.

61 Griffiths R. (1970). *The Abilities of Babies.* London, England: University of London Press.

62 Bayley N. (1993). *The Bayley Scales of Infant Development*, 2nd edn. New York, NY: Psychological Corporation.

63 Amess PN, Penrice J, Wylezinska M, et al. (1999). Early brain proton magnetic resonance spectroscopy and neonatal neurology related to neurodevelopmental outcome at 1 year in term infants after presumed hypoxic–ischaemic brain injury. *Dev Med Child Neurol*, **41**, 436–445.

64 Mercuri E, Ricci D, Cowan FM, et al. (2000). Head growth in infants with hypoxic–ischemic encephalopathy: correlation with neonatal magnetic resonance imaging. *Pediatrics*, **106**, 235–243.

65 Rutherford MA, Pennock JM, Counsell SJ, et al. (1998). Abnormal magnetic resonance signal in the internal capsule predicts poor neurodevelopmental outcome in infants with hypoxic–ischemic encephalopathy. *Pediatrics*, **102**, 323–328.

66 Barkowich AJ, Hajnal BL, Vigneron D, et al. (1998). Prediction of neuromotor outcomes in perinatal asphyxia: evaluation of MR scoring systems. *Am J Neuroradiol*, **19**, 143–149.

67 Huang C-C, Wang S-T, Chang Y-C, et al. (1999). Measurement of the urinary lactate: creatinine ratio for the early identification of newborn infants at risk for hypoxic–ischemic encephalopathy. *N Engl J Med*, **341**, 328–335.

68 Gaffney G, Flavell V, Johnson A, et al. (1994). Cerebral palsy and neonatal encephalopathy. *Arch Dis Child*, **70**, F195–F200.

69 Gaffney G, Flavell V, Johnson A, et al. (1995). Model to identify potentially preventable cerebral palsy of intrapartum origin. *Arch Dis Child*, **74**, F106–F108.

70 Yudkin PL, Johnson A, Clover LM, Murphy KW. (1995). Assessing the contribution of birth asphyxia in term singletons. *Pediatr Perinat Epidemiol*, **9**, 156–170.

71 Gaffney G, Sellers S, Flavell V, et al. (1994). Case-control study of intrapartum care, cerebral palsy, and perinatal death. *Br Med J*, **308**, 743–750.

72 Watt JM, Robertson CMT and Grace MGA. (1989). Early prognosis for ambulation of neonatal intensive care survivors with cerebral palsy. *Dev Med Child Neurol*, **31**, 766–773.

73 Rutherford MA, Pennock JM, Murdock-Eaton DM, et al. (1992). Athetoid cerebral palsy with cysts in the putamen after hypoxic–ischemic encephalopathy. *Arch Dis Child*, **67**, 846–850.

74 Rosenbloom L. (1994). Dyskinetic cerebral palsy and birth asphyxia. *Dev Med Child Neurol*, **36**, 285–289.

75 Saint-Hilaire MH, Burke RE, Bressman SB, et al. (1991). Delayed-onset dystonia due to perinatal and early childhood asphyxia. *Neurology*, **216**, 22.

76 Govaert P, Matthys E, Zecic A, et al. (2000). Perinatal cortical infarction within middle cerebral artery trunks. *Arch Dis Child Fetal Neonatal Edn*, **82**, F59–F63.

77 Sreenan C, Bhargava R and Robertson CMT. (2000). Cerebral infarction in the term newborn: clinical presentation and long-term outcome. *J Pediatr*, **137**, 351–355.

78 Estan J, Hope P. (1997). Unilateral neonatal cerebral infarction in full term infants. *Arch Dis Child*, **76**, F88–F93.

79 Koelfen W, Freund M and Varnholt V. (1995). Neonatal stroke involving the middle cerebral artery in term infants: clinical presentation, EEG and imaging studies, and outcome. *Dev Med Child Neurol*, **37**, 204–212.

80 Blair E and Stanley F. (1985). Interobserver agreement in the classification of cerebral palsy. *Dev Med Child Neurol*, **27**, 615–622.

81 Pharoah POD, Cooke T, Johnson MA, et al. (1988). Epidemiology of cerebral palsy in England and Scotland, 1984–9. *Arch Dis Child Fetal Neonatal Edn*, **79**, F21–F25.

82 Robertson CMT, Svenson LW and Joffres MR. (1998). Prevalence of cerebral palsy in Alberta. *Can J Neurol Sci*, **25**, 117–122.

83 Prechtl HFR. (1997). State of the art of a new functional assessment of the young nervous system. An early predictor of cerebral palsy. *Early Hum Dev*, **50**, 1–11.

84 Prechtl HF, Einspieler C, Cioni G, et al. (1997). An early marker for neurological deficits after perinatal brain lesions. *Lancet*, **349**, 1361–1363.

85 Weindling AM, Hallam P, Gregg J, et al. (1996). A randomized controlled trial of early physiotherapy for high-risk infants. *Acta Paediatr*, **85**, 1107–1111.

86 Sola DA and Grant AD. (1995). Prognosis for ambulation in cerebral palsy. *Dev Med Child Neurol*, **37**, 1020–1026.

87 Palisano R, Rosenbaum P, Walter S, et al. (1997). Development and reliability of a system to classify gross motor function in children with cerebral palsy. *Dev Med Child Neurol*, **30**, 214–223.

88 Rosenbloom L. (1995). Diagnosis and management of cerebral palsy. *Arch Dis Child*, **72**, 350–354.

89 American Psychiatric Association. (2000). *Diagnostic and Statistical Manual of Mental Disorders (DSM-IV-TR)*, 4th edn, *Test Revision*, pp. 41–49, 85–93. Washington, DC: American Psychiatric Association.

90 Richardson SA and Koller H. (1994). Mental retardation. In *The Epidemiology of Childhood Disorders*, ed. Pless IB, pp. 277–303. New York: Oxford University Press.

91 Shankaran S, Woldt E, Koepke T, et al. (1991). Acute neonatal morbidity and long-term central nervous system sequelae of perinatal asphyxia in term infants. *Early Hum Dev*, **25**, 135–148.

92 Roth SC, Baudin J, Cady E, et al. (1997). Relation of deranged neonatal cerebral oxidative metabolism with neurodevelopmental outcome and head circumference at 4 years. *Dev Med Child Neurol*, **39**, 718–725.

93 Prechtl HFR, Ferrari F and Cioni G. (1993). Predictive value of general movements in asphyxiated full term infants. *Early Hum Dev*, **35**, 91–120.

94 Robertson CMT. (1999). Can hypoxic–ischemic encephalopathy (HIE) associated with term birth asphyxia lead to mental disability without cerebral palsy? *Can J Neurol Sci*, **2**, 36.

95 Mizrahi EM and Kellaway P. (1987). Characterization and classification of neonatal seizures. *Neurology*, **37**, 1837–1844.

96 Evans DJ and Levene MI. (2000). Anticonvulsants for preventing mortality and morbidity in full term newborns with perinatal asphyxia. *Cochrane Database System Rev*, CD001240.

97 van Hof-van Duin J and Mohn G. (1984). Visual defects in children after cerebral hypoxia. *Behav Brain Res*, **14**, 147–155.

98 Mercuri E, Atkinson J, Braddick O, et al. (1997). Basal ganglia damage and impaired visual function in the newborn infant. *Arch Dis Child*, **77**, F111–F114.

99 Cioni G, Fazzi B, Ipata AE, et al. (1996). Correlation between cerebral visual impairment and magnetic resonance imaging in children with neonatal encephalopathy. *Dev Med Child Neurol*, **38**, 120–132.

100 Atkinson JJ and van Hof-van Duin J. (1993). Assessment of normal and abnormal vision during the first year of life. In *Management of Visual Handicap in Childhood*, eds. Fielder A and Bax M, pp. 9–39. London: Mac Keith Press.

101 Mercuri E, Atkinson J, Braddick O, et al. (1997). Visual function in full-term infants with hypoxic–ischemic encephalopathy. *Neuropediatrics*, **28**, 155–161.

102 Mercuri E, Haataja L, Guzzetta A, et al. (1999). Visual function in term infants with hypoxic–ischemic insults: correlation with neurodevelopment at 2 years of age. *Arch Dis Child Fetal Neonatal Edn*, **80**, F99–F104.

103 Lambert SR, Hoyt CS, Jan JE, et al. (1987). Visual recovery from hypoxic cortical blindness during childhood. Computed tomographic and magnetic resonance imaging predictors. *Arch Ophthalmol*, **105**, 1371–1377.

104 Jiang ZD. (1995). Long-term effect of perinatal and postnatal asphyxia on developing human auditory brainstem responses: peripheral hearing loss. *Int J Pediatr Otorhinolaryngol*, **33**, 225–238.

105 Joint Committee on Infant Hearing. (1991). 1990 position statement. *J Am Speech Hearing Assoc*, **33** (suppl. 5), 3–6.

106 D'Souza SW, McCartney E, Nolan M, et al. (1981). Hearing, speech, and language in survivors of severe perinatal asphyxia. *Arch Dis Child*, **56**, 245–252.

107 Borg E. (1997). Perinatal asphyxia, hypoxia, ischemia and hearing loss. *Scand Audiol*, **26**, 77–91.

108 The Neonatal Inhaled Nitric Oxide Group. (2000). Inhaled nitric oxide in term and near-term infants: neurodevelopmental follow-up of the Neonatal Inhaled Oxide Study Group (NINOS). *J Pediatr*, **136**, 611–617.

109 Cheung P-Y, Magathan-Haluschak M, Finer NN, et al. (1996). Sensorineural hearing loss in survivors of neonatal extracorporeal membrane oxygenation. *Early Hum Dev*, **44**, 225–233.

110 Cheung P-Y, Tyebkhan JM, Peliowski A, et al. (1999). Prolonged use of pancuronium bromide and sensorineural hearing loss in childhood survivors of congenital diaphragmatic hernia. *J Pediatr*, **135**, 233–239.

111 Kileny P, Connolly C and Robertson C. (1980). Auditory brainstem responses in perinatal asphyxia. *Int J Ped Otorhinolaryngol*, **2**, 147–159.

112 Jiang ZD and Tierney TS. (1996). Long-term effect of perinatal and postnatal asphyxia on developing human auditory brainstem responses: brainstem impairment. *Int J Pediatr Otorhinolaryngol*, **34**, 111–127.

113 Badawi N, Kurinczuk JJ and Blair EE. (1994). Early prediction of the development of microcephaly after hypoxic–ischemic encephalopathy in the full-term newborn. *Pediatrics*, **93**, 703–707.

114 Mercuri E, Ricci D, Cowan FM, et al. (2000). Head growth in infants with hypoxic–ischemic encephalopathy: correlation with neonatal magnetic resonance imaging. *Pediatrics*, **106**, 235–243.

115 Cordes I, Roland EH, Lupton BA, et al. (1994). Early prediction of the development of microcephaly after hypoxic–ischemic encephalopathy in the full-term newborn. *Pediatrics*, **93**, 703–707.

116 Lupton B, Hill A, Roland EH, et al. (1988). Brain swelling in the asphyxiated term newborn: pathogenesis and outcome. *Pediatrics*, **82**, 139–146.

117 Dennis J, Johnson A, Mutch L, et al. (1989). Acid–base status at birth and neurodevelopmental outcome at four and one half years. *Am J Obstet Gynecol*, **161**, 213–220.

118 Goodwin TM, Belai I, Hernandez P, et al. (1992). Asphyxial complications in the term newborn with severe umbilical acidemia. *Am J Obstet Gynecol*,**162**, 1506–1512.

119 Yadkin PL, Johnson A, Clover LM, et al. (1994). Clustering of perinatal markers of birth asphyxia and outcome at age five years. *Br J Obstet Gynaecol*, **101**, 774–781.

120 Ingemarsson J, Herbst A and Thorngren-Jerneck K. (1997). Long term outcome after umbilical artery acidaemia at term birth: influence of gender and duration of heart rate abnormalities. *Br J Obstet Gynaecol*, **104**, 1123–1127.

121 Korst LM, Phelon JP, Wang YM, et al. (1998). Acute fetal asphyxia and permanent brain injury: a retrospective analysis of current indicators. *J Matern Fetal Med*, **8**, 101–106.

122 Bzoch KR and League R. (1991). *Receptive–Expressive Emergent Language Scale*, 2nd edn Austin, TX: Pro-ed.

123 Corah NL, Anthony EJ, Painter P, et al. (1965). Effects of perinatal anoxia after seven years. Psychological monographs: general and applied. *Am Psychol Assoc*, **79**, 1–34.

124 Stevenson RD, Roberts CD and Vogtle B. (1993). The effects of non-nutritional factors on growth in cerebral palsy. *Dev Med Child Neurol*, **37**, 124–130.

125 Stallings VA, Charney EB, Davies JC, et al. (1993). Nutrition-related growth failure of children with quadriplegic cerebral palsy. *Dev Med Child Neurol*, **35**, 126–138.

126 Robertson CMT and Grace MGA. (1992). Validation of prediction of kindergarten-age school-readiness scores of nondisabled survivors of moderate neonatal encephalopathy. *Can J Public Health*, **2** (suppl.), 51–57.

127 Touwen BCL. (1979). *Examination of the Child with Minor Neurological Dysfunction, Clinics in Developmental Medicine*, no. 71, 2nd edn. London: William Heinemann Medical Books.

128 Bruininks RH. (1978). *Bruininks–Oseretsky Test of Motor Proficiency*. Circle Pines, Minnesota: American Guidance Service.

129 Painter MJ, Scott M, Hirsch RP, et al. (1988). Fetal heart rate patterns during labour: neurologic and cognitive development at six to nine years of age. *Am J Obstet Gynecol*, **159**, 854–858.

130 Gottfried A. (1973). Intellectual consequences of perinatal anoxia. *Psychol Bull*, **80**, 231–252.

131 Scott H. (1976). Outcome of very severe birth asphyxia. *Arch Dis Child*, **51**, 712–716.

132 Seidman DS, Paz I, Laor A, et al. (1991). Apgar scores and cognitive performance at 17 years of age. *Obstet Gynecol*, **77**, 875–878.

133 Thomson AJ, Searle M and Russell G. (1977). Quality of survival after severe birth asphyxia. *Arch Dis Child*, **52**, 620–626.

134 Handley-Derry M, Low JA, Burke SO, et al. (1997). Intrapartum fetal asphyxia and the occurrence of minor deficits in 4- to 8-year old children. *Dev Med Child Neurol*, **39**, 508–514.

135 Wechsler D. (1974). *Manual for the Wechsler Intelligence Scale for Children*, revised. New York: Psychological Corporation.

136 McCracken RA. (1966). *Standard Reading Inventory.* Klamath Falls, Oregon: Klamath.

137 Connolly A, Nachtman W and Pritchell E. (1982). *Keymath Diagnostic Arithmetic Test,* Canadian edn. Markham, Ontario, Canada: Psycan.

138 Woodcock RW and Mather N. (1989). Woodcock-Johnson – Revised (WJ-R) tests of achievement. In *Woodcock-Johnson Psycho-educational Battery,* revised. eds. Mather N and Jaffe LE. Allen, Texas: D.L.M. Teaching Resources.

139 Koppitz EM. (1963). *The Bender–Gestalt Test for Young Children.* New York: Grune & Stratton.

140 Roswell FG and Chall JS. (1962). *Roswell–Chall Diagnostic Reading Test.* New York: Essay Press.

141 Wepman JM. (1973). *The Auditory Discrimination Test.* Chicago: Language Research Associates.

142 Baker HJ and Leland B. (1967). *Detroit Tests of Learning Aptitude.* Indianapolis, IN: Bobbs-Merrill.

143 Kirk SA, McCarthy JJ and Kirk WD. (1961). *The Illinois Test of Psycholinguistic Abilities.* Urbana, IL: University of Illinois Press.

144 Semel-Mintz E and Wiig EH. (1969). *Clinical Evaluation of Language Function, Diagnostic Battery.* Columbus, OH: Charles E. Merrill.

145 Keith RW. (1988). Tests of auditory function. In *Auditory Disorders in School Children,* ed. Keith RW, pp. 33–52. Houston, Texas: College-Hill Press.

146 Musiek FE. (1985). Application of central auditory tests: an overview. In *Handbook of Clinical Audiology,* ed. Katz J, pp. 321–336. Baltimore: Williams and Wilkins.

147 Williford JA and Burleigh JM. (1985). Learning disorders, the auditory process of language. In *Handbook of Central Auditory Processing Disorders in Children,* ed. Williford JA and Burleigh JM, pp. 1–19. Orlando: Grune and Stratton.

148 Williford JA. (1985). Assessment of central auditory disorders in children. In *Assessment of Central Auditory Dysfunction, Foundations and Clinical Correlations,* eds. Pinheiro ML and Musiek FE, pp. 239–255. Baltimore: Williams and Wilkins.

149 Bradley L and Bryant P. (1985). *Rhyme and Reason in Reading and Spelling.* Ann Arbor, Michigan: University of Michigan Press.

150 Hurford DP. (1990). Training phonemic segmentation ability with phonemic discrimination intervention in second and third grade children with reading disabilities. *J Learn Disabil,* **23**, 564–569.

151 Talley JL. (1990). *Children's Auditory Verbal Learning Test.* Odessa, Florida: Psychological Assessment Resources.

152 Musiek FE and Pinheiro ML. (1985). Dichotic speech tests in detection of central auditory dysfunction. In *Assessment of Central Auditory Dysfunction, Foundations and Clinical Correlations,* eds. Pinheiro ML and Musiek FE, pp. 201–218. Baltimore: Williams and Wilkins.

153 Musiek FE. (1983). Assessment of central auditory dysfunction: the dichotic digit test revisited. *Ear Hear,* **4**, 79–83.

154 Pinheiro ML and Musiek FE. (1985). Sequencing and temporal ordering in the auditory system. In *Assessment of Central Auditory Dysfunction, Foundations and Clinical Correlations,* eds. Pinheiro ML and Musiek FE, pp. 219–238. Baltimore: Williams and Wilkins.

155 Hodge MM and Wellman L. (1999). Management of children with dysarthria. In *Clinical Management of Motor Speech Disorders in Children,* eds. Caruso A and Strand E, pp. 209–280. New York: Thieme Medical.

156 Bennett S and Netsell RW. (1999). Possible roles of the insula in speech and language processing: directions for research. *J Med Speech Language Pathol,* **7**, 255–272.

157 Chen CY, Zimmerman RA, Faro S, et al. (1995). MR of the cerebral operculum: topographic identification and measurement of interopercular distances in healthy infants and children. *Am J Neurol Radiol,* **16**, 1677–1687.

158 Wulfeck BB, Trauner DA and Tallal PA. (1999). Neurologic, cognitive, and linguistic features of infants after early stroke. *Pediatr Neurol,* **7**, 266–269.

159 Kiessling LS, Denckla MB and Carlton M. (1983). Evidence for differential hemispheric function in children with hemiplegic cerebral palsy. *Dev Med Child Neurol,* **25**, 727–734.

160 Feldman HM, Holland AL, Kemp SS, et al. (1992). Language development after unilateral brain injury. *Brain Lang,* **42**, 89–102.

161 Squire LR and Knowlton BJ. (1996). Memory, hippocampus, and brain system. In *The Cognitive Sciences.* ed. Gazzaniga MS, pp. 825–846. Cambridge, MA: Massachusetts Institute of Technology Press.

162 Kinney HC and Armstrong DD. (1997). Perinatal neuropathology. In *Greenfield's Neuropathology,* 6th edn, eds. Graham DI and Lantos PL, pp. 535–599. London: Oxford University Press.

163 Gadian DG, Aicardi J, Watkins KE, et al. (2000). Developmental amnesia associated with early hypoxic–ischemic injury. *Brain,* **123**, 499–507.

164 Temple CM, Dennis J, Carny R, et al. (1995). Neonatal seizures: long-term outcome and cognitive development among normal "survivors". *Dev Med Child Neurol,* **37**, 109–118.

165 Williams K and Alderman E. (1998) Survival in cerebral palsy: the role of severity and diagnostic labels. *Dev Med Child Neurol,* **40**, 376–379.

166 Crichton JU, MacKinnon M and White CP. (1995). The life-expectancy of persons with cerebral palsy. *Dev Med Child Neurol*, **37**, 567–576.

167 Hutton JL, Cooke T and Pharoah POD. (1994). Life expectancy in children with cerebral palsy. *Br Med J*, **309**, 431–435.

42

Appropriateness of intensive care application

Ernlé W.D. Young

Stanford University, Palo Alto, CA, USA

The real question, it seems to me, is When may the application of intensive care be said to be inappropriate? rather than When is it appropriate? If it is not possible to specify circumstances in which or conditions for which intensive care is inappropriate, it is meaningless to speak of an appropriate application of the technology of the modern intensive care nursery. Unless saying no to aggressive interventions at times and for good reason is a genuine option, saying yes is emptied of all significance.

But this raises a second question: Who is to decide that the application of intensive care is inappropriate? Is this for the experts to determine – perinatologists, nurses, social workers, and other members of the perinatal team – or is it up to the parents of the neonate, the courts, or society at large?

Two questions then confront us in this chapter: What is inappropriate neonatal intensive care, and who decides that it is inappropriate? These questions seem straightforward enough, but they are fraught with difficulty, conceptual as well as emotional, and, depending on where one happens to live, practice, have children, and care for them, the answers to them will be quite different.[1]

Starting with the second, in a country like Sweden, for example, where the provision of medical care is the responsibility of the state, and where savings in one area can effectively be allocated to provide needed services elsewhere, the government, acting on the advice of experts in the field and after paying attention to lobbyists (parents and people with disabilities), ultimately decides when providing neonatal intensive care is inappropriate. In the USA, which does not have a centralized system and where there is no effective mechanism for transferring savings achieved in one sector to another where an infusion of resources could be of obvious benefit, authority for deciding when intensive care is inappropriate and for what reasons is more diffuse. The experts may line up on one side of the issue to find themselves opposed by parents or other experts, on the other, with the state remaining neutral.

Two cases that made headline news illustrate how diffuse decision making is in the USA and how difficult it is to arrive at a consensus that the application of intensive care is inappropriate and, therefore, contraindicated. In short, these cases remind us how almost impossible it is to say no.

The first, reported in the *New York Times*,[2] is the story of Ryan Nguyen, born "six weeks before his due date, asphyxiated, and with barely a heart beat." The initial resuscitation attempt was successful, but weeks later the infant's physicians at Sacred Heart Medical Center in Spokane, Washington, when confronted with Ryan's multiple medical problems, including "kidney failure, bowel obstructions, and brain damage," decided that aggressive medical treatments "would only prolong his suffering and that he would never survive infancy. They suggested that his life support be withdrawn." Clearly, they had concluded that the continued application of intensive care technology was inappropriate, for two reasons: even with intensive care, the child would not survive beyond infancy, and applying the technology was cruel, since the burdens imposed by treatment would be disproportionately massive relative to any possible benefits. Other medical experts (from the Children's Hospital and Medical Center in Seattle) concurred with this assessment by the child's neonatologists at Sacred Heart Medical Center. This suggests that the initial recommendation to forgo further intensive care was not impulsive or arbitrary but was carefully considered and had the unequivocal support of colleagues in the field.

However, even as one group of physicians was attempting (for what seemed to them good reason) to say no to the continued application of intensive care, another group was willing to say yes. Neonatologists "at a medical center in Portland, Oregon [Legacy Emmanuel Children's Hospital], reading about the baby in a newspaper, said they were willing to treat him and that he was likely to survive. Almost immediately, Ryan was transferred to their care." The parents' wishes, reinforced by their pro-life lawyer and a court order requiring continued hemodialysis for the infant's kidney failure (obtained before the baby's transfer from Spokane to Portland) prevailed over the professional judgment (and integrity) of the original perinatal team and their consultants. Five months after admission to the Portland hospital, Ryan was discharged home and was reported to be doing well.

The second is the now infamous "Baby K" case.[5] This anencephalic child was born at Fairfax Hospital in Falls Church, Virginia, on 13 October 1992. Nationally, the standard of care for anencephalic infants requires only the provision of comfort measures: nutrition, hydration, and warmth. Ordinarily they are so treated, held, cared for, and allowed to die. When they experience respiratory distress they are not offered mechanical ventilation and are allowed to succumb from respiratory failure.

In this case, however, the child's mother, believing that "all life should be protected,"[4] wanted her child to have cardiopulmonary resuscitation and mechanical ventilation when she had trouble breathing. The hospital filed a declaratory judgment action to determine its obligations to provide this kind of emergency medical treatment to Baby K, "since the hospital and physician concluded that such treatment was medically and ethically inappropriate."[5] Although Baby K was eventually weaned from the ventilator and discharged to a nursing home, she required readmission on several occasions.

A panel of the Fourth Circuit Court of Appeals ruled, by a margin of two to one, "that federal patient anti-dumping law, EMTALA [Emergency Treatment and Active Labor Act of 1986], required that all patients with emergency conditions be treated and stabilized, even when the medical standard was not to treat."

The hospital argued against an application of the statutory language of EMTALA on four grounds:

1. EMTALA only requires uniform treatment of patients with the same condition, making it basically an antidiscrimination standard.
2. Congress did not intend to require treatments that were outside the prevailing medical standard of care.
3. EMTALA cannot be read to force a physician to provide treatments that he or she considers medically inappropriate.
4. EMTALA only applies to patients transferred from a hospital in an unstable condition.

The court rejected all four arguments. Legal analysts were dismayed. Barry Furrow, professor at the Widener University School of Law in Wilmington, Delaware, writes:

> The court's focus on stabilization under the Act, in the case of an anencephalic newborn, misses the point of the Act . . . Since Baby K is not a case of "patient dumping" for economic reasons, and the standard of care is generally accepted as to non-treatment, this is a better case for a judicial interpretation of the statute that is not stubbornly literal, but rather attentive to both medical practice and the congressional intent in passing EMTALA.[3]

Baby K, aka Stephanie Harrell, died in 1995 after her sixth return to the Emergency Department at Fairfax Hospital for resuscitation because of respiratory distress.

Other similar anecdotes could be adduced, such as the Florida case in which Sarasota Memorial Hospital sent home brain-dead 13-year-old Teresa Hamilton on a ventilator (at the hospital's expense) because the child's family did not want mechanical ventilation stopped. The child's father, Frederick Hamilton, an unemployed oil engineer who emigrated to Florida from Scotland, "said the family had been contacted by many people who recovered after being declared brain-dead and urged them not to lose hope."[6] Teresa's death was formally recognized 6 months later.

Cases such as these lead to the conclusion that in practice it is sometimes impossible to refuse to provide intensive care because it is felt that doing so is inappropriate. Is defining, or attempting to define "appropriate" applications of intensive care technology then largely an academic exercise, even an exercise in futility?

Holding that it is may be to take too pessimistic a view. Research conducted in two adult intensive care units by Prendergast and Luce in two separate 1-year periods (1987–88 and 1992–93)[7] indicates that, while the majority of intensive care unit deaths (90% in the more recent period studied, up from 51% in the previous period) follow the withdrawal of artificial support systems on the recommendation of the treating physicians, in only a very few instances (eight out of 179 in the group more recently studied, or 4.8%) are physicians' recommendations refused by family members or surrogates. Extrapolating from their data, one has to hope that cases such as those cited above, frustrating as they must have been to the physicians involved who attempted to limit aggressive treatment, are exceptional rather than commonplace.

Therefore, to answer our first question, it may still be useful and important to attempt to define, from an ethical perspective, limits to the appropriate application of neonatal intensive care technology. Some of the factors indicating that initiating or continuing with an aggressive course is inappropriate were alluded to, either explicitly or implicitly, in the cases already mentioned. Others may also be delineated.

Ethical arguments for limiting the application of neonatal intensive care technology

For purposes of this discussion, I will assume that, with few exceptions, the "default" mode (using computer language) in neonatal intensive care is initially to treat in order to stabilize the infant and then to evaluate his or her situation. Only after these goals have been accomplished will the question of continuing with or stopping an aggressive course come up for consideration. Even in cases where there are suspected chromosomal or genetic abnormalities, until these suspicions are confirmed by cytogenetic studies, measures will usually be taken to assure the stabilization of the infant. Until there is a definitive diagnosis, the question of limiting or forgoing treatments already in place typically will not arise.

One of the exceptions to this characterization (and there are several) is the anencephalic infant, as in the case of Baby K. Here, a national standard of care generally warrants the withholding of aggressive treatment – at the outset. That this did not happen in the case of this particular baby is not due to any lack of a medical or ethical consensus, but to a legal technicality that allowed that consensus to be circumvented.

In many respects, emergency medicine is quite similar. Generally, the rule is to treat in order to stabilize, and only then to evaluate the patient's overall situation. Questions may then arise about withdrawing modalities already in place or forgoing those that could yet be offered. Withholding these treatments at the outset is done only in quite specific circumstances. These circumstances may include patients with available advance directives clearly specifying treatments they do not want to receive, or conditions for which cardiopulmonary resuscitation is contraindicated on the basis of extensive outcome data.

Other exceptions to the "default" mode where there is a national standard that warrants an initial withholding of intensive care because this is inappropriate include extreme prematurity (with the infant's lungs being developmentally incapable of exchanging blood gases), birth weight so low as to make survival unprecedented, and conditions such as agenesis of the kidneys that make it virtually certain that the infant will not survive even if treated aggressively and vigorously. Mildred Stahlman, for example, asserts, "At the present state of our medical skill and technology, less than 24 completed weeks' gestation and less than 500 g birth weight in a normally grown (not small for dates) infant are considered to be at the lower limits of *ex utero* visibility."[8]

Neonatologists must themselves more carefully describe these exceptions. But that apart, the question remains: How are we to determine that continuing with an aggressive course already initiated is no longer appropriate, and that the time has come to shift the focus to palliative and comfort care at the end of life? I will suggest four lines along which it might be possible to do this. Following these ethical guidelines, either separately or in combination, may lead a physician or a neonatal team to recommend that the continued application of intensive care technology is inappropriate. Generalizing on the basis of Prendergast's and Luce's data, these recommendations will, for the most part, be accepted by parents or family members when they are presented clearly, consistently, firmly, and with reasoned arguments to support them. In some cases where parents or family members refuse or resist medical recommendations, there may be strategies for building consensus. Some of these will also be explored below. But in a minority of cases, no meeting of the minds will occur, despite all good-faith efforts. Until society decides somehow to set limits to the power of idiosyncratic beliefs (and the demands to which they give rise), and thus to override in the name of the common good what some individuals unreasonably insist on, the recommending physician or team simply may have to be reconciled to the fact that there are always no-win situations – as in the cases of Ryan Nguyen, Baby K, and Teresa Hamilton.

At least four factors suggesting that intensive care is no longer appropriate will be described. Seldom do these occur in isolation from one another. Usually, some or all of them converge, serving to reinforce one another. However, for purposes of clarity, they will be treated separately.

The infant has virtually no chance of surviving, even with intensive care

The key word here is "virtually." The second usage of "virtually" in the *Oxford English Dictionary* (second edition) is: "In effect, though not formally or explicitly; practically, to all intents, as good as." While it may seldom be possible to assert, with absolute certainty, that an infant has no chance of surviving, even with continued intensive care, it may be said that the probability of surviving is so low as to make death practically, or to all intents, or as good as, certain.

Although, in theory, probability can approach but never be synonymous with certainty, in practice the effect or result of causal factors with an extremely high level of probability may be almost always the same as certainty. Hence my use of the term "virtually" no chance of surviving – even with intensive care.

A determination that a given outcome is virtually certain has to be based on empirical data, not subjective belief or bias alone. This is why physicians often find themselves at odds with nurses in the intensive care nursery. Nurses, at the bedside for 24 h a day, 7 days a week, tend to intuit sooner than physicians (who attend their tiny patients more episodically) that an infant is or is not "going to make it." Physicians have to be persuaded of this by empirical evidence: not only the evidence the particular infant is providing, but also its corroboration by similar findings by their peers in similar circumstances as documented in the medical literature. This is how a "national standard of care" comes to be developed, on the basis of repeated and consistent empirical clinical findings.

Mildred Stahlman argues that:

> The decision to withhold or withdraw life-sustaining treatment can be justified only if one has a set of medical (not social or emotional) circumstances whose outcomes can be predicted with accuracy. This accuracy has been significantly increased by certain types of modern technology, and by long-term follow-up studies on medical and behavioral outcomes of a wide variety of neonatal conditions, including extreme prematurity, chronic lung disease, and many congenital abnormalities.[12]

Where these findings, in the case of a given individual neonatal patient with specific medical complications or conditions, suggest that survival is unprecedented – the application of neonatal intensive care technology notwithstanding – a physician may with confidence (and in good conscience) recommend that aggressive treatments be withdrawn. The use of the term "virtually no chance of survival," with the implication that the recommendation is based on probability rather than absolute certainty, may prompt some few parents to refuse the recommendation and to insist on continued aggressive treatments. Statistical probability applies to groups and has little to say about discrete individuals. As one adult cardiosurgical patient, who had been told by his surgeons that his chances of not surviving open heart surgery were one in 10000 put it to me: "They said I have a fifty–fifty chance of not making it." When I asked him how he got from one in 10000 to fifty–fifty, his reply was: "Either I die on the table, or I don't." Even odds of winning as low as one in several million do not deter multitudes of people from buying lottery tickets. Nevertheless, most reasonable people accept the fact that a prognosis of "virtually" no chance of survival is to all intents indistinguishable from one where there is "absolutely" no chance at all.

In the Nguyen case, not all the physicians consulted agreed that little Ryan had virtually no prospect of surviving his multiple medical problems. There was also no generally agreed-upon standard of care for babies in his condition. Although, as the case of Baby K brings home, having a national standard of care is not an infallible means of limiting aggressive treatments considered inappropriate, it is more often true that the lack of a medical consensus is commonly the reason why doing this is so difficult and, at times, impossible. The challenge to academic neonatal medicine, in particular, is to establish national standards of care for patients in more and more categories. One of the positive benefits of managed care and its emphases on cost-effectiveness, outcome assessment, and evidence-based medicine is that it is driving research of this kind. Without the backing of a community standard or, even better, a national standard of care, the individual neonatologist who is convinced that an infant has virtually no chance of surviving even with continued aggressive treatments and that these are now inappropriate, and who accordingly recommends their withdrawal, is out on a limb – very much at the mercy of the whims and wants of parents or family members.

In the adult arena, two states, California and Texas, have enacted legislation allowing health-care institutions and physicians to forgo treatments they consider ineffective or nonbeneficial. Several hospitals have developed "medically ineffective treatment" policies in response to these legal developments, "creating a pathway for cautiously but deliberately reaching the conclusion that life-sustaining treatments may be withdrawn, even against the objections of the family."[9,10] Although there have as yet been no court challenges to test these enactments, they offer some hope that the days may finally be numbered when idiosyncratic demands for futile therapies prevail over medical judgment and common sense.

The effort to enable the infant to survive is inflicting harms massively disproportional to any hoped-for benefits

Between the two cardinal biomedical ethical principles of nonmaleficence (requiring that, above all else, the physician do no harm) and beneficence (mandating the attempt to benefit or to help the patient) there is the moral notion of proportionality. Every attempt to help entails some risk of harm. Every intervention, however safe and efficacious it may be in the majority of cases, will sometimes prove neither safe nor effective. Vaccination provides a good example of this. While millions of children benefit from being vaccinated, there are rare exceptions – children who develop damaging and sometimes lethal reactions to the vaccines.

For the most part in neonatal medicine, the risk or probability of harm is outweighed by the prospect of benefiting the patient. However, there comes a time in the aggressive treatment of some patients when the balance shifts. Harms, mostly iatrogenic in nature, begin to outweigh the help that is being afforded. The harms become disproportionately burdensome relative to the meager benefits. At this juncture it is not merely ethically permissible to stop treating the infant aggressively, it is obligatory. To continue on an aggressive course that is doing more harm than good is cruel. This is morally as well as medically reprehensible.

But how are harms to be defined? The infant has no language, except body language, with which to communicate. The assessment of harms and benefits, of necessity, must be made by those caring for the infant rather than by the patient him- or herself. Adult observers will rely on both subjective and objective indicators of harm, and these may be in conflict with one another. Nurses are commonly the first to protest that an infant is being harmed rather than helped by aggressive treatments, claiming that their tiny patients are "being tortured." Physicians, on the other hand, may dismiss these assertions as overly subjective, as emotional rather than empirical deductions, because they see objective signs of improvement in the data being provided by their patients. While acknowledging the unfortunate side-effects of their treatments, they may continue to insist that these are more than outweighed by the actual and hoped-for benefits.[11] This is particularly likely to happen when clinicians are also investigators, and have enrolled their patients in clinical trials. In a recent study, Anita Joy Catlin found that "despite awareness of the high morbidity and mortality, 96% of the physicians [interviewed] offered resuscitation to all ELBW neonates in the delivery room. The main factors affecting their decisions were "the role of physician;" having been "trained to save lives;" the belief that "if called, I resuscitate;" the inability to determine gestational age; requests from parents to "do everything;" and the need to move from a "chaotic" delivery room to a controlled neonatal intensive care unit.[11]

How can these opposing points of view be reconciled in the best interests of the patient being treated? One criticism of the claim that infants are not being harmed because there are objective signs of improvement is that those making this claim are looking at isolated trees, but not at the forest as a whole. The infant's renal function may be somewhat improved, or her lungs may appear marginally better, or the intracranial bleed may seem slowly to be resolving, but the *patient* may not be getting better at all. Treatments may have effects without necessarily providing benefits. The tendency to focus on isolated organ systems rather than the whole person can blind even the most objective observer to the fact that, overall, less good than harm is being done. The role of the nurse as advocate for a holistic view of the patient may be to teach physicians, who are generally more oriented to an objective perspective, how to observe the subtle nuances of the infant's body language over time. This body language may eloquently proclaim the disproportionality of harms to benefits. The same may be true for parents who visit their child infrequently and continue unrealistically to insist, despite all evidence to the contrary, that the child is getting better and that aggressive treatments cannot be forgone. Requiring these parents to spend uninterrupted time at their child's bedside is often the most effective way of breaking through their denial, and winning their agreement that the time has come to switch from a curative to a palliative course.

Rotating the nursing staff with primary responsibility for a neonatal patient can provide a valuable safeguard against an overly subjective assessment of an infant's distress. If not one nurse but every nurse who spends a shift of 8 or 12 h with a patient agrees that, on balance, the infant is being harmed rather than helped, this admittedly subjective point of view becomes powerfully compelling. Those who dispute it on the basis of the objective data being monitored have to be challenged to spend as much time at the infant's bedside as those who claim that the moment has arrived when shifting from an aggressive to a more palliative course is warranted. Besides, the subjective view may correlate well with the aggregate data, if not with the indications for particular organ systems.

The key to discerning the infant's best interest, and to implementing the moral notion of proportionality in the trade-off between harms and benefits, is teamwork. As Stevenson and I put it elsewhere:

> The fact that there is a treatment team, rather than a solitary treating physician, can be a useful check and balance against

overly subjective interpretations – one way or the other. In this respect, many heads (and hearts) are better than one. When a consensus begins to emerge among all who are participating in the care of an infant that the harms of continued treatment (or non-treatment) are outweighed by the benefits, then it becomes difficult for any one member of the group to make claims to the contrary; increasingly persuasive arguments in support of such claims will be necessary.[12]

Should the infant survive, his or her capacities for personal life will be profoundly diminished

E. Haavi Morreim pointed out in an important article[13] that the so-called futility debate "turns on intractable conflicts of deeply held beliefs about the value of life." On the one hand are the "vitalists," who believe that all life is fully, even infinitely, valuable, regardless of its quality. On the other are those whom Morreim describes as "qualitists" (for want of a better term) "who believe that there are some conditions under which a life is no longer of value to the person who has it – that such a person would be better off, or at least not worse off, dead."

Central to this controversy is the fact that vitalists conflate the meanings of "human life" and "personal life," while qualitists insist on distinguishing the two concepts.

To equate human life with personal life fosters the view that simply by being a member of the human species (having human DNA), a fertilized egg, a fetus, a severely neurologically impaired neonate, or – at the other end of the life cycle – a permanently vegetative adult, are all persons. Persons are sacred; their right to life is inviolable. Therefore, except in the case of those with afflictions incompatible with survival, everything that can be done technologically must be done to insure their survival. Withholding and withdrawing life-sustaining treatments are not seen as moral options.

Incidentally, this view is adopted as de facto policy in many state institutions for those who are profoundly neurologically impaired, whether developmentally or as the result of some insult to the brain after the child is born. Once a child is admitted to such a state institution, typically not even attempted cardiopulmonary resuscitation in the event of cardiac arrest may be withheld. Quality-of-life considerations are not allowed to enter into, let alone inform, the decision-making process. This is not necessarily because the state departments and professional staff involved support the vitalist position; it may reflect society's judgment that not to protect the lives of the most vulnerable of its wards by doing everything possible for them would be a first step on to a slippery slope at the downward end of which lies a return to the Third Reich.

There was a good example of the vitalist view recently in the press. An appeals court in London ruled that 8-week-old twins joined at the pelvis must be separated in an operation the babies' parents oppose. Unless they are separated, both will die. If they are separated, one will die; the other will possibly survive. Writing in the *New York Times*,[14] Robert Sirico remarks: "Here, as in the case of abortion, one simple principle applies: There is no justification for deliberately destroying innocent life. In this case, the court has turned its back on a tenet that the West has stood by: Life, no matter how limited, should be protected." It comes as no surprise to the reader to learn that Robert Sirico is a Roman Catholic priest. He exemplifies the vitalist position perfectly.

At the opposite extreme are those who do not regard the terms "human life" and "personal life" as synonymous and attempt to emphasize what to them seems to be an important distinction. We are human by virtue of our membership of the human species (by having human DNA). But we are persons only as we have actual or potential capacities for sentience (being able to experience pain or pleasure), responding to external and internal stimuli, relating to our environments and to one another, and for being, at least in some slight measure, self-determining moral agents. These capacities, so far as we can tell, depend entirely on neocortical function. If neocortical function is absent, or has been lost irretrievably, we cease to be persons, though we continue to be human beings.

The two views of what constitutes personal life may be further described, respectively, as passive and active. The vitalist view is passive: personhood is acquired simply by virtue of being a member of the human species. The qualitist sees it differently: we become persons, not merely by being endowed with human genes, but by becoming actively involved in reacting and responding to stimuli within our various environments, forming relationships, and, eventually, making choices. Ronald Dworkin refers to this as the "investment" each of us has made, is making, and will continue to make to become the persons we are.[15] If these kinds of activity are preempted because the neocortex is either absent or has been destroyed, personhood either is not or is no longer possible. For example, Dworkin writes: "The life of a single human organism commands respect and protection . . . because of the complex creative investment it represents and because of our wonder at the divine or evolutionary processes that produce new lives from old ones, at the processes of nation and community and language through which a human being will come to absorb and continue hundreds of generations of cultures and forms of life and value, and, finally, when mental life has begun and flourishes, at the process of internal personal creation and judgment by which a person will make and remake himself, a mysterious, inescapable process in which we all participate, and which is therefore the most powerful and inevitable source of empathy and communion we have with every other creature who faces the same frightening challenge."[15]

These are the broad lines of the debate between the two camps. As Morreim observes: "At every juncture, each side's argument presupposes as true its distinctive view about the value of fetal [or neonatal] life."[13] The debate hinges on deeply held beliefs, and the values to which they give rise. These may not be amenable to rational persuasion. They may have to be accepted as givens by which people in both groups live and for which, if necessary, they might be prepared to fight and die.

The vitalists gained the upper hand during the "Baby Doe" era. The Federal Rehabilitation Act of 1973 was invoked to warn health-care providers that to withhold services from handicapped infants (the term then in vogue) that ordinarily would be provided to others would constitute a violation that could render their institutions ineligible for federal financial assistance. In order to implement the threat of action under the Rehabilitation Act, the Department of Heath and Human Services issued an "interim rule" in March 1983; the final rules were promulgated in January 1984. These regulations (named for "Baby Doe," from whom life-sustaining treatments had been withheld in 1982 at the request of the parents), and eventually struck down by the Supreme Court, expressly excluded "quality of life" from the decisional process in the intensive care nursery.[16] However, their legacy endures in the Federal Child Abuse Amendments of 1984 and, more significantly, in the Americans With Disabilities Act of 1990. The Americans With Disabilities Act expands the Rehabilitation Act in several respects. As Hank Greely points out: "Perhaps most importantly, it includes physicians along with other health-care providers as 'public accommodations' under the Act who, subject to a few limitations, have to make services available regardless of a patient's disability."[17,18] (Marisa et. al. comment: "In the United States, the American Academy of Pediatrics does support forgoing life-sustaining treatment when physicians consider the treatment not in the newborn's best interest. However . . . a US survey found that physicians frequently felt pressure to overtreat infants because of federal regulations, and technological developments. They believed that the regulations did not allow adequate consideration of infants' suffering and interfered with parents' right to determine which course of action is in the best interest of their child.")

Despite these developments, there is a widespread consensus among adults that supports the qualitist position. Notwithstanding the Helga Wanglies (those in a permanent vegetative state) of this world, many, if not most, of us would not want biological existence extended mechanically (in our own case) when personal life, as we understand it, is no longer possible. The fear that this could happen as a result of physicians mindlessly subscribing to the technological imperative gave impetus to the so-called "right to die" movement; so-called because, strictly speaking, death is not so much a right as a destiny. What the term "right to die" means is the right to die with some measure of control, dignity, and humanity. This right is now recognized and may be expressed in legally binding advance directives, such as the Durable Power of Attorney for Health Care or California's Advance Health Care Directive (or its equivalent in other states), which allow competent adults to specify, beforehand, that they desire life-sustaining treatments to be withheld or withdrawn when these will merely maintain biological existence in the absence of qualities they deem necessary for a personal life.

Although infants are incapable of defining for themselves an acceptable (or unacceptable) quality of life, it seems not unreasonable to allow their parents a degree of freedom to do this for them. After all, parents are at liberty to impart their values to their children in virtually every other aspect of their lives. If infants either lack or are likely not to have those capacities (for responsiveness to stimuli, for relationships, and for self-determination) that their parents believe necessary for the attainment of personhood, it is arguably their right to forgo the artificial support systems that will not restore these capacities but merely prolong biological existence. Peterson and colleagues[19] conclude from their data that preterm birth is associated with regionally specific, long-term reductions in brain volume and that the morphological abnormalities are, in turn, associated with poorer cognitive outcome. This is an important finding, in providing objective criteria for asserting that a child's prognosis is one of profoundly diminished life.

This right was the view of the President's Commission,[20] whose members recommended that infants' parents be regarded as the principal decision makers, particularly in borderline cases. The Baby Doe regulations swept this recommendation aside. That does not necessarily invalidate it, considering the vitalist ideology that gave rise to the regulations in the first place. However, the legacy of these regulations, mentioned earlier, makes it more difficult (and legally hazardous) to follow it.

Implementing the recommendation that parents be regarded as the principal decision makers for their infants will require a high degree of unanimity among all the nursery staff that, in a given case, an infant's capacities for personal life are so profoundly diminished that the parents' request to forgo life-sustaining treatment is appropriate and ought to be respected. In the absence of unanimity there could be repercussions, both for the attending neonatologists and for the institution, not only in terms of litigation but also, and this is of perhaps greater concern, unwanted media attention and the adverse publicity that can be associated with it. These practical considerations may in the end prevail over the moral and medical judgment of the physicians and, hence, the parents.

The cost of providing neonatal intensive care to some infants may be disproportionally large relative to the meager, hoped-for benefits

However much one may deplore the intrusion of economics into health-care policy, one cannot ignore this development. If the percentage of the gross domestic product (GDP) expended on medical care is to be held more or less constant so that limited public funds can also be allocated to other desired social goods such as education, rehabilitation, housing, entitlement programs, defense, maintaining the country's infrastructure, and reducing the national debt, then economic constraints on medicine become inescapable. Within a finite budget, it is impossible simultaneously to realize both goals of utilitarianism: providing the greatest good for the greatest number. Either the greatest good will be made available to fewer than the greatest number (roughly the situation at present, with an estimated 43 million Americans, or between 16 and 17% of the US population, the working poor, having no health insurance at the beginning of 2001[21]), or less than the greatest good will be provided to the greatest number (the goal of universal access to a decent minimum of medical care).

Economic realities are compelling health-care professionals to face the issue of cost-effective treatment as never before. Not only must the proportionality of benefits and burdens be weighed (the traditional obligation incumbent on physicians) but now, as well, the proportionality of benefits to costs. To provide treatments the costs of which are disproportionally massive relative to their meager benefits is increasingly recognized as morally irresponsible – an affront to the ethical principle of distributive justice.

An article in the *New England Journal of Medicine*[22,23] makes the plea that:

> We need more sophisticated quantitative approaches with which to characterize the status of newborns as they enter neonatal intensive care units and to document in greater detail the value of techniques of neonatal care. These approaches are now being developed . . . [and] will help identify the most cost-effective methods, reduce inappropriate variation among units, and make clearer which children are unlikely to benefit from continued intervention.[22]

Much of the impetus for doing this will come from managed care. The shift from fee-for-service medicine to capitation is having far-reaching effects on treatment decisions. In the fee-for-service era, the more services hospitals and physicians delivered, the more money they made. There was a built-in incentive to use the available technology indiscriminately, even inappropriately. This has been turned around completely by the system of capitation. Now, the fewer services hospitals and physicians provide, the more money they make. There is a built-in incentive to use the available technology with greater discernment, and only when appropriate. The power of financial incentives to alter treatment decisions cannot be exaggerated. It is this that will drive the demand for more rigorous outcome assessment and cost-effectiveness data.

In perinatal medicine, there are at least two areas where this is beginning to occur. One is that of prenatal care. Traditionally, public spending on prenatal care has been justified by the claim, taken by many to be axiomatic, that for every dollar spent preventively, between $1.70 and $3.38 will be saved. This received wisdom is now being questioned. Huntington and Connell subject it to close scrutiny.[24] Their conclusion is that "The evidence that prenatal care pays for itself is simply not strong enough to merit the virtual certainty with which this claim has been espoused." They continue: "We should make every effort to evaluate the costs and benefits of medical care before it becomes established in the profession's or the public's mind as the standard of care. This is as true for potentially widespread preventive programs, such as prenatal care, as it is for a new drug or medical technology." Yet, in the end, the question may be not, How much does this save? but, rather, How much is this worth? These authors suggest that the worth of prenatal care may have to be demonstrated on the basis of its inherent value rather than by making cost-effectiveness comparisons between preventive and high-technology medicine.

This paper notwithstanding, many more studies summarized in a report from the Office of Technology Assessment have shown that there is an inverse relationship between the provision of prenatal care and low birth weight and neonatal mortality.[25] Mothers who receive prenatal care have 50% fewer low-birth-weight babies; this, in turn, reduces neonatal deaths (two-thirds of all neonatal deaths occur in infants with a birth weight of less than 2500 g) as well as neonatal morbidity (low-birth-weight babies are two to three times more likely to have lifelong disabilities than are babies of normal weight.[26]

As Birt Harvey points out, "to demonstrate conclusively that low birth weight and high infant mortality rate are caused by – rather than associated with – lack of prenatal care, a randomized, prospective, controlled study with defined frequency and content of care would be required."[27] This may not be feasible. The alternative, according to Harvey, "is to utilize non-randomized observational studies and retrospectively collected data comparing women receiving or not receiving prenatal care. Such studies can be controlled for many demographic and medical risk factors; alternatively, the instrumental variable technique can be used to attempt to correct for selection bias." It is likely that this alternative will be more rigorously pursued as managed care demands more precise outcome data and greater accountability in the area of prenatal care.

Second, in the arena of high-technology medicine, better cost-effectiveness data are needed with respect to extremely premature babies weighing less than 750 g with a gestational age of 24–26 weeks. One study,[28] presenting data from six neonatal centers, suggests that in this category of infants the mean survival rate was 33.5%; of those infants surviving, an average of 31% were left with significant neurodevelopmental disabilities. The cost of neonatal intensive care for these infants was presented: "The mean length of stay among the survivors was 137 days (range 71–221 days), and the mean cost of care per infant was $158 880 (range $72 110 to $524 110)." As Stevenson and I commented elsewhere, "These figures require adjustment for inflation and do not, in any case, include the long-term, life-long costs of caring for those with residual handicapping disabilities."[29] When these additional expenditures are taken into account, it is clear that the costs of treating infants in this particular category are exorbitant and the benefits marginal, at best.

These figures cause Harvey pointedly to ask: "Do we provide unlimited resources to achieve the lowest possible mortality and morbidity for the smallest of newborns?"[27] His response to his own question is that:

> rationing decisions do not belong in the hands of the individual physician. Physicians should do all they can for the individual patient within the constraints imposed by society. It is the responsibility of society through elected policy- makers to make programmatic decisions that provide the boundaries within which the physician may provide diagnosis and treatment services, and which the patient must ultimately accept.

Harvey may be too sanguine in assuming that policy-makers will have the will to make programmatic decisions; the way in which the 1992 attempts at structural health-care reform fizzled out illustrates the lengths to which our elected leaders will go to avoid doing this. Nevertheless, what the politicians appear unwilling to accomplish, the financiers behind the managed-care movement seem likely to attempt. It is not unrealistic to expect third-party payers to begin, sooner rather than later, to classify neonatal intensive care for this category of infants to be inappropriate (and therefore not reimbursable) on the basis of cost-effectiveness considerations.

Outcome data have led the Fetus and Newborn Committee of the Canadian Paediatric Society to recommend that, for infants born at 22 weeks or less and with a birth weight of less than 500 g, only comfort care be given; for those born at 23 or 24 weeks they suggest flexibility with respect to resuscitation, with careful consideration of the views of the family and the condition of the infant at birth. For infants born at 25–26 weeks, they accept that full resuscitation is warranted."[29]

In summary, if an infant has virtually no chance of surviving, even with aggressive treatment, or if the attempt to enable the infant to survive is inflicting iatrogenic harm massively disproportional to any hoped-for benefits, or if the infant should survive his or her capacities for personal life are likely to be profoundly diminished, or where the financial cost of providing neonatal intensive care to some infants is so exorbitant relative to marginal, hoped-for benefits, then, for any one or more of these reasons, an intensive care nursery team may recommend that life-sustaining treatments already in place be withdrawn and that others that could be offered be withheld. By describing these applications of intensive care as inappropriate, I recognize that in all other applications the "default" mode (presuming aggressive treatment) is appropriate.

In the overwhelming majority of cases, it is likely that such a recommendation, when clearly presented and explained with reasoned arguments, will be accepted by the parents. In a small minority of cases, the recommendation will be flatly refused by the parents and, in the absence of a court ruling or specific legislative authority (such as California's AB 871, which allows physicians and health-care institutions to refuse to provide treatments deemed medically ineffective), it will be impossible to withdraw or withhold life-sustaining treatments. And in some cases, even if the initial treatment team recommendation that intensive care is not or is no longer appropriate meets with initial parental resistance, there are strategies that can be used for successfully building an eventual consensus. In closing, I turn to a brief description of these.

Strategies for building consensus

In regional intensive care centers, many parents may live at some considerable distance from the nursery. Because of responsibilities at work or to other children at home, these parents may be able to visit their hospitalized newborns only infrequently. When the parents opposing the team's suggestion that intensive care is no longer appropriate fall into this category, one way to build consensus is to encourage them to spend more time at the infant's bedside. Once they do this, and experience at first hand what professionals are describing as the disproportionality of harms to benefits or the infant's profoundly diminished capacity for personal life, they frequently come to see that their insistence on aggressive treatment is unreasonable. What is not evident to such parents when they visit the child from afar for an hour or two a month rapidly becomes apparent when they can be persuaded to be at the bedside for days at a stretch. This is not manipulative. It merely allows the power of reality to dispel the illusions of fantasy.

Some parents oppose the suggestion that continued intensive care is no longer appropriate because of religious beliefs. They accept the fact that the situation is desperate, but they have faith in God, in the power of prayer, and in the provision of miracles. Because they are awaiting a miracle for their child, they refuse to sanction the withholding or withdrawing of life-sustaining treatments. Such beliefs present the nursery team with a particularly difficult challenge, one dimension of which is the reluctance of professionals to show any disrespect for the beliefs and values of their patient's parents, however seemingly unrealistic or idiosyncratic these may appear to be.

Including in the nursery team trained hospital chaplains who are able to win the trust of such parents, on the one hand, and, on the other, to begin to explore and probe the theology underlying their expectations, can be invaluable in such situations. It is especially important that all the nursery personnel – registered nurses, physicians, social workers, and chaplains – present the parents with the same factual information, reinforcing one another's attempts to temper the parents' hopes for their child with greater realism. When the parents belong to religious groups not represented in the hospital's chaplaincy service (fundamentalists of various sorts, for example), the hospital chaplain may need to work with a pastor or minister from the community who represents the parents' denomination or sect. Such alliances occasionally can bring the parents to the point where they will be willing to entrust their child to the wisdom, love, and healing power of God and at the same time agree to forgo medically inappropriate treatments.

Other parents who refuse medical recommendations do so because they are in a denial phase of a natural grieving process. Whether the neonatal team is aware of this or not, these parents are grieving the loss of the normal, healthy baby they had expected and are coming to terms with the fact that they either have a baby who is not going to survive or will survive only with major deficits. While the human emotions that are evoked in the course of grieving occur randomly and repeatedly, rather than in neat, sequential "stages," the phenomenon of denial can for a time predominate over other feelings such as sadness, anger, guilt, depression, fear, envy, and resignation. One paradoxical element in what is often thought to be denial is the will to live, the resolve to fight on, to make every effort to turn a seemingly hopeless situation around. It is this that often underlies parental refusal of medical recommendations to limit further aggressive measures. Again, having social workers and chaplains on the neonatal intensive care team who are skilled in grief counseling and in facilitating "grief work" can be invaluable in helping parents move away from denial towards acceptance – both of the reality of the situation and of the team's recommendation.

Finally, a long-term strategy for resolving conflicts between parents and providers may lie at the policy level. Parents with infants in neonatal intensive care nurseries generally are shielded from any direct responsibility for meeting the costs of their infants' care. Third-party payers, federal and state Medicaid funds, and children's services typically absorb all or most of the hospital's charges, separately or together. So long as parents are exempt from financial responsibility, they are at liberty to demand even those treatments considered inappropriate (for any of the reasons delineated earlier). However, if they were to be confronted, personally and directly, with but a small fraction of the costs incurred in complying with their demands, this would inject a healthy dose of realism into their otherwise often unrealistic view of their infant's prognosis.

It seems consistent with the principle of distributive justice to require those demanding treatments considered inappropriate to pay for these themselves – at least in part in the form of small copayments. None of us has the right to appropriate public funds for our own private purposes; yet this, in fact, is what parents in the category we are discussing may actually be doing. At the policy level, it seems fair to urge that once parents have crossed the line between reasonable requests and unreasonable demands, the burden of meeting the costs incurred should shift from society to them, even if only symbolically.

It is to be expected that the prolife lobby will oppose this. Yet, logically, their opposition would be highly inconsistent. Opponents of abortion typically argue against the public funding of abortion. They hold that, while abortion may be legal, there is a large segment of the population morally opposed to this procedure and that, therefore, public monies should not be used to pay for it. Precisely the same argument can be made with respect to parental demands for treatments deemed inappropriate by the professionals involved in the care of babies in the four categories we have delineated in this chapter.

REFERENCES

1 Rebagliato M, Cuttini M, Broggin L, et al. (2000). Neonatal end-of-life decision making: physicians' attitudes and relationship with self-reported practices in 10 European countries. *Journal of the American Medical Association*, **284**, 2451–2459.

2 Anonymous. (1994). Battle over a baby's future raises hard ethical issues. *New York Times*, December 27, A1.

3 Anonymous. (1994). *ASLME Briefings: The Newsletter of the American Society of Law, Medicine, and Ethics*, no. 10, summer, p. 1, 5.

4 Anonymous. (1994). Court order to treat baby with partial brain prompts debate on costs and ethics. *New York Times*, February 20, p. 20.

5 Anonymous. (1994). In the matter of baby K, *1994 U.S.App.LEXIS 215*, C.A. 4th Cir., February 10.

6 Anonymous. (1994). Brain-dead Florida girl will be sent home on life support. *New York Times*, February 19.

7 Prendergast TJ and Luce John M. (1996). Increasing incidence of withholding and withdrawal of life support from the critically ill. *American Journal of Respiratory and Critical Care Medicine*, 15.

8 Stahlman M. (1995). Withholding and withdrawing therapy and actively hastening death. In *Ethics and Perinatology*, eds. Goldworth A, Silverman W, Stevenson DK, et al., pp. 163, 165. New York: Oxford University Press.

9 Truog RD. (2000). Futility in pediatrics: from case to policy. *Journal of Clinical Ethics*, **11**, 136–141.

10 Orr RD. (2000). Comment: will futility policies make a difference? *Journal of Clinical Ethics*, **11**, 142–144.

11 Catlin AJ. (1999). Physicians' neonatal resuscitation of extremely low-birth-weight preterm infants. *Image: Journal of Nursing Scholarship*, **31**, 269–275.

12 Goldworth A, Silverman W, Stevenson DK, et al. (eds) (1995). *Ethics and Perinatology*, p. 6. New York: Oxford University Press.

13 Morreim EH. (1994). Profoundly diminished life: the casualties of coercion. *Hastings Center Report*, **24**, 33–42.

14 Sirico RA. (2000). An unjust sacrifice. *New York Times*, September 28, A31.

15 Dworkin R. (1993). *Life's Dominion: An Argument About Abortion, Euthanasia, and Individual Freedom*. New York: Alfred A. Knopf.

16 Stevenson DK, Ariagno RL, Kutner JS, et al. (1986). The 'baby Doe' rule. *Journal of the American Medical Association*, **225**, 1909–1912.

17 Greely HT. (1995). Baby Doe and beyond: the past and future of government regulations in the United States. In *Ethics and Perinatology*, eds. Goldworth A, Silverman W, Stevenson DK, et al., pp. 296–306. New York: Oxford University Press.

18 Matrisa R, et al. (1995). In *Ethics and Perinatology*, eds. Goldworth A, Silverman W, Stevenson DK, et al. New York: Oxford University Press.

19 Petersen B, Vohr B, Staib LH, et al. (2000). Regional brain volume abnormalities and long-term cognitive outcome in preterm infants. *Journal of the American Medical Association*, **284**, 1939–1947.

20 President's Commission for the Study of Ethical Problems in Medicine and Behavioral Research. (1983). *Deciding to Forgo Life-sustaining Treatment,* pp. 6–8, 197–229. Washington, DC: US Government Printing Office.

21 Inglehart JK. (2001). Will new leadership address the issue of the uninsured? *Health Affairs* **20**, 6.

22 McCormick MC. (1994). Survival of very tiny babies – good news and bad news. *New England Journal of Medicine,* **331**, 802–803.

23 Fulbrook P and Foxcroft D. (1999). Measuring the outcome of paediatric intensive care. *Intensive and Critical Care Nursing,* **15**, 44–51.

24 Huntington J and Connell F. (1994). For every dollar spent – the cost-savings argument for prenatal care. *New England Journal of Medicine* **331**, 1303–1307.

25 Minor AF. (1989). *The Cost of Maternity Care and Childbirth in the United States, 1989,* Washington, DC: Health Insurance Association of America.

26 Shapiro S, McCormick MC, Starfield BH, et al. (1980). Relevance of correlates of infant deaths for significant morbidity at 1 year of age. *American Journal of Obstetrics and Gynecologists,* **136**, 363–373.

27 Harvey B. (1995). Financing perinatal care in the US. In *Ethics and Perinatology,* eds. Goldworth A, Silverman W, Stevenson DK, et al., pp. 341–354. New York: Oxford University Press.

28 Young EWD and Stevenson DK. (1990). Limiting treatment for extremely premature, low-birth-weight infants (500 to 750 g). *American Journal of Diseases of Childhood,* **144**, 549–552.

29 Hack M and Faranoff AA. (1989). Outcomes of extremely low-birthweight infants between 1982 and 1988. *New England Journal of Medicine,* **321**, 660–664.

30 Fetus and Newborn Committee of the Canadian Paediatric Society and the Maternal–Fetal Medicine Committee of the Society of Obstetricians and Gynecologists Canada Statement. (1993). *Approach to the Woman with Threatened Birth of an Extremely Low Gestational Age Infant (22–26 Completed Weeks).* Ottawa, Ontario: Canadian Paediatric Society.

Medicolegal issues in perinatal brain injury

David Sheuerman

Sheuerman, Martini & Tabari, Attorneys at Law, San Jose, CA, USA

Perinatal hypoxic–ischemic brain injury is an important and often troublesome medicolegal problem for practicing physicians. Brain injury to infants occurring during the perinatal period is probably the most common cause of severe long-term neurological deficit in patients, consequently the incentive for legal action is high.

Although vast advances in care have taken place during the past several decades in the practice of perinatal medicine, the incidence of brain injury and its sequelae has not seen a significant decline. Litigation involving these types of injuries has remained a constant over many years despite endeavors in education of both physicians and patients, and improvements in care. This chapter will attempt to explore and explain the manner in which legal principles are applied to complex medical issues in the medicolegal examination of perinatal brain injury.

The term "medical malpractice," often misused and frequently misunderstood, refers to any professional act or omission to act that encompasses or represents an unreasonable lack of knowledge, care, or skill in carrying out one's professional duties. As used herein the term "medical malpractice" is synonymous with medical "negligence."

Although there are a number of legal theories which may be brought against a physician for allegedly fault-worthy conduct in perinatal or other medical context, the vast majority of such legal actions are based on allegations that a physician or other practitioner was negligent – that is, that he or she did not perform in a reasonable manner as compared to other practitioners of similar standing acting under the same or similar circumstances.

Duty

The first element of the theory of negligence as malpractice is a duty which is created by the physician–patient relationship. In certain instances, whether such a "duty" has been created is a contested legal issue. Such circumstances might include where an informal communication which might be construed as a consultation takes place or where a physician volunteers to help in an emergency situation. This duty calls for the practitioner to possess and utilize that degree of knowledge, care, and skill exercised by a reasonable and prudent physician under the same or similar circumstances. A physician owes the patient a duty to act in a manner consistent with the standards established by his or her profession, commonly referred to as the "standard of care."

There is no clear or precise definition of the duty of a particular physician under each factual scenario. Thus, because most medical malpractice cases, especially those in the perinatal area, are highly technical, the standard of care is defined by witnesses who profess to carry special medical qualifications and who are asked to provide guidance to the judge or jury. In general, the finder of fact is instructed to base its decision solely on the opinions of such experts in deciding whether the physician in question acted with ordinary prudence[1] (Box 43.1). Instructions are also given to the jury on physician duty[2] (Box 43.2).

Box 43.1 Medical negligence – standard of care determined by expert testimony

You must determine the standard of professional learning, skill, and care required of the defendant only from the opinions of the physicians (including the defendant) who have testified as expert witnesses as to such standard.

You should consider each such opinion and should weigh the qualifications of the witness and the reasons given for his or her opinion. Give each opinion the weight to which you deem it entitled.

(You must resolve any conflict in the testimony of the witnesses by weighing each of the opinions expressed against the others, taking into consideration the reasons given for the opinion, the facts relied upon by the witness, and the relative credibility, special knowledge, skill, experience, training, and education of the witness.)

Box 43.2 Duration of physician's responsibility

Once a physician has undertaken to treat a patient, the employment and duty as a physician to the patient continues until (the physician withdraws from the case after giving the patient notice and a reasonable time to employ another doctor) (or) (the condition of the patient is such that the physician's services are no longer reasonably required).

(A physician may limit (his) (or) (her) obligation to a patient by undertaking to treat the patient (only for a certain ailment of injury) (or) (only) (at a certain time or place). If the employment is so limited, the physician is not required to treat the patient (for any other ailment or injury) (or) (at any other time or place).)

Breach of duty

The second element of a cause of action for medical malpractice is proof, beyond a preponderance of the evidence, that the physician did not comply with the duty described above. It is thus alleged that the physician breached his or her duty by failing to act within the applicable standard of care. This is obviously a vigorously contested issue in each medicolegal case with a variety of criteria to be examined in supporting the plaintiff or the defense case mostly surrounding the opinions of the various experts. In the perinatal arena, consensus statements and guidelines such as those published by the American College of Obstetricians and Gynecologists (ACOG) and the American Academy of Pediatrics (AAP) are frequently utilized to clarify the standard of care in the community. Of course, it is not possible for any consensus statement or clinical practice guideline to encompass or anticipate each clinical scenario or to speak to the important aspect of physician judgment employed in each case. The jury is instructed by the court to utilize a specific framework in evaluating whether the physician deviated from the standard of care[3] (Box 43.3).

Box 43.3 Duty of physician

A physician, performing professional services for a patient, owes that patient the following duties of care:

1. The duty to have that degree of learning and skill ordinarily possessed by reputable physicians, practicing in the same or a similar locality and under similar circumstances;
2. The duty to use the care and skill ordinarily exercised in like cases by reputable members of the profession practicing in the same or a similar locality under similar circumstances; and
3. The duty to use reasonable diligence and (his) (her) best judgment in the exercise of skill and the application of learning.

A failure to perform any one of these duties is negligence.

Medical perfection not required

A physician is not necessarily negligent because (he) or (she) errs in judgment or because (his) or (her) efforts prove unsuccessful. The physician is negligent if the error in judgment or lack of success is due to a failure to perform any of the duties as defined in these instructions.

Physicians asked to consult on a given case and to render their opinion whether the practitioner(s) met the standard of care commonly apply very different standards in the application of the "standard of care" to a given set of facts and circumstances. Many consultants are misled into believing that if the practitioner in question acted in a manner which deviated from the treatment the consultant believes he or she would have given, the standard must have been breached. This is clearly an incorrect application of the law, which provides that different methods may be employed by different practitioners and where no uniformity of opinion exists, the physician is not negligent merely because he or she chooses a method different from or not favored by other physicians.

A generally accurate description by a testifying expert witness is "a physician must use the care a reasonable physician might employ in the same or similar circumstances." An error in judgment does not constitute negligence. Intentionally, and by necessity, the legal definition of the "standard" to be met is vague. The author proposes that if one may logically surmise the practitioner has demonstrated adequate knowledge to apply the necessary skills and has utilized that knowledge in a logical manner in an attempt to achieve the desired result, the physician has met the standard of care, regardless of the outcome of the treatment.

Causation

The third element that must be proved by the plaintiff, again by a preponderance of the evidence, is that the act or omission said to be negligent by the physician was a cause of the resulting injury. The closeness of this connection is described as "legal" or "proximate" cause. In the law, the concept of causation differs markedly from the concept of etiology in medicine. The law requires only that a particular act or omission be a "substantial factor" and not necessarily the major or most immediate cause of the injury as a physician would apply the term to describe the etiology of an injury.

Physicians involved in the legal process, whether as defendants, retained experts, or treating physicians, often confuse (or allow themselves to be confused) when they are being cross-examined regarding their opinions on causation. Plaintiffs' burden of proof to show something did or did not happen by a "preponderance" of the evidence requires only that the "likelihood" of the occurrence or nonoccurrence is greater than 50%. Thus, words such as "probably" or "likely" have critical meaning in the legal forum. Physicians are to be cautioned that use of these words in an answer (or a response linked to a question containing these words) constitutes a medical opinion which may make or break the legal case. The jury receives instruction on causation[4] (Box 43.4).

Box 43.4 Cause – substantial factor test

The law defines cause in its own particular way. A cause of injury, damage, loss, or harm is something that is a substantial factor in bringing about an injury, damage, loss, or harm.

There may be more than one cause of an injury. When ((negligent) (or) (wrongful) conduct of two or more persons) contribute(s) concurrently as (a) cause(s) of an injury, (the conduct of) each is a cause of the injury regardless of the extent to which each contributes to the injury. A cause is concurrent if it was operative at the moment of injury and acted with another cause to produce the injury. (It is no defense that the (negligent) (wrongful) conduct of a person not joined as a party was also a cause of the injury.)

Causation is a critical element in the evaluation of most perinatal brain injury cases. Numerous criteria are evaluated in an attempt to prove the likelihood or lack of causation in the perinatal period, including epidemiology, indicators of intrauterine injury, evaluation of fetal heart monitor tracings, consideration of alternate causes of brain injury to those occurring in the perinatal period, correlation of clinical findings and timing of the hypoxic–ischemic event by use of Apgar scores, blood gases, brain imaging, placental pathology, hematologic markers such as nucleated red blood cells,[5] and the like.

Damages

The fourth element of the medical malpractice lawsuit is plaintiffs' proof of the nature and extent of damages. During the perinatal brain injury case, damages may include a wide range of financial, physical, and emotional injury to the patient.

General or noneconomic damages are awarded for pain and suffering, mental anguish, grief, and emotional conditions which are thought to flow inevitably from the injury caused by the defendant as a natural and foreseeable consequence of the injury.

"Special" or "economic" damages in the perinatal brain injury case are presented by a team of experts on each side, which has grown into a cottage industry, often thought by the defense to represent extreme departures from reason. The plaintiffs' bar, on the other hand, argue defense experts are hired to reduce unreasonably just compensation for legitimate injuries. Economic damages in a severe perinatal injury case will generally include:

- Health-care services, often including those of a pediatrician, internist, dentist, podiatrist, nutritionist, vision specialist, occupational and physical therapist, speech therapist, psychological services, behavioral intervention, therapeutic recreation, lab, emergency room, case manager, financial manager, and acute hospitalization;
- Medical supplies, including medications, bowel and bladder supplies, gastrostomy supplies, respiratory supplies and equipment, medical equipment including wheelchair, orthotics, mechanical bedding, bedside equipment and supplies;
- Diagnostic testing, chest, hips, spine, and other X-rays, neurodiagnostic studies such as magnetic resonance imaging/computed tomography of the head, electroencephalograms, and various laboratory work are claimed as intermittent needs;
- Attendant care, often alleged to be necessary around the clock can, alone, easily generate damages of several hundred thousand dollars per year for life. The level of care required is a frequently contested issue, often involving millions of dollars, depending on whether the jury finds care should be provided by a trained attendant, a licensed vocational nurse, or a registered nurse;
- Home modifications, such as access ramps, widened hallways, lowered cabinets, and specialized bathroom facilities are commonly prescribed.

In many cases, such lifetime damages are funded by the purchase of an annuity, generally at a small fraction of the expenses projected by the plaintiffs. An exemplar of such damages can be found as part of a typical life care plan[6] (Box 43.5).

Documentation

No discussion of medicolegal issues in any area of medicine can ignore the critical importance of careful and accurate charting. One must recognize that the practitioner's primary responsibility is to provide quality care to the patient, even if that endeavor detracts from accurate charting. The ability to time precisely particular events or to record all "significant" information is highly dependent on clinical circumstances. However, when trying to defend one's actions best reflected by the chart years after an event has taken place, failure to record, as recommended by obstetric and nursing organizations, makes it far more likely that a lay jury will infer a negative event is represented by lack of documentation. Often the issue in a perinatal case brought years after the event involves when the status of the fetus was compromised. Long time periods of undocumented fetal heart rates often simply reflect long periods of fetal well-being. Plaintiffs will argue, perhaps supported by suboptimal blood gases or low Apgar scores, that the lack of documentation reflects lack of adequate monitoring. Both ACOG and NAACOG (the organization for obstetric, gynecologic and neonatal nurses) have published standards requiring specific frequency of recording as well as specifying the characteristics required to be noted. For instance, ACOG provides that auscultated fetal heart rates should be recorded in the chart after *each* observation.[7] The practitioner must recognize the events of labor, delivery, or neonatal care often are not even examined by lawyers or consulting experts until several years after the events. Substandard record keeping alone, where the actual care was adequate, has led to many malpractice suits.

Accurate and consistent use of terms (or the reverse) is often the difference between the filing or the successful prosecution of cases alleging substandard perinatal care. The term "fetal distress" is most commonly misapplied in medical charts to the reaction of the fetus to the stress of labor, and the term's indiscriminate use can lead to confusion or worse.

ACOG has stated: "Terms such as asphyxia,

Box 43.5 Exemplar: future medical needs: neonatal brain injury

I **Future medical care**

A. *Physicians*

1. Internist: four times a year over life expectancy after age 18.
2. Pediatrician: four to six times a year until age 18.
3. Other (neurologist, ophthalmologist, immunologist, gastroenterologist, hematologist, pulmonologist, rehabilitation medicine, orthopedist, etc): 10–12 visits per year over the patient's life expectancy.

B. *Ancillary medical care*

1. Dentist: cleaning 3–4 times per year. Currently, seeing a special pediatric "special needs" dentist. Because of oral tactile defensiveness, as patient ages, will likely need examination and cleaning under anesthesia.
2. Podiatrist: one to two times per year over the patient's life expectancy.
3. Nutritionist: two times per year over the patient's life expectancy.
4. Low-vision specialist: one time per year until age 18.

C. *Counseling*

1. Individual counseling for mother six times per year over the patient's life expectancy.
2. Family counseling for parents as a couple six times per year over the patient's life expectancy.
3. Sibling (5-year-old brother) four times per month for 3 months, then one time per month until age 18.

D. *Behavioral intervention*

1. A behavioral specialist to assist with a program of environmental and behavioral modification to extinguish negative self-mutilating behavior and the behavior of kicking, pinching, and biting others. Initial intervention at 6–12 sessions for the first 6 months, supervised by a psychologist. Thereafter, two visits per year over the patient's life expectancy.

II **Diagnostic testing**

A. *Routine blood chemistry*

1. Complete blood count: six times per year on average over the patient's life expectancy, exclusive of inpatient lab.
2. Sequential multiple analyzer count (SMAC) 20: two times per year over the patient's life expectancy.
3. Valproic acid levels: two times per year over the patient's life expectancy.
4. Immunoglobulin G levels.

III **Neurodiagnostic studies**

A. Magnetic resonance imaging/computed tomography head scans: four to six more over the patient's life expectancy.

B. Electroencephalogram: four to six more over the patient's life expectancy.

IV **Radiologic studies**

A. *Chest X-ray*

Two to four per year over the patient's life expectancy. Based on this track record thus far, this is a conservative estimate.

B. *Joint X-ray/spine X-ray*

Approximately one to two per year over the patient's life expectancy to follow scoliosis; rule out fractures/dislocation secondary to anticipated falls.

V **Gastrointestinal studies**

A. *Upper gastrointestinal endoscopy*

Four to six per year over the patient's life expectancy for recurrent obstruction, gastrointestinal bleeding, and vomiting.

Box 43.5 *(cont.)*

VI Rehabilitation therapy

A. *Physical therapy*

One time per week until age 18. Then, four times per year over the patient's life expectancy to reevaluate lower-extremity range of motion, mobility status, and equipment.

B. *Occupational therapy*

Two times per week until age 18. Thereafter, four times a year to reevaluate equipment, upper-extremity range of motion, and self-care potential.

C. *Speech therapy*

One time per week until age 18. Thereafter, reevaluations are appropriate once every 3–5 years.

D. *Therapeutic recreation*

One time per year over the patient's life expectancy to assist with the selection of developmentally appropriate recreational activities.

VII Equipment

A. *Feeding supplies*

1. Gastrostomy tubes (Mic Key buttons with adapters for both J-tube site and separate G-tube site). Buttons are changed every 3–4 months.
2. Feeding bags with tubing.
3. Intravenous pole.
4. Feeding pump.
5. Syringe.
6. 2×2 dressings for both G-tube and J-tube sites.
7. Stockinette (wrapped around abdomen to secure G-tube and J-tube dressings).

B. *Incontinent supplies*

1. Diaper wipes.
2. Diapers (approximately eight per day).
3. A&D ointment.
4. Gloves.
5. Bactroban ointment.

C. *Respiratory equipment*

1. Suction machine, portable.
2. Yankauer suction handle.
3. Pulse oximeter.
4. Pulmoaide.

D. *Mobility aids*

1. Wheelchair: pediatric manual Quickie wheelchair with: head rest; lateral trunk and lateral thigh supports; hip abduction wedge; detachable foot rests; antitip bars; heavy-duty wheels; back support with lumbar insert; chest and lap belts; handles on back for parents to push chair.
2. Bilateral ambulatory foot orthotics: will require a new pair every 12 months until age 18. Thereafter, replace every 2–3 years.

E. *Equipment*

1. Hospital bed.
2. Bath equipment: (shower chair and hand-held shower hose will be needed after age 8–10 years. Currently, parents lift him in and out of bathtub.

Box 43.5 *(cont.)*

F. *Safety equipment*

1. Restraint jacket to use in any bad conditions (traveling).
2. Helmet.
3. Vail bed enclosure.
4. Bilateral arm splints to hold elbows in extension to prevent self-mutilation.
5. Other: Porto-Cath, implanted. Change? How often?

VIII **Medications**

A. *See attached.*

In addition, is frequently on antibiotics several times per year. These include Keflex, Septra, etc., per J-tube and Rocephin, intramuscularly as an outpatient.

IX **Tube feeding**

A. Vivonex via J-tube at 65 ml/h × 24 h/day.

X **Transportation**

A. Vab wutg wheelchair left currently being used.

XI **Personal needs**

A. *Financial manager:* potential future need.

B. *Conservator.*

XII **Long-term placement**

A. Home

1. Licensed vocational nurse/registered nurse-level of care since patient needs 24-h/day monitoring secondary to apnea, potential for seizures, 24-h/day tube feeding, and medication delivery via J-tube.
2. Medical case manager: four hours per month over the patient's life expectancy. In the event of parental death/disability, case manager services would likely increase.

XIII **Home modifications**

XIV **Hospitalizations**

A. Possible complications include: G-tube/J-tube malfunction, recurrent duodenal obstruction, recurrent erosive gastritis, recurrent aspiration pneumonia, uncontrolled seizures, complications of falls (head trauma, fractures). Anticipate 14 days of hospitalization per year over the patient's life expectancy.

XV **Emergency Room visits**

A. Anticipate two to three Emergency Room visits per year for seizures, G-tube or J-tube malfunction or dislodgement, falls, fever, etc.

hypoxia, and fetal distress should not be applied to continued electronic fetal monitoring or auscultations."[8]

Practitioners have been cautioned by ACOG against indiscriminate use of the term "fetal distress;" instead, the term "nonreassuring fetal status" is recommended.[9]

Another term used with consistent imprecision is "perinatal asphyxia." According to ACOG, "long usage prevents its abandonment."[10] The current AAP and ACOG guidelines state that "asphyxia" should be reserved to describe neonates with *all* the following conditions:

1. Acidemia, pH below 7.0 on arterial cord blood;
2. Apgar score of 0–3 for longer than 5 min;
3. Objective neonatal neurological signs and symptoms (seizures, coma, hypotonia, etc.)
4. Multisystem organ dysfunction (cardiovascular, gastrointestinal, hematologic, pulmonary, or renal).[11]

It should be noted, effective in 1998, the International Classification of Diseases (ICD) dropped "all inclusion terms" for "fetal distress" except metabolic acidemia.

Case study – obstetrics/labor and delivery

In a case alleging negligent care by two obstetricians, the hospital nursing staff and the anesthesiologist, the minor plaintiff brought this action for severe brain injury following uterine rupture.

Mother of baby was a 25-year-old gravida 3 para 1 with a relatively uncomplicated prenatal course admitted to the subject hospital for induction at 40 4/7 weeks' gestational age due to a low amniotic fluid index. The patient had no known risk factors for the eventual complication, a uterine rupture. She had previously delivered a 3500+ g infant by uncomplicated vaginal delivery.

The patient was in the hospital for induction for approximately 12 h on the day prior to delivery. During that time she received oxytocin augmentation which was discontinued around midnight to allow her to rest overnight. On the following day, the obstetricians began a trial of misoprostol for induction. After approximately 7 h of relatively normal, albeit slow progress of labor (there was dispute whether the fetal monitors reflected fetal well-being and whether there was evidence of hyperstimulation), the mother requested her labor epidural. She testified, as compared with her previous pregnancy, that she felt delivery was imminent.

The external fetal monitor belt was removed for placement of the epidural. A few minutes after the epidural was in, the mother reported a tearing sensation and severe pain, which the experienced nursing staff interpreted as labor pain. The fetal monitoring Doppler was being reattached; however, the nurses had not obtained a fetal heart beat since attempting to replace the external fetal monitor belt following the epidural. The next 6–8 min passed as the nursing staff attempted to obtain a fetal heart rate, without success. The obstetrician was called, arrived within 5 min and delivered the baby from the abdomen by cesarean section within 20 min of her arrival.

Allegations vs prenatal obstetrician

Plaintiff alleged the prenatal care was negligent in that the position of the baby at 29 weeks was confirmed as transverse and that no accurate testing regarding presentation was done thereafter until the uterine rupture occurred. Plaintiff complained the obstetricians did not assess the position of the fetus sonographically on several visits leading up to the delivery and failed to document that the fetus was in vertex position throughout the period of induction at the hospital.

Plaintiff complained various drugs were used to promote cervical ripening and dilatation without any descent of the fetus and without dilatation in the mother. Plaintiff claimed these drugs, rather than promoting ripening, induced hypercontractility. Plaintiff alleged the prenatal obstetrician was negligent in failing to confirm a vertex presentation during the last few prenatal visits. That obstetrician testified he most probably conducted a Leopold's maneuver to determine fetal presentation given the mother's excessive weight gain and the fact that the first baby was nearly macrosomic. However, that obstetrician failed to document in the medical record that he had performed a Leopold's maneuver nor did he document fetal presentation. Plaintiff alleged, had the examination been performed, it would have likely diagnosed a transverse lie requiring cesarean rather than vaginal delivery.

Plaintiff further claimed that the patient was not adequately informed concerning the risks and benefits of oxytocin under the circumstances of having a low amniotic fluid index and that the obstetricians further failed to explain the risks involved in the use of misoprostol.

Allegations vs labor obstetrician

Plaintiff complained the obstetrician managing the labor and delivery was negligent in failing to consider the potential for uteroplacental insufficiency, and thereby discontinue the use of misoprostol; failing to confirm fetal presentation before ordering the use of misoprostol; and failing to observe the patient adequately to "insure" normal fetal heart rate and uterine contraction patterns in a patient laboring under misoprostol induction. Plaintiff alleged the mother of baby was hyperstimulated and that according to misoprostol protocols the patient's dosage should have been reduced or discontinued.

Allegations vs anesthesiologist

Plaintiff claimed the anesthesiologist was negligent in ignoring complaints of severe pain at the time the epidural was administered despite two preceding doses of narcotic medications without relief; plaintiff alleged removal of the fetal monitor during epidural administration was negligent in the face of "abnormalities" present on the fetal heart rate monitor and with contractions occurring every 1–2 min.

Plaintiff contended it was the responsibility of the anesthesiologist practicing in the labor and delivery department to know the status of both mother and fetus and to be "sure" that both were stable at all times. Plaintiff complained of the anesthesiologist that he made no inquiries of the status of the fetus and that he prematurely left the patient's room shortly after giving the epidural. Plaintiff alleged the standard of care required the anesthesiologist to remain in the room for 15–20 min following epidural administration. Had he done so, plaintiff alleged, he would have been aware of the report by the mother of baby that she felt a rip or tearing pain and that this would have alerted him to the occurrence of a uterine rupture. Plaintiff complained that when the nurse, following the epidural, was unable to obtain a fetal heart rate, the anesthesiologist should have immediately contacted the obstetrician rather than allowing the nursing staff to evaluate the reasons for loss of fetal heart rate.

Allegations vs hospital (nursing staff)

Plaintiff alleged the hospital nursing staff failed to determine fetal position on vaginal exams, failed to contact the obstetrician to report decelerations in the absence of uterine contraction, failed to detect hyperstimulation, failed to administer terbutaline to reduce the frequency of contractions, failed to evaluate the patient's complaints of pain described as hallmarks of uterine rupture, and delayed contacting the obstetrician once the fetal heart tones were found to be undetectable.

The prenatal obstetrician defended his actions by arguing he did in fact determine this fetus was in a vertex presentation based on the fact he had written in his record the location of the fetal heart rate and had performed an abdominal examination. An ultrasound examination was done shortly before admission for the primary purpose of determining the amniotic fluid volume. He argued that he certainly would not have scheduled the patient for an induced labor had there been a transverse lie at the time of his examination. He testified he utilized four methods to determine the vertex presentation on his final prenatal visit: (1) location of the fetal heart rate in the lower quadrant; (2) palpating the fetal back through the abdominal wall; (3) vaginal examination with palpation of vertex; (4) ultrasound confirmation of vertex presentation. However, only heart sound location was documented.

He testified that misoprostol is a synthetic prostaglandin E_1 analog which can be administered intravaginally or orally for cervical ripening and induction; it had been studied in randomized clinical trials, and had been found to be an effective agent for induction of labor. Reports of uterine rupture in use of misoprostol had occurred, he argued, only in patients with prior cesarean section.

The labor and delivery obstetrician argued that she most likely did discuss the risks of induction with the patient despite the fact that she had made no note of such. She also argued that fetal presentation was vertex at the time of her initial evaluation although, again, she did not make a note of that. She argued that the fetal heart rate and contraction patterns were adequate and reassuring. She saw no evidence of hyperstimulation. She argued that she was paged stat and that she arrived in 5 min time. The baby was delivered within 20 min of her arrival.

The anesthesiologist defended his case by responding to the plaintiff's contention that he should have "questioned the indication for the epidural" by pointing to the mother's own testimony that she did feel as though she was in labor at the time of the epidural and had compared this labor to her previous delivery. He argued that the nursing staff, far more experienced in managing labor than he, also felt the patient was in labor.

The anesthesiologist responded to the plaintiff's criticism that the fetal heart monitor should not have been moved during epidural administration by pointing to the fact that there is no standard or guideline requiring such monitoring in the face of many hours of a reassuring heart rate pattern. He argued that it would be substandard either not to remove or to move the fetal monitor strap to place the epidural and such would violate the sterile field. The nursing staff would then have been free to position the Doppler on the patient's abdomen during placement of the epidural if that was felt to be warranted.

The anesthesiologist argued that he did not prematurely exit the patient's bedside and that his chart reflected he recorded the patient's blood pressures every 5 min from the time he first saw her until the time of delivery. Thus, he argued, the plaintiff's testimony that he left the room and did not return was due to faulty memory.

The anesthesiologist responded to the allegation that he had failed to contact an obstetrician under emergency circumstances by arguing that the nurses were making constant attempts to locate the fetal heart rate and that the normal interaction between the obstetrician and the staff is that the notification to obtain an obstetrician for a problem is made by the nurses, not the anesthesiologist. He argued it is not the role of the anesthesiologist to assume the tasks of the labor and delivery nurses, whose roles are carefully coordinated with certain responsibilities assigned to them.

Discussion

This case points out several common areas in which plaintiffs may make allegations of substandard care. First, failure to document adequately fetal presentation by the obstetricians left them open to claims that the baby was inappropriate for induction despite the logical inference that trained obstetrical personnel, including physicians and nurses, would not induce a patient for vaginal delivery in a transverse lie. In fact, the prenatal obstetrician would not have even been in the case had he documented fetal position. The physicians' and nurses' failure to document their informed consent discussions or even the fact that such discussions took place with the patient left them open for criticism that they had not advised the patient as to the risks of induction with a low amniotic fluid index. Informed consent should always be documented. In many jurisdictions, the jury is instructed that a failure to give informed consent may subject the physician to liability for any injury caused by the treatment, even if the treatment itself is provided appropriately[12] (Box 43.6).

Serious questions arose in this case as to the time of the uterine rupture and the ability of the team to respond to this catastrophic event. The defendants argued that the baby and the placenta were both extruded into the abdomen at the time of the rupture. Thus, regardless of whether the baby had a heart rate at that time, the rupture of the placenta resulted in complete and total asphyxia of the child from the point of rupture. Utilizing the mother's testimony and the chart to establish this timing, it became difficult to conceive of a scenario where this child could have been delivered without having suffered severe brain damage unless an obstetrician was present at the time of the rupture.

Demonstrating their awareness of this weakness in their case, the plaintiffs were highly motivated to

Box 43.6 Duty of disclosure

It is the duty of the physician to disclose to the patient all material information to enable the patient to make an informed decision regarding the proposed treatment.

Material information is information which the physician knows or should know would be regarded as significant by a reasonable person in the patient's position when deciding to accept or reject a recommended medical procedure. To be material a fact must also be one which is not commonly appreciated.

When a procedure inherently involves a known risk of death or serious bodily harm it is the physician's duty to disclose to the patient the possibility of such outcome and to explain in lay terms the complications that might possibly occur.

Even though the patient has consented to a proposed treatment or operation, the failure of the physician to inform the patient as stated in this instruction before obtaining such consent is negligence and renders the physician subject to liability for *any* injury caused by the treatment if a reasonably prudent person in the patient's position would not have consented to the treatment if he or she had been adequately informed of all the significant perils. (Italics added.)

find flaws in the prenatal care and in the early labor pattern to circumvent the causation defense which became operative at the time of rupture. Thus, the plaintiff was motivated to focus less on the delay in diagnosis after the rupture had occurred. This was an area that was problematic for the defense where substantial delays took place between the time of the apparent rupture and notification to the obstetrician.

This case also illustrates how allegations of negligence may shift in focus if, for instance, at a particular time, causation cannot be proven to be linked with a particular act or mission. Here, it was likely that the infant suffered severe irreparable brain damage within 8–10 min of the rupture, making a therapeutic response to the event virtually impossible. Delay in notification to the obstetrician was thus less significant. The focus of the case therefore shifted to the weaker negligence arguments, such as the allegation that a 29-week prenatal ultrasound showing the baby was transverse indicated the baby was transverse at the time of induction.

The case against the hospital and the anesthesiologist settled before trial with approximately 80% of the payment coming from the hospital. The case went to trial against the two obstetricians. There was a finding of negligence by the jury, who also concluded this negligence (by the prenatal obstetrician) was *not* a cause of injury to the child. The resulting judgment was for the physicians.

Case study – obstetric discharge/pediatric follow-up

This action was brought by a 5-year-old child with severe athetoid cerebral palsy from bilirubin encephalopathy which developed between 3 and 5 days after birth. Plaintiff alleged "early discharge" resulted in missed hyperbilirubinemia.

Plaintiff was delivered with Apgars of 9/9 at approximately 36 weeks' gestational age (a few days short of the AAP definition of "term"). The child was observed for approximately 32 h in the hospital without any indication of jaundice. During that time, the child voided and stooled normally, had normal feeding habits, normal laboratory values, including hematocrit and hemoglobin levels, had frequent normal vital signs, normal skin color, normal activity, and normal tone. A cephalohematoma of unspecified size was noted.

Mother and child were discharged by the obstetrician with instructions to the mother to observe for color, feeding, activity, sleep, voiding, stools, and signs of illness. The mother was shown a video tape with similar instructions, which included a section on jaundice. At the time of discharge the mother was instructed to return to the pediatrician's office in "1–2 days."

The medical records and the mother's deposition testimony reflect that the child did well at home until approximately 3 days following discharge. The medical records and the mother's testimony also reflected the child exhibited symptoms of opisthotonos, the hallmark of bilirubin encephalopathy, on the third evening following discharge. The testimony demonstrated the mother had not returned to the pediatrician's office during that 1–2-day period as instructed at the time of discharge.

The records indicated the mother called the pediatrician's office for the first time 4 days postdischarge. The child was seen by the pediatrician at approximately midday on the fifth day of life. The pediatrician charted a relatively benign newborn exam, except that the child was jaundiced to the midabdomen. The pediatrician sent the patient to the hospital laboratory for a bilirubin level, which came back in approximately 2½h, revealing a bilirubin level of 32mg/dl. In light of the relatively benign physical examination, the pediatrician elected to order a retest stat to determine if there was lab error. The entire process between the completion of the pediatrician's first exam and the completion of the second blood test was approximately 4h. When the retest came back at the same level, the parents were sent immediately to the nearest neonatal intensive care unit. In the meantime, the pediatrician called the neonatologist at the neonatal intensive care unit for the purpose of preparing the staff for accepting the child for treatment. The neonatologist in charge ordered blood from the blood bank and began preparations for treatment. Because of the time required to obtain the blood, the transfusion did not take place for approximately an additional 4h.

Allegations vs obstetrician

Plaintiff's experts alleged the obstetrician had violated the standard of care in the "early" discharge because the patient was at increased risk for potential elevated concentration of free ("toxic") bilirubin due to: (1) prematurity; (2) cephalohematoma; (3) breast-feeding; (4) mother's receipt of oxytocin during labor; and (5) Asian ancestry. Plaintiff also alleged the obstetrician deviated from the standard of care in failing to educate the mother "vigorously" regarding her need to watch for jaundice, contending that the baby had a 50% increased risk of hyperbilirubinemia at the time of discharge. Plaintiff relied heavily on ACOG and AAP literature advocating against "early discharge."

Allegations vs pediatrician

Plaintiff alleged the pediatrician was negligent because he failed to: (1) obtain a complete history of symptoms in a baby at "very high risk" for hyperbilirubinemia, and therefore did not conduct the appropriate physical examination; (2) did not order the initial bilirubin test stat; (3) did not inform the lab to phone with the results of the bilirubin in the initial order; and (4) that he reordered the bilirubin test after receiving the result of 32mg/dl, without having the mother stay at the hospital to receive the results.

The plaintiff's attorney retained two experts on the subject of hyperbilirubinemia. One, a nationally recognized expert in the pathophysiology of hyperbilirubinemia, with extensive writings on the subject, was called to express opinions only on causation. This physician gave testimony which contradicted much of the causation testimony of the second plaintiff expert. The defense argued that had the mother followed the obstetrician's instructions to return the baby to the pediatrician in 1–2 days, the treatment would have been available. Plaintiff expert 1 admitted that had this child been treated with the standard therapies in the 3 days following discharge, she would have had no great injury whatsoever. Plaintiff expert 1 also acknowledged that, based on the serum bilirubin lab values taken at the time of the first test, the child's level had either peaked or was on its way down when the pediatrician first examined the child. This expert further admitted that if the child was truly exhibiting opisthotonic movements, characterized by back-arching on the previous evening, this would be an indication of bilirubin brain toxicity even before the pediatrician saw the child.

Plaintiff expert 2, a retired physician, clearly was an advocate for the plaintiff. Causation was strenuously contested throughout the cross-examination of this expert. Plaintiff expert 2 refused to acknowledge that the back-arching movements witnessed by the parents before the child was seen at the pediatrician's office were characteristic of opisthotonos. This expert claimed that most, or all, of the brain damage would have been avoided and/or reversed if treatment had been initiated by the pediatrician on the first visit. Plaintiff expert 2 produced a self-generated "table" of neonatal signs of bilirubin-induced neurological dysfunction progressing to kernicterus, purporting to correlate clinical signs in three stages, with those stages being: (1) reversible; (2) partially reversible; and (3) irreversible. This table was not the product of any controlled studies, nor had it been submitted for publication. Both plaintiff experts admitted that bilirubin encephalopathy does occur at levels over 20%. Expert 1, along with the defense experts, testified that the bilirubin level had peaked or was on the way down at the time the mother presented the child to the pediatrician's office. Thus, the bilirubin level on the morning before the child arrived at the pediatrician's office was approximately 30 mg/dl. Bilirubin toxicity to the brain cells, it was acknowledged, may occur even before clinical symptoms are present. Following the expert depositions, the plaintiff dismissed the case and refiled it in a different jurisdiction before the running of the statute of limitations. Plaintiff's expert 1 was not to be called in the refiled case. Thereafter, the case was settled for a small fraction of the proffered damages.

Discussion

The defense had legitimate fears of how the jury might react to specialty society (e.g., ACOG, AAP) guidelines advocating against early discharge. While the practitioners here sought to balance the discharge with early pediatric follow-up, deviations from such guidelines can be devastating at trial.

The hospital staff had documented (twice) the discharge instructions to the mother, to return the child to the pediatrician's office in 1–2 days. Moreover, they had the mother sign the discharge instructions, acknowledging receipt and understanding. That follow-up instructions were given is frequently denied by plaintiffs. Signed instructions are a valuable and effective way to rebut such denials. However, the doctor is protected from liability only for injury resulting *solely* from the negligent failure of the patient to follow instructions[13] (Box 43.7).

Box 43.7 Patient's duty to follow instructions

A patient has a duty to follow all reasonable and proper advice and instructions regarding care, activities, and treatment given by such patient's doctor.

A doctor is not liable for any injury resulting *solely* from the negligent failure of the patient to follow such advice and instructions.

However, if the negligence of the doctor is a cause of injury to the patient, the contributory negligence of the patient, if any, in not following such advice and instructions does not bar recovery by the patient against the doctor but the total amount to which the patient would otherwise be entitled shall be reduced in proportion to the negligence attributable to the patient. (Italics added)

This case illustrates the enormous impact a thorough analysis of the causation elements of the case may have on the ultimate result. Objective evidence utilizing the natural progression of the bilirubin levels led to a strong conclusion that the child's encephalopathy had occurred before the visit to the pediatrician' s office. This strong causation defense again caused the plaintiffs to focus arguments against the obstetrician, which may not have been made otherwise. The fact of the serious contradictory testimony between the two plaintiff experts also weighed heavily on the ultimate outcome of the case.

REFERENCES

1 California BAJI Jury Instructions, 6.30
2 California BAJI Jury Instructions, 6.05
3 California BAJI Jury Instructions, 6.00.1, 6.02
4 California BAJI Jury Instructions, 3.76, 3.77
5 The earliest case controlled study of the obstetrical importance of nucleated red blood cells occurred around 1990. It showed a sufficient numerical increase of nucleated red blood cells indicates risk or perinatal asphyxia. Perhaps more importantly, there is a correlation between fetal growth retardation, increased fetal erythropoietin, increased placental and peripheral blood nucleated red blood cells, and fetal asphyxia. Altshuler, G., 1995, *Seminars in Pediatric Neurology*, Vol.2, No. 1, pp. 90–99.

6 Exemplar: Future Medical Needs – Neonatal Brain Injury
7 ACOG Tech Bulletin #207
8 ACOG Tech Bulletin #132
9 ACOG Comm Opinion #104
ACOG Comm Opinion #137
ACOG Comm Opinion #207, 1995 (However, later publications from ACOG have used the term "fetal distress.")
10 ACOG Tech Bulletin #163
11 American Academy of Pediatrics and American College of Obstetrics/Gynecology (1992) *Guidelines for Perinatal Care* (3rd Edition), (ed. R.L. Poland and R.K. Freeman) pp 221–224. American Academy of Obstetrics/Gynecology (1994). *Utility of Umbilical Cord Blood Acid- Base Assessment.* ACOG Committee Opinion: Committee on OB Practice No 138, April 1994.
12 California BAJI Duty of Disclosure 6.11 (revised)
13 California BAJI, 6.28, Duty of Patient

Index